Priorities in

CRITICAL CARE NURSING

http://evolve.elsevier.com/Urden/priorities/

Priorities in
CRITICAL CARE NURSING

FIFTH EDITION

Linda D. Urden, DNSc, RN, CNA-BC, FAAN
Executive Director, Nursing Quality, Education and Research
Palomar Pomerado Health
Escondido, California
Coordinator, Executive Nurse Leader Program
University of San Diego
San Diego, California

Kathleen M. Stacy, MS, RN, CNS, CCRN, PCCN, CCNS
Clinical Nurse Specialist–Intermediate Care Unit
Nursing Quality, Education and Research
Palomar Pomerado Health
Escondido, California
Adjunct Faculty Member
School of Nursing, College of Health and Human Services
San Diego State University
San Diego, California

Mary E. Lough, MS, RN, CNS, CCRN, CNRN
Clinical Nurse Specialist, Medical/Surgical/Neuro/Trauma ICU
Stanford University Hospital and Clinics
Stanford, California
Associate Clinical Professor
Department of Physiological Nursing
University of California, San Francisco
San Francisco, California

With 160 *illustrations*

MOSBY
ELSEVIER

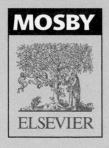

MOSBY
ELSEVIER

11830 Westline Industrial Drive
St. Louis, Missouri 63146

Priorities in Critical Care Nursing ISBN-13: 978-0-323-05259-7

Notice

Knowledge and best practice in this field are constantly changing. As new research and experience broaden our knowledge, changes in practice, treatment, and drug therapy may become necessary or appropriate. Readers are advised to check the most current information provided (i) on procedures featured or (ii) by the manufacturer of each product to be administered, to verify the recommended dose or formula, the method and duration of administration, and contraindications. It is the responsibility of the practitioner, relying on their own experience and knowledge of the patient, to make diagnoses, to determine dosages and the best treatment for each individual patient, and to take all appropriate safety precautions. To the fullest extent of the law, neither the Publisher nor the Authors assume any liability for any injury and/or damage to persons or property arising out or related to any use of the material contained in this book.

The Publisher

Previous editions copyrighted 2004, 2000, 1996, 1992

ISBN-13: 978-0-323-05259-7

Executive Publisher: Barbara Nelson Cullen
Managing Editor: Maureen R. Iannuzzi
Senior Developmental Editor: Jennifer Ehlers
Publishing Services Manager: John Rogers
Senior Project Manager: Beth Hayes
Design Direction: Teresa McBryan

Printed in Canada

Last digit is the print number: 9 8 7 6 5 4 3

Contributors

Kara L. Adams, RN, MS, CCRN
Clinical Nurse Specialist
University Medical Center
Tucson, Arizona
Trauma

Beverly Carlson, MS, RN, CNS
Lecturer, School of Nursing
San Diego State University
San Diego, California
Shock and Multiple Organ Dysfunction Syndrome

Joni L. Dirks, MS, RN, CCRN
Critical Care Educator
Sacred Heart Medical Center
Spokane, Washington
Cardiovascular Therapeutic Management

Lorraine Fitzsimmons, DNS, RN, FNP, CS
Chair
Advanced Practice Nursing of Adults and Elderly
Director
Adult and Geriatric Nurse Practitioner Program
San Diego State University School of Nursing
San Diego, California
Shock and Multiple Organ Dysfunction Syndrome

Celine Gelinas, RN, PhD
School of Nursing
McGill University
Montreal, Quebec, Canada
Pain Management

Karen Johnson, RN, PhD, CCRN
Associate Professor
University of Maryland School of Nursing
Baltimore, Maryland
Trauma

Karin T. Kirchhoff, PhD, RN, FAAN
Rodefer Chair and Professor
School of Nursing
University of Wisconsin
Madison, Wisconsin
End-of-Life Issues

Mary E. Lough, MS, RN, CNS, CCRN, CNRN
Clinical Nurse Specialist, Medical/Surgical/Neuro/Trauma ICU
Stanford University Hospital and Clinics
Stanford, California
Associate Clinical Professor
Department of Physiological Nursing
University of California, San Francisco
San Francisco, California
Sedation, Agitation, and Delirium Management
Cardiovascular Assessment and Diagnostic Procedures
Cardiovascular Disorders
Renal Disorders and Therapeutic Management
Endocrine Assessment and Diagnostic Procedures
Endocrine Disorders and Therapeutic Management

Jeanne M. Maiden, RN, CNS, PhD(c)
Associate Professor
Point Loma Nazarene University
San Diego, California
Pulmonary Assessment and Diagnostic Procedures

Barbara Mayer, BSN, MS, RN
Director of Nursing Education
Palomar Pomerdo Health
Escondida, California
Hematologic and Oncologic Issues

Colleen O'Leary-Kelley, PhD, RN, CCRN, CNSN
Associate Professor
School of Nursing
San Jose State University
San Jose, California
Nutrition Alterations

Laura Pagano, MS, ANP-GNP, CNS, CCRN, CDR
LCDR
U.S. Navy Nurse Corps
Shock and Multiple Organ Dysfunction Syndrome

Karen L. Rice, MSN, APRN, BC
Adult Nurse Practitioner/Clinical Specialist
Ochsner Clinic Foundation
New Orleans, Louisiana
Gerontologic Alterations

Mary Schira, PhD, APRN, BC, ACNP
Associate Clinical Professor and Director
Acute Care and Emergency Nurse Practitioner Programs
The University of Texas at Arlington School of Nursing
Arlington, Texas
Renal Assessment and Diagnostic Procedures

Kathleen M. Stacy, MS, RN, CNS, CCRN, PCCN, CCNS
Clinical Murse Specialist–Intermediate Care Unit
Nursing Quality, Education and Research
Palomar Pomerdo Health
Escondido, California
School of Nursing, College of Health and Human Services
San Diego State University
San Diego, California
Pulmonary Assessment and Diagnostic Procedures
Pulmonary Disorders
Pulmonary Therapeutic Management
Neurologic Assessment and Diagnostic Procedures
Neurologic Disorders and Therapeutic Management
Gastrointestinal Disorders and Therapeutic Managment

Sheila Cox Sullivan, PhD, RN
Associate Professor
College of Nursing
Harding University
Searcy, Arkansas
Sleep Alterations

Linda D. Urden, DNSc, RN, CNA-BC, FAAN
Executive Director, Nursing Quality, Education and Research
Palomar Pomerdo Health
Escondido, California
Coordinator, Executive Nurse Leader Program
University of San Diego
San Diego, California
Caring for the Critically Ill Patient
Ethical and Legal Issues
Patient and Family Education
Psychosocial Alterations

To my three sweet girls, Maggie, Lightning, and Annie,
who are always there for me.

LDU

To Linda Urden—you have had a profound influence on my life.
Thank you for helping me achieve my professional goals.

KMS

To the nurses of the Stanford medical/surgical/neuro/trauma ICU
who give such high-quality care every day. I have learned so much
from working with all of you.

MEL

Preface

We are grateful to the many students, nurses, and educators who made the first four editions of *Priorities in Critical Care Nursing* successful. We actively solicited input from users of the fourth edition and incorporated their comments and suggestions regarding format, content, and organization for this book. The emphasis continues to be on priorities for the critical care nurse. We believe that prioritizing conditions and issues will assist critical care nurses in quickly assessing and intervening in the most efficient and effective manner.

ORGANIZATION

Organizationally, the book comprises nine major units, with two appendixes. The chapter content of Unit One, *Foundations of Critical Care Nursing Practice*, forms the basis of practice regardless of the physiologic alterations of the critically ill patient. Although chapters in this book may be studied in any sequence, we recommend that Chapter 1, Caring for the Critically Ill Patient, be studied first because it clarifies the major assumptions on which the book is based.

Unit Two, *Common Problems in Critical Care*, examines potential critical care practice problems and is divided into seven chapters: Psychosocial Alterations, Sleep Alterations, Nutritional Alterations, Gerontologic Alterations, Pain Management, Sedation Assessment and Management, and End-of-Life Issues.

Unit Three, *Cardiovascular Alterations*, and Unit Four, *Pulmonary Alterations*, are each organized according to the following three-chapter format:

Assessment and Diagnostic Procedures
Disorders
Therapeutic Management

This organization permits easy retrieval of information for students and clinicians and provides flexibility for the educator to individualize teaching methods by assigning chapters that best suit student needs.

Unit Five, *Neurologic Alterations;* Unit Six, *Renal Alterations;* Unit Seven, *Gastrointestinal Alterations;* and Unit Eight, *Endocrine Alterations*, are each organized according to the following two-chapter format:

Assessment and Diagnostic Procedures
Disorders and Therapeutic Management

Unit Nine, *Multisystem Alterations*, addresses disorders that affect multiple body systems and necessitate discussion as a separate category. Unit Nine is organized in a three-chapter format:

Trauma
Shock and Multiple Organ Dysfunction Syndrome
Hematologic and Oncologic Issues

Appendix A, *Nursing Management Plans of Care*, contains the core of critical care nursing practice in a nursing process format: signs and symptoms, nursing diagnosis, outcome criteria, and nursing interventions. The Nursing Management Plans of Care are referenced throughout the book within the Nursing Diagnosis Priorities boxes.

Finally, Appendix B, *Physiologic Formulas for Critical Care*, features commonly encountered hemodynamic and oxygenation formulas and other calculations presented in easily understood terms.

NURSING DIAGNOSIS AND MANAGEMENT

The power of research-based critical care practice has been incorporated into nursing interventions. To foster critical thinking and decision making, a boxed menu of nursing diagnoses complete with specific etiologic or related factors accompanies each medical disorder and major medical treatment discussion and directs the learner to the section of the book where appropriate nursing management is detailed.

In keeping with the emphasis on priorities in critical care, Nursing Diagnosis Priorities boxes list the most urgent potential nursing diagnoses to be addressed. To facilitate student learning, the Nursing Management Plans of Care incorporate nursing diagnoses, etiologic or related factors, clinical manifestations, and interventions with rationales. The Nursing Management Plans of Care are liberally cross-referenced throughout the book for easy retrieval by the reader.

NEW TO THIS EDITION

New to this edition are the following chapters:

Chapter 10, End-of-Life Issues
Chapter 28, Hematologic and Oncologic Issues

Chapter 10 provides an overview of conditions and

nursing interventions for caring for patients at the end of life. Special attention is focused on both physiologic interventions and psychosocial approaches for patients and families. Chapter 28 focuses on hematologic and oncologic conditions that may be seen in the critical care or intermediate care areas. These conditions may be primary admission diagnoses or complications of other health conditions.

New to this edition are Patient Safety Priorities, which serve to alert the nurse to special evidence-based considerations to specific practices and interventions that will ensure safe patient care and the best outcomes. Another new feature is Concept Maps, which appear throughout the book and link pathophysiologic processes, clinical manifestations, and medical and nursing interventions.

LEARNER ENHANCEMENTS

To accompany *Priorities in Critical Care Nursing*, the teaching and learning package has been revised for this edition. The Instructor's Resource provides a variety of aids to help enhance the course instruction. It is available online on the Evolve website. Included are sample course outlines with teaching strategies, a test bank of more than 500 questions with answers and rationales, and PowerPoint lecture slides of key text, tables, boxes, and figures.

This edition of *Priorities in Critical Care Nursing* is web-active, with open-book quizzes available on the Student Resource portion of the Evolve website. Students can test their knowledge and review key issues using this helpful study tool.

Priorities in Critical Care Nursing, fifth edition, represents our continued commitment to bringing you the best in all things a textbook can offer: the best and brightest in contributing and consulting authors; the latest in scientific research befitting the current state of health care and nursing; an organizational format that exercises diagnostic reasoning skills and is logical and consistent; and outstanding artwork and illustrations that enhance student learning. We pledge our continued commitment to excellence in critical care education.

ACKNOWLEDGMENTS

The talent, hard work, and inspiration of many people have produced the fifth edition of *Priorities in Critical Care Nursing*. We appreciate the assistance of our managing editor, Maureen Iannuzzi, and our developmental editor, Jennifer Ehlers. We are also grateful to our project manager, Beth Hayes, for her scrupulous attention to detail.

Linda D. Urden
Kathleen M. Stacy
Mary E. Lough

Contents

CHAPTER 1

Caring for the Critically Ill Patient

LINDA D. URDEN

OBJECTIVES

- Describe critical care nursing roles.
- Discuss the importance of holistic care for the critically ill patient and family.
- Articulate nursing's unique role in health care.
- List and discuss the six phases of the nursing process in critical care.
- Compare and contrast interdisciplinary critical care management models and tools.
- Explain safety issues in the critical care environment.

CONTEMPORARY CRITICAL CARE

Critical care today is provided to patients by a multidisciplinary team of health care professionals who have in-depth education in the specialty field of critical care. The team consists of physician intensivists, specialty physicians, nurses, advanced-practice nurses and other specialty nurse clinicians, pharmacists, respiratory therapy practitioners, other specialized therapists and clinicians, social workers, and clergy. Critical care is provided in specialized units or departments, with a focus on the continuum of care and efficient transition of care from one setting to another.

CRITICAL CARE NURSING ROLES

Nurses provide and contribute to the care of critically ill patients in a variety of roles. The most prominent role for the professional registered nurse (RN) is that of direct care provider. Other nurse clinicians also contribute to patient care, including patient educators, cardiac rehabilitation specialists, physician's office nurses, and infection control specialists. The specific types of expanded-role nursing positions are determined by individual organizational resources and needs.

Advanced-practice nurses (APNs) have met educational and clinical requirements beyond the basic nursing educational requirements for all nurses. The APNs in critical care areas are predominantly the clinical nurse specialist (CNS) and the nurse practitioner (NP) or acute care nurse practitioner (ACNP). APNs have a broad depth of knowledge and expertise in their specialty area and manage complex clinical and systems issues. The organizational system and existing resources of an institution determine what roles may be needed and how these roles function.

CNSs serve in specialty roles that require their clinical, teaching, research, leadership, and consultative abilities. They work in direct clinical roles and systems or administrative roles and in various other settings in the health care system. They may be organized by specialty, such as cardiovascular, or function, such as cardiac rehabilitation. CNSs also may be designated as case managers for specific patient populations.

NPs and ACNPs manage clinical care of a group of patients and have various levels of prescriptive authority, depending on the state and practice area in which they work. They also provide care consistency, interact with families, plan for patient discharge, and provide teaching to patients, families, and other members of the heath care team.[1]

CRITICAL CARE NURSING STANDARDS

The American Association of Critical-Care Nurses (AACN) has established nursing standards to provide a framework for critical care nurses. The standards are authoritative statements that describe the level of care and performance by which the quality of nursing care can be judged. Standards serve as descriptions of expected nursing roles and responsibilities.[2] The six AACN Standards of Care for Acute and Critical Care Nursing are prescriptive of a competent level of nursing practice (Box 1-1). The AACN also provides eight standards of professional practice (Box 1-2).

EVIDENCE-BASED NURSING PRACTICE

Much of early medical and nursing practice was based on nonscientific traditions that resulted in variable and haphazard patient outcomes.[3] These traditions and rituals, which were based on folklore, gut instinct,

Box 1-1

AACN Standards of Care for Acute and Critical Care Nursing

Standard of Care I: Assessment
The nurse caring for acute and critically ill patients collects relevant patient health data.

Standard of Care II: Diagnosis
The nurse caring for acute and critically ill patients analyzes the assessment data in determining diagnoses.

Standard of Care III: Outcome Identification
The nurse caring for acute and critically ill patients identifies individualized, expected outcomes for the patient.

Standard of Care IV: Planning
The nurse caring for acute and critically ill patients develops a plan of care that prescribes interventions to attain expected outcomes.

Standard of Care V: Implementation
The nurse caring for acute and critically ill patients implements interventions identified in the plan of care.

Standard of Care VI: Evaluation
The nurse caring for acute and critically ill patients evaluates the patient's progress toward attaining expected outcomes.

From American Association of Critical-Care Nurses: *Standards of care for acute and critical care nursing,* Aliso Viejo, Calif, 1998, The Association.
AACN, American Association of Critical-Care Nurses.

trial and error, and personal preference, were often passed down from one generation of practitioners to another.[3-5] Examples of non–scientific-based critical care nursing practice include suctioning artificial airways every 2 hours, using iced saline injectable when measuring a cardiac output, always using lead II for cardiac monitoring, stripping chest tubes every 2 hours, and limiting visiting hours for all patients.[4]

The dramatic and multiple changes in health care and the ever-increasing presence of managed care in all geographic regions have placed greater emphasis on demonstrating the effectiveness of treatments and practices on outcomes.[6,7] In addition, emphasis is greater on efficiency, cost-effectiveness, quality of life, and patient satisfaction ratings.[8] It has become essential for nurses to use the best data available to make patient care decisions and carry out the appropriate nursing interventions.[8] By means of a scientific basis, with its ability to explain and predict, nurses are able to provide research-based interventions with consistent, positive outcomes. The content of this book is research based, with the most current, cutting-edge research abstracted and placed throughout the chapters as appropriate to topical discussions.

The increasingly complex and changing health care system presents multiple challenges for creating an evidence-based practice. Not only must appropriate research studies be designed to answer clinical questions, but also research findings must be used to make necessary changes for implementation in practice.[9] Multiple evidence-based practice and research utilization models exist to guide practitioners in the use of existing research findings. One such model is the *Iowa Model of Evidence-Based Practice to Promote Quality Care,* which incorporates both evidence and research as the basis for practice.[10] Inquisitive practitioners who strive for best practices using valid and reliable data will demonstrate quality outcomes-driven care and practices.[11]

The American Association of Critical-Care Nurses (AACN) has promulgated several practice summaries

Box 1-2

AACN Standards of Professional Practice for Acute and Critical Care Nursing

Standard of Professional Practice I: Quality of Care
The nurse caring for acute and critically ill patients systematically evaluates the quality and effectiveness of nursing practice.

Standard of Professional Practice II: Individual Practice Evaluation
The nurse caring for acute and critically ill patients reflects knowledge of current professional practice standards, laws, and regulations.

Standard of Professional Practice III: Education
The nurse caring for acute and critically ill patients maintains current knowledge and competency in the care of acute and critically ill patients.

Standard of Professional Practice IV: Collegiality
The nurse caring for acute and critically ill patients interacts with and contributes to the professional development of peers and other health care providers as colleagues.

Standard of Professional Practice V: Ethics
The nurse's decision and actions on behalf of acute and critically ill patients are determined in an ethical manner.

Standard of Professional Practice VI: Collaboration
The nurse caring for acute and critically ill patients collaborates with the team, consisting of patient, family, and health care providers, in providing patient care in a healing, humane, and caring environment.

Standard of Professional Practice VII: Research
The nurse caring for acute and critically ill patients uses clinical inquiry in practice.

Standard of Professional Practice VIII: Resource Utilization
The nurse caring for acute and critically ill patients considers factors related to safety, effectiveness, and cost in planning and delivering patient care.

From American Association of Critical-Care Nurses: *Standards of care for acute and critical care nursing,* Aliso Viejo, Calif, 1998, The Association.
AACN, American Association of Critical-Care Nurses.

in the form of a "Practice Alert." These alerts are short directives that can be used as a quick reference for practice areas (e.g., oral care, noninvasive blood pressure monitoring, ST segment monitoring). They are succinct and supported by evidence and address both nursing and multidisciplinary activities. Each alert includes the clinical information, followed by references that support the practice.[12] Practice Alerts may be found throughout the book, as appropriate.

HOLISTIC CARE

The high-technology–driven critical care environment is fast paced and directed toward monitoring and treating life-threatening changes in patient conditions. For this reason, attention is often focused on the technology and treatments necessary for maintaining stability in the physiologic functioning of the patient. Great emphasis is placed on technical skills and professional competence and responsiveness to critical emergencies. Concern has been voiced about the lesser emphasis on the caring component of nursing in this fast-paced, highly technologic health care environment.[13,14] Nowhere is this more evident than in areas where critical care nursing is practiced. Keeping the care in nursing care is one of our greatest challenges.[14] The critical care nurse must be able to deliver high-quality care skillfully, using all appropriate technologies, while incorporating psychosocial and other holistic approaches as appropriate to the time and the patient's condition.

The caring aspect between nurses and patients is fundamental to the nurse-patient relationship and to the health care experience. Holistic care focuses on human integrity and stresses that the body, mind, and spirit are interdependent and inseparable. Thus, all aspects need to be considered in planning and delivering care.[15,16]

Health care providers clearly understand that a patient's physical condition progresses in fairly predictable stages, depending on the presence or absence of comorbid conditions. Less clearly understood is the effect of psychosocial issues on the healing process. For this reason, special consideration must be given to determining the unique interventions that will positively impact each individual patient and help the patient progress toward desired outcomes.

An important aspect in the care delivery to and recovery of critically ill patients is the personal support of family members and significant others. The value of both patient-centered and family-centered care should not be underestimated.[17] It is important for families to be included in care decisions and to be encouraged to participate in the care of the patient as appropriate for the patient's level of needs and the family's level of ability.

Cultural diversity in health care is not a new topic but is gaining emphasis and importance as the world becomes more accessible to all as the result of increasing technologies and interfaces with places and peoples. Diversity includes not only ethnic sensitivity but also sensitivity and openness to differences in lifestyles, opinions, values, and beliefs.

Unless cultural differences are taken into account, optimal health care cannot be provided. More attention has been directed recently at determining the physiologic and disease development and progression differences among various ethnic groups. Mortality rates from cardiovascular disease are significantly higher for both black men and black women than for white men and white women. The prevalence of coronary heart disease is highest in black women, followed by Mexican American men.[18] An increased sensitivity to the health care needs and vulnerabilities of all groups must be developed by care providers.

Cultural competence is one way to ensure that individual differences related to culture are incorporated into the plan of care.[19,20] Nurses must possess knowledge about biocultural, psychosocial, and linguistic differences in diverse populations to make accurate assessments. Interventions must then be tailored to address the uniqueness of each patient and family.

As persons search for meaning and guidance in critical, emergent, and unexpected tragic circumstances, spirituality becomes more important.[21,22] Likewise, health care practitioners turn to their own spirituality to manage stress and find answers to the health care issues that they face on an intense, daily basis. Spiritual practices consist of meditation, prayer, and spiritual materials and are based on personal values and beliefs. Holt-Ashley[21] describes how to incorporate prayer into the critical care unit, concentrating on both patients and families and the nurse. The author also offers strategies for creating an environment that is conducive to spiritual well-being for both patients and staff.

NURSING'S UNIQUE ROLE IN HEALTH CARE

Nursing is dynamic and responds to the changing nature of societal needs.[23] Four key features of contemporary nursing practice are described as follows[23]:

1. Attention to the full range of human experiences and responses to health and illness without restriction to a problem-focused orientation
2. Integration of objective data with knowledge gained from an understanding of the patient's or group's subjective experience
3. Application of scientific knowledge to the processes of diagnosis and treatment
4. Provision of a caring relationship that facilitates health and healing

The phenomena of concern to nurses are human experiences and responses to birth, illness, and death. Specifically, nursing care focuses on the following areas[23]:

- Physiologic and pathophysiologic processes
- Care and self-care processes
- Physical and emotional comfort, discomfort, and pain
- Emotions related to experiences of birth, health, illness, and death
- Meanings ascribed to health and illness
- Decision-making and choice-making abilities
- Perceptual orientations
- Relationships, role performance, and change processes within relationships

Box 1-3
Format for Nursing Diagnoses

Actual Problem (Three-Part Statement)
Part 1: Nursing Diagnosis
Ineffective Tissue Perfusion: Myocardial

Part 2: Etiologic Factors (Related to:)
Acute myocardial ischemia secondary to CAD

Part 3: Defining Characteristics
Angina >30 min but <6 hr
ST-segment elevation on 12-lead ECG
Elevation of CK and CK-MB enzymes
Apprehension

Risk Problem (Two-Part Statement)
Part 1: Nursing Diagnosis
Risk for Aspiration

Part 2: Etiologic Factors (Related to:)
Impaired laryngeal sensation or reflex
Impaired laryngeal peristalsis or tongue function
Impaired laryngeal closure or elevation
Increased gastric volume
Increased intragastric pressure
Decreased lower esophageal sphincter pressure
Decreased antegrade esophageal propulsion

CAD, Coronary artery disease; *ECG,* electrocardiogram; *CK,* creatine kinase; *CK-MB,* MB isoenzyme of creatine kinase.

THE NURSING PROCESS

The nursing process is a method for making clinical decisions. It is a way of thinking and acting in relation to the clinical phenomena of concern to nurses. The nursing process is a systematic decision-making model that is cyclic, not linear. By virtue of its evaluation phase, the nursing process incorporates a feedback loop that maintains quality control of its decision-making outputs. Similar to a problem-solving method, the nursing process begins with an assessment phase and offers an organized, systematic approach to clinical problems. Unlike a problem-solving method, however, the nursing process is continuous, not episodic.

Nursing Diagnosis

NANDA International has supported the continued development and evolution of research-based nursing diagnoses.[24] With nursing diagnosis as a component of their decision-making methods, nurses necessarily become more systematic in the collection and interpretation of data and accomplish a change in the substance of clinical nursing operations, from symptom management to problem solving. The most essential and distinguishing feature of any nursing diagnosis is that it describes a health condition primarily resolved by nursing interventions or therapies.

Some nursing diagnoses need accompanying qualifiers or specifiers based on the characteristics of the health problem as it manifests itself in a particular patient (Box 1-3). For example, the diagnosis Fear needs specification as to the object of the patient's particular fear, such as death, pain, disfigurement, or malignancy.

Outcome Identification

The emphasis on patient outcomes has become increasingly important in the provision of quality care and services. It is important that nurse-sensitive outcomes are delineated so that nursing care and services can be described and understood by all health care professionals, consumers, and payers.[25,26] Outcome statements consist of highly specific indicators that will be used by the nurse in the evaluation phase as criteria that either (1) the actual diagnosis has been resolved or reduced or (2) the risk diagnosis has not occurred. An outcome statement is a projection of the expected influence that the nursing intervention will have on the patient in relation to the identified diagnosis.

Outcome criteria should be measurable, desirable, and attainable, with full consideration given to patient/nurse resources. Measurable outcome criteria consist of recognizable patient behaviors, statements, and physiologic parameters. Many of the phenomena that critical care nurses diagnose and treat are readily measurable, such as adequacy of spontaneous ventilation, cardiac output, and tissue perfusion. Outcome statements are made further measurable by indicating the date and time of anticipated attainment. The individual patient's baseline and patterns and the available nurse/patient resources are the dominant considerations in a projection of desired outcome versus normative values.

Planning

During the planning phase, comprehensive planning of all care and services for the patient is done. The process consists of collaboration by the nurse with all appropriate health care providers, the patient, and family members as well as significant others.

Implementation

Implementation is the action component of planning. The nursing treatment plan is carried out in this phase of the nursing process. Assessment and evaluation are continuous throughout the implementation phase.

Nursing Interventions

Also known as nursing orders or nursing prescriptions, nursing interventions constitute the treatment approach to an identified health alteration. Interventions are selected to satisfy the outcome criteria and prevent or resolve the nursing diagnosis. Interventions have the greatest impact when they are directed at the etiologic/related factors of the diagnosis or, in the case of a risk diagnosis, the risk factors. This approach stipulates that the etiologic factors of a problem can be modified by nursing management.

Evaluation

Evaluation of attainment of the expected patient outcomes occurs formally at intervals designated in the outcome criteria. Informal evaluation occurs continuously. The evaluation phase and the associated activities may be the most important dimensions of the nursing process.

INTERDISCIPLINARY CRITICAL CARE MANAGEMENT

The managed care environment has placed emphasis on examining methods of care delivery and processes of care by all health care professionals. Partnerships have been formed or strengthened, with a focus on increasing quality of care and services while containing or decreasing costs. Coordination of care in critical care units has been demonstrated to influence patient outcomes significantly.[27]

Thornby[28] discussed the importance of skilled communication as essential to excellent patient care and a climate of safety. Ineffective nurse-physician communication has been related to adverse patient events, as well as nurse burnout and turnover.[29] Gerardi and Fontaine[30] described a model of true collaboration that could be used to improve interdisciplinary communications and ultimately to have a positive impact on patient outcomes. In this model, there is a continuum of collaboration that has seven components: self-awareness, information sharing, negotiation, feedback, conflict engagement, conflict resolution, and forgiveness and reconciliation. Successfully working through these stages will result in a collaborative environment.

Case Management

Case management is the process of overseeing the care of patients and organizing services in collaboration with the patient's physician or primary health care provider. The case manager may be a nurse, allied health care provider, or the patient's primary care provider. Case managers are usually assigned to a specific population group, and they facilitate effective coordination of care services as patients move in and out of different settings. Ideally, the case manager oversees the care of the patient across the continuum of care.

Outcomes Management

Outcomes management refers to a model aimed at managing the outcomes of care by the use of various tools, quality improvement processes, and interdisciplinary team involvement and action. Specifically, emphasis is placed on consistent standards of care, measurement of disease-specific clinical outcomes as well as patient functioning and well-being, and assessment of clinical and outcome data for the specific conditions.[31] Outcomes management also takes place in multiple settings across the continuum of care. Professional nurse outcomes managers ensure that variances from the plan of care are addressed in a timely manner. They also examine aggregate information with the team for quality improvement in the interdisciplinary plan of care.

Care Management Tools

Many quality improvement tools are available to providers for care management.

Clinical Pathway

The clinical pathway presents an overview of the entire multidisciplinary plan of care for routine patients. It focuses on the critical elements in the care of certain patient populations and may track variances from the pathway. Pathways are developed by a multidisciplinary team based on a specific diagnosis or condition and integrated with the most recent research and best practices from the literature. Pathways are ideal for high-volume diagnosis groups that are amenable to standardization. Many pathways are incorporated into the medical record or computerized, making them a permanent part of the clinical record.

Algorithm

An algorithm is a stepwise decision-making flowchart for a specific care process or processes. Algorithms are more focused than clinical pathways and guide the clinician through the "if, then" decision-making process, addressing patient responses to particular treatments. Well-known examples of algorithms are the advanced cardiac life support (ACLS) algorithms published by the American Heart Association.

Practice Guideline

A practice guideline is usually developed and written by a team of experts representing professional organizations (e.g., AACN, Society of Critical Care Medicine, American College of Cardiology) or a governmental agency to provide recommendations to care providers. Recommendations are given for managing care and treatments for specific diseases and are based on research or expert opinions.[32] Practice guidelines are generally written in text prose, rather than in the flowchart format of pathways and algorithms. Practice guidelines are used as resources in formulating the pathway or algorithm. An example is a ventilator-associated pneumonia clinical practice guideline that was developed with major implications for nursing practice: head-of-bed elevation, hand hygiene, oral care, glove use, and ventilator tubing condensate removal.[33]

Protocol

A protocol is a common tool in research studies. Protocols are more directive and rigid than pathways or guidelines, and providers should not vary from a protocol. Patients are screened carefully for specific entry criteria before being started on a protocol. The many national research protocols include those for cancer and chemotherapy studies. Protocols are helpful when built-in "alerts" signal the provider to potentially serious problems. Computerization of protocols assists providers in being more proactive to dangerous drug interactions, abnormal laboratory values, and other untoward effects that are preprogrammed into the computer.

Order Set

An order set consists of preprinted provider orders that are used to expedite the order process once a standard has been validated through analytic review of practice and research. Order sets complement and increase compliance with existing practice standards. Sets can also be used to represent the algorithm or protocol in order format.

REGULATORY ISSUES IN CRITICAL CARE

SAFETY

Patient safety has become a major focus of attention by health care consumers as well as providers of care and administrators of health care institutions. The Institute of Medicine publication *Crossing the Quality Chasm: A New Health System for the 21st Century* was released in 2001 and has been the impetus for debate and actions to improve the safety of health care environments. In this report, information and details were given indicating that health care harms patients too frequently and routinely fails to deliver its potential benefits.[34] Oftentimes, the definitions of medical errors and approaches to resolving patient safety issues differ among nurses, physicians, administrators, and other health care providers.[35]

Patient safety has been described as an ethical imperative, and one that is implied in health care professionals' actions and interpersonal processes.[36] Critical care units are prime examples of where errors may occur due to the hectic, complex environment where the margins of error are narrow and the demands for safety are crucial.[37] In this environment, patients are particularly vulnerable due to their compromised physiologic status, multiple technologic and pharmacologic interventions, and multiple care providers who frequently work at a fast pace. It is essential that care delivery processes that minimize the opportunity for errors are designed and that a "safety culture" rather than a "blame culture" is created.[38,39] When an injury or inappropriate care occurs, it is crucial that health care professionals promptly give an explanation of how the injury or mistake occurred and the short- or long-term effects to the patient and family. They should be informed that the factors involved in the injury will be investigated so that steps can be taken to reduce or avoid the likelihood of similar injury to other patients.

The Joint Commission has approved 2007 National Patient Safety Goals (NPSGs)[40] that are to be implemented in health care organizations (Box 1-4).

The Safe Medical Device Act (SMDA) requires that hospitals report serious or potentially serious device-related injuries or illness of patients and/or employees

Box 1-4

2007 National Patient Safety Goals

- Improve the accuracy of patient identification
- Improve the effectiveness of communication among caregivers
- Improve the safety of using medications
- Reduce the risk of health care–associated infections
- Accurately and completely reconcile medications across the continuum of care
- Reduce the risk of patient harm resulting from falls
- Encourage patients' active involvement in their own care as a patient and safety strategy
- Ensure that the organization identifies safety risks inherent in its patient population

to the manufacturer of the device, and if death is involved, to the U.S. Food and Drug Administration (FDA). In addition, implantable devices must be documented and tracked.[41] This reporting serves as an "early warning system" so that the FDA can obtain information on device problems. Failure to comply with the act will result in civil action.

PRIVACY AND CONFIDENTIALITY

In 1996 a landmark law was passed to provide consumers with greater access to health care insurance, promote more standardization and efficiency in the health care industry, and protect the privacy of health care data.[42] The Health Insurance Portability and Accountability Act of 1996 (HIPAA) has created additional challenges for health care organizations and providers due to the stringent requirements and additional resources needed in order to meet the requirements of the law. Most specific to critical care clinicians is the privacy and confidentiality related to protection of health care data. This has implications when interacting with family members as well as others, and the oftentimes very close work environment, tight working spaces, and emergent situations. Clinicians are referred to their organizational policies and procedures for specific procedures for their organizations.

evolve To test your mastery of this chapter, try the Open-Book Quiz at http://evolve.elsevier.com/Urden/priorities/

REFERENCES

1. Kleinpell R: Reports of role descriptions of acute care nurse practitioners, *AACN Clin Issues* 9(2):290, 1998.
2. American Association of Critical-Care Nurses: *Practice resources,* http://www.aacn.org.
3. Omery A, Williams RP: An appraisal of research utilization across the United States, *J Nurs Adm* 29(12):50, 1999.
4. Wojner AW: Why do we do the things we do? Stop the carnage of nursing research, *AACN News* 17(4):2, 12, 2000.
5. Mick D: Folklore, personal preference, or research-based practice, *Am J Crit Care* 9(1):6, 2000.
6. Rosswurm MA, Larrabee JH: A model for change to evidence-based practice, *Image J Nurs Sch* 31(4):317, 1999.
7. Fineout-Overholt E, Melnyk B: Building a culture of evidence-based practice, *Nurse Leader,* p. 26, December 2005.
8. McPheeters M, Lohr KN: Evidence-based practice and nursing: commentary, *Outcomes Manag Nurs Pract* 3(3):99, 1999.
9. Newhouse RP: Examining the support for evidence-based practice, *J Nurs Adm* 36(7/8):337, 2006.
10. Titler MG et al: The Iowa model of evidence-based practice to promote quality care, *Crit Care Nurs Clin North Am* 13(4):497, 2001.
11. Hopp L: Talk to me about evidence-based practice, *AACN Adv Crit Care* 17(23):250, 2006.
12. American Association of Critical-Care Nurses: *Practice alert,* http://www.aacn.org/AACN/practiceAlerts.nsf/vwdoc/pa2, accessed April 7, 2007.
13. Panting K: Intensive care/intensive cure: the future of critical care? *Crit Care Nurse* 15(12):100, 1995.
14. Miller KL: Keeping the care in nursing care: our biggest challenge, *J Nurs Adm* 25(11):29, 1995.
15. Marlano C: Holistic ethics, *Am J Nurs* 101(1):24A, 2001.
16. Holistic healing methods positively advance patient care, *Nurs Manage,* p. 30, July 2006.
17. Powers PH et al: The value of patient- and family-centered care, *Am J Nurs* 100(5):84, 2000.
18. Alspach G: Time for sensitivity training: cultural diversity in cardiovascular disease, *Crit Care Nurse* 20(3):14, 2000.
19. Gonzales R, Gooden M, Porter C: Eliminating racial and ethnic disparities in health care, *Am J Nurs* 100(3):56, 2000.
20. Leonard B, Plotnikoff GA: Awareness: the heart of cultural competence, *AACN Clin Issues* 11(1):51, 2000.
21. Holt-Ashley M: Nurses pray: use of prayer and spirituality as a complementary therapy in the intensive care setting, *AACN Clin Issues* 11(1):60, 2000.
22. Bensing K: Prayer and healing, part II. *Advance for Nurses,* p. 10, June 12, 2006.
23. American Nurses Association: *Nursing's social policy statement,* Washington, DC, 1995, The Association.
24. North American Nursing Diagnosis Association: Nursing diagnosis: definitions and classification, Philadelphia, 1999, The Association.
25. Brooten D, Naylor M: Nurses' effect on changing patient outcomes, *Image J Nurs Sch* 27(2):95, 1995.
26. Himali U: A unified nursing language: the missing link in establishing nursing-sensitive patient outcomes, *Am Nurs* 27(2):23, 1995.
27. Knaus W et al: An evaluation of outcome from intensive care in major medical centers, *Ann Intern Med* 104:410, 1986.
28. Thornby D: Beginning the journey to skilled communication, *AACN Adv Crit Care* 17(3):266, 2006.
29. Arford PH: Nurse-physician communication: an organizational accountability, *Nurs Econ* 23(2):72, 2005.
30. Gerardi D, Fontaine DK: True collaboration: envisioning new ways of working together, *AACN Adv Crit Care* 18(1):10, 2007.
31. Wojner A: Outcomes management: an interdisciplinary search for best practice, *AACN Clin Issues* 7(1):133, 1996.
32. Hedges C: Show me the guidelines, *AACN Adv Crit Care* 18(1):88, 2007.
33. Abbott CA et al: Adoption of a ventilator-associated pneumonia clinical practice guideline, *Worldviews Evid Based Nurs* 3(4):139, 2006.
34. Institute of Medicine: *Crossing the quality chasm: a new health system for the 21st century,* Washington, DC, 2001, National Academy Press.
35. Cook A et al: An error by any other name, *Am J Nurs* 104(6):32, 2004.
36. White GB: Patient safety: an ethical imperative, *Nurs Econ* 20(4):195, 2002.
37. Benner P: Creating a culture of safety and improvement: a key to reducing medical error, *Am J Crit Care* 10(4):281, 2001.

38. Smith AP: In search of safety: an interview with Gina Pugliese, *Nurs Econ* 20(1):6, 2002.
39. Kalisch BJ, Aebersold M: Overcoming barriers to patient safety, *Nurs Econ* 24(3):143, 2006.
40. The Joint Commission: *National patient safety goals*, http://www.jointcommission.org/PatientSafety/NationalPatientSafetyGoals/07_hap_cap_nps, accessed April 7, 2007.
41. Jensen JR: FDA's safe medical device act, *Risk Manag Rep* 1(2):1, 1997.
42. Centers for Medicare & Medicaid Services: *Health Insurance Portability and Accountability Act (HIPAA)—administrative simplification*, http://www.cms.hhs.gov.

CHAPTER 2

Ethical and Legal Issues

LINDA D. URDEN

OBJECTIVES

- Discuss ethical principles as they relate to critical care patients.
- Discuss strategies to address moral distress in critical care nursing.
- Discuss the concept of medical futility.
- Describe what constitutes an ethical dilemma.
- List steps for making ethical decisions.
- Identify legal and professional obligations of critical care nurses.
- Describe the elements of certain torts that may result from critical care nursing practice.
- Identify and discuss specific legal issues in critical care nursing practice.

MORALS AND ETHICS

Morals are the "shoulds," "should nots," "oughts," and "ought nots" of actions and behaviors and have been related closely to sexual mores and behaviors in Western society. Religious and cultural values and beliefs largely mold a person's moral thoughts and actions. Morals form the basis for action and provide a framework for evaluation of behavior.

Ethics is concerned with the "why" of the action rather than with whether the action is right or wrong, good or bad. Ethics implies that an evaluation is being made and is theoretically based on or derived from a set of standards.

MORAL DISTRESS

Moral distress has recently been discussed in the literature as a serious problem for nurses. It occurs when one knows the ethically appropriate action to take but cannot act upon it. It also presents when one acts in a manner contrary to personal and professional values. As a result, there can be significant emotional and physical stress that leads to feelings of loss of personal integrity and dissatisfaction with the work environment.[1] Relationships with both co-workers and patients are affected and can negatively impact the quality of care. There is also a great impact on personal relationships and family life. It is therefore important that nurses recognize moral distress and actively seek strategies to address the issue through institutional, personal, and professional organizational resources. Knowledge and application of ethical principles and guidelines will assist the nurse in daily practice when ethical dilemmas occur. The American Association of Critical-Care Nurses (AACN)[1,2] has created a framework to support those nurses who are experiencing moral distress (Figure 2-1).

ETHICAL PRINCIPLES

Certain ethical principles were derived from classic ethical theories that are used in health care decision making. *Principles* are general guidelines that govern conduct, provide a basis for reasoning, and direct actions. The six ethical principles discussed here are autonomy, beneficence, nonmaleficence, veracity, fidelity, and justice (Box 2-1).

AUTONOMY

The concept of autonomy appears in all ancient writings and early Greek philosophy. In health care,

Box 2-1
Ethical Principles in Critical Care

- Autonomy
- Beneficence
- Nonmaleficence
- Veracity
- Fidelity
  - Confidentiality
  - Privacy
- Justice/allocation of resources

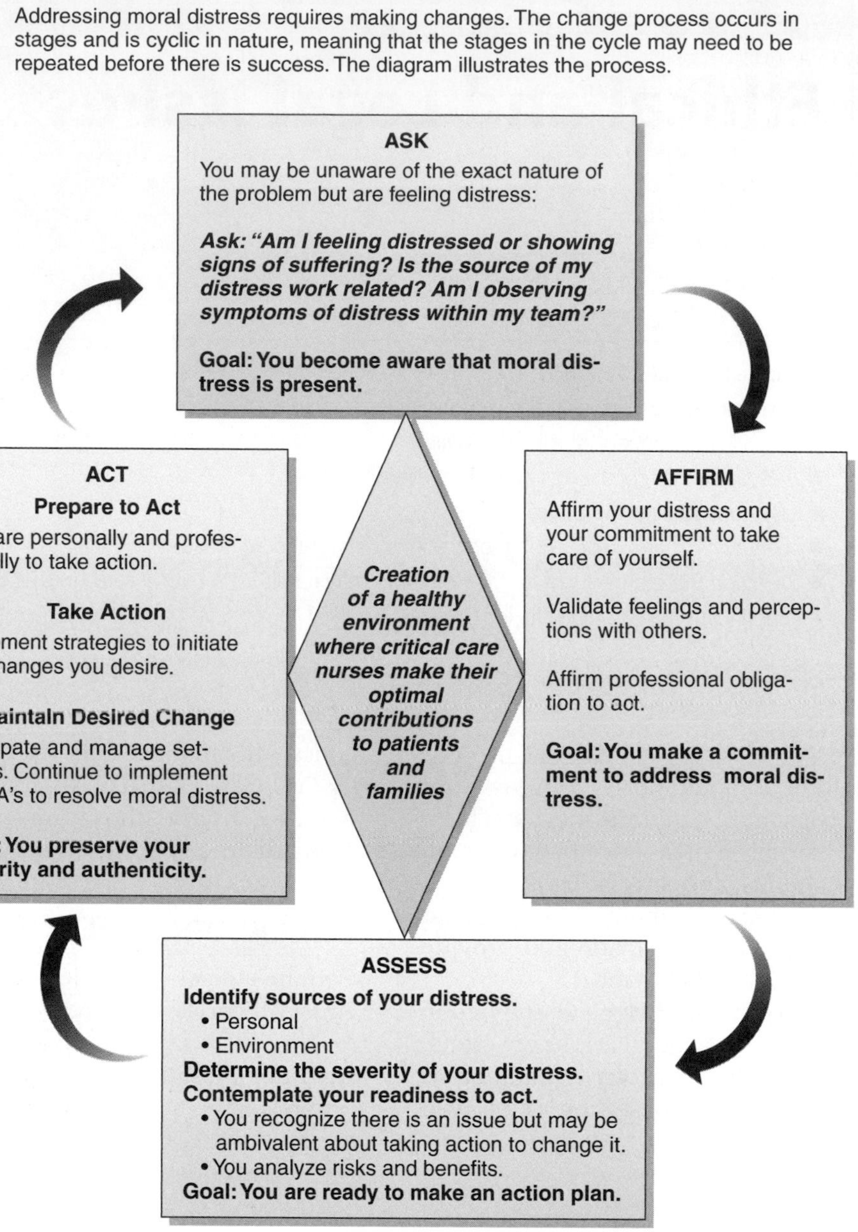
Addressing moral distress requires making changes. The change process occurs in stages and is cyclic in nature, meaning that the stages in the cycle may need to be repeated before there is success. The diagram illustrates the process.
ASK
You may be unaware of the exact nature of the problem but are feeling distress:
Ask: "Am I feeling distressed or showing signs of suffering? Is the source of my distress work related? Am I observing symptoms of distress within my team?"
Goal: You become aware that moral distress is present.
AFFIRM
Affirm your distress and your commitment to take care of yourself.
Validate feelings and perceptions with others.
Affirm professional obligation to act.
Goal: You make a commitment to address moral distress.
ASSESS
Identify sources of your distress.
• Personal
• Environment
Determine the severity of your distress.
Contemplate your readiness to act.
• You recognize there is an issue but may be ambivalent about taking action to change it.
• You analyze risks and benefits.
Goal: You are ready to make an action plan.
ACT
Prepare to Act
Prepare personally and professionally to take action.
Take Action
Implement strategies to initiate the changes you desire.
Maintain Desired Change
Anticipate and manage setbacks. Continue to implement the 4A's to resolve moral distress.
Goal: You preserve your integrity and authenticity.
Creation of a healthy environment where critical care nurses make their optimal contributions to patients and families

FIGURE 2-1. The 4A's to rise above moral distress. (From American Association of Critical-Care Nurses, Aliso Viejo, Calif, 2004.)

autonomy can be viewed as the freedom to make decisions about one's own body without the coercion or interference of others. Autonomy is a freedom of choice or a self-determination that is a basic human right. It can be experienced in all human life events.

The critical care nurse is often "caught in the middle" in ethical situations, and promoting autonomous decision making is one of those situations. As the nurse works closely with patients and families to promote autonomous decision making, another crucial element becomes clear. Patients and families must have all the information about a particular situation before they can make a decision that is best for them. They not only should be given all the pertinent information and facts but also must have a clear understanding of what was presented.[3] In this situation the nurse assumes one of the most important roles of the health care team, that is, as *patient advocate,* providing more information as needed, clarifying points, reinforcing information, and providing support during the decision-making process.

Beneficence

The concept of doing good and preventing harm to patients is a sine qua non for the nursing profession. However, the ethical principle of beneficence, which requires that one *promote* the well-being of patients, indicates the importance of this duty for the health care professional. The principle of beneficence presupposes that harms and benefits are balanced, leading to positive or beneficial outcomes.

In approaching issues related to beneficence, conflict with the principle of autonomy is common. Paternalism exists when the nurse or physician makes a decision for the patient without consulting the patient.

Traditional health care has been based on a paternalistic approach to patients. Many patients are still more comfortable in deferring all decisions about care and treatment to their health care provider. Active involvement by various organizations and agencies in regard to health care has demonstrated a trend toward the public's need and desire for more information about health care in general, as well as more about alternative treatments and providers. Paternalism, or *maternalism* in the case of female providers, may always be a possibility in the health care setting, but enlightened consumers are causing a change in this practice of health care professionals.

NONMALEFICENCE

The ethical principle of nonmaleficence, which dictates that one prevent harm and correct harmful situations, is a prima facie duty for the nurse. Thoughtfulness and care are necessary, as is balancing risks and benefits. Beneficence and nonmaleficence are on two ends of a continuum and are often adhered to differently, depending on the views of the practitioner.

VERACITY

Veracity, or truth telling, is an important ethical principle that underlies the nurse-patient relationship. Communication trust, or the trust of disclosure, is rooted in respect and based on veracity.[4]

Veracity is important when soliciting informed consent because the patient needs to be aware of all potential risks of and benefits to be derived from specific treatments or alternative therapies.[5-7] Again, the critical care nurse may be in the middle of a situation where all the facts and information about a particular treatment option are not disclosed. Sometimes information has been given accurately to the patient and family but has been delivered with bias or in a misleading way. Veracity must guide all areas of practice for the nurse, that is, in colleague relationships and employee relationships, as well as in the nurse-patient relationship.

FIDELITY

Fidelity, or faithfulness and promise keeping to patients, is also a sine qua non for nursing. It forms a bond between individuals and is the basis of all relationships, both professional and personal. Regardless of the amount of autonomy that patients have in the critical care areas, they still depend on the nurse for many types of physical care and emotional support. A trusting relationship that establishes and maintains an open atmosphere is positive for all involved.[8] Making a promise to a patient is voluntary for the nurse, whereas having respect for a patient's decision making is a moral obligation.[9]

Fidelity extends to the family of the critical care patient. When a promise is made to the family that they will be called if an emergency arises or that they will be informed of any other special events concerning the patient, the nurse must make every effort to follow through on the promise. Fidelity not only will uphold the nurse-family relationship but also will reflect positively on the nursing profession as a whole and on the institution where the nurse is employed.

Confidentiality is one element of fidelity that is based on traditional health care professional ethics. Confidentiality is described as a right whereby patient information can be shared only with those involved in the care of the patient. An exception to this guideline might be when the welfare of others will be put at risk by keeping patient information confidential. Again in this situation, the nurse must balance ethical principles and weigh risks with benefits. Special circumstances, such as the existence of mandatory reporting laws, will guide the nurse in certain situations.

Privacy also has been described as being inherent in the principle of fidelity. Privacy may be closely aligned with confidentiality of patient information and a patient's right to privacy of his or her person, such as maintaining privacy for the patient by pulling the curtains around the bed or making sure that the patient is adequately covered.

JUSTICE

The principle of justice is often used synonymously with the concept of *allocation of scarce resources.* With escalating health care costs, expanded technologies, an aging population with their own special health care needs, and in some cases a scarcity of health care personnel, the question of how to allocate health care becomes even more complex.

The application of the justice principle in health care is concerned primarily with divided or portioned allocation of goods and services, which is termed distributive justice. As health care resources become increasingly scarce, allocation of resources to certain programs and rationing of resources within certain programs will become more evident.

MEDICAL FUTILITY

The concept of medical futility has resulted in various discussions and proposed criteria and formulas to predict outcomes of care.[10-12] Medical futility has both a qualitative and a quantitative basis and can be defined as "any effort to achieve a result that is possible but that reasoning or experience suggests is highly improbable and that cannot be systematically reproduced."[13]

Therapy or treatment that achieves its predictable outcome and desired effect is, by definition, effective. Effect must be distinguished from benefit, however; although predictable and desired, the effect is nonetheless futile if it is of no benefit to the patient.

ETHICAL FOUNDATION FOR NURSING PRACTICE

Traditional theories of professions include a code of ethics upon which the practice of the profession is based. It is by adherence to a code of ethics that the professional fulfills an obligation to provide quality practice to society.

A professional ethic is based on three elements: (1) the professional code of ethics, (2) the purpose of the profession, and (3) the standards of practice of the professional. The code of ethics developed by the profession is the delineation of its values and relationships with and among members of the profession and society. The need for the profession and its inherent promise to provide certain duties form a contract between nursing and society. The professional standards describe specifics of practice in a variety of settings and subspecialties. Each element is dynamic, and ongoing evaluations are necessary as societal expectations change, technologies increase, and the profession evolves.

NURSING CODE OF ETHICS

The American Nurses Association (ANA) provides the major source of ethical guidance for the nursing profession. The *Code of Ethics for Nurses* serves as the basis for nurses in analyzing ethical issues and decision making (Box 2-2).[14]

Box 2-2

Code of Ethics for Nurses

1. The nurse, in all professional relationships, practices with compassion and respect for the inherent dignity, worth, and uniqueness of every individual, unrestricted by considerations of social or economic status, personal attributes, or the nature of health problems.
2. The nurse's primary commitment is to the patient, whether an individual, family group, or community.
3. The nurse promotes, advocates for, and strives to protect the health, safety, and rights of the patient.
4. The nurse is responsible and accountable for individual nursing practice and determines the appropriate delegation of tasks consistent with the nurse's obligation to provide optimum patient care.
5. The nurse owes the same duties to self as to others, including the responsibility to preserve integrity and safety, to maintain competence, and to continue personal and professional growth.
6. The nurse participates in establishing, maintaining, and improving health care environments and conditions of employment conducive to the provision of quality health care and consistent with the values of the profession through individual and collective action.
7. The nurse participates in the advancement of the profession through contributions to practice, education, administration, and knowledge development.
8. The nurse collaborates with other health care professionals and the public in promoting community, national, and international efforts to meet health needs.
9. The profession of nursing, as represented by associations and their members, is responsible for articulating nursing values, for maintaining the integrity of the profession and its practice, and for shaping social policy.

From American Nurses Association: *Code of ethics for nurses with interpretive statements,* Washington, DC, 2002, The Association.

WHAT IS AN ETHICAL DILEMMA?

In general, ethical cases are not always clear-cut or "black and white." The most common ethical dilemmas encountered in critical care are forgoing treatment and allocating the scarce resources of critical care. Before the application of any decision model is made, it must be determined whether a true ethical dilemma exists. Thompson and Thompson[15] delineate the following three criteria for defining moral and ethical dilemmas in clinical practice:

1. An awareness of the different options
2. An issue that has different options
3. Two or more options with true or "good" aspects, with the choice of one option over the other compromising the option not chosen

STEPS IN ETHICAL DECISION MAKING

To facilitate the ethical decision-making process, a model or framework must be used so that all parties involved will consistently and clearly examine the multiple ethical issues that arise in critical care (Box 2-3).

Step One

First, the major aspects of the medical and health problems must be identified. In other words, the scientific basis of the problem, potential sequelae, prognosis, and all data relevant to the health status must be examined.

Box 2-3

Steps in Ethical Decision Making

1. Identify the health problem.
2. Define the ethical issue.
3. Gather additional information.
4. Delineate the decision maker.
5. Examine ethical and moral principles.
6. Explore alternative options.
7. Implement decisions.
8. Evaluate and modify actions.

Step Two

The ethical problem must be clearly delineated from other types of problems. *Systems problems* result from failures and inadequacies in the health care facility's organization and operation or in the health care system as a whole and are often misinterpreted as ethical issues. *Social problems* arising from conditions in the community, state, or country as a whole also are occasionally confused with ethical issues. Social problems can lead to *systemic problems,* which can constrain responses to ethical problems.

Step Three

Although categories of necessary additional information will vary, whatever is missing in the initial problem presentation should be obtained. If not already known, the health prognosis and potential sequelae should be clarified. Usual demographic data (e.g., age, ethnicity, religious preferences, educational/economic status) may be considered in the decision-making process. The role of the family or extended family and other support systems needs to be examined. Any desires that the patient may have expressed about the treatment decision, either in writing or in conversation, must be obtained.

Step Four

The patient is the primary decision maker and autonomously makes these decisions after receiving information about the alternatives and sequelae of treatments or lack of treatment. In many ethical dilemmas the patient is not competent to make a decision, however, as when the patient is comatose or otherwise physically or mentally unable to make a decision. In these cases, surrogates are designated or court appointed because the urgency of the situation requires a quick decision.

Others who are involved in the decision also need to be identified at this time, such as family, nurse, physician, social worker, clergy, and members of other disciplines in close contact with the patient. The role of the nurse must be examined. It may not be necessary for the nurse to make a decision at all; rather, the nurse's role may be simply to provide additional information and support to the decision maker.

Step Five

Personal values, beliefs, and moral convictions of all persons involved in the decision process need to be known. Whether actually achieved through a group meeting or through personal introspection, values clarification facilitates the decision-making process.

General ethical principles also need to be examined in regard to the case at hand. For example, are veracity, informed consent, and autonomy being promoted? Beneficence and nonmaleficence will be analyzed as they relate to a patient's condition and desires. Close examination of these principles will reveal any compromise of ethical or moral principles for either the patient or the health care provider and will assist in decision making.

Step Six

After the identification of alternative options, the outcome of each action must be predicted. This analysis helps the person select the option with the best "fit" for the specific situation or problem. Both short-range and long-range consequences of each action must be examined, and new or creative actions must be encouraged. Consideration also must be given to the "no action" option, which is another choice.

Step Seven

When a decision has been reached, it is usually after much thought and consideration.

Step Eight

Evaluation of an ethical decision serves both to assess the decision at hand and to provide a basis for future ethical decisions. If outcomes are not as predicted, it may be possible to modify the plan or to use an alternative that was not originally chosen.

LEGAL RELATIONSHIPS

When a professional nurse commences employment in a critical care facility, three legal relationships are formed. First, on accepting employment, the relationship between the nurse and the *employer* is formed. Second, on assuming the care of a patient, a relationship is created between the patient and nurse. Third, every state has a law that mandates the entry-level educational requirements that must be met for a person to become licensed to practice nursing. The act of licensing creates a legal relationship between the nurse and the *state.*

These relationships impose legal obligations. The nurse owes a patient the duty of reasonable and prudent care under the circumstances. The nurse owes

Box 2-4
Classification of Torts

Intentional Torts
Assault
Battery
False imprisonment
Trespass
Infliction of mental or emotional distress

Specific Torts
Defamation
Slander
Libel
Invasion of privacy

Unintentional Torts
Negligence
Medical/nursing treatment torts
Professional malpractice
Abandonment

Strict Liability
Product liability

the employer the duty of competency and the ability to follow policies and procedures; other contractual duties may exist as well. The nurse owes the state and public the duty of safe, competent practice as legally defined by practice standards.

The critical care nurse's legal duties are enforceable, and the nurse can be held legally accountable for breach or violation through a variety of laws and legal processes. Nurses, hospitals, patients, and other health care providers can be involved in a variety of legal disputes, including negligence and professional malpractice, incompetence, unauthorized practice, unprofessional or illegal conduct, workers' compensation, and contract and labor disputes.

Tort Liability

The area of civil law is divided into many categories, two of which are contracts and torts. The law of contracts contains a set of rules governing the creation and enforcement of an agreement between two or more parties (entities or individuals). For example, contract law may apply to a dispute between the nurse, as employee, and an institution, as employer. In contrast, a *tort* is a type of civil wrong or injury that results from a breach of a legal duty. Tort law is generally divided into intentional and unintentional torts, strict liability, and specific torts (Box 2-4).

Intentional torts involve (1) a mind-set indicative of purpose and (2) an act. Intent exists when the person forms a mental design to achieve a particular outcome and consequence. Assault, battery, false imprisonment, trespass, and intentional infliction of emotional distress are all examples of intentional torts. In each of these torts, a specific act is required, and there is purposeful interference with a person or property.

In *assault* the act is a behavior that places the *plaintiff* (person being wronged who later sues) in fear or apprehension of offensive physical contact; in civil law the *defendant* is the person being sued for wronging another. *Battery* is the unlawful or offensive touching of or contact with the plaintiff or something attached to the plaintiff. *False imprisonment* is detaining, confining, or restraining another against the person's will. The two types of *trespass* involve (1) a person's land and (2) an individual's personal property. These acts are defined as "unauthorized entry onto land of another" or "unauthorized handling of another's personal property." In addition, the law protects a person's interest in peace of mind through the tort claim of *infliction of mental or emotional distress.* The act in this case, however, must involve extreme misconduct or outrageous behavior.

Unintentional torts involve failures or breach of nursing duties that lead to harm, including negligence, malpractice, and abandonment. *Negligence* is the failure to meet an ordinary standard of care, resulting in injury to the patient or plaintiff. *Malpractice* is a type of professional liability based on negligence and includes professional misconduct, breach of a duty or standard of care, illegal or immoral conduct, or failure to exercise reasonable skill, all of which lead to harm (see later discussion). *Abandonment* is a type of negligence in which a duty to give care exists, is ignored, and results in harm to a patient. It is the absence of care and the failure to respond to a patient that may give rise to an allegation of abandonment.

Specific torts involve privacy and reputation interests and include invasion of privacy and defamation. *Defamation* is composed of two torts: *slander* (oral defamation) and *libel* (written defamation). Defamation is not the mere statement or writing of words that injures a person's reputation or good name; the words also must be communicated to another. If the words are true, this may provide a defense against a defamation claim. *Invasion of privacy* involves the violation of a person's right to privacy. Nurses can invade another's privacy by revealing confidential information without authorization or by failing to follow the patient's health care decisions.

Nurses can avoid allegations of these specific claims by (1) making statements about another's reputation only when necessary and substantiated by fact and (2) respecting another's privacy and autonomy and maintaining a confidential relationship with the patient.

Administrative Law and Licensing Statutes

A second type of law and legal process in which nurses are involved is administrative law and the regulatory process. This area of law governs the nurse's relationship with the *government,* either state or federal. Administrative law involves the rules of the government's activities in regulating health care delivery and practice; the rules of investigation, procedure, and evidence differ from those of civil and criminal law. Several government health care agencies are involved in such regulation.

A state has the power to regulate nursing because the state is responsible for the health, safety, and welfare of its citizens. Therefore, establishing minimal entry-level requirements, standards of nursing practice, and educational requirements are acceptable state actions. State legislatures create laws governing nursing practice, generally termed nurse practice acts, and a unit of the state government within the executive branch is responsible for the enforcement of nursing laws. This unit is often called the *State Board of Nursing* or *Board of Nurse Examiners;* however, the name varies by state. Standards also vary by state, which is another important reason that nurses should seek advice from counsel licensed to practice law in their own state. Because law is the minimum expected behavior, the profession oftentimes sets a higher standard. Additional methods to ensure competency are continuing education for renewal of license, work-based orientation programs, and certification in specialty practice areas. Self-reflection and assessment of one's current competencies and level of technical knowledge can serve to elevate practice.[16]

Negligence and Malpractice

As defined earlier, negligence is an unintentional tort involving a breach of duty or failure (through an act or an omission) to meet a standard of care, causing personal harm. Malpractice is a type of professional liability based on negligence in which the defendant is held accountable for breach of a duty of care involving special knowledge and skill. These torts have several elements, all of which the plaintiff has the burden of proving.

The law recognizes four elements of negligence and malpractice. The first element, a *duty,* or legal obligation, requires the person ("actor") to conform to a certain standard of conduct for the protection of others against unreasonable risks. The critical care nurse's legal duty is to act in a reasonable and prudent manner, as any other critical care nurse would act under similar circumstances. The standard is that of a critical care nurse, a professional with special knowledge and skill in critical care. The standard is that owed at the time the incident or injury occurred, not at the time of litigation. In most jurisdictions the standard of care is a national standard, as opposed to a local or community standard. General critical care nursing duties are implied by statute and administrative rules and regulations and are stated explicitly in judicial decisions (Box 2-5).

Box 2-5
Legal Duties of Critical Care Nurses

- Observe.
- Assess.
- Conduct ongoing observations and assessments.
- Recognize significance of information.
- Report.
- Plan, implement, and evaluate care.
- Respond to changes.
- Interpret and carry out orders.
- Take reasonable measures to ensure patient safety.
- Exercise professional judgment.
- Properly perform procedures.
- Follow hospital policies and procedures.
- Record and document.

The second element, *breach of duty,* involves a failure on the actor's part to conform to the standard required. *Causation,* the third element, involves proving that the actor's breach was reasonably close or causally connected to the resulting injury. This is also referred to as *proximate cause.* The fourth element, *injury* or damages, must involve an actual loss or damage to the plaintiff or his or her interest. A plaintiff may claim different types of damages, such as compensatory and punitive. Patient injury can range in value, depending on what happened to the patient. The plaintiff must produce evidence of the damages and their value. If the nurse breaches a standard of care that leads to injury, the plaintiff must show what amount of money will compensate for his or her injuries. The goal of the compensation is to provide the amount of money that will return the plaintiff to the position that existed before the injury occurred.

Res ipsa loquitur, "the thing speaks for itself," is a rule of evidence used by plaintiffs in negligence or malpractice litigation. It is a rebuttable presumption or inference of negligence by the defendant, which arises on the plaintiff's proof that (1) the injury is one that ordinarily does not happen in the absence of negligence and (2) the instrumentality causing the injury was in the defendant's exclusive management and control. The burden then shifts to the defendant to prove absence of negligence. For example, negligence can be inferred when muscle ischemia and necrosis occur as a result of improper body positioning and the application of splints or restraints. Negligence can also be inferred from a foreign object left in a patient's body cavity after surgery.

Because critical care nurses deal with life-threatening situations, any patient injury is potentially severe or may result in death. Should the injury occur as a result of alleged negligence, the nurse may be held liable

Box 2-6

Select Critical Care Nursing Actions in Negligence Lawsuits

General

Failure to advise physician/supervisor of change in patient's health status
Failure to monitor patients at requisite intervals
Failure to adhere to established institutional protocols
Failure to assess patients' clinical status adequately
Failure to respond to alarms
Failure to maintain accurate, timely, and complete medical records
Failure to carry out treatment and evaluate treatment results properly
Failure to use safe, functional equipment

Specific

Failure to provide supplemental oxygen when the ventilator cannot be promptly reattached
Failure to use intravenous (IV) infusion equipment properly, causing extensive fluid extravasation
Failure to monitor IV infusions, recognize infiltration, and discontinue IV therapy
Failure to recognize signs of intracranial bleeding
Failure to investigate patient's complaint of pain and discover hematoma under blood pressure cuff

for the patient's death and also for the resulting loss to surviving family members. All states have "wrongful death" acts, and a number of states have both "death" acts and "survival" acts, which are prosecuted concurrently. With the two causes of action, the expenses, pain and suffering, and loss of earnings of the decedent up to the time of death are allocated to the survival action, and loss of benefits to the survivors is allocated to the wrongful death action.

Specific critical care nursing actions have resulted in litigation (Box 2-6). In such cases the nurse's action is central to the lawsuit. However, nurses are named as sole defendant or codefendant in a comparatively small percentage of cases. Although this pattern is changing, physicians and hospitals are generally named as defendants.

Typically, nursing negligence cases involve breach or failure in six general categories (Box 2-7). The first category includes the use of defective equipment or the failure to perform safety and maintenance assessments. Nurses have made errors in drug identification, administration, and dosages. Nurses have failed to report changes in patient status to physicians in a timely manner. Nurses have not communicated to supervisors a physician's failure to respond to the nurse's communication. Failure to supervise and assist patients who subsequently fall is also a source of nursing negligence. Improper wound care with resulting infection and incorrect instrument and sponge counts in the surgical setting have also led to patient injury and lawsuits.

Box 2-7

Six General Categories of Nursing Negligence

1. Improper administration of treatments
2. Improper administration of medications
3. Inadequate or false written and verbal communication
4. Insufficient supervision of patients
5. Improper postoperative treatment and wound care
6. Incorrect perioperative instrument and sponge counts

It is important to report and document any adverse event or unexpected outcome in an honest and genuine manner. Disclosure should take place as soon after the event has been identified as possible. This information needs to be orally discussed with the patient and family, as well as documented. Documentation, also upon identification of the issue, needs to include the date, time, place, and all individuals involved, including the discussion with the patient and family. Document the discussion with the patient and family (use quotations of any key statements of anyone involved), the follow-up plan, and any subsequent discussions. The documentation must be accurate and concise with no admission of guilt or negligence.[17]

Legal Doctrines and Theories of Liability

In tort law the nurse's action may be examined and legal duties defined according to the following theories of liability:

- Personal liability
- Vicarious liability: *respondeat superior*
- Corporate liability
- Other liability doctrines (e.g., temporary or borrowed servant, captain of the ship)

Under the theory of *personal liability,* each individual is responsible for his or her own actions, including the critical care nurse, supervisor, physician, hospital, and patient. Each has responsibilities that are uniquely his or her own. In contrast to personal liability, the individual may be afforded the protection of personal immunity.

Vicarious liability is indirect responsibility, such as the liability of an employer for the acts of the employee. Under the doctrine of *respondeat superior,* a "master" is liable for certain wrongful acts of a "servant," as is a principal for those of an agent. An employer may be liable for an employee's acts that are performed within the legitimate scope of employment. In critical care the nurse typically is an employee of a hospital. However, nurses may be independent contractors with the hospital through critical care nursing agencies or businesses. If the latter is the case, the nurse is not an employee of the hospital, and the hospital is not vicariously liable for the nurse's action.

Corporate liability is the liability attached to the corporate entity (e.g., the hospital) for its own corporate activities and decisions.

Other doctrines, such as *temporary servant* or *borrowed servant* and *captain of the ship,* may apply to the critical care nurse and the critical care unit. These doctrines are used when the plaintiff argues that the physician is responsible for the nurse's actions, even though the nurse is an employee of the hospital, not of the physician. If it can be shown that the nurse acted under the direction and control of the physician, the physician may be accountable for the nurse's actions. However, these doctrines are becoming increasingly uncommon. What viability remains is typically found in cases involving nurse anesthetists and operating room nurses.

NURSE PRACTICE ACTS

The practice of nursing is regulated by the state. As a general rule, the state's police power to regulate prevails, as long as the state's actions are not arbitrary or capricious. All nurses must be licensed to practice under their individual state's licensure statutes. Licensure authorizes (1) the right to practice and (2) access to employment. Therefore licensure is a property right that is constitutionally protected. Every state has legislation that defines the legal scope of nursing practice and defines unprofessional and illegal conduct that may lead to investigation and disciplinary action by the state and sanctions on the right to practice. The state nurse practice act establishes entry requirements, definitions of practice, and criteria for discipline. Although licensure is mandatory for registered nurses (RNs), statutory content varies among the states.

Generally, state law contains two definitions of nursing: one for the RN (or professional nurse) and one for the licensed practical (or vocational or technical) nurse. These definitions determine titles that may be used by nurses, the scope of nursing practice, and requirements for entering the nursing profession. In some states, advanced RN practice, prescriptive authority for certain nurses, and third-party reimbursement are also defined by statute.

Mandatory continuing education requirements are also defined by statute in most states. The state authorizes its board of nursing to monitor practice, implement standards of care, enforce rules and regulations, and issue sanctions. Sanctions include additional education, restricted practice, supervised practice, license suspension, and license revocation. Some form of disciplinary action generally occurs as a result of unauthorized practice, negligence or malpractice, incompetence, chemical or other impairment, criminal acts, or violations of specific nurse practice act provisions.

The scope of medical practice is also statutorily defined, and in most states a physician is given broad discretion to delegate tasks to others. Physicians may delegate to critical care nurses through written protocols or standing orders, which must be written, dated, and signed by the physician; standing orders and protocols must be updated regularly. The nurse must be adequately prepared to follow the protocol and perform with a reasonable degree of skill, care, and diligence as performed by similar nurses under similar circumstances. Protocol and standing orders should identify unambiguously the corresponding roles of hospital administrators, nurses, and physicians. Within a state's jurisdiction, however, the scope of medical practice and the scope of nursing practice often overlap because each practice may authorize the same functions. Such overlapping creates problems at the regulatory level and will expand as the role of nursing continues to evolve.

Chemical impairment is a common reason for disciplinary action. In some states the impaired nurse may avoid serious sanctions by voluntarily suspending practice and entering a rehabilitation program. This must be done with the advice of counsel (the nurse's own lawyer). Generally, this option is available as long as no patient has been harmed because of the nurse's impairment.

SPECIFIC PATIENT CARE ISSUES

Myriad legal issues and controversies exist in the field of critical care. Concerns often arise in the areas of (1) informed consent and authorization for treatment and (2) the patient's right to accept or refuse medical treatment.

INFORMED CONSENT AND AUTHORIZATION FOR TREATMENT

There are two types of consent: express and implied. *Express consent* may be written or verbal and is the consent given specifically for nonroutine procedures. *Implied consent* may be implied in fact, an assumption based on patient behavior (e.g., patient extending arm for venipuncture or nodding approval), or may be implied in law (e.g., unconscious, hemorrhaging patient in emergency department). This discussion summarizes the elements of valid informed consent, the adequacy of consent and negligent nondisclosure, and exceptions to consent requirements and the duty to disclose.

Valid consent must be (1) voluntary, (2) obtained, and (3) informed. Although consent can be verbal or written, most hospital policies require that informed, voluntary consent to nonroutine procedures be obtained and confirmed in writing, as signed and dated by the patient, physician, and witness (if required).

Most informed consent statutes provide that a consent in writing to a medical or surgical procedure that meets the consent and disclosure requirements of the statute creates a legal presumption that informed consent was given.

In the vast majority of jurisdictions the decision maker (person giving consent) must be a legally competent adult (i.e., having reached age of majority, or age 18 years in most states). Competence is a legal judgment, and as a general rule, there is a legal presumption of patient competence.[18] A person is mentally incompetent (thereby rendering a consent invalid) if adjudicated incompetent. A person must likewise have the capacity (a medical and nursing judgment) to give consent. The patient must be oriented and understand what he or she has been told, and current medications must be documented. For adults legally adjudicated incompetent, the guardian may give consent if the guardian has been given this authority.

Minors are legally incompetent, and consent is obtained from the parent or guardian. In many jurisdictions, however, there are two important exceptions to this rule: (1) mature minors may consent to treatment for substance abuse, sexually transmitted disease, and matters involving contraception and reproduction; and (2) emancipated minors may consent to treatment in general. Minors are considered "emancipated" if married or divorced before the age of majority, if in the military service, or if living independently with parental consent.

Consent must also be informed and timely. The physician has a duty to disclose the diagnosis, condition, prognosis, material risks/benefits associated with the treatment or procedure, explanation of the treatment, providers of the treatment (who is performing, supervising, and assisting in procedure), material risks and benefits of alternative therapy, and the probable outcome (including material risks/benefits) if the patient refuses the treatment or procedure. Failure to disclose such information or inadequate disclosure with resultant injury may constitute negligence and give rise to tort claims of malpractice, battery, negligent nondisclosure, and abandonment. Consent is generally valid for 7 to 30 days. However, the time at which consent expires must be explicitly stated in the institutional policy and procedure manual.

There are many exceptions to consent requirements and the duty to disclose, and clearly the exceptions vary according to jurisdiction. Emergencies constitute one exception, unless the patient refuses treatment or has previously made a competent and informed refusal. States vary significantly in the following treatment situations: endangered fetal viability, alcohol or other drug detoxification, emergency blood transfusion, cesarean birth, and substance abuse during pregnancy. Jurisdictions also vary on the issue of sources of consent (informal directives) for the incompetent patient or the patient in an emergency who has no legal guardian. Alternatives include consensus from as many next of kin as possible, with evidence that (1) the treatment is reasonable and necessary and (2) the family's decision would not be contrary to the patient's wishes, known as *substituted judgment* (made by a surrogate decision maker). Another alternative is a court order for treatment. In the absence of substituted judgment, many courts use the "best interests" standard.

Right to Accept or Refuse Medical Treatment

The right to consent and informed consent includes the right to refuse treatment. In most cases a competent adult's decision to refuse even life-sustaining treatment is honored.[19-23] The underlying rationale is that the patient's right to withdraw or withhold treatment is not outweighed by the state's interest in preserving life. The right to refuse treatment is *not* honored in some situations, including (but not limited to) the following:

1. The treatment relates to a contagious illness that threatens the health of the public.
2. Innocent third parties will suffer (e.g., parent's wish to refuse blood transfusion to child most likely would be overruled to save child's life).
3. The refusal violates ethical standards.
4. Treatment must be instituted to prevent suicide and to preserve life.

When patients refuse treatment, complex ethical, legal, and practical problems arise. Hospitals should have specific policies to guide nurses in these areas, and nurses' participation in hospital or institutional ethics committees is strongly advised.

Withholding and Withdrawing Treatment

As stated, an adult has the right to refuse treatment, even treatment that sustains life. This right means that the critical care nurse may participate in the withholding or withdrawing of treatment. Historically, the distinction between withholding and withdrawing treatments was considered the issue of importance, but this is no longer the case. Health care decisions become most complex when patients lose competency and capacity to make their own decisions personally.

Advance Directives

The U.S. Congress passed landmark legislation known as the Patient Self-Determination Act/Omnibus Budget Reconciliation Act (OBRA) of 1990.[24-33] The statute requires that all adults must be provided written information on an individual's rights under state law to make medical decisions, including the right to refuse treatment and the right to formulate advance directives.

The law mandates that providers of health care services under Medicare and Medicaid must comply with requirements relating to patient advance directives, which are written instructions recognized under state law for provisions of care when persons are incapacitated. Providers may not be reimbursed for the care they provide unless the requirements of this provision are met.

Providers must have written policies and procedures (1) to inform all adult patients at initiation of treatment of their right to execute an advance directive and of the provider's policies on the implementation of that right, (2) to document in the medical record whether an individual has executed an advance directive, (3) *not* to condition care and treatment or otherwise discriminate on the basis of whether a patient has executed an advance directive, (4) to comply with state laws on advance directives, and (5) to provide information and education to staff and the community on advance directives.

Patients themselves can provide clear direction by preparing in advance written documents that specify their wishes.[34] These documents are termed *advance directives* and include the living will and durable power of attorney for health care. To be effective in a jurisdiction, both these directives must be statutorily or judicially recognized. The *living will* specifies that if certain circumstances occur, such as terminal illness, the patient will decline specific treatment, such as cardiopulmonary resuscitation and mechanical ventilation. The living will does not cover all treatment; in some states, for example, nutritional support may not be declined through a living will. The *durable power of attorney for health care* is a directive through which a patient designates an "agent," someone who will make decisions for the patient if the patient becomes unable to do so. Critical care nurses whose patients have executed advance directives must follow state law provisions and the hospital's policies and require education regarding advance directives and their important role in patient advocacy.[35]

Orders Not to Resuscitate

Hospital policies that address orders to withhold or withdraw treatment should exist in all critical care units. For example, orders not to resuscitate, typically referred to as *do-not-resuscitate* (DNR) orders, should be governed by written policies, including (but not limited to) the following:

1. DNR orders should be entered in the patient's record with full documentation by the responsible physician about the patient's prognosis and the patient's agreement (if he or she is capable) or, alternatively, the family's consensus.
2. DNR orders should have the concurrence of another physician designated in the policy.
3. Policies should specify that orders are reviewed periodically (some policies require daily review).
4. Patients with capacity must give their informed consent.
5. For patients without capacity, that incapacity must be thoroughly documented, along with the diagnosis, prognosis, and family consensus.
6. Judicial intervention before writing a DNR order is usually indicated when the patient's family does not agree or there is uncertainty or disagreement about the patient's prognosis or mental status. As a general rule, however, in the absence of conflict or disagreement, DNR orders are legal in a majority of jurisdictions if executed clearly and properly.
7. Policies should specify who is to be contacted and notified within the hospital administration.

Other orders to withhold or withdraw treatment may involve mechanical ventilation, dialysis, nutritional support, hydration, and medications such as antibiotics. The legal and ethical implications of these orders for each patient must be carefully considered. Hospitals should have written policies on all orders to withhold and withdraw treatment. Policies must cover how decisions will be made, who will decide, and what roles the patient, family, health care providers, and the institution will play. Policies must be developed that consider state laws and judicial opinions.

evolve To test your mastery of this chapter, try the Open-Book Quiz at http://evolve.elsevier.com/Urden/priorities/

REFERENCES

1. American Association of Critical-Care Nurses: *Position statement: moral distress,* Aliso Viejo, Calif, July 8, 2004, The Association.
2. Rushton CH, American Association of Critical-Care Nurses: Defining and addressing moral distress, *AACN Adv Crit Care* 17(6):4, 2000.
3. Correll N: Identifying patient's needs helps with ethical dilemmas, *AACN News* 17(6):4, 2000.
4. Rushton CH, Reina ML, Reina DS: Building trustworthy relationships with critically ill patients and families, *AACN Adv Crit Care* 18(1):19, 2007.
5. Dennis BP: The origin and nature of informed consent: experiences among vulnerable groups, *J Prof Nurs* 15(5):285, 1999.
6. Crow KG, Matheson L, Steed A: Informed consent and truth telling: cultural direction of healthcare providers, *J Nurs Adm* 30(3):148, 2000.
7. Michael JE: Stay in-the-know regarding informed consent, *Nurs Manage* 33(5):22, 2002.
8. Washington G: Trust: a critical element in critical care nursing, *Focus Crit Care* 17(5):418, 1990.
9. Aroskar M: Fidelity and veracity: questions of promise keeping, truth telling and loyalty. In Foweler M, Levine-Ariff J, editors: *Ethics at the bedside,* Philadelphia, 1987, Lippincott.

10. Ewer MS: The definition of medical futility: are we trying to define the wrong term? *Heart Lung* 30(1):3, 2001.
11. Angelucci PA: Grasping the concept of medical futility, *Nurs Manage* 37(2):12, 2006.
12. Pfeifer GM: Understanding medical futility, *Am J Nurs* 106(5):25, 2006.
13. Schneiderman LJ, Jecker NS, Jonsen AR: Medical futility: its meaning and ethical implications, *Ann Intern Med* 112(12):949, 1990.
14. American Nurses Association: *Code of ethics for nurses with interpretive statements,* Washington, DC, 2002, The Association.
15. Thompson J, Thompson H: *Bioethical decision-making for nurses,* Norwalk, Conn, 1985, Appleton-Century-Crofts.
16. Ludwick R: Ethical thoughtfulness and nursing competency, *Online J Issues Nurs,* December 10, 1999, http://www.nursingworld.org/ojin/ethicol/ethics_2.htm.
17. Monson MS: Disclosing adverse events: you said it, now write it. *Nurs Manage* 37(8):16, 2006.
18. Northrop CE, Kelly ME: *Legal issues in nursing,* St Louis, 1987, Mosby.
19. *Bouvia v Superior Court,* 225 Cal Rptr 297; 179 C.A.3d 1127, review denied (Cal App 1986).
20. *In re Farrell,* 529 A.2d 404 (NJ 1987).
21. *McKay v Bergstedt,* 801 P.2d 617 (Nev 1990).
22. *State v McAfee,* 385 S.E.2d 651 (Ga 1989).
23. Wilson-Clayton ML, Clayton MA: Two steps forward, one step back: *McKay v Bergstedt, Whittier Law Rev* 12:439, 1991.
24. *Advance directives for health care: deciding today about your care in the future,* Des Moines, 1991, Iowa Hospital Association, Iowa Medical Society, Iowa State Bar Association.
25. *Put it in writing: a guide to promoting advance directives,* Chicago, 1991, American Hospital Association (800-242-2626).
26. Cate FH, Gill BA: *The Patient Self-Determination Act: implementation issues and opportunities,* Washington, DC, 1991, Annenberg Washington Program.
27. *Advance directive protocols and the Patient Self-Determination Act: a resource manual for the development of institutional protocols,* New York, 1991, Choice in Dying (212-366-5540; formerly Society for the Right to Die/Concern for Dying).
28. Emanuel L, Emanuel E: The medical directive: a new comprehensive advance care document, *JAMA* 261(22):3, 288, 1989.
29. *The Patient Self-Determination Act of 1990: implementation in Iowa hospitals,* Des Moines, 1991, Iowa Hospital Association (515-288-1955).
30. *Advance medical directives,* Arlington, Va, 1991, National Hospice Organization (703-243-5900).
31. *The patient self-determination directory and resources guide,* Washington, DC, 1991, National Health Lawyers Association (202-833-1100).
32. Patient Self-Determination Act/Omnibus Budget Reconciliation Act of 1990, Pub L No 101-508, Sec 4206, 42 USC Sec 1395cc(a)(1) (1990).
33. *Advance directives,* Des Moines, Iowa, 1991, Unisys (800-776-6045).
34. Douglas R, Brown HN: Patients' attitudes toward advance directives, *J Nurs Scholarsh* 34(1):61, 2002.
35. Ryan CJ et al: Perceptions about advance directives by nurses in a community hospital, *Clin Nurse Spec* 15(6):246, 2001.

CHAPTER 3

Patient and Family Education

LINDA URDEN

OBJECTIVES

- Adapt and apply teaching-learning theory to the critical care setting.
- Perform a learning needs assessment.
- Construct a teaching plan for patients in the critical care unit.
- Discuss four methods of instruction and the appropriateness of each to the critical care setting.
- Describe informational needs of families of critically ill patients.

ADULT LEARNING PRINCIPLES

Central to successful implementation of an education plan in the critical care and telemetry environment is the incorporation of the principles of adult learning theory.[1] Adults must be ready to learn, having moved from one developmental or educational task to the next. They need to know why it is important to learn something before they can actually learn it. Inherent in their attitudes is a responsibility for their own decisions. Consequently, they may resent when others try to force different beliefs on them. Adults bring a wealth of experience to the learning environment that must be recognized and promoted in educational techniques. Because their orientation to learning is life centered, the tasks being taught should focus on current problem resolution. Finally, motivation for the adult learner arises out of internal pressures such as self-esteem and quality of life.

TEACHING-LEARNING PROCESS

The teaching-learning process is a dynamic, continuous activity (Box 3-1). Teaching is not just the passing of facts and information from one person to another. Learning is both growth and development. It is an active process that occurs internally over time and cannot be forced. Learning involves altering behavior to produce changes in one or more of the three learning domains: knowledge, attitudes, and skills.[2]

Assessment

Assessment is the gathering of information for the purposes of identifying actual or potential learning needs. It identifies gaps in the knowledge, attitudes, and skills the patient or family has regarding the illness, environment, or lifestyle (Box 3-2). Knowing this information will allow the nurse to develop a collaborative, individualized, need-targeted education plan of care. The assessment process does not stop after the completion of the admission assessment; it is continuous and ongoing.

Patients and families may be so overwhelmed by what they see or have already been told that they may

Box 3-1
Steps in the Education Process

Step 1: Assessment: Information Gathering
Patient/family: culture, age-specific considerations
Actual and potential learning needs
Possible barriers to the teaching learning-process

Step 2: Education Plan Development
Identify needs and write expected outcomes
Design interventions: information to be taught, removal of barriers
Mobilize resources as needed to remove barriers and enhance communication of information

Step 3: Implementation
Implement interventions for information sharing, learner participation in education process
Use written plan to structure the teaching encounter, cover essential information, and communicate outcomes between practitioners

Step 4: Evaluation
Evaluate learner response to the encounter, any need for follow-up teaching to attain goals
Evaluate learner comfort level with information: coping and adaptation

Step 5: Documentation
Document interventions used, resources used, information taught, and outcome of teaching encounter

Box 3-2

Assessment Questions for the Critically Ill Patient and Family

- What brings you to the hospital? Can you tell me what happened? Can you tell me more?
- What have you been told so far about your (your family member's) condition and plan of care?
- What is the most important thing for you to know right now?
- What would you like to know? What information can I give you right now?
- Who are your main support people?
- Has anything like this ever happened to you (your family) before?
- Have you (your family) ever been in an intensive care unit or hospital before?
- Do you have any special concerns that we need to address right now?

Modified from Reeder J: *AACN Clin Issues* 2:188, 1991.

be unable to identify their own learning needs. The bedside nurse is responsible for involving both the patient and the family in the assessment process and discovering what they want and need to know. Involving patients and families in this process gives value to their needs and assists them in gaining some control over a situation in which they may feel powerless. Active participation and control stimulate the motivation to receive information, as well as make the overall education process more satisfying; in essence, the patient/family will learn more.

Assessing ability, willingness, and readiness to learn is an essential part of developing and implementing an education plan of care. Readiness to learn is the motivation to try out new concepts and behaviors.[3] The ability to learn is the capacity of the learner to understand, pay attention, and comprehend the material being taught. Willingness to learn describes the learner's openness to new ideas and concepts. Several factors affect ability, willingness, and readiness to learn as well as the ability to cope and adapt to the current situation. These factors include physiologic, psychologic, sociocultural, financial, and environmental aspects.[2-4]

Development of Education Plan

The education plan must be ongoing, interactive, and consistent with the patient's plan of care and education level (Box 3-3). Information gathered from the assessment must be analyzed and used to prioritize educational needs, formulate a nursing diagnosis, and develop an education plan of care. The nurse also must consider the patient's clinical and emotional status when setting education priorities. The education plan should include (1) expected outcomes, (2) objectives, (3) content to be taught, (4) interventions, (5) available educational materials, and (6) appropriate teaching strategies. Box 3-4 provides a sample education plan for patients undergoing coronary artery bypass surgery. Refer to the Nursing Management Plan for Deficient Knowledge (p. A-18).

Box 3-3

Essential Critical Care Information for the Patient/Family

- Orientation to the various care providers and the services they deliver
- Orientation to the unit environment (e.g., call light, bed controls)
- Orientation to unit routines and plan of care: visiting hours, frequency of monitoring and nurse assessments, venipunctures to obtain blood specimens, daily weights, special shift routines
- Explanations regarding reasons for equipment, monitors, and associated alarms (e.g., cardiac monitor, ventilator, intravenous [IV] lines, IV pumps, pacemaker, pulse oximetry)
- Explanation of all procedures and expected sensations/discomforts both in and off the unit
- Medications given: drug name, reason for receiving, side effects to report to nurse/others
- Immediate plan of care
- Transition to next level of care: reason for transfer, environment, staffing, availability of care providers
- Discharge plan: medications, diet, activity, pathophysiology of disease, symptom management, special procedures and associated equipment, when to call health care provider, available community resources

Establish Education Phases and Priorities

It can be a difficult task to prioritize the multitude of learning needs that practitioners are required to address during a period in acute care. Learning needs in the intensive care unit (ICU), the progressive care, or the telemetry setting can be separated into six different categories to help set teaching priorities in each phase of the hospitalization (Table 3-1). Learning needs during the initial contact or first hours of hospitalization can be predicted. Education during this time frame should be directed toward the reduction of immediate stress, anxiety, and fear rather than future lifestyle alterations or rehabilitation needs. The plan should focus on survival skills, orientation to the environment and equipment, communication of prognosis, procedure explanations, and the immediate plan of care.

As the hospital length of stay increases, patients and families begin to adapt to the situation and learning needs change. The patient/family develop positive

Box 3-4
Teaching Plan for Patient Undergoing Coronary Artery Bypass Surgery

Preoperative Phase

During preoperative educational interactions the nurse should assess the patient/family's level of anxiety and the effect on the ability or desire to learn. Preoperative education should be individualized to prepare the patient appropriately for the surgery, to provide education about postoperative care, and to minimize anxiety. Before the teaching-learning experience, the nurse should do the following:

- Assess the patient's level of anxiety and desire to learn about the upcoming surgery.
- Individualize the preoperative teaching plan based on assessment findings.

Areas to Consider in Teaching Session

- Review of coronary artery bypass graft (CABG) procedure
- Time leaving room for surgery, length of surgery, location of family waiting area
- Surgical preparation and shave
- Nothing by mouth (NPO) after midnight
- What to expect when awakening from anesthesia
- Sights and sounds of recovery room/critical care unit
- Tubes and drains: chest tubes, hemodynamic monitoring lines, Foley catheter, intravenous lines, pacemaker wires (if appropriate), endotracheal tube (inability to speak with tube in place)
- Discomfort to expect from incisions; availability of pain medication
- Coughing/deep breathing practice
- Use of incentive spirometer
- When, how long, and how often family can visit
- Usual length of critical care unit stay

Other Nursing Actions

- Reassure patient/family that many staff members and much activity around bedside are normal and do not indicate complications.
- Elicit and answer any specific questions that patient/family may have at this time.
- Determine specific needs and desires for day of surgery (e.g., patient needs hearing aid or glasses as soon as possible).
- Meet with family alone to offer support and address concerns that they may not want to express to the patient.

Critical Care Unit Phase

Patient/family education is designed to meet immediate needs and reduce anxiety in the critical care unit phase. Appropriate content to address at this time includes the following:

- Basic explanation of bedside equipment
- Review of tubes and drains
- Turning, coughing, deep breathing
- Use of incentive spirometry
- Use of oxygen equipment
- Orientation to time, place, and situation
- Explanation of procedures
- Basic purpose of medications
- Explanation of normal progression in early postoperative period
- Basic range-of-motion (ROM) exercises (e.g., ankle circles, point and flex)

Other Nursing Actions

- Reassure patient/family of normal progression.
- Repeat and reinforce information as necessary.
- Answer questions as they arise.
- Begin early to prepare patient for transfer to prevent transfer anxiety.
- Determine family learning needs, and address these needs with patient or in separate teaching sessions as appropriate.

Step-Down Unit Phase

After transfer from the critical care unit, patient/family educational needs increase. Short daily educational sessions should be planned to cover the following content:

- Basic pathophysiology of coronary artery disease (CAD)
- Review of CABG procedure
- Risk factors for CAD
- Upper extremity ROM exercises
- Dietary recommendations (salt-modified diet, fat/cholesterol-modified diet)
- Taking of own pulse
- Recognition and treatment of angina (use of nitroglycerin)

Other Nursing Actions

- Use audiovisual materials in teaching sessions or as reinforcement of content.
- Provide printed take-home materials outlining important content.
- Answer questions as they arise.

Discharge Teaching

Before discharge the following content should be covered with the patient and family:

- Activity guidelines
- Lifting restrictions
- Incision care
- Possibility of patient being extremely fatigued or depressed after discharge
- Guidelines for return to work, driving, and sexual activity
- Medication safety and administration

Other Nursing Actions

- Reassure patient that "ups and downs" are normal.
- If necessary, reassure patient/family that likelihood of cardiac emergencies at home is minimal.
- Provide printed material for further study by patient/family.
- Answer questions as they arise.
- Provide phone number for patient/family to call when further questions arise.

Table 3-1

Education Phases and Priorities

PHASE	EDUCATION PRIORITIES
Initial contact/first visit Focus on immediate needs	Preparation for the visit: patient representatives or nurses can prepare the family and patient for the first visit • What to expect in the environment • How long the visit will last • What the patient may look like (e.g., tubes, IV lines) Orientation to unit/environment: call light, bed controls, waiting rooms, unit contact numbers Orientation to unit policies/hospital policies • HIPAA, advance directives, visitation policies Equipment orientation: monitors, IV pumps, pulse oximetry, pacemakers, ventilators Medications: rationale, effects, side effects What to do during the visit: talk to the patient, hold patient's hand, length of visits (if applicable) Patient status: stable or unstable and what that terminology means What treatments and interventions are being done for the patient Upcoming procedures When the doctor visited or is expected to visit Disciplines involved in care and the services they provide Immediate plan of care (next 24 hours) Mobilization of resources for crisis intervention
Continuous care	Day-to-day routine: meals, laboratory visits, doctor visits, frequency of monitoring (VS), nursing assessments, daily weights, and shift routines Explanation of any procedures: expected sensations or discomforts (e.g., chest tube removal, arterial sheath removal) Plan of care: treatments, progress, patient accomplishments (e.g., extubation) Medications: name, why the patient is receiving them, side effects to report to the nurse or health care team Disease process: what it is and how it will affect life, symptoms to report to health care team How to mobilize resources to assist the patient/family in coping with stress and crisis: pastoral care, social workers, case managers, victim assistance, domestic violence Gifts: When a loved one is ill, it is traditional to send flowers, balloons, or cards; if your unit has any restrictions on gifts, make the family aware Begin teaching self-management skills and discuss aftercare information
Transfer to a different level of care	**Sending Unit** Acknowledge positive move out of critical care When the transfer will occur Why the transfer is occurring What to expect in the different unit Name of the new caregiver Availability of care provider Visiting hours Directions, how to get there; the new room number and phone number **Receiving Unit** Orientation to environment, visitation policies, visitors Unit routine, meals, shift changes, doctor visits Expectations about patient self-care; ADLs Medication and diagnostic testing routine times
Planning for aftercare, discharge planning	Self-care management: symptom management, medication administration, diet, activity, durable medical equipment, tasks or procedures What to do for an emergency What constitutes an emergency or when to call the physician How to care for incisions or procedure sites
Completed throughout the hospital stay	Return appointment: name of physician practice, practice phone numbers and contacts Obtaining medications: prescriptions, pharmacy, special drug ordering information Required lifestyle changes: mobility and safety issues for the paraplegic or stroke victim, activities of daily living issues relative to medications or symptoms Potential risk modifications: smoking cessation, diet modifications, exercise Resources: cardiac rehabilitation, support groups, home health care agencies
End-of-life care	End-of-life care: participation in care, services available, mobilizing resources Palliative care Hospice

HIPAA, Health Insurance Portability and Accountability Act of 1996; *IV,* intravenous; *VS,* vital signs; *ADLs,* activities of daily living.

feelings of relief and happiness in the fact that survival has been achieved. Because lower-level, physiologic needs are met, the patient's efforts can be concentrated on modifying behavior to meet higher-level needs such as self-concept and self-actualization. Teaching during the continuous phase of nursing care is aimed at answering patient or family questions about the treatment plan or how the acute illness will impact their day-to-day lives. Education on lifestyle modification and self-management skills should be presented during this phase of nursing care. Discharge planning is also part of the education process and should start with admission to the hospital. Instructions for home health care, also known as aftercare, should be accomplished before the day of discharge to avoid decreased retention of education that occurs with information overload.

Implementation of Education Plan

Patients in the critical care environment are educated in many informal interactions with the nurse, and the knowledge gained fosters patient understanding and well-being. Educational opportunities can be present during various nursing care activities, such as bathing and administration of medication. Each encounter with the patient/family must be viewed as a teaching opportunity. At times during the hospitalization, however, more formal or structured educational experiences may be required.

Learning Environment

As discussed, patient barriers to learning are related to physiologic, emotional, and motivational factors. To structure a successful teaching-learning experience in a critical care area, the nurse must also carefully assess the environmental and iatrogenic barriers that affect the interaction. Bright lights, unpleasant odors, unfamiliar noises, and untidy surroundings can distract patients and add to cognitive impairment. Control of these factors can facilitate the learning process. Factors that cannot be controlled must be explained to the patient to alleviate anxiety and facilitate a trusting relationship between patient and nurse.

Teaching Methods

There are three basic methods of teaching: lecture, discussion, and demonstration. The selection of the methods will be determined by various factors, including patient clinical status, readiness to learn, cognitive abilities, learning style, instructional time, and availability of teaching materials and resources. In addition, innovative methods of teaching and presentation of educational materials must be developed and used efficiently to maximize existing resources.[5]

Lecture. Lecture is the presentation of information in a highly structured format to a group. In this method the teacher provides a great deal of material but may not provide ample opportunities for teacher-learner interaction. This style of teaching is inappropriate for acutely ill patients in the critical care unit, although it may be useful in the telemetry unit. Optimally, the group size should be arranged to enable the learners to ask questions and receive appropriate feedback on content presented.

Discussion. Discussion is less structured than lecturing and allows an exchange and feedback between the teacher and learner. The teacher can adapt the material to meet the needs of the individual or group. Discussion groups can be effective with hospitalized patients when a group with similar problems and at similar stages of adaptation can be gathered. Individual discussion with patients/families is appropriate and valuable during the acute phase of illness because it allows them to express their feelings and interpretations.

Demonstration. Demonstration involves acting out a procedure while giving appropriate explanations to provide the learner with a clear idea of how to perform a task. Patients can then practice the skill and can be given feedback about their performance. This method is often used in the acute care setting, as when coughing/deep breathing or taking one's own pulse is taught.

Other Methods of Instruction

In addition to the three basic methods, several other approaches are available to deliver or augment information in a patient teaching program. These methods include commercially prepared or custom-designed printed materials, bedside videotape programs, and computer-assisted patient education programs.

Written Materials. Written materials can be very useful tools in patient/family education. These materials allow repetition and reinforcement of content and provide basic information in printed form for reference later. To be useful, however, the content must be accurate and current, and the patient/family must be able to read and understand it.

Low literacy levels are considered to be a barrier to successful patient/family education and the teaching-learning process.[6] Typical patient education materials are written at or above the eighth-grade or ninth-grade reading level and may be out of reach for many people.[3,7] Almost 20% of the U.S. adult population have low literacy skills and read at or below the fifth-grade reading level.[8] To help overcome the problem of low literacy, it is recommended that patient education materials be written at or below the fifth-grade reading level[7,9] (Box 3-5).

Audiovisual Media. Using media devices can be an excellent method of instruction. Use of overhead projectors, slides, pictures, videos, and closed-circuit patient education TV channels are the most frequently

Box 3-5

Example of Different Reading Levels in Critical Care Education

College Reading Level
Consult your physician immediately with the onset of chest discomfort, shortness of breath, or increased perspiration.

Twelfth-Grade Reading Level
Call your physician immediately if you experience chest discomfort, shortness of breath, or increased sweatiness.

Eighth-Grade Reading Level
Call your doctor immediately if you start having chest pain or shortness of breath or feel sweaty.

Fourth-Grade Reading Level
Call your doctor right away if you start having chest pain, can't breathe, or feel sweaty.

used audiovisual media strategies. These methods entertain the learners as much as "tell" them important information they should know. This type of media can provide "nice to know" information as well as "need to know" information. Viewing a video alone does not ensure retention of material or knowledge acquisition. Patient education channels and videos should not replace nurse interaction and should be used jointly. The nurse must review with the learner the content presented to reiterate key points and evaluate the outcome.

Closed-circuit television (CCTV) is a common service in many health care settings. CCTV is best used as one component of a comprehensive educational program and is not intended to be used alone. CCTV allows for viewing of the session at a time that best suits the patient/family and can be stopped, restarted, or repeated as necessary.

Computer-Assisted Instruction. Computer-assisted instruction (CAI) is new in the patient/family education arena. Although personal computers are now commonplace, this learning medium may not be suitable for some individuals because comfort levels with technical aspects of the computer vary. The learner must pay attention to the material being presented and must not be preoccupied with learning how to use the "mouse." Many computer systems available to the general public for learning purposes have "touch screens" that are easy to use and do not depend on the learner being familiar with computers. These CAI programs are generally easy to use, self-directed, and presented in a pleasurable, colorful format.

Internet Websites. Patients and families often use Internet websites to research information regarding the illness or condition of concern. Websites contain a wealth of information, but not all the information is accurate. The nurse must advise the patient/family of this fact and ask them to print out and bring in such material so that it can be discussed.

EVALUATION

What to Evaluate

The evaluation process helps the nurse determine the effectiveness of patient/family education interventions. The nurse must decide how well the learner has met the expected outcomes and objectives. Evaluation should be done as each intervention is carried out to allow the nurse to give feedback to the patient/family and revise the education plan of care to accommodate continued learning needs. It is also important to assess the patient/family's response to the process. The response to the teaching-learning interaction includes the level of interest, willingness to learn, and level of participation.

How to Evaluate

There are several ways to determine the effectiveness of the teaching-learning process. Evaluating knowledge can be done through verbal questioning or written testing on the topic. Questioning provides an interactive avenue for the nurse to assess whether the learner has retained the information taught. Verbal questioning should occur not only immediately after the teaching event but also later to assess knowledge retention. Some CAI programs include a posttest that provides participants with immediate feedback on their learning. Written tests may also be administered to assess knowledge retention but are infrequently used in the critical care setting.

Observation and return demonstration represent the evaluation of choice for the skills-learning domain. For the patient/family to be "checked off" on a particular skill, they should be able to perform it independently, using the nurse only as a resource for questions. Endotracheal suctioning, placing condom catheters, and performing dressing changes are common tasks that patients and families may be asked to learn. Because of the increasingly complex care patients now require at home after discharge, these skills may be the entire focus of teaching before discharge.

It is important to remember that not every teaching moment is a success, and the nurse should not have feelings of guilt or failure when the learner has not achieved the desired objective. Revisiting and revising the goals and objectives during the teaching-learning session may be necessary to meet the ever-changing needs of the patient or family.

DOCUMENTATION

Documentation of the teaching-learning process is multifaceted and should reflect each component in the education plan of care. Whenever a teaching-learning encounter has been completed, the interaction, material taught, and learner response must be recorded.[10] The assessment documentation should include assessment of patient/family learning needs, abilities, preferences, and readiness to learn as well as potential barriers to learning. The remainder of the documentation should include the expected outcome/goals, objectives, interventions, who was taught, what was taught, materials used, patient/family response to teaching, and any follow-up education or materials needed.

SEDATED AND UNCONSCIOUS PATIENTS

Patient education should not be reserved for the conscious and coherent patient only; it should be provided to the unconscious or sedated patient as well. Addressing the learning needs of this critically ill population of patients is challenging. These patients cannot communicate their educational needs, nor can they interact and participate in the learning process. Whereas it is truly not known what the unconscious or sedated patient hears or remembers, it is known that some sedated patients undergoing surgery remember discussions that took place among physicians and staff during the procedure. Therefore, one should not ignore unconscious or sedated patients during the education process. These patients may not be able to respond or participate, and the effectiveness of the teaching process cannot be evaluated, but providing information regarding environment, procedures, sensations, and time of day is benevolent and may help to decrease immediate physiologic stress.

INFORMATIONAL NEEDS OF FAMILIES IN CRITICAL CARE

Family members and significant others of critically ill patients are integral to the recovery of their loved ones. When planning for the overall care of patients, nurses and other caregivers need to consider the informational and emotional support needs of this group.[11] Families of critically ill patients report their greatest need is for information.[12] Flexible visiting hours and informational booklets regarding the critical care experience are recommended to meet this need (Box 3-6).[13]

Box 3-6

Informational Requirements of Families With a Critically Ill Patient

- Have questions answered honestly.
- Know the facts about the patient's prognosis.
- Know the results of procedures as soon as possible.
- Have staff inform family members of the patient's status.
- Know why things are being done.
- Know about possible complications.
- Receive explanations that can be understood.
- Know exactly what is being done.
- Know about the staff providing care.
- Receive directions about what to do during a procedure.

Modified from Miracle VA, Hovenkamp G: *Am J Crit Care* 3(3):155, 1994.

PREPARATION OF PATIENT/FAMILY FOR TRANSFER FROM CRITICAL CARE

When patients are more stable, requiring less hemodynamic monitoring and close observation, they are frequently transferred to another level of care in a different geographic hospital setting. They may be transferred to an intermediate care unit (also called step-down, intermediate care area, or telemetry). While on these units, patients receive optimal care to their level of requirement, a lower nurse-to-patient ratio, and less expensive technological monitoring in a quieter environment.[14-15]

Transferring a patient from the critical care unit to a step-down unit may result in anxiety and stress. At this time, patients and families have become dependent on the monitors, equipment, constant nursing attention, and abundant information received while in the critical care unit. The patient has become secure knowing that immediate physiologic and emotional needs are being met. A strong bond has often developed between the staff and the family. Many patients and families are reluctant to give up that bond and believe that their needs will not be met as well on a step-down unit. To avoid anxiety and provide the patient and family with some control over the event, nurses need to prepare them for the transfer process.

Preparation for transfer should start after the patient has been stabilized and the life-threatening event that resulted in hospitalization has subsided. The stressor at this point is not the now-familiar critical care environment but the unfamiliar step down environment. Explanations as to where the patient will be transferred, the reason for transfer, and the name of the nurse who will be providing care should be provided as soon as known. Before transfer, information about changes in care, expectations for self-care, and visiting hours should be provided to the patient/family. Family members should also be contacted concerning exactly when the patient will be transferred so they can be present during the transfer or made aware of the patient's new location.

The education plan of care and tips learned by the critical care staff about that particular patient and family should be communicated to the step-down unit staff. Most of the patient transfers made from the critical care unit to a step-down unit are planned events. At times, however, unplanned or unexpected transfers occur, usually when the critical care unit requires bed space for a more seriously ill patient. In this situation the transfer occurs quickly, either during the day or often at night. Families may be present in the hospital or may have gone home for the evening. This sudden need to transfer the patient can produce as much anxiety as the initial event, primarily because the patient/family may not feel ready for the transfer or may think they have lost control of the situation. Providing the patient/family with concrete evidence of improvement, such as more favorable vital signs or the need for fewer medications or tubes, can assure them of improvement in the patient's condition before unplanned transfers occur. Increased communication and providing consistent information to patients and families also increases satisfaction with care and services.[16]

evolve To test your mastery of this chapter, try the Open-Book Quiz at http://evolve.elsevier.com/Urden/priorities/

REFERENCES

1. Hansen M, Fisher JC: Patient-centered teaching from theory to practice, *Am J Nurs* 98(1):56, 1998.
2. Phillips LD: Patient education: understanding the process to maximize time and outcomes, *J Intraven Nurs* 22(1):19, 1999.
3. Rankin S, Stallings K: *Patient education: issues, principles, practices,* ed 3, Philadelphia, 1996, Lippincott.
4. Ruzicki D: Realistically meeting the educational needs of hospitalized acute and short-stay patients, *Nurs Clin North Am* 24(3):629, 1989.
5. Barnes LP: The illiterate client: strategies in patient teaching, *MCN Am J Matern Child Nurs* 17(3):127, 1992.
6. Quirk P: Screening for literacy and readability: implications for the advanced practice nurse, *Clin Nurse Spec* 14(1):26, 2000.
7. Doak C, Doak L, Root J: *Teaching patients with low literacy skills,* ed 2, Philadelphia, 1996, Lippincott.
8. Doak C et al: Improving comprehension for cancer patients with low literacy skills: strategies for clinicians, *CA Cancer J Clin* 48(3):151, 1998.
9. Klingbeil C, Speece M, Schubiner H: Readability of pediatric patient education materials, *Clin Pediatr (Phila)* 34(2):96, 1995.
10. Casey F: Documenting patient education: a literature review, *J Contin Educ Nurs* 26(6):257, 1995.
11. Doering LV, McGuire AW, Rourke D: Recovering from cardiac surgery: what patients want to know, *Am J Crit Care* 11(4):333, 2002.
12. Henneman EA, McKenzie JB, Dewa CS: An evaluation of interventions for meeting the information needs of families of critically ill patients, *Am J Crit Care* 1(3):85, 1993.
13. Miracle VA, Hovenkamp G: Needs of families of patients undergoing invasive cardiac procedures, *Am J Crit Care* 3(3):155, 1994.
14. White SK, Edwards RJ: Visitation guidelines promote safe, satisfying environments. *Nurs Manage* 37(8):21, 2006.
15. Radtke A: Telemetry monitoring: a preferred solution for intermediate care. *Nurs Manage* 37(12):52A, 2006.
16. Mages ME: Helping patients, helping families, *Healthc Exec* 11(4):40, 2006.

CHAPTER 4

Psychosocial Alterations

LINDA D. URDEN

OBJECTIVES

- Explain the following coping strategies as they relate to critically ill patients: regression, suppression, denial, hope, trust, religious beliefs, and family support.
- Describe the needs and coping mechanisms of families of critically ill patients.
- Explain interventions and nursing management for patients with coping alterations.
- Identify situations that increase the risk of disturbances of self-concept.

EFFECTS OF STRESS

Patients requiring critical care must cope with a variety of stressors. A patient's response to these stressors depends on individual differences, such as age, gender, social support, cultural background, medical diagnosis, current hospital course, and prognosis. A person's perceptions of self and relationships with others, of spiritual values, and of self-competency in social roles also play a major role in how he or she will respond to stress and illness.

The intensive care unit (ICU) environment can be frightening. Technologic equipment can control one's breathing and prevent speaking. Invasive procedures, abrupt or continual noises, loss of privacy, sleep interruptions, pain, medications, isolation, and minimal contact with significant support persons all create feelings of powerlessness and loss of control. Disorientation, which is common for patients in the ICU, is influenced by several factors, including the severity of the physical problem, chemical imbalances, sensory overload or deprivation, and previous experiences with the health care system. In addition to these factors are personal variables (i.e., biologic factors, social roles, and the person's emotional responses of anxiety, confusion, or depression).[1-2] However, for some individuals the ICU is perceived as a safe environment where lifesaving procedures are immediately at hand and administered by highly competent caregivers.

ANXIETY AS A RESPONSE TO STRESS

Anxiety is a normal subjective human response to a perceived or actual threat to self-integrity, which can range from a vague, generalized feeling of discomfort to a state of panic and loss of control. The initial emotional responses of excitement and heightened awareness diminish as anxiety levels increase, the individual's perceptual field narrows, and problem-solving and coping skills are lost. Prolonged stress can exhaust available resources.

An acute or chronic illness, facing a real or anticipated loss, being hospitalized, and any other event that is perceived as stressful can be triggers for anxiety. Anxiety elicits changes in the neurohumoral release patterns involving the neurotransmitters, including acetylcholine, norepinephrine, dopamine, serotonin, and their corresponding receptors. The complex and elusive integration of these responses within the central nervous system relies on communication between the cerebral cortex, the limbic system, the thalamus, the hypothalamus, the pituitary gland, and the reticular activating system.

SELF-CONCEPT

The human self-concept is a major concern for nurses because nursing interventions that do not consider the individual in his or her wholeness, including the self-concept, will probably not be effective. The self-concept comprises attitudes about oneself; perceptions of personal abilities, body image, and identity; and a general sense of worth. The stressors imposed by physical illness, trauma, and surgical procedures can cause disturbances in the self-concept. A person's response to these stressors depends on a variety of individual differences (Box 4-1).

The terms *self-concept* and *self-esteem* have often been used synonymously, with no clear-cut definitions made. However, theoretic models used in the development of measurements refer to the self-concept as the "self-schema," or knowledge, of abilities, beliefs, and values that influence behavior during interactions

Box 4-1

Stressors in the Critical Care Setting

Patients' experience of critical illness and care will vary. However, each patient must cope with at least some of the following stressors:

- Threat of death
- Threat of survival, with significant residual problems related to the illness/injury
- Pain or discomfort
- Lack of sleep
- Loss of autonomy over most aspects of life and daily functioning
- Loss of control over environment, such as loss of privacy and exposure to light, noise, and general activity of the critical care unit, including the care of other patients
- Daily hassles or common frustrations
- Loss of usual role, and with that, loss of the arena in which usual coping mechanisms serve the patient
- Separation from family and friends
- Loss of dignity
- Boredom, broken only by brief visits, threatening stimuli, and frightening thoughts
- Loss of ability to express self verbally when intubated

Effects and response to the stressors depend on the individual's perception of the intensity of the stress and the following factors:

- Acute/chronic duration of stressors
- Cumulative effect of simultaneous stressors
- Sequence of stressors
- Individual's previous experience with stressors and coping effectiveness
- Amount of social support

with others in the social and cultural environments. Self-esteem is most closely linked to one's sense of self-worth.[3-5] Although relatively stable, the self-concept can be modified by the developmental phases and social roles a person experiences over a lifetime.[5,6] Any event with unpredictable body changes and functions requires adjustments in the self-concept, as well as a realistic readjustment to the role limitations that are imposed. These adjustment stages are complex and highly individualized.

A person faced with an intolerable situation may panic, may display behavior that distorts reality, and may exhibit excessive demands or may be suspicious of motives and methods of the caregivers. Depression and anxiety are common reactions as the person experiences a loss of control and worries over outcomes.[7,8] The illness experience may have different meanings for individuals from different cultures and ethnic groups. Assessment of their needs can be elicited through use of tools that include questions that are sensitive to cultural values.[4,8-10] Patients in critical care units usually do not have time to adjust to the illness conditions and may exhibit signs of shock, numbness, and avoidance of reality and may be unable to understand clearly the implications of the situation.[11,12] The patient is usually transferred to an intermediate care unit before a true acknowledgment phase occurs.

Disturbed Body Image

Body image is the mental picture an individual has of his or her body and its physical functioning at any given time. It includes one's attitudes and feelings about one's body in reference to appearance, build, health, performance ability, and gender-related concepts.[7] The body image develops over time from internal sensations of postural changes, contact with people and objects in the environment, emotional experiences, and fantasies. The ability to project possible images of one's self in the future that are highly desirable or feared may play a powerful role in motivating and regulating goal-directed behavior.[3]

Disturbances in body image arise when the person fails to perceive or adapt to the changes that are imposed by age, disease, trauma, or surgery. In some cases the person may feel betrayed by the body, which no longer seems "normal." Body image may also be altered by the need to incorporate a prosthetic device or a donated body part.[11,13] The disease or problem may be corrected by surgery and treatments, but when the result is visible to the patient and others, the change in body image can arouse intense feelings of anger, frustration, depression, and powerlessness.[11,14] The critical care nurse often begins the process of helping the patient live with this permanent alteration. Interventions by the nurse and other health team members focus on helping the person manage the physical changes and the psychosocial alterations.

Disturbances in Self-Esteem

Self-esteem, or self-measurement of one's worth, develops as a part of self-concept through the perceived appraisals of significant others.[3] The need for self-esteem is a part of the hierarchy of human needs postulated by Maslow.[15] Having high self-esteem helps a person deal with the environment and face the maturational and situational crises of life more easily. Persons with a well-developed self-esteem are at less risk for disturbances of self-esteem than those with poorly developed self-esteem.[6,13]

Self-esteem has been studied in a variety of contexts and is an important concept for nurses, who have a significant impact on ill patients' understanding.[7,13,16] Illness can rob the person of perspective and shrinks both the familiar world and the one of possibility, often leading to low self-esteem, powerlessness, helplessness, and depression.[7,8,17] A low self-regard impairs one's ability to adapt. The person may refuse to participate in self-care, may exhibit self-destructive behavior, or may be too compliant, asking no questions and permitting others to make all decisions.[18] Refer to the Nursing Management Plan for Situational Low Self-Esteem (p. A-47).

POWERLESSNESS

Powerlessness, as a nursing diagnosis, is defined as the perception of the individual that one's own action will not significantly affect an outcome.[8,19,20] Unrelieved powerlessness may result in hopelessness (see Coping Mechanisms).

The causes of powerlessness include factors in the health care environment, interpersonal interactions, one's culture and religious beliefs, illness-related regimen, and a lifestyle of helplessness. The range in levels of powerlessness varies and depends on the person's perceived sense of control, the amount of losses experienced, and the availability of social support. Powerlessness can be manifested by delayed decision making or refusal to make decisions and by expressions of self-doubt in role performance. Frustration, anger, and resentment over being dependent on others often manifest as verbal expressions of dissatisfaction with care.[10]

Individuals vary in the amount of control they prefer.[18,21] The critical care unit routines may oppose or preclude any control by the patient. The person for whom control is important should be helped to continue to control as many areas of life as possible. On the other hand, a patient must be given the opportunity to choose not to control.

Rotter's early research[22] on human behavior and perception of control has helped explain the variability of responses from persons in similar situations. He proposed two major concepts of internal versus external locus of control. Individuals who have internal locus of control perceive themselves to be responsible for the outcome of events. Individuals with external locus of control believe their actions will have no effect on outcomes of a situation. The scale to measure internal/external locus of control developed by Rotter is useful in assessing this personality trait, which is a relatively stable tendency.

Another aspect of powerlessness is learned helplessness, or excessive dependence.[23] A person who repeatedly experiences uncontrollable situations loses the motivation for making decisions about life events. Some people assume a "martyr" role and accept the illness state as their fate, thus doing nothing to improve their status. Others may find the sick role a gratifying means for gaining control over others by using their symptoms to gain attention.[24] Setting limits on these behaviors, encouraging independence and participation in self-care, providing counseling, and involving family members in establishing realistic goals are helpful strategies to assist the person in abandoning this manipulative behavior.

Critically ill patients generally have experienced a rapid onset of illness without time to acquire the illness role. If "control" is defined as the ability to determine the use of time, space, and resources, admission to a critical care unit strips away this power. On admission, persons lose their independent status and become patients. Choice of clothing and use of other personal belongings are usually restricted in a critical care unit. Patients cannot decide who enters the room, who provides personal care, or who intrudes with painful treatments. Hospital rules usually are not open to modification. Patients may feel anxious because they are separated from a familiar environment and have restrictions on who may visit them.[25]

Poor interactions with the health care providers may make the situation worse. Patients may react aggressively, may try bargaining, or may refuse to comply with diagnostic and treatment regimens. They may resent the close scrutiny of the nurses and physicians and the invasion of their privacy. By virtue of their experiences with critical illness and care, people may lose sight of areas of influence they still do retain over themselves because so much control has been taken from them. Nursing emphasizes the patient's influence on control and thus helps to preserve it.[12,16] Refer to the Nursing Management Plan for Powerlessness (p. A-44).

SPIRITUAL DISTRESS

Spiritual distress has been defined as the disruption in the life principle that pervades one's being and that integrates and transcends one's biologic and psychosocial nature.[19,20] Adherence to a particular philosophic, psychologic, sociologic, or political belief may bring a sense of one's value and of life's meaning. Threats imposed by any physiologic or psychologic illness and prolonged pain and suffering can challenge a person's spirituality.[26] Life-threatening illness causes a person to face his or her mortality. The provision of holistic nursing care is not limited to meeting a person's religious needs; it also encompasses all that provides meaning to life.

A person in spiritual distress may question the meaning of suffering and death in relation to a personal belief system. The person may express anger toward God or other supreme being, feelings of self-blame, or regret over inability to practice belief rituals. Individuals may even question the necessity for the therapeutic regimen. Spiritual care is described as health-promoting interventions that relieve the responses to stress affecting spiritual perspectives of individuals or groups.[27]

ACUTE CONFUSION AND DELIRIUM

Acute confusion, which encompasses global cognitive impairment, has not been clearly or consistently defined.[27,28] Synonyms include delirium (the medical term), ICU psychosis, postcardiotomy delirium, and acute brain failure.[29] Additional terms are acute mental status change, acute organic reaction, metabolic encephalopathy, and reversible cognitive dysfunction. Orientation to person, time, or place and the ability to reason, follow directions, process incoming stimuli, or maintain concentration are lost. Confused persons may be aware of these disturbances and fear that they are "losing their minds." The confused state is a secondary response to organic causes, that is, hypoxia, drugs, or fluid and electrolyte imbalances, or to inorganic causes such as stress and sleep deprivation. Onset is abrupt, and duration can be shortened if early diagnosis and treatment are initiated. It is estimated that confusion develops in 50% of hospitalized elderly patients; however, it is often misdiagnosed because of inaccurate assessment and assumptions that a mental deterioration is the result of the effects of aging.[30,31] More than 80% of reports of confused status in the elderly are attributed to organic causes; dehydration and recent falls, hip fractures, and polypharmacy are additional risk factors for confusion. Behavioral symptoms may be subtle and varied. Prodromal symptoms include insomnia, distractibility, drowsiness, anxiety, and nightmares. Symptoms of acute confusion resemble those of dementia, which makes differentiation between the two conditions more difficult. However, dementia, which cannot be reversed, has a gradual onset and is of long duration.

Approximately 10% to 15% of all hospitalized medical-surgical patients experience symptoms of delirium. This percentage is increased by 30% to 40% in the critical care setting. Hospital stays are prolonged for this population.[27] An increased level of confusion may be the first indicator of a biologic problem or may be the result of environmental stressors. The nurse must continually assess cognitive function. Several tools for assessing this are available. The Mini-Mental State Examination (MMSE), developed by Folstein, Folstein, and McHugh,[32] is the most popular and easy to administer. Items included on the examination relate to orientation, comprehension, recall, and following commands.

ETIOLOGY

Understanding the causes and symptoms of delirium, knowing the people who are at risk for developing delirium, and using appropriate measures to minimize causal factors are primary aspects of the critical care nurse role. The majority of the time, the exact etiology is unknown.

Three predisposing contributors to the development of delirium are (1) age 60 years or over, (2) presence of brain damage, and (3) presence of a chronic brain disorder, such as Alzheimer's disease. Cognitive dysfunctions are believed to occur when "there is a widespread reduction of cerebral oxidative metabolism and an imbalance of neuro-transmission"[27,28,33] (Box 4-2).

Drugs that are commonly used in the ICU contribute to delirium. Some of these are digitalis, antibiotics, steroids, β-blockers, and respiratory stimulants. Additional causes of delirium include sleep deprivation, sensory deprivation or overload, and immobilization, all of which are events commonly encountered in the ICU.[34]

The patient in the ICU is deprived of the restorative benefits of deep sleep and the rapid eye movement (REM) phase of sleep because of frequent interruptions by equipment noises, voices, and procedures. Constant, bright overhead lights, the absence of day-night cycles, immobility, pain, and medications contribute to the patient's disorientation to time and place. Daytime napping, complaints of fatigue, slurred speech, as well as depression, cognitive impairment, and hallucinations can result. Delayed recovery, increased length of hospital stay, and the seriousness of sleep deprivation are closely related.

ASSESSMENT

Three forms of delirium have been identified—hyperactive, hypoactive, and a mixture of both forms.[27-29] The patient with the hyperactive form may become violent; remove intravenous lines, dressings, and catheters; be extremely restless and try to get out of bed; pick at things in the air; and call out to persons who are not there. Sympathetic nervous system responses of tachycardia, dilation of pupils, diaphoresis, and facial flushing are evident. In the hypoactive form, persons complain of extreme fatigue, are slow to respond, and have hypersomnolence that can progress to loss of consciousness. At times these individuals are absorbed in a dreamlike state, mumble to themselves, experience vivid hallucinations, and make inappropriate gestures. The third form is a mixture of agitation and hypoactive behaviors that can vary throughout the day. Symptoms and hallucinations seem to worsen during the night—often referred to as *sundowner syndrome*—with more lucid intervals occurring during the day.

MENTAL STATUS EXAMINATION

The mental status examination is a full, criteria-based assessment of the patient's cognitive function and thought processes. Although the examination is rarely conducted in its entirety in the critical care setting,

Box 4-2

Defining Characteristics of Delirium/Acute Confusion and Etiologic Factors

Defining Characteristics

Displays at least two of the following:

Early Signs/Symptoms

- Sudden onset of global cognitive function impairment (from hours to days)
- Restlessness, agitation, combative behavior
- Drowsiness—can lead to loss of consciousness
- Slurred speech, inappropriate statements, or "word salad," and mumbling
- Inappropriate gestures, short attention span—needs questions repeated; inability to learn new material
- Disordered awake-sleep cycle
- Disorientation to person, time, place, situation
- Difficulty in separating dreams from reality—may experience bizarre dreams/nightmares
- Anger at staff for continued questions about his or her orientation

Later Signs/Symptoms

- Symptoms tend to fluctuate throughout the day and night
- Early symptoms continue—may be more frequent and of longer duration
- Illusions
- Hallucinations
- Extreme agitation—attempts to climb out of bed, pull out catheters, rip off dressings
- Calling out in loud voice; may swear; attempt to bite or hit people who approach person

Etiologic Factors

- Fluid and electrolyte imbalances
- Potential for organ dysfunction (hepatic, renal, gastrointestinal, cardiac, respiratory) because of oxygenation
- Delay in metabolism and excretion of drugs, thus prolonging half-life and increasing drug's effect or interaction with other drugs
- Immune-suppressant drugs' side effects
- Narcotic analgesics
- Hypersensitivity to drugs
- Surgical time (or on by-pass equipment) more than 4 hours
- Stressors in ICU (also refer to Box 4-1)
- Physical and mental status of patient before surgery—preexisting medical conditions (e.g., diabetes, epilepsy, neoplasm)
- Withdrawal symptoms (e.g., alcohol, drugs, amphetamines)
- Minimal accessibility to social-spiritual/family support

Data from Geary S: *Crit Care Nurs Q* 17(1):51, 1994; Hall G, Wakefield B: Acute confusion in the elderly: what to do when the clouds roll in, *Nursing CE Handbook* (on-line), March 1998, Springhouse; and American Psychiatric Association: *Diagnostic and statistical manual of mental disorders–DSM-IV-TR,* ed 4, Washington, DC, 2000, The Association.

Box 4-3

The Mental Status Examination

General Observations

- Appearance
- Reaction to interviewer
- Behavior and psychomotor activity

Sensorium and Intelligence

- Level of consciousness
- Orientation
- Memory
- Intellectual function
- Judgment
- Comprehension

Thought Processes

- Form of thought
- Content of thought
- Mood
- Affect
- Insight

knowledge of its main components will enhance the nurse's effectiveness in collecting data to document findings by using accepted terminology and identifying issues that need further assessment (Box 4-3).

MANAGEMENT

The American Psychiatric Association[35] has developed a practice guideline for the treatment of patients with delirium. Psychiatric consultation and management are preferred, with communication among the primary treatment team, the critical care nurse, and the family. The treatment of choice is to diagnose and treat the underlying medical condition that is causing the delirium. Once this is done, it is important to treat the ongoing symptoms that are distressing the patient. Sedation is prescribed for patients with hyperactive delirium. A neuroleptic drug such as haloperidol, commonly used for neurotic and personality disorders, is useful in the treatment of delirium. Currently haloperidol is considered to be the drug of choice, and a regular dosing schedule is preferred rather than waiting until symptoms recur before giving another dose. A typical regimen is as follows: *mild agitation,* 1 to 3 mg; *moderate agitation,* 5 to 7 mg; and *severe agitation,* 10 mg or more.[36] "However, haloperidol may have a paradoxical effect on some patients, worsening the delirium." If continued dosing increases agitation, administration should be discontinued. A combination of haloperidol and lorazepam, a benzodiazepine drug that produces sedative effects, allows lower doses of each drug to be given, is very effective, and produces fewer side effects. Benzodiazepine monotherapy should be avoided unless the delirium is attributable to sedative or alcohol withdrawal.

The newer atypical antipsychotics appear to provide similar efficacy and are better tolerated; however, few randomized and controlled trials have been reported. Risperidone, olanzapine, quetiapine, and ziprasidone have been shown to be effective for the treatment of delirium in retrospective case reports.

When delirium is considered to be secondary to pain, narcotics can be administered. However, the paradoxical effects of depressed respirations and cardiac output can exacerbate the delirium. The elderly patient particularly benefits from smaller doses given on a regular basis.[28] The use of barbiturates is no longer recommended as routine treatment, but they are used in the treatment of barbiturate withdrawal–induced delirium.

Finally, neuromuscular blocking agents are sometimes used for severely agitated patients who are on mechanical ventilation to effect a decrease in oxygen consumption, to promote synchrony with the ventilator, and to increase tissue oxygenation. These complex drugs can be dangerous but do not affect consciousness, cognition, or pain levels; thus sedatives or analgesics should be added as appropriate.[27,28]

COPING MECHANISMS

When a patient copes effectively, what he or she is doing to cope often goes unnoticed. Emotionally the patient seems relatively comfortable, is a cooperative recipient of care, and exhibits nonproblematic behavior. The patient may be using multiple appropriate coping mechanisms that help to manage a problem or stressful situation. Refer to the Nursing Management Plan for Powerlessness (p. A-44) for specific nursing interventions.

REGRESSION

Regression is an unconscious defense mechanism that involves a retreat, in the face of stress, to behavior characteristic of an earlier developmental level.[37] Regression allows the patient to give up his or her usual role, autonomy, and privacy to become the passive recipient of medical and nursing care. In fact, the patient who does not regress jeopardizes his or her care. Conversely, the patient who becomes too regressed presents another problem. Regression is a normal reaction to severe burns, and the person may become childlike in interactions with staff, whining, clinging to staff, and attempting to keep the nurse at the bedside. In both cases the patient must know the limits set on behavior if he or she is to receive essential care. The patient is best served when limits are set in a supportive manner.

Although the behavior of these patients can provoke confrontations or reprimands, such responses should be avoided. These responses from staff may only worsen a situation in which a patient is already struggling with issues of dependence and autonomy.

SUPPRESSION

Suppression is a conscious, intentional process in which patients push ideas, problems, or desires out of their conscious thoughts.[37] Patients often use suppression when their problems are overwhelming and they are in no position to resolve them. Before becoming ill, for example, an individual may have been struggling to meet financial obligations but now uses suppression to postpone dealing with this concern until later in the recovery phase.

DENIAL

According to NANDA International, denial includes both conscious and unconscious attempts to disavow knowledge or the meaning of an event. This text uses the psychoanalytic definition of denial, "an unconscious defense mechanism that reduces anxiety by eliminating or reducing the seriousness of the perceived threat," to allow for the distinction between denial and suppression. When used by a critically ill patient, denial reduces the anxiety and the threat of the illness.[19] The degree to which denial is used varies among patients and may vary in the same patient at different times. Patients also may deny different aspects of the illness.

TRUST

Trust manifests in the critical care patient as the belief that the staff will see the patient through the illness, managing any untoward event that might occur. Trust is an unconscious process in which the patient transfers the trust learned in early significant relationships onto caregivers in the present.[25,38]

HOPE

Although hope has long been recognized as a significant factor in patient recovery and survival, the phenomenon receives little attention until the patient becomes hopeless. Hope is the expectation that a desire will be fulfilled. It can exist even in the face of a realistic appraisal of a grim situation.[38] Hope supports the patient and helps the patient endure the physical and psychologic insults of the daily experience. Hope is central to resilience and spiritual strength.[8,17,39,40]

SPIRITUAL BELIEFS AND PRACTICES

Spiritual beliefs and practices may provide the patient with some measure of acceptance of an illness, a sense of mastery and control, a source of hope and trust beyond the limits the staff can provide, and the strength to endure the current stress. A patient may discuss personal beliefs and concerns openly or view the subject as a private and personal matter.[8,26,41]

Use of Family Support

The patient may use the presence of a supportive family to cope with critical illness. The patient with a supportive family knows that family members share a past and hope for a future with the patient. They love the patient as a person and member of the family. The patient also realizes that family members know him or her in ways the staff cannot. With family the patient may know that his or her experience is truly understood, even when little is said. Family members also may be involved in the patient's personal care and may attend to the practical problems the patient cannot, such as managing finances.[42] Family members can help the nurse to understand and know the patient especially when patients are unable to communicate themselves.

Sharing Concerns

Sharing concerns with a caring and understanding listener can relieve some of the patient's spiritual and emotional distress. The patient is consoled knowing that he or she is not alone and that someone knows and cares about what the patient is experiencing.[16,38] The patient may share concerns with family members. However, the patient may be reluctant to upset loved ones further or may have a family for whom such communication is not the norm. A patient who relies on this coping mechanism will benefit from a nurse who recognizes when a patient needs to talk and who knows how to listen.

COPING ASSESSMENT

Ineffective coping may be suggested in patient behaviors. Overt hostility, severe regression, and noncompliance with treatment may suggest ineffective coping. The patient may also report such problems as severe anxiety, despondence, and despair. The nurse who suspects that coping is ineffective should consider a number of factors before questioning the patient directly.

It is not always clear whether the patient's coping is truly ineffective and intervention by the nurse is indicated. Witnessing problematic behavior can be very uncomfortable, especially when that behavior is directed at the caregiver. Careful evaluation of one's reaction to the behavior is needed to discover whether patient care can continue to be provided objectively by the nurse alone or whether consultation with other team members is needed to alleviate the problem.[10,11,25,26]

COPING ENHANCEMENT

Some patients remember well their time in the ICU, whereas others have few memories of the experience. A recent study revealed that the overall psychosocial need of ICU patients was a feeling of safety. Nurses providing emotional support and encouragement, supplying information about patients' progress, helping them regain some control and independence, instilling a sense of hope, and building a close trusting relationship with family members made the patients feel safe. The patients felt reassured by the nurses' professional skill performance and sensitivity to their emotional and spiritual needs.[12,16,42] Essential techniques for effective interventions include an attitude of caring; openness and warmth; and withholding judgment until the nurse "knows" the patient (has an understanding of the individual's perception about self), the current illness or problem, and the type of social support available. Assessment skills are essential, as is a willingness to become involved when the potential for, or use of, ineffective coping mechanisms exists.

Teaching the patient new coping skills may be impossible, because individuals have a repertoire of defense and coping mechanisms, both conscious and unconscious, that they automatically bring into play when facing stressful situations. A person who is experiencing extreme psychologic stress cannot learn new methods to manage these defense mechanisms. However, the nurse may help to reduce the level of anxiety by employing active listening, encouraging support from family members and other caregivers, and introducing changes in the environment as appropriate. In this way the nurse can facilitate the changes the patient must make. It is extremely important that the patient express an interest in learning and recognize a personal need for help.[8,40] An individualized education program can be effective in decreasing the anxiety of both patients and families when patients are transferred to another unit.[43]

A patient's trust in the nurse's competence in the physical and technical aspects of care aids in the patient's participation. Hope is instilled when the nurse and other caregivers display a sense of realistic optimism regarding the patient's progress. Patients must receive honest feedback because they are keen observers of their caregivers and read them well. Trust and hope are easily lessened when inappropriate information is given.[42] Refer to the Nursing Management Plan for Anxiety (p. A-9) and Ineffective Coping (p. A-38) for specific nursing interventions.

Supporting Family Members

Patient-centered care is also family-centered care. Consideration of nonbiologic or nonlegal partners of the patient as members of the patient's support system

Box 4-4

Interventions to Support Family Members

1. Identify a family spokesperson and support persons.
2. Identify a primary nursing contact for the family.
3. Establish a mechanism for family access to the patient.
4. Promote access to the patient, and ensure consistency in adhering to unit routines.
5. Establish a mechanism to contact the family and to update on changes in patient status.
6. Provide information based on family needs.
7. Ensure support services are available, and refer to specialized services as needed.
8. Explain all procedures using understandable terms.
9. Include family in providing care.
10. Provide a comfortable environment for the family.
11. Include family in end-of-life planning, and provide palliative care and support for terminally ill patients and families.

Modified from Twibell RS: *Dimens Crit Care Nurs* 17(2):100, 1998.

is also necessary in providing holistic care. The nurse's support of family members at the bedside can enhance the value of the visits for the patient,[40-42] and other supportive interventions should be considered (Box 4-4).44 Patients often look to the family for love, understanding, support, and care in matters they cannot attend to themselves.

SUPPORTING SPIRITUAL CARE

There is a certain amount of uncertainty in all illness experiences, and it affects a person's adaptation and outcomes. Uncertainty has been defined as a multidimensional concept related to the inability to determine the meaning of illness-related events.[14,37] Self-reflection, with a focus on examining issues that attack the self, is a component of the search for meaning.[45] Separation from religious rituals/ties and intense suffering can induce spiritual distress for patients and their families. Using a spiritual assessment tool to identify a person/family's perception of their current situation, inner strengths, self-concept, and beliefs helps the nurse in supporting spiritual care.[8,26,45]

evolve To test your mastery of this chapter, try the Open-Book Quiz at http://evolve.elsevier.com/Urden/priorities/

REFERENCES

1. Benner P, Tanner C, Chesla C: *Expertise in nursing practice*, New York, 1998, Springer.
2. Motzer SA et al: Natural killer cell function and psychological distress in women with and without irritable bowel syndrome, *Biol Res Nurs* 4(1):31, 2002.
3. Stein K, Rose R, Markus H: Self-schemas and possible selves as predictors and outcomes of risky behaviors in adolescents, *Nurs Res* 47(2):96, 1998.
4. Mendyka B: Exploring culture in nursing: a theory-driven practice, *Holistic Nurs Pract* 15(1):32, 2000.
5. Coopersmith S: *The antecedents of self-esteem*, San Francisco, 1967, Freeman.
6. Judge T et al: Are measures of self-esteem, neuroticism, locus of control and generalized self-efficacy indicators for a common core construct? *J Pers Soc Psychol* 83(3):693, 2002.
7. Polusky S: Street music or the blues? The lived experience and social environment of depression, *Public Health Nurs* 17(4):292, 2000.
8. Bay E et al: Chronic stress, sense of belonging, and depression among survivors of traumatic brain injury, *J Nurs Scholarsh* 34(3):221, 2002.
9. Beck AT et al: The measurement of pessimism: the hopelessness scale, *J Consult Clin Psychol* 42(6):861, 1974.
10. National Institute of Mental Health: *Depression*, 2002, available from www.nimh.nih.gov.
11. Kaba E, Thompson D, Burnard P: Coping after heart transplantation: a descriptive study of heart transplant recipients' methods of coping, *J Adv Nurs* 32(4):930, 2000.
12. Hupcey J: Feeling safe: the psychosocial needs of ICU patients, *J Nurs Scholarsh* 32(4):361, 2000.
13. Shaffer R, Corish C: Cardiac surgery and women: cardiac surgery. II. Recovery, *J Cardiovasc Nurs* 12(4):14, 1998.
14. McCormick K: A concept analysis of uncertainty in illness, *J Nurs Scholarsh* 34(2):127, 2002.
15. Maslow H: *Motivation and personality*, New York, 1954, Harper & Row.
16. Whittemore R: Consequences of not "knowing the patient," *Clin Nurs Spec* 14(2):75, 2000.
17. Gibson J, Kenrick M: Pain and powerlessness: the experience of living with peripheral vascular disease, *J Adv Nurs* 24(4):737, 1998.
18. Colling K: A taxonomy of passive behaviors in people with Alzheimer's, *J Nurs Scholarsh* 32(3):239, 2000.
19. North American Nursing Diagnosis Association: *Nursing diagnosis: definitions and classifications*, St Louis, 2001-2002, The Association.
20. Ackley B, Ladwig G: *Nursing diagnosis handbook: a guide to planning care*, St Louis, 2001, Mosby.
21. Hustey F, Meldon S: The prevalence and documentation of impaired mental status in elderly emergency department patients, *Ann Emerg Med* 39(3):248, 2002.
22. Rotter JB: Generalized expectancies for internal versus external control of reinforcement, *Psychol Monogr* 80(609):1, 1966.
23. Janis IL, Rodin J: Attribution, control, and decision-making: social psychology and health care. In Stone GC, Adler NC, editors: *Health psychology: a handbook*, San Francisco, 1979, Jossey-Bass.
24. Seligman ME: *Helplessness: on depression, development and death*, San Francisco, 1975, Freeman.
25. Grendell R: Psychologic aspects of physiologic illness. In Fortinash K, Holoday-Worret P, editors: *Psychiatric mental health nursing*, ed 2, St Louis, 2000, Mosby.
26. Dossey B, Dossey L: Holistic modalities and healing moments, *Am J Nurs* 98(6):44, 1998.
27. Geary S: Intensive care unit psychosis revisited: under-

standing and managing delirium in the critical care setting, *Crit Care Nurs Q* 17(1):51, 1994.
28. Hall G, Wakefield B: Acute confusion in the elderly: what to do when the clouds roll in, *Nursing CE handbook* (on-line), March 1998, Springhouse.
29. Stuart G: A stress adaptation model of psychiatric nursing care. In Stuart GW, editor: *Principles and practices of psychiatric nursing,* ed 6, St Louis, 2004, Mosby.
30. Mentes J et al: Acute confusion indicators: risk factors and prevalence using MDS data, *Res Nurs Health* 22:95, 1999.
31. Burke MM, Laramie J: *Primary care of the older adult,* St Louis, 2004, Mosby.
32. Folstein MF, Folstein SE, McHugh PR: "Mini-mental state": a practical method for grading the cognitive state of patients for the clinician, *J Psychiatr Res* 12(3):189, 1975.
33. Porth C: *Pathophysiology: concepts of altered health states,* ed 5, Philadelphia, 1998, Lippincott.
34. Doenges ME, Moorhouse MF: *Nurse's pocket guide: diagnoses, interventions, and rationales,* ed 7, Philadelphia, 2004, FA Davis.
35. American Psychiatric Association: Practice guidelines for the treatment of patients with delirium, *Am J Psychiatry* 156(suppl 5):1, 1999.
36. Barber JM. Pharmacologic management of integrative brain failure, *Crit Care Nurs Q* 26(3):192, 2003.
37. Holoday-Worret P: Foundations of psychiatric mental health nursing. In Fortinash K, Holoday-Worret P, editors: *Psychiatric mental health nursing,* ed 3, St Louis, 2004, Mosby.
38. Gelling L: The role of hope for relatives of critically ill patients: a review of the literature, *Nurs Stand* 4(1):33, 1999.
39. Roberts S, Johnson L, Kelly B: Fostering hope in the elderly congestive heart patient in critical care, *Geriatr Nurs* 20(4):195, 1999.
40. Morse J, Penrod J: Linking concepts of enduring, uncertainty, suffering, and hope, *Image J Nurs Sch* 31(2):145, 1999.
41. Taylor K: Standards of holistic nursing practice, *AORTN* 72(6):1080, 2000.
42. Hupcey JE: Establishing the nurse-family relationship in the intensive care unit, *West J Nurs Res* 20(2):180, 1998.
43. Tel H, Tel H: The effect of individualized education on the transfer anxiety of patients with myocardial infarction and their families, *Heart Lung* 35(2):101, 2006.
44. Twibell RS: Family coping during critical illness, *Dimens Crit Care Nurs* 17(2):100, 1998.
45. Carson V, Green H: Spiritual well-being: a predictor of hardiness in patients with acquired immunodeficiency syndrome, *J Prof Nurs* 8(4):209, 1992.

CHAPTER

5 Sleep Alterations

SHEILA COX SULLIVAN

OBJECTIVES

- Define the stages of sleep.
- Explain the physiologic effects that occur during rapid eye movement (REM) sleep.
- Describe changes in sleep resulting from the aging process.
- Name three commonly prescribed critical care medications that decrease REM sleep.
- Describe evidence-based practice methods for promoting sleep in critical care.

SLEEP PHYSIOLOGY

Humans spend about one third of their lives engaged in a process known as sleep. Although little is known at present about the physiologic process or the degree to which sleep affects us, researchers are learning more about sleep every day. The behavioral definition of sleep is a reversible behavioral state of perceptual disengagement from and unresponsiveness to the environment.[1] Research involving simultaneous monitoring using the electroencephalogram (EEG), electrooculogram (EOG), and electromyogram (EMG) has shown that there are two distinct stages of sleep: *nonrapid eye movement* (NREM) and *rapid eye movement* (REM).

SLEEP STAGES

NONRAPID EYE MOVEMENT SLEEP

Humans experience three states of being. They are either awake (Figure 5-1), in REM sleep, or in NREM sleep, which can be further divided into stages 1 through 4, with each stage a progressively deeper sleep state. Adults usually enter sleep through NREM *stage 1* sleep (Figure 5-2), which is a transitional, lighter sleep state from which the patient can be easily aroused by light touch or softly calling his or her name. Stage 1 is demonstrated by an EEG pattern of low-voltage, mixed-frequency waveforms with vertex sharp waves. A patient with severely disrupted sleep may experience an increase in the amount of stage 1 sleep throughout the sleep cycle. As a patient makes the transition from awake to asleep, a brief memory impairment may result.[1] Patients may experience muscle jerks and recall vivid images on awakening. These reactions, called *hypnic myoclonia,* are not pathologic conditions but can cause the patient to awaken feeling frightened.

In NREM *stage 2,* sleep deepens, and the patient is more difficult to arouse. As stage 2 continues, high-voltage, slow-wave activity begins to appear. When these slow waves represent 20% of the EEG activity per page, they meet the criteria for NREM *stage 3* sleep. Stage 3 slow waves continue to develop until 50% of the EEG waveforms are slow wave, which meets the criteria for *stage 4* sleep. Stages 3 and 4 often are combined and referred to as *slow-wave sleep,* or *delta sleep* (Figure 5-3). Delta sleep has the highest arousal threshold.

NREM sleep is dominated by the parasympathetic nervous system. The body tries to maintain a homeostatic regulation, resulting in a decreased level of energy expenditure. Blood pressure, heart and respiratory rates, and metabolic rate return to basal levels. EMG activity is lower in NREM versus wake states but not as low as that in REM sleep. A patient may experience sweating or shivering with temperature extremes in NREM sleep, but this ceases during REM sleep.[1]

During slow-wave sleep, 80% of growth-stimulating hormone is released, stimulating protein synthesis while sparing catabolic breakdown. The release of other hormones, such as prolactin and testosterone, suggests that anabolism is occurring during slow-wave sleep. Cortisol release peaks during early-morning hours, whereas melatonin is released only during darkness, and thyroid-stimulating hormone is inhibited during sleep. Activities associated with NREM stage 4 sleep include protein synthesis and tissue repair, such as the repair of epithelial and specialized cells of the brain, skin, bone marrow, and gastric mucosa.[2] Some propose that NREM sleep is a restorative period that relieves the stresses of waking activities, whereas REM sleep serves to refuel creative brain stores. Table 5-1 lists the time spent in sleep stages for normal adults.

Rapid Eye Movement Sleep

Although REM sleep is also called the "dream stage," dreaming is not the exclusive property of any one stage. REM can be viewed as a highly active brain in a paralyzed body. REM sleep is frequently referred to as *paradoxical sleep* because some areas of the brain remain very active while others are suppressed. EMG waveforms are relatively slow low voltage with saw-tooth waves present. Increased cortical activity occurs, with the EEG pattern resembling that of the awake state (Figure 5-4).

The sympathetic nervous system predominates during REM sleep.[3] Oxygen consumption increases, and blood pressure, cardiac output, and respiratory/heart rates become variable. The body's response to decreased oxygen levels and increased carbon dioxide levels is lowest during REM sleep. Cardiac efferent vagus nerve tone is generally suppressed during REM sleep, and irregular breathing patterns can lead to oxygen reduction, particularly in patients with pulmonary and cardiac disease. An increase in premature ventricular contractions and tachydysrhythmias may be associated with respiratory pauses during REM sleep.[3] Arterial pressure surges and increases in heart rate, coronary arterial tone, and blood viscosity may cause the combination of plaque rupture and hypercoagulability in patients with cardiac disease.[4]

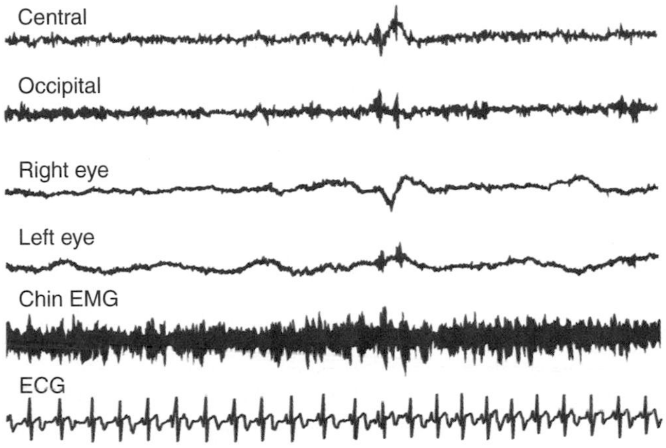

FIGURE 5-1. Awake. *EMG,* Electromyogram; *ECG,* electrocardiogram; upper tracings are electroencephalogram (EEG) and electrooculogram (EOG) measurements.

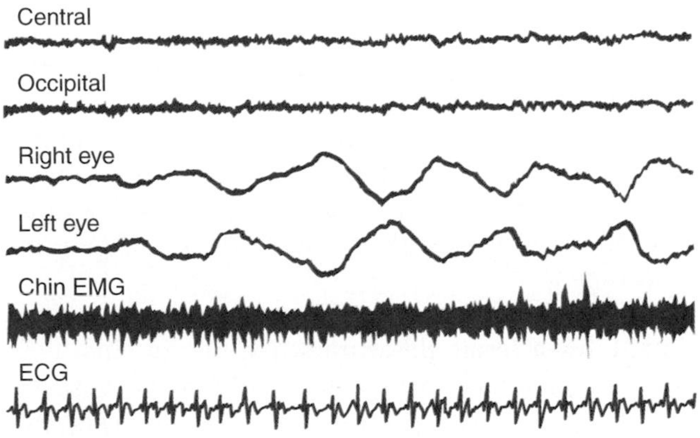

FIGURE 5-2. NREM stage 1 sleep.

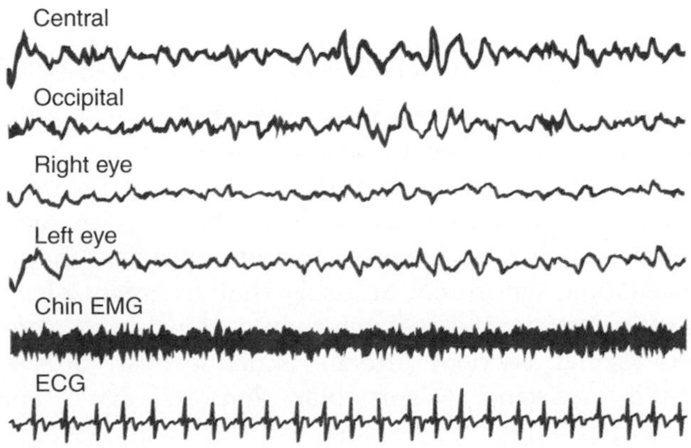

FIGURE 5-3. Delta sleep.

SLEEP CYCLES

NREM and REM sleep cycles alternate throughout the night. Sleep onset usually occurs in stage 1 sleep, progressing through stages 2 to 4 and then going back

Table 5-1

Time Spent in Sleep Stages for Normal Adults

STAGE	PERCENT OF NOCTURNAL SLEEP
1	2-5
2	45-55
3	3-8
4	10-15
REM	20-25

REM, Rapid eye movement.

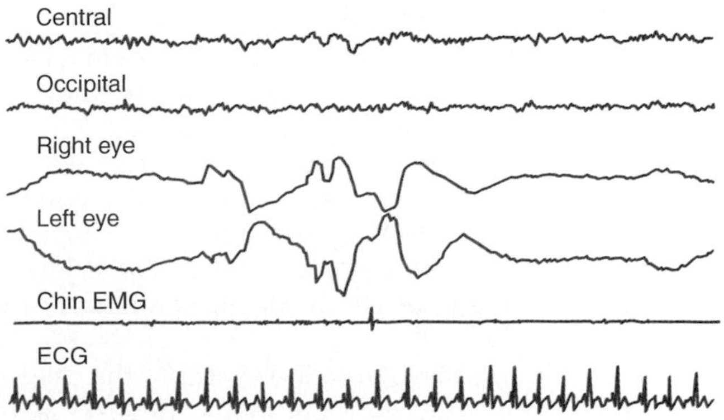

FIGURE 5-4. Rapid eye movement (REM) sleep.

to stage 2, at which time the person usually enters REM. This first cycle usually takes about 70 to 100 minutes, with later cycles lasting 90 to 120 minutes. Four to five cycles are completed during normal adult sleep. NREM sleep predominates during the first third of the night, whereas REM is more prominent during the last third. Brief episodes of wakefulness (usually less than 5%) tend to intrude later into the night and are usually not remembered the next morning.

The amount of sleep required is still debated. No set number of hours has been established, and sleep length may be determined by many factors, including genetic predisposition. A sufficient amount of sleep has been achieved when the person awakens without the alarm and proceeds through the day without feeling sleepy.

SLEEP CHANGES WITH AGE

Elderly persons most often complain about either excessive sleepiness or insomnia, and current research offers justification for both these complaints.[5] Sleep pattern changes in older adults include fewer episodes of stages 3 and 4 NREM and REM sleep.[6] Elderly persons also report that they do not sleep as soundly or feel as rested after awakening,[7] possibly because they do not consolidate their sleep into one session. They may go to bed, awake 4 hours later, stay awake for an extended period, then go back to sleep, resulting in fragmented sleep patterns.[8] Many of the diseases associated with aging may contribute to these nocturnal arousals, including diabetes, nocturia, cardiovascular symptoms, chronic pain, and depression.[8-10] In addition, sleep-related respiratory disorders and increased incidence of periodic leg movements in elders may further disrupt their sleep.[11] Increasing age brings many physical and social changes with which the elder must cope. Assessment of elderly patients must always include sleep history as an indicator of mental health because depression is a common struggle for this population.[12]

SLEEP AND DISEASE

Lack of sufficient, restful sleep is at an epidemic proportion in American society. According to the National Sleep Foundation's 2005 *Sleep in America* poll, 71% of adult Americans sleep less than 8 hours per night.[13] Failure to gain adequate sleep in sufficient amounts is linked with impaired glucose tolerance,[14] weight gain in women,[15] hypertension,[16] and increased levels of C-reactive protein, a risk factor for coronary heart disease (CHD).[17]

Conversely, disease processes affect the sleep quality of those with the conditions. Redeker and Stein[18] found that participants with heart failure had poorer sleep quality and more daytime sleepiness than a control group without heart failure. Study subjects suffering from idiopathic pulmonary fibrosis[19] identified sleep disruption as a factor in coping with their disease process. Further, adequate treatment of disease processes, such as lung volume reduction in subjects with emphysema, can positively affect sleep.[20]

PHARMACOLOGY AND SLEEP

Many drugs essential to treatment of critically ill patients impact sleep quality (Table 5-2).[21-24] It is important to understand the relationship between various medications and the sleep of patients in the critical care unit. Pathophysiology and age may profoundly affect not only medication absorption and elimination but also how patients cope with their illness and their ability to maintain health.

SLEEP APNEA SYNDROMES

Sleep apnea syndrome, sometimes called *sleep-disordered breathing,* occurs when airflow is absent or reduced. Apneas during sleep can be divided into three types: obstructive, central, and mixed. In obstructive apnea the absence of airflow is caused by an obstruction in the upper airway. Complete obstruction lasting 10 seconds or longer is referred to as *obstructive apnea,* whereas a partial obstruction is known as *hypopnea.* In *central apnea,* airflow is absent because of lack of ventilatory muscle effort. The third type of sleep apnea syndrome, *mixed,* occurs when a combination of both obstructive and central patterns occurs in one apneic event. An apnea-hypopnea index (number of apneic and hypopneic episodes per hour divided by hours of sleep) of 5 or greater is diagnostic of sleep apnea syndrome.[25]

All types of sleep apnea syndrome are accompanied by arterial desaturation and potentially by hypoxemia, which may cause pulmonary vasoconstriction and increased systemic vascular resistance. However, desaturation and hypoxemia are most severe in the obstructive type.

OBSTRUCTIVE SLEEP APNEA-HYPOPNEA SYNDROME

Obstructive sleep apnea-hypopnea syndrome (OSAHS) occurs when obstruction in the upper airway causes at least five apneic or hypopneic events per hour of sleep. The incidence of OSAHS is believed to increase with age. Consequences include chronic hypoventilation syndrome, arousals that fragment sleep, cardiovascular changes such as hypertension,[26,27] cerebrovascular accident (stroke), ischemic heart disease, insulin resistance, ventricular hypertrophy,[28] and nocturnal angina.[29] Because of the cardiovascular complications and accidents caused by sleepiness, OSAHS is a significant condition that should be thoroughly evaluated.

Table 5-2

Pharmacologic Management: Select Drugs That Affect Sleep and Wakefulness

CLASS	DRUG	EFFECT	COMMENTS
Hypnotics			
Benzodiazepines		↓ SWS, ↑ TST, ↓ WASO, ↓ stage 1 sleep, mild REM suppression	↑ Apnea, ↑ daytime residual sedation, mild respiratory depression, ↓ psychomotor function
Immediate-acting	Quazepam	Half-life 20-120 hr	
	Temazepam	Half-life 8-20 hr	
Long-acting	Flurazepam, HCl	Half-life 40-250 hr	
Rapid-acting	Triazolam	Half-life 2-6 hr	
	Estazolam	Half-life 8-24 hr	Rebound insomnia
Nonbenzodiazepines		No effect on REM or SWS	
Rapid-acting	Zolpidem	Half-life 1 hr	
	Zaleplon	Half-life 1 hr	No cognitive or performance impairment; ↓ abuse potential; can be taken in middle of night
	Eszopiclone (Lunesta)	Half-life 6 hr, ↓ SL, ↓ WASO	Unpleasant taste and headache
Stimulants			
	Nicotine	↑ SL, ↓ TST, ↓ REM	
	Amphetamines	↓ REM, ↓ SWS, ↓ TST, ↑ WASO	Less daytime fatigue
Nonsympathomimetics	Xanthine derivatives: coffee, chocolate, tea; scopolamine; strychnine; pentylenetetrazol; modafinil	↓ TST, ↓ REM, ↓ SWS, ↑ SL, ↑ WASO	
Direct sympathomimetics	Isoproterenol, epinephrine, norepinephrine, phenylephrine, phenylpropanolamine, apomorphine	↑ Wake, ↑ REM onset, ↓ fatigue, ↓ sleepiness	↑ Blood pressure, ↓ heart rate
Indirect sympathomimetics	Amphetamine, methamphetamine, cocaine, piperacillin (Pipradrol), methylphenidate, tyramine	↑ WASO, ↑ daytime SL, ↓ sleepiness	Narcolepsy treatment, ↑ cognitive tasks
	Pemoline		Possible liver damage
Antihypertensives			
β-Antagonists	Propranolol, metoprolol	↑ Wake, TWT, SL, ↓ REM	Insomnia, nightmares
α_2-Agonists	Atenolol, clonidine	↓ REM, ↓ TST in hypertensives, ↑ TST in normal subjects	Nightmares, sedation, ↓ concentration, mental slowing
	Methyldopa	↑ REM, ↑ TST	Sedation, insomnia, nightmares
Diuretics	Hydrochlorothiazide, chlorthalidone, indapamide	No data	CNS effects unlikely
Vasodilators	Hydralazine	No data	Depression, insomnia, anxiety
Catecholamine depletors	Reserpine	↑ REM and stage shifts	
Calcium antagonists	Verapamil, nifedipine, diltiazem, amlodipine, felodipine, nisoldipine	No data	Insomnia, nightmares, depression, sedation, difficulty concentrating
Antihistamines			
Histamine H_1-receptor antagonists	H_1 antihistamines (*chem. class:* selective histamine H_1-receptor antagonist) (e.g., diphenhydramine, hydroxyzine, triprolidine)	↑ Drowsiness, ↓ SL	Impaired daytime performance
	H_1 antihistamines (*chem. class:* ethanolamine derivative H_1-receptor antagonist) (e.g., loratadine, terfenadine)	No sedation effects	

Continued

Table 5-2

Pharmacologic Management: Select Drugs That Affect Sleep and Wakefulness—*cont'd*

CLASS	DRUG	EFFECT	COMMENTS
Histamine H_2-receptor antagonists	Histamine$_2$ antagonists (e.g., cimetidine, ranitidine)	May cause insomnia or somnolence	Drowsiness in patients; renal impairment
Antidepressants			
Tricyclic antidepressants	Amitriptyline, doxepin, imipramine (trimipramine), clomipramine, desipramine, nortriptyline, protriptyline	↑ TST, ↓ wake	↓ Psychomotor and cognitive performance and daytime drowsiness
Selective serotonin reuptake inhibitors	Fluoxetine	↑ TST, ↑ wake, ↑ stage 1, ↑ SEM	Mild ↑ in psychomotor performance
	Paroxetine	↑ Wake, ↓ TST, ↑ stage 1, ↑ SL	
	Sertraline	No data	Insomnia (7%-16%)
	Fluvoxamine	↓ TST, ↑ wake, ↑ stage 1, ↑ SL	
	Citalopram	No change	Insomnia, no impairment in performance
	Trazodone	Variable, ↑ TST possible, ↓ SL	↓ Cognitive performance in elderly
Monoamine oxidase inhibitors	Phenelzine, tranylcypromine, moclobermide, brofaromine	↑ Daytime sleepiness because of ↓ TST, ↑ wake	Some improved psychomotor performance

↓, Decreased; ↑, increased; *SWS*, slow-wave sleep; *TST*, total sleep time; *WASO*, wake after sleep onset; *REM*, rapid eye movement; *SL*, sleep latency; *TWT*, total wake time; *CNS*, central nervous system; *SEM*, slow eye movement.

The cause of OSAHS is not entirely understood, although upper airway structure, hormonal balance, and neural control are implicated. Factors that contribute to OSAHS are (1) anatomic narrowing of the upper airway, (2) increased compliance of the upper airway tissue, (3) reflexes affecting upper airway caliber, and (4) pharyngeal inspiratory muscle function.[30] Computed tomography scans of awake subjects have shown that patients with OSAHS have narrower airways than normal subjects. The narrower the airway, the more easily it becomes obstructed.

Unstable control of the respiratory nerves of the diaphragmatic, intercostal, and upper airway muscles can cause sleep apnea.[30] Hypothyroidism can alter respiratory controls and therefore contribute to OSAHS. Other contributing disorders are exogenous obesity, kyphoscoliosis, and autonomic dysfunction.

The patient with OSAHS develops cycles of hypoxemia, hypercapnia, and acidosis with each episode of apnea until the patient is aroused and airflow resumes. Alveolar hypoventilation accompanies each apneic episode and results in hypercapnia. Between episodes, alveolar ventilation improves, so there is no net retention of carbon dioxide.

With obstruction, inspiratory subatmospheric intrathoracic pressures are abnormally elevated. This increased pressure promotes a tendency for airways to collapse, resulting in both hemodynamic and electrocardiographic changes. The extremely elevated pressures in OSAHS patients who have apneic episodes in both REM and NREM stages cause systemic and pulmonary hypertension. Systemic pressures of 200/120 mm Hg (awake control: 130/80 mm Hg) and pulmonary artery pressures of 80/54 mm Hg (awake control: 30/20 mm Hg) have been reported.[29] Cardiac dysrhythmias associated with obstructive apnea include bradycardias, sinus arrest, and occasionally, second-degree heart blocks. After resumption of airflow, tachycardias typically occur. Thus bradycardia-tachycardia syndrome is associated with OSAHS.[29]

Assessment and Diagnosis

Careful monitoring of oxygen saturation and breathing patterns can help the critical care nurse identify OSAHS and assist in its diagnosis and treatment. Patients at risk for OSAHS may have the following: snoring; obesity; short, thick neck circumference; cardiovascular disease; systemic hypertension; pulmonary hypertension; sleep fragmentation; gastroesophageal reflux; and an impaired quality of life.

OSAHSs frequently end in brief EEG arousals. Patients may experience hundreds of arousals and not even realize they awaken hundreds of times during the night. These arousals cause the patient to experience sleep fragmentation, causing excessive daytime sleepiness. This cardinal symptom of OSAHS may lead to irritability, poor job performance, troubled relationships, depression, and impaired quality of life. Further, OSAHS is highly correlated to cardiovascular disease[28] and hypertension.[26,27]

Diagnosis of OSAHS is made with *polysomnography*, an overnight sleep study. Polysomnography is used to determine the number and length of apnea episodes and sleep stages, number of arousals, airflow, respiratory effort, and oxygen desaturation.

Medical Management

For patients with mild OSAHS (apnea-hypopnea index of 5 to 10), weight loss, sleeping on the side if apneas are associated with sleeping on the back, avoidance of sedative medications and alcohol before bedtime, and avoidance of sleep deprivation may be sufficient. Patients with moderate to severe levels of apnea may be treated with mechanical, surgical, or pharmacologic therapy. Treatment may vary depending on the type and severity of illness.

Continuous positive airway pressure (CPAP) via nasal mask is the treatment of choice. When a patient cannot tolerate CPAP, *bimodal* positive airway pressure (BiPAP), which provides separate pressures for inspiration and expiration, may be used.

Various surgical treatments are available for treatment of apnea and snoring. Patients with mild OSAHS or snoring alone may undergo an outpatient procedure called *laser uvulopalatopharyngoplasty* (LAUP), which uses lasers to remove excess tissue at the soft palate level. For patients who snore but do not have apnea, somnoplasty may provide relief. Somnoplasty involves inserting a small electrode into the soft palate and heating the tissue, causing the area to shrink and tighten.[31]

Uvulopalatopharyngoplasty (UPPP) was one of the first surgical procedures used to treat OSAHS. Essentially a large tonsillectomy is performed with all redundant tissue removed. Only about 50% of patients experience sleep apnea improvement.[31] Complications include speech impairment, inability to eat, hemorrhage, and infection. Although tracheostomy was the original procedure used to treat OSAHS, it is now used only in patients with the most severe forms of apnea who do not respond to other treatments.

Treatment of OSAHS with medication is usually a last resort and has proved to be very disappointing. *Protriptyline* has been shown to decrease apnea and reduce excessive daytime sleepiness by decreasing REM sleep apnea frequency that increases during REM sleep. Oxygen may be used to lower hypoxemia and nocturnal desaturations.

Nursing Management

The nurse's role in the management of OSAHS includes educating the patient and family about the syndrome and the consequences of noncompliance with treatment regimens. This education may also include preoperative teaching for surgical procedures such as UPPP. Monitoring of patients with OSAHS while in critical care should include assessment of the breathing patterns, hours of sleep, and pulse oximetry. Refer to the Nursing Management Plan for Insomnia (p. A-43).

If patients are admitted to the critical care unit with a history of OSAHS, they need to use their home CPAP mask and equipment as part of their regular sleep routine. The nurse can promote compliance with the CPAP system through specific interventions for these patients (Box 5-1).

Box 5-1

Nursing Care for Patients Using CPAP

- Make sure that the mask fits snugly.
- Maintain the prescribed airway pressure.
- Ensure that air is not leaking, especially to the eye area.
- Monitor skin integrity under the mask.
- Make sure that the patient does not experience gastric insufflation.
- Encourage compliance at home.

Postoperative monitoring after UPPP includes risk of aspiration, pain management, anxiety relief, patient education, and monitoring for respiratory complications, hemorrhage, infection, impaired speech, nutritional concerns, and sleep disturbances.

Central Sleep Apnea

Central sleep apnea can be seen on polysomnography as an absence of airflow and respiratory effort for at least 10 seconds. Complete loss of EMG activity in respiratory muscles would be expected because central sleep apnea is defined as a pause in respiration without ventilatory effort.[32]

Central sleep apnea is not a single disease but rather a group of disorders in which breathing ceases momentarily during sleep because of the transient withdrawal of central nervous system drive to the muscles of respiration.[33] A patient with central sleep apnea may also experience obstructive events.

Central sleep apnea may result from many physiologic and pathophysiologic events.[32] Possible causes of *nonhypercapnic* central sleep apnea include periodic breathing at high altitude, renal/metabolic disturbances, Cheyne-Stokes breathing, and idiopathic central apnea seen at sea level. *Hypercapnic* central sleep apnea may occur in many neuromuscular conditions, including spinal cord or brain injury, encephalitis, brain stem neoplasm or infarcts, muscular dystrophy, myasthenia gravis, bulbar poliomyelitis, and post-polio syndrome.

Assessment and Diagnosis

Clinical characteristics of hypercapnic central sleep apnea include respiratory failure, cor pulmonale, peripheral edema, polycythemia, daytime sleepiness, and snoring. Patients with nonhypercapnic central sleep apnea have clinical features very similar to those of OSAHS. Nonhypercapnic central sleep apnea characteristics include daytime sleepiness, insomnia or poor sleep, mild or intermittent snoring, and awakenings accompanied by choking or feeling short of breath. Frequently the patients are of normal body weight. Diagnosis is made by overnight polysomnography or sleep study, which will determine the respiratory and sleep patterns of the patient.

Medical Management

Because there are two types of central sleep apnea, two therapeutic approaches are available depending on the cause of the apnea. The hypercapnic patient who has worsening hypoventilation during sleep is best served by nocturnal ventilation. Most of these patients experience some respiratory muscle failure. One treatment for patients with nonhypercapnic apnea or heart failure is nasal CPAP, which also may provide a beneficial cardiovascular effect. Nocturnal oxygen supplementation may be effective as well. If CPAP is not tolerated, pharmacologic management may be used. *Medroxyprogesterone,* a respiratory stimulant, may improve ventilation in selected patients.[32] *Acetazolamide,* a carbonic anhydrase inhibitor that can result in metabolic acidosis, also may decrease frequency of apneic episodes.

Nursing Management

For the nurse caring for a patient with central sleep apnea, patient and family education about the patient's condition and treatment regimen can help ensure patient compliance. The nurse needs to address any fear or anxiety about going to sleep. Nurses should caution patients to avoid alcohol or sedative medications. Weight loss is recommended if the patient is obese. The nurse must carefully monitor and assess the patient's respiratory status.

SLEEP PROMOTION IN CRITICAL CARE

Critical care nurses may promote sleep by determining potential causes of sleep disruption and addressing these causes directly. For example, patients with anxiety or pain may be soothed by nursing interventions that promote relaxation or comfort, such as massage.[34] Relaxing sounds[35] or music therapy, open visitation policies, and controlling noise and light in the unit environment may also promote rest. Finally, nurses should control the flow of interventions to allow times of consolidated nocturnal sleep.[36]

evolve To test your mastery of this chapter, try the Open-Book Quiz at http://evolve.elsevier.com/Urden/priorities/

REFERENCES

1. Carskadon MA, Dement WC: Normal human sleep: an overview. In Kryger MH, Roth T, Dement WC, editors: *Principles and practice of sleep medicine,* ed 3, Philadelphia, 2000, Saunders.
2. Davidhizar RE, Poole VL, Giger JN: What nurses need to know about sleep, *J Nurs Sci* 1:61, 1995.
3. Douglas NJ: Respiratory physiology: control of ventilation. In Kryger MH, Roth T, Dement WC, editors: *Principles and practice of sleep medicine,* ed 3, Philadelphia, 2000, Saunders.
4. Krachman SL, D'Alonzo GE, Criner GJ: Sleep in the intensive care unit, *Chest* 107(6):1713, 1995.
5. Ancoli-Israel S et al: Identification and treatment of sleep problems in the elderly, *Sleep Med Rev* 1:3, 1997.
6. Ancoli-Israel S: Sleep problems in older adults: putting myths to bed, *Geriatrics* 52(1):20, 1997.
7. Buysse DJ et al: Napping and 24-hour sleep/wake patterns in healthy elderly and young adults, *J Am Geriatr Soc* 40(8):779, 1992.
8. Vitiello MV: Normal versus pathologic sleep changes in aging humans. In Kuna ST, editor: *Sleep and respiration in aging,* New York, 1991, Elsevier Science.
9. Bliwise DL: Normal aging. In Kryger MH, Roth T, Dement WC, editors: *Principles and practice of sleep medicine,* ed 3, Philadelphia, 2000, Saunders.
10. Bliwise DL, King AC, Harris RB: Habitual sleep durations and health in a 50-65 year old population, *J Clin Epidemiol* 47(1):35, 1994.
11. Sloan E, Flint A: Circadian rhythms and psychiatric disorders in the elderly, *J Geriatr Psychiatry Neurol* 9(4):164, 1996.
12. Zarit S, Zarit J: *Mental disorders in older adults,* New York, 1998, Guilford Press.
13. National Sleep Foundation: 2005 *Sleep in America* poll, http://sleepfoundation.org/atf/cf/%7BF6BF2668-A1B4-4FE8-8D1A-A5D39340D9cB%7D/2005_summary_of_findings.pdf. 2005.
14. Gottlieb DJ et al: Association of sleep time with diabetes mellitus and impaired glucose intolerance, *Arch Intern Med* 165:863, 2005.
15. Patel SR et al: Association between reduced sleep and weight gain in women, *Am J Epidemiol* 164:947, 2006.
16. Kato M et al: Effects of sleep deprivation on neural circulatory control, *Hypertension* 35:1173, 2000.
17. Meier-Ewert HK et al: Effect of sleep loss on C-reactive protein, an inflammatory marker of cardiovascular risk, *J Am Coll Cardiol* 42:678, 2004.
18. Redeker NS, Stein S: Characteristics of sleep in patients with stable heart failure versus a comparison group, *Heart Lung* 35:252, 2006.
19. Swigris JJ et al: Patients' perspectives in how idiopathic pulmonary fibrosis affects the quality of their lives, *Health Qual Life Outcomes* 3:61, 2005.
20. Krachman S et al. Effects of lung volume reduction surgery on sleep quality and nocturnal gas exchange in patients with severe emphysema, *Chest* 128(5):3221, 2005.
21. Henderson WB: Hypnotics: basic mechanisms and pharmacology. In Kryger M, Roth T, Dement WC, editors: *Principles and practice of sleep medicine,* ed 3, Philadelphia, 2000, Saunders.
22. Schweitzer PK: Drugs that disturb sleep and wakefulness. In Kryger M, Roth T, Dement WC, editors: *Principles and practice of sleep medicine,* ed 3, Philadelphia, 2000, Saunders.
23. Obermeyer WH, Benca RM: Effects of drugs on sleep, *Neurol Clin* 14:827, 1996.

24. Nolen TM: Sedative effects of antihistamines: safety, performance, learning, and quality of life, *Clin Ther* 19:39, 1997.
25. Kryger MH: Management of obstructive sleep apnea-hypopnea syndrome: overview. In Kryger MH, Roth T, Dement WC, editors: *Principles and practice of sleep medicine,* ed 3, Philadelphia, 2000, Saunders.
26. Peppard P et al: Prospective study of the association between sleep-disordered breathing and hypertension, *N Engl J Med* 342:1378, 2000.
27. Nieto F et al: Sleep disordered breathing and neuropsychological deficits, *Am J Respir Crit Care Med* 156:1813, 1997.
28. Moore T et al: Sleep-disordered breathing in men with coronary artery disease, *Chest* 109:659, 1996.
29. Weiss JW, Launois SH, Anand A: Cardiorespiratory changes in sleep-disordered breathing. In Kryger MH, Roth T, Dement WC, editors: *Principles and practice of sleep medicine,* ed 3, Philadelphia, 2000, Saunders.
30. Hudgel DW: Mechanisms of obstructive sleep apnea, *Chest* 101(2):541, 1992.
31. Krug P: Snoring and obstructive sleep apnea, *AORN J* 69:792, 1999.
32. White DP: Central sleep apnea. In Kryger MH, Roth T, Dement WC, editors: *Principles and practice of sleep medicine,* ed 3, Philadelphia, 2000, Saunders.
33. Bradley T, Phillipson E: Central sleep apnea, *Clin Chest Med* 13(3):493, 1992.
34. Richards KC, Gibson R, Overton-McCoy AL: Effects of massage in acute and critical care, *AACN Clin Issues* 11(1):77, 2000.
35. Williamson JW: The effects of ocean sounds on sleep after coronary artery bypass graft surgery, *Am J Crit Care* 1(1):91, 1992.
36. Olsen DM et al: Quiet time: a nursing intervention to promote sleep in neurocritical care units, *Am J Crit Care* 10(2):74, 2001.

CHAPTER 6

Nutritional Alterations

COLLEEN O'LEARY-KELLEY

OBJECTIVES

- Describe the adverse effects of nutritional impairments on critically ill patients.
- Assess the nutritional status of critically ill patients with cardiovascular, pulmonary, neurologic, renal, gastrointestinal, and endocrine alterations.
- Recognize nutritional alterations associated with cardiovascular, pulmonary, neurologic, renal, gastrointestinal, and endocrine alterations.
- Collaborate with a multidisciplinary team in designing a nutrition program for critically ill patients.
- Identify complications of nutrition support and nursing interventions for prevention and management of these complications.

METABOLIC RESPONSE TO STARVATION AND STRESS

Critically ill patients are at risk for a combination of starvation and the physiologic stress resulting from injury, trauma, major surgery, and sepsis. Starvation occurs because the person must have nothing by mouth (NPO) for surgical procedures, may be unable to eat because of disease-related factors, and may be hemodynamically too unstable to be fed. The physiologic stress causes an increased metabolic rate (hypermetabolism) that results in a rise in oxygen consumption and energy expenditure.

The hypermetabolic process results from hormonal changes caused by the stressful event. The sympathetic nervous system is stimulated, causing the adrenal medulla to release catecholamines (epinephrine and norepinephrine). Other hormones released in response to stress include glucagon, adrenocorticotropic hormone (ACTH), and antidiuretic hormone (ADH), as well as glucocorticoids and mineralocorticoids (e.g., cortisol, aldosterone). All these hormonal changes cause nutrient substrates, primarily amino acids, to move from peripheral tissues (e.g., skeletal muscle) to the liver for gluconeogenesis.

Unfortunately, this mobilization of substrates occurs at the expense of body tissue and function at a time when the needs for protein synthesis (e.g., for wound healing and acute-phase proteins) also are high. Hyperglycemia results from the effects of increased catecholamines, glucocorticoids, and glucagon. Loss of protein results in a negative nitrogen balance and weight loss.

UNDERNUTRITION: IMPLICATIONS FOR THE SICK OR STRESSED PATIENT

As many as 12% to 55% of hospitalized patients are at risk for malnutrition.[1-5] Although illness or injury is the major factor contributing to development of malnutrition, other possible contributing factors are lack of communication among the nurses, physicians, and dietitians responsible for the care of these patients; frequent diagnostic testing and procedures, which lead to interruption in feeding medications and other therapies that cause anorexia, nausea, or vomiting and thus interfere with food intake; insufficient monitoring of nutrient intake; and inadequate use of supplements, tube feedings, or total parenteral nutrition (TPN) to maintain the nutritional status of these patients.

Nutritional status tends to deteriorate during hospitalization unless appropriate nutrition support is started early and continually reassessed. Malnutrition in hospitalized patients is associated with a wide variety of adverse outcomes. Wound dehiscence, pressure ulcers, sepsis, infections, respiratory failure requiring ventilation, longer hospital stays, and death are more common among malnourished patients.[6-8] Decline in nutritional status during hospitalization is associated with higher incidences of complications, mortality, and increased length of stay and higher hospital costs.

ASSESSING NUTRITIONAL STATUS

A nutrition screening should be conducted on every patient. A brief questionnaire to be completed by the patient or significant other, the nursing admission form, or the physician's admission note usually provides enough information to determine whether the patient is at nutritional risk (Box 6-1). Any patient judged to be nutritionally at risk needs a more thorough nutrition assessment.

Box 6-1

Patients at Risk for Malnutrition

- Involuntary loss or gain of a significant amount of weight (>10% of usual body weight in 6 months, >5% in 1 month), even if the weight achieved by loss or gain is appropriate for height
- Weight 20% more or less than ideal body weight, or body mass index <18.5 or >25
- Chronic disease
- Chronic use of a modified diet
- Increased metabolic requirements
- Illness or surgery that may interfere with nutritional intake
- Inadequate nutrient intake for >7 days
- Regular use of three or more medications
- Poverty

The nutrition assessment can be performed by or under the supervision of a registered dietitian or by a nutrition care specialist (e.g., a nurse with specialized expertise in nutrition). See Figure 6-1 to assess the route of administration of specialized nutrition support.

Biochemical Data

A wide range of laboratory tests can provide information about nutritional status, including blood and urine tests often used in the clinical setting (Table 6-1). No diagnostic tests for evaluation of nutrition are "perfect," and care must be taken in interpreting the results of the tests.

Clinical and Physical Manifestations

A thorough physical examination is an essential part of nutrition assessment. In assessing the patient for altered nutritional state, the nurse especially checks for signs of muscle wasting, loss of subcutaneous fat, skin or hair changes, and impaired wound healing (Box 6-2).

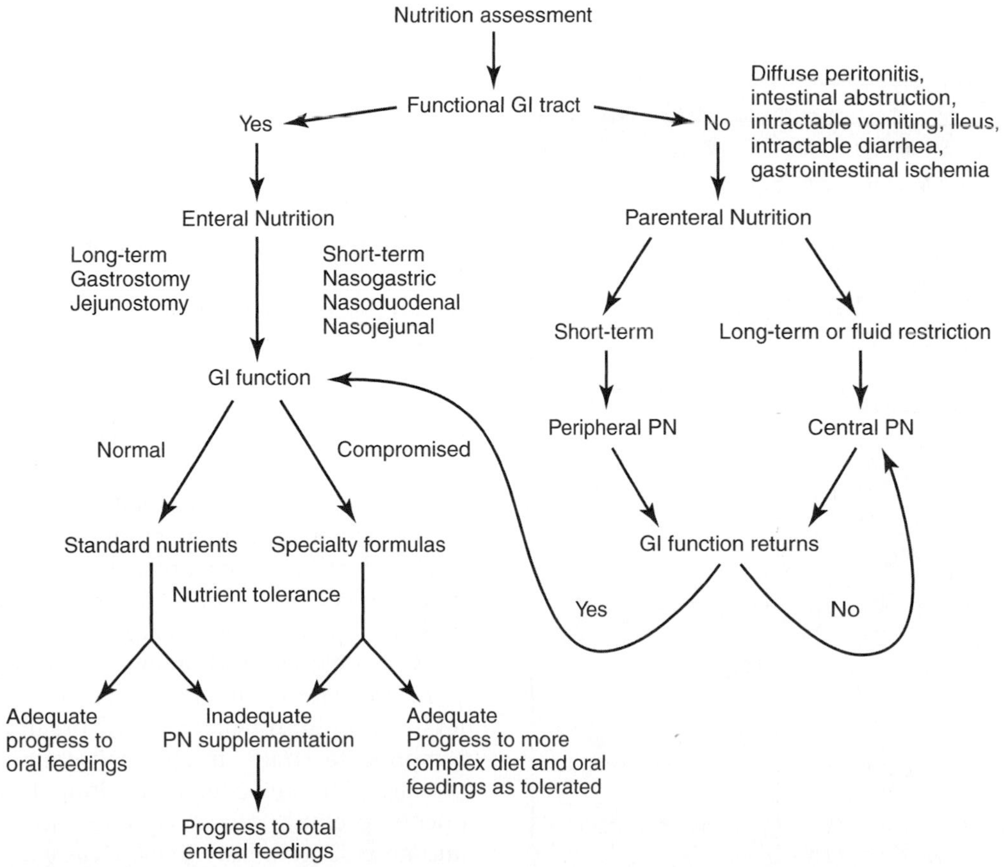

FIGURE 6-1. Route of administration of specialized nutrition support. (From ASPEN, Board of Directors, and the Clinical Guidelines Task Force: *JPEN J Parenter Enteral Nutr* 26[suppl 1]:8SA, 2002.)

Table 6-1

Common Blood and Urine Tests Used in Nutrition Assessment

TEST	COMMENTS/LIMITATIONS
Serum Proteins	
Albumin or prealbumin	Levels decrease with protein deficiency but also in liver failure; albumin levels are slow to change in response to malnutrition and repletion; prealbumin levels fall in response to trauma and infection
Hematologic Values	
Anemia	
Normocytic (normal MCV, MCHC)	Common with protein deficiency
Microcytic (decreased MCV, MCH, MCHC)	Indicative of iron deficiency (can be from blood loss)
Macrocytic (increased MCV)	Common in folate and vitamin B_{12} deficiency
Lymphocytopenia	Common in protein deficiency

MCV, Mean corpuscular volume; *MCHC,* mean corpuscular hemoglobin concentration; *MCH,* mean corpuscular hemoglobin.

Box 6-2

Clinical Manifestations of Nutritional Alterations

Manifestations That May Indicate Protein-Calorie Malnutrition
- Hair loss; dull, dry, brittle hair; loss of hair pigment
- Loss of subcutaneous tissue; muscle wasting
- Poor wound healing; decubitus ulcer
- Hepatomegaly
- Edema

Manifestations Often Present in Vitamin Deficiencies
- Conjunctival and corneal dryness (vitamin A)
- Dry, scaly skin; follicular hyperkeratosis, in which the skin appears to have gooseflesh continually (vitamin A)
- Gingivitis; poor wound healing (vitamin C)
- Petechiae; ecchymoses (vitamin C or K)
- Inflamed tongue, cracking at the corners of the mouth (riboflavin [vitamin B_2], niacin, folic acid, vitamin B_{12}, or other B vitamins)
- Edema; heart failure (thiamine [vitamin B_1])
- Confusion; confabulation (thiamine [vitamin B_1])

Manifestations Often Present in Mineral Deficiencies
- Blue sclerae; pale mucous membranes; spoon-shaped nails (iron)
- Hypogeusia, or poor sense of taste; dysgeusia, or bad taste; eczema; poor wound healing (zinc)

Manifestations Often Observed With Excessive Vitamin Intake
- Hair loss; dry skin; hepatomegaly (vitamin A)

Box 6-3

Nutrition History Information

Inadequate Intake of Nutrients
Alcohol abuse
Anorexia, severe or prolonged nausea or vomiting
Confusion, coma
Poor dentition
Poverty

Inadequate Digestion or Absorption of Nutrients
Previous gastrointestinal surgeries, especially gastrectomy, jejunoileal bypass, and ileal resection
Certain medications, especially antacids and histamine H_2-receptor antagonists (reduce upper small bowel acidity), cholestyramine (binds fat-soluble nutrients), and anticonvulsants

Increased Nutrient Losses
Blood loss
Severe diarrhea
Fistulae, draining abscesses, wounds, decubitus ulcers
Peritoneal dialysis or hemodialysis
Corticosteroid therapy (increased tissue catabolism)

Increased Nutrient Requirements
Fever
Surgery, trauma, burns, infection
Cancer (some types)
Physiologic demands (pregnancy, lactation, growth)

Diet and Health History

Information about dietary intake and significant variations in weight is a vital part of the history (Box 6-3). Dietary intake can be evaluated in several ways, including a diet record, a 24-hour recall, and a diet history.

Evaluating Assessment Findings

A patient rarely exhibits a lack of only one nutrient. Nutritional deficiencies usually are combined, with the patient lacking adequate amounts of protein, calories, and possibly vitamins and minerals. A common form of combined nutritional deficit among hospitalized patients is *protein-calorie malnutrition* (PCM). Two types of PCM are kwashiorkor and marasmus.

Kwashiorkor results in low levels of the serum proteins albumin, transferrin, and prealbumin; low total lymphocyte count; impaired immunity; loss of hair or hair pigment; edema resulting from low plasma oncotic pressure caused by a loss of plasma proteins; and an enlarged, fatty liver. *Marasmus* is recognizable by weight loss, loss of subcutaneous fat, and muscle wasting. In the marasmic person, creatinine excretion in the urine is low, an indication of loss of muscle mass. Because PCM weakens muscles, increases vulnerability

Table 6-2

Estimating Energy Needs

CATEGORY	DESCRIPTION	cal/kg	cal/lb
Obese	More than 40% over ideal body weight, or BMI >30	21	9.5
Sedentary	Relatively inactive individual without regular aerobic exercise; hospitalized patient without severe injury or sepsis	25-30	11-13.5
Moderate activity or injury	Individual obtaining regular aerobic exercise plus routine activities; patient with trauma or sepsis	30-35	13.5-16
Very active or severe injury	Manual laborer or athlete in very active training; patient with major burns or trauma	40	18

Box 6-4

Common Findings in Patients With Cardiovascular Disease

- Overweight/obesity, underweight (cardiac cachexia)
- Abdominal fat: increased risk of cardiovascular disease with waist measurement >102 cm (>40 inches) for men and >88 cm (>35 inches) for women
- Elevated total serum cholesterol, LDL cholesterol, and triglycerides
- Wasting of muscle and subcutaneous fat (cardiac cachexia)
- Sedentary lifestyle
- Excessive intake of saturated fat, cholesterol, salt, and alcohol
- Angina, respiratory difficulty, fatigue during eating
- Medications that impair appetite (e.g., digitalis preparations, quinidine)

LDL, Low-density lipoprotein.

to infection, and can prolong hospital stays, the health care team should diagnose this serious disorder as quickly as possible so that appropriate nutritional intervention can be implemented.

Calorie and protein needs of patients are often estimated using formulas that provide allowances for increased nutrient usage associated with injury and healing. Although indirect calorimetry is considered the most accurate method to determine energy expenditure, estimates using formulas have demonstrated reasonable accuracy.[9,10] Commonly used formulas can be found in Appendix B. Some "rules of thumb" are also available to provide a rough estimate of caloric needs so that nurses and other caregivers can quickly determine if patients are being seriously overfed or underfed (Table 6-2).

The goal of nutrition assessment is to obtain the most accurate estimate of nutritional requirements. Both underfeeding and overfeeding must be avoided during critical illness. Overfeeding results in excessive production of carbon dioxide, which can be a burden in the person with pulmonary compromise. In addition, overfeeding increases fat stores, which can contribute to insulin resistance and hyperglycemia. Hyperglycemia increases the risk of postoperative infections in both diabetic and nondiabetic individuals.[11-13] Therefore hyperglycemia is a complication to be avoided if at all possible.

NUTRITION AND CARDIOVASCULAR ALTERATIONS

Diet and cardiovascular disease may interact in a variety of ways. On the one hand, excessive nutrient intake, manifested by overweight or obesity and a diet rich in cholesterol and saturated fat, is a risk factor for development of arteriosclerotic heart disease. On the other hand, the consequences of chronic myocardial insufficiency may include malnutrition.

Nutrition Assessment

A nutrition assessment provides the nurse and other health care team members with the information necessary to plan the cardiovascular patient's nutrition care and education (Box 6-4). The major nutritional concerns relate to appropriateness of body weight and the levels of serum lipids and blood pressure.

Nutrition Intervention

Myocardial Infarction

The following guidelines will assist the nurse in providing appropriate nutritional care for the patient in the immediate post–myocardial infarction period:

- Limit meal size for the patient with severe myocardial compromise or postprandial angina.
- Monitor the effect of caffeine on the patient, if caffeine is included in the diet.
- Use caution in serving foods at temperature extremes.

Hypertension

A substantial number of individuals with hypertension are "salt sensitive," with their disorder improving when sodium intake is limited. Therefore restriction of sodium intake, usually to 2.5 g/day or less, is often advised to help control hypertension.[14] One teaspoon of salt provides about 2.3 g of sodium. Most salt substitutes contain potassium chloride and may be used with the physician's approval by the patient who has no renal impairment. A diet rich in fruits, vegetables, and low-fat dairy products (the DASH, or Dietary Approaches to Stopping Hypertension, diet) combined with a sodium restriction is often more effective than sodium restriction alone.[15]

Heart Failure

Nutrition intervention for the patient with heart failure is designed to reduce fluid retained within the body and thus reduce the preload. Because fluid accompanies sodium, limitation of sodium is necessary to reduce fluid retention. Specific interventions include limiting salt intake, usually to 5 g/day or less, and limiting fluid intake as appropriate. If fluid is restricted, the daily fluid allowance is usually 1.5 to 2 L/day, to include both fluids in the diet and those given with medications and for other purposes.

Cardiac Cachexia

The severely malnourished cardiac patient often develops heart failure. Therefore sodium and fluid restriction, as previously described, is appropriate. It is important to concentrate nutrients into as small a volume as possible and to serve small amounts frequently, rather than three large meals daily. The individual should be encouraged to consume calorie-dense foods and supplements. Good choices include meats and poultry, cheeses, yogurt, frozen yogurt, and ice cream.

Because the patient is likely to tire quickly and to suffer from anorexia, enteral tube feeding may be necessary. Typical tube feeding formulas provide 1 calorie per milliliter (cal/ml), but more-concentrated products are available to provide adequate nutrients in a smaller volume. The nurse must monitor the fluid status of these patients carefully when they are receiving nutrition support. Assessing breath sounds and observing for presence and severity of peripheral edema and changes in body weight are performed daily or more frequently. A consistent weight gain of more than 0.11 to 0.22 kg (0.25 to 0.5 lb) per day usually indicates fluid retention rather than gain of fat and muscle mass.

NUTRITION AND PULMONARY ALTERATIONS

Malnutrition has extremely adverse effects on respiratory function, decreasing surfactant production, diaphragmatic mass, vital capacity, and immunocompetence. Patients with acute respiratory disorders find it difficult to consume adequate oral nutrients and can rapidly become malnourished. Individuals who have an acute illness superimposed on chronic respiratory problems are also at high risk. Almost three fourths of patients with chronic obstructive pulmonary disease (COPD) have had weight loss. Patients with undernutrition and end-stage COPD, however, often cannot tolerate the increase in metabolic demand that occurs during refeeding. In addition, they are at significant risk for development of cor pulmonale and may fail to tolerate the fluid required for delivery of enteral or parenteral nutrition support. Prevention of severe nutritional deficits, rather than correction of deficits once they have occurred, is important in nutritional management of these patients.

Nutrition Assessment

Common findings in nutrition assessment related to pulmonary alterations are summarized in Box 6-5. The patient with respiratory compromise is especially vulnerable to the effects of fluid volume excess and must be assessed continually for this complication, particularly during enteral and parenteral feeding.

Nutrition Intervention

Prevent or Correct Undernutrition/Underweight

The nurse and dietitian work together to encourage oral intake in the undernourished or potentially undernourished patient who is capable of eating. Small, frequent feedings are especially important because a very full stomach can interfere with diaphragmatic movement. Mouth care should be provided before meals and snacks to clear the palate of the taste of sputum and medications. Administering bronchodilators with food can help to reduce the gastric irritation caused by these medications.

Because of anorexia, dyspnea, debilitation, or need for ventilatory support, however, many patients will require enteral tube feeding or TPN. It is especially important for the nurse to be alert to the risk of pulmonary aspiration in the patient with an artificial airway. To reduce the risk of pulmonary aspiration during enteral tube feeding, the nurse should (1) keep the patient's head elevated at least 45 degrees during feedings, unless contraindicated; (2) discontinue feedings 30 to 60 minutes before any procedures that require lowering the head; (3) keep the cuff of the artificial airway inflated during feeding, if possible; (4) monitor the patient for increasing abdominal distention; and (5) check tube placement before each feeding

Box 6-5

Common Findings in Patients With Pulmonary Disease

- Underweight
- Elevated carbon dioxide partial pressure related to overfeeding
- Edema, dyspnea, signs of pulmonary edema related to fluid volume excess
- Poor food intake related to dyspnea
- Unpleasant taste in mouth from sputum production or bronchodilator therapy
- Endotracheal intubation preventing oral intake

(if intermittent) or at least every 4 to 8 hours if feedings are continuous.

Avoid Overfeeding

Overfeeding increases the production of carbon dioxide (CO_2). This is unlikely to be significant in the patient who is eating foods. Instead, it is an iatrogenic complication of TPN or enteral feeding. Arterial CO_2 tension ($Pa{CO_2}$) may rise sufficiently to make it difficult to wean a patient from the ventilator. A balanced regimen with both lipids and carbohydrates providing the nonprotein calories is optimal for the patient with respiratory compromise, and the patient needs to be reassessed continually to ensure that caloric intake is not excessive.

Prevent Fluid Volume Excess

Pulmonary edema and failure of the right side of the heart, which may be precipitated by fluid volume excess, further worsen the status of the patient with respiratory compromise. Maintaining careful intake and output records allows for accurate assessment of fluid balance. Usually the patient requires no more than 35 to 40 ml/kg/day of fluid. For the patient receiving nutrition support, fluid intake can be reduced by (1) using 20% or 30% lipid emulsions as a source of calories, (2) using tube feeding formulas providing at least 2 cal/ml (the dietitian can recommend appropriate formulas), and (3) choosing oral supplements that are low in fluid.

NUTRITION AND NEUROLOGIC ALTERATIONS

Because neurologic disorders such as stroke and closed head injury tend to be long-term problems, these patients require good nutritional care to prevent nutritional deficits and promote well-being.

NUTRITION ASSESSMENT

Nutrition-related assessment findings vary widely in the patient with neurologic alterations, depending on the type of disorder present (Box 6-6).

Box 6-6

Common Findings in Patients With Neurologic Alterations

- Hyperglycemia (with corticosteroid use)
- Wasting of muscle and subcutaneous fat related to disuse or to poor food intake
- Poor food intake related to altered state of consciousness
- Dysphagia or other chewing/swallowing difficulties
- Ileus resulting from spinal cord injury or use of pentobarbital
- Hypermetabolism resulting from head injury
- Decubitus ulcers

NUTRITION INTERVENTION: PREVENT OR CORRECT NUTRITION DEFICITS

Oral Feedings

Patients with dysphagia or weakness of the swallowing musculature often experience the greatest difficulty in swallowing dry foods and thin liquids (e.g., water) that are difficult to control.

Tube Feedings and Total Parenteral Nutrition

Patients who are unconscious or unable to eat because of severe dysphagia, weakness, ileus, or other reasons require tube feedings or TPN. Prompt initiation of nutrition support must be a priority in the patient with neurologic impairment. Needs for protein and calories are increased by infection and fever, as in the patient with encephalitis or meningitis. Needs for protein, calories, zinc, and vitamin C are increased during wound healing, as in trauma patients and those with decubitus ulcers.

Patients with neurologic deficits have an increased risk of certain complications (particularly pulmonary aspiration) during tube feeding and therefore require especially careful nursing management. Patients of most concern are (1) those with an impaired gag reflex, such as some patients with cerebrovascular accident (stroke); (2) those with delayed gastric emptying, such as patients in the early period after spinal cord injury and patients with head injury treated with barbiturate coma; and (3) those likely to experience seizures. To help prevent pulmonary aspiration, the patient's head is kept elevated, if not contraindicated; when elevation of the head is not possible, administering feedings with the patient in the prone or lateral position will allow free drainage of emesis from the mouth and decrease the risk of aspiration.

Administering phenytoin with enteral formulas decreases the absorption of the drug and the peak serum level achieved and thus may increase the risk of seizures. The phenytoin dosage must be adjusted appropriately. Phenytoin levels should be monitored carefully in patients receiving enteral feedings.[16]

Hyperglycemia is a common complication in patients receiving corticosteroids. Regular monitoring of blood glucose is an important part of their care. They may require insulin to control the hyperglycemia.

Prompt use of nutrition support is especially important for patients with head injuries because head injury causes marked catabolism, even in patients who receive barbiturates, which should decrease metabolic demands. Head-injured patients rapidly exhaust glycogen stores and begin to use body proteins to meet energy needs, a process that can quickly lead to PCM. The catabolic response is partly a result of corticosteroid therapy in head-injured patients. However, the hypermetabolism and hypercatabolism are also caused by dramatic hormonal responses to this type of injury.[17] Levels of cortisol, epinephrine, and norepinephrine increase as much as seven times normal. These hormones increase the metabolic rate and caloric demands, causing mobilization of body fat and proteins to meet the increased energy needs. Furthermore, head-injured patients undergo an inflammatory response and may be febrile, creating increased needs for protein and calories. Improvement in outcome and reduction in complications have been observed in head-injured patients who receive adequate nutrition support early in the hospital course.[18]

NUTRITION AND RENAL ALTERATIONS

Providing adequate nutrition care for the patient with renal disease can be extremely challenging. Although renal disturbances and their treatments can greatly increase needs for nutrients, necessary restrictions in intake of fluid, protein, phosphorus, and potassium make delivery of adequate calories, vitamins, and minerals difficult. Thorough nutrition assessment provides the basis for successful nutrition management in patients with renal disease.

Nutrition Assessment

Some common assessment findings in individuals with renal disease are listed in Box 6-7.

Nutrition Intervention

The goal of nutrition interventions is to administer adequate nutrients, including calories, protein, vitamins, and minerals, while avoiding excesses of protein, fluid, electrolytes, and other nutrients with potential toxicity.

Protein

The kidney is responsible for excreting nitrogen from amino acids or proteins in the form of *urea*. Thus, when urinary excretion of urea is impaired in renal failure, blood levels of urea rise. Excessive protein intake may worsen uremia. However, the patient with renal failure often has (1) other physiologic stresses that actually increase protein/amino acid needs; (2) losses from dialysis, wounds, and fistulae; (3) use of corticosteroid drugs that exert a catabolic effect; (4) increased endogenous secretion of catecholamines, corticosteroids, and glucagon, all of which can cause or aggravate catabolism; (5) metabolic acidosis, which stimulates protein breakdown; and (6) catabolic conditions (e.g., trauma, surgery, sepsis). Therefore patients with acute renal failure need adequate amounts of protein to avoid catabolism of body tissues. Approximately 1.5 to 1.7 g/kg/day has successfully maintained adequate protein nutrition in these patients.[19,20]

During hemodialysis and arteriovenous hemofiltration, amino acids are freely filtered and lost, but proteins such as albumin and immunoglobulin are not lost. Both proteins and amino acids are removed during peritoneal dialysis, creating a greater nutritional requirement for protein. Protein needs are estimated at approximately 1.0 to 1.2 g/kg/day for stable patients receiving hemodialysis or hemofiltration and 1.2 to 1.3 g/kg/day for those receiving peritoneal dialysis.[21,22] Patients in the process of wound healing and those with ongoing protein losses have greater needs.

Box 6-7

Common Findings in the Patient With Renal Failure

- Underweight (may be masked by edema)
- Electrolyte imbalances
- Hypoalbuminemia related to protein restriction and amino acid losses in dialysis
- Anemia related to inadequate erythropoietin production and blood loss with hemodialysis
- Hypertriglyceridemia related to use of glucose as osmotic agent in dialysis and use of carbohydrates to supply needed calories
- Wasting of muscle and subcutaneous tissue (may be masked by edema)
- Poor dietary intake related to protein and electrolyte restrictions

Fluids

The patient with renal insufficiency usually does not require a fluid restriction until urine output begins to diminish. Patients receiving hemodialysis are limited to a fluid intake resulting in a gain of no more than 0.45 kg (1 lb) per day on the days between dialysis. This generally means a daily intake of 500 to 750 ml plus the volume lost in urine. With the use of continuous peritoneal dialysis, hemofiltration, or hemodialysis, the fluid intake can be liberalized.[23] This more liberal fluid allowance permits more adequate nutrient delivery, whether by oral, tube, or parenteral feedings. Enteral formulas containing 1.5 to 2.0 cal/ml or more provide a concentrated source of calories for tube-fed patients who require fluid restriction. Intravenous lipids, particularly 20% emulsions, can be used to supply concentrated calories for the TPN patient. Intradialytic TPN can be used to supply an additional source of nutrients at a time when the fluid can be rapidly removed in dialysis.[24,25]

Energy (Calories)

Energy needs are not increased by renal failure, but adequate calories must be provided to avoid catabolism.[19] It is essential that the renal patient receive an adequate number of calories to prevent catabolism of body tissues to meet energy needs. Catabolism not only reduces the mass of muscle and other functional body tissues but also releases nitrogen that must be excreted by the kidney. Adults with renal insufficiency need about 30 to 35 cal/kg/day, compared with the 25 to 30 cal/kg/day needed by healthy adults, to prevent catabolism and ensure that all protein consumed is used for anabolism rather than to meet energy needs.[19] After renal transplantation, when the patient initially receives large doses of corticosteroids, it is especially important to ensure that caloric intake is adequate (usually 25 to 35 cal/kg/day) to prevent undue catabolism.

Hypertriglyceridemia is found in a substantial number of patients with renal disorders. This condition is worsened by excessive intake of simple refined sugars, such as sucrose (table sugar) or glucose. Glucose in the peritoneal dialysate may be a significant calorie source and a contributing factor in hypertriglyceridemia. Approximately 70% of the glucose instilled during peritoneal dialysis to serve as an osmotic agent may be absorbed, and this must be considered part of the patient's carbohydrate intake. The glucose monohydrate used in intravenous and dialysate solutions supplies 3.4 cal/g. Thus, if a patient receives 4.25% glucose (4.25 g glucose per 100 ml solution) in the dialysate, the patient receives the following:

$$42.5 \text{ g/L} \times 70\% \times 3.4 \text{ cal/g} = 101 \text{ cal/L of dialysate}$$

To help control hypertriglyceridemia, only about 30% to 35% of the patient's calories should come from carbohydrates, including glucose from the dialysate, with the major portion of dietary carbohydrate coming from complex carbohydrates (starches and fibers).

NUTRITION AND GASTROINTESTINAL ALTERATIONS

Because the gastrointestinal (GI) tract is so inherently related to nutrition, it is not surprising that impairment of the GI tract and its accessory organs has a major impact on nutrition. Two of the most serious GI-related illnesses seen among critical care patients are hepatic failure and pancreatitis.

NUTRITION ASSESSMENT

Common assessment findings in patients with GI disease are listed in Box 6-8.

NUTRITION INTERVENTION

Hepatic Failure

Because the diseased liver has impaired ability to deactivate hormones, levels of circulating glucagon, epinephrine, and cortisol are elevated. These hormones promote catabolism of body tissues and cause glycogen stores to be exhausted. Release of lipids from their storage depots is accelerated, but the liver has decreased ability to metabolize them for energy. Furthermore, inadequate production of bile salts by the liver results in malabsorption of fat from the diet. Therefore body proteins are used for energy sources, producing tissue wasting.

The *branched-chain amino acids* (BCAAs)—leucine, isoleucine, and valine—are especially well used for energy, and their levels in the blood decline. Conversely, levels of the *aromatic amino acids* (AAAs)—phenylalanine, tyrosine, and tryptophan—rise as a result of tissue catabolism and impaired ability of the liver to clear them from the blood. The AAAs are precursors for neurotransmitters in the central nervous system (serotonin and dopamine). Rising levels of AAAs may alter nerve activity within the brain, leading to symptoms of encephalopathy. In addition, the damaged liver cannot clear ammonia from the circulation adequately, and ammonia accumulates in the brain. The ammonia may contribute to the encephalopathic symptoms and also to brain edema.[26,27]

Monitoring Fluid and Electrolyte Status. Ascites and edema occur because of a combination of factors. There is decreased colloid osmotic pressure in the plasma, because of the reduction of production of albumin and other plasma proteins by the diseased liver, increased portal pressure caused by obstruction, and renal sodium retention from secondary hyperaldosteronism. To control the fluid retention, restriction of sodium (usually 2000 mg) and fluid (1500 ml or less daily) is generally necessary, in conjunction with administration of diuretics. Patients are weighed daily to evaluate the success of treatment. Physical status and laboratory data must be closely monitored for deficiencies of potassium, phosphorus, and vitamins A, D, E, and K, and zinc.[28]

Provision of a Nutritious Diet and Evaluation of Response to Dietary Protein. PCM and nutritional deficiencies are common in hepatic failure. The causes of malnutrition are complex and usually related to

Box 6-8

Common Findings in Patients With Gastrointestinal Disease

- Underweight related to malabsorption (from inadequate production of bile salts and pancreatic enzymes), anorexia, or poor intake (from pain caused by eating)
- Hypoalbuminemia (may result primarily from liver damage, not malnutrition)
- Hypocalcemia related to steatorrhea
- Hypomagnesemia related to alcohol abuse
- Anemia related to blood loss from bleeding varices
- Wasting of muscle and subcutaneous fat
- Confusion, confabulation, nystagmus, and peripheral neuropathy related to thiamine deficiency caused by alcohol abuse (Wernicke-Korsakoff syndrome)
- Steatorrhea

decreased intake, malabsorption, maldigestion, and abnormal nutrient metabolism. Nutrition intervention is individualized and based on these metabolic changes. A diet with adequate protein helps to suppress catabolism and promote liver regeneration. Stable patients with cirrhosis usually tolerate 0.8 to 1 g protein/kg/day. Patients with severe stress or nutritional deficits have increased needs—as much as 1.2 to 2 g/kg/day.[29] Aggressive treatment with medications, including lactulose, neomycin, or metronidazole, is considered first-line therapy in the management of acute hepatic encephalopathy. In a minority of patients, pharmacotherapy may not be effective, and protein restriction to as little as 0.5 g/kg/day or less may be necessary for brief periods. Chronic protein restriction is not recommended as a long-term management strategy for patients with liver disease.[28,29]

Anorexia may interfere with oral intake, and the nurse may need to provide much encouragement to the patient to ensure intake of an adequate diet. Prospective calorie counts may need to be instituted to provide objective evidence of oral intake. Small, frequent feedings are usually better tolerated by the anorexic patient than are three large meals daily. Soft foods are preferred because the patient may have esophageal varices that might be irritated by high-fiber foods. If patients are unable to meet their caloric needs, they may require oral supplements or enteral feeding. Small-bore nasoenteric feeding tubes can be used safely without increasing risk of variceal bleeding.[29] TPN should be reserved only for patients who are absolutely unable to tolerate enteral feeding.[28] Diarrhea from concurrent administration of lactulose should not be confused with feeding intolerance.

A diet adequate in calories (at least 30 cal/kg daily) is provided to help prevent catabolism and to prevent the use of dietary protein for energy needs.[30] In cases of malabsorption, medium-chain triglycerides (MCTs) may be used to meet caloric needs. Pancreatic enzymes may also be considered for malabsorption problems.

BCAA-enriched products have been developed for enteral and parenteral nutrition of patients with hepatic disease. These products may be used in patients with acute hepatic encephalopathy who do not tolerate standard diets or enteral formulas, or who are unresponsive to lactulose. However, no substantial evidence exists showing BCAAs are superior to standard formulas in regard to nitrogen balance or as treatment for encephalopathy.[28,29] The patient who undergoes successful liver transplantation is usually able to tolerate a regular diet with few restrictions. Intake during the postoperative period must be adequate to support nutritional repletion and healing; 1 to 1.2 g protein/kg/day and approximately 30 cal/kg/day are usually sufficient. Immunosuppressant therapy (corticosteroids and cyclosporine or tacrolimus) contributes to glucose intolerance. Dietary measures to control glucose intolerance include (1) obtaining approximately 30% of dietary calories from fat; (2) emphasizing complex sources of carbohydrates; and (3) eating several small meals daily. Moderate exercise often helps to improve glucose tolerance.

Pancreatitis

The pancreas is an exocrine and endocrine gland required for normal digestion and metabolism of proteins, carbohydrates, and fats. Acute pancreatitis is an inflammatory process that occurs as a result of autodigestion of the pancreas by enzymes normally secreted by that organ. Food intake stimulates pancreatic secretion and thus increases the damage to the pancreas and the pain associated with the disorder. Patients usually present with abdominal pain and tenderness and elevations of pancreatic enzymes. A mild form of acute pancreatitis occurs in 80% of patients requiring hospitalization, and severe acute pancreatitis occurs in the other 20%.[31] Patients with the mild form of acute pancreatitis do not require nutrition support and generally resume oral feeding within 7 days. Chronic pancreatitis may develop and is characterized by fibrosis of pancreatic cells. This results in loss of exocrine and endocrine function because of the destruction of acinar and islet cells. The loss of exocrine function leads to malabsorption and steatorrhea. In chronic pancreatitis, the loss of endocrine function results in impaired glucose tolerance.[31]

Prevention of Further Damage to the Pancreas and Preventing Nutritional Deficits. Effective nutritional management is a key treatment for patients with acute pancreatitis or exacerbations of chronic pancreatitis. The concern that feeding may stimulate the production of digestive enzymes and perpetuate tissue damage has led to the widespread use of TPN and bowel rest. Recent data suggest that enteral nutrition infused into the distal jejunum bypasses the stimulatory effect of feeding on pancreatic secretion and is associated with fewer infectious and metabolic complications compared to TPN.[32,33]

The results of randomized studies comparing TPN with total enteral nutrition (TEN, or enteral tube feeding) indicate that TEN is preferable to TPN in patients with severe acute pancreatitis, reducing costs and the risk of sepsis and improving clinical outcome.[32-34] Patients unable to tolerate TEN should receive TPN, and some patients may require a combination of TEN and TPN to meet nutritional requirements.[35,36] Low-fat enteral formulas and those with fat provided by MCTs are more readily absorbed than formulas that are high in long-chain triglycerides (e.g., corn or sunflower oil).

When oral intake is possible, small frequent feedings of low-fat foods are least likely to cause discomfort.[33] Alcohol intake should be avoided because it worsens the tissue damage and the pain associated with pancreatitis. Guidelines for treatment of diabetes (see following sections) are appropriate for the care of the person with glucose intolerance or diabetes related to pancreatitis.

NUTRITION AND ENDOCRINE ALTERATIONS

Endocrine alterations have far-reaching effects on all body systems and thus affect nutritional status in a variety of ways. One of the most common endocrine problems, both in the general population and among critically ill patients, is diabetes mellitus.

NUTRITION ASSESSMENT

Common assessment findings in individuals with endocrine alterations are listed in Box 6-9. Because of the prevalence of patients with non–insulin-dependent (type 2) diabetes mellitus among the hospitalized population, the acute nutritional problems most often noted in patients with endocrine alterations are related to glycemic control.

NUTRITION INTERVENTION

Nutrition Support and Blood Glucose Control

Patients with insulin-dependent (type 1) diabetes mellitus or endocrine dysfunction caused by pancreatitis often have weight loss and malnutrition as a result of tissue catabolism because they cannot use dietary carbohydrates to meet energy needs. Although patients with type 2 diabetes are more likely to be overweight than underweight, they too may become malnourished as a result of chronic or acute infections, trauma, major surgery, or other illnesses. Nutrition support should not be neglected simply because a patient is obese, because PCM develops even in these patients. When a patient is not expected to be able to eat for at least 5 to 7 days or when inadequate intake persists for that period, initiation of tube feedings or TPN is indicated. No disease process benefits from starvation, and development or progression of nutritional deficits may contribute to complications such as decubitus ulcers, pulmonary or urinary tract infections, and sepsis, which prolong hospitalization, increase the costs of care, and may even result in death.

Box 6-9

Common Findings in Patients With Endocrine Disease

- Hyperglycemia related to poor diabetic control, infection, trauma/burns, or glucocorticoid use
- Elevated hemoglobin A_{1c} related to chronic poor diabetic control
- Hypoglycemia related to vomiting or poor food intake without adjustment of the dosage of insulin or oral hypoglycemic agents

Blood glucose control is especially important in the care of surgical patients. Hyperglycemia in the early postoperative period is associated with increased rates of nosocomial infection. To maintain tight control of blood glucose, glucose levels are monitored regularly, usually several times a day until the patient is stable. Regular insulin added to the solution is the most common method of managing hyperglycemia in the patient receiving TPN. Multiple injections of regular insulin may be used to maintain tight control of blood glucose in the enterally fed patient.

In patients receiving enteral tube feedings, the postpyloric route (via nasoduodenal, nasojejunal, or jejunostomy tube) may be the most effective, because gastroparesis may limit tolerance of intragastric tube feedings.[37] Postpyloric feedings are given continuously because dumping syndrome and poor absorption may occur if feedings are given rapidly into the small bowel. Continuous enteral infusions are associated with improved control of blood glucose. Fiber-enriched formulas may slow the absorption of the carbohydrate, producing a more delayed and sustained glycemic response. Most standard formulas contain balanced proportions of carbohydrate, protein, and fats appropriate for diabetic patients. Specialized diabetic formulas have not shown improved outcomes compared to standard formulas.[38]

Severe Vomiting or Diarrhea in the Patient With Type 1 Diabetes Mellitus. When insulin-dependent patients experience vomiting and diarrhea severe enough to interfere significantly with oral intake or result in excessive fluid and electrolyte losses, adequate carbohydrates and fluids must be supplied. Nausea and vomiting should be treated with antiemetic medication.[37] Delayed gastric emptying is common in diabetes and may improve with administration of prokinetic agents.[37] Small amounts of food or liquids taken every 15 to 20 minutes are generally the best tolerated by the patient with nausea and vomiting. Foods and beverages containing approximately 15 g of carbohydrate include $^1/_2$ cup regular gelatin, $^1/_2$ cup custard, $^3/_4$ cup regular ginger ale, $^1/_2$ cup regular soft drink, and $^1/_2$ cup orange or apple juice. Blood glucose levels should be monitored at least every 2 to 4 hours.

ADMINISTERING NUTRITION SUPPORT

ENTERAL NUTRITION

Whenever possible, the enteral route is the preferred method of feeding. Patients with abdominal trauma in particular have lower morbidity and mortality rates if fed enterally rather than parenterally.

There are a variety of commercial enteral feeding products, some of which are designed to meet the specialized needs of the critically ill. Products designed for the stressed patient with trauma or sepsis are usually rich in glutamine, arginine, and antioxidant nutrients (e.g., vitamins C, E, and A; selenium). The antioxidants help to reduce oxidative injury to the tissues (e.g., from reperfusion injury). Some products can be consumed orally, but it can be difficult for the critically ill patient to consume enough orally to meet the increased needs associated with stress. Refer to Table 6-3 for enteral formulas.

Oral Supplementation

Oral supplementation may be necessary for patients who can eat and have normal digestion and absorption but simply cannot consume enough regular foods to meet caloric and protein needs. Patients with mild to moderate anorexia, burns, or trauma may be included in this category.

Tube Feeding

Tube feedings are used for patients who have at least some digestive and absorptive capability but are unwilling or unable to consume enough by mouth. Patients with profound anorexia and those experiencing severe stress (e.g., major burns, trauma) that greatly increases their nutritional needs often benefit from tube feedings. Individuals who require elemental formulas because of impaired digestion or absorption or specialized formulas for altered metabolic conditions such as renal or hepatic failure usually require tube feeding because the unpleasant flavors of the free amino acids, peptides, or protein hydrolysates used in these formulas are very difficult to mask.

Location and Type of Feeding Tube

Nasal intubation is the simplest and most common route for gaining access to the GI tract; this method allows access to the stomach, duodenum, or jejunum. *Tube enterostomy*—a gastrostomy or jejunostomy—is used primarily for long-term feedings (6 to 12 weeks or more) and when obstruction makes the nasoenteral route inaccessible. Tube enterostomies may also be used for the patient who is at risk for tube dislodgment because of severe agitation or confusion. A conventional gastrostomy or jejunostomy is often performed at the time of other abdominal surgery. The *percutaneous endoscopic gastrostomy* (PEG) tube has become extremely popular because it can be inserted without the use of general anesthetics. Percutaneous endoscopic jejunostomy (PEJ) tubes are also used.

Transpyloric feedings via nasoduodenal, nasojejunal, or jejunostomy tubes are typically used when there is a risk of pulmonary aspiration, because theoretically the pyloric sphincter provides a barrier that lessens the risk of regurgitation and aspiration. If nasogastric tubes are used, choosing the smallest possible tube diameter reduces the risk of gastroesophageal reflux and pulmonary aspiration. Transpyloric feedings have an advantage over intragastric feedings for patients with delayed gastric emptying, such as those with head injury, gastroparesis associated with uremia or diabetes, or postoperative ileus. Small bowel motility returns more quickly than gastric motility after surgery, and thus it is often possible to deliver transpyloric feedings within a few hours of injury or surgery.[39] Promotility agents such as metoclopramide may improve feeding tolerance. See Figure 6-2 for location of tube feeding sites.[40]

Nursing Management

The nurse's role in delivery of tube feedings usually includes (1) insertion of the tube, if a temporary tube is used; (2) maintenance of the tube; (3) administration of the feedings; (4) prevention and detection of complications associated with this form of therapy; and (5) participation in assessment of the patient's response to tube feedings.

Tube Placement. Critical care nurses are usually familiar with tube insertion, and therefore this topic is not discussed here. However, it is well to remember that if transpyloric positioning is desirable, administration of metoclopramide or erythromycin before tube insertion increases the likelihood of tube passage through the pylorus.[41]

Correct tube placement must be confirmed before initiation of feedings and regularly throughout the course of enteral feedings. Radiographs are the most accurate way of assessing tube placement, but repeated radiographs are costly and can expose the patient to excessive radiation. An inexpensive and relatively accurate alternative method involves assessing the pH of fluid removed from the feeding tube; some tubes are equipped with pH monitoring systems.

If the pH is less than 4.0 in patients not receiving gastric acid inhibitors, or less than 5.5 in patients who are receiving acid inhibitors, the tube tip is likely to be in the stomach.[42] Intestinal secretions usually have a pH greater than 6.0, and respiratory tract fluids usually have a pH greater than 5.5. The esophagus may have an acid pH, which may cause confusion between esophageal and gastric placement. However, other clues can help in identifying a tube that has its distal tip in the esophagus: it may be especially difficult to aspirate fluid out of the tube; a large portion of the tube may extend out of the body (although a tube inserted to the proper length could be coiled in the esophagus); and belching often occurs immediately after air is injected into the tube.[42]

Assessing both the pH and the *bilirubin* concentration of fluid aspirated from the feeding tube is a promising new method for confirming tube placement.[43] The bilirubin concentration in tracheobron-

Table 6-3
Enteral Formulas

FORMULA TYPE	NUTRITIONAL USES	CLINICAL EXAMPLES	EXAMPLES OF COMMERCIAL PRODUCTS (MANUFACTURER)
Formulas Used When GI Tract Is Fully Functional			
Polymeric (standard): Contains whole proteins (10%-15% of calories), long-chain triglycerides (25%-40% of calories), and glucose polymers or oligosaccharides (50%-60% of calories); most provide 1 calorie/ml	Inability to ingest food Inability to consume enough to meet needs	Oral or esophageal cancer Coma, stroke Anorexia resulting from chronic illness Burns or trauma	Ensure (Ross) NuBasics (Nestlé) IsoSource (Novartis) Pediasure (Ross), for children ages 1-10 Boost (Mead Johnson)
High-nitrogen: Same as polymeric except protein provides >15% of calories	Same as polymeric, plus mild catabolism and protein deficits	Trauma or burns Sepsis	IsoSource HN (Novartis) Osmolite HN (Ross) Ultracal (Mead Johnson)
Concentrated: Same as polymeric except concentrated to 2 cal/ml	Same as polymeric, but fluid restriction needed	Heart failure Neurosurgery COPD Liver disease	Deliver 2.0 (Mead Johnson) TwoCal HN (Ross) Nutren 2.0 (Nestlé)
Formulas Used When GI Function Is Impaired			
Elemental or predigested: Contains hydrolyzed (partially digested) protein, peptides (short chains of amino acids), and/or amino acids, little fat (<10% of calories) or high MCT, and glucose polymers or oligosaccharides; most provide 1 cal/ml	Impaired digestion and/or absorption	Short bowel syndrome Radiation enteritis Inflammatory bowel disease	Criticare HN (Mead Johnson) Vital High Nitrogen (Ross) Reabilan HN (Nestlé)
Diets for Specific Disease States*			
Renal failure: Concentrated in calories; low sodium, potassium, magnesium, phosphorus, and vitamins A and D; low protein for renal insufficiency; higher protein formulas for dialyzed patients	Renal insufficiency Dialysis	Predialysis Hemodialysis or peritoneal dialysis	Suplena (Ross) Renalcal (Nestlé) Nepro (Ross) Magnacal Renal (Mead Johnson)
Hepatic failure: Enriched in BCAA; low sodium	Protein intolerance	Hepatic encephalopathy	NutriHep (Nestlé) Hepatic-Aid II (B Braun+ McGaw)
Pulmonary dysfunction: Low carbohydrate, high fat, concentrated in calories	Respiratory insufficiency	Ventilator dependence	NutriVent (Nestlé) Pulmocare (Ross)
Glucose intolerance: High fat, low carbohydrate (most contain fiber and fructose)	Glucose intolerance	Individuals with diabetes mellitus whose blood sugar is poorly controlled with standard formulas	Glucerna (Ross) Choice dm (Mead Johnson) Diabeti Source (Novartis) Glytrol (Nestlé)
Critical care, wound healing: High protein; most contain MCT to improve fat absorption; some have increased zinc and vitamin C for wound healing; some are high in antioxidants (vitamin E, β-carotene); some are enriched with arginine, glutamine, and/or omega-3 fatty acids	Critical illness	Severe trauma or burns Sepsis	Immun-Aid (B Braun+McGaw) Impact (Novartis) Perative (Ross) Crucial (Nestlé) TraumaCal (Mead Johnson)

*These diets may be beneficial for selected patients; costs and benefits must be considered.

GI, Gastrointestinal; *COPD,* chronic obstructive pulmonary disease; *MCT,* medium-chain triglyceride; *BCAA,* branched chain–enriched amino acid.

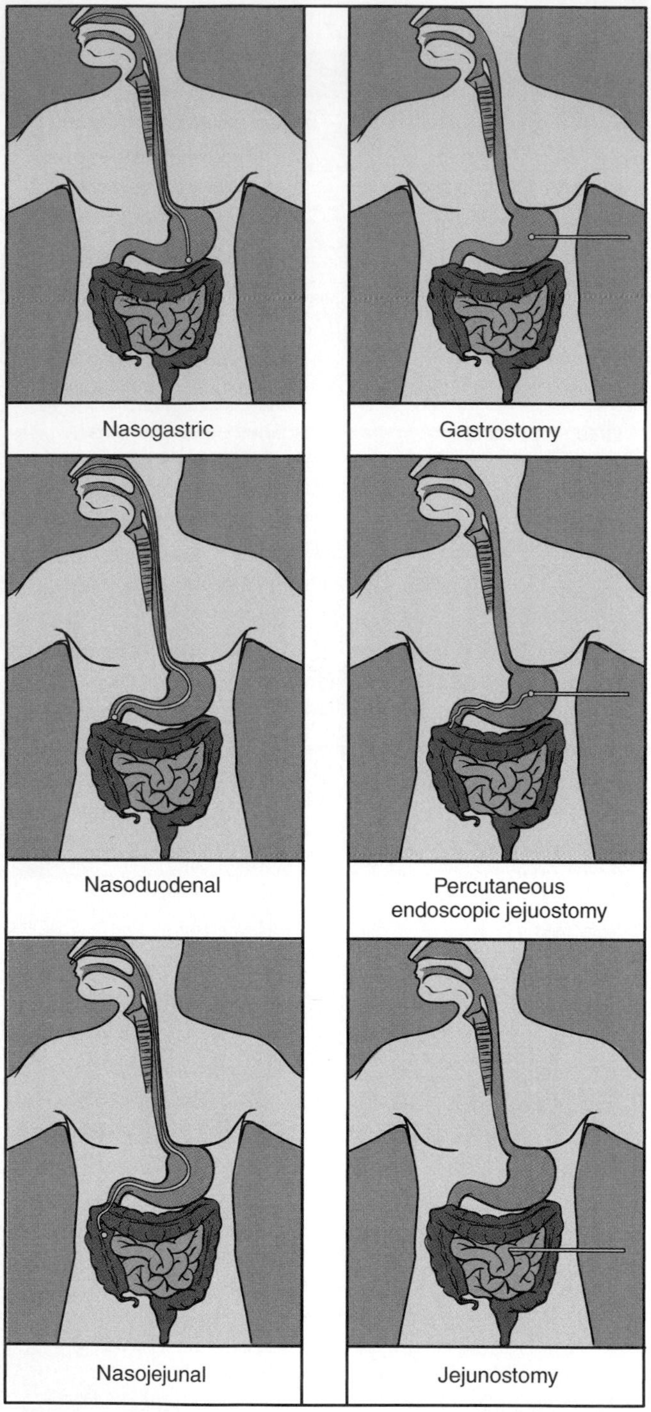

FIGURE 6-2. Tube feeding sites.

chial and pleural fluid and in the stomach is approximately 90% less than in the intestine. Therefore the nurse who obtains fluid with a pH greater than 5.0 and a low bilirubin concentration from a feeding tube can be relatively sure that the distal tip of the tube is in the pulmonary system.[43] Measurement of end-tidal CO_2 also shows promise for confirming tube placement in ventilated patients. Refer to Box 6-10 for verification of feeding tube placement as described in the American Association of Critical-Care Nurses (AACN) Practice Alert.

Formula Delivery. Careful attention to administration of tube feedings can prevent many complications. Very clean or aseptic technique in the handling and administration of the formula can help prevent bacterial contamination and a resultant infection. The optimal schedule for delivery of feedings also is important. Tube feedings may be administered intermittently or continuously.

Bolus feedings, which are intermittent feedings delivered rapidly into the stomach or small bowel, are likely to cause distention, vomiting, and dumping syndrome with diarrhea. Instead of using bolus feedings, nurses can gradually drip intermittent feedings, with each feeding lasting 20 to 30 minutes or longer, to promote optimal assimilation. The question of which feeding schedule—continuous or intermittent—is superior in critically ill patients remains unanswered.

Prevent or Correct Complications. Some of the more common complications of tube feeding are pulmonary aspiration, diarrhea, constipation, tube occlusion, and gastric retention (Table 6-4).

Total Parenteral Nutrition

TPN refers to the delivery of all nutrients by the intravenous (IV) route. TPN is used when the GI tract is not functional or when nutritional needs cannot be met solely via the GI tract. Likely candidates for TPN include patients who have a severely impaired absorption (as in short bowel syndrome, collagen-vascular diseases, and radiation enteritis), intestinal obstruction, peritonitis, and prolonged ileus. In addition, some postoperative, trauma, and burn patients may need TPN to supplement the nutrient intake they are able to tolerate via the enteral route.

Types of Parenteral Nutrition

TPN involves administration of highly concentrated dextrose that ranges from 25% to 70%, providing a rich source of calories. Such highly concentrated dextrose solutions are hyperosmolar, as much as 1800 mOsm/L, and therefore must be delivered through a central vein.[44] Peripheral parenteral nutrition (PPN) has a glucose concentration of 5% to 10% and may be delivered safely through a peripheral vein. PPN solution delivers nutrition support in a large volume that cannot be tolerated by patients who require fluid restriction. It provides short-term nutrition support for a few days to less than 2 weeks.

Regardless of the route of administration, both PPN and TPN provide glucose, fat, protein, electrolytes, vitamins, and trace elements. Although dextrose–amino acid solutions are commonly thought of as good growth media for microorganisms, they actually suppress the growth of most organisms usually associated

Box 6-10
Verification of Feeding Tube Placement

Expected Practice:

- Obtain radiographic confirmation of correct tube placement on all critically ill patients who are to receive feedings or medications via blindly inserted gastric or small bowel tubes prior to initial use.
- Mark and document the tube's exit site from the nose or mouth immediately after radiographic confirmation of correct tube placement; observe the mark to assess for a change in length of the external portion of the tube.
- Use bedside techniques to assess tube location at regular intervals to determine if the tube has remained in its intended position. No one single technique has been shown to be reliable for continually assessing tube placement:
  - Review routine chest and abdominal x-rays to determine if they refer to tube location
  - Helpful bedside techniques include measuring the pH and observing the appearance of fluid withdrawn from the tube.
  - Do not rely on the auscultatory method to determine tube location.

Supporting Evidence:

- Radiographic confirmation is the only reliable method to date of confirming enteral tube placement. The pH and appearance of an aspirate from the newly inserted tube, while not 100% reliable, are highly suggestive of gastric or small bowel placement and can be used as an initial indicator of placement. However, radiographic confirmation should always be done.
  - An aspirate from a gastric tube often has a pH of 5 or less and is usually grassy-green or clear and colorless, with off-white to tan mucus shreds.[1-10]
  - An aspirate from a small bowel tube often has a pH of 6 or greater and is usually bile-stained (ranging in color from light to golden yellow or brownish-green). In addition, the aspirate is usually thicker and more translucent than fluid withdrawn from a gastric tube. [1-10]
  - An aspirate from a tube inadvertently positioned in the tracheobronchial tree or the pleural space typically has a pH of 6 or greater. An aspirate from a tube in the tracheobronchial tree usually has the appearance of fluid obtained during tracheal suctioning. An aspirate from a tube in the pleural space is usually straw-colored and watery, perhaps tinged with bright-red blood (caused by perforation of the pleura by the tube).[1-10]
- There are numerous anecdotal reports of blindly-inserted tubes entering the respiratory tract undetected. In most of these cases, the auscultatory method falsely assured that the tube was correctly positioned in the stomach.[11–16] There is also a report of the auscultatory method failing to detect inadvertent placement of a nasogastric tube in the brain.[17] The auscultatory method was found to have a sensitivity of only 34% in differentiating between gastric and small bowel tube placement in 85 acutely ill adults.[18] In another study auscultation for insufflated air was found to have a sensitivity of only 45% in determining whether 134 tube insertions resulted in placement above or below the diaphragm.[19]
- It is not uncommon for a feeding tube to dislocate from its intended site, either after being tugged at by a confused patient or during the delivery of care.[20–21] An increase in the external portion of tubing extending from the nose or mouth can signal that the tube's distal tip has dislocated upward in the gastrointestinal tract (such as from the small bowel into the stomach or esophagus, or from the stomach into the esophagus).[22]
- Measuring the pH of fluid aspirated from tubes of fasting patients is helpful in differentiating between gastric and respiratory placement, and gastric and small bowel placement.[1-7]
- Observing the appearance of fluid aspirated from tubes of fasting patients is helpful in differentiating between gastric and respiratory placement, and gastric and small bowel placement.[7-10]
- Observing the pH and appearance of aspirates from feeding tubes when continuous feedings are in progress is less helpful than when the patient is fasting; nonetheless, these methods are occasionally of benefit in distinguishing between gastric and small bowel tube location.[23]
- A sudden increase in residual volume from a feeding tube in the small bowel may signal upward displacement of the tube into the stomach. Aspirates from small-bowel feeding tubes are usually less than 10 ml; an increase to 50 ml or higher may signal upward displacement of the tube into the stomach.[22]
- Injecting 30 ml of air into the tube via a 60 ml syringe immediately before pulling back of the plunger facilitates the withdrawal of fluid from small-diameter tubes.[24]
- Flushing the tube with 30 ml of water (or normal saline, if indicated for patients with hyponatremia) after residual volume measurements prevents the tube from clogging.[25, 26]

What You Should Do:

- Obtain an x-ray that visualizes the newly inserted tube to ensure that it is in the desired position (either the stomach or small bowel) before administering formula or medications via the tube for the first time.
- Ensure that your critical care unit has written practice documents such as a policy, procedure or standard of care that include when the initial x-ray should be obtained, a method of making the feeding tube, where to document the exit site, and the frequency of the documentation.
- If documentation of tube placement is not currently a part of the routine interpretation of chest and/or abdominal x-rays, from a collaborative team including a radiologist, pulmonologist, staff nurse, and risk manager to develop strategies for implementing this practice.

Need More Information or Help?

- Talk with a clinical practice specialist for additional information/assistance at www.aacn.org then select PRN.

References:

1. Metheny NA, Williams P, Wiersema L, Wehrie MA, Eisenberg P, McSweeney M. Effectiveness of pH measurements in predicting feeding tube placement. Nurs Res 1989; 38(5):280-285.

Continued

Box 6-10

Verification of Feeding Tube Placement—*cont'd*

2. Metheny NA, Reed L, Wiersema L, McSweeney M, Wehrie MA, Clark J. Effectiveness of pH measurements in predicting feeding tube placement: An update. Nurs Res 1993; 42(6):324-331.
3. Metheny NA, Stewart BJ, Smith L, Yan H, Diebold M, Clouse RE. pH and concentrations of pepsin and trypsin in feeding tube aspirates as predictors of tube placement. JPEN 1997; 21(5):279-285.
4. Metheny NA, Clouse RE, Clark JM, Reed L, Wehrle MA, Wiersema L. Techniques & procedures. pH testing of feeding-tube aspirates to detrmine placement. Nutr Clin Pract 1994;9(5):185-190.
5. Metheny NA, Stewart BJ, Smith L, Yan H, Diebold M, Clouse RE. pH and concentration of bilirubin in feeding tube aspirates as predictors of tube placement. Nurs Res 1999; 48(4):189-197.
6. Griffith DP, McNally AT, Battey CH et al. Intravenous erythromycin facilitates bedside placement of postpyloric feeding tubes in critically ill adults: a double-blind, randomized, placebo-controlled study. Crit Care Med 2003; 31(1):39-44.
7. Gharpure V, Meert KL, Samaik AP, Metheny NA. Indicators of postpyloric feeding tube placement in children. Crit Care Med 2000; 28(8):2962-2966.
8. Metheny N, Reed L, Berglund B, Wehrie MA. Visual characteristics of aspirates from feeding tubes as a method for predicting tube location. Nurs Res 1994; 43(5):282-287.
9. Harrison AM, Clay B, Grant MJ et al. Nonradiographic assessment of enteral feeding tube position. Crit Care Med 1997; 25(12):2055-2059.
10. Welch SK, Hanlon MD, Waits M, Foulks CJ. Comparison of four bedside indicators used to predict duodenal feeding tube placement with radiography. JPEN 1994; 18(6):525-530.
11. Metheny NA, Dettenmeier P, Hampton K, Wiersema L, Williams P. Detection of inadvertent respiratory placement of small-bore feeding tubes: A report of 10 cases. Heart Lung 1990; 19(6):631-638.
12. Lipman TO, Kessler T, Arabian A. Nasopulmonary intubation with feeding tubes: Case reports and review of the literature. JPEN 1985; 9(5):618-620.
13. Hendry PJ, Akyurekli Y, McIntyre R, Quarrington A, Keon WJ. Bronchopleural complications of nasogastric feeding tubes. Crit Care Med 1986; 14(10):892-894.
14. Metheny NA, Meert K. Invited Review. Monitoring feeding tube placement. Nutrition in Clinical Practice. 2004 Vol 19, No. 5, pages 487-496.
15. el Gamel A, Watson DC. Transbronchial intubation of the right pleural space: A rare complication of nasogastric intubation with a polyvinylchloride tube–a case study. Heart Lung 1993; 22(3):224-225.
16. Nakao MA, Killam D, Wilson R. Pneumothorax secondary to inadvertent nasotracheal placement of a nasoenteric tube past a cuffed endotracheal tube. Crit Care Med 1983; 11(3):210-211.
17. Metheny NA. Inadvertent intracranial nasogastric tube placement. Am J Nurs 2002; 102(8):25-27.
18. Metheny NA, McSweeney M, Wehrie MA, Wiersema L. Effectiveness of the auscultatory method in predicting feeding tube location. Nurs Res 1990; 39(5):262-267.
19. Keams PJ, Donna C. A controlled comparison of traditional feeding tube verification methods to a bedside, electromagnetic technique. JPEN 2001; 25(4):210-215.
20. Metheny NA, Spies M, Eisenberg P. Frequency of nasoenteral tube displacement and associated risk factors. Res Nurs Health 1986; 9(3):241-247.
21. Ellett MLC, Maahs J, Forsee S. Prevalence of feeding tube placement errors & associated risk factors in children. MCN 1998; 23(5):234-239.
22. Metheny NASchnelker R, McGinnis J et al. Indicators of tubesite during feedings. J Neurosc Nurs; (in press).
23. Metheny NA, Stewart BJ. Testing feeding tube placement during continuous tube feedings. Applied Nursing Research 2002; 15(4): 254-258.
24. Metheny NA, Reed L, Worseck M, Clark J. How to aspirate fluid from small-bore feeding tubes. Am J Nurs 1993; 93(5):86-88.
25. Metheny NA, Eisenberg P, McSweeney M. Effect of feeding tube properties and three irrigants on clogging rates. Nurs Res 1988; 37(3):165-169.
26. Schallom L, Stewart J, Nuetzel G, Schnelker R, Gardner R, Ludwig J, Metheny N. Abstract. Testing a protocol for measuring gastrointestinal residual volumes in tube-fed patients. American Journal of Critical Care. 2004; 13(3)265-266.

American Association of Critical Care Nurses: practice alert: verification of feeding tube placement. Issued May 2005.

with catheter-related sepsis, except yeasts. However, because the many manipulations required to prepare solutions increase the possibility of contamination, TPN solutions are best used with caution. They should be prepared under laminar flow conditions in the pharmacy, with avoidance of additions on the nursing unit. Solution containers need to be inspected for cracks or leaks before hanging, and solutions must be discarded within 24 hours of hanging. An in-line 0.22-μm filter, which eliminates all microorganisms but not endotoxins, may be used in administration of solutions. Use of the filter, however, cannot be substituted for good aseptic technique.

Nursing Management of Potential Complications

Nursing management of the patient receiving TPN includes catheter care, administration of solutions, prevention or correction of complications, and evaluation of patient responses to IV feedings. Refer to Table 6-5 for nursing management of TPN complications.

Because TPN requires an indwelling catheter in a central vein, it carries an increased risk of sepsis as

Table 6-4
Nursing Management of Enteral Tube Feeding Complications

COMPLICATION	CONTRIBUTING FACTOR(S)	PREVENTION/CORRECTION
Pulmonary aspiration	Feeding tube positioned in esophagus or respiratory tract	Check tube placement before intermittent feeding and every 4-6 hr during continuous feedings by checking the pH of fluid aspirated from the tube (usually gastric juice pH is <3.5).
	Regurgitation of formula	Elevate head to 45 degrees during feedings unless contraindicated; if head cannot be raised, position patient in lateral (especially right lateral, which facilitates gastric emptying) or prone position to improve drainage of vomitus from the mouth. Keep cuff of endotracheal or tracheostomy tube inflated during feedings, if possible. Metoclopramide may improve gastric emptying and decrease the risk of regurgitation. Evaluate feeding tolerance every 2 hr initially, then less frequently as condition becomes stable; intolerance may be manifested by bloating, abdominal distention and pain, lack of stool and flatus, diminished or absent bowel sounds, tense abdomen, increased tympany, nausea and vomiting, residual volume >200 ml aspirated from an NG tube or >100 ml aspirated from a gastrostomy tube (but a high residual volume in the absence of other abnormal findings may not be grounds for stopping feedings); (measuring residual volumes is a controversial practice; see the section on tube occlusion that follows); if intolerance is suspected, abdominal radiographs may be done to check for distended gastric bubble, distended loops of bowel, or air/fluid levels.
Diarrhea	Medications with GI side effects (antibiotics, digitalis, laxatives, magnesium-containing antacids, quinidine, caffeine, and many others)	Evaluate the patient's medications to determine their potential for causing diarrhea, consulting the pharmacist if necessary.
	Hypertonic formula or medications (e.g., oral suspensions of antibiotics, potassium, or other electrolytes), which cause dumping syndrome	Evaluate formula administration procedures to be sure that feedings are not being given by bolus infusion; administer the formula continuously or by slow intermittent infusion. Dilute enteral medications well.
	Bacterial contamination of the formula	Use scrupulously clean technique in administering tube feedings; prepare formula with sterile water if there are any concerns about the safety of the water supply or if the patient is seriously immunocompromised; keep opened containers of formula refrigerated, and discard them within 24 hr; discard enteral feeding containers and administration sets every 24 hr; hang formula no more than 4-8 hr unless it comes prepackaged in sterile administration sets.
	Fecal impaction with seep-age of liquid stool around the impaction	Perform a digital rectal examination to rule out impaction; see guidelines for prevention of constipation that follow.
Constipation	Low-residue formula, creating little fecal bulk	Consult with the physician regarding the possibility of using a fiber-containing formula.
Tube occlusion	Medications administered via tube (which either physically plug the tube or coagulate the formula, causing it to clog the tube)	If medications must be given by tube, avoid use of crushed tablets; consult with the pharmacist to determine whether medications can be dispensed as elixirs or suspensions; irrigate tube with water before and after administering any medication; never add any medication to the formula unless the two are known to be compatible.
	Sedimentation of formula	Irrigate tube every 4 hr during continuous feedings and after every intermittent feeding.
	Aspirating gastric contents to measure residual volumes (acidified protein from the formula clots in the tube)	It has been suggested that aspiration of gastric residuals be avoided with small-bore feeding tubes (8 Fr) and that patient tolerance be assessed by physical examination; if residuals are measured, flush the tube thoroughly after returning the formula to the stomach.
Gastric retention	Delayed gastric emptying related to head trauma, sepsis, diabetic or uremic gastroparesis, electrolyte balance, or other illness	The cause must be corrected if possible; consult with the physician about use of postpyloric feedings or metoclopramide to stimulate gastric emptying; encourage patient to lie in right lateral position frequently, unless contraindicated.

Modified from Moore MC: *Pocket guide to nutritional care,* ed 4, St Louis, 2000, Mosby.
NG, Nasogastric; *GI,* gastrointestinal.

Table 6-5
Nursing Management of TPN Complications

COMPLICATION	CLINICAL MANIFESTATIONS	PREVENTION/CORRECTION
Catheter-related sepsis	Fever, chills, glucose intolerance, positive blood culture	Use aseptic technique when handling catheter, IV tubing, and TPN solutions; hang a bottle of TPN no longer than 24 hr, lipid emulsion no longer than 12-24 hr; use an in-line 0.22-μm filter with TPN to remove microorganisms; avoid drawing blood, infusing blood or blood products, piggybacking other IV solutions into TPN IV tubing, or attaching manometers or transducers via the TPN infusion line, if at all possible. If catheter-related sepsis is suspected, remove catheter or assist in changing the catheter over a guidewire and administer antibiotics as ordered.
Air embolism	Dyspnea, cyanosis, apnea, tachycardia, hypotension, "millwheel" heart murmur; mortality estimated at 50% (depends on quantity of air entering)	Use Luer-Lok connections; use an in-line air-eliminating filter; have patient perform Valsalva maneuver during tubing changes; if the patient is on a ventilator, change tubing quickly at end expiration; maintain occlusive dressing over catheter site for at least 24 hr after removing catheter to prevent air entry through catheter tract. If air embolism is suspected, place patient in left lateral decubitus and Trendelenburg positions (to trap air in the apex of the right ventricle, away from the outflow tract) and administer oxygen and CPR as needed; immediately notify physician, who may attempt to aspirate air from the heart.
Pneumothorax	Chest pain, dyspnea, hypoxemia, hypotension, radiographic evidence, needle aspiration of air from pleural space	Thoroughly explain catheter insertion procedure to patient, because when a patient moves or breathes erratically he or she is more likely to sustain pleural damage; perform x-ray examination after insertion or insertion attempt. If pneumothorax is suspected, assist with needle aspiration or chest tube insertion, if necessary.
Central venous thrombosis	Edema of neck, shoulder, and arm on same side as catheter; development of collateral circulation on chest; pain in insertion site; drainage of TPN from the insertion site; positive findings on venogram	Follow measures to prevent sepsis; repeated or traumatic catheterizations are most likely to result in thrombosis. If thrombosis is confirmed, remove catheter and administer anticoagulants and antibiotics as ordered.
Catheter occlusion or semiocclusion	No flow or a sluggish flow through the catheter	If infusion is stopped temporarily, flush catheter with saline or heparinized saline. If catheter appears to be occluded, attempt to aspirate the clot; if this is ineffective, physician may order thrombolytic agent such as streptokinase, alteplase (t-PA) instilled in the catheter.
Hypoglycemia	Diaphoresis, shakiness, confusion, loss of consciousness	Infuse TPN within 10% of ordered rate; monitor blood glucose until stable after discontinuance of TPN. If hypoglycemia is present, administer oral carbohydrate; if the patient is unconscious or oral intake is contraindicated, the physician may order a bolus of IV dextrose.
Hyperglycemia	Thirst, headache, lethargy, increased urinary output	Administer TPN within 10% of ordered rate; monitor blood glucose level at least daily until stable; the patient may require insulin added to the TPN if hyperglycemia is persistent; sudden appearance of hyperglycemia in a patient who was previously tolerating the same glucose load may indicate onset of sepsis.

Modified from Moore MC: *Pocket guide to nutritional care,* ed 4, St Louis, 2000, Mosby.
IV, Intravenous; *TPN,* total parenteral nutrition; *CPR,* cardiopulmonary resuscitation.

well as potential insertion-related complications such as pneumothorax and hemothorax. Air embolism is also more likely with central vein TPN. Patients requiring multiple IV therapies and frequent blood sampling usually have multilumen central venous catheters, and TPN is often infused via these catheters.

Some clinical studies have reported that catheter-related sepsis is higher with multilumen catheters; others have found no difference compared with single-lumen catheters.[45] Clearly, patients requiring multilumen catheters are likely to be very ill and immunocompromised, and scrupulous aseptic technique is essential in maintaining multilumen catheters. The manipulation involved in frequent changes of IV fluid and obtaining blood specimens through these catheters increases the risk of catheter contamination. Peripherally inserted central catheters (PICCs) allow central venous access through long catheters inserted in peripheral sites. This reduces the risk of complications associated with percutaneous cannulation of the subclavian vein and provides an alternative to PPN.[46]

The indwelling central venous catheter provides an excellent nidus for infection. Catheter-related infections arise from endogenous skin flora, contamination of the catheter hub, seeding of the catheter by organisms carried in the bloodstream from another site, or contamination of the infusate. Good hand washing and scrupulous aseptic technique in all aspects of catheter care and TPN delivery are the primary steps for prevention of catheter-related infections. Other measures to reduce the incidence of catheter-related infections include using maximal barrier precautions (i.e., cap, mask, sterile gloves, sterile drape) at the time of insertion, tunneling the catheter underneath the skin, use of a 2% chlorhexidine preparation for skin cleansing, no routine replacement of the central venous catheter for prevention of infection, and use of antiseptic/antibiotic-impregnated central venous catheters.[47]

Metabolic complications associated with parenteral nutrition include glucose intolerance and electrolyte imbalance. Slow advancement of the rate of TPN (25 ml/hr) to goal rate will allow pancreatic adjustment to the dextrose load. Capillary blood glucose should be monitored every 4 to 6 hours. Insulin can be added to the TPN solution or can be infused as a separate drip to control glucose levels. Rapid cessation of TPN may not lead to hypoglycemia; however, tapering the infusion over 2 to 4 hours is recommended.[48]

Serum electrolyte levels are obtained upon starting TPN. During critical illness, levels should be monitored and corrected daily, and then weekly or twice weekly once the patient is more stable. The refeeding syndrome is a potentially lethal condition characterized by generalized fluid and electrolyte imbalance. It occurs as a potential complication after initiation of oral, enteral, or parenteral nutrition in malnourished patients. During chronic starvation, several compensatory metabolic changes occur. The reintroduction of carbohydrates and amino acids leads to increased insulin production. This creates an anabolic environment that increases intracellular demand for phosphorus, potassium, magnesium, vitamins, and minerals.[49] These metabolic demands result in severe shifts from the extracellular compartment. Increased insulin levels also result in fluid retention. Severe hypophosphatemia, hypokalemia, and hypomagnesemia result in altered cardiac, gastrointestinal, and neurologic function. In particular, hypophosphatemia causes a decrease in 2,3-diphosphosoglycerate (2,3 DPG) and also limits the many reactions that require ATP. As a result, hypophosphatemia and other electrolyte deficiencies may lead to respiratory failure, congestive heart failure, and dysrhythmias.

It is important to anticipate refeeding syndrome in patients who may be at risk. Patients with chronic malnutrition or underfeeding, chronic alcoholism, or anorexia nervosa or those maintained NPO for several days with evidence of stress are at risk for refeeding syndrome.[50] In high-risk patients, nutrition support should be started cautiously at 25% to 50% of required calories and slowly advanced over 3 to 4 days as tolerated. Close monitoring of serum electrolyte levels before and during feeding is essential. Normal values do not always reflect total body stores. Correction of preexisting electrolyte imbalances are necessary before initiation of feeding. Continued monitoring as well as supplementation with electrolytes and vitamins is necessary throughout the first week of nutrition support.[50]

Lipid Emulsion

Lipids or intravenous fat emulsions (IVFE) provide calories for energy and prevent essential fatty acid depletion. In contrast to dextrose–amino acid solutions, IVFE provide a rich environment for the growth of bacteria and fungi including *Candida albicans*. Furthermore, IVFE cannot be filtered through an in-line 0.22-μm filter, because some particles in the emulsions have larger diameters than this. Lipids may be infused into the TPN line downstream from the filter. No other drugs should be infused into a line containing lipids or TPN. Lipid emulsions are handled with strict asepsis, and they must be discarded within 12 to 24 hours of hanging. There is a trend toward mixing lipid emulsions with dextrose–amino acid TPN solutions; these are called 3-in-1 solutions or total nutrient admixtures (TNA). Consolidating the nutrients in one container is more economical and saves nursing time, although TNA solutions may be less stable.[44]

EVALUATING RESPONSE TO NUTRITION SUPPORT

A multidisciplinary approach is required in evaluating the effects of nutrition support on clinical outcomes. Assessment of response to nutrition support is an ongoing process that involves anthropometric measurements, physical examination, and biochemical evaluation. Daily monitoring of nutritional intake is an important aspect of critical care and is a key element in preventing problems associated with underfeeding and overfeeding. Daily weights and the maintenance of accurate intake-and-output records are crucial for evaluating nutritional progress and the state of hydration in the patient receiving nutrition support. Serum levels of electrolytes, calcium, phosphorus, and magnesium serve as a guide to the amount of these nutrients that has to be supplied; blood urea nitrogen and creatinine levels reflect the adequacy of renal function to handle nutrition support; blood glucose is an indicator of the patient's tolerance of the carbohydrate; prealbumin is an indicator of the adequacy of nutrition support; and serum triglyceride concentrations (in patients receiving intravenous lipid emulsions) reflect the ability of the tissues to metabolize the lipids.

evolve To test your mastery of this chapter, try the Open-Book Quiz at http://evolve.elsevier.com/Urden/priorities/

REFERENCES

1. Huang YC et al: Nutritional status of mechanically ventilated critically ill patients: comparison of different types of nutrition, *Clin Nutr* 19(2):101, 2000.
2. Kelly IE et al: Still hungry in hospital: identifying malnutrition in acute hospital admissions, *QJM* 93:93, 2000.
3. Waitzberg DL, Caiaffa WT, Correia MI: Hospital malnutrition: the Brazilian national survey (IBRANUTRI): a study of 4000 patients, *Nutrition* 17(7):573, 2001.
4. Pirlich M et al: Prevalence of malnutrition in hospitalized medical patients: impact of underlying disease, *Dig Dis* 21(3):245, 2003.
5. Kyle UG et al: Prevalence of malnutrition in 1760 patients at hospital admission: a controlled population study of body composition, *Clin Nutr* 22(5):473, 2003.
6. Braunschweig C, Gomez S, Sheehan PM: Impact of declines in nutritional status on outcomes in adult patients hospitalized for more than 7 days, *J Am Diet Assoc* 100:1316, 2000.
7. Mathus-Vliegen EMH: Nutritional status, nutrition and pressure ulcers, *Nutr Clin Pract* 16:286, 2001.
8. Rubinson L et al: Low caloric intake is associated with nosocomial bloodstream infections in patients in the medical intensive care unit, *Crit Care Med* 32:350, 2004.
9. Cheng CH et al: Measured versus estimated energy expenditure in mechanically ventilated critically ill patients, *Clin Nutr* 21(2):165, 2002.
10. Alberda CL et al: Energy requirements in critically ill patients: how close are our estimates? *Nutr Clin Pract* 17(1):38, 2002.
11. Van den Berghe G et al: Intensive insulin therapy in critically ill patients, *N Engl J Med* 345:1359, 2001.
12. Rassias AJ et al: Insulin increases neutrophil count and phagocytic capacity after cardiac surgery, *Anesth Analg* 94:1113, 2002.
13. Clement S et al: Management of diabetes and hyperglycemia in hospitals, *Diabetes Care* 27:553, 2004.
14. National Education Programs Working Group: Report on the management of patients with hypertension and high blood cholesterol, *Ann Intern Med* 114:224, 1991.
15. Vollmer WM et al: Effects of diet and sodium intake on blood pressure: subgroup analysis of the DASH-sodium trial, *Ann Intern Med* 135:1019, 2001.
16. Yeung SC, Ensom MH: Phenytoin and enteral feedings: does evidence support an interaction? *Ann Pharmacother* 34(7-8):895, 2000.
17. Wilson RF, Tyburski JG: Metabolic responses and nutritional therapy in patients with severe head injuries, *J Head Trauma Rehabil* 13:11, 1998.
18. Taylor SJ et al: Prospective, randomized, controlled trial to determine the effect of early enhanced enteral nutrition on clinical outcome in mechanically ventilated patients suffering head injury, *Crit Care Med* 27:2525, 1999.
19. Kierdorf HP: The nutritional management of acute renal failure in the intensive care unit, *New Horiz* 3:699, 1995.
20. Bellomo R et al: A prospective comparative study of moderate versus high protein intake for critically ill patients with acute renal failure, *Ren Fail* 19:111, 1997.
21. Mitch WE, Maroni BJ: Factors causing malnutrition in patients with chronic uremia, *Am J Kidney Dis* 33:176, 1999.
22. Kopple J: Therapeutic approaches to malnutrition in chronic dialysis patients: the different modalities of nutritional support, *Am J Kidney Dis* 33:180, 1999.
23. Riella MC: Nutrition in acute renal failure, *Ren Fail* 19:237, 1997.
24. Brewer ED: Pediatric experience with intradialytic parenteral nutrition and supplemental tube feeding, *Am J Kidney Dis* 33:205, 1999.
25. Cato Y: Intradialytic parenteral nutrition therapy for the malnourished hemodialysis patient, *J Intraven Nurs* 20:130, 1997.
26. Hazell AS, Butterworth RF: Hepatic encephalopathy: an update of pathophysiologic mechanisms, *Proc Soc Exp Biol Med* 222:99, 1999.
27. Albrecht J, Jones EA: Hepatic encephalopathy: molecular mechanisms underlying the clinical syndrome, *J Neurol Sci* 170:138, 1999.
28. August D et al: Guidelines for the use of parenteral and enteral nutrition in adult and pediatric patients, *JPEN J Parenter Enteral Nutr* 26:18SA, 2002.
29. Patton KM, Aranda-Michel J: Nutritional aspects in liver disease and liver transplantation, *Nutr Clin Pract* 17:332, 2002.
30. Florez DA, Aranda-Michel J: Nutritional management of acute and chronic liver disease, *Semin Gastrointest Dis* 13(3):169, 2002.
31. Khokhar AS, Seidner DL: The pathophysiology of pancreatitis, *Nutr Clin Pract* 19:5, 2004.
32. Avgerinos C et al: Nutritional support in acute pancreatitis, *Dig Dis* 21(3):214, 2003.
33. Russell MK: Acute pancreatitis: a review of pathophysiology and nutrition management, *Nutr Clin Pract* 19:16, 2004.
34. Al-Omran M, Groof A, Wilke D: Enteral versus parenteral nutrition for acute pancreatitis, *Cochrane Database Syst Rev* 1:1, 2003.
35. Dejong CH, Greve JW, Soeters PB: Nutrition in patients with acute pancreatitis, *Curr Opin Crit Care* 7(4):251, 2001.
36. Abou-Assi S, O'Keefe SJ: Nutrition support during acute pancreatitis, *Nutrition* 18:938, 2002.
37. Jones MP: Management of diabetic gastroparesis, *Nutr Clin Pract* 19:145, 2004.
38. Charney P, Hertzler SR: Management of blood glucose and diabetes in the critically ill patient receiving enteral feeding, *Nutr Clin Pract* 19:129, 2004.

39. Braga M et al: Artificial nutrition after major abdominal surgery: impact of route of administration and composition of the diet, *Crit Care Med* 26:24, 1998.
40. Booth CM, Heyland DK, Paterson WG: Gastrointestinal promotility drugs in the critical care setting: a systematic review of the evidence, *Crit Care Med* 30:1429, 2002.
41. Lord LM et al: Comparison of weighted vs. unweighted enteral feeding tubes for efficacy of transpyloric intubation, *JPEN J Parenter Enteral Nutr* 17:71, 1993.
42. Metheny NA et al: pH testing of feeding-tube aspirates to determine placement, *Nutr Clin Pract* 9:185, 1994.
43. Metheny NA et al: pH and concentration of bilirubin in feeding tube aspirates as predictors of tube placement, *Nurs Res* 48:189, 1999.
44. Worthington P, Gilbert KA, Wagner BA: Parenteral nutrition for the acutely ill, *AACN Clin Issues* 11(4):559, 2000.
45. Dobbins BM et al: Each lumen is a potential source of central venous catheter-related bloodstream infection, *Crit Care Med* 31(6):1688, 2003.
46. Orr ME: The peripherally inserted central catheter: what are the current indications for its use? *Nutr Clin Pract* 17:99, 2002.
47. O'Grady NP et al: Guidelines for the prevention of intravascular catheter-related infections, *Infect Control Hosp Epidemiol* 23(12):759, 2002.
48. Speerhas R et al: Maintaining normal blood glucose concentrations with total parenteral nutrition: is it necessary to taper total parenteral nutrition? *Nutr Clin Pract* 18: 414, 2003.
49. Crook MA, Hally V, Panteli JV: The importance of the refeeding syndrome, *Nutrition* 17:632, 2001.
50. Hearing SD: Refeeding syndrome, *BMJ* 328(7445):908, 2004.

CHAPTER

7 Gerontologic Alterations

KAREN L. RICE

OBJECTIVES

- Describe the age-associated physiologic changes that occur in the cardiovascular, respiratory, renal, gastrointestinal, hepatic, integumentary, immune, and central nervous systems.
- State the clinical significance of age-related physiologic changes and the expected nursing considerations or interventions used in caring for older critical care patients.
- Relate the age-related changes in hepatic function and the accompanying pharmacokinetic changes to the administration of various cardiovascular medications.

Patients in critical care units include an increasing number of older adults. Early in this decade, the United States population older than 65 years reached 35.6 million, accounting for 12.3% of the overall population. Those in the 65- to 74-year age-group numbered 18.3 million, 75- to 84-year-olds accounted for 12.7 million, and those in the 85-year or older age-group numbered 6 million. This latter group is expected to reach 9.6 million by 2030.[1] In 2001 a 65-year-old woman had a life expectancy of 19.4 more years, whereas men could expect to live another 16.4 years.[1]

The process of senescence (growing old) is characterized by tissue and organ changes. This, in combination with the prevalence of chronic conditions in the older adult, contributes to increased morbidity and mortality in the critical care unit. Aging is accompanied by physiologic changes in the cardiovascular, respiratory, renal, gastrointestinal (GI), hepatic, integumentary, immune, and central nervous systems. With advancing age the incidence of disease increases, with cardiovascular and neoplastic diseases being the most common causes of death.[2] However, although physiologic decline and disease processes influence each other, physiologic decline occurs independently of disease and is responsible for the development of symptoms at an earlier stage of disease in older adults than in their younger counterparts.[2] Therefore changes in physiologic function are important to consider when caring for the older adult patient.

CARDIOVASCULAR SYSTEM

Advancing age has many effects on the cardiovascular system. With advancing age both the myocardium and the vascular system undergo a multitude of anatomic and cellular changes that alter the function of both the myocardium and peripheral vascular system.[3] These changes in cardiovascular function significantly impact critical illness in the older adult because of the age-related effects on cardiovascular structure and function. In addition, because age is a major risk factor for cardiovascular disease in the older adult, this high-risk population will encounter more cardiovascular events when admitted for noncardiac problems to the critical care unit.[4]

Age-Related Changes in Myocardial Structure and Function

Myocardial collagen content increases with age.[5,6] Collagen is the principal noncontractile protein occupying the cardiac interstitium.[7] Increased myocardial collagen content renders the myocardium less compliant; therefore a decrease in myocardial compliance can adversely affect diastolic filling (through decreased distensibility and dilation) and myocardial relaxation. Consequently, the left ventricle must develop a higher filling pressure for a given increase in ventricular volume. Decreased left ventricular compliance may be evident in the older adult by the presence of an S_4 heart sound.[8]

The functional consequence of these changes could be an increase in myocardial oxygen consumption. Under normal physiologic conditions, an increase in myocardial oxygen demand is met with a corresponding increase in coronary artery blood flow. However, in the presence of coronary artery disease, coronary artery blood flow can be limited because of atherosclerotic-mediated narrowing of the coronary arteries. Hence the older patient is at risk for developing myocardial ischemia and/or infarction. Clinical manifestations of myocardial ischemia include electrocardiographic (ECG) changes and chest pain. However, the sensation

Table 7-1

Age-Related Changes in Electrocardiographic Variables

	AGE (YEARS)			
ECG VARIABLE	YOUNGER THAN 30	30-39	40-49	OLDER THAN 49
R-wave amplitude (mm)	10.43	10.53	9.01	9.25
S-wave amplitude (mm)	15.21	14.21	12.22	12.42
Frontal plane axis (degrees)	48.93	48.13	36.50	38.83
PR duration (ms)	15.89	16.23	16.04	16.25
QRS duration (ms)	7.64	7.51	7.36	8.00
QT duration (ms)	37.83	37.50	37.99	39.58
T-wave amplitude (ms)	5.21	4.57	4.31	4.42

Data from Bachman S, Sparrow D, Smith LK: *Am J Cardiol* 48:513, 1981.
ECG, Electrocardiogram.

of chest pain may be altered in the older adult. Atypical symptoms, such as dyspnea, confusion, and failure to thrive are frequently the only symptoms associated with myocardial infarction in this high-risk population.[9]

The aging heart also undergoes a modest degree of hypertrophy that is similar to pressure overload–induced hypertrophy. Such hypertrophy entails a thickening of the left ventricular wall without appreciable changes in left ventricular cavity size.[10] However, increases in left ventricular cavity size associated with aging occur only in men.[9] The increase in left ventricular wall thickness is a result primarily of an increase in muscle cell size. In older individuals the myocardial hypertrophy may be caused by corresponding increases in aortic impedance and systemic vascular resistance.[11]

Myocardial contractility depends on numerous factors. However, the most important determinants of myocardial contraction are the intracellular level of free calcium and the sensitivity of the contractile proteins for calcium.[11,12] Because peak contractile force in the senescent myocardium is unaltered, this suggests that neither the amount of intracellular free calcium during systole nor the sensitivity of the contractile proteins for calcium is altered. The prolonged duration of contraction (systole) is caused in part by a slowed or delayed rate of myocardial relaxation, which may be an adaptive mechanism to preserve contractile function compromised by age-related increases in afterload.[3,12]

Age-Associated Changes in Hemodynamics and the Electrocardiogram

Resting (supine) heart rate decreases with age.[13,14] Cinelli et al[13] reported a decrease in the resting heart rate from 78.8 beats/min in young adults to 62.3 beats/min in older adults. Heart rate is an important determinant of cardiac output (CO), and the normal resting heart beats approximately 70 times a minute. At rest or with minimal activity, the older adult probably will not experience any untoward cardiovascular effect (i.e., a decrease in CO) with a heart rate of 62 beats/min. However, if the heart rate response is attenuated during exercise, the older person's capacity for exercise may be limited.

Resting CO and stroke volume (SV) are not changed with advancing age. At rest, left ventricular end-diastolic volume (LVEDV, preload), end-systolic volume, and the ejection fraction are not affected by age.[15] In the elderly human myocardium, the early diastolic filling period and isovolumic phase of myocardial relaxation are prolonged.[15-17] However, these changes, although suggestive of diastolic dysfunction, do not translate into decreases in end-diastolic volume or stroke volume.[16,17] Finally, aging is associated with a moderate increase in pulmonary artery pressure.[18]

Advancing age produces changes in the ECG. R-wave and S-wave amplitude significantly decrease in persons older than 49 years, whereas QT duration increases[19] (Table 7-1). The incidence of asymptomatic cardiac dysrhythmias increases in elderly patients.[20] The most common dysrhythmia occurring in older individuals is the premature ventricular contraction (PVC). Carom et al[21] and Fleg and Kennedy[22] report that 70% to 80% of all patients older than 60 years experience PVCs. Other common types of dysrhythmias are sinus node dysfunction (atrial fibrillation, atrial flutter, or paroxysmal supraventricular tachycardia) and atrioventricular conduction disturbances.[15,19,20] Because the majority of patients are asymptomatic, the use of antidysrhythmics is generally not recommended. The side effects and toxic effects of antidysrhythmics impose more of a risk, as compared with the risk of mortality or morbidity related to the dysrhythmia.[20,23]

In contrast, for patients who are symptomatic and have malignant ventricular dysrhythmias (sustained ventricular tachycardia and/or fibrillation), pharmacologic therapy is warranted.[20,23]

AGE-RELATED CHANGES IN BARORECEPTOR FUNCTION

Baroreceptor reflex function is altered with aging.[24] Baroreceptors, located at the bifurcation of the common carotid artery and aortic arch, are mechanoreceptors that respond to stretch and other changes in the blood vessel wall.[25] Impulses arising in the baroreceptor region project to the vasomotor center (nucleus of tractus solitarius) in the medulla. Abrupt changes in blood pressure caused by increases in peripheral resistance, CO, or blood volume are sensed by the baroreceptors, resulting in an increase in the impulse frequency to the vasomotor center within the medulla. This increase inhibits vasoconstrictor impulses arising from the vasoconstrictor region within the medulla.[25] The result is a decrease in heart rate (HR) and peripheral vasodilation; both these effects return the blood pressure to within normal limits.

Postural hypotension was once thought to occur more frequently in elderly persons and to be related to age. However, recent studies have shown that the prevalence of postural hypotension is quite low in elderly persons.[26,27] The prevalence of orthostatic hypotension is greater in institutionalized elderly patients who are receiving antihypertensive medications.[28]

LEFT VENTRICULAR FUNCTION

In most individuals, aging is associated with a decline in exercise performance. The thickening of the left ventricular wall along with stiffening of the aortic and mitral valves makes the aging heart less able to provide adequate contractile strength.[29] With advancing age the maximal HR achieved during exercise is attenuated; however, the decreased HR response is accompanied by an increase in LVEDV and SV. This augmentation in LVEDV and SV offsets the attenuated HR response and maintains CO in exercise.

Healthy older persons have no age-associated decline in CO during exercise, but other factors (e.g., neural functioning, skeletal/joint functioning, pulmonary function) may limit an older individual's ability to exercise.

PERIPHERAL VASCULAR SYSTEM

The effects of aging on the peripheral vascular system are reflected in the gradual but linear rise in systolic blood pressure.[30,31] Diastolic blood pressure is less affected by age and generally remains the same or decreases.[31]

Important determinants of systolic blood pressure include the compliance of the vasculature and the blood volume within the vascular system. Similar to the heart, the compliance of the vasculature is determined by its cell type and tissue composition. With advancing age the intimal layer thickens, principally because of an increase in smooth muscle cells that have migrated from the medial layer, and the amount of connective tissue (collagen, elastic tissue) increases.[30] These changes occur in the intima of the large and distal arteries. This gradual decrease in arterial compliance, or "stiffening of the arteries," is known as arteriosclerosis. Arteriosclerotic and atherosclerotic processes cause the arteries to become progressively less distensible, altering the vascular pressure-volume relationship. These changes are clinically significant because small changes in intravascular volume are accompanied by disproportionate increases in systolic blood pressure. The decrease in arterial compliance and disproportionate increase in systolic blood pressure may lead to an increase in afterload and the development of concentric (pressure-induced) ventricular hypertrophy in the elderly patient.[32]

Arterial pressure is also governed by the amount of blood volume, which in turn is regulated by plasma levels of sodium and water and the activity of the renin-angiotensin system.[33] Plasma renin activity declines with age, and aging per se has no appreciable effect on sodium and water homeostasis.[34,35] As noted later, however, age-related changes occur in renal tubular function, and the glomerular filtration rate (GFR) decreases, both of which can affect overall sodium and water homeostasis. Circulating levels of sodium-regulating hormones, such as natriuretic hormone, aldosterone, and antidiuretic hormone (ADH), are not appreciably altered by advancing age.[35,36] However, a delayed natriuretic response after sodium loading and plasma volume expansion and a diminished renal response to ADH secretion have been reported in elderly persons.[36]

CARDIOVASCULAR SYSTEM SUMMARY

- Aorta and other arteries become stiff and less pliable, leading to increased workload on the heart to perfuse tissue.
- Systolic and diastolic pressures increase, along with an increase in systemic vascular resistance and a decrease in cardiac output.
- There is a loss of capacity in the myocardium and arterial system and decreased ability to respond and recover from periods of physiologic and psychologic stress.
- A decreased myocardial efficiency results in less relaxation during diastole.
- The alteration in baroreceptor function leads to changes in compensatory responses.

Table 7-2

Progressive Changes in Arterial Oxygen Tension (Pao_2) and Carbon Dioxide Tension ($Paco_2$)

AGE-GROUP (YEARS)	Pao_2 (mm Hg)	$Paco_2$ (mm Hg)
<30	94	39
31-40	87	38
41-50	84	40
51-60	81	39
>60	74	40

Modified from Sorbini CA et al: *Respiration* 25:3, 1968.

PULMONARY SYSTEM

Many of the changes in the pulmonary system that occur with aging are reflected in pulmonary function tests and include changes in thoracic wall expansion and respiratory muscle strength, morphology of alveolar parenchyma, and decreases in arterial oxygen tension (Pao_2)[37] (Table 7-2). These changes occur progressively as age advances and should not alter the elderly person's ability to breathe effortlessly. However, factors such as repeated exposure to environmental pollutants, cigarette smoking, and frequent pulmonary infections can accelerate age-related changes, thereby making it difficult to identify the age-associated changes in pulmonary function.

Thoracic Wall and Respiratory Muscles

Upper airway changes include weakening support of upper and lower cartilage, predisposing elderly persons to obstructive changes. Submucosal glands decrease production of mucus, leading to dryness and thickened secretions.[38] With advancing age the chest wall (thoracic skeleton) and vertebrae undergo a small degree of osteoporosis, and at the same time the costal cartilages that connect the rib cage together become calcified and stiff. These changes may produce kyphosis and reduce chest wall compliance, respectively.[37,39,40] The functional effect is a decrease in thoracic wall excursion. Other factors, such as an increase in abdominal girth and change in posture, also decrease thoracic excursion. These anatomic changes are reflected by an increase in residual volume and decrease in vital capacity.

The strength of the respiratory muscles (diaphragm, external/internal intercostal muscles) gradually decreases. Respiratory muscle weakness begins as early as age 55 years.[41] During aging, skeletal muscle progressively atrophies and its energy metabolism decreases, which may partially explain the declining strength of the respiratory muscles.[42,43] In addition, an age-associated decrease occurs in the effectiveness of the cough reflex, possibly caused by a decrease in ciliary responsiveness and motion.[44]

Alveolar Parenchyma

With advancing age a diminished recoil (or increased compliance) of the lung occurs.[45] The reduced recoil results from the increase in the ratio of elastin to collagen content that occurs with advancing age.[46] Collagen, elastin, and reticulin are the primary connective tissue proteins of the lung tissue.[47,48] They are responsible for the elasticity and performance of the airways of the lung. Whereas total lung collagen remains unaltered, the amount of elastin increases with age in the interlobular septa and pleura and possibly within the bronchi and their vessels. These anatomic changes are reflected by an increase in residual volume and a decrease in forced expiratory volume. With changes in cartilage the trachea and bronchi become stiffer and less compliant.[38] Also, the size of the alveolar ducts increases after age 40 years.[37] The bronchial enlargement displaces inhaled air volume away from the alveoli that line the alveolar ducts (Figure 7-1).

Ventilation and oxygen/carbon dioxide exchange (diffusion) depend on numerous factors, including the surface area available for diffusion. A displacement of inhaled air volume away from the alveoli limits the surface area available for gas exchange. This may partly explain the progressive and linear decrease in the pulmonary diffusion capacity, which depends on both surface area and capillary blood volume. Capillary blood volume and surface area have been reported to decrease with advancing age.[49]

Pulmonary Gas Exchange

The arterial oxygen tension (Pao_2) decreases with age, such that the median Pao_2 for healthy persons older than 60 years is 74.3 mm Hg, as compared with 94 mm Hg for younger adults.[50] In contrast, arterial carbon dioxide ($Paco_2$) does not change with advancing age (see Table 7-2).[50] The decrease in Pao_2 may be the result of an increase[51,52] Consequently, dependent lung zones may be ventilated intermittently, leading to regional differences in ventilation. It is possible that alterations in blood volume and vascular resistance within the pulmonary circulation may also contribute to ventilation/perfusion (V/Q) mismatching. Other factors, such as smoking and pulmonary disease, also have an impact on the level of arterial oxygenation.

Lung Volumes and Capacities

With advancing age, total lung capacity and tidal volume do not change.[39] Residual volume (RV) increases with age, paralleling the decrease in chest wall compliance and reduced strength of the respiratory

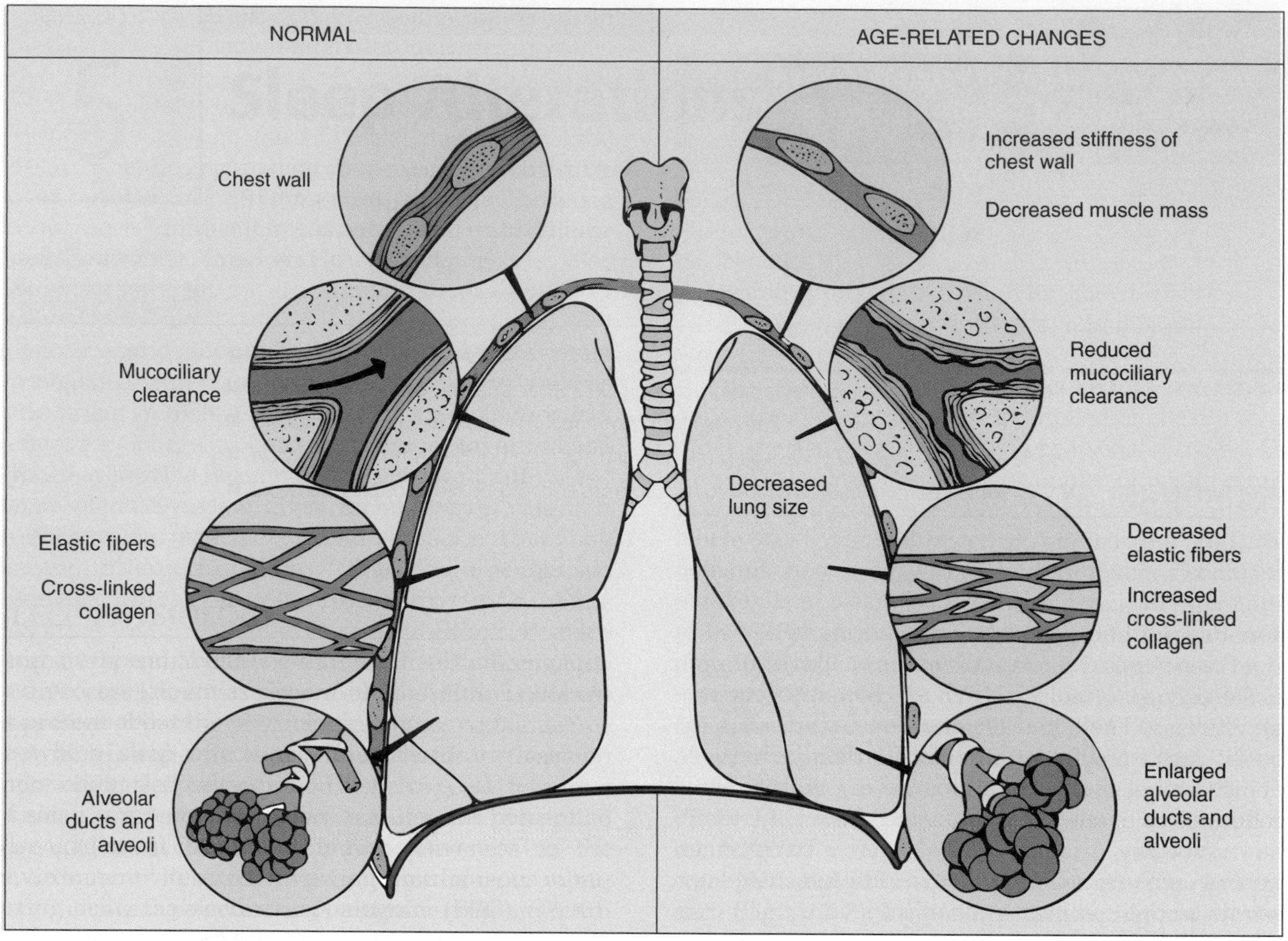

FIGURE 7-1. Age-related changes in human respiratory system. With advancing age, compliance of the chest wall and lung tissue changes, with reduced clearance of mucus by cilia that line the pulmonary tree and enlargement of alveolar ducts and alveoli.

muscles. The increase in RV may also add to the diminished strength of the inspiratory muscles by stretching the diaphragm and altering the tension-length relationship.

Pulmonary System Summary

- Lung tissue stiffens.
- Diffusion of gases is impaired by 8% per year after age 65.
- There is a decrease in vital capacity and maximal breathing capacity.
- Increased weakness of diaphragm and abdominal and accessory muscles leads to decreased ability to inhale and exhale.

RENAL SYSTEM

Aging produces changes in renal structure and function, many of which begin at approximately 30 to 40 years of age.[53,54] One of the prominent changes is a decrease in the number and size of the nephrons, which begins in the cortical regions and progresses toward the medullary portions of the kidney.[55] The decrease in the number of nephrons corresponds to a 20% decrease in the weight of the kidney between 40 and 80 years of age.[55] Initially this loss of nephrons does not appreciably alter renal function because of the large renal reserve: the kidney contains approximately 2 million to 3 million nephrons, all of which are not needed to maintain adequate fluid and acid-base homeostasis. However, with time the geriatric patient also loses this renal reserve.[55] Nephron loss is caused by a gradual reduction in blood flow to the glomerular capillary tuft.[56] Total renal blood flow declines after the fourth decade of life[53] because of hyaline arteriosclerosis.[56,57] The etiology of this vascular lesion within the glomerular tuft is unknown. By the eighth decade of life, 50% of the glomeruli are lost as a result of this arteriolar hyalinization.[55]

Fluid Filtration

GFR decreases with advancing age.[58,59] In elderly persons the decrease in GFR is most likely caused by the decrease in nephron number as well as decreased renal blood flow.[58]

Even though the remaining nephrons adapt to the loss of nephrons by glomerular hyperfiltration and increased solute load per nephron, the reduced GFR predisposes the elderly patient to adverse drug reactions and drug-induced renal failure. Some drugs are excreted unchanged in the urine, whereas other drugs have active or nephrotoxic metabolites that are excreted in the urine. In addition, the senescent kidney is more susceptible to injury by hypotensive episodes because of the age-related decrease in renal blood flow and reduced pressure gradient across the afferent arteriole.[60]

Age-related changes also occur in tubular function. The age-related changes in tubular function become apparent when extreme changes occur in the body fluid composition or acid-base balance. For example, with systemic acidosis the rate and amount of total acid excretion (bicarbonate, titratable acid, ammonium) are reduced.[58,60] This predisposes the elderly patient to metabolic acidosis, volume depletion, and hyperchloremia. At a normal pH level, however, the kidney of an elderly person can maintain acid-base homeostasis.

The senescent kidney has diminished capability to excrete a free water load, conserve water during periods of dehydration, and conserve sodium during periods of low salt intake.[58] Elderly persons are at high risk for dehydration because of these renal changes, along with decreased overall total body water, decreased concentrating ability, and decreased thirst perception.[61] Age-related changes also occur in extrarenal mechanisms, such as the decreased activity and responsiveness of the senescent kidney to the sympathetic nervous system and renin-angiotensin-aldosterone system, which are important in integrating overall fluid homeostasis and maintaining blood pressure in response to changes in body position.[34]

Renal System Summary

- A decreased renal blood flow leads to a decrease in glomerular filtration and decreased renal tubule function.
- There is decreased elimination of physiologic substances (blood urea nitrogen [BUN] and creatinine).

GASTROINTESTINAL SYSTEM

Age-related gastrointestinal changes occur in the processes of swallowing, motility, and absorption.[62,63] Swallowing may be difficult for the elderly person because of incomplete mastication of food.[63] Deteriorating dentition, diminished lubrication (secondary to salivary dysfunction), and poorly fitting dentures result in insufficient mastication of food within the oral cavity, predisposing the elderly patient to aspiration.[62] In addition, the number and velocity of the peristaltic contractions of the elderly person's esophagus decrease, and the number of nonperistaltic contractions increases.[63]

These changes in esophageal motility are referred to as presbyesophagus. These changes may predispose the patient to erosion of the esophageal wall (recurrent esophagitis) because food remains in the esophagus longer. In addition, bed rest and reclining in a supine position for a prolonged period can cause esophageal reflux, which also can lead to esophagitis.

The aging process produces thinning of the smooth muscle within the gastric mucosa.[64] The epithelial layer of the gastric mucosa, which contains the chief and parietal cells, undergoes a modest degree of atrophy, resulting in the hyposecretion of pepsin and acid, respectively.[65]

Mucin secretion from the mucous cells decreases, thereby altering the protective function of the gastric mucosal (bicarbonate) barrier. Because of this, the stomach wall is more susceptible to acid injury, thus increasing the incidence of gastric ulcerations.[66] Aging does not appreciably alter gastric emptying of solid foods. Alterations within the small intestine include a decrease in intestinal weight after age 50 and a flattening and shortening of jejunal villi.[67] Age produces no change in the small intestine's absorption of fats and proteins; however, decreased carbohydrate absorption has been reported.[68,69] There is essentially no change in vitamin or mineral absorption, except for a decrease in calcium absorption from the aged duodenum.[63]

Liver

With advancing age, both hepatocyte number and liver weight decrease.[70] Total liver blood flow decreases by 50% between 25 and 65 years of age.[70-72] The liver has many complex functions, including carbohydrate storage, ketone body formation, reduction/conjugation of adrenal and gonadal steroid hormones, synthesis of plasma proteins, deamination of amino acids, storage of cholesterol, urea formation, and detoxification of toxins and drugs. Despite changes in hepatocyte number and blood flow, however, liver function is not appreciably altered.[72] Several liver function tests, including serum bilirubin, alkaline phosphatase, and aspartate aminotransferase (AST) levels, are not altered with advancing age. However, because of the decrease in total liver blood flow, first-pass clearance of drugs is somewhat reduced. The most important age-related change in liver function is the decrease in the liver's capacity to metabolize drugs.[73,74] Although liver function tests do not reflect this change in metabolism, it is well recognized that drug side effects and toxic effects occur more frequently in older adults than in young adults.[74]

Gastrointestinal System Summary

- Gastric emptying, splenic blood flow, and GI motility are decreased; GI pH and thinning or reduction of absorptive surface of the gut are increased.
- Absorption rates are decreased.
- Bacterial colonization of duodenum is increased.
- There is a decline in drug metabolism by hepatic enzymes.

CENTRAL NERVOUS SYSTEM

Cognitive Functioning

Cognitive functioning involves the process of transforming, synthesizing, storing, and retrieving sensory input. Additional components include perception, attention, thinking, memory, and problem solving. For the aging individual, cognition is altered by the speed at which information is processed and retrieved.[75] Performance on timed tests declines slowly after age 20 years. Intelligence remains fairly stable after age 30 until the mid-80s. Although the rate at which complex tasks are completed may be diminished, these age-related changes are not synonymous with cognitive impairment.

Marked deterioration of any component of cognitive functioning is not a normal expectation of the aging process.[76] Cognitive impairment in older adults more often results from acute and chronic etiologies. Acute problems such as infection, electrolyte imbalance, and pharmacologic toxicity are generally reversible once identified. Long-term chronic impairment develops from more organic causations, such as multi-infarct dementia or Alzheimer's disease.[77]

Changes in Structure and Morphology

The brain decreases approximately 20% in size between 25 and 95 years of age (Figure 7-2).[78] The reduced brain weight may be related in part to the overall decrease in the number of neurons that occurs with advancing age. Neurons are lost from the hippocampus, amygdala, and cerebellum and from areas of the brain stem such as the locus ceruleus, dorsal motor nucleus of vagus nerve, and substantia nigra.[75] In contrast, very few neurons disappear with advancing age in areas such as the hypothalamus.[77] In addition, portions of the cerebral cortex atrophy, principally the frontal (superior frontal gyrus) and temporal (superior temporal gyrus) cortical association areas.[78]

The cerebral ventricles enlarge and develop an asymmetric appearance. Cerebrospinal fluid (CSF) also accumulates in the ventricles, although total brain CSF is not increased.[79] Accompanying the loss of neurons are changes in the ultrastructure and intracellular structures of the neuron.[80] Also, neuron shrinkage and degenerative changes in the cell bodies and axons of certain acetylcholine-secreting neurons have been reported. There are also increases in norepinephrine and dopamine synthesis.[81] These changes may explain alterations in processing and receiving information.[77]

In the senescent brain, synaptogenesis (synaptic regeneration) still occurs after partial nerve degeneration. After a nerve fiber is damaged, neighboring undamaged neurons often sprout new fibers and form new connections. However, synaptogenesis occurs at a slower rate in the older brain.[80]

Cerebral Metabolism and Blood Flow

Cerebral blood flow decreases with advancing age. This decrease parallels the decrease in brain weight and is most likely caused by the reduction in neuron number and metabolic needs of the cerebral tissue.[82]

Central Nervous System Summary

- The dilation of the ventricle results in a decrease in the number of Purkinje cells and loss of cells in the vestibular system.
- There are changes in neurotransmitter synthesis and function, and there is degeneration of the blood-brain barrier.
- Abnormal changes in gyral function, senile plaque formation, formation of neurofibrillary tangles, and a decrease in brain volume may occur.

Communication problems associated with tracheal intubation and age-related changes in visual acuity and hearing may affect the accurate assessment of cognitive and neurological status.[83,84]

IMMUNE SYSTEM

Several changes in immune function render the older adult more susceptible to infections.[83-88] Infections in the geriatric population are associated with higher rates of mortality.[88] Common infections in the older adult include bacterial pneumonia, urinary tract infection, intraabdominal infections, gram-negative bacteremia, and decubitus ulcers.[88] The reasons for the increased susceptibility are multifactorial and include changes in cell- and humoral-mediated immunity; breakdown in physical barriers, such as the skin and oral mucosa; and changes in nutrition.

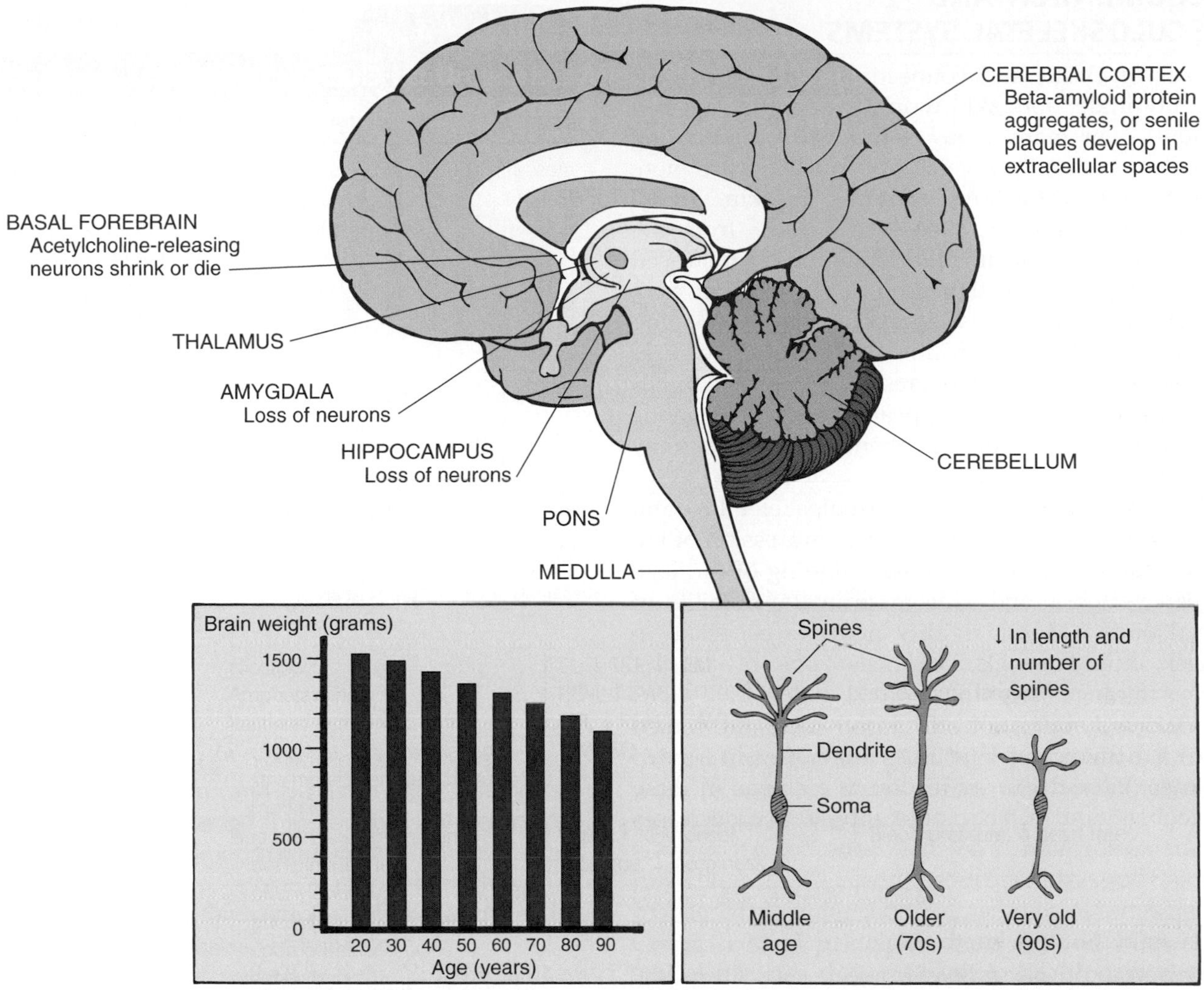

FIGURE 7-2. Summary of age-related changes in the brain. (From Selkoe DJ: *Sci Am* 267:135, 1992.)

Cell-Mediated and Humoral-Mediated Immunity

Immune system function depends on many cell types with distinct functions. T cells are the primary effector of cell-mediated immunity, whereas bone marrow–derived B cells produce antibodies that are the effector cells of humoral-mediated immunity.[83,85,87] With aging, cell-mediated immunity declines. Even though the total number of T cells remains unchanged with advancing age, T-cell function decreases.[85,87] For example, there is a decrease in T-cell production of interleukin-2 (IL-2) and in differentiation of T cells into effector cells. IL-2 is essential for activating B cells, which eventually differentiate into antibody-secreting cells. Subsets of T cells mature into cytotoxic cells, whereas other T cells activate B cells and stimulate B-cell proliferation. Changes in B-lymphocyte function are not as well understood, even though with age the ability of B cells to produce antibodies into new antigens declines.[83,85]

Furthermore, inadequate emptying of urine secondary to bed rest, obstruction, or side effects from anticholinergic medications can result in stagnation of urine and recurrent urinary tract infections. Long-term placement of urinary catheters is a significant source of bacteriuria. However, treatment with antibiotic therapy is not indicated unless the patient becomes symptomatic with anorexia or cognitive impairment or has a history of a chronic illness such as diabetes or chronic obstructive pulmonary disease.[83,88,91]

Immune System Summary

- The number of gamma and helper T cells increases; suppressor/cytotoxic T lymphocytes decrease; germinal centers of lymph nodes decrease; and plasma cells and lymphocytes in the bone marrow increase.
- Cell surface characteristics of lymphocytes change.
- There are impaired humoral immune and antibody responses.

INTEGUMENTARY AND MUSCULOSKELETAL SYSTEMS

The loss of elastic and connective tissue causes the skin to wrinkle; both skin wrinkles and sagging may be found over many areas of the body. Underlying structures, such as the veins and muscles, are more visible because of the transparency of the skin.

Multiple ecchymotic areas may result from decreased protective subcutaneous tissue layers, increased capillary fragility, and flattening of the capillary bed, all of which predispose elderly persons to developing ecchymosis.[92-95] In conjunction with frequent aspirin use, these physiologic factors result in increased bleeding tendencies and the appearance of ecchymotic areas. However, areas of unexplained ecchymosis may also indicate elder abuse.

Changes that occur in the musculoskeletal system are a decrease in lean body mass, compression of the spinal column resulting from the thinning of cartilage between vertebra, and a decrease in the mobility of skeletal joints.[96] Muscle rigidity increases, especially in the neck, shoulders, hips, and knees,[97] possibly causing changes in range of motion.

Bone demineralization affects both men and women as they age but occurs four times more often in women than men. Bone demineralization refers to an increase in osteoblast and osteoclast activity, which decreases calcium absorption into the bone.[96] Osteoporosis produces bones that are more "porous" or fragile. With extensive bone demineralization, an elderly patient may sustain multiple fractures.

INTEGUMENTARY AND MUSCULOSKELETAL SYSTEMS SUMMARY

- Loss of elasticity and connective tissue
- Decreased protective subcutaneous tissue layers
- Decrease in lean body mass
- Compression of the spinal column
- Decrease in mobility of skeletal joints
- Bone demineralization

CHANGES IN PHARMACOKINETICS AND PHARMACODYNAMICS

The many benefits of modern advancements in pharmacologic therapy are frequently counterbalanced by adverse drug effects, medication interactions, and therapeutic failure.[84] Adverse drug effects and medication interactions are related to pharmacokinetics and pharmacodynamics. There are many age-related changes in drug pharmacokinetics, which is the manner in which the body absorbs, distributes, metabolizes, and excretes a drug.[84,98,99] The aging process is associated with changes in gastric acid secretion, which can alter the ionization or solubility of a drug and hence its absorption[98,99] (Table 7-3).

Table 7-3
Age-Related Changes in Pharmacokinetics

ACTION	DEFINITION	CHANGES
Absorption	Receptor-coupled or diffusional uptake of drug into tissue	Decreased absorptive surface area of small intestine Decreased splanchnic blood flow Increased gastric acid pH Decreased gastrointestinal motility
Distribution	Theoretic space (tissue) or body compartment into which free form of drug distributes	Decreased lean body mass and total body water Increased total body fat Decreased serum albumin level Increased α_1-acid glycoprotein
Metabolism	Chemical change in drug that renders it active or inactive	Decreased liver mass Decreased activity of microsomal drug-metabolizing enzyme system Decreased total liver blood flow
Excretion	Removal of drug through an eliminating organ, often the kidney; some drugs are excreted in bile or feces, in saliva, or through the lungs	Decreased renal blood flow and glomerular filtration rate Decreased distal renal tubular secretory function

Data from Gilman AG et al, editors: *Goodman and Gilman's the pharmacological basis of therapeutics,* ed 8, London, 1990, Pergamon; and Vestal RE, Cusack BJ: In Schneider EL, Rowe JW, editors: *Handbook of the biology of aging,* San Diego, 1990, Academic Press.

Drug distribution depends on body composition, as well as the physiochemical properties of the drug. With advancing age, fat content increases, lean body mass decreases, and total body water decreases, which can alter the drug disposition.[99] For example, because of the increase in the ratio of body fat content to body weight, lipophilic drugs have a greater volume of distribution per body weight in older adults as compared with younger adults. Other age-related factors[98,100] affecting drug disposition are listed in Table 7-3.

As noted, the senescent liver and kidneys are less able to metabolize and excrete drugs, which also affects clinical outcomes. For example, the rate of absorption, time to peak plasma concentration, and clearance of loop diuretics is reduced in older adults, which may necessitate high dosing regimens in order to facilitate diuresis.[101,102] This poses an increased risk of metabolic acidosis, because the higher diuretic dose increases competition for the organic acid transport pathway at the proximal tubule. Using the example of diuretics, bioavailability between agents may also be variable. For instance, bumetanide has a fairly consistent bioavailability in advanced age, whereas that of furosemide varies from 20% to 80%.[102]

Similarly, other drugs associated with management of common disorders seen in critically ill patients—such as digoxin, angiotensin II–converting enzyme (ACE) inhibitors, and angiotensin II–receptor blockers (ARBs)[100]—have delayed excretion, increased serum concentration, and more prolonged duration of action because their excretion parallels GFR (which decreases with age).[100] See Table 7-3 for age-related changes in drug pharmacokinetics and Table 7-4[101-110] for the potential side effects, nursing interventions, and/or special considerations for frequently used pharmacologic agents in the elderly patient in the critical care unit.

Age-related changes in pharmacodynamics have also been reported. Pharmacodynamics refers to the pharmacologic or physiologic response to a drug that occurs after the drug interacts with its receptor on the plasma membrane. The chronotropic and inotropic effects of β-adrenergic agonists reportedly decrease in elderly patients.[111,112] There also are reports that age produces no change in heparin-stimulated increases in partial thromboplastin time, whereas the effects of warfarin (Coumadin) are very susceptible to medication interactions.

The use of multiple medications in the presence of multiple comorbidities has been associated with an increase in adverse drug reactions. Although this is not always avoidable, it is important to avoid choosing an agent for its side effect profile (e.g., diphenhydramine for sedative effects) and monitor the effects of the chosen agent. A major cause of therapeutic failure is the underuse or inappropriate use of drug therapy that is indicated for the treatment of a particular problem. It is not uncommon for delirium not associated with a withdrawal syndrome to be treated with benzodiazepines in critical care. However, this frequently makes agitation worse, once the sedative effects are gone, in comparison to a low-dose antipsychotic agent.[113,114]

Box 7-1

Effects of Aging on Various Laboratory Values

Values That Do Not Change With Age
- Hemoglobin/hematocrit
- Platelet count
- White blood cell count with differential
- Serum electrolytes
- Coagulation profile
- Liver function tests
- Thyroid function tests
- ↔ or ↓ Blood urea nitrogen
- ↔ or ↓ Creatinine

Values That Change With Age But Have Little Clinical Significance
- ↓ Calcium
- ↑ Uric acid

Values That Change With Age and Have Clinical Significance
- ↓ Erythrocyte sedimentation rate
- ↓ Arterial oxygen tension (partial pressure)
- ↑ Blood glucose
- ↓ or ↑ Serum lipid profile
- ↓ Albumin

From Duthie EH, Abbasi AA: *Geriatrics* 46:41, 1991.
↔, No change; ↓, decreased; ↑, increased.

SUMMARY

The elderly patient requires more intense observation and consideration in the critical care unit. The patient's system has become less adaptable to stress and illness, and changes in laboratory values may be clinically significant[115,116] (Box 7-1). The major changes in the various systems require specific clinical considerations (Table 7-5).[117] Many physiologic changes occur with advancing age, and each change may render a particular system less adaptable to stress (Figure 7-3). In addition, a change in one system may affect another system in the presence of disease.

evolve To test your mastery of this chapter, try the Open-Book Quiz at http://evolve.elsevier.com/Urden/priorities/

Table 7-4

Pharmacologic Management: Gerontologic Patients

PHARMACOLOGIC AGENT	DRUG ACTIONS	ADVERSE DRUG EFFECTS*	NURSING INTERVENTIONS AND/OR SPECIAL CONSIDERATIONS
ACE Inhibitors			
Captopril Enalapril	Inhibits the conversion of angiotensin I to angiotensin II	Hypotension, especially in patients taking diuretics Hypokalemia	Monitor HR and BP Monitor serum creatinine level Monitor serum K^+ level Excreted by the kidney so the dosage is reduced if the GFR is reduced
Diuretics			
Bumetanide			
Furosemide	Inhibits Na^+ and Cl^- absorption from the proximal tubule and loop of Henle	Hypokalemia Volume depletion	Reduced rate of clearance and magnitude of the diuretic response
Cardiac Glycosides			
Digoxin	Inhibits the sarcolemmal Na^+/K^+-ATPase	Digitalis toxicity	Monitor HR and serum K^+ and serum digoxin levels
Dopamine	α_1-Adrenergic agonist, dopaminergic agonist	Ectopic beats, hypotension	Verapamil, quinidine, and amiodarone increase serum digoxin levels
Dobutamine	Sympathomimetic, β_1-adrenergic agonist		
Antidysrhythmics			
Procainamide	Decreases myocardial conduction velocity and excitability and prolongs myocardial refractoriness	Procainamide toxicity	Procainamide is converted to its active metabolite, N-acetylprocainamide (NAPA), in the liver; NAPA may accumulate and cause side effects, even though the procainamide plasma level is within therapeutic range
Lidocaine	Decreases automaticity (especially in Purkinje fibers) and prolongs conduction and refractoriness	Dizziness, paresthesia, and drowsiness at lower plasma concentrations	Can be administered only parenterally
Calcium Channel Blockers			
Verapamil	Blocks the entry of Ca^{++} through voltage-dependent Ca^{++} channels and decreases SA automaticity and AV conduction	Constipation May alter liver function	Monitor liver function tests Contraindicated in heart failure, sick sinus syndrome, or first-degree AV block
Nifedipine		Headaches, tachycardia, palpitations, flushing, and ankle edema	Calcium channel blockers have a negative inotropic effect, but nifedipine produces less of a negative inotropic effect as compared with verapamil
Diltiazem		Constipation	Monitor liver function tests Contraindicated in heart failure, sick sinus syndrome, or first-degree AV block
Narcotic Analgesics			
Meperidine	Blocks the transmission of pain and inhibits the release of substance P; site of action is within the CNS	Respiratory depression and oversedation Tremors and muscle twitches related to effects of the metabolite normeperidine	Accumulation of normeperidine can produce CNS hyperexcitability
Morphine	Synthetic analgesic; mechanism similar to meperidine	Respiratory depression and oversedation	The volume of distribution for morphine is small; hence plasma and tissue levels are greater at a specific plasma concentration

Data modified from Creasy WA et al: *J Clin Pharmacol* 26:264, 1986; Gilman AG et al, editors: *Goodman and Gilman's the continued pharmacologic basis of therapeutics,* London, 1990, Pergamon; Hockings N, Ajayi AA, Reid JL: *Br J Pharmacol* 21:341, 1986; Lynch RA, Horowitz LN: *Geriatrics* 46:41, 1991; Pederson KE: *Acta Med Scan* 697(suppl 1):1, 1985; Vidt GD, Borazanian RA: *Geriatrics* 46:28, 1991; Wall RT: *Clin Geriatr Med* 6:345, 1990; and Watters JM, McClaran JC. In Wilmore DW et al, editors: *Care of the surgical patient,* vol 7, Special problems, New York, 1990, Scientific American.

HR, Heart rate; *BP,* blood pressure; *GFR,* glomerular filtration rate; *Na^+,* sodium; *Cl^-,* chloride; *K^+*, potassium; *Ca^{++}*, calcium; *SA,* sinoatrial; *AV,* atrioventricular; *CNS,* central nervous system.

*Not all side effects are listed for each drug.

Table 7-5

Summary of Age-Related Physiologic Changes and Related Clinical Considerations

AGE-RELATED EFFECT	CLINICAL CONSIDERATIONS
Cardiovascular System	
↓ Inotropic and chronotropic response of myocardium to catecholamine stimulation	The increase in CO achieved during stress or exercise is achieved by an increase in diastolic filling (increased dependence on Starling's law of the heart)
↑ Myocardial collagen content	Leads to a decrease in the compliance of the ventricle (higher filling pressures are needed to maintain stroke volume)
↓ Baroreceptor sensitivity	↑ Tendency for orthostatic hypotension after prolonged bed rest or if patient is taking antihypertensive medication or has systolic hypertension
Prolonged rate of relaxation	May predispose the elderly patient to hemodynamic derangements in the presence of tachydysrhythmias, hypertension, or ischemic heart disease
↓ Compliance of blood vessels	↑ Peripheral vascular resistance and blood pressure
Respiratory System	
↓ Strength of the respiratory muscles, recoil of lungs, chest wall compliance, and efficiency and number of cilia in airways	↑ Susceptibility to aspiration, atelectasis, and pulmonary infection Patient may require more frequent deep breathing, coughing, and position change
↓ Pao_2 level	↓ Ventilatory response to hypoxia and hypercapnia ↑ Sensitivity to narcotics
Renal System	
↓ GFR	Careful observation of patient when administering aminoglycosides, antibiotics, and contrast dyes
↓ Ability to concentrate and conserve water	May predispose patient to development of dehydration and hypernatremia, especially if patient is fluid-restricted and insensible losses are high (e.g., during mechanical ventilation or fever)
↓ Ability to excrete salt and water loads, as well as urea, ammonia, and drugs	Observe for clinical manifestations of fluid overload and drug reactions
↓ Response to an acid load	After an acid load (i.e., metabolic acidosis) the elderly patient may be in a state of uncompensated metabolic acidosis for a longer period
Liver	
↓ Total liver blood flow	Adverse drug reactions, especially with polypharmacy
Gastrointestinal System	
Diminished ability to swallow Impaired esophageal motility Delayed emptying of liquids ↓ Stool weight and transit time	May predispose elderly patient to aspiration pneumonia Assess for proper fit of dentures and ability to chew Flex head forward 45 degrees Develop awareness for complaints of food or medications "sticking in throat" Assess for complaints of heartburn or epigastric discomfort Avoid prolonged supine position Examine abdomen for distention Investigate complaints of anorexia Obtain thorough bowel history and note routine use of laxatives Increase intake of dietary fiber and assess for fecal incontinence and impaction
Neurologic System	
↑ Cranial dead space	Elderly persons may sustain a significant amount of hemorrhage before symptoms are apparent
↓ Number of neurons and dendrites and length of dendrite spines	Delayed or impaired processing of sensory and motor information
Delay in the rate of synaptogensis Changes in neurotransmitter turnover	May cause desynchronization of neurotransmission

Modified from Rebenson-Piano M: *Crit Care Q* 12:1, 1989.
CO, Cardiac output; *GFR,* glomerular filtration rate.

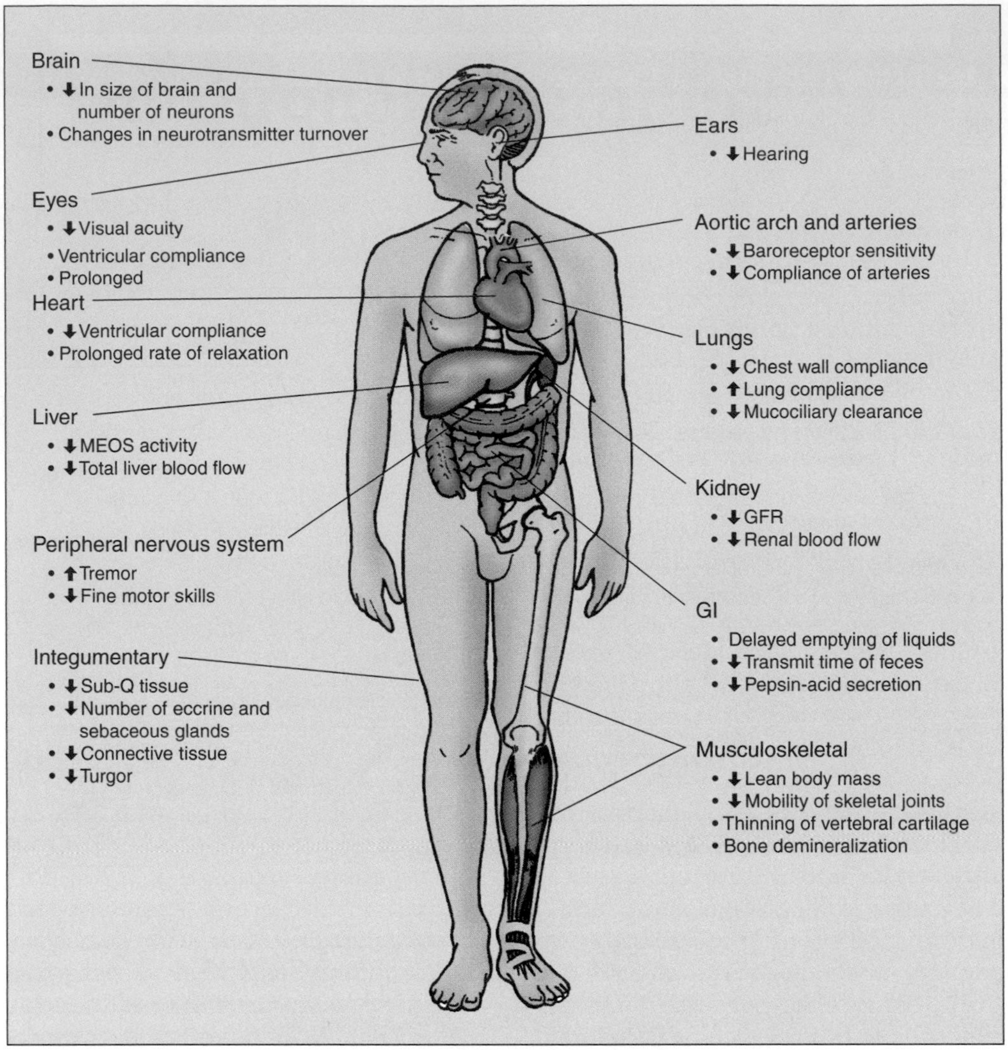

FIGURE 7-3. Summary of physiologic changes that occur in all systems and that the critical care nurse must consider in caring for elderly patients in the critical care unit. *MEOS,* Microsomal enzyme oxidative system; *GFR,* glomerular filtration rate; *GI,* gastrointestinal; *Sub-Q,* subcutaneous.

REFERENCES

1. *Profile of Older Americans,* 2003, Administration on Aging, US Department of Health and Human Services, http://www.aoa.dhhs.gov/aoa/stats/profile/default.html.
2. Resnick NM: Geriatric medicine. In Braunwald E et al, editors: *Harrison's principles of internal medicine,* ed 15, New York, 2001, McGraw Hill.
3. Levine BS, Craven RF: Physiologic adaptations with aging. In Woods SL et al, editors: *Cardiac nursing,* ed 5, Philadelphia, 2005, Lippincott Williams & Wilkins.
4. Polanczyk C et al: Impact of age on perioperative complications and length of stay in patients undergoing noncardiac surgery, *Ann Intern Med* 134:637, 2001.
5. Eghbali M et al: Collagen accumulation in heart ventricles as a function of growth and aging, *Cardiovasc Res* 23:723, 1989.
6. Wegelius O, von Knorring J: The hydroxyproline and hexosamine content in human myocardium at different ages, *Acta Med Scand Suppl* 412:233, 1964.
7. Katz AM: Heart failure. In Fozzard HA et al, editors: *The heart and cardiovascular system,* New York, 1991, Raven.
8. Eaton L: Cardiovascular function. In Lueckenotte AG, editor: *Gerontologic nursing,* ed 2, St Louis, 2000, Mosby.
9. Lakatta EG, Schulman SP, Gerstenblith G: Cardiovascular aging in health and therapeutic considerations in older patients with cardiovascular diseases. In Fuster V et al, editors: *Hurst's the heart,* ed 10, New York, 2001, McGraw-Hill.
10. Gerstenblith G et al: Echocardiographic assessment of normal adult aging population, *Circulation* 56:273, 1977.
11. Opie LH: *The physiology of the heart and metabolism,* New York, 1991, Raven.
12. Lakatta EG et al: Prolonged contraction duration in the aged myocardium, *J Clin Invest* 55:61, 1975.
13. Cinelli P et al: Effects of age on mean heart rate variability, *Aging* 10:146, 1987.

14. Ribera JM et al: Cardiac rate and hyperkinetic rhythm disorders in healthy elderly subjects: evaluation by ambulatory electrocardiographic monitoring, *Gerontology* 35:158, 1989.
15. Aronow WS: Effects of aging on the heart. In Tallis RC, Fillit HM, editors: *Brocklehurst's textbook of geriatric medicine and gerontology,* ed 6, London, 2003, Churchill Livingstone.
16. Bonow RO et al: Effects of aging on asynchronous left ventricular regional function and global ventricular filling in normal human subjects, *J Am Coll Cardiol* 11:50, 1988.
17. Miller TR et al: Left ventricular diastolic filling and its association with age, *Am J Cardiol* 58:531, 1986.
18. Davidson WR, Fee WC: Influence of aging on pulmonary hemodynamics in a population free of coronary artery disease, *Am J Cardiol* 65:1454, 1990.
19. Bachman S, Sparrow D, Smith LK: Effect of aging on the electrocardiogram, *Am J Cardiol* 48:513, 1981.
20. Horwitz LN, Lynch RA: Managing geriatric arrhythmias. I. General considerations, *Geriatrics* 46:31, 1991.
21. Carom AJ et al: The rhythm of the heart in active elderly subjects, *Am Heart J* 99:598, 1980.
22. Fleg JL, Kennedy HL: Cardiac arrhythmias in 9 healthy elderly population: detection by a 24-hour ambulatory electrocardiography, *Chest* 81:638, 1982.
23. Aronow WS: Cardia arrhythmias. In Tallis RC, Fillit HM, editors: *Brocklehurst's textbook of geriatric medicine and gerontology,* ed 6, London, 2003, Churchill Livingstone.
24. Docherty JR: Cardiovascular responses in ageing: a review, *Pharmacol Rev* 42:103, 1990.
25. Opie LH: *The physiology of the heart and metabolism,* New York, 1991, Raven.
26. Smith JJ et al: The effect of age on hemodynamic response to graded postural stress in normal men, *J Gerontol* 42:406, 1987.
27. Dambrink JHA, Wieling W: Circulatory response to postural change in healthy male subjects in relation to age, *Clin Sci* 72:335, 1987.
28. Applegate WB et al: Prevalence of postural hypotension at baseline in the Systolic Hypertension in the Elderly Program (SHEP) cohort, *J Am Geriatr Soc* 39:1057, 1991.
29. Stanley JA: Congestive heart failure in the elderly, *Geriatr Nurs* 20:180, 2000.
30. Bierman EL: Arteriosclerosis and aging. In Finch CE, Schneider EL, editors: *Handbook of the biology of aging,* New York, 1985, Van Nostrand Reinhold.
31. Schoenberger JA: Epidemiology of systolic and diastolic systemic blood pressure elevation in the elderly, *Am J Cardiol* 57:45, 1986.
32. Rowe JW: Clinical consequences of age-related impairments in vascular compliance, *Am J Cardiol* 60:68, 1987.
33. Rose BD: *Clinical physiology of acid-base and electrolyte disorders,* New York, 1989, McGraw-Hill.
34. Hall JE, Coleman TG, Guyton AC: The renin-angiotensin system: normal physiology and changes in older hypertensives, *J Am Geriatr Soc* 37:801, 1989.
35. Crane MG, Harris JJ: Effect of aging on renin activity and aldosterone excretion, *J Lab Clin Med* 87:947, 1976.
36. Sica DA, Harford A: Sodium and water disorders in the elderly. In Zawada ET, Sica DA, editors: *Geriatric nephrology and urology,* Littleton, Mass, 1985, PSG.
37. Webster JR, Kadah H: Unique aspects of respiratory disease in the aged, *Geriatrics* 46:31, 1991.
38. Sheahan SL, Musialowski R: Clinical implications of respiratory system changes in aging, *J Gerontol Nurs* 27(5):26, 2001.
39. Levitzky MG: Effects of aging on the respiratory system, *Physiologist* 27:102, 1984.
40. Mittman C et al: Relationship between chest wall and pulmonary compliance and age, *J Appl Physiol* 20:1211, 1965.
41. Anderson WM, Tockman MS: Aging and the lungs. In Beers MH, Berkow R, editors: *Merck manual of geriatrics,* http://www.merck. com/pubs/mm_geriatrics.
42. Rizzato G, Marazzine L: Thoracoabdominal mechanisms in elderly men, *J Appl Physiol* 28:457, 1970.
43. Gutmann E, Hanzlikova V: Fast and slow motor units in ageing, *Gerontology* 22:280, 1976.
44. Pontoppidan HH, Beecher HK: Progressive loss of protective reflexes in the airway with advance of age, *JAMA* 1974:229, 1960.
45. Knudson RJ et al: Changes in the normal maximal expiratory flow-volume curve with growth and aging, *Am Rev Respir Dis* 127:725, 1983.
46. Turner JM, Mead J, Wohl ME: Elasticity of human lungs in relation to age, *J Appl Physiol* 25:664, 1968.
47. Pierce JA, Hocott JB: Studies on the collagen and elastin content of the human lung, *J Clin Invest* 39:8, 1960.
48. Pierce JA, Ebert RV: Fibrous network of the lung and its change with age, *Thorax* 20:469, 1965.
49. Semmens M: The pulmonary artery in the normal aged lung, *Br J Dis Chest* 64:65, 1970.
50. Sorbini CA et al: Arterial oxygen tension in relation to age in healthy subjects, *Respiration* 25:3, 1968.
51. LeBlanc P, Ruff F, Milic-Emili J: Effects of age and body position on "airway closure" in man, *J Appl Physiol* 28: 448, 1970.
52. Holland J et al: Regional distribution of pulmonary ventilation and perfusion in elderly subjects, *J Clin Invest* 47:81, 1968.
53. Weder AB: The renally compromised older hypertensive: therapeutic considerations, *Geriatrics* 46:36, 1991.
54. Maddox DA, Alavi FK, Zawada ET: The kidney and aging. In Massry SG, Glassock RJ, editors: *Textbook of nephrology,* ed 4, Philadelphia, 2001, Lippincott Williams & Wilkins.
55. Gilbert BR, Vaughan ED: Pathophysiology of the aging kidney, *Clin Geriatric Med* 6(1):12, 1990.
56. Kasiske BL: Relationship between vascular disease and age-associated changes in the human kidney, *Kidney Int* 31:1153, 1987.
57. Anderson S, Brenner BM: Effects of aging on the renal glomerulus, *Am J Med* 80:435, 1986.
58. Weder AB: The renally compromised older hypertensive: therapeutic considerations, *Geriatrics* 46:36, 1991.
59. Gilbert BR, Vaughan ED: Pathophysiology of the aging kidney, *Clin Geriatr Med* 6:12, 1990.
60. Watters JM, McClaran JC: The elderly surgical patient. In Wilmore DW et al, editors: *Care of the surgical patient,* vol 7, Special problems, New York, 1990, Scientific American.
61. Bennett JA: Dehydration: Hazards and benefits, *Geriatr Nurs* 21:84, 2000.

62. Brandt LJ: Gastrointestinal disorders in the elderly. In Rossman I, editor: *Clinical geriatrics,* ed 3, Philadelphia, 1986, Lippincott.
63. Williams SA, Fogel RP: Common gastrointestinal problems in the elderly, *JAMA* 87:29, 1989.
64. Altman DF: Changes in gastrointestinal, pancreatic, biliary and hepatic function in aging, *Gastroenterol Clin North Am* 19:227, 1990.
65. Thomson AB, Keelan M: The aging gut, *Can J Physiol Pharmacol* 64:30, 1986.
66. Bansal SK et al: Upper gastrointestinal hemorrhage in the elderly: a record of 92 patients in a joint geriatric/surgical unit, *Age Aging* 16:279, 1987.
67. Schuster MM: Disorders of the aging GI system, *Hosp Prac* 11:95, 1976.
68. Curran J: Overview of geriatric nutrition, *Dysphagia* 5:72, 1990.
69. Ausman LM, Russel RM: Nutrition and aging. In Schneider EL, Rowe JW, editors: *Handbook of the biology of aging,* San Diego, 1990, Academic Press.
70. Sato TG, Miwa T, Tauchi H: Age changes in the human liver of the different races, *Gerontology* 16:368, 1970.
71. Bach B et al: Disposition of antipyrine and phenytoin correlated with age and liver volume in man, *Clin Pharmacokinet* 6:389, 1981.
72. Kampmann JP, Sinding J, Moller-Jorgensen I: Effect of age on liver function, *Geriatrics* 30:91, 1975.
73. Schmucker DL, Wang RK: Age-related changes in liver drug metabolism: structure versus function, *Proc Soc Exp Biol Med* 165:178, 1980.
74. Vestal RE, Cusack BJ: Pharmacology and aging. In Schneider EL, Rowe JW, editors: *Handbook of the biology of aging,* San Diego, 1990, Academic Press.
75. Katzman R: Human nervous system. In Masoro EJ, editor: *Handbook of physiology: aging,* New York, 1995, Oxford University Press.
76. Foreman MD, Grabowski R: Diagnostic dilemma: cognitive impairment in the elderly, *J Gerontol Nurs* 18:5, 1992.
77. Arriagada P et al: Neurofibrillary tangles but not senile plaques parallel duration and severity of Alzheimer's disease, *Neurology* 42:631, 1992.
78. Selkoe DJ: Aging brain, aging mind, *Sci Am* 267:134, 1992.
79. Morris JC, McManus DQ: The neurology of aging: normal versus pathologic change, *Geriatrics* 46:47, 1991.
80. Lytle LD, Altar A: Diet, central nervous system, and aging, *Fed Proc* 38:2017, 1979.
81. Stuart-Hamilton IA: Normal cognitive aging. In Tallis RC, Fillit HM, editors: *Brocklehurst's textbook of geriatric medicine and gerontology,* ed 6, London, 2003, Churchill Livingstone.
82. Gottstein U, Held K: Effects of aging on cerebral circulation and metabolism in man, *Acta Neurol Scand Suppl* 72:54, 1979.
83. Gravenstein S, Fillit HM, Ershler WB: Clinical immunology of aging. In Tallis RC, Fillit HM, editors: *Brocklehurst's textbook of geriatric medicine and gerontology,* ed 6, London, 2003, Churchill Livingstone.
84. Hanlon JT et al: Geriatric pharmacotherapy. In Tallis RC, Fillit HM, editors: *Brocklehurst's textbook of geriatric medicine and gerontology,* ed 6, London, 2003, Churchill Livingstone.
85. Miller RA: Immune system. In Masoro EJ, editor: *Handbook of physiology: aging,* New York, 1995, Oxford University Press.
86. Terpenning MS, Bradley SF: Why aging leads to increased susceptibility to infection, *Geriatrics* 46:77, 1991.
87. Miller RA: The aging immune system: primer and prospectus, *Science* 273:70, 1996.
88. Rajagopalan S, Moran D: Infectious disease emergencies in older adults, *Clin Geriatr* 9:1, 2001, http://www.mmhc.com/engine.pl?station=mmhc&template=cgfull.html&id=1003.
89. Happ MB, Tate J, Garrett K. Nonspeaking older adults in the ICU, *Am J Nurs* 106(3):29, 2006.
90. McAdams JL, Puntillo KA. Older adults in the ICU, *Am J Nurs* 106(5):30, 2006.
91. President's Commission for the Study of Ethical Problems in Medicine and Biomedical and Behavioral Research: *Deciding to forgo life-sustaining treatment: a report on the ethical, medical and legal issues on treatment decisions,* 1993, Washington, DC, US Government Printing Office.
92. Jones PL, Millman A: Wound healing and the aged patient, *Nurs Clin North Am* 25:263, 1990.
93. Kelly L, Mobily PR: Iatrogenesis in the elderly, *J Gerontol Nurs* 17(9):24, 1991.
94. Shenefelt PD, Fenske NA: Aging and the skin: recognizing and managing common disorders, *Geriatrics* 45(10):57, 1990.
95. Wenger NK: Cardiovascular disease in the elderly, *Curr Probl Cardiol* 17(10):609, 1992.
96. Kalu DN: Bone. In Masoro EJ, editor: *Handbook of physiology: aging,* New York, 1995, Oxford University Press.
97. Exton-Smith AN: Mineral metabolism. In Finch CE, Schneider EL, editors: *Handbook of the biology of aging,* New York, 1985, Van Nostrand Reinhold.
98. Guay DRP et al: The pharmacology of aging. In Tallis RC, Fillit HM, editors: *Brocklehurst's textbook of geriatric medicine and gerontology,* ed 6, London, 2003, Churchill Livingstone.
99. Yuen GJ: Altered pharmacokinetics in the elderly, *Clin Geriatric Med* 6:257, 1990.
100. Schwertz DW, Bushmann MT: Pharmacogeriatics, *Crit Care Q* 12:26, 1989.
101. Gilman AG et al, editors: *Goodman and Gilman's the pharmacological basis of therapeutics,* ed 8, London, 1990, Pergamon.
102. Gillespie ND, Struthers AD: Chronic cardiac failure. In Tallis RC, Fillit HM, editors: *Brocklehurst's textbook of geriatric medicine and gerontology,* ed 6, London, 2003, Churchill Livingstone.
103. Watters JM, McClaran JC: The elderly surgical patient. In Wilmore DW et al, editors: *Care of the surgical patient,* vol 7, Special problems, New York, 1990, Scientific American.
104. The SCOPE Study Group: The study on cognition and prognosis in the elderly (SCOPE): principal results of a randomized double-blind intervention trial, *J Hypertension* 21:875, 2003.
105. Mooradian AD: An update of the clinical pharmacokinetics, therapeutic monitoring techniques and treatment recommendations, *Clin Pharmacokinet* 18:165, 1988.

106. Creasy WA et al: Pharmacokinetics of captopril in elderly healthy male volunteers, *J Clin Pharmacol* 26:264, 1986.
107. Hockings N, Ajayi AA, Reid JL: Age and the pharmacodynamics of angiotensin converting enzyme inhibitors, enalapril and enalaprilat, *Br J Pharmacol* 21:341, 1986.
108. Pederson KE: Digoxin interactions: the influence of quinidine and verapamil on the pharmacokinetics and receptor binding of digitalis glycosides, *Acta Med Scand* 697(suppl 1):1, 1985.
109. Lynch RA, Horowitz LN: Managing geriatric arrhythmias. II. Drug selection and use, *Geriatrics* 46:41, 1991.
110. Vidt GD, Borazanian RA: Calcium channel blockers in geriatric hypertension, *Geriatrics* 46:28, 1991.
111. Bertel O et al: Decreased beta-adrenoreceptor responsiveness as related to age, blood pressure and plasma catecholamines in patients with essential hypertension, *Hypertension* 2:130, 1980.
112. Kendall MJ et al: Responsiveness to beta-adrenergic receptor stimulation: the effects of age are cardioselective, *Br J Clin Pharmacol* 14:821, 1982.
113. Pompei P: Delirium. In Tallis RC, Fillit HM, editors: *Brocklehurst's textbook of geriatric medicine and gerontology,* ed 6, London, 2003, Churchill Livingstone.
114. Litton KA: Delirium in the critical care patient: what the professional staff needs to know, *Crit Care Nurs Q* 26:208, 2003.
115. Cavalieri TA et al: When outside the room is normal: interpreting lab data in the aged, *Geriatrics* 47(5):66, 1992.
116. Kane RL et al: *Essentials of clinical geriatrics,* ed 3, New York, 1994, McGraw-Hill.
117. Rebenson-Piano M: The physiologic changes that occur with aging, *Crit Care Q* 12:1, 1989.

CHAPTER

8 Pain and Pain Management

CELINE GELINAS

OBJECTIVES

- Explain the physiology of pain.
- Discuss how to perform a pain assessment in the critically ill patient.
- Identify patient and health care professional barriers to a pain assessment.
- Describe the pharmacologic and nonpharmacologic interventions for pain management.
- Describe nursing interventions that are essential in the treatment of acute pain.

Pain is an important stressor for patients in critical care settings.[1-5] Many sources of pain have been identified such as acute illness, surgery, trauma, invasive equipment, nursing and medical interventions, and immobility.[6-8] Moderate to severe pain is experienced by patients in critical care, which reinforces the importance of providing attention to pain.[2,3,9-15]

IMPORTANCE OF PAIN ASSESSMENT

Because pain is an important problem in critical care, its detection is a priority. To detect pain, it has to be adequately assessed. Recently, clinical guidelines and recommendations specific to the critically ill for the assessment and the management of pain were made.[16,17] They reinforce McCaffery and Pasero's suggestion[18] that the patient's self-report of pain be obtained as often as possible because it represents the most valid measure of pain. Unfortunately in critical care, many factors affect verbal communication with patients: the administration of sedative agents, mechanical ventilation, and the patient's change in level of consciousness.[6,19,20] These obstacles make pain assessment more complex. Nevertheless, except for being unable to speak, many intubated patients can communicate that they have pain by using facial expressions or hand motions or by seeking attention with other movements.[2] Pain scales have also been used with intubated patients, who point on them to communicate about their pain.[3,11,12] When the patient is unable to verbally communicate, observable indicators clustered as behavioral and physiologic cues become unique indices for pain assessment.[6,7,19,21-23] Indeed, behavioral alterations caused by pain are valuable forms of self-report and should be considered as alternative measures of pain in uncommunicative patients.[24]

Moreover, pain assessment is an important part of the quality of care provided to critically ill patients and an essential part of nursing practice.[25] Because nurses are at the patient's bedside on a continuous basis, they play a major role in pain assessment and management.[26] Despite the growing body of research conducted in the field of pain in critical care, pain is still undertreated.* Lack of education regarding pain, as well as underestimation of patients' pain, and incomplete and difficult pain assessment have been identified as significant barriers to adequate pain management.[15,25,27,30-34]

Undetected and untreated pain can lead to many complications involving the cardiovascular, pulmonary, and neurologic systems.[11,19,23,35-37] Conversely, an adequate pain assessment can lead to better treatment and a decrease in the risks of complications in critically ill patients.[38]

The American Association of Critical-Care Nurses (AACN) identified pain as a priority area for nursing research, and many nursing professional organizations have developed pain management position statements.[39-40] Many health care agencies have increased their vigilance regarding the patient's pain and its management, including designating pain assessment as the fifth vital sign.[41] With the frequency of the diagnosis of pain and the professional responsibility to manage pain, the critical care nurse must understand the mechanisms, assessment process, and appropriate therapeutic measures for managing pain.

A DEFINITION AND DESCRIPTION OF PAIN

Pain is an unpleasant sensory and emotional experience associated with actual or potential tissue damage.[42] Pain is recognized as a subjective and multidimensional experience.[43-45] Its subjective characteristic implies that pain is whatever the experiencing person says it is and

*References 3, 9, 10, 12, 14, 15, 27-30

exists whenever he or she says it does.[18] Its multidimensional characteristics include physiologic, sensory, affective, cognitive, and behavioral components.[46] The physiologic component refers to nociception and the stress response. The sensory component is the perception of many characteristics of pain such as intensity, location, and quality. The affective component includes negative emotions such as anxiety and fear that may be associated with the experience of pain. The cognitive component refers to the interpretation of pain by the person who experiences it. Finally, the behavioral component includes the strategies used by the person to express, avoid, or control pain.

The major types of pain are acute and chronic. Acute pain is short-lasting, usually less than 6 months in duration, and implies tissue damage that is usually from an identifiable cause.[47,48] Acute nociceptive pain is associated with the inflammatory process[49] caused by trauma, surgery, or an acute illness.[47] If undertreated, acute pain can become chronic pain.[50] Chronic pain persists over time, following the process of healing from the original injury, and may or may not be associated with an illness.[48] Chronic pain develops when the healing process is incomplete or when there is permanent damage to the nervous system. It has also been associated with a prolonged stress response.[51]

Both acute and chronic pain can be divided into somatic, visceral, or neuropathic origin. Somatic pain involves superficial tissues such as the skin, muscles, joints, and bones. Its location is well defined. Visceral pain involves organs such as the heart, stomach, and liver. Its location is diffuse and can be referred. Finally, neuropathic or deafferentation pain is described as an abnormal sensory process caused by changes in the excitability of nerve cells. These changes are associated with the acute inflammatory process or with nociceptive nerve damage that can be caused by surgery or an illness process.[52-54] The origin of the pain may be peripheral or central. Neuralgia and phantom pain are peripheral deafferentation pains. Cerebrovascular accidents can cause central deafferentation pain. Neuropathic pain can be difficult to manage and frequently requires a multimodal approach.[18]

PHYSIOLOGY OF PAIN

NOCICEPTION

Nociception refers to the mechanism of pain and engages the sensory, emotional, and cognitive processing areas of the brain.[55] Four processes are involved in nociception[18]:

1. Transduction
2. Transmission
3. Perception
4. Modulation

Illustrations of the four processes are provided in Figures 8-1 and 8-2.

Transduction

Transduction refers to mechanical (e.g., surgical incision), thermal (e.g., burn), or chemical (e.g., toxic substance) stimuli that damage tissues. In critical care many nociceptive stimuli exist, including the patient's acute illness condition, technology used for patients, and multiple interventions that have to be done for them. These stimuli, also called stressors, stimulate the liberation of many chemical substances such as prostaglandins, bradykinin, serotonin, histamine, glutamate, and substance P.[35] These neurotransmitters stimulate peripheral nociceptive receptors and thus serve to initiate nociceptive transmission.

Transmission

As a result of transduction, an action potential is produced and is transmitted by nociceptive nerve fibers in the spinal cord that reach higher centers of the brain. This is called transmission and represents the second process of nociception. The principal nociceptive fibers are the Aδ and C fibers. Small-diameter, myelinated Aδ fibers transmit well-localized, sharp pain. Small-diameter, unmyelinated C fibers transmit diffuse, dull, and aching pain. These fibers transmit the noxious sensation from the periphery to the dorsal route of the spinal cord. With the liberation of substance P, these fibers then synapse with ascending spinothalamic fibers to the central nervous system (CNS). These spinothalamic fibers are clustered into two specific pathways: neospinothalamic (NS) and paleospinothalamic (PS). Generally, the Aδ fibers transmit the pain sensation to the brain within the NS pathway, whereas the C fibers use the PS pathway.[56]

Through synapsing of nociceptive fibers with motor fibers in the spinal cord, muscular rigidity can appear because of a reflex activity.[35] Muscular rigidity can be a behavioral indicator associated with pain. It can contribute to immobility and decrease diaphragmatic excursion. This can lead to hypoventilation and hypoxemia.[35,38] Hypoxemia can be detected by monitoring pulse oximetry (Spo_2) and oxygen arterial pressure (Pao_2). In intubated patients, the alarms of the ventilator could also indicate the presence of pain.[21,57,58]

Perception

The pain message is transmitted by the spinothalamic pathways to centers in the brain where it is perceived. Pain sensation transmitted by the NS pathway reaches the thalamus, whereas the pain sensation transmitted by the PS pathway reaches brain stem, hypothalamus, and thalamus.[56] These parts of the CNS contribute to the initial perception of pain. Projections to the limbic system allow for the expression of the affective component of pain.[45,59] From these lower parts of the CNS, many projections reach higher parts of the CNS. More specifically, projections to the sensory cortex located in the parietal lobe allow the patient to describe

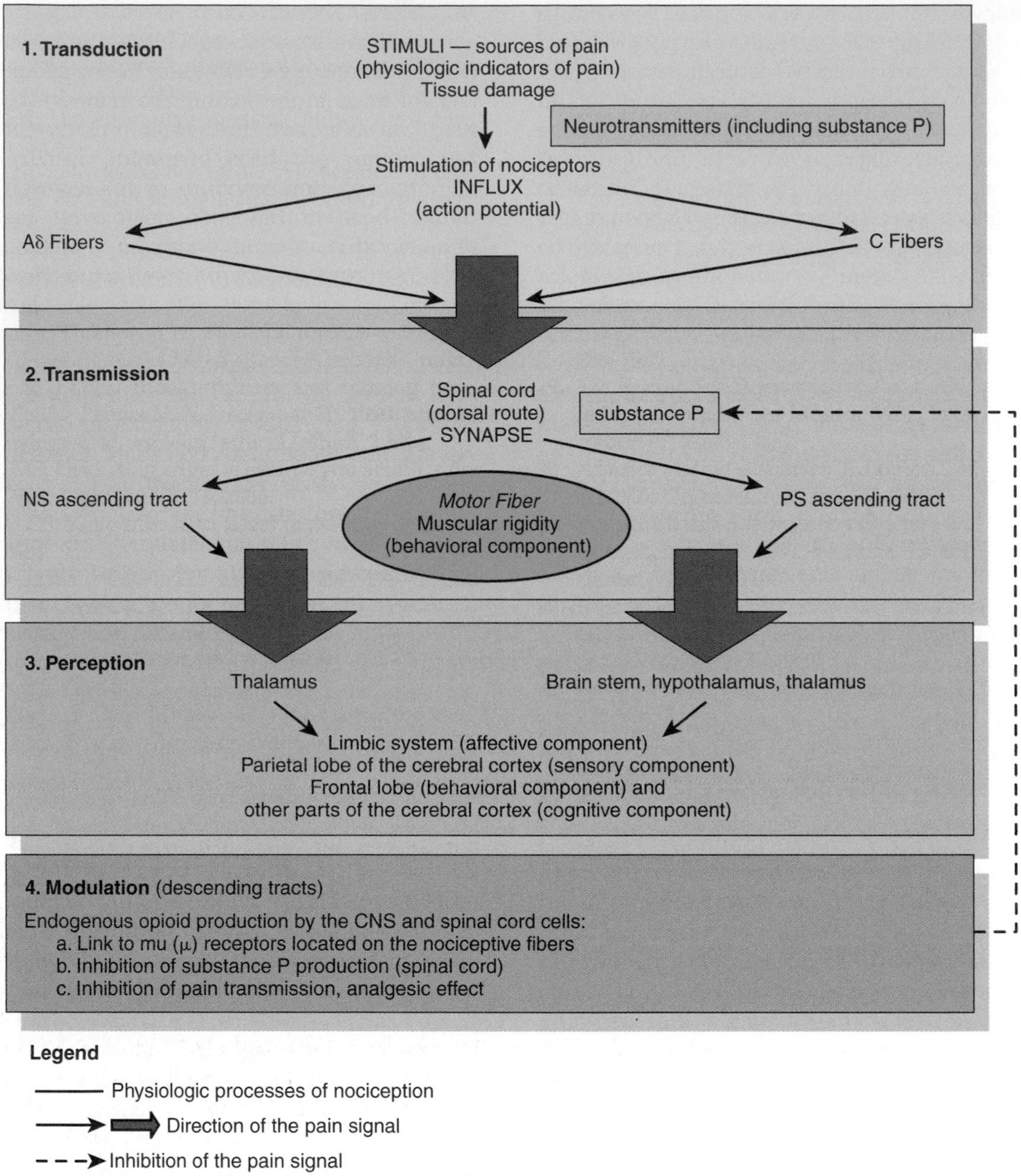

FIGURE 8-1. Integration of pain assessment in the four processes of nociception. (Courtesy Celine Gelinas, School of Nursing, McGill University, Canada.)

the sensory characteristics of his or her pain, such as location, intensity, and quality.[45,56,60] The cognitive component of pain involves many parts of the cerebral cortex and is complex. These three components (affective, sensory, and cognitive) represent the subjective interpretation of pain. Parallel to this subjective process, certain facial expressions and body movements are behavioral indicators of pain occurring as a result of pain fiber projections to the motor cortex located in the frontal lobe.[44,61]

Modulation

Modulation is the liberation of endogenous opioids by the CNS such as β-endorphins, enkephalins, and dynorphins. Endogenous opioids inhibit through the descending pathways the transmission of pain sensation in the spinal cord and produce analgesia. These substances link to mu receptors located on nociceptive fibers, inhibiting the liberation of substance P and blocking the transmission of the pain sensation.[44,56]

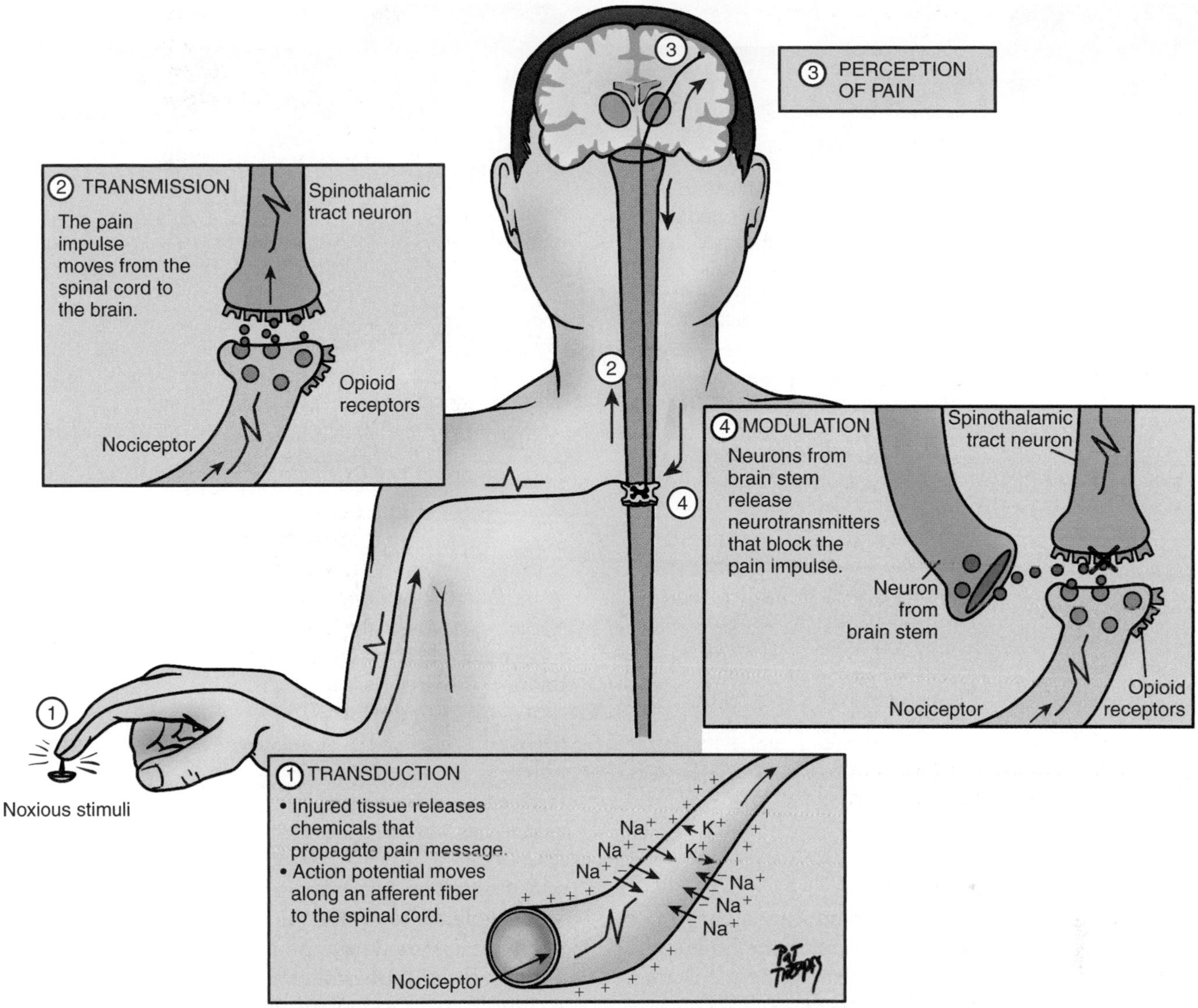

FIGURE 8-2. Illustration of the four processes of nociception. (From Jarvis C: *Physical examination and health assessment*, ed 4, Philadelphia, 2004, Saunders.)

PAIN ASSESSMENT

Pain assessment has two major components: nonobservable/subjective and observable/objective. The complexity of pain assessment requires the use of multiple strategies by critical care clinicians.

Pain Assessment: The Subjective Component

Pain is recognized as a subjective experience. Pain is whatever the patient says it is and exists whenever the patient says it does.[18] Thus the subjective component of pain assessment refers to the patient's self-report of pain about his or her sensorial, affective, and cognitive experience of pain. Because it is the most valid measure of pain, the patient's self-report must be obtained as often as possible.[7,16,62] Mechanical ventilation should not prevent nurses from documenting patients' self-reports of pain. Many intubated patients can communicate having pain[2] or can use pain scales by pointing on them.[3,11,12] Before concluding that a patient is unable to self-report, three attempts to ask the patient about pain are recommended.[7] Sufficient time should be allowed for the patient to respond with each attempt.

If sedation and cognition levels allow the patient to give more information about pain, a multidimensional assessment can be documented. Multidimensional pain assessment tools, including the sensorial, affective, and cognitive components, are available (e.g., Brief Pain Inventory,[63] Initial Pain Assessment Tool,[18] and the short-form McGill Pain Questionnaire[64]). Because intubated patients receive sedative and analgesic agents, a tool must be short enough to be completed. For instance, the short form McGill Pain Questionnaire takes 2 to 3 minutes to complete[64] and has been used with intubated patients.[3,11,12]

Table 8-1

Description of the PQRSTU and Examples of Questions

	DESCRIPTION	EXAMPLES OF QUESTIONS
P	Provocative or palliative/aggravating factors	What caused you pain? What were you doing when the pain appeared? What helps you relieve the pain? What makes the pain worse?
Q	Quality	Describe the pain sensation (e.g., dull, aching, sharp, burning, stabbing).
R	Region or location, radiation	Where do you feel pain? Does the pain spread somewhere else? The patient may answer by pointing to the pain location.
S	Severity and other symptoms	How intense is your pain? Many pain intensity scales are available (see Figure 8-3). Do you feel other discomforts besides pain (e.g., shortness of breath, nausea, anxiety, fatigue)?
T	Timing	When did the pain appear? How long have you been feeling pain? Is pain constant or intermittent?
U	Understanding	What do you think is your pain related to? Have you felt this pain before? If yes, what was the problem?

Table 8-2

Behavioral and Physiologic Indicators for Pain Assessment

INDICATOR FOR PAIN ASSESSMENT	DESCRIPTION
Behavioral	
Facial expression	Grimacing, frowning, wincing, eyes squeezed closed, teeth clenched, wrinkled brow, teary/crying
Body movements	Immobile, slow/cautious movements, touching the pain site or tubes, seeking attention through movements, restlessness
Muscular tension	Rigid, tense, stiff, splinting
Compliance with the ventilator	Coughing, turning the alarms on, fighting the ventilator
Sounds or vocalizations	Groaning, moaning, sighing, sobbing, grunting
Physiologic	
Heart rate	Increase or decrease
Blood pressure	Increase or decrease
Respiratory status	Increase or decrease rate, decrease depth
Spo_2	Decrease
End-tidal CO_2	Increase or decrease
Perspiration	General
Pallor	Skin
Pupil	Dilation

The patient's self-report of pain can also be obtained by questioning the patient using the mnemonic PQRSTU[65] (Table 8-1). Because of the patient's change in communication, lack of concentration secondary to sedation therapies, and the life-or-death immediacy of most actions in the critical care environment, pain assessment may be reduced to one question: Do you have pain? When unable to respond verbally (e.g., intubated), the patient may answer by head nodding or other signs.

Pain Assessment: The Observable/Objective Component

When the communication with the patient is impossible, the nurse can rely on observation of behavioral and physiologic indicators. Table 8-2 lists behavioral and physiologic indicators that may be associated with pain.[2,57,58,66-68]

Facial expressions of pain have been widely studied in adults. There are four primary facial movements:

1. Brow lowering
2. Orbit tightening
3. Levator contraction (deepening of the nasolabial furrow)
4. Eyelid closing[69]

The presence of the first three facial movements may suggest moderate pain, whereas the presence of all four facial movements may suggest severe pain.[69] A higher pain intensity is related to an increased number of facial movements. Physicians and critical care nurses recognize facial expression (e.g., frowning, eye tightening, grimacing, tears) as an important indicator for pain assessment.[70] The facial expression of grimacing is an indicator often recorded by critical care nurses[68] that has been related to patient-reported pain intensity.[66,71]

Other nonverbal patterns are used by critically ill patients to communicate their pain to nurses.[2] Muscle tension has been related to patient-reported pain intensity.[66,67,71] When a patient is tense, rigid, spastic, and resistive to being turned, critical care nurses have noted this as an indicator of pain.[70] Conscious patients may remain immobile in order to protect themselves from pain associated with movement.[70] However, restlessness is also a body movement associated with pain.[34,66-68] Ventilator dyssynchrony in an intubated patient may be associated with pain.[70,71]

Patients' sounds or vocalizations may be used for pain assessment in critically ill extubated patients.[66-68] Pain-related vocalizations include sighing, groaning, moaning, crying, or sobbing.[66,67] These types of vocal-

Table 8-3

Description of the Critical-Care Pain Observation Tool (CPOT)

INDICATOR	DESCRIPTION	MEASUREMENT SCALE	
Facial expression	No muscular tension observed	Relaxed, neutral	0
	Presence of frowning, brow lowering, orbit tightening, and levator contraction	Tense	1
	All previous facial movements plus eyelid tightly closed	Grimacing	2
Body movements	Does not move at all (doesn't necessarily mean absence of pain)	Absence of movements	0
	Slow, cautious movements, touching or rubbing the pain site, seeking attention through movements	Protection	1
	Pulling tube, attempting to sit up, moving limbs/thrashing, not following commands, striking at staff, trying to climb out of bed	Restlessness	2
Muscular tension	No resistance to passive movements	Relaxed	0
Evaluation by passive flexion and extension of upper limbs	Resistance to passive movements	Tense, rigid	1
	Strong resistance to passive movements, incapacity to complete them	Very tense or rigid	2
Compliance with the ventilator (intubated patients)	Alarms not activated, easy ventilation	Tolerating movements	0
	Alarms stop spontaneously	Coughing but tolerating	1
	Asynchrony: blocking ventilation, alarms frequently activated	Fighting ventilator	2
or			
Vocalization (extubated patients)	Talking in normal tone or no sound	Talking in normal tone or no sound	0
	Sighing, moaning	Sighing, moaning	1
	Crying out, sobbing	Crying out, sobbing	2

From Gelinas C et al: *Am J Crit Care* 15:420, 2006.

izations were found to be related to patient-reported pain intensity.[66,67,71] Patient vocalization was the third-most recorded pain indicator by critical care nurses in their pain assessments.[68]

Physiologic indicators associated with pain are shown in Table 8-2. Because pain is a stressor, hormones from the stress response are released, contributing to increased vital signs, which are common signs of acute pain.[58,68] However, physiologic indicators are not sensitive for discriminating pain from other sources of distress. They should never be used alone but rather considered as a cue for further assessment of pain.[16]

Some of these observable indicators were included in tools developed and validated for clinical use in critical care: PACU Behavioral Pain Rating Scale (PACU BPRS),[66] Pain Assessment and Intervention Notation (PAIN),[68] Behavioral Pain Scale (BPS),[58] and Critical-Care Pain Observation Tool (CPOT)[57] (Table 8-3). Although these tools have limitations, they may help support pain assessment in critical care, especially in uncommunicative patients. Research is still needed to improve the use of observable indicators for pain assessment in critically ill patients. It is also important to remember that absence of observable indicators (behavioral and physiologic) does not mean absence of pain.[68] Pain is considered the fifth vital sign,[72] and including pain assessment with other routinely documented vital signs may help ensure that pain is assessed and controlled for all patients on a regular basis.[73] Recommendations of information to include in complete pain assessment documentation are proposed in Table 8-4.

PATIENT BARRIERS TO PAIN ASSESSMENT AND MANAGEMENT

Difficulty in Communicating

The most obvious patient barrier to the assessment of pain in the critical care population is an alteration in the ability to communicate. The patient who is intubated cannot verbalize a description of the pain. If the patient can communicate in any way, such as by head nodding or pointing, then pain may be reported in that manner. With uncommunicative patients, the nurse relies on behavioral and physiologic clues. If there is absolutely no observable evidence to support a diagnosis of pain, the clinician needs to use the concept that if the trauma, disease, injury, or procedure is painful for most patients, it is painful for this patient, too.[16,18]

Altered Level of Consciousness

The patient in a coma presents a dilemma for the critical care nurse. Because pain recognition depends on cortical response, there is the mistaken belief that the patient without higher cortical function has no perception of pain.[74,75] Interviews with 100 patients who experienced being unconscious revealed that 27% of

Table 8-4

Components to Include for Complete Pain Assessment Documentation

PAIN DOCUMENTATION	DESCRIPTION		
Sources of pain	Admission diagnosis (acute illness, trauma, surgery) Invasive equipment (e.g., endotracheal tube, venous lines, chest tube) Nursing interventions (e.g., positioning, endotracheal suctioning) Medical interventions Immobility		
Patient's self-report	**Sensory** 1. Intensity (pain scale)* 2. Location 3. Quality 4. Aggravating/alleviating factors 5. Onset/time *The first pain information to focus on in the patient's self-report.	**Affective** 1. Emotions	**Cognitive** 1. Meaning of pain 2. Impact of pain
Observable indicators	**Physiologic** 1. Blood pressure (BP) 2. Heart rate (HR) 3. Respiratory rate (RR)	**Behavioral** 1. Facial expressions 2. Body movements 3. Muscular tension, rigidity (posture) 4. Compliance with the ventilator (intubated patients) 5. Vocalizations (extubated patients)	
Intervention for pain	Always conduct pain assessment before and after an intervention for pain (pharmacologic and nonpharmacologic) is undertaken as an ongoing assessment.		

Courtesy Celine Gelinas, School of Nursing, McGill University, Canada.

them could hear, understand, and respond emotionally to what was being said while they were unconscious.[76]

THE ELDERLY

Many elderly patients do not complain much about pain. Some misconceptions, such as believing that pain is a normal consequence of aging or being afraid to disturb the health care team, are barriers to pain expression for the elderly.[77,78] Delirium, dementia, or cognitive deficits present additional barriers to pain assessment. In a study by Ferrell, Ferrell, and Rivera,[79] it was found that 83% of elderly patients with moderate to severe cognitive deficits could communicate their pain by using an intensity scale. Most elderly patients with or without cognitive deficits are able to give a self-report of pain. Pain intensity scales are easily understood by this group of patients, and their use is recommended (Figure 8-3).[80]

CULTURAL INFLUENCES

Another barrier to accurate pain assessment is cultural influences on pain and pain reporting.[81] These cultural influences may be compounded if the patient speaks a language other than that of the health care team members. In order to facilitate communication, the use of a pain intensity scale in the patient's language is relevant. The 0 to 10 numeric pain scale has been translated into many different languages.[18]

LACK OF KNOWLEDGE

A relatively overlooked patient barrier to accurate pain assessment is the public knowledge deficit regarding pain and pain management. Many patients and their families are frightened by the risk of addiction to pain medication. They fear that addiction will occur if the patient is medicated frequently or with amounts of opiates necessary to relieve the pain. This concern is so powerful for some that they will deny or deliberately underreport the frequency or intensity of pain. Another misconception held by some patients is the expectation that unrelieved pain is simply part of a critical illness or procedure.[82] Many patients have no memory of receiving an explanation of their pain management plan.[27] With that in mind, it is important that the critical care nurse teach both the family and the patient about the importance of pain control and the use of opioids in treating the critically ill patient.

HEALTH PROFESSIONAL BARRIERS TO PAIN ASSESSMENT AND MANAGEMENT

The health professional's beliefs and attitudes about pain and pain management are frequently a barrier to accurate and adequate pain assessment. This can lead to poor management practices.[18,83,84] It is well documented that the study of pain assessment and management is lacking in most nursing schools and in nursing textbooks.[82,83] Multiple studies have documented nurses' misconceptions or lack of knowledge

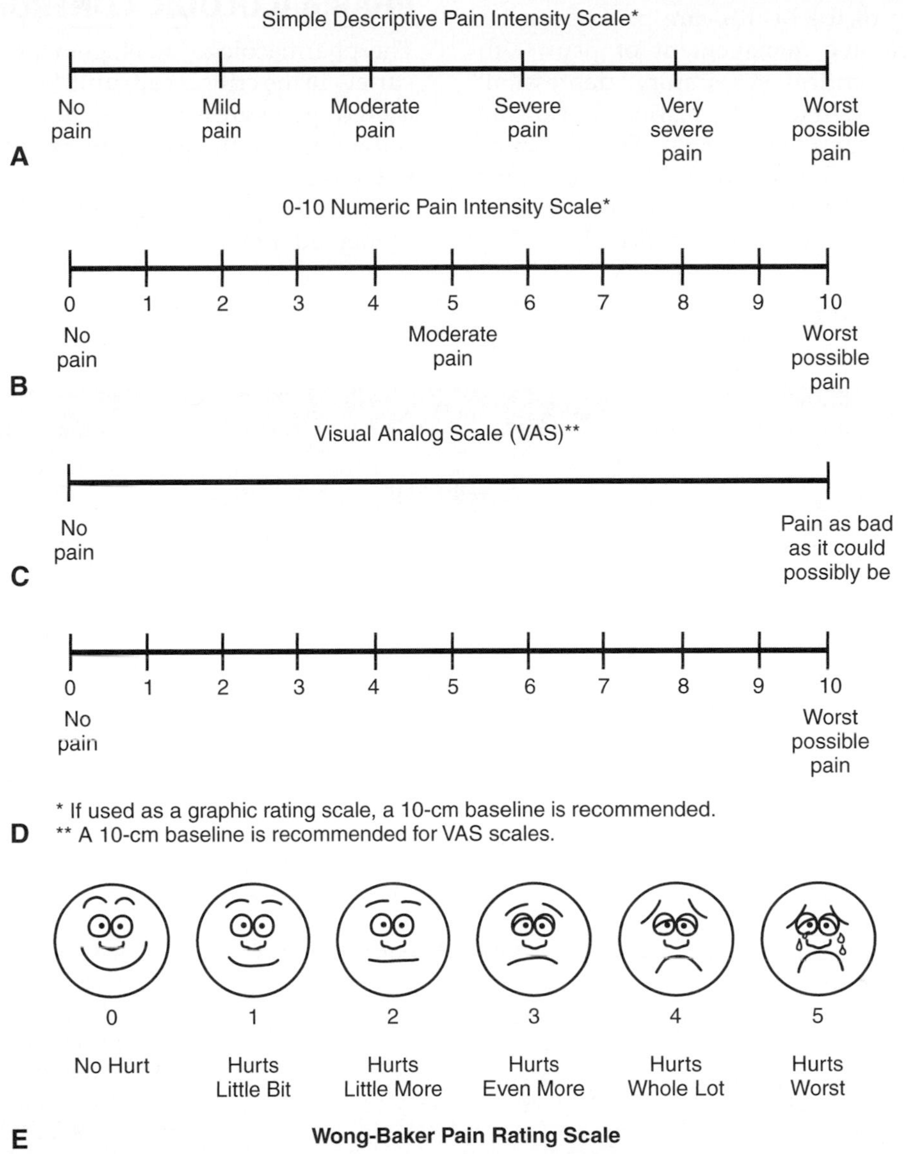

FIGURE 8-3. Pain intensity scales. **A,** Simple Descriptive Pain Intensity Scale. **B,** Numeric Pain Intensity Scale. **C,** Visual analog scale. **D,** Simple Descriptive Pain Intensity Scale. **E,** Wong-Baker FACES Pain Rating Scale. (**E** From Hockenberry MJ: *Wong's essentials of pediatric nursing,* ed 7, St Louis, 2004, Mosby.)

regarding addiction, physiologic dependence, drug tolerance, and respiratory depression.[18] The problematic misconception on the part of nurses is that the patient must have a physiologic and behavioral response to pain that matches the nurse's concept of what a patient in pain looks like (i.e., the patient must have a marked change in vital signs and be moaning, writhing, and crying to truly be in pain). This hampers appropriate management of the patient's pain. The critical care nurse must remember that pain is what the patient states it is and that no additional finding is necessary to treat the patient's pain.[18]

Nursing concerns with addiction can contribute to misinterpretation of signs during the pain assessment process. Addiction rates for patients in acute pain who receive opioid analgesics are less than 1%.[18] Some of the false beliefs that surround addiction result from a lack of knowledge about the terms *addiction* and *tolerance.* Addiction is defined by a pattern of compulsive drug use that is characterized by an incessant longing for an opioid and the need to use it for effects other than pain relief. Tolerance is defined as a diminution of opioid effects over time. Physical dependence and tolerance to opioids may develop if the drug is given over a long period. Physical dependence is manifested by withdrawal symptoms when the opioid is abruptly stopped.[18] If this is an anticipated problem, withdrawal may be avoided by simply weaning the patient from the opioid slowly to allow the brain to reestablish neurochemical balance in the absence of the opioid.

Another concern of the health care professional is the fear that aggressive management of pain with opioids will cause critical respiratory depression. Opioids can cause respiratory depression, but in the critically ill this is a rare phenomenon. The incidence of respiratory depression is less than 1%. Respiratory depression from the administration of opioids can be managed with diligent assessment practices.[85]

PHARMACOLOGIC CONTROL OF PAIN

The pharmacologic management of pain has infinite variety in the critical care unit. Some commonly administered agents are listed in Table 8-5. Pain pharmacology is divided into three categories of action:

- Opioid agonists (morphine, fentanyl, hydromorphone, meperidine, codeine, and methadone)

Table 8-5

Pharmacologic Management: Pain

DRUG	DOSAGE	ONSET (min)	DURATION (hr)	AVAILABLE ROUTES	PROPERTIES	SIDE EFFECTS AND COMMENTS
Morphine	1-4 mg IV bolus 1-10 mg IV infusion	5-10	3-4	PO, SL, R, IV, IM, Sub-Q, EA, IA	Analgesia Antianxiety	Standard for comparison Side effects: sedation, respiratory depression, euphoria/dysphoria, hypotension, nausea, vomiting, pruritus, constipation, urinary retention M6G can accumulate in renal failure or hepatic dysfunction patients
Fentanyl	25-100 mcg IV bolus 25-200 mcg IV infusion	1-5	0.5-4	OTFC, IV, IM, TD, EA, IA	Analgesia Antianxiety	Same side effects as morphine Rigidity with high doses
Hydromorphone (Dilaudid)	0.2-1 mg IV bolus 0.2-2 mg IV infusion	5	3-4	PO, R, IV, IM, Sub-Q, EA, IA	Analgesia Antianxiety	Same side effects as morphine
Meperidine (Demerol)	75-100 mg IM	5-10	2-4	PO, IV, IM, Sub-Q, EA, IA	Analgesia	Seem to cause less constipation, urinary retention, pruritus, sedation and nausea than morphine Neurotoxicity (normeperidine) High doses may cause agitation, muscle jerking, seizures, or hypotension Use with care in patients with renal failure, convulsive disorders, and dysrhythmias
Codeine	15-30 mg IM, Sub-Q	10-20	3-4	PO, IM, Sub-Q	Analgesia (mild-to-moderate pain)	Lacks potency (unpredictable absorption, and not all patients convert it to an active form to achieve analgesia) Most common side effects: light-headedness, dizziness, shortness of breath, sedation, nausea, and vomiting
Methadone (Dolophine)	5-10 mg IV	10	4-8	PO, SL, R, IV, Sub-Q, IM, EA, IA	Analgesia	Usually less sedating than morphine but repeated doses can result in accumulation and can cause serious sedation (2-5 days)
Acetaminophen	650 mg Maximum 4 g/day	20-30	4-6	PO, R	Analgesia Antipyretic	Rare side effects Hepatotoxicity
Ketorolac (Toradol)	15-30 mg IV	<10	6-8	PO, IM, IV	Analgesia Minimum anti-inflammatory effect	Short term (<5 days) Side effects: gastric ulceration, bleeding, exacerbation of renal insufficiency Use with care in elderly and renal failure patients

IV, Intravenous; *PO,* oral; *SL,* sublingual; *R,* rectal; *IM,* intramuscular; *Sub-Q,* subcutaneous; *EA,* Epidural analgesia; *IA,* intrathecal analgesia; *M6G,* morphine-6-glucuronide; *OTFC,* oral transmucosal fentanyl citrate; *TD,* transdermal.

- Nonopioids (acetaminophen, nonsteroidal antiinflammatory drugs [NSAIDs])
- Adjuvants (anticonvulsants, antidepressants, local anesthetics)

Opioid agonists are the most commonly used and are recommended as first-line analgesics. As a clinical practice guideline, scheduled opioid doses or a continuous infusion is preferred over an "as needed" regimen to ensure consistent analgesia in critically ill patients.[17] Also, the use of nonopioids in combination with an opioid is now recommended in selected critical care patients.[17] They may reduce opioid requirement and provide greater analgesic effect, through their action at the peripheral and central levels (Figure 8-4).[86,87] Even if not widely mentioned in the critical care literature, adjuvants can be helpful for pain relief in patients with complex pain syndromes such as neuropathic pain or for other specific purposes (e.g., procedural pain).[18]

How pain is approached and managed is a progression or combination of the available agents, the type of pain, and the patient response to the therapy. Figure 8-4 illustrates the analgesic action sites in relation to nociception.

DELIVERY METHODS

The most common route for drug administration is the intravenous (IV) route—via continuous infusion, bolus administration, or patient-controlled analgesia (PCA). Traditionally the choice has been IV bolus administration. The benefits of this method are the rapid onset of action and the ease of titration. The major disadvantage is the rise and fall of the serum level of the opioid, leading to periods of pain control with periods of breakthrough pain (Figure 8-5).[88]

Continuous infusion of opioids via an infusion pump provides constant blood levels of the ordered opioid. This promotes a consistent level of comfort. It is a particularly helpful method of administration during sleep because the patient awakens with an adequate level of pain relief.[89] It is important that the patient be given the loading dose that relieves the pain and also raises the circulating dose of the drug. After the basal rate is established, the patient maintains a steady state of pain control unless there is additional pain from a procedure, an activity, or a change in the patient's condition. Orders for additional boluses of opioid must be available.

Patient-Controlled Analgesia

PCA is a method of delivery, via the IV route and an infusion pump, that allows the patient to self-administer small doses of analgesics. Different opioids can be used, but the most extensively used is morphine.[88] This method of medication delivery allows the patient to control the level of pain and sedation and to avoid the peaks and valleys of intermittent dosing by the health care professional (see Figure 8-5). The patient can self-administer a bolus of medication the moment the pain begins, thus acting preemptively.

Certain patients are not candidates for PCA. Alterations in the level of consciousness or mentation preclude the patient's understanding the use of the equipment. The very elderly or patients with renal or hepatic insufficiency may require careful screening for PCA.

Allowing the patient to self-administer opioid doses does not diminish the role of the critical care nurse in pain management. The nurse advises for necessary changes to the prescription and continues to monitor the effects of the medication and doses. The patient is closely monitored during the first 2 hours of therapy and after every change in the prescription. If the patient's pain does not respond within the first 2 hours of therapy, a total reassessment of the pain state is essential. The nurse monitors the number of boluses the patient delivers. If the patient is pressing the PCA button to administer boluses more often than the prescription, the dose may be insufficient to maintain pain control. Naloxone must be readily available to reverse any episode of opiate respiratory depression. Ideally the patient undergoing an elective procedure requiring opioid analgesia postoperatively is instructed in the use of PCA during preoperative teaching. This allows the patient to become comfortable with the concept of self-medication before use.

Intraspinal Pain Control

Intraspinal anesthesia uses the concept that the spinal cord is the primary link in nociceptive transmission. The goal is to mimic the body's endogenous opioid pain modification system by interfering with the transmission of pain and providing an opiate-receptor binding agent directly into the spinal cord. The benefits of the intraspinal route include good to excellent pain control particularly in the thorax, upper abdomen, and lower extremities, with typically lower doses of opioids, increased patient mobility, minimal sedation, and increased patient satisfaction.[90] Also, the hemodynamic status of the patient changes very little.

Epidural Analgesia

Epidural analgesia is commonly used in the critical care unit after major abdominal surgery, nephrectomy, thoracotomy, and major orthopedic procedures. Certain conditions preclude the use of this pain control method: systemic infection, anticoagulation, and increased intracranial pressure. Epidural delivery of opiates provides longer-lasting pain relief with lower doses of opiates. When delivered into the epidural

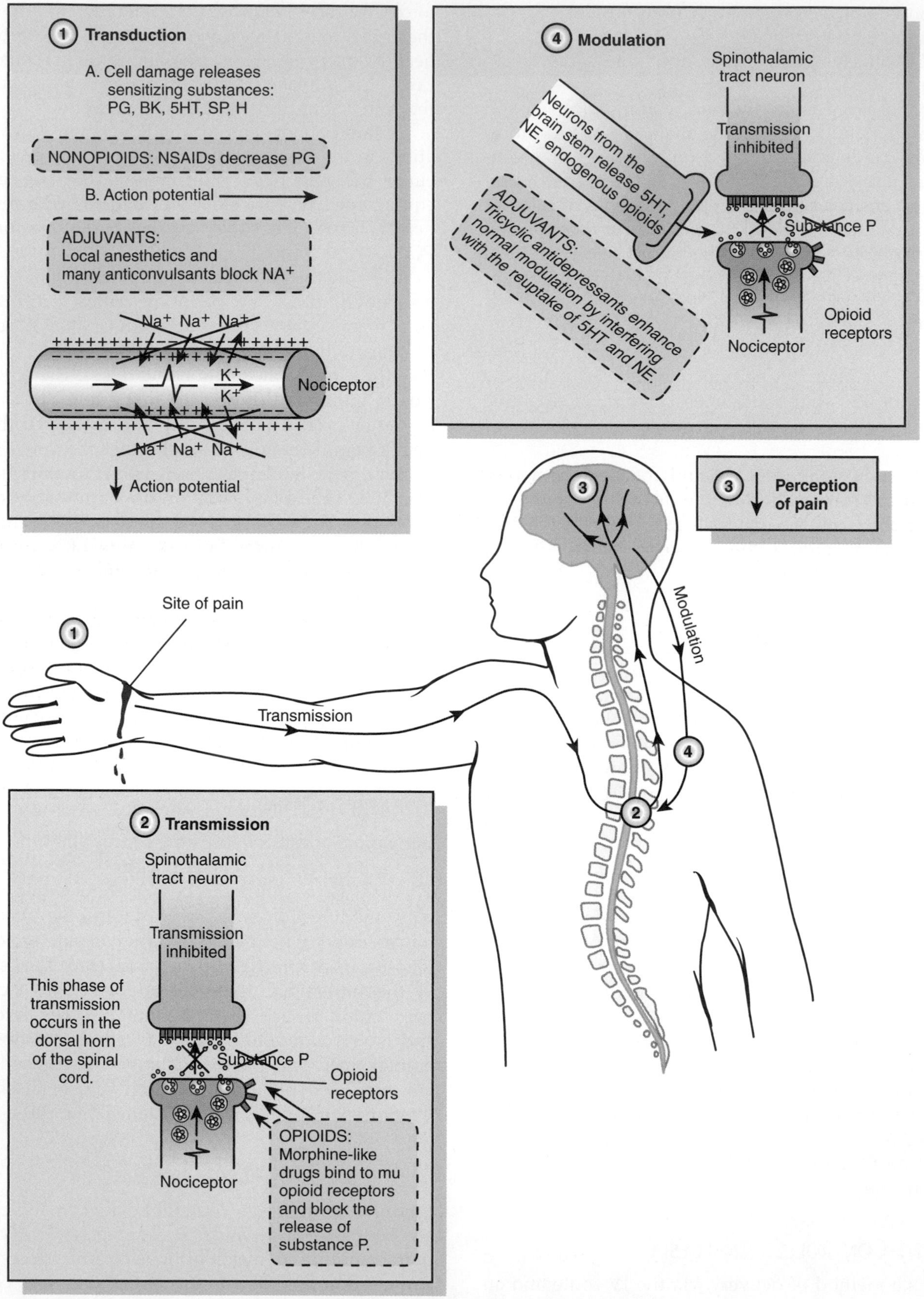

FIGURE 8-4. Nociception and analgesic action sites. (From McCaffery M, Pasero C: *Pain: clinical manual for nursing practice*, ed 2, St Louis, 1999, Mosby.)

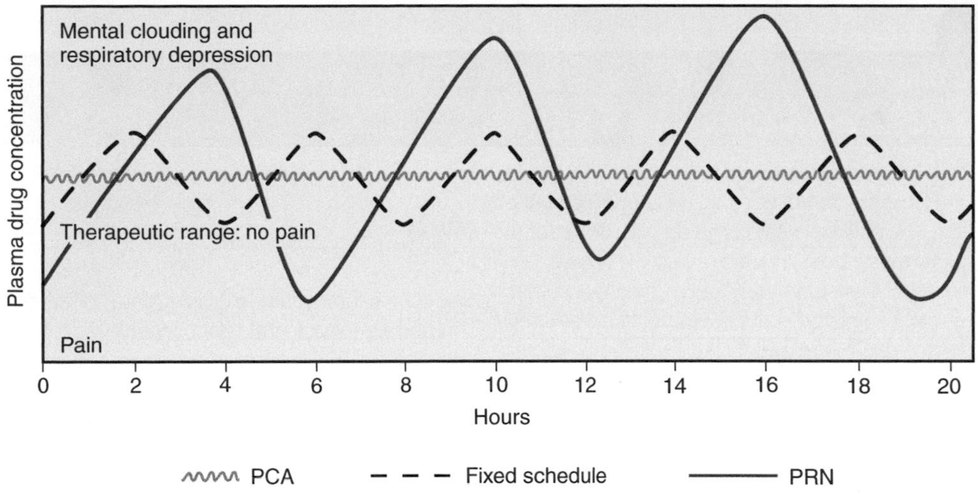

FIGURE 8-5. Fluctuations in opioid blood levels seen with three dosing procedures. (From Lehne RA: *Pharmacology for nursing care,* ed 5, Philadelphia, 2004, Saunders.)

space, 5 mg of morphine may be effective for 6 to 24 hours, compared with 3 to 4 hours when delivered IV. Drugs delivered epidurally may be administered as a bolus or continuously infused. Opioids infused in the epidural space are more unpredictable than those administered intrathecally. The epidural space is filled with fatty tissue and is external to the dura mater. The fatty tissue interferes with uptake, and the dura acts as a barrier to diffusion, making diffusion rate difficult to predict.

The rapidity of the drug diffusion is determined by the type of medication. The drugs are either hydrophilic or lipophilic. Hydrophilic drugs are water soluble and penetrate the dura slowly, giving them a longer onset and duration of action. Morphine is hydrophilic. Lipophilic drugs are lipid soluble; they penetrate the dura rapidly and therefore have a rapid onset of action but a shorter duration of action.[18] Fentanyl is lipophilic.

The nurse must assess the patient for respiratory depression. This phenomenon may occur early in the therapy or as late as 24 hours after initiation. Naloxone must be readily available to reverse adverse opiate respiratory effects. The epidural catheter also puts the patient at risk for infection. The efficiency of this pain control method and the increased mobility of the patient does not diminish the nurse's responsibility to monitor and evaluate the outcomes of the pain management protocol in use.

EQUIANALGESIA

At some point in the patient's recovery, strong opioids are replaced by more moderate agents. In doing any conversion the goal is to provide equal analgesic effects with the new agents. This concept is referred to as *equianalgesia*. The critical care nurse is the practitioner most likely to convert the patient from parenteral medication to oral medication in preparation for a change in the level of care or for discharge. There is the misconception that when a patient is able to take oral medication the pain is less severe. The change to oral medications does not indicate a need for less medication.

The nurse needs to practice equianalgesia when converting the patient. Because of the variety of agents and routes, the professional pain organizations have developed equianalgesia charts for use by the health care professional. All critical care units need to have a chart posted for easy referral. Table 8-6 provides the equianalgesia dose for different drugs used in clinical practice.

NONPHARMACOLOGIC METHODS OF PAIN MANAGEMENT

Numerous methods of pain management other than drugs appear in the critical care literature.[91,92] In most instances these therapies augment and enhance the pharmacologic management of the patient's pain. Stimulating other nonpain sensory fibers (alpha-beta) present in the periphery modifies pain transmission.[44] These fibers are stimulated by thermal changes, as in the application of heat or cold, and by simple massage. The use of massage has been a mainstay in the nursing management of the patient in pain. It is an appropriate pain management technique for most critically ill patients.

TRANSCUTANEOUS ELECTRICAL NERVE STIMULATION

The nonpain sensory fibers (alpha-beta) in the periphery are stimulated by the action of transcutaneous electrical nerve stimulation (TENS). The use of TENS has contraindications in the critical care unit. Because the

Table 8-6

Equianalgesic Chart

Approximate Equivalent Doses of Opioids for Moderate-to-Severe Pain

ANALGESIC	PARENTERAL (IM, Sub-Q, IV) ROUTE[1,2] (mg)	PO ROUTE[1] (mg)	COMMENTS
Mu Opioid Agonists			
Morphine	10	30	Standard for comparison; multiple routes of administration; available in immediate-release and controlled-release formulations; active metabolite M6G can accumulate with repeated dosing in renal failure
Codeine	130	200 NR	IM has unpredictable absorption and high side effect profile; used PO for mild-to-moderate pain; usually compounded with nonopioid (e.g., Tylenol No. 3)
Fentanyl	100 mcg/hr parenterally and transdermally ≅ 4 mg/hr morphine parenterally; 1 mcg/hr transdermally ≅ 2 mg/24 hr morphine PO	—	Short half-life, but at steady state, slow elimination from tissues can lead to a prolonged half-life (up to 12 hr); start opioid-naïve patients on no more than 25 mcg/hr transdermally; transdermal fentanyl NR for acute pain management; available by oral transmucosal route
Hydromorphone (Dilaudid)	1.5	7.5	Useful alternative to morphine; no evidence that metabolites are clinically relevant; shorter duration than morphine; available in high-potency parenteral formulation (10 mg/ml) useful for Sub-Q infusion; 3 mg rectal ≅ 650 mg aspirin PO; with repeated dosing (e.g., PCA), it is more likely than 2-3 mg parenteral hydromorphone = 10 mg parenteral morphine
Levorphanol (Levo-Dromoran)	2	4	Longer-acting than morphine when given repeatedly; long half-life can lead to accumulation within 2-3 days of repeated dosing.
Meperidine	75	300 NR	No longer preferred as a first-line opioid for the management of acute or chronic pain due to potential toxicity from accumulation of metabolite, normeperidine; normeperidine has 15-20 h half-life and is not reversed by naloxone; NR in elderly or patients with impaired renal functions; NR by continuous IV infusion
Methadone (Dolophine)	10	20	Longer-acting than morphine when given repeatedly; long half-life can lead to delayed toxicity from accumulation within 3-5 days; start PO dosing on PRN schedule; in opioid-tolerant patients converted to methadone, start with 10%-25% of equianalgesic dose
Oxycodone	—	20	Used for moderate pain when combined with a nonopioid (e.g., Percocet, Tylox); available as single entity in immediate-release and controlled-release formulations (e.g., OxyContin); can be used like PO morphine for severe pain
Oxymorphone (Numorphan)	1	10 rectal	Used for moderate-to-severe pain; no PO formulation
Agonist-Antagonist Opioids: Not recommended for severe, escalating pain. If used in combination with mu agonists, may reverse analgesia and precipitate withdrawal in opioid-dependent patients.			
Buprenorphine (Buprenex)	0.4	—	Not readily reversed by naloxone; NR for laboring patients
Butorphanol (Stadol)	2	—	Available in nasal spray
Dezocine (Dalgan)	10	—	
Nalbuphine (Nubain)	10	—	
Pentazocine (Talwin)	60	180	

[1]Duration of analgesia is dose dependent; the higher the dose, usually the longer the duration.

[2]IV boluses may be used to produce analgesia that lasts approximately as long as IM or Sub-Q doses. However, of all routes of administration, IV produces the highest peak concentration of the drug, and the peak concentration is associated with the highest level of toxicity, e.g., sedation. To decrease the peak effect and lower the level of toxicity, IV boluses may be administered more slowly, e.g., 10 mg of morphine over a 15 minute period, or smaller doses may be administered more often, e.g., 5 mg of morphine every 1-1.5 hours.

NR, Not recommended; ≅, roughly equal to.

Data from Pasero C, Portenoy RK, McCaffery M: Opioid analgesics, pp. 161-299. In McCaffery M, Pasero C: *Pain: clinical manual,* St Louis, 1999, Mosby, pp 241-243.

American Pain Society (APS): *Principles of analgesic use in the treatment of acute and cancer pain,* ed 3, Glenview, Ill, 1992, APS.

Table 8-6
Equianalgesic Chart—*cont'd*

Lawlor P, Turner K, Hanson J, et al: Dose ratio between morphine and hydromorphone in patients with cancer pain: a retrospective study, *Pain* 72(1,2):79, 1997.
Manfredi PL, Borsook D, Chandler SW, et al: Intravenous methadone for cancer pain unrelieved by morphine and hydromorphone: clinical observations, *Pain* 70:99, 1997.
Portenoy RK: Opioid analgesics. In Portenoy RK, Kanner RM, editors: *Pain management: theory and practice,* Philadelphia, 1996, FA Davis Company, pp. 249.
IM, Intramuscular; *IV,* intravenous; *M6G,* morphine-6-glucuronide; *NR,* not recommended; *PCA,* patient-controlled analgesia; *PO,* by mouth; *PRN, pro re nata* (as needed); *Sub-Q* subcutaneous.

Approximate Equivalent Doses of PO Nonopioids and Opioids for Mild-to-Moderate Pain

ANALGESIC	PO DOSAGE (mg)
Nonopioids	
Acetaminophen	650
Aspirin (ASA)	650
Opioids*	
Codeine	32-60
Hydrocodone†	5
Meperidine (Demerol)	50
Oxycodone‡	3-5
Propoxyphene (Darvon)	65-100

*Often combined with acetaminophen; avoid exceeding maximum total daily dose of acetaminophen (4000 mg/day).
†Combined with acetaminophen, e.g., Vicodin, Lortab.
‡Combined with acetaminophen, e.g., Percocet, Tylox. Also available alone as controlled-release OxyContin and immediate-release formulations.

A Guide to Using Equianalgesic Charts

- Equianalgesic means approximately the same pain relief.
- The equianalgesic chart is a guideline. Doses and intervals between doses are titrated according to individual's response.
- The equianalgesic chart is helpful when switching from one drug to another, or switching from one route of administration to another.
- Dosages in the equianalgesic chart for moderate-to-severe pain are not necessarily starting doses. The doses suggest a ratio for comparing the analgesia of one drug to another.
- For elderly patients, initially reduce the recommended adult opioid dose for moderate to severe pain by 25% to 50%.
- The longer the patient has been receiving opioids, the more conservative the starting dose of a *new* opioid.

Data from McCaffery M, Portenoy RK: Nonopioids: acetaminophen and nonsteroidal antiinflammatory drugs, pp. 241-243. In McCaffery M, Pasero C: *Pain: clinical manual,* St Louis, 1999, Mosby, p. 133, American Pain Society (APS): *Principles of analgesic use in the treatment of acute pain and cancer pain,* ed. 3, Glenview, IL, APS, 1992, Kaiko R et al: Analgesic efficacy of controlled-release (CR) oxycodone and CR morphine, *Clin Pharmacol Ther* 59:130, 1996.

device is controlled by the patient, mentation must be intact. TENS is also contraindicated in patients with pacemakers or automatic implantable defibrillators, because these devices may recognize and erroneously interpret the TENS electrical signal. TENS therapy is efficient, patient-controlled pain management for orthopedic, obstetric, and some postoperative pain states.

Cognitive Techniques

Using the cortical interpretation of pain as the foundation, a number of interventions are known to reduce the patient's pain report. These modalities include cognitive techniques: patient teaching, relaxation, distraction, guided imagery, and music therapy.[18,91,92]

Relaxation

Relaxation is a well-documented method for reducing the distress associated with pain. Although not a substitute for pharmacology, relaxation is an excellent adjunct for controlling pain.[93,94] Relaxation decreases oxygen consumption and muscle tone and can decrease heart rate and blood pressure. It can give the patient a sense of control and reduce muscle tension and anxiety. Not all patients are interested in relaxation therapy. For those patients, deep-breathing exercises may be helpful and frequently lead to relaxation.[18]

Distraction

The patient and family may provide information about other sources of distraction for the patient. Determining what distraction therapies the patient normally uses may provide a clue to which might work during the illness. Some persons are distracted by television; however, for others television is a source of increased anxiety.

Guided Imagery

Guided imagery is a technique that uses the imagination to provide control over pain. It can be used to distract or relax. Guiding a patient to a place in his or her imagination that is pain free and relaxing takes a considerable time commitment on the part of the nurse. Although this may be a challenge in the critical care environment, it may be beneficial.[92]

Music Therapy

Music therapy is a commonly used intervention for relaxation. Music that is pleasing to the patient may have soothing effects.[95] Ideally the music should be supplied by a small set of headphones. This method also serves to minimize the distracting and anxiety-producing noises of a critical care unit. It is important to educate the patient and family regarding the role of music in relaxation and pain control and also to provide music of the patient's choice.

SUMMARY

Today's health care environment mandates that patients experience positive outcomes as rapidly as possible. Because pain is a major barrier to early mobility and rapid return to a preillness state, pain management is of paramount importance to the critical care nurse. Because the critically ill patient is the most difficult to assess and manage, the critical care nurse must develop the skill and intervention techniques necessary to manage complex pain states. As patient advocate the nurse assumes the responsibility for establishing pain control as a priority for the health care team. The nurse's role and responsibility become more important as the regulating agencies and professional bodies focus more attention on the area of patient pain. The nurse's knowledge and understanding of pain and its implications for patients are the foundations for meeting patients' pain needs safely and efficiently.

evolve To test your mastery of this chapter, try the Open-Book Quiz at http://evolve.elsevier.com/Urden/priorities/

REFERENCES

1. Hallenberg B, Bergbom-Engberg I, Haljamäe H: Patients' experiences of postoperative respirator treatment—influence of anaesthetic and pain treatment regimens, *Acta Anaesthesiol Scand* 34:557, 1990.
2. Puntillo KA: Pain experience of intensive care unit patients, *Heart Lung* 19:526, 1990.
3. Puntillo KA: Dimensions of procedural pain and its analgesic management in critically ill surgical patients, *Am J Crit Care* 3:116, 1994.
4. Turner JS et al: Patients' recollection of intensive care unit experience, *Crit Care Med* 18:966, 1990.
5. Wilson VS: Identification of stressors related to patients' psychologic responses to the surgical intensive care unit, *Heart Lung* 16:267, 1987.
6. Christoph SB: Pain assessment: the problem of pain in the critically ill patient, *Crit Care Nurs Clin North Am* 3:11, 1991.
7. Kwekkeboom KL, Herr K: Assessment of pain in the critically ill, *Crit Care Nurs Clin North Am* 13:181, 2001.
8. Murray MJ: Pain problems in the ICU, *Crit Care Clin* 6:235, 1990.
9. Desbiens NA et al: Pain and satisfaction with pain control in seriously ill hospitalized adults: findings from the SUPPORT research investigations, *Crit Care Med* 24:1953, 1996.
10. Ferguson J, Gilroy D, Puntillo K: Dimensions of pain and analgesic administration associated with coronary artery bypass grafting in an Australian intensive care unit, *J Adv Nurs* 26:1065, 1997.
11. Puntillo KA, Weiss SJ: Pain: its mediators and associated morbidity in critically ill cardiovascular surgical patients, *Nurs Res* 43:31, 1994.
12. Puntillo KA et al: Patients' perceptions and responses to procedural pain: results from Thunder Project II, *Am J Crit Care* 10:238, 2001.
13. Stanik-Hutt J et al: Pain experiences of traumatically injured patients in a critical care setting, *Am J Crit Care* 10:252, 2001.
14. Valdix SW, Puntillo KA: Pain, pain relief and accuracy of their recall after cardiac surgery, *Prog Cardiovasc Nurs* 10:3, 1995.
15. Whipple JK et al: Analysis of pain management in critically ill patients, *Pharmacotherapy* 15:592, 1995.
16. Herr K et al: Pain assessment in the nonverbal patient: position statement with clinical practice recommendations, *Pain Manag Nurs* 7:44, 2006.
17. Jacobi J et al: Clinical practice guidelines for the sustained use of sedatives and analgesics in the critically ill adult, *Crit Care Med* 30:119, 2002.
18. McCaffery M, Pasero C: *Pain: clinical manual for nursing practice,* ed 2, St Louis, 1999, Mosby.
19. Hamill-Ruth RJ, Marohn L: Evaluation of pain in the critically ill patient, *Crit Care Clin* 15:35, 1999.
20. Shannon K, Bucknall T: Pain assessment in critical care: what have we learned from research, *Intensive Crit Care Nurs* 19:154, 2003.
21. Kaiser KS: Assessment and management of pain in the critically ill trauma patient, *Crit Care Nurs Q* 15:14, 1992.
22. Mlynczak B: Assessment and management of the trauma patient in pain, *Crit Care Nurs Clin North Am* 1:55, 1989.
23. Puntillo KA: Pain in the critically ill: assessment and management, Gaithersburg, Md, 1991, Aspen.
24. Anand KJS, Craig KD: New perspectives on the definition of pain, *Pain* 67:3, 1996.
25. Ferrell B, Wheden M, Rollins B: Pain and quality assessment/improvement, *J Nurs Care Qual* 9:69, 1995.
26. Bellinger K et al: The impact of nursing on pain management. In Weiner R, editor: *Pain management: a practical guide for clinicians,* Sonora, Calif, 1998, CRC Press.
27. Carroll KC et al: Pain assessment and management in critically ill postoperative and trauma patients: a multisite study, *Am J Crit Care* 8:105, 1999.
28. Maxam-Moore VA, Wilkie DJ, Woods SL: Analgesics for cardiac surgery patients in critical care: describing current practice, *Am J Crit Care* 3:31, 1994.
29. Puntillo KA et al: Practices and predictors of analgesic interventions for adults undergoing painful procedures, *Am J Crit Care* 11:415, 2002.

30. Tittle M, McMillan SC: Pain and pain-related side effects in an ICU and on a surgical unit: nurses' management, *Am J Crit Care* 3:25, 1994.
31. Stannard D et al: Clinical judgment and management of postoperative pain in critical care patients, *Am J Crit Care* 5:433, 1996.
32. Manias E, Botti M, Bucknall T: Observation of pain assessment and management—the complexities of clinical practice, *J Clin Nurs* 11:724, 2002.
33. Sullivan LM: Factors influencing pain management: a nursing perspective, *J Post Anesth Nurs* 9:83, 1994.
34. Gelinas C et al: Pain assessment and management in critically ill intubated patients: a retrospective study, *Am J Crit Care* 13:126, 2004.
35. Carr DB, Goudas LC: Acute pain, *Lancet* 353:2051, 1999.
36. O'Gara PT: The hemodynamic consequences of pain and its management, *J Intensive Care Med* 3:3, 1988.
37. Wild L: Transition from pain to comfort: managing the haemodynamic risks, *Crit Care Nurs Q* 15:46, 1992.
38. Cheever KH: Reducing the effects of acute pain in critically ill patients, *Dimensions Crit Care Nurs* 18:14, 1999.
39. American Nurses Association: *Position statement: promotion of comfort and relief in the dying patient*, Washington, DC, 1992, The Association.
40. Lindquist R, Banasik J, Barnsteiner J: Determining AACN's research priorities for the 90s, *Am J Crit Care* 2:110, 1993.
41. Joint Commission on Accreditation of Healthcare Organizations: *Comprehensive accreditation manual for hospitals*, Oakbrook Terrace, Ill, 2000, JCAHO.
42. International Association for the Study of Pain (IASP), Subcommittee on Taxonomy: Pain terms: a list with definitions and notes on usage, *Pain* 6:249, 1979.
43. Loeser JD, Cousins MJ: Contemporary pain management, *Med J Aust* 153:208, 1990.
44. Melzack R, Wall PD: Pain mechanisms: a new theory, *Science* 150:971, 1965.
45. Melzack R, Casey KL: Sensory, motivational, and central control determinants of pain: a new conceptual model. In Kenshalo D, editor: *The skin senses*, Springfield, Ill, 1968, Charles C Thomas.
46. McGuire D: Comprehensive and multidimensional assessment and measurement of pain, *J Pain Symptom Manage* 7:312, 1992.
47. Cousins M: Acute and postoperative pain. In Wall PD, Melzack R, editors: *Textbook of pain*, New York, 1994, Churchill Livingstone.
48. Marchand S: *Le phénomène de la douleur* [The phenomenon of pain], Montreal, 1998, Chenelière/McGraw-Hill.
49. Levine J, Taiwo Y: Inflammatory pain. In Wall PD, Melzack R, editors: *Textbook of pain*, New York, 1994, Churchill Livingstone.
50. Katz J et al: Acute pain after thoracic surgery predicts long-term post-thoracotomy pain, *Clin J Pain* 12:50, 1996.
51. Melzack R: Pain and stress: a new perspective. In Gatchel RJ, Turk DC, editors: *Psychological factors in pain*, New York, 1999, Guilford Press.
52. Hayes C, Molloy AR: Neuropathic pain in the perioperative period, *Int Anesthesiol Clin* 35:67, 1997.
53. Siddall PJ, Cousins MJ: Neurobiology of pain, *Int Anesthesiol Clin* 35:1, 1997.
54. Woolf CJ, Mannion RJ: Neuropathic pain: aetiology, symptoms, mechanisms, and management, *Lancet* 353:1959, 1999.
55. Charlton JE: *Core curriculum for professional education in pain*, ed 3, Seattle, 2005, IASP Press.
56. Melzack R, Wall PD: *The challenge of pain*, ed 2, London, 1996, Penguin.
57. Gelinas C et al: Validation of the Critical-Care Pain Observation Tool in adult patients, *Am J Crit Care* 15:420, 2006.
58. Payen JF et al: Assessing pain in the critically ill sedated patients by using a behavioral pain scale, *Crit Care Med* 29:2258, 2001.
59. McKenna JE, Melzack R: Analgesia produced by lidocaine microinjection into the dentate gyrus, *Pain* 49:105, 1992.
60. Bromm B: Consciousness, pain, and cortical activity. In Bromm B, Desmedt JE, editors: *Pain and the brain: from nociception to cognition*, New York, 1995, Raven Press.
61. Behbehani MM: Physiology and mechanisms of pain. In Parker MM, Shapiro MJ, Porembka DT, editors: *Critical care: state of the art*, Anaheim, Calif, 1995, Society of Critical Care Medicine.
62. Agency for Health Care Policy and Research: Acute pain management: operative or medical procedures and trauma, part I, *Clin Pharm* 1:309, 1992.
63. Daut RL, Cleeland CS: The prevalence and severity of pain in cancer, *Cancer* 50:1913, 1982.
64. Melzack R: The short form McGill Pain Questionnaire, *Pain* 30:191, 1987.
65. Jarvis C: *Physical examination and health assessment*, ed 4, Philadelphia, 2004, Saunders.
66. Mateo OM, Krenzischek DA: A pilot study to assess the relationship between behavioral manifestations and self-report of pain in postanesthesia care unit patients, *J Post Anesth Nurs* 7:15, 1992.
67. Webb MR, Kennedy MG: Behavioral responses and self-reported pain in postoperative patients, *J Post Anesth Nurs* 9:91, 1994.
68. Puntillo KA et al: Relationship between behavioral and physiological indicators of pain, critical care self-reports of pain, and opioid administration, *Crit Care Med* 25:1159, 1997.
69. Prkachin KM: The consistency of facial expressions of pain: a comparison across modalities, *Pain* 51:297, 1992.
70. Gelinas C et al: Les indicateurs de la douleur en soins critiques [Pain indicators in critical care], *Perspective Infirmière* 2(4):12, 2005.
71. Gelinas C et al: *Observable indicators of pain in cardiac surgery ICU patients*, Oral presentation, National Teaching Institute (NTI), American Association of Critical-Care Nurses (AACN), Annual Congress, Orlando, Fla, May 15-20, 2004, http://www.aacn.org/AACN/NTIPoster.nsf/vwdoc/ 2004RESCGelinas?opendocument.
72. Lynch M: Pain as the fifth vital sign, *J Intraven Nurs* 24:85, 2001.
73. Wild LR: Pain management: an organizational perspective, *Crit Care Nurs Clin North Am* 13:297, 2001.
74. Caillet R: *Pain: mechanisms and management*, Philadelphia, 1993, Davis.
75. Halloran T, Pohlman A: Managing sedation in the critically ill patient, *Crit Care Nurse* 5(suppl 4):1, 1995.

76. Lawrence M: The unconscious experience, *Am J Crit Care* 4:227, 1995.
77. Forrest J: Assessment of acute and chronic pain in older adults, *J Gerontol Nurs* 21(10):15, 1995.
78. Gibson MC: Improving pain control for the elderly patient with dementia, *Am J Alzheimers Dis Other Demen,* p 10, January/February, 1998.
79. Ferrell BA, Ferrell BR, Rivera L: Pain in cognitively impaired nursing home patients. *J Pain Symptom Manage* 10:591, 1995.
80. Herr KA, Mobily PR: Complexities of pain assessment in the elderly: clinical considerations, *J Gerontol Nurs* 17:12, 1991.
81. Bozeman M: Cultural aspects of pain management. In Salerno E, Willens J, editors: *Pain management handbook: an interdisciplinary approach,* St Louis, 1996, Mosby.
82. Ulmer J: Identifying and preventing pain mismanagement. In Salerno E, Willens J, editors: *Pain management handbook: an interdisciplinary approach,* St Louis, 1996, Mosby.
83. Alpen M, Titler M: Pain management in the critically ill: what do we know and how can we improve? *AACN Clin Issues Crit Care Nurs* 5:159, 1994.
84. Sun X, Weissman C: The use of analgesics and sedatives in the critically ill patient: physician's order versus medication administered, *Heart Lung* 23:169, 1994.
85. Pasero CL, McCaffery M: Avoiding opioid-induced respiratory depression, *Am J Nurs* 94(2):25, 1994.
86. Joint Commission on Accreditation of Healthcare Organizations: *Pain: current understanding of assessment, management, and treatments,* Oakbrook Terrace, Ill, 2001, The Commission.
87. Levine RL: Pharmacology of intravenous sedatives and opioids in critically ill patients, *Crit Care Clin* 10:709, 1994.
88. Lehne RA: *Pharmacology for nursing care,* ed 5, Philadelphia, 2004, Saunders.
89. Collins P, Spunt A, Huml M: Symptom management. In Salerno E, Willens J, editors: *Pain management handbook: an interdisciplinary approach,* St Louis, 1996, Mosby.
90. Dyble K: Epidural and intrathecal methods of analgesia in the critically ill. In Puntillo K, editor: *Pain in the critically ill: assessment and management,* Gaithersburg, Md, 1991, Aspen.
91. Rietman L: Pain management. In Chulay M, Guzzetta C, Dossey B, editors: *AACN handbook of critical care nursing,* Stamford, Conn, 1997, Appleton & Lange.
92. Gujol M: A survey of pain assessment and management practices among critical care nurses, *Am J Crit Care* 3:123, 1994.
93. Miller KM, Perry PA: Relaxation technique and postoperative pain in patients undergoing cardiac surgery, *Heart Lung* 19:136, 1990.
94. Houston S, Jesurum J: The quick relaxation technique: Effect on pain associated with chest tube removal, *Appl Nurs Res* 12:196, 1999.
95. Broscious SK: Music: An intervention for pain during chest tube removal after open heart surgery, *Am J Crit Care* 8:410, 1999.

CHAPTER 9

Sedation, Agitation, and Delirium Management

MARY E. LOUGH

OBJECTIVES

- Explain the differences among light, moderate, and deep levels of sedation.
- Describe the role of standardized assessment tools to determine sedation requirements.
- Compare and contrast the pharmacologic agents used to provide sedation.
- List the risk factors for development of delirium in critical illness.

PATIENT AGITATION AND NEED FOR SEDATION/ANALGESIA

One of the challenges facing clinicians is how to provide a therapeutic environment for patients in the alarm-filled, emergency-focused critical care unit. Rest and relaxation can be difficult to find. As many as 74% of critical care patients demonstrate some degree of agitation during their critical care hospitalization.[1] Many patients report upsetting dreams, hallucinations, nightmares, and flashbacks once they are recovered. The many causes of this agitation include painful procedures, invasive tubes, sleep deprivation, fear, anxiety, and the stress associated with critical illness. Some patients experience posttraumatic stress disorder (PTSD) after prolonged hospitalization.[1]

The goal of recent clinical practice guidelines is to increase the awareness of these issues within the medical and nursing community.[2] When the sedation assessment, as with the pain assessment, is recognized as a *fifth vital sign,* nurses may be able to decrease the incidence of agitation and delirium in critically ill patients.

The need for analgesics and sedatives to maintain patient safety and comfort is important, but it is increasingly recognized that excessive sedation can prolong the duration of mechanical ventilation, create physical and psychologic dependence, and increase the length of the hospital stay.[3] The goal is to find a balance between providing compassionate patient care and avoiding oversedation.

ASSESSING LEVEL OF SEDATION

SEDATION SCALES

The use of scoring systems to assess and record levels of sedation and agitation is now strongly recommended.[2] Four frequently used scales are the Ramsey Scale, the Riker Sedation-Agitation Scale (SAS), the Motor Activity Assessment Scale (MAAS), and the Richmond Agitation-Assessment Scale (RAAS) (Table 9-1).[3,4] If a scale is not available, the sedation level is sometimes conveyed by the words "light," "moderate," and "deep" as listed in Box 9-1.[2,3] Collaboratively, the critical care team must decide which level of sedation is most appropriate for an individual patient.[2,3]

The first step in assessing the agitated patient is to rule out any sensations of pain.[3] Clinical assessment is more challenging when the patient is mechanically[5] ventilated. If the patient can communicate, the 0 to 10 verbal pain scale is very useful. If the patient is intubated and cannot vocalize, assessing pain becomes considerably more complex. Once medication for pain has been provided, the next step is to determine the minimum level of sedation required. If deep or moderate sedation is being applied, it is essential that all members of the health care team are qualified and have appropriate credentials to manage sedative medications and any potential patient complications that arise.[2,3]

CONTINUOUS NERVOUS SYSTEM MONITORING

In an attempt to clarify clinical assessment of depth of consciousness some hospitals use continuous monitoring of the electroencephalogram (EEG) for sedated, mechanically ventilated patients. The United States Food and Drug Administration (FDA) has approved two modified continuous EEG monitoring systems. The first, and most widely used, system in critical care units is the bispectral index (BIS).[6,7] The BIS system uses sensor electrodes on a single band placed on the patient's forehead. The other continuous EEG moni-

Table 9-1
Sedation Scales

SCORE	DESCRIPTION	DEFINITION
Riker Sedation-Agitation Scale (SAS)[1]		
7	Dangerous agitation	Pulls at endotracheal tube (ETT), tries to remove catheters, climbs over bedrail, strikes at staff, thrashes side to side
6	Very agitated	Does not calm despite frequent verbal reminding of limits, requires physical restraints, bites ETT
5	Agitated	Anxious or mildly agitated, attempts to sit up, calms down to verbal instructions
4	Calm and cooperative	Calm, awakens easily, follows commands
3	Sedated	Difficult to arouse, awakens to verbal stimuli or gentle shaking but drifts off again, follows simple commands
2	Very sedated	Arouses to physical stimuli, but does not communicate or follow commands, may move spontaneously
1	Unarousable	Minimal or no response to noxious stimuli, does not communicate or follow commands
Motor Activity Assessment Scale (MAAS)[2]		
6	Dangerously agitated	No external stimulus required to elicit movement; is uncooperative, pulls at tubes/catheters, thrashes side to side, strikes at staff, tries to climb out of bed, does not calm down when asked
5	Agitated	No external stimulus required to elicit movement; attempts to sit up or move limbs out of bed, does not consistently follow commands (e.g., will lie down when asked, but soon reverts back to attempts)
4	Restless and cooperative	No external stimulus required to elicit movement; picks at sheets/tubes or uncovers self, follows commands
3	Calm and cooperative	No external stimulus required to elicit movement; adjusts sheets/clothes purposefully, follows commands
2	Responsive to touch or name	Opens eyes, raises eyebrows, or turns head toward stimulus; or moves limbs when touched or when name loudly spoken
1	Responsive only to noxious stimulus	Opens eyes, raises eyebrows, or turns head toward stimulus; or moves limbs with noxious stimulus
0	Unresponsive	Does not move with noxious stimulus
Ramsey Scale[3]		
1	Awake	Anxious and agitated or restless, or both
2		Cooperative, oriented, and tranquil
3		Responds only to commands
4	Asleep	Brisk response to light glabellar tap or loud auditory stimulus
5		Sluggish response to light glabellar tap or loud auditory stimulus
6		No response to light glabellar tap or loud auditory stimulus
Richmond Agitation-Sedation Scale (RASS)[4,5]		
4	Combative	Overly combative or violent, immediate danger to staff
3	Very agitated	Pulls on or removes tubes or catheters or has aggressive behavior toward staff
2	Agitated	Frequent nonpurposeful movement or patient-ventilator dyssynchrony
1	Restless	Anxious or apprehensive but movements not aggressive or vigorous
0	Alert and calm	
−1	Drowsy	Not fully alert, but has sustained—more than 10 seconds—awakening with eye contact to voice
−2	Light sedation	Briefly, less than 10 seconds, awakening with eye contact to voice
−3	Moderate sedation	Any movement, but no eye contact to voice
−4	Deep sedation	No response to voice, but any movement to physical stimulation
−5	Unresponsive	No response to voice or physical stimulation

References

1. Riker RR, Picard JT, Fraser GL: Prospective evaluation of the Sedation-Agitation Scale for adult critically ill patients, *Crit Care Med* 27(7):1325, 1999.
2. Devlin JW et al: Motor Activity Assessment Scale: a valid and reliable sedation scale for use with mechanically ventilated patients in an adult surgical intensive care unit, *Crit Care Med* 27(7):1271, 1999.
3. Ramsey MA et al: Controlled sedation with alphaxalone-alphadolone, *Br Med J* 2:656, 1974.
4. Sessler CN et al: The Richmond Agitation-Sedation Scale: validity and reliability in adult intensive care unit patients, *Am J Respir Crit Care Med* 166(10):1338, 2002.
5. Ely EW et al: Monitoring sedation status over time in ICU patients: reliability and validity of the Richmond Agitation-Sedation Scale (RASS), *JAMA* 289(22):2983, 2003.

Box 9-1

Levels of Sedation

Light Sedation (Minimal Sedation, Anxiolysis)
Drug-induced state during which patients respond normally to verbal commands. Although cognitive function and coordination may be impaired, ventilatory and cardiovascular functions are unaffected.

Moderate Sedation With Analgesia (Conscious Sedation, Procedural Sedation)
Drug-induced depression of consciousness during which patients respond purposefully to verbal commands, either alone or accompanied by light tactile stimulation. No interventions are required to maintain a patent airway, and spontaneous ventilation is adequate. Cardiovascular function is usually maintained.

Deep Sedation and Analgesia
Drug-induced depression of consciousness during which patients cannot be easily aroused but respond purposefully after repeated or painful stimulation. The ability to maintain ventilatory function independently is impaired. Patients require assistance in maintaining a patent airway, and spontaneous ventilation may be inadequate. Cardiovascular function is usually maintained.

General Anesthesia
Drug-induced loss of consciousness during which patients are not arousable, even by painful stimulation. The ability to maintain ventilatory function independently is impaired, and assistance in maintaining a patent airway is required. Positive-pressure ventilation may be required because of depressed spontaneous ventilation or drug-induced depression of neuromuscular function. Cardiovascular function may be impaired.

Data from Joint Commission on Accreditation of Healthcare Organizations: *Comprehensive accreditation manual for hospitals,* Oakbrook Terrace, Ill, 2000, The Commission; and Jacobi J et al: *Crit Care Med* 30(1):119, 2002.

toring system monitors a "Patient State Index" (PSI) via an electrode array that is also placed on the forehead.[8] Both systems analyze the patient's EEG signals to detect the effect of sedatives, hypnotics, and analgesics on the brain. These technologies have been successfully used in the operating room when the patient is under general anesthesia and are increasingly used in the critical care unit for ventilated patients who are deeply sedated or are sedated and pharmacologically paralyzed. Both systems calculate a number on a scale from 0 to 99 or 100. A value greater than 95 indicates wakefulness, and a value less than 50 to 60 indicates the patient is unconsciousness or deeply sedated with a low probability of mental recall of events. A value below 20 denotes an extremely deep level of sedation sufficient to cause brain-wave suppression. Unless the goal is to achieve a level of sedation equivalent to a barbiturate coma, brain wave suppression is not desirable. Both systems incorporate an electromyogram (EMG) sensor to filter out erroneous muscle movement that may distort the numerical sedation value.[6-8] Continuous nervous system monitoring via EEG may have a role for critically ill patients who are deeply sedated, are receiving opiate analgesia, and are pharmacologically paralyzed, although research outside the operating room is limited at this time.[9]

It is recommended that all critically ill, intubated, mechanically ventilated patients have a stated goal for analgesia and sedation (Figure 9-1).[3] Once the sedation goal is articulated and documented, the ongoing use of a validated assessment scale is recommended to facilitate consistency between all critical care practitioners (see Table 9-1).

COMPLICATIONS OF SEDATION

Oversedation is recognized as a state of unintended patient unresponsiveness in which the patient resides in a state of suspended animation that resembles general anesthesia.[10] Prolonged deep sedation is associated with significant complications of immobility, including pressure ulcers, thromboemboli, gastric ileus, hospital-acquired pneumonia, and delayed weaning from mechanical ventilation.

Too little sedation is equally hazardous. Most nurses have experienced the challenge of caring for a patient who unexpectedly removes the endotracheal or nasogastric tube. Unplanned extubation in restless, anxious, agitated patients occurs in 8% to 10% of intubated patients. Of self-extubations, 6% cause significant complications including aspiration, dysrhythmias, bronchospasm, and bradycardia.[10]

SELECTING MEDICATIONS FOR SEDATION

Several categories of sedatives are commercially available. None of these medications has any analgesic properties. Therefore, if the patient is experiencing pain, analgesia must be administered in addition to any sedative agents. Sedative agents include the benzodiazepines, anesthetic agents such as propofol, and the central α-agonists (Table 9-2).[3]

BENZODIAZEPINES

Benzodiazepines are sedative-hypnotics with powerful amnesic properties that inhibit reception of new sensory information.[3,10] Benzodiazepines do not have analgesic properties. The most frequently used critical care benzodiazepines are *diazepam* (Valium), *midazolam* (Versed), and *lorazepam* (Ativan). Midazolam is recommended for control of acute short-term agitation because of an intravenous (IV) onset of action of under 3 minutes.[3,10] However, when midazolam is administered for longer than 24 hours as a continuous infusion, the sedative effect is prolonged by active metabolites.[3]

When long-term sedation is required, converting to a continuous infusion of lorazepam is recommended

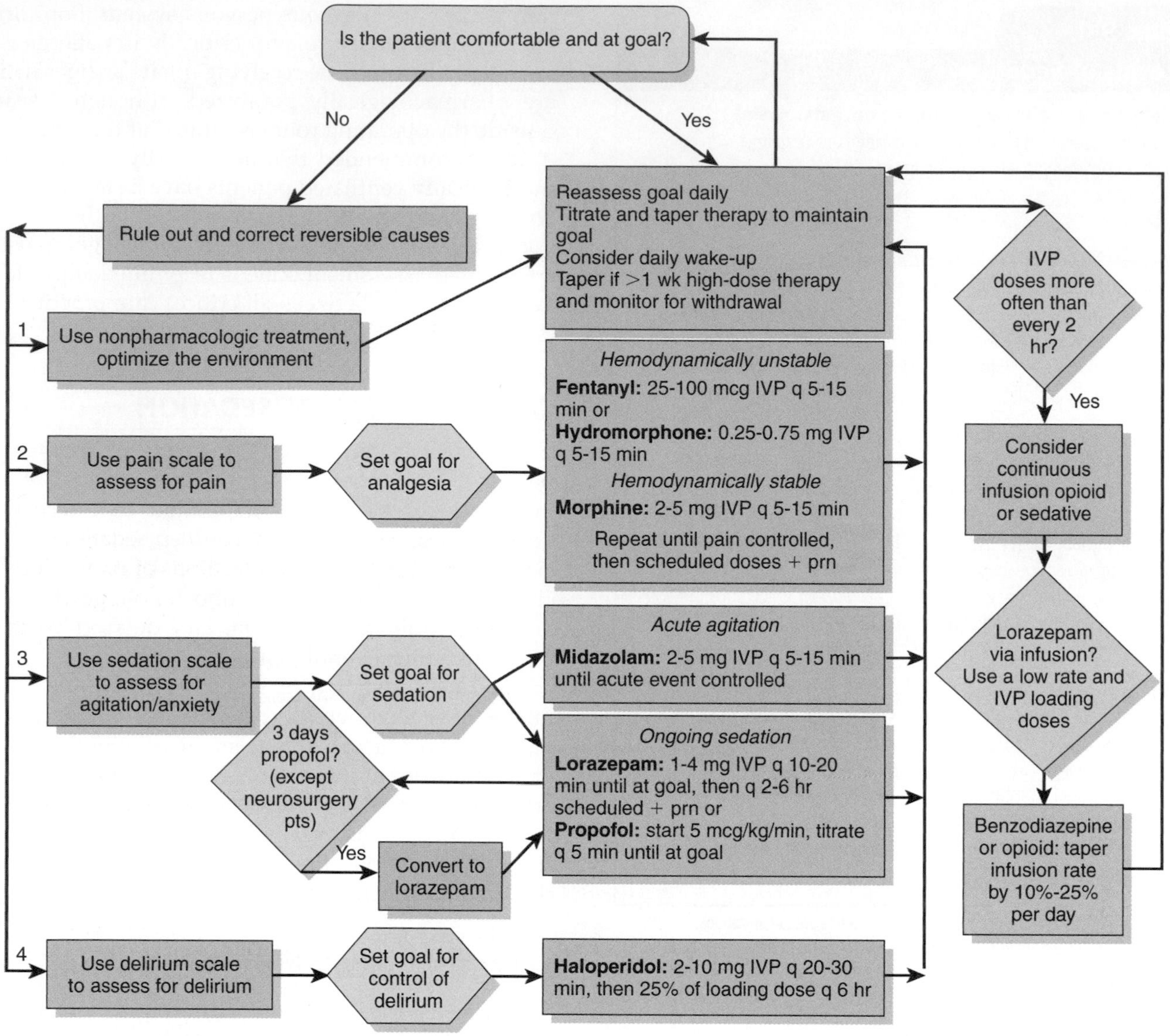

FIGURE 9-1. General guidelines for sedation and analgesia management of mechanically ventilated critical care patients. Doses are approximate for a 70-kg (154-pound) adult. *IVP,* Intravenous push; *q,* every; *prn,* as needed. (From Jacobi J et al: *Crit Care Med* 30(1):119, 2002.)

(see Figure 9-1). One advantage of lorazepam for long-term sedation is that it does not have active metabolites that contribute to the overall sedative effect. Lorazepam has a slow onset, which makes it unsuitable for the treatment of acute agitation. As would be expected, the recovery time from a sedated state takes longer when infusing lorazepam (Ativan) compared with midazolam (Versed); the higher the dose infused, the longer the recovery time for both drugs.[11] Mechanically ventilated patients who were sedated with a continuous infusion of lorazepam for 72 hours emerged from light sedation in 11.9 hours, whereas recovery from deep sedation took 31.1 hours. By contrast, in the same research study, patients who were sedated with a continuous midazolam infusion emerged from light sedation in 3.6 hours and from deep sedation in 14.9 hours.[11] Clearly, even within the class of benzodiazepines it is important to select the sedative agent carefully, anticipating how long the patient will be sedated and how long it will take to recover from the sedative state.

Benzodiazepine Antidote

The major unwanted side effects associated with the benzodiazepines are dose-related respiratory depression and hypotension.[10] If needed, *flumazenil* (Romazicon) is the antidote used to reverse benzodiazepine overdose in symptomatic patients.[10] Flumazenil should be avoided in patients with benzodiazepine dependence because rapid withdrawal can induce seizures.[10]

Sedative-Hypnotic Agents

Propofol (Diprivan) is an IV-delivered sedative-hypnotic.[3,12,13] At high doses (greater than 100 to 200 mcg/kg/min), propofol is intended to produce a

Table 9-2
Pharmacologic Management: Sedation

DRUGS	DOSAGE	ACTIONS	SPECIAL CONSIDERATIONS
Benzodiazepines			
Diazepam	0.03-0.1 mg/kg every 0.5-6 hr (slow IV intermittent doses)	Anxiolysis Amnesia Sedation	*Onset:* 2-5 min following IV administration. *Side effects:* Hypotension, respiratory depression. *Half-life of parent compound:* long, from 20-120 hr. Contains active sedative metabolites that also contribute to prolonged sedative effect. *Drug tolerance:* Physical tolerance develops with prolonged use, and more drug is required to achieve same effect over time. Slow wean required from diazepam after continuous prolonged use. Phlebitis in peripheral IV.
Lorazepam	0.02-0.06 mg/kg every 2-6 hr (slow IV intermittent doses) 0.01-0.1 mg/kg/hr (continuous infusion)	Anxiolysis Amnesia Sedation	*Onset:* 5-20 min following IV administration. *Side effects:* Hypotension, respiratory depression. *Half-life of parent compound:* Relatively long, ranges from 8-15 hr. Sedative effect is also prolonged. *Drug tolerance:* Physical tolerance develops with use, and higher drug dosage is required to achieve same effect over time. Slow wean required from lorazepam after continuous prolonged use. Solvent-related acidosis/renal failure at high doses.
Midazolam	0.02-0.08 mg/kg every 0.5-2 hr (slow IV intermittent doses) 0.04-0.2 mg/kg/hr (continuous infusion)	Anxiolysis Amnesia Sedation	*Onset:* 2-5 min following IV administration. *Side effects:* Hypotension, respiratory depression. *Half-life of parent compound:* Ranges from 3-11 hr. Sedative effect prolonged when midazolam infusion has continued for many days. This is due to presence of active sedative metabolites. Sedative effect also prolonged in renal failure. *Drug tolerance:* Physical tolerance develops with prolonged use, and higher drug dosage is required to achieve same effect over time. Slow wean required from midazolam after prolonged use.
Sedative-Hypnotic Agents			
Propofol	5-80 mcg/kg/min (continuous infusion)	Anxiolysis Amnesia Sedation	*Onset:* 1-2 min, very rapid onset following IV administration. *Side effects:* Hypotension, respiratory depression (patient must be intubated and mechanically ventilated to eliminate this complication). *Half-life of parent compound:* 2-8 min when used as a short-term agent. *Sedative effect:* Can range from 26-32 hr with prolonged continuous IV infusion. Effective short-term anesthetic agent, useful for rapid "wake-up" of patients for assessment. If continuous infusion is used for many days, emergence from sedation can take hours or days. Sedative effect is dependent upon dose of drug administered, depth of sedation, and length of time sedated. Change IV infusion tubing every 12 hr. Requires a dedicated IV catheter and tubing (do not mix with other drugs). Monitor serum triglyceride levels.
Neuroleptic Agents			
Haloperidol	0.03-0.15 mg/kg every 0.5-6 hr (IV intermittent doses) 0.04-0.15 mg/kg/hr (continuous infusion)	Antipsychotic Antidelirium	*Onset:* 3-20 min following IV administration. *Half-life of parent compound:* 18-54 hr. Used in management of delirium. Sedation is an unintended side effect. Measure QT interval at baseline and periodically during haloperidol infusion. Active metabolites may cause extrapyramidal symptoms (EPS). Anticholinergic agent may be administered if EPS occur.
Alpha-Adrenergic Receptor Agonists			
Dexmedetomidine	1 mcg/kg initial loading dose over 20 min 0.2-0.7 mcg/kg/hr (continuous infusion)	Anxiolysis Analgesia Sedation	*Half-life:* Approximately 2 hr. Duration of infusion up to 24 hr only. Bolus dosing is not recommended. Maintenance infusion is adjusted to achieve desired level of sedation.

IV, Intravenous; *EPS,* extrapyramidal symptoms.

state of general anesthesia in the operating room.[13] In the critical care unit, propofol is generally prescribed at lower doses to induce a state of deep sedation (5 to 50 mcg/kg/min).[13] The clinical advantage of propofol is its very short half-life and rapid elimination from the body. It does not have active metabolites.[12,13] This drug is especially suitable for management of the agitated neurologic patient with brain injury. Propofol quickly crosses the blood-brain barrier, slows cerebral metabolism, and decreases elevated intracranial pressure (ICP).[13]

With short-term administration the drug infusion can be turned off, and the patient can be fully alert within 30 minutes. The half-life is 2 to 4 minutes with short-term use.[13] If propofol is infused for several days, the wake-up time is also prolonged.[12,14] If propofol is infused for over 10 days, the half-life extends to 1 to 3 days.[13] Propofol is not a reliable amnesic, and patients sedated with only propofol can have vivid recollections of their experiences. It is therefore important to add an opiate such as *fentanyl* to ensure adequate amnesia.[12]

Significant disadvantages of propofol are mainly related to the high lipid content. It comes packaged in a glass container and has the appearance of milk. Propofol is emulsified in a soybean Intralipid emulsion that delivers 1.1 kcal/ml as fat. These calories must be taken into account when assessing nutritional intake.[13] Propofol can elevate serum triglyceride levels and has been associated with pancreatitis. The lipid emulsion can also act as a potential medium for bacterial growth. Administration requires a dedicated IV line, and the IV solution and tubing must be changed every 12 hours.[13] Propofol shares with other sedatives the propensity for hypotension when delivered rapidly.[12,13]

Propofol infusion syndrome (PIS) is a rare complication of prolonged, high-dose propofol administration. It occurs more commonly in children than in adult critically ill patients. The syndrome includes cardiac arrest, myocardial failure, metabolic acidosis, rhabdomyolysis, and hyperkalemia that occur on day 4 or 5 following very high-dose propofol infusion.[15,16] Clinicians are advised not to administer dosages above 5 mg/kg/hr for longer than 48 hours. Propofol is prescribed only for intubated patients.[15,16]

Central α-Agonists

Two central α-adrenergic agonists are available for sedation: clonidine (often prescribed as a Catapres patch) and dexmedetomidine (Precedex as a continuous infusion). *Clonidine* is prescribed for patients experiencing withdrawal syndromes. *Dexmedetomidine* is a newer α_2-agonist recently approved for use as a short-term sedative (less than 24 hours) for the mechanically ventilated patient. It is prescribed in some hospitals to wean patients from short-term ventilation after cardiac surgery.[17,18] At this time there is not enough information to determine whether dexmedetomidine will have a wider role in sedation therapy lasting more than 24 hours.[3]

SEDATIVE SELECTION

The choice of sedative is both patient and situation specific. If the need is for *short-term* sedation (less than 24 hours), the most frequently used sedatives are midazolam or propofol.[3,10-14] Both these drugs may be combined with a short-acting opioid analgesic (e.g., fentanyl). If the need is for *intermediate-term* sedation (1 to 3 days), the most frequently prescribed drugs again are propofol and midazolam, plus an opiate analgesic. If the need is for *long-term* sedation, the recommended agent is lorazepam.[3] Research using continuous EEG monitoring has shown that patients who receive continuous sedative infusions are more deeply sedated than patients who are given sedatives as an IV bolus; patients receiving continuous infusions are also more likely to become oversedated.[19]

SEDATION VACATION

One innovative strategy to avoid pitfalls of sedative dependence and withdrawal is a planned "daily drug holiday." This means that all sedative agents are turned off once a day and the patient is allowed to awaken.[20,21] The patient is carefully monitored, and when consciousness and awareness are attained, an assessment of level of consciousness and neurologic function is performed. When using protocols that incorporate daily interruption of sedative infusions, it is imperative that any neurological assessments be performed and documented during the wake-up period. Also, if the patient becomes agitated, it is essential that a protocol be in place for the nurse to restart the sedatives, plus opiates if applicable.[20,21] One protocol scheduled the daily interruption of sedatives in the morning and, after a full assessment, recommended restarting the sedative and opiate infusions at 50% of the previous morning dose and adjusting upward until the patient was comfortable.[20,21] The intubated patients who were woken up daily by turning off the sedative infusions experienced a lower rate of complications and lower levels of PSTD.[21-23] For patients with coronary artery disease, there was no change in myocardial ischemia during the daily sedation vacation.[24]

AGITATION

The question of which sedatives and opiates to use to minimize agitation once the drugs are discontinued is complex. Long-term patients are frequently mechanically ventilated and often seriously ill for weeks. To

Table 9-3
Signs and Symptoms of Sedative/Analgesic Drug Withdrawal*

SYSTEM	OPIATE WITHDRAWAL	BENZODIAZEPINE WITHDRAWAL†
Neurologic	Delirium, tremors, seizures	Agitation, anxiety, delirium, tremors, myoclonus, headache, seizures, fatigue, paresthesias, sleep disturbances
Hemodynamic	Tachycardia, hypertension (SNS stimulation)	Tachycardia, hypertension (SNS stimulation)
Sensory	Dilation of pupils, teary eyes, irritability, increased sensitivity to pain, sweating, yawning	Increased sensitivity to light/sound, sweating
Musculoskeletal	Cramps, muscle aches	Muscle cramps
Gastrointestinal	Vomiting, diarrhea	Nausea, diarrhea
Respiratory	Tachypnea	Tachypnea

*Data on propofol is limited, but withdrawal symptoms after prolonged use similar to those of the benzodiazepines.[3]
†Not all symptoms are seen in all patients.[3,25]
SNS, Sympathetic nervous system.

tolerate the ventilator and other procedures, patients must receive sedation and analgesia. When it is time to decrease the sedation, many patients have become physically tolerant, and as the drug dosage is reduced, they become highly agitated.

Physical symptoms of agitation can include increased heart rate, blood pressure, and respiratory rate. Other notable symptoms include lack of self-awareness, unawareness of surroundings, very short-term memory for information, irritability, anxiety, confusion, delirium, and even seizures.[3] Patients may pull at the tubes and attempt to climb out of bed and can represent a danger to themselves, the nurse, and family visitors. The temptation to resedate is powerful, because it is hard to watch someone become disorientated and agitated.

An important nursing responsibility is to prevent the patient from coming to harm during drug withdrawal (Table 9-3). Some movement in bed is expected, but extreme restlessness increases myocardial oxygen consumption and work of breathing and activates the sympathetic nervous system. If the patient is seriously agitated, it is vital to consult with the physician and pharmacist to establish an effective treatment plan that will allow weaning from these agents without harm. The approach to avoid sedative and opiate tolerance and withdrawal symptoms is not yet fully delineated but clearly requires a multidisciplinary effort with ongoing evaluation using an established assessment scale (see Table 9-1).

Box 9-2
Causes of Delirium in Critically Ill Patients

Metabolic
Acid-base disturbance
Electrolyte imbalance
Hypoglycemia

Intracranial
Epidural/subdural hematoma
Intracranial hemorrhage
Meningitis
Encephalitis
Cerebral abscess
Tumor

Endocrine
Hyperthyroidism/hypothyroidism
Addison's disease
Hyperparathyroidism
Cushing's syndrome

Organ Failure
Liver encephalopathy
Uremic encephalopathy
Septic shock

Respiratory
Hypoxemia
Hypercarbia

Drug Related
Alcohol withdrawal
Drug-induced
Heavy metal poisoning

Modified from Szokol JW, Vender JS: *Crit Care Clin* 17(4):821, 2001.

ASSESSING FOR DELIRIUM

Delirium is described as a reversible global impairment of cognitive processes, usually of sudden onset, coupled with disorientation, impaired short-term memory, altered sensory perceptions (hallucinations), abnormal thought processes, and inappropriate behavior. Delirium is probably more prevalent than generally recognized and is difficult to diagnose in the critically ill patient. The incidence ranges from 30% to 70% in medical-surgical critical care patients (Box 9-2).[3,25] Delirium increases both hospital stay and mortality in patients who are mechanically ventilated.[26] The increase in mortality remains true even after controlling for associated variables such as coma, sedatives, and analgesic administration.[26]

When patients are agitated, restless, and pulling at tube and lines, they are often identified as delirious. In this scenario, delirium may be described as *ICU psychosis*. However, the delirious patient is not always agitated, and it is much more difficult to detect delirium when the patient is apparently calm.[3,25,27] The major categories to assess include (1) acute onset of mental status changes or fluctuating course, (2) inattention, (3) disorganized thinking, and (4) altered level of consciousness, which can include any level of consciousness other than "alert". Routine assessment for the presence of delirium is recommended in critical care patients.[27] Specific scoring scales are available to assess for delirium, and an experienced psychiatric consultant can be helpful.[27]

EVIDENCE-BASED COLLABORATIVE PRACTICE

Sedation in the Critically Ill

The key recommendations from the clinical practice guideline for the sustained use of sedatives and analgesia in the critically ill adult, based upon research and expert panel opinion, are as follows:

Assessment, Communication, and Documentation

1. Frequent assessment of critically ill patients is mandated to determine if sedation and analgesia are required and appropriate as part of the plan of care.
2. A sedation goal or endpoint should be established for each patient at the beginning of therapy; for example, "a calm patient that can be easily aroused with maintenance of the normal sleep-wake cycle." Some patients may require deep sedation to facilitate synchrony with mechanical ventilation.
3. Need for sedation should be reevaluated on a frequent basis as the clinical condition of the patient changes.
4. Sedation regimens should be written with the flexibility to allow titration to the desired endpoint, anticipating fluctuations in sedation requirements throughout the day.
5. Use of a validated sedation assessment scale to standardize assessment among clinicians and document the patient's level of sedation and response to sedatives is recommended. Vital signs such as blood pressure or heart rate are not sufficiently specific or sensitive to serve as indicators of sedation effectiveness.
6. Sedation and analgesia goals must be communicated to all caregivers and to the patient and family.
7. Due to insufficient research, using sedation monitors that interpret EEG data are not endorsed for monitoring critical care patients.

Agitation

8. Sedation of agitated critically ill patients should be started only after providing adequate analgesia and providing treatment for reversible physiologic causes of agitation.
9. Cautious use of sedatives is warranted for patients not yet intubated because of the risk of respiratory depression.

Drug Therapy

10. Midazolam or diazepam should be used for rapid sedation of acutely agitated patients.
11. Propofol is the preferred sedative when rapid awakening for rapid neurologic assessment or extubation is important.
12. Midazolam is recommended for short-term use only, because it provokes unpredictable awakening and time to extubation when infusions continue longer than 48 to 72 hours.
13. Lorazepam is the recommended sedative when prolonged mechanical ventilation is required, via intermittent IV administration or continuous infusion.

Avoidance of Complications

14. The titration of the sedative dose to a defined endpoint is recommended with systemic tapering of the dose, or daily interruption with retitration to minimize prolonged sedative effects.
15. Triglyceride concentrations should be monitored after 2 days of propofol infusion, and total caloric intake from lipids should be included in the nutrition support prescription.
16. The potential for opioid, benzodiazepine, and propofol withdrawal should be considered after high doses of more than approximately 7 days of continuous therapy. Doses should be tapered systematically to prevent withdrawal symptoms.

Delirium

17. Routine assessment for the presence of delirium is recommended. The CAM-ICU is noted as a promising assessment tool for delirium.
18. Haloperidol is the preferred agent for the treatment of delirium in critically ill patients.
19. ECG monitoring for detection of potential QT interval prolongation and dysrhythmias is recommended when haloperidol is administered.

Sleep

20. Sleep promotion should include optimization of the environment and nonpharmacologic methods to promote relaxation with adjunctive use of hypnotics.

Data from Jacobi J et al: *Crit Care Med 30*(1):119, 2002.

EEG, Electroencephalogram; *IV*, intravenous; *CAM-ICU*, Confusion Assessment Method-ICU instrument; *ECG*, electrocardiogram.

The *nonpharmacologic* strategies used to prevent agitation and delirium include back massage, music therapy, noise reduction in the environment, decreasing lights at night to promote sleep, clustering nursing care to provide some uninterrupted rest periods, and speaking in a calm, quiet, and gentle voice.* Reorientation to the environment and the use of a person's hearing aid or glasses, if these are normally used, can lower the incidence of delirium.[27]

SELECTING MEDICATIONS FOR MANAGING DELIRIUM

Unfortunately, the medications typically prescribed for sedation and analgesia may exacerbate the symptoms of delirium. Sedatives make delirious patients confused, less responsive, and more obtunded,[23] thus creating a situation that can also lead to a paradoxical increase in agitation. The neuroleptic drug haloperidol (Haldol) is frequently prescribed. This antipsychotic agent stabilizes cerebral function by blocking dopamine-mediated neurotransmission at the cerebral synapses and in the basal ganglia. Delirium is reduced, but the patient tends to have a flat affect and diminished interest in surroundings and with higher doses becomes sedated. Electrocardiographic (ECG) monitoring is recommended because neuroleptic agents produce dose-dependent QT interval prolongation, with an increased incidence of ventricular dysrhythmias.[10]

COLLABORATIVE MANAGEMENT

Collaborative management of anxiety, agitation, and sedation is a responsibility shared by all members of the health care team (see Evidence-Based Collaborative Practice: Sedation in the Critically Ill).

Recognition of the problem is the first step toward a solution to establish a more effective standard of patient care in sedation/analgesia management. It is important to involve families and significant companions in the plan of care for effective management of both pain and sedation.

evolve To test your mastery of this chapter, try the Open-Book Quiz at http://evolve.elsevier.com/Urden/priorities/

REFERENCES

1. Fraser GL, Riker RR: Monitoring sedation, agitation, analgesia, and delirium in critically ill adult patients, *Crit Care Clin* 17(4):967, 2001.
2. Joint Commission on Accreditation of Healthcare Organizations: Standards and intents for sedation and analgesia care in the revisions to anesthesia care standards. In *Comprehensive accreditation manual for hospitals*, Oakbrook Terrace, Ill, 2000, The Commission.

*References 2, 3, 9, 10, 12, 13, 27, 28.

3. Jacobi J et al: Clinical practice guidelines for the sustained use of sedatives and analgesics in the critically ill adult, *Crit Care Med* 30(1):119, 2002.
4. Consensus conference on sedation assessment: a collaborative venture by Abbott Laboratories, American Association of Critical-Care Nurses, and Saint Thomas Health System, *Crit Care Nurse* 24(2):33, 2004.
5. Payen JF et al: Current Practices in Sedation and analgesia for mechanically ventilated artically ill patients, Anesthesiology 106(4):687, 2007.
6. Arbour R: Continuous nervous system monitoring, EEG, the bispectral index, and neuromuscular transmission, *AACN Clin Issues* 14(2):185, 2003.
7. Arbour R: Using bispectral index monitoring to detect potential breakthrough awareness and limit duration of neuromuscular blockade, *Am J Crit Care* 13(1):66, 2004.
8. Drover DR et al: Patient State Index: titration of delivery and recovery from propofol, alfentanil, and nitrous oxide anesthesia, *Anesthesiology* 97(1):82, 2002.
9. McGaffigan PA: Advancing sedation assessment to promote patient comfort, *Crit Care Nurse* 22(suppl):29, 2002.
10. Young CC, Prielipp RC: Benzodiazepines in the intensive care unit, *Crit Care Clin* 17(4):843, 2001.
11. Barr J et al: A double-blind, randomized comparison of IV lorazepam versus midazolam for sedation of ICU patients via a pharmacologic model, *Anesthesiology* 95(2):286, 2001.
12. Angelini G, Ketzler JT, Coursin DB: Use of propofol and other nonbenzodiazepine sedatives in the intensive care unit, *Crit Care Clin* 17(4):863, 2001.
13. Whitcomb JJ, Huddleston MC, McAndrews KL: The use of propofol in the mechanically ventilated medical/surgical intensive care patient: is it the right choice? *Dimens Crit Care Nurs* 22(2):60, 2003.
14. Barr J et al: Propofol dosing regimens for ICU sedation based upon an integrated pharmacokinetic-pharmacodynamic model, *Anesthesiology* 95(2):324, 2001.
15. Cremer OL et al: Long-term propofol infusion and cardiac failure in adult head-injured patients, *Lancet* 357(9250):117, 2001.
16. Kang TM: Propofol infusion syndrome in critically ill patients, *Ann Pharmacother* 36(9):1453, 2002.
17. Coursin DB, Maccioli GA: Dexmedetomidine, *Curr Opin Crit Care* 7(4):221, 2001.
18. Herr DL, Sum-Ping ST, England M: ICU sedation after coronary artery bypass graft surgery: dexmedetomidine-based versus propofol-based sedation regimens, *J Cardiothorac Vasc Anesth* 17(5):576, 2003.
19. de Wit M, Epstein SK: Administration of sedatives and level of sedation: comparative evaluation via the Sedation-Agitation Scale and the Bispectral Index, *Am J Crit Care* 12(4):343, 2003.
20. Kress JP et al: Daily interruption of sedative infusions in critically ill patients undergoing mechanical ventilation, *N Engl J Med* 342(20):1471, 2000.
21. Schweickert WD et al: Daily interruption of sedative infusions and complications of critical illness in mechanically ventilated patients, *Crit Care Med* 32(6):1272, 2004.
22. Kress JP et al: The long-term psychological effects of daily sedative interruption on critically ill patients, *Am J Respir Crit Care Med* 168(12):1457, 2003.

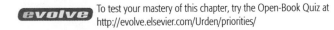

23. Carson SS et al: A randomized trial of intermittent lorazepam versus propofol with daily interruption in mechanically ventilated patients, *Crit Care Med* 34(5):1326, 2006.
24. Kress JP et al: Daily sedative interruption in mechanically ventilated patients at risk for coronary artery disease, *Crit Care Med* 35(2):365, 2007.
25. Szokol JW, Vender JS: Anxiety, delirium, and pain in the intensive care unit, *Crit Care Clin* 17(4):821, 2001.
26. Ely EW et al: Delirium as a predictor of mortality in mechanically ventilated patients in the intensive care unit, *JAMA* 291(14):1753, 2004.
27. Pandharipande P et al: Delirium: acute cognitive dysfunction in the critically ill, *Curr Opin Crit Care* 11:360, 2005.
28. Honkus VL: Sleep deprivation in critical care units, *Crit Care Nurs Q* 26(3):179, 2003.

CHAPTER 10

End-of-Life Issues

KARIN T. KIRCHHOFF

OBJECTIVES

- Describe the impact of advance directives and advance care planning on provision of end-of-life care in the intensive care unit (ICU).
- Discuss the concepts of patient and family-centered decision making.
- Explain the need for symptom assessment and management during end-of-life care in the ICU.
- Discuss the role of collaborative practice in end-of-life care in the ICU.

End of life has not been thought of as an important clinical topic in critical care. Because the primary purpose of admission of patients to a critical care unit is for aggressive, lifesaving care, the death of a patient is generally regarded as a failure. Because the culture is that of saving lives, the language around end of life is stated in negative terms such as forgoing life-sustaining treatments, do not resuscitate (DNR), and withdrawal of life support. At times the phrase *withdrawal of care* is used—imagine the impact of that phrase on families. Content on end of life in critical care textbooks, both medical[1] and nursing,[2] is minimal; further, the first textbook on end of life in critical care was only published in 1998[3] and the second in 2001.[4]

More attention is being given to the quality of the end-of-life experience of the critically ill with recognition of the numbers of patients who die in critical care units. The focus of the content in this chapter will be on the evidence we have for the care we are rendering to the dying critical care patient and his or her family, and care that is recommended by evidence, research reports, and summaries of research and guidelines.

END-OF-LIFE EXPERIENCE IN CRITICAL CARE

This attention to end of life in hospitalized patients has increased since the publication of the Study to Understand Prognoses and Preferences for Outcomes and Risks of Treatments (SUPPORT).[5] In this major report, more than 9000 seriously ill patients in five medical centers were studied. Despite an intervention to improve communication, shortcomings were found, aggressive treatment was frequent, only one half of physicians knew their patients' preferences to avoid cardiopulmonary resuscitation (CPR), more than one third of patients who died spent at least 10 days in a critical care unit, and for 50% of conscious patients, family members reported moderate to severe pain at least half of the time.

Following closely after the publication of the SUPPORT study, the Institute of Medicine (IOM) released a report, *Approaching Death: Improving Care at the End of Life.*[6] The group detailed deficiencies in care and gave seven recommendations to improve care:

1. Patients with fatal illnesses and their family should receive reliable, skillful, and supportive care.
2. Health professionals should improve care for the dying.
3. Policymakers and consumers should work with health professionals to improve quality and financing of care.
4. Health profession education should include end-of-life content.
5. Palliative care should be developed, possibly as a medical specialty.
6. Research on end of life should be funded.
7. The public should communicate more about the experience of dying and options available.

In SUPPORT and in the IOM report, critical care patients were included with other hospitalized patients. In order to describe the number of deaths in critical care units, Angus et al[7] reviewed hospital discharge data from six states and the National Death Index. Of the more than 500,000 deaths studied, 38.3% were in hospitals, and 22% (59% of all hospital deaths) occurred after admission to the critical care unit. Terminal admissions associated with critical care accounted for 80% of all terminal hospitalization costs.[7] The likelihood of dying in hospital increased from age 25 to 74, and the likelihood of dying after critical care unit admission remained 25% of all deaths for each age category. Although 90% of people would prefer to die in their own homes,[6] more than 20% of those who died in this review received high-tech aggressive care before they died.

ADVANCE DIRECTIVES

Although advance directives, also known as a *living will* or a *health care power of attorney,* were encouraged to ensure patients received the care they desired, the enactment has been less than desired. Like other preventive measures, it is underused, even though it is inexpensive and potentially effective.[8] Prevalence rates of advance directives were 30% or less in a group 65 years or older, but only 15% had discussed their wishes with their primary physician, which is a bigger issue.[9] Even when advance directives are present, the question arises as to whether they are applicable; in other words, "Is this a terminal illness?"

ADVANCE CARE PLANNING

Cultural influences in the United States discourage discussion of death. To actually plan for decisions to be made when one is incompetent is difficult, however helpful they would be for those families members left to make those decisions. Advance care planning for those with chronic illness would be advantageous for all involved, especially where there are repeated critical care unit admissions involved. Communication of the patient's wishes between primary care providers and intensivists is critical. If patients have stated desires, those should be communicated when patients are transferred. If the patient has not specified his or her preferences, that too is important and should be communicated to new health care providers; if patients desire aggressive care, it should be offered as appropriate. If aggressive care is not how the patient wishes to be managed, then patients, families, and care providers could be so informed and families would not be left in emergency situations trying to decide what to do.

ETHICAL/LEGAL ISSUES

Legal and ethical principles guide many of our decisions in caring for the dying patient and the family. The patient is respected as autonomous and able to make his or her own decisions. When the patient is unable to make decisions, the same respect should be accorded to surrogates. These wishes may have been put in writing by the patient as an advance directive. The Patient Self-Determination Act supports the patient's right to control future treatment in the event the individual cannot speak for himself or herself.

Two of the basic ethical principles underlying the provision of health care are beneficence and nonmaleficence. Beneficence is the principle of intending to benefit the other through one's actions. Nonmaleficence means to do no harm. Sometimes, at end of life, these are seen in conflict, such as when resuscitation is attempted under beneficence but does cause harm.

COMFORT CARE

The decision to withdraw life-sustaining treatments and switch to comfort care at end of life should be made with as much involvement of the patient as possible, including physical presence of the patient in decision making or procuring paper documents if the patient is not able to be present. If neither is available, the patient's intent as understood from discussions or knowledge of the patient should guide the decision whether or not to withdraw treatment. Withholding and withdrawing are considered to be morally and legally equivalent.[10] However, families have more stress in withdrawing treatments than in withholding them,[11] so treatments should not be started that the patient would not want or that would not be beneficial.

The goal of withdrawal of life-sustaining treatments is to remove treatments that are not beneficial and may be uncomfortable. Any treatment in this circumstance may be withheld or withdrawn. Once the goal of comfort has been chosen, each procedure should be evaluated to see if it is necessary or if it causes discomfort. If discomfort is caused, those treatments do not need to be continued. Forgoing life-sustaining treatments is not the same as active euthanasia or assisted suicide. Killing is an action causing another's death, whereas allowing dying is avoiding any intervention that interferes with a natural death following illness or trauma.[3]

IMPACT OF DO-NOT-RESUSCITATE ORDERS

A DNR order should prevent the initiation of CPR. In a review of 25 years since the DNR was established, Burns et al[12] found that those with a DNR order sometimes received less care, and some treatments were withheld[13] without those changes being specified in the DNR order. DNR is sometimes thought to mean Do Not Care, but that is not the intent. DNR orders should be written before withdrawal of life support; this will prevent any unfortunate errors in unwanted resuscitation during the time period between initiation of withdrawal and the actual death.

PROGNOSTICATION

Why patients who will die soon receive life-prolonging therapy shortly before their death can be partially explained by a series of studies. Physicians' ability to prognosticate has been found to be limited;[14,15] in general, time to death is overestimated. Patients' wishes are usually not known, or when known, are vague[16] or change over the course of an illness.[17] Care is often not in accord with patient wishes, and this is more prevalent when comfort care is desired over aggressive care.[18] Skills in communication and end-of-life care are not emphasized in medical curricula.[19,20] The very skills that would enable assessment of patient wishes are not well developed.

Cardiopulmonary Resuscitation

One decision to be made as death approaches, the do-not-resuscitate order, is frequently delayed.[21] However, the benefits of resuscitation may be overestimated both for survival and for the more relevant outcome of functional status. In a meta-analysis of 51 studies, Ebell et al[22] found that the overall survival to discharge after in-hospital CPR was 13.4%. A decreased rate of immediate survival was found for patients with acquired immune deficiency syndrome (AIDS), those with a hematocrit above 35%, and those who were male. Decreased survival to discharge was related to sepsis on the day before resuscitation, cancer with or without metastasis, dementia, elevated serum creatinine level, African American race, and dependent status. CPR was originally developed for those with coronary artery disease, and they are the most likely to survive resuscitation to discharge, as well as those who suffer cardiac arrest in the critical care unit.[22] FitzGerald et al[23] found that functional status among almost one half of the survivors of in-hospital CPR had deteriorated compared with their condition 2 months before the event. After 6 months, 30% of those patients had died, and two thirds continued to lose function. Despite these dismal statistics, CPR is offered as an option without fully informing patients or families of the low possibility of survival, the pain and suffering involved during and after the procedure, and the potential for decline in functional status.

Prognostic Tools

There are two common tools for estimating critical care unit mortality: Acute Physiology and Chronic Health Evaluation (APACHE) and multiple organ dysfunction score (MODS).[24] However, when these were compared to physician estimates of intensive care unit survival less than 10%, the physician estimate was associated with subsequent life-support limitation. Physician estimate was more powerful in predicting mortality than illness severity, organ dysfunction, and use of inotropes or vasopressors.[25]

Despite this information and these tools, uncertainty remains a major issue in decision making, not only for physicians but for patients and families[17] as well. Because one is never sure, and because a few patients who were never thought likely to survive actually do return to visit a critical care unit, professionals are not confident about issues of survivability. In addition, many families cling to small hopes of survival and recovery.

COMMUNICATION AND DECISION MAKING

Communication with the patient and family is critically important.

Patient Communication

Patients' capacity for decision making is limited by illness severity; they are too sick or are hampered by the therapies or medications used to treat them.[26] As decision making is required, the patient is the first person to be approached. When the patient is not able to safely make health care decisions, because of disease progression or the therapy used for treatment, written documents such as a living will or a health care power of attorney should be obtained when possible. Without those documents, wishes of the patient should be ascertained from those closest to the patient. Some states have a legal order of priority for surrogates.

Family Communication

How questions are asked of surrogates is extremely important. The question is not, "What do you want to do about (patient's name)?" but rather, "What would (patient's name) want if he knew he were in this situation?" The consequences of the questions for the family are vastly different. The former has a greater likelihood of engendering guilt over "pulling the plug." The latter question gives more the sense of fulfilling what the patient wanted. Sometimes this discussion is held in the family meeting where a general sense of goals can be discussed. As families make decisions, they appreciate support of those decisions, and that support can reduce the burden they experience.

Family members have reported dissatisfaction with communication and decision making.[27] Increasing the frequency of communication and sharing concerns early in the hospitalization will make subsequent discussions easier for both the patient and family and the health professional. Having the entire critical care unit team present for morning rounds is one method of improving communication.[28]

CULTURE AND RELIGIOUS INFLUENCES

Cultural and religious influences on attitudes and beliefs about death and dying differ dramatically. Those cultures of the predominant religions commonly seen in the surrounding community should be familiar to the local health care team. These differences may affect how the health care team is viewed, how decisions are made, whether aggressive treatment is preferred, how death is met, and how grieving will occur.[29,30] One's own attitude toward the specific practices of a culture should be that of assessment[31] and respect. Interpreters are necessary when the patient or the family do not speak English.

HOSPICE

Although hospice care has been available, patients and families frequently view that method of support during the last months of a patient in end-stage illness as "giving up." Health professionals can assist patients and families by providing information about the hospice benefit. Some hospices are offering to partner with critical care units in the provision of end-of-life care and in the process of withdrawal of ventilatory support.

WITHDRAWAL OR WITHHOLDING OF TREATMENT

Discussions about the potential for impending death are never held early enough. Usually the first discussion is around the discontinuation of life support. The late timing of that first discussion is an issue, because sometimes families have arrived at the notion of withdrawal before physicians.[26,32] Physicians could give families time to adjust by providing discussions early on about prognosis, goals of therapy, and patient's wishes.[33]

Proactive Approach

Once a poor prognosis is established, a length of time can elapse before end-of-life treatment goals are established. Campbell and Guzman[34] recommended a proactive case-finding approach by palliative care personnel to decrease hospital length of stay for patients with multiorgan system failure and global cerebral ischemia. They shortened the time between identifying the poor prognosis and establishing comfort care goals, decreased length of critical care unit stay for patients with multisystem organ dysfunction, and reduced the cost of care.

Disagreement and Distress for Caregivers

Nurses and doctors frequently disagree about the futility of interventions. Sometimes nurses consider withdrawal before physicians and patients and feel as though the care they are giving is unnecessary and possibly harmful. Nurses in one study were found to be more pessimistic but more often correct than physicians in the prognosis of dying patients, but the nurses proposed treatment withdrawal in some very sick patients who survived.[35] This issue is a serious one for critical care nurses, because the score on the emotional exhaustion subscale of the Maslach Burnout Inventory and the score on the frequency subscale on the Moral Distress Scale were found to correlate in a group of 60 critical care nurses.[36]

Barriers to Dying

Many barriers to diagnosing dying are present in the critical care unit: hope for the patient to improve, unclear diagnosis, pursuance of futile interventions, disagreement about the patient's condition, failure to recognize key signs and symptoms, poor ability to communicate, fears about foreshortening life, concerns about withdrawal and withholding, and medicolegal issues.[37] Further, prognostic models are used to predict mortality rates for groups of critical care patients, rather than to guide specific decisions to forego treatment.[38]

Steps Toward Comfort Care

If a series of interventions is to be withdrawn, usually dialysis is discontinued first along with diagnostic procedures and vasopressors. Next, intravenous (IV) fluids, monitoring, laboratory tests, and antibiotics are stopped.[38] Withdrawal of specific treatments may have effects necessitating symptom management. Withdrawal of dialysis may cause dyspnea from volume overload, which may necessitate the use of opioids or benzodiazepines. Efforts to discontinue artificial feeding may be met with concern from the family, because offering food has high social significance.

PALLIATIVE CARE

Those patients who are identified as being near the end of life require aggressive care for their symptom management, provided by a team of health professionals. The most relevant clinical goal should be to palliate these unpleasant situations by assessing for them and implementing appropriate interventions.[3] Palliative care guidelines have been released by a consortium of organizations concerned with palliative care and end-of-life care, and these may provide guidance when the usual first-line treatments do not promote comfort for critically ill patients who are near death.[39] Palliative care has been thought of as desirable only when the patient nears death or when several interventions have been tried for management of symptoms without success. However, recent publications such as these guidelines and the IOM report *Improving Palliative Care for Cancer*[40] stated that palliative care ideally begins at the time of diagnosis of a life-threatening illness and continues through cure or until death and into the family's bereavement period.

Pain Management

Because many critical care patients are not conscious, assessment of pain and other symptoms becomes more difficult.[41] Gelinas et al[42] recommended using signs of body movements, neuromuscular signs, facial expressions, or response to physical examination for pain assessment in patients with altered consciousness (see Chapter 8). Foley,[43] while acknowledging the usual three-step approach of the World Health Organization, admitted that in critical care units, step 3 is frequently used because of the intensity of the pain. Nonopioid drugs are the first-line approach, followed by adding an opioid for additional analgesia when relief is not obtained. Because opioids provide seda-tion and anxiolysis as well as analgesia, they are particularly beneficial in the ventilated patient. Morphine is the drug of choice, and there is no upper limit in dosing.[3] In nonventilated patients, sedation may cause respiratory depression,[43] and nonopioids or specific anesthetic agents may be more appropriate. The Society of Critical Care Medicine (SCCM) has published a guideline for the sustained use of sedatives and analgesia[44] (see Chapter 9).

Symptom Management

Symptom assessment is necessary for the patient who is near death and should include dyspnea, nausea and vomiting, edema and pulmonary edema, anxiety and delirium, metabolic derangements, skin integrity, and anemia and hemorrhage.[3]

Dyspnea

Campbell[45] recently published a review of terminal dyspnea and respiratory distress. Dyspnea is best managed with close evaluation of the patient and the use of opioids, sedatives, and nonpharmacologic interventions (oxygen, positioning, and increased ambient air flow). Morphine reduces anxiety and muscle tension and increases pulmonary vasodilation. Benzodiazepines may be used in patients who are not able to take opioids, or for whom the respiratory effects are minimal. Benzodiazepines and opioids should be titrated to effect.

Nausea and Vomiting

Nausea and vomiting are common and should be treated with antiemetics. The cause of nausea and vomiting may be intestinal obstruction. Treatment for decompression may be uncomfortable in dying patients, so its use should be weighed using a benefit/burden ratio.

Fever and Infection

Fever and infection will necessitate assessment of the benefits of continuing antibiotics so as not to prolong the dying process.[3] Management of the fever with antipyretics may be appropriate for patient comfort, but other methods such as ice or hypothermia blankets should be balanced against the amount of distress the patient would experience.

Edema

Edema may cause discomfort, and diuretics may be effective if kidney function is intact. Certainly dialysis would not be warranted at end of life. The use of fluids may contribute to the edema when kidney function is impaired and the body is slowing its functions.[46]

Anxiety

Anxiety should be assessed verbally, if possible, or by changes in vital signs or restlessness. Benzodiazepines, especially midazolam with its rapid onset and short half-life, are frequently used.

Delirium

Delirium is commonly observed in the critically ill and in those approaching death. Haloperidol is recommended as useful, and restraints should be avoided. Kehl[47] has published a review of available literature. She concluded that despite the recommendations of most authors to use neuroleptic medications as a treatment for restlessness, a number of studies demonstrated the effectiveness of other medications such as benzodiazepines (notably midazolam and lorazepam) or phenothiazines, either alone or in combination.

Metabolic Derangement

Treatments for metabolic derangements, skin problems, anemia, and hemorrhage should be tempered with concerns for patient comfort. Only those interventions promoting comfort should be performed. Patients do not necessarily feel better "when the lab values are right," if they had to have invasive treatments to get there.

Providing Comfort

The nursing interventions at end of life should focus on the provision of comfort care as an active, desirable, and important service. Unnecessary checks of vital signs, laboratory work, and any treatment that does not promote comfort should be avoided. Positioning the patient who is actively dying has comfort as its purpose. A positioning schedule to promote skin integrity is not warranted. Coordinating this care with the many members of the critical care team is important to ensure consistency across disciplines and across shifts. When symptom management is not successful in ensuring comfort, the services of the pain team or the palliative care service may be required.

NEAR-DEATH AWARENESS

Two hospice nurses have described a phenomenon of near-death awareness.[48] The same behaviors may be seen in conscious critical care patients near death. Having an awareness of the phenomenon will allow for more careful assessment of behaviors that could be interpreted as delirium, acid-base imbalance, or other metabolic derangements. These behaviors include communicating with someone who is not alive, preparing for travel, describing a place they can see, or even knowing when death will occur.[49]

WITHDRAWAL OF MECHANICAL VENTILATION

During the family meeting where a decision to withdraw life support is made, a time to initiate withdrawal is usually established. For example, a distant family member may need to arrive, and then the procedure will occur. Where possible, the patient should be moved to a separate or special room. It is helpful if noninvolved staff are alerted to the fact that a withdrawal is occurring. A neutral sign hung on the door or use of a special room may caution staff to avoid loud conversations and laughter, which is quite upsetting to families present.

Pacemakers or implantable cardioverter-defibrillators should be turned off to prevent patient distress from their firing[50] and to avoid interfering with the pronouncement of death.[38] Neuromuscular blocking agents should be discontinued, because paralysis precludes the assessment of patient discomfort and the means of the patient to communicate with loved ones. Time for clearance of the medication should be included in the schedule.[38]

The removal of monitors is usually recommended.[10] However, physicians may use the monitor to assess the distress of the patient during the withdrawal process to adjust the amount of medication needed. Families may glance at the monitor to verify that electrical activity has ceased because the appearance of death may be too subtle to detect. If not needed, monitors should be removed to make the room appear as normal as possible.

Opioids and Sedatives

Opioids and benzodiazepines are the most commonly administered medications, because dyspnea and anxiety are the usual symptoms related to ventilator withdrawal. Campbell[3] stated that brain-dead patients do not require sedation and patients with brain stem activity only may not show signs of distress or need sedation. Von Gunten and Weissman[51] recommended sedating all patients, even those who are comatose. They recommend a bolus dose of morphine, 2 to 10 mg IV, and a continuous morphine infusion at 50% of the bolus dose per hour. Midazolam, 1 to 2 mg IV, is given, followed by an infusion at 1 mg/hour. The intent is to provide good symptom control so that doses accelerate until patient comfort is achieved. Additional medication should be available at the bedside for immediate administration when patient discomfort is observed.

Ventilator Settings

After patient comfort is achieved, reduction of ventilator settings occurs. An experienced physician, a respiratory therapist, and a nurse should be present during this time. Ventilator alarms should be turned off. Which method of withdrawal is adopted is usually up to clinician preference. The choice of terminal wean as opposed to extubation is made based on considerations of access for suctioning, appearance of the patient for the family, how long the patient will survive off the ventilator, and whether the patient has the ability to communicate with loved ones at the bedside.

If terminal wean is used, first positive end-expiratory pressure (PEEP) is reduced to normal, then the mode is set to patient control. Next the FiO_2 is reduced to 0.21 (21%). Alternatively, the ventilator may be set to continuous positive airway pressure (CPAP) with pressure support (PS) increased to overcome symptoms of dyspnea. All of these steps are taken slowly while observing the patient for distress or anxiety. If extubation is used immediately, rather then at the end of the terminal wean, the family should be prepared for airway compromise and a change in the appearance of the patient.

All patients do not require the same ventilator weaning or extubation protocols. For example, Campbell[3] recommends turning off the ventilator and extubating patients who are brain dead, placing patients who have brain stem–only injuries on a T-piece, and using terminal weaning for those with altered consciousness or those who are conscious. The terminal wean offers the most control over secretions, respiratory noises, and gasping.

PROFESSIONAL ISSUES/HEALTH CARE SETTINGS

Professional issues surround the provision of palliative care within traditional acute and clinical settings. In critical care units, care may be managed by an intensivist or by a "committee" of specialists, seldom by the family physician who knows the patient. The use of consultants may be limited. Palliative care specialists might be advisable at times, but they are considered to be "outsiders" and are infrequently invited. How the consultation is arranged may vary by institution. "Turf" issues should not be the reason patients do not get the care they need.

Emotional Support for the Nurse

Nurses who care for the dying patient need to have that work as valued as the "high-tech" functions in the critical care unit. At times, critical care units have several nurses who seem to be the ones who are relied upon to give end-of-life care or to assist with withdrawal of life support. When there are several deaths together in time, those nurses may be called on frequently. Some consideration in assignment should be given when a nurse has more than one death in a shift or a week. Taking a new admission is also difficult immediately following a death, sometimes before the family has left the unit. Nurse administrators can provide some additional resources, debriefing, or time off when the burden has been high. Critical care nurses have reported that colleagues' comments of support are also helpful.[52]

Organ Donation

The Social Security Act, section 1138, requires that hospitals have written protocols for the identification of potential organ donors.[53] The Joint Commission has a standard on organ donation, LD.3.110.[54] All hospitals must have a written agreement with an organ procurement organization (OPO), which must include agreement with at least one tissue bank and one eye bank. Although an impending death marks a difficult time for family members, the nurse must notify the OPO to approach the family with a donation request. Those individuals have training to make a supportive request and are the ones to decide if a family should not be approached based on the patient's disease. Although organ donation may not be appropriate in some cases, tissue donation remains a consideration.

Brain Death

Death may be pronounced when the patient meets a list of neurologic criteria. However, there are differences among hospital policies for certification of brain death, which may permit differences among the circumstances under which patients are pronounced dead in different U.S. hospitals.[55] Families do not understand the meaning of brain death, and they are less likely to donate organs when they believe the patient will not be dead until the ventilator is turned off and the heart stops.[56] How these conversations are held will determine families' understanding and positively affect donation. Campbell[3] recommended not suggesting that the organs are alive while the brain is dead, but rather that the organs are functioning as a result of the machines used.

FAMILY CARE

In this chapter, the term *family* means whatever the patient states is the family. An integral part of the patient-family dyad, families expect a "cure" for any condition the patient may have; they do not expect to receive "bad news." They look for the good news in any message received from caregivers and are surprised when told that death is the only outcome possible.[52] Families need assistance in forming their expectations about outcomes. It is preferable to have ongoing communication about patient progress, rather than waiting until the patient is near death and then communicating with the family.

Communication Needs

Families have complained about infrequent physician communication,[57] unmet communication needs in the shift from aggressive to end-of-life care,[58] and lacking or inadequate communication.[59] Sometimes families are not ready to receive the prognosis and engage in decision making.[60] Communication seems to be the most common source of complaint in families across studies and should be at the center of efforts to improve end-of-life care.

The health care team can reinforce to the family the legitimacy of expressing feelings of disappointment, sadness, and loss. It is important that the family is made aware that the patient was more than simply a clinical disease and that he or she was recognized as an individual while in the critical care unit. It is important to final ways to address the cultural, social, and emotional issues surrounding the expression of grief at end of life.

Waiting for "Good News"

Patients and families do not come to the critical care unit with the expectation of death. Even those who have had previous admissions expect to be "saved." They tend to listen to imparted information looking for good news; even when "bad news" is given, they may initially deny it or have great difficulty taking it in.[59] Having this in mind while talking to families may assist professionals in interpreting families' responses.

Preparing families for changes in the patient as the health condition deteriorates helps them make plans. They need to know if other family members should be called, if someone should spend the night, or if financial arrangements should be changed before an impending death (e.g., to enable the widow to have access to funds). Anticipated changes can be described to prepare families.

Families may refuse to forgo life-supporting treatments and want "everything done" because of mistrust of health professionals, poor communication, survivor guilt, or religious/cultural reasons.[26] Effective communication throughout the hospitalization, as well as providing information throughout the stay, predisposes the family to better acceptance of "news" as the patient deteriorates.

Family Meetings

Families may experience a sense of crisis as emergencies occur or as the patient deteriorates or dies. There will be various responses to the news of the death. They could show anger or quiet, emotions or stoicism. Culture or religious beliefs may affect their response to news. It is helpful to ask if they would like to see a chaplain or a social worker. Quiet and calm, some privacy, and support are always appreciated.

Family meetings in the presence of the critical care team have been one method used to arrive at a common understanding of the patient's prognosis and goals for future care.[61,62] An analysis of the amount of opportunity families had to speak in these meetings revealed that when families had greater opportunity to talk, their satisfaction with physician communication increased and their ratings of conflict with the physician decreased. Abbott et al[63] discussed families' descriptions, 1 year after decisions about withdrawal of life support, of conflict centering on communication and the behavior of the staff. After the patient's death, greater family satisfaction with withdrawal of life support was associated with the following measures:

- The process of withdrawal of life support being well explained
- Withdrawal of life support proceeding as expected
- Patient appearing comfortable
- Family/friends prepared
- Appropriate person initiating discussion
- Adequate privacy during withdrawal of life support
- A chance to voice concerns[64]

Family Presence During Cardiopulmonary Resuscitation

To be helpful, family presence during procedures or resuscitative attempts[65] should be coupled with staff support. Critical care nurses and emergency nurses have taken family members to the bedside for resuscitation or invasive procedures, but most did not have written policies for family presence.[66] At times these experiences provide opportunities for the family to be supportive of the patient. At other times the family may become more aware of what is involved in decisions they have made on behalf of the patient. Seeing the steps of resuscitation may make clearer the impact of decisions made or delayed.

Visiting Hours

Providing the visiting time to help family members say good-bye is an important function. Family members may have difficulty in seeing the person they knew among all the tubes. Coaching can be provided about how to approach the patient and that the patient may still be able to hear despite appearing to be nonresponsive. Visitors should be permitted to the extent possible, not interfering with other patients' privacy or rest. Children, unless they represent a significant source of infection, should be able to say good-bye as well, but they may need adult assistance in understanding the situation. Families may have religious or cultural ceremonies that are important for them to perform before the patient dies or experiences withdrawal of life support. These should be encouraged and facilitated as much as possible.

Continuity of care by the same nurse is important. As the patient nears death, nurses have sometimes stayed with the family after the end of a shift when death was imminent, so that they would not need to adjust to another person at this difficult time.[52]

Following Death

Following the death, the family may wish to spend time at the bedside. The family's time with the body should be unhurried and private. They need adequate room to sit and spend time. They can be asked if they need assistance or resources and whether they wish to be alone or have someone nearby. Frequently the bed is needed for another patient, and juggling is required to ensure that the family has sufficient time even as another patient needs to be admitted. Supporting families after a death involves immediate bereavement support, information on what to do about the death, bereavement support for the future, contact with the family after death, and assessment of the quality of care the patient experienced.[67] Having material already prepared with the necessary after-death information is quite helpful at this time. Nurses need to be aware of their own judgment on what is an appropriate response, because individuals respond differently to the same news, even within the same family.

COLLABORATIVE CARE

The ability to provide collaborative, compassionate end-of-life care is the responsibility of all clinicians who work with the critically ill (see Evidence-Based Collaborative Practice: End-of-Life Care).

EVIDENCE-BASED COLLABORATIVE PRACTICE

End-of-Life Care

The key recommendations of the guidelines for *end-of-life care in the intensive care unit,* based on research and expert panel review, are as follows:

The management of patients at the end of life can be divided into two phases:

1. The first phase concerns the pursuit of shared decision making that leads from the pursuit of cure or recovery to the pursuit of comfort and freedom from pain.
2. The second phase concerns the actions that are taken once this shift in goals has been made and focuses on both the humanistic and technical skills that must be enlisted to ensure that the needs of the patient and family are met.

This guideline focuses predominantly on the second phase.

Needs of the Patient, Family, and Clinical Team

1. Needs of the patient

   Many patients have lost consciousness before the decision is made to move to palliative care. The following are five patient-centered domains of good end-of-life care:
   - Receiving adequate pain and symptom management
   - Avoiding inappropriate prolongation of dying
   - Achieving a sense of control
   - Relieving burden
   - Strengthening relationships with loved ones
2. Needs of the family

   The 10 most important needs of families of critically ill dying patients are the following:
   - To be with the dying person
   - To be helpful to the dying person
   - To be informed of the dying person's changing condition
   - To understand what is being done to the patient and why
   - To be assured of the patient's comfort
   - To vent emotions
   - To be assured that their decisions were right
   - To find meaning in the dying of their loved one
   - To be fed, hydrated, and rested
3. Needs of the clinical team
   - Multidisciplinary teamwork
   - Administrative support that values intensive palliative care
   - Opportunity for bereavement and debriefing

Comfort and Freedom From Pain

4. Clinical assessments and interventions
   - Assessment of pain
   - Assessment of suffering
   - Use of medications to relieve pain and suffering
   - Alleviation of symptoms such as dyspnea, nausea and vomiting, thirst, skin irritation, anxiety, and delirium
   - Avoiding use of restraints
5. Terminal weaning versus extubation
   - Terminal wean
   - Extubation

   Decisions about how to discontinue ventilatory support depend on the patient's clinical condition, the patient's wishes, if known, family concerns, and the prior experiences of the clinical team.

Sensitivity After the Death

6. Procedures
   - Cultural or religious requests
   - Organ donation
   - Autopsy

   Sometimes families may have specific requests related to religion or culture. Also, there are several procedures that may occur following the death of a patient, and the family must be approached with sensitivity and a consciousness that they are grieving the loss of a loved one.

Data from Truog RD et al: *Crit Care Med* 29(12):2332, 2001.

In 2001 the Society of Critical Care Medicine published "Recommendations for End-of-Life Care in the Intensive Care Unit" to provide guidance for end-of-life care.[68] The Robert Wood Johnson Foundation (RWJF) Critical Care End-of-Life Peer Workgroup identified seven end-of-life care domains for use in the intensive care unit:

1. Patient- and family-centered decision making
2. Communication
3. Continuity of care
4. Emotional and practical support
5. Symptom management and comfort care
6. Spiritual support
7. Emotional and organizational support for intensive care unit clinicians[69]

SUMMARY

Recently individuals[70] and groups[71] have developed websites of online tools to improve end-of-life care. Critical care unit staff will be able to assess the quality of their end-of-life care by assessing perceptions of families and staff, auditing documentation,[72] or making observations of care. We need to put the same attention into improving our end-of-life care that we do into our skills of electrocardiogram (ECG) interpretation or hemodynamic monitoring.

evolve To test your mastery of this chapter, try the Open-Book Quiz at http://evolve.elsevier.com/Urden/priorities/

REFERENCES

1. Rabow MW et al: End-of-life care content in 50 textbooks from multiple specialties, *JAMA* 283(6):771, 2000.
2. Kirchhoff KT et al: Analysis of end-of-life content in critical care nursing textbooks, *J Prof Nurs* 19(6):372, 2003.
3. Campbell ML: Forgoing life-sustaining therapy: How to care for the patient who is near death, Aliso Viejo, Calif, 1998, AACN.
4. Curtis JR, Rubenfeld GD, editors: *Managing death in the intensive care unit: the transition from cure to comfort,* Oxford, 2001, Oxford University Press.
5. The SUPPORT Principal Investigators: A controlled trial to improve care for seriously ill hospitalized patients: the study to understand prognoses and preferences for outcomes and risks of treatments (SUPPORT), *JAMA* 274(20):1591, 1995.
6. Field MJ, Cassell CK, editors: *Approaching death: improving care at the end of life,* Washington, DC, 1997, National Academy Press.
7. Angus DC et al: Use of intensive care at the end of life in the United States: an epidemiologic study, *Crit Care Med* 32(3):638, 2004.
8. Gillick MR: Advance care planning, *N Engl J Med* 350(1):7, 2004.
9. Gordon NP, Shade SB: Advance directives are more likely among seniors asked about end-of-life care preferences, *Arch Intern Med* 159(7):701, 1999.
10. Rubenfeld GD, Crawford SW: Withdrawal of life-sustaining treatment. In Curtis JR, Rubenfeld, GD, editors: *Managing death in the intensive care unit: the transition from cure to comfort,* Oxford, 2001, Oxford University Press.
11. Tilden V et al: Family decision-making to withdraw life-sustaining treatments from hospitalized patients, *Nurs Res* 50(2):105, 2001.
12. Burns JP et al: Do-not-resuscitate order after 25 years, *Crit Care Med* 31(5):1543, 2003.
13. Keenan CH, Kish SK: The influence of do-not-resuscitate orders on care provided for patients in the surgical intensive care unit of a cancer center, *Crit Care Nurs Clin North Am* 12(3):385, 2000.
14. Christakis NA, Lamont EB: Extent and determinants of error in doctors' prognoses in terminally ill patients: prospective cohort study, *BMJ* 320(7233):469, 2000.
15. Lynn J et al.: Prognoses of seriously ill hospitalized patients on the days before death: implications for patient care and public policy, *New Horiz* 5(1):56, 1997.
16. McDonald DD et al: Communicating end-of-life preferences, *West J Nurs Res* 25(6):652-666, discussion 667, 2003.
17. Fried TR, Bradley EH: What matters to seriously ill older persons making end-of-life treatment decisions? A qualitative study, *J Palliat Med* 6(2):237, 2003.
18. Teno JM et al: Medical care inconsistent with patients' treatment goals: association with 1-year Medicare resource use and survival, *J Am Geriatr Soc* 50(3):496, 2002.
19. Mularski RA et al: Educational agendas for interdisciplinary end-of-life curricula, *Crit Care Med* 29(2 suppl): N16, 2001.
20. Wood EB et al: Enhancing palliative care education in medical school curricula: implementation of the palliative education assessment tool, *Acad Med* 77(4):285, 2002.
21. Covinsky KE et al: Communication and decision-making in seriously ill patients: findings of the SUPPORT project—the study to understand prognoses and preferences for outcomes and risks of treatments, *J Am Geriatr Soc* 48(5 suppl): S187, 2000.
22. Ebell MH et al: Survival after in-hospital cardiopulmonary resuscitation: a meta-analysis, *J Gen Intern Med* 13(12):805, 1998.
23. FitzGerald JD et al: Functional status among survivors of in-hospital cardiopulmonary resuscitation: SUPPORT investigators study to understand progress and preferences for outcomes and risks of treatment, *Arch Intern Med* 157(1):72, 1997.
24. Marshall JC et al: Multiple organ dysfunction score: a reliable descriptor of a complex clinical outcome, *Crit Care Med* 23(10):1638, 1995.
25. Rocker G et al: Clinician predictions of intensive care unit mortality, *Crit Care Med* 32(5):1149, 2004.
26. Prendergast TJ, Puntillo KA: Withdrawal of life support: intensive caring at the end of life, *JAMA* 288(21):2732, 2002.
27. Baker R et al: Family satisfaction with end-of-life care in seriously ill hospitalized adults, *J Am Geriatr Soc* 48(5 suppl): S61, 2000.
28. Curtis JR: Communicating about end-of-life care with patients and families in the intensive care unit, *Crit Care Clin* 20(3):363, 2004.
29. Lipson JG et al: *Culture & nursing care: a pocket guide,* San Francisco, 1996, UCSF Nursing Press.
30. Degenholtz HB et al: Race and the intensive care unit: disparities and preferences for end-of-life care, *Crit Care Med* 31(5 suppl):S373, 2003.
31. Crawley LM et al: Strategies for culturally effective end-of-life care, *Ann Intern Med* 136(9):673, 2002.
32. Breen CM et al: Conflict associated with decisions to limit life-sustaining treatment in intensive care units, *J Gen Intern Med* 16(5):283, 2001.
33. Curtis JR, Patrick DL: How to discuss dying and death in the ICU. In Curtis JR, Rubenfeld GD, editors: *Managing death in the intensive care unit: the transition from cure to comfort,* Oxford, 2001, Oxford University Press.
34. Campbell ML, Guzman JA: Impact of a proactive approach to improve end-of-life care in a medical ICU, *Chest* 123(1):266, 2003.
35. Frick S et al: Medical futility: predicting outcome of intensive care unit patients by nurses and doctors—a prospective comparative study, *Crit Care Med* 31(2):456, 2003.
36. Meltzer LS, Huckabay LM: Critical care nurses' perceptions of futile care and its effect on burnout, *Am J Crit Care* 13(3):202, 2004.
37. Ellershaw J, Ward C: Care of the dying patient: the last hours or days of life, *BMJ* 326(7379):30, 2003.
38. Faber-Langendoen K, Lanken PN: Dying patients in the intensive care unit: forgoing treatment, maintaining care, *Ann Intern Med* 133(11):886, 2000.
39. National Consensus Project for Quality Palliative Care: *Clinical Practice Guidelines for Quality Palliative Care,* 2004, http://www.nationalconsensusproject.org/index.html.

40. Foley KM, Gelband H, editors: *Improving palliative care for cancer,* Washington, DC, 2001, National Academy Press.
41. Mularski RA: Pain management in the intensive care unit, *Crit Care Clin* 20(3):381, 2004.
42. Gelinas C et al: Pain assessment and management in critically ill intubated patients: a retrospective study, *Am J Crit Care* 13(2):126, 2004.
43. Foley KM: Pain and symptom control in the dying ICU patient. In Curtis JR, Rubenfeld GD, editors: *Managing death in the intensive care unit: the transition from cure to comfort,* Oxford, 2001, Oxford University Press.
44. Jacobi J et al: Clinical practice guidelines for the sustained use of sedatives and analgesics in the critically ill adult [erratum appears in *Crit Care Med* 30(3):726, 2002], *Crit Care Med* 30(1):119, 2002.
45. Campbell ML: Terminal dyspnea and respiratory distress, *Crit Care Clin* 20(3):403, 2004.
46. Viola RA et al: The effects of fluid status and fluid therapy on the dying: a systematic review, *J Palliative Care* 13(4):41-52, 1997.
47. Kehl KA: Treatment of terminal restlessness: a review of the evidence, *J Pain Palliat Care Pharmacother* 18(1):5, 2004.
48. Callanan M, Kelley P: *Final gifts: understanding the special awareness, needs, and communications of the dying,* New York, 1997, Bantam.
49. Marchand L: *Fast fact and concepts #118: near death awareness,* 2004, End of Life Physician Education Resource Center (EPERC), www.eperc.mcw.edu/.
50. Mueller PS et al: Ethical analysis of withdrawal of pacemaker or implantable cardioverter-defibrillator support at the end of life, *Mayo Clin Proc* 78(8):959, 2003.
51. von Gunten C, Weissman DE: *Fast facts and concepts #34: symptom control for ventilator withdrawal in the dying patient, part II,* 2001, End of Life Physician Education Resource Center (EPERC), available from www.eperc.mcw.edu/.
52. Kirchhoff KT et al: Intensive care nurses' experiences with end-of-life care, *Am J Crit Care* 9(1):36, 2000.
53. Social Security Administration: Hospital protocols for organ procurement and standards for organ procurement agencies, http://www.ssa.gov/OP_Home/ssact/title11/1138.htm.
54. Joint Commission on the Accreditation of Healthcare Organizations: *2004 Comprehensive accreditation manual for hospitals,* Chicago, 2004, The Commission.
55. Powner DJ et al: Variability among hospital policies for determining brain death in adults, *Crit Care Med* 32(6):1284, 2004.
56. Siminoff LA et al: Families' understanding of brain death, *Prog Transplant* 13(3):218, 2003.
57. Heyland DK et al: Family satisfaction with care in the intensive care unit: results of a multiple center study, *Crit Care Med* 30(7):1413, 2002.
58. Norton SA et al: Life support withdrawal: communication and conflict, *Am J Crit Care* 12(6):548, 2003.
59. Kirchhoff KT et al: The vortex: families' experiences with death in the intensive care unit, *Am J Crit Care* 11(3):200, 2002.
60. Murphy PA et al: Under the radar: contributions of the SUPPORT nurses, *Nurs Outlook* 49(5):238, 2001.
61. Ambuel B, Weissman D: *Fast fact and concept #16: conducting a family conference,* 2001, End of Life Physician Education Resource Center (EPERC), www.eperc.mcw.edu/.
62. Curtis JR et al: The family conference as a focus to improve communication about end-of-life care in the intensive care unit: opportunities for improvement, *Crit Care Med* 29(2 suppl):N26, 2001.
63. Abbott KH et al: Families looking back: one year after discussion of withdrawal or withholding of life-sustaining support, *Crit Care Med* 29(1):197, 2001.
64. Keenan SP et al: Withdrawal of life support: how the family feels, and why, *J Palliat Care* 16(suppl):S40, 2000.
65. Emergency Nurses' Association: *Family presence at the bedside during invasive procedures and resuscitation,* Des Plaines, Ill, 2001, The Association.
66. MacLean SL et al: Family presence during cardiopulmonary resuscitation and invasive procedures: practices of critical care and emergency nurses, *Am J Crit Care* 12(3):246, 2003.
67. Shannon SE: Helping families cope with death in the ICU. In Curtis JR, Rubenfeld GD, editors: *Managing death in the intensive care unit: the transition from cure to comfort,* Oxford, 2001, Oxford University Press.
68. Truog RD et al: Recommendations for end-of-life care in the intensive care unit: the Ethics Committee of the Society of Critical Care Medicine, *Crit Care Med* 29(12):2332, 2001.
69. Clarke EB et al: Quality indicators for end-of-life care in the intensive care unit, *Crit Care Med* 31(9):2255, 2003.
70. Curtis JR: *End-of-life care research program,* 2004, http://depts.washington.edu/eolcare/currentprojects/.
71. Promoting Excellence in End-of-Life Care: *Promoting excellence tools,* 2004, http://www.promotingexcellence.org/.
72. Kirchhoff KT et al: Assessment of documentation on withdrawal of life support in adult ICU patients, *Am J Crit Care* 13(4):328, 2004.

CHAPTER 11

Cardiovascular Assessment and Diagnostic Procedures

MARY E. LOUGH

OBJECTIVES

- Identify the components of a cardiovascular history.
- Describe inspection, palpation, percussion, and auscultation of the patient with cardiovascular dysfunction.
- Discuss the clinical significance of selected laboratory tests used in the assessment of cardiovascular disorders.
- Describe key diagnostic procedures used in assessment of the patient with cardiovascular dysfunction.
- Discuss the nursing management of a patient undergoing a cardiovascular diagnostic procedure.
- Illustrate the correct placement of the electrodes for accurate bedside electrocardiographic (ECG) monitoring.
- Outline the steps in analyzing an ECG rhythm strip.
- Explain the significance of normal and abnormal ECG findings
- Describe nursing actions for management of significant atrial, ventricular, and junctional dysrhythmias.
- Describe the use of arterial, central venous, and pulmonary artery catheters for bedside hemodynamic monitoring.
- Outline the steps to interpret a change in $Scvo_2$/Svo_2 values.

Physical assessment of the cardiovascular patient is a skill that must not be lost amidst the technology of the critical care setting. Data collected from a thorough, thoughtful history and examination contribute to both the nursing and the medical decisions for therapeutic interventions.

HISTORY

The patient history is important for providing data that contribute to the cardiovascular diagnosis and treatment plan. For a patient in acute distress, the history is curtailed to just a few questions about the patient's chief complaint, the precipitating events, and current medications. For a patient without obvious distress, the history focuses on the following four areas:

1. Review of the patient's present illness
2. Overview of the patient's general cardiovascular status, including previous cardiac diagnostic studies, interventional procedures, cardiac surgeries, and current medications (cardiac, noncardiac, and herbal)
3. Examination of the patient's general health status, including family history of coronary artery disease (CAD), hypertension, diabetes, peripheral arterial disease, or stroke
4. Survey of the patient's lifestyle, including risk factors for CAD

One of the unique challenges in cardiovascular assessment is identifying when "chest pain" is of cardiac origin and when it is not. The following safety information should always be considered:

- If there is any evidence of CAD or risk of heart disease, assume that the chest pain is caused by myocardial ischemia until proven otherwise.
- Questions to elicit the nature of the chest pain cover five basic areas: quality, location, duration of pain, factors that provoke the pain, and factors that relieve the pain.[1]
- There may be little correlation between the severity of chest discomfort and the gravity of its cause. This is a result of the subjective nature of pain and the unique presentation of ischemic disease in women, elderly patients, and individuals with diabetes.
- Subjective descriptors vary greatly between individuals. Not all patients use the word pain; some may describe "pressure," "heaviness," "discomfort," or "indigestion."[1]
- There is not always a correlation between the location of chest discomfort and its source because of *referred pain*. For example, in patients with

gastroesophageal reflux disease (GERD), esophageal spasm can also present with visceral substernal chest pain that radiates to the left arm and jaw.[2,3]
- Other nonpainful symptoms that may signal cardiac dysfunction are dyspnea, palpitations, cough, fatigue, edema, ischemic leg pain, nocturia, syncope, and cyanosis.

In a recent meta-analysis of the evaluation of stable, intermittent chest pain, a patient's description of chest pain was found to be the most important predictor of underlying coronary disease.[4] In the evaluation of acute chest pain, the 12-lead electrocardiogram (ECG) was the most useful bedside predictor for a diagnosis of ST-elevation myocardial infarction (STEMI).[4]

PHYSICAL EXAMINATION

A comprehensive physical assessment is fundamental to achievement of an accurate diagnosis. The nurse who has developed the skills of inspection, palpation, and auscultation will be confident when assessing patients with cardiovascular disease. Percussion is not employed when assessing the cardiovascular system.

INSPECTION

The priorities for inspection of the patient with cardiovascular dysfunction are (1) assessing the general appearance, (2) evaluating jugular veins, (3) observing the apical impulse, and (4) examining the extremities.

Assessing General Appearance

The face is observed for the color of the skin (cyanotic, pale, or jaundiced) and for apprehensive or painful expressions. The skin, lips, tongue, and mucous membranes are inspected for pallor or cyanosis. *Central cyanosis* is a bluish discoloration of the tongue and sublingual area. Multiracial studies indicate that the tongue is the most sensitive site for observation of central cyanosis, which must be recognized and treated as a medical emergency. Pulse oximetry, arterial blood gas analysis, and treatment with 100% oxygen must be instituted immediately. Body posture is observed to indicate the amount of effort it takes to breathe. For example, sitting upright to breathe may be necessary for the patient with acute heart failure, and leaning forward may be the least painful position for the patient with pericarditis. The patient is observed for signs of confusion or lethargy that may indicate hypotension, low cardiac output (CO), or hypoxemia.

Examining the Extremities

The nail beds are inspected for signs of discoloration or cyanosis. *Clubbing* in the nail bed is a sign of longstanding central cyanotic heart disease or pulmonary disease with hypoxemia. Clubbing describes a nail that has lost the normal angle between the finger and the nail root; the nail becomes wide and convex. The terminal phalanx of the finger also becomes bulbous and swollen. Clubbing is rare and a sign of severe central cyanosis (Figure 11-1). *Peripheral cyanosis,* a bluish discoloration of the nail bed, is more commonly seen. Peripheral cyanosis occurs as a result of a reduction in the quantity of oxygen in the peripheral extremities secondary to arterial disease or decreased cardiac output. Clubbing never occurs as a result of peripheral cyanosis.

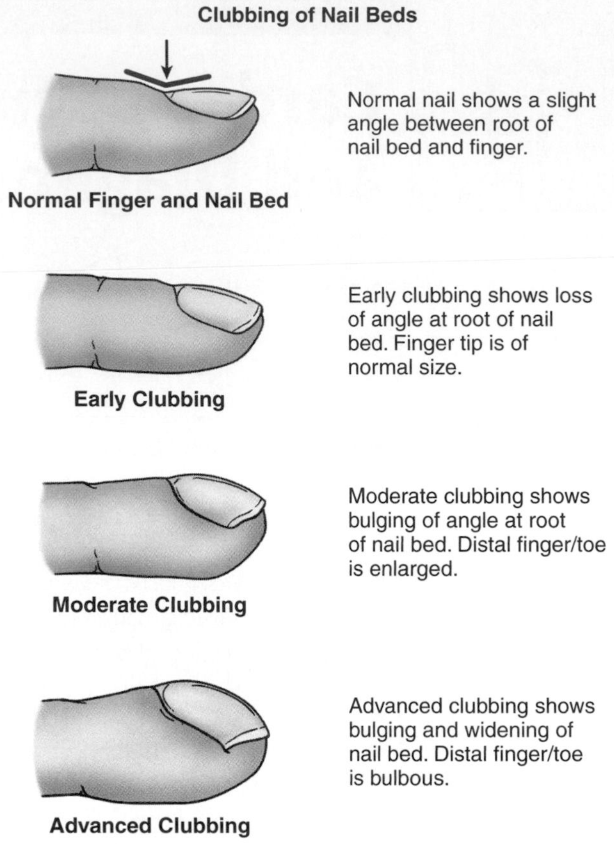

FIGURE 11-1. Clubbing of the nail beds.

The legs are inspected for signs of peripheral arterial or venous vascular disease. The visible signs of arterial vascular disease include pale, shiny legs with sparse hair growth. Venous disease creates an edematous limb with deep red rubor, brown discoloration, and frequently leg ulceration. A comparison of peripheral arterial disease and peripheral venous disease is presented in Table 11-1.

Evaluating Jugular Veins

The jugular veins of the neck are inspected for a noninvasive estimate of intravascular volume and pressure. The external jugular veins are observed for jugular vein distention (JVD) (Figure 11-2 and Box 11-1). *Jugular venous distention* occurs when central venous pressure is elevated, which occurs with fluid volume overload

Table 11-1

Inspection and Palpation of Extremities: Comparison of Arterial and Venous Disease

CHARACTERISTICS	PERIPHERAL ARTERIAL DISEASE	PERIPHERAL VENOUS DISEASE
Hair loss	Present	Absent
Skin texture	Thin, shiny, dry	Flaking, stasis, dermatitis, mottled
Ulceration	Located at pressure points, painful, pale, dry with little drainage; well-demarcated with eschar or dried; surrounded by fibrous tissue; granulation tissue scant and pale	Usually at the ankle; painless, pink, moist with large amount of drainage; irregular, dry, and scaly; surrounded by dermatitis; granulation tissue healthy
Skin color	Elevational pallor, dependent rubor	Brown patches, rubor, mottled cyanotic color when dependent
Nails	Thick, brittle	Normal
Varicose veins	Absent	Present
Temperature	Cool	Warm
Capillary refill	Greater than 3 seconds	Less than 3 seconds
Edema	None or mild, usually unilateral	Usually present foot to calf, unilateral or bilateral
Pulses	Weak or absent (0 to 1+)	Normal, strong, and symmetric

Modified from Krenzer ME: *AACN Clin Issues* 6(4):631, 1995.

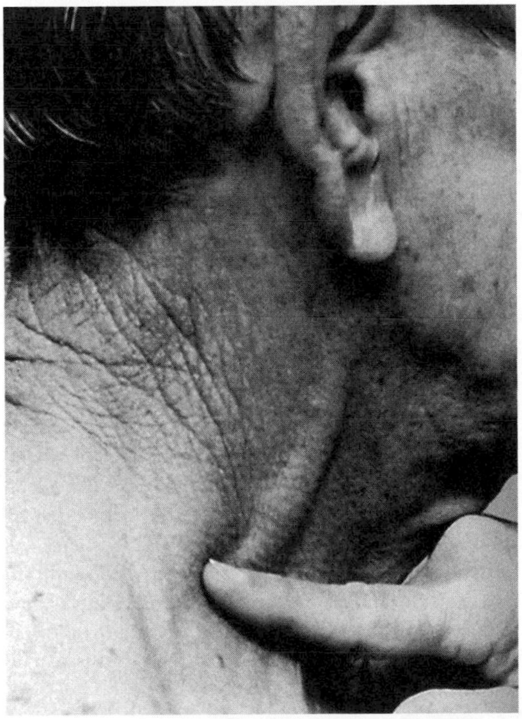

FIGURE 11-2. Assessment of jugular vein distention (JVD). Applying light finger pressure over the sternocleidomastoid muscle, parallel to the clavicle, helps identify the external jugular vein by occluding flow and distending it. Release the finger pressure, and observe for true distention. If the patient's trunk is elevated to 30 degrees or more, JVD should not be present.

Box 11-1

Procedure for Assessing Jugular Vein Distention

1. Patient reclines at a 30- to 45-degree angle.
2. Examiner stands on patient's right side and turns patient's head slightly toward the left.
3. If jugular vein is not visible, light finger pressure is applied across sternocleidomastoid muscle just above and parallel to clavicle. This pressure will fill external jugular vein by obstructing flow (see Figure 11-2).
4. Once location of vein has been identified, pressure is released and presence of jugular vein distention (JVD) assessed.
5. Because inhalation decreases venous pressure, JVD should be assessed at end-exhalation.
6. Any fullness in the vein extending more than 3 cm above sternal angle is evidence of increased venous pressure. Generally the higher the sitting angle of the patient when JVD is visualized, the higher the central venous pressure.
7. *Documentation:* JVD is reported by including angle of the head of the bed at the time JVD was evaluated (e.g., "presence of JVD with head of bed elevated to 45 degrees").

and right ventricular dysfunction. The right internal jugular vein can be used for measurement of central venous pressure (CVP) in centimeters of water (cm H_2O) (Figure 11-3 and Box 11-2).[5,6]

Observing Apical Impulse

The anterior thorax is inspected for the *apical impulse,* sometimes referred to as the *point of maximal impulse* (PMI). The apical impulse occurs as the left ventricle contracts during systole and rotates forward, causing the left ventricular apex of the heart to hit the chest wall. The apical impulse is a quick, localized, outward movement normally located just lateral to the left midclavicular line at the fifth intercostal space in the adult patient. The apical impulse is the only normal pulsation visualized on the chest wall. In the patient without cardiac disease, PMI may not be noticeable (Figure 11-4).

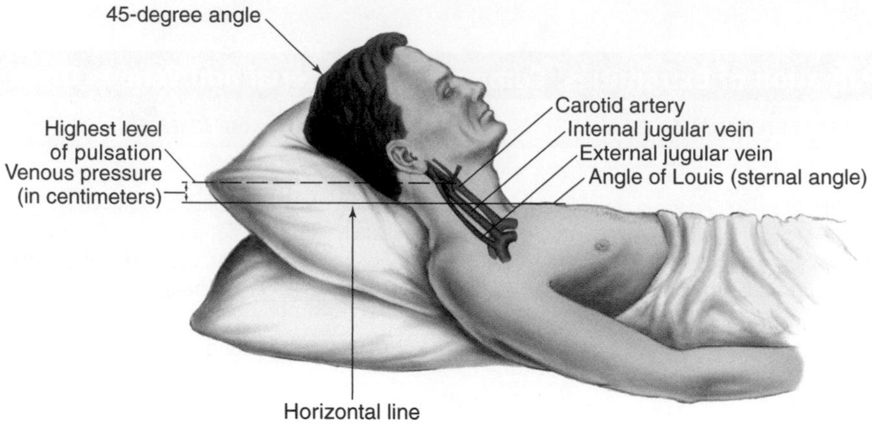

FIGURE 11-3. Position of internal and external jugular veins. Pulsation in the internal jugular vein can be used to estimate central venous pressure. (Modified from Thompson JM et al: *Mosby's clinical nursing,* ed 5, St Louis, 2002, Mosby.)

Box 11-2

Procedure for Assessing Central Venous Pressure

1. Patient reclines in bed. Highest point of pulsation in the internal jugular vein is observed during exhalation.
2. Vertical distance between this pulsation (at top of fluid level) and the sternal angle is estimated or measured in centimeters (cm).
3. This number is then added to 5 cm for an estimation of central venous pressure (CVP). The 5 cm is the approximate distance of sternal angle above level of right atrium (see Figure 11-3).
4. *Documentation:* Degree of elevation of patient is included in report (e.g., "CVP estimated at 13 cm, using internal jugular vein pulsation, with head of bed elevated 45 degrees").

Palpation

The priorities for palpation of the patient with cardiovascular dysfunction are (1) assessing arterial pulses, (2) evaluating capillary refill, (3) estimating edema, and (4) assessing for signs of deep vein thrombosis.

Assessing Arterial Pulses

Seven pairs of bilateral arterial pulses are palpated. The examination incorporates bilateral assessment of the carotid, brachial, radial, ulnar, popliteal, dorsalis pedis, and posterior tibial arteries. The pulses are palpated separately and compared bilaterally to check for consistency. Pulse volume is graded on a scale of 0 to 3+ (Box 11-3). The abdominal aortic pulse can also be palpated.

A diminished or absent pulse may indicate low CO or arterial stenosis or occlusion proximal to the site

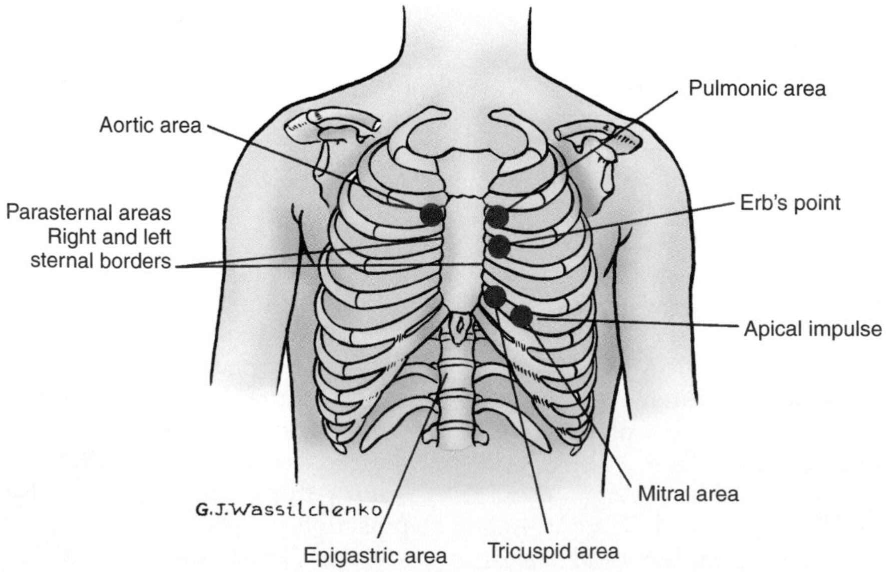

FIGURE 11-4. Thoracic palpation and auscultation points.

Box 11-3

Pulse Palpation Scale

0	Not palpable
1+	Faintly palpable (weak and thready)
2+	Palpable (normal pulse)
3+	Bounding (hyperdynamic pulse)

of the examination. An abnormally strong or bounding pulse suggests the presence of an aneurysm or an occlusion distal to the examination site. If a distal pulse cannot be palpated using light finger pressure, a Doppler ultrasound stethoscope is often helpful. It is important to mark the location of the audible signal with an indelible ink marker pen for future evaluation of pulse quality.

The Allen test is an evaluation of blood flow and pulse quality to the hand by assessing the radial and ulnar arterial pulses.[7] This test is performed before insertion of an arterial line and is described in Box 11-4. Note that if a critically ill patient is unable to repeatedly make a fist the Allen test, results may be inaccurate.[7]

Evaluating Capillary Refill

Capillary refill assessment is a maneuver that uses the patient's nail beds to evaluate both arterial circulation to the extremity and overall perfusion. The nail bed is compressed to produce blanching, and the release of the pressure should result in a return of blood flow and baseline nail color in less than 3 seconds. The severity of arterial insufficiency is directly proportional to the amount of time necessary to reestablish flow and color.

Estimating Edema

Edema is fluid accumulation in the extravascular spaces of the body. The dependent tissues within the legs and sacrum are particularly susceptible. Note whether the edema is dependent, unilateral or bilateral, and pitting or nonpitting. The amount of edema is quantified by measuring the circumference of the limb or by pressing the skin of the feet, ankles, and shins against the underlying bone. Edema is a symptom associated with several diseases, and further diagnostic evaluation is required to determine the cause. Although no universal scale for pitting edema exists, one such scale uses 0 to 4+ (Table 11-2).

AUSCULTATION

The priorities for auscultation of the patient with cardiovascular dysfunction are (1) measuring blood pressure, (2) detecting bruits, (3) assessing normal heart sounds, and (4) identifying abnormal heart sounds, murmurs, and pericardial rubs.

Box 11-4

Procedure for Assessment of Arterial Blood Supply to the Hand—The Allen Test

Before a radial artery is punctured or cannulated, the Allen test is performed to assess blood flow to the hand and ensure that it is adequate.

If the patient is alert and cooperative, the procedure is as follows:

Allen Test by Visual Inspection

1. The patient is requested to repeatedly make a tight fist to squeeze the blood out of his or her hand.
2. The radial artery is compressed with firm thumb pressure by the examiner.
3. The patient is requested to open the hand, palm side up, while the radial artery is still occluded.
4. Pressure is released, and the time it takes for the color to return to the hand is noted.

If the ulnar artery is patent, the color will return within 3 seconds. The patient may describe a tingling in the palm as blood flow returns. Delayed color return (a "failed" Allen test) implies that the ulnar artery is inadequate; therefore the radial artery is the only source of blood flow to the hand and must not be punctured or cannulated.

Allen Test With Pulse Oximetry

1. If the patient is unable to cooperate to make a fist, an alternative approach is to use a pulse oximeter that displays a pulse waveform.
2. Place the pulse oximeter on the middle finger, and establish an adequate pulse amplitude display on the monitor.
3. Simultaneously compress the radial and ulnar arteries until the waveform clearly decreases or vanishes.
4. Release pressure off the ulnar artery only. If the ulnar artery is patent, the pulse amplitude recovers its normal appearance.
5. Repeat the procedure with the radial artery.
6. Only when there is adequate blood supply to the hand can arterial catheterization of the radial artery be accomplished safely.

Table 11-2

Pitting Edema Scale

		INDENTATION DEPTH		
SCALE	EDEMA	INCHES	METRIC	TIME TO BASELINE
0	None present	0	0	
1+	Trace	0-1/4	<6.5 mm	Rapid
2+	Mild	1/4-1/2	6.5-12.5 mm	10-15 sec
3+	Moderate	1/2-1	12.5 mm-2.5 cm	1-2 min
4+	Severe	>1	>2.5 cm	2-5 min

Measuring Blood Pressure

Blood pressure (BP) measurement is an essential component of every complete physical examination.[8] Hypertension is diagnosed as a systolic BP of 140 mm Hg or higher or a diastolic BP of 90 mm Hg or above.[9] The incidence of hypertension in the United States has increased dramatically as a result of an aging population and obesity. In 1999 to 2000, 65 million adults in the United States were hypertensive, compared with 50 million in 1988 through 1994—an increase of 30%.[10]

Detecting Vascular Bruits

The carotid and femoral arteries are auscultated for bruits. A bruit, a high-pitched "sh-sh," is an extracardiac vascular sound that vacillates in volume with systole and diastole. An abnormal bruit is produced as blood flows through a partially occluded vessel. The auscultation of a bruit can expedite the diagnosis of suspected arterial obstruction. To auscultate for the presence of a bruit place the diaphragm of the stethoscope at the site of major pulses: carotid, abdominal aorta, and femoral arteries.

Assessing Normal Heart Sounds

Auscultation of the heart is the most challenging part of the cardiac physical examination and, in an era of increasing technologic demands, is daunting to new clinicians. To summarize the advice given by most experts, the examiner must do the following:

1. Auscultate systematically across the precordium
2. Visualize the cardiac anatomy under each point of auscultation, expecting to hear the physiologically associated sounds
3. Memorize the cardiac cycle to enhance the ability to hear abnormal sounds
4. Practice, practice, practice[11]

First and Second Heart Sounds. Normal heart sounds are referred to as the *first heart sound* (S_1) and the *second heart sound* (S_2). S_1 is the sound associated with mitral and tricuspid valve closure and is heard most clearly in the mitral and tricuspid areas. S_2 (aortic and pulmonic closure) can be heard best at the second intercostal space to the right and left of the sternum. Both sounds are high-pitched and heard best with the diaphragm of the stethoscope. Each sound is loudest in an auscultation area located "downstream" from the actual valvular component of the sound.

Identifying Abnormal Heart Sounds, Murmurs, and Pericardial Rubs

Third and Fourth Heart Sounds. The abnormal heart sounds are labeled as the *third heart sound* (S_3) and the *fourth heart sound* (S_4) and are referred to as *gallops* when auscultated during an episode of tachycardia. These low-pitched sounds occur during diastole and are best heard with the bell of stethoscope positioned lightly over the apical impulse. The presence of S_3 may be normal in children and young adults because of rapid filling of the ventricle in a young, healthy heart. However, an S_3 in the presence of cardiac symptoms is an indication of increased ventricular volume suggestive of heart failure with fluid overload.[5,6] Auscultation of an S_4—also referred to as an "atrial gallop"—also leads the examiner to suspect heart failure and decreased ventricular compliance.

Box 11-5

Grading of Cardiac Murmurs

I/VI	Very faint; may be heard only in a quiet environment
II/VI	Quiet, but clearly audible
III/VI	Moderately loud
IV/VI	Loud; may be associated with a palpable thrill
V/VI	Very loud; thrill easily palpable
VI/VI	Very loud; may be heard with stethoscope off the chest; thrill palpable and visible

Heart Murmurs. *Heart valve murmurs* are prolonged extra sounds that occur during systole or diastole. Murmurs are produced by turbulent flood flow through the chambers of the heart causing vibrations that occur during systole or diastole. Valvular murmurs may be described as systolic or diastolic, depending on when the murmur is audible in the cardiac cycle (Table 11-3). Most murmurs are caused by structural cardiac changes. Heart murmurs are characterized by specific criteria as follows:

1. *Timing*—place in the cardiac cycle (systole/diastole)
2. *Location*—where it is auscultated on the chest wall (mitral/aortic area)
3. *Radiation*—how far the sound spreads across chest wall
4. *Quality*—whether the murmur is blowing, grating, or harsh
5. *Pitch*—whether the tone is high or low
6. *Intensity*—the loudness is graded on a scale using roman numerals I to VI; the higher the number, the louder the murmur, as shown in Box 11-5

Pericardial Friction Rub. A *pericardial friction rub* is a sound that can occur within 2 to 7 days of an MI. The friction rub results from pericardial inflammation *(pericarditis)*. Classically a pericardial friction rub is a grating or scratching sound that is both systolic and diastolic, corresponding with cardiac motion within the pericardial sac. It is often associated with chest pain, which can be aggravated by deep inspiration, coughing, swallowing, and changing position. It is important to differentiate pericarditis from acute myocardial ischemia, and the detection of the pericardial friction rub through auscultation can assist in this differentiation, leading to effective diagnosis and treatment.

Table 11-3
Characteristics of Some Murmurs

DEFECTS	TIMING IN THE CARDIAC CYCLE	PITCH, INTENSITY, QUALITY	LOCATION, RADIATION
Systolic Murmurs			
Mitral regurgitation	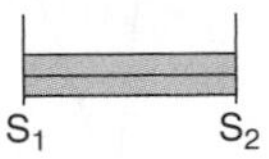	High Harsh Blowing	Mitral area May radiate to axilla
Tricuspid regurgitation	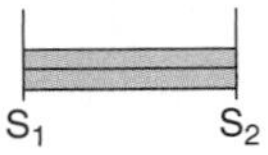	High Often faint, but varies Blowing	Tricuspid RLSB, apex, LLSB, epigastric areas Little radiation
Ventricular septal defect	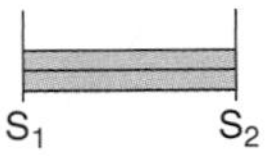	High Loud Blowing	Left sternal border
Aortic stenosis	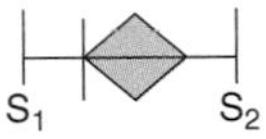	Chhhh hh Medium Rough, harsh	Aortic area to suprasternal notch, right side of neck, apex
Pulmonary stenosis	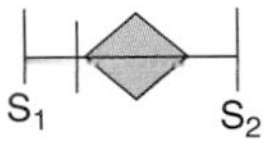	Low to medium Loud Harsh, grinding	Pulmonic area No radiation
Diastolic Murmurs			
Mitral stenosis	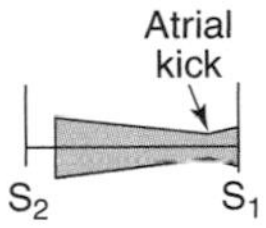	Low Quiet to loud with thrill Rough rumble	Mitral area Usually no radiation
Tricuspid stenosis	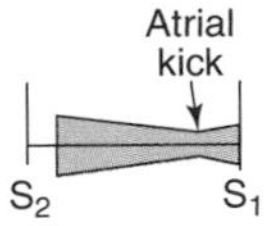	Medium Quiet; louder with inspiration Rumble	Tricuspid area or epigastrium Little radiation
Aortic regurgitation	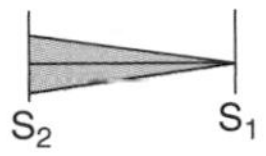	High Faint to medium Blowing	Aortic area to LLSB and aorta Erb's point
Pulmonic regurgitation	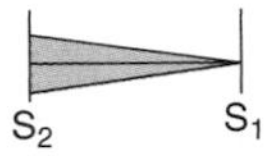	Medium Faint Blowing	Pulmonic area No radiation

RLSB, Right lower sternal border; *LLSB,* left lower sternal border.

LABORATORY ASSESSMENT

The priorities for laboratory assessment for the patient with cardiovascular dysfunction focus on (1) interpreting serum electrolyte levels and safely replacing electrolyte deficiencies, (2) monitoring cardiac biomarkers, (3) trending hematologic studies, (4) assessing coagulation values, and (5) evaluating the serum lipid profile.

Interpreting Serum Electrolyte Levels

Potassium

During depolarization and repolarization of nerve and muscle fiber, potassium and sodium exchange occurs intracellularly and extracellularly. The potassium gradient across the cell membrane determines conduction velocity and helps confine pacing activity to the sinus node. Thus either excess or deficiency of potassium can alter myocardial muscle function. Normal serum potassium levels are 3.5 to 4.5 mEq/L.

Hyperkalemia. Elevated serum potassium level, termed *hyperkalemia,* can be caused by a variety of conditions that include excess potassium administration, extensive skeletal muscle destruction (rhabdomyolysis),[12,13] tumor lysis syndrome,[14] renal failure,[15] and some drugs.[16] Drugs that may induce hyperkalemia include potassium-sparing diuretics, angiotensin-converting enzyme (ACE) inhibitor drugs, and angiotensin receptor–blocker (ARB) drugs.[16] Hyperkalemia elicits significant changes in the ECG because it decreases the rate of ventricular depolarization, shortens repolarization, and also depresses atrioventricular (AV) conduction.[17] As the serum levels of potassium rise above normal (greater than 4.5 mEq/L), evidence of these phenomena is clearly seen on the ECG (Figure 11-5, *A*). Tall, peaked T waves are usually, although not uniquely, associated with early hyperkalemia and are followed by prolongation of the PR interval, loss of the P wave, widening of the QRS complex, and asystole. Severely elevated serum potassium level (greater than

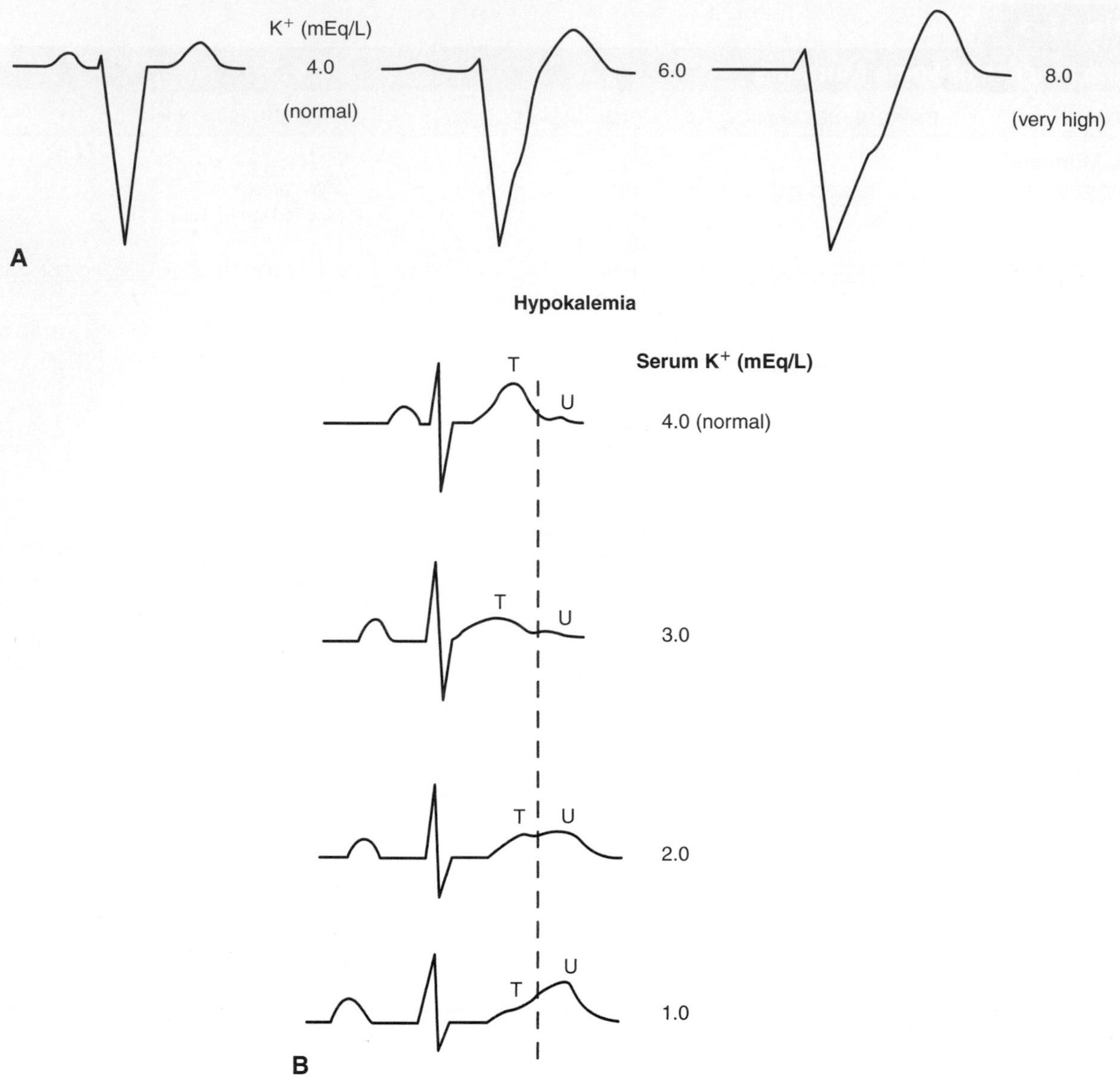

FIGURE 11-5. A, Effects of hyperkalemia. Stages in hyperkalemia from normal potassium levels to plasma levels of 8 mEq/L. At approximately 6 mEq/L, the P wave flattens, the QRS broadens, and the ST segment disappears, with the S wave flowing into the tall, tented T wave. **B,** Effects of hypokalemia. Variable ST segment patterns may be seen ranging from a slight flattening to the appearance of U waves, sometimes with ST depression or T-wave inversions.

8 mEq/L) will cause a wide QRS tachycardia that will lead to ventricular fibrillation or cardiac standstill.

This life-threatening condition can be acutely managed with an intravenous (IV) insulin/glucose infusion that drives the potassium inside the cell and temporarily out of the serum. Potassium is permanently removed from the serum by cation-exchange resin products, such as Kayexalate, placed into the gastrointestinal (GI) tract, or removed directly from the blood by hemodialysis. Coexisting low serum sodium, calcium, or pH levels potentiate the cardiac effects of hyperkalemia.

Hypokalemia. A low serum potassium level, called *hypokalemia* (less than 3.5 mEq/L), is commonly caused by GI losses, diuretic therapy with insufficient replacement, or chronic steroid therapy. Hypokalemia is also reflected by changes on the ECG (Figure 11-5, *B*). The earliest ECG change is often premature ventricular contractions (PVCs), which can deteriorate into ventricular tachycardia (VT) or ventricular fibrillation (VF) without appropriate potassium replacement.

Hypokalemia impairs myocardial conduction and prolongs ventricular repolarization. This can be seen by a prominent U wave (a positive deflection following the T wave on the ECG). The U wave is not totally unique to hypokalemia, but its presence is a signal for the clinician to check the serum potassium level. In the critical care unit, where patients are receiving diuretics and/or have nasogastric tubes to suction, the serum potassium is checked frequently by the critical care nurse and replaced intravenously to normal levels to prevent dysrhythmias. Great care must be taken when replacing potassium intravenously, to ensure it is diluted sufficiently and administered slowly to prevent accidental overdose. Potassium is considered a "high-alert medication," and additional safety procedures are recommended for this drug (see Patient Safety Priorities: Medication Administration). If concomitant hypomagnesemia exists, successful replenishment of potassium deficit cannot be accomplished until the hypomagnesemia is reversed.

Box 11-6

Chemistry Values That Affect Cardiac Contractility and Conduction

	NORMAL RANGES		
	mEq/L	mg/dl	mmol/L
Potassium (K^+)	3.5-4.5		
Ionized calcium (Ca)		4.0-5.0	1.05-1.30
Total calcium (Ca^{++})		8.5-10.5	2.00-2.60
Magnesium (Mg^{++})	1.5-2.0	1.8-2.4	0.7-1.1

NOTE: Laboratory values may be reported as either mEq/L, mg/dl, or mmol/L. Each measurement parameter used will produce a different value. Some electrolytes are reported with more than one reference value.
Different clinical laboratories use different reference values. Cited reference values may vary slightly between hospital laboratories.

Calcium

Calcium (Ca^{++}) is an important cation in the body. Calcium metabolism is controlled by many factors including normal parathyroid hormone (PTH) function, calcitonin, and vitamin D acting on target organs such as the kidney, bone, and the GI tract.[18] Calcium is an important mediator of many cardiovascular functions because of its effect on vascular tone, myocardial contractility, and cardiac excitability.[18] Serum calcium values are recorded in three possible ways, depending on the hospital laboratory: milliequivalents per liter (mEq/L), milligrams per deciliter (mg/dl), or millimoles per liter (mmol/L) (Box 11-6).

In the bloodstream, 55% of calcium is bound to protein (primarily albumin) and found in complexes with anions such as chloride and phosphate. As such it is not physiologically available to the body.[7] The remaining 45% of calcium is biologically active and is called the *ionized calcium.*[7] The only accurate way to determine the level of ionized calcium—described as physiologically active, "unbound," or "free"—is to measure the serum value with a laboratory assay. The mathematically calculated values that extrapolate from total calcium and serum albumin levels are severely inaccurate and variable and should no longer be used.[18,19]

Hypercalcemia. Hypercalcemia is defined as increased amounts of ionized calcium (greater than 4.8 mg/dl or 1.30 mmol/L) or increased amounts of total serum calcium (greater than 10.5 mg/dl or 2.60 mmol/L). Serum calcium levels are increased by bone tumors; primary hyperparathyroidism caused by elevated PTH levels; excessive intake of supplemental calcium and vitamin D, usually in oral antacids; hypomagnesemia; and as a complication of kidney failure from decreased renal excretion of calcium.[7] Hypercalcemia affects multiple organs, causes smooth muscle relaxation, and can lead to neurologic changes such as lethargy, confusion, and even coma.[18] Elevated serum calcium level has the cardiovascular effect of strengthening contractility and shortening ventricular repolarization, demonstrated on the ECG by a shortened QTc interval.[18] Rhythm disturbances may include bradycardia; first-, second-, and third-degree heart block; and bundle branch block (BBB). Hypercalcemia can potentiate the effects of digitalis, precipitate digitalis toxicity, and cause hypertension.[18,20]

Hypocalcemia. *Hypocalcemia* is defined as an *ionized calcium* level below normal (below 4 mg/dl or below 1.05 mmol/L) or a low total serum calcium level. Hypocalcemia (measured by ionized calcium) is a common finding and is reported to occur in 26% to 88% of critically ill patients, depending on the admitting diagnosis.[21] The more severe the patient's illness, the greater the risk of developing hypocalcemia.[21] Transfusions of blood from the blood bank lower serum calcium levels because the citrate used as an anticoagulant in banked blood binds to the calcium. This is called *citrate chelation.* If citrate is used during hemodialysis or plasmapheresis, it will have the same calcium-binding (chelating) effect.[21] Phosphate also binds to calcium and will lower the serum calcium level.[18] Metabolic alkalosis often coexists with hypocalcemia.[18] The cardiovascular effects of hypocalcemia include decreased myocardial contractility, decreased cardiac output, and hypotension. Rhythm disturbances with severe hypocalcemia are variable, ranging from bradycardia to ventricular tachycardia and asystole. When the ionized calcium is low, the ECG may show a

PATIENT SAFETY PRIORITIES

Medication Administration

1. Accurate patient identification
   - Use at least two patient identifiers (not patient's room number) whenever taking blood samples or administering medications or blood products. Examples include patient name, date of birth, or hospital record number.
2. Effective communication among caregivers
   - Hospitals should have (or implement) a process for taking verbal or telephone orders that requires a verification "read-back" of the complete order by the person receiving the order.
   - Because thousands of brand name and generic drugs are available, there is always potential for error. Similar drug names, either written or spoken, account for approximately 15% of all medication error reports to the *U.S. Pharmacopeia* (USP) Medication Errors Reporting program.
   - In March 2001 the USP released "Use Caution, Avoid Confusion," an updated list highlighting hundreds of confusing drug name sets and identifying more than 750 unique drug names that have been reported to the Medication Errors Reporting program. A poster and a laminated, quick-reference card are available for health care professionals free of charge from the USP by contacting USP's Practitioner and Product Experience department at 800-487-7776, or the list may be accessed from USP's website at http://www.usp.org/reporting/review/.
   - An organizational method to decrease the number of medication errors is the use of *computerized physician order entry* (CPOE), as advocated by the Leapfrog Group: http://www.leapfroggroup.org.
   - Standardize the abbreviations, acronyms, and symbols used throughout the organization, including a list of abbreviations, acronyms, and symbols not to use.
   - Examples of problematic abbreviations include "U" for "units" and "μg" for "micrograms." When handwritten, "U" can be mistaken for a zero; in numerous case reports, an insulin dosage in "U" was interpreted as "0." Using the abbreviation "μg" instead of "mcg" for micrograms is also problematic; when handwritten, the symbol "μ" can look like an "m."
   - Use of "trailing zeros" (e.g., 2.0 versus 2) and a "leading decimal point without a leading zero" (e.g., .2 instead of 0.2) are also dangerous prescription-writing practices. Misinterpretation of such abbreviations has caused and could lead to tenfold dosing errors.
3. High-alert medication safety
   - Remove concentrated electrolytes (including but not limited to potassium chloride, potassium phosphate, and hypertonic sodium chloride) from patient care units.
   - Standardize and limit the number of drug concentrations available in the organization.
   - In the first 2 years after enacting a "sentinel event" reporting mechanism, the most common category was medication errors, and the most frequently implicated drug was potassium chloride (KCl). The Joint Commission reviewed 10 incidents of patient death resulting from misadministration of KCl. Eight were the result of direct infusion of concentrated KCl. In six of the eight cases the KCl was mistaken for another medication, primarily due to similarities in packaging and labeling. Most often KCl was mistaken for sodium chloride, heparin, or furosemide (Lasix).
   - The Joint Commission suggests that health care organizations NOT make concentrated KCl available outside the pharmacy unless appropriate, specific safeguards are in place.
4. Infusion pump safety
   - Ensure free-flow protection on all general-use and patient-controlled analgesia (PCA) intravenous (IV) infusion pumps used in the organization.
   - Infusion pumps that do not provide protection from the free flow of IV fluid or medication into the patient are hazardous. USP reported six cases in which a patient died because an IV pump did not provide protection from free flow of the IV solution. (October 1991 to November 1999: four additional cases resulted in near-death.)
   - *Free flow* occurs when IV solution flows freely, under force of gravity, without being controlled by the infusion pump. Free flow typically occurs after the administration set is temporarily removed from the pump to transfer a patient to another area, change a patient's gown, or place a patient on a radiography table. Clinicians can greatly reduce this risk by using administration sets with set-based anti–free-flow mechanisms that prevent gravity free flow by closing off the IV tubing to prohibit flow when the administration set is removed from the pump.

Information related to this feature can be accessed on the websites of the following organizations:
The Joint Commission:http://www.jointcommission.org
Institute for Healthcare Improvement:http://www.ihi.org
The Leapfrog Group:http://www.leapfroggroup.org

prolonged QTc interval that predisposes a patient to the life-threatening ventricular dysrhythmia called torsades de pointes.

Management of hypocalcemia, especially when the ionized calcium level is low, involves infusion of IV calcium chloride or IV calcium gluconate. Calcium chloride is generally used to raise calcium levels because it contains more calcium for the same volume[18]:

- Calcium chloride provides 27 mg elemental calcium per milliliter.
- Calcium gluconate provides 9 mg elemental calcium per milliliter.

Magnesium

Magnesium (Mg^{++}) is essential for many enzyme, protein, lipid, and carbohydrate functions in the body and is critical for the production and use of energy. The body stores most magnesium in bone (53%), muscle (27%), and soft tissues (19%); only a tiny proportion resides within the bloodstream—red blood cells contain 0.5% and serum contains 0.3%.[22] As with other electrolytes (see foregoing discussion of calcium), the ionized portion of the serum magnesium is the biologically active component that is available for biochemical processes. Serum magnesium is 67% ionized, 19% protein bound, and 14% complexed.[22] The serum magnesium is what is normally measured in a routine blood test. Serum magnesium can be reported either in mEq/L, mg/dl, or mmol/L, depending on the laboratory running the analysis. The normal serum range is from 1.5 to 2 mEq/L; 1.8 to 2.4 mg/dl; or 0.7 to 1.1 mmol/L. These represent the same serum level of magnesium despite different measurement guidelines used in the report. It is important to anticipate that normal reference values will vary between different hospital laboratories.

Hypermagnesemia. The incidence of hypermagnesemia is rare in comparison with hypomagnesemia, and it occurs secondary to kidney failure, tumor lysis syndrome, or iatrogenic overtreatment.

Hypomagnesemia. A total serum magnesium concentration below 1.5 mEq/L defines *hypomagnesemia.* It is commonly associated with other electrolyte imbalances, most notably alterations in potassium, calcium, and phosphorus. Low serum magnesium level can stem from many causes. Hypomagnesemia is caused by insufficient intake in the diet or in total parental nutrition (TPN) and is associated with chronic alcohol abuse. In the critical care unit, aggressive diuresis with loop diuretics will lower both serum potassium and magnesium levels.[22] Diarrhea can be a significant cause of magnesium loss because lower GI fluids contain up to 15 mEq/L magnesium; vomiting or gastric suction causes less depletion because the upper GI fluids contain about 1 mEq/L.[22] Another cause of magnesium depletion is rapid administration of citrated blood products, which causes the citrate to bind to the magnesium, a condition known as *citrate chelation.* In chronic hypomagnesemia the serum levels will be replenished from the bone stores.[22]

Both hypokalemia and hypocalcemia are likely to be unresponsive to replacement therapy until the hypomagnesemia is corrected.[18,22] Expected cardiac-related changes with hypomagnesemia include hypertension and vasospasm, including coronary artery spasm. Some studies have linked magnesium depletion to sudden cardiac death, to an increased incidence of acute myocardial infarction (MI), and to the occurrence of ventricular dysrhythmias.[22] IV magnesium sulfate is the treatment of choice for torsades de pointes. It is important to evaluate kidney function when administering magnesium to avoid precipitating hypermagnesium states.

Table 11-4

Serum Biomarkers After Acute Myocardial Infarction

SERUM BIOMARKER	TIME TO INITIAL ELEVATION (Hours)*	PEAK ELEVATION† (Hours)*	RETURN TO BASELINE (Hours/Days)*
Troponin I (TnI)	3-6	24	5-10 days
Troponin T (TnT)	3-6	12-48	5-14 days
CK-MB	4-18	24	2-3 days
Myoglobin	1-4	6-7	24 hours

CK, Creatine kinase.
*Time periods represent average reported values.
†Does not include patients who have had reperfusion therapy.

Monitoring Cardiac Biomarkers

Cardiac Biomarkers

Cardiac biomarkers, previously described by the term *cardiac enzymes,* are proteins that are released from severely damaged myocardial tissue cells.[23,24] When myocardial cells are damaged, they release detectable proteins into the bloodstream so that a rise in biomarkers can be correlated with myocardial cellular damage. Biomarkers are divided into *cardiac-specific*—present only in cardiac muscle—and *nonspecific*—present in many muscles of the body. The biomarkers that are routinely measured include the cardiac-specific *troponin I (TnI)* and *CK-MB,* and the nonspecific muscle biomarkers *myoglobin, creatine kinase (CK),* and *troponin T (TnT).* See Table 11-4 for a summary of this information.[25] Unfortunately, in many hospitals the laboratory turnaround time for results of cardiac biomarkers is between 60 and 90 minutes, which limits the usefulness of the biomarkers in the emergency department when the patient is first admitted with symptoms of acute coronary syndrome.[25] If point-of-care testing at the bedside is used, the results are available more quickly and may be more helpful in the clinical decision-making process.[25]

CK and CK-MB

The traditional "gold standard" for diagnosing MI is the rise and fall of the serum MB fraction of the enzyme CK within 24 hours after the onset of symptoms. The CK-MB serum levels rise 4 to 8 hours after MI, peak at 15 to 24 hours, and remain elevated for 2 to 3 days (see Table 11-4). Serial samples are drawn routinely at 6- or 8-hour intervals, and three samples are usually sufficient to support or rule out the diagnosis of MI. CK-MB is rarely an isolated test; it is frequently performed in conjunction with cardiac troponin levels.

Troponin T and Troponin I

The *troponins* are a structurally related group of proteins found in both cardiac and skeletal muscle. In cardiac muscle the troponin complexes (cTnI and cTnT) are mostly bound to the thin actin filament, which is disrupted when the muscle is deprived of oxygen (infarction). Either cTnI or cTnT can be used as markers of acute MI, both in centralized laboratory tests and in bedside point-of-care testing.[25] Several different methods of laboratory assay are currently in use, which means that "normal" serum levels will vary between different clinical settings, although cardiac serum troponin levels (cTnI and cTnT) are low in the absence of myocardial muscle damage.

The initial elevation of troponin (cTnI and cTnT) and CK-MB occurs 3 to 6 hours after the acute myocardial damage has occurred. This means that if an individual comes to the emergency department as soon as chest pain is experienced, the enzymes will not have risen. For this reason, it is current clinical practice to diagnose an acute MI by 12-lead ECG and clinical symptoms, without waiting for results of cardiac biomarkers.[24]

Myoglobin

Myoglobin is a nonspecific indicator of myocardial cell damage because it is identical in both cardiac and skeletal muscle. It is useful because it is the biomarker that rises earliest in the serum. Myoglobin begins to rise about 1 to 4 hours after myocardial injury. It is never used alone but can be used in conjunction with other more cardiac-specific biomarkers.

Trending Hematologic Studies

Hematologic laboratory studies that are routinely ordered for the management of patients with altered cardiovascular status are red blood cell (RBC or erythrocyte) level, hemoglobin (Hgb) level, hematocrit (Hct) level, and white blood cell (WBC or leukocyte) level.

Red Blood Cells

The normal amount of RBCs in a person varies with age, gender, environmental temperature, altitude, and exercise. Males produce 4.5 million to 6 million RBCs per cubic millimeter, whereas the normal level for females is 4 million to 5.5 million per cubic millimeter.

Hemoglobin

Hgb levels normally range from 14 to 18 g/dl in males and from 12 to 16 g/dl in females.

Hematocrit

Hct is the volume percentage of RBCs in whole blood—40% to 54% for males and 38% to 48% for females.

White Blood Cells

Most inflammatory processes that produce necrotic tissue within the heart muscle, such as rheumatic fever, endocarditis, and MI, increase the WBC level. White blood cells are also known as leukocytes, and a WBC test may be called a serum leukocyte count. The normal WBC level for both genders is 5000 to 10,000 per cubic millimeter.

Platelets

The normal platelet count is 150,000 to 400,000 cells per cubic millimeter (cmm). Less commonly the normal platelet count range will be written as 150 to 400 × 10^9/L. If the platelet count is low, this is termed *thrombocytopenia*.

Assessing Blood Coagulation Studies

Coagulation studies are ordered to determine blood-clotting effectiveness. Anticoagulants—most notably heparin, direct thrombin inhibitors, warfarin, and platelet inhibitory agents—are administered daily in critical care units for a myriad of clinical reasons.[26-28] It is essential for the nurse to understand the laboratory tests that are used to monitor the effectiveness of therapeutic anticoagulation. In addition, many new anticoagulants are under development that will require close clinical surveillance of these specialized laboratory tests.[29]

Prothrombin Time

Most coagulation study results are reported as the length of time in seconds it takes for blood to form a clot in the laboratory test tube. The *prothrombin time* (PT) is no longer directly used to determine the therapeutic dosage of warfarin (Coumadin) necessary to achieve anticoagulation. The PT is not standardized between laboratories, so the result of this test is always reported as a standardized *international normalized ratio* (INR).[30]

International Normalized Ratio

The INR was developed by the World Health Organization (WHO) in 1982 to standardize PT results among clinical laboratories worldwide.[30] Table 11-5 illustrates target INR ranges for different cardiovascular conditions that require anticoagulation.[30] It is recommended that the INR be used to guide anticoagulation therapy with warfarin rather than the PT, especially if the PT results are analyzed at more than one laboratory.[30]

When a patient is first started on warfarin, it is important to know that it can take 72 hours or more to achieve a therapeutic level of anticoagulation. This is because the half-life of prothrombin is between 60 and 72 hours.[30] This delay in anticoagulation effectiveness

Table 11-5

Therapeutic Coagulation Values

TEST	CLINICAL CONDITION	NORMAL VALUE	THERAPEUTIC ANTICOAGULANT TARGET VALUE
INR	Normal coagulation	Less than 1.0	
INR	Chronic atrial fibrillation	2.0-3.0	
INR	Treatment of DVT/PE	2.0-3.0	
INR	Mechanical heart valve(s)	2.5-3.5	
aPTT	Normal coagulation	28-38 sec	1.5-2.5 times normal
PTT	Normal coagulation	60-90 sec	1.5-2.0 times normal
ACT*	Normal coagulation	0-120 sec	150-300 sec

INR, International normalized ratio; *DVT,* deep vein thrombosis; *PE,* pulmonary embolism; *aPPT,* activated partial thromboplastin time; *PTT,* partial thromboplastin time; *ACT,* activated coagulation time.
*ACT normal, therapeutic values may vary with type of activator used.

also occurs if a patient is being converted from heparin anticoagulation to warfarin anticoagulation. To ensure a safe transition, a delay of 4 days or more must be anticipated and PT/INR values must be assessed before the heparin is discontinued.[30] For patients who are to undergo surgery and have a high risk of thromboembolism and thus require anticoagulation, the steps are reversed. The warfarin is stopped 4 days before surgery and when the INR has returned to normal the patient is started on therapeutic unfractionated heparin (UFH) or low-molecular-weight heparin (LMWH).[26]

Activated Partial Thromboplastin Time

The *activated partial thromboplastin time* (aPTT) is used to measure the effectiveness of IV or subcutaneous heparin administration. Coagulation monitoring is required with heparin, although not with subcutaneous LMWH, because of lower levels of plasma protein binding.[29] In cases of over-anticoagulation with heparin the antidote is protamine sulfate.

Activated Coagulation Time

An additional test of heparin effect is the *activated coagulation time* (ACT). The ACT can be performed outside of the laboratory setting in areas such as the cardiac catheterization laboratory, the operating room, or specialized critical care units. Normal and therapeutic values for all of these coagulation studies are shown in Table 11-5.

Evaluating Serum Lipid Studies

Four primary blood lipid levels are important in evaluating an individual's risk of developing and/or having progression of coronary artery disease: total cholesterol, low-density lipoprotein cholesterol (LDL-C), triglycerides, and high-density lipoprotein cholesterol (HDL-C). When levels of cholesterol low-density lipoproteins (LDLs) and triglycerides are elevated or the level of high-density lipoproteins (HDLs) is low, the patient is considered "at risk" for developing or having progression of coronary artery disease and is offered intensive interventions in diet therapy, exercise prescription, and/or drug therapy.[31,32]

Table 11-6

Desirable Lipid Levels

LIPID	DESIRABLE LEVEL
Total cholesterol	<200 mg/dl
LDL-C	<130 mg/dl without CAD
	<100 mg/dl with CAD but not considered "high-risk"
	<70 mg/dl with CAD and considered "high risk" for future coronary events
Triglycerides	<150 mg/dl
HDL-C	>40 mg/dl (male)
	>50 mg/dl (female)

Data from Executive Summary of the Third Report of the National Cholesterol Education Program (NCEP) Expert Panel on Detection, Evaluation, and Treatment of High Blood Cholesterol in Adults (Adult Treatment Panel III), *JAMA* 285(19):2486-2497, 2001; and Grundy SM et al: *Circulation* 110:227, 2004.
LDL-C, Low-density lipoprotein cholesterol; *CAD,* coronary artery disease; *HDL-C,* high-density lipoprotein cholesterol.

Total Cholesterol

Cholesterol is a fatlike substance (lipid) that is present in cell membranes; produced by the liver, it is a precursor of bile acids and steroid hormones. The cholesterol level in the blood is determined partly by genetics and partly by acquired factors such as diet, calorie balance, and level of physical activity. Cholesterol in excess amounts (more than 200 mg/dl) in the serum forces the progression of atherosclerosis (atherogenesis). See Table 11-6 for desirable lipid levels to lower the risk of CAD and to reduce morbidity and mortality in patients with established CAD.

Low-Density Lipoproteins

About 60% to 70% of the total serum cholesterol is carried in the bloodstream, complexed as *LDL-C*. Both the LDL-C and total serum cholesterol levels are directly correlated with risk for CAD, and high levels of each are significant predictors of future acute MI in persons with established coronary artery atherosclerosis. LDL-C is the major atherogenic lipoprotein and thus is the primary target for cholesterol-lowering efforts.[31-33] Current guidelines recommend maintaining an LDL-C level below 130 mg/dl for the patient with no history of atherosclerotic disease. A patient with known coronary artery disease but who is not high risk should aim for an LDL-C level below 100 mg/dl. The recommended target LDL-C level for high-risk patients with CAD has recently been lowered to 70 mg/dl.[32]

Very-Low-Density Lipoproteins and Triglycerides

The *very-low-density lipoproteins* (VLDLs) contain 10% to 15% of the total serum cholesterol along with most of the triglycerides in fasting serum. Elevated triglyceride levels are often associated with reduced HDL-C levels.[31,32]

High-Density Lipoproteins

HDLs are particles that carry 20% to 30% of the total serum cholesterol. A low HDL-C level (less than 35 mg/dl) is another independent, significant risk factor for CAD. Several studies also support the finding that HDL-C helps protect against atherogenesis, and a level greater than 50 mg/dl may act as a "shield" against the risk of CAD.[31,32]

DIAGNOSTIC PROCEDURES

An overview of the various diagnostic procedures used to evaluate cardiovascular dysfunction is provided in Table 11-7.

Nursing Management

The nursing management of a patient undergoing a diagnostic procedure involves a variety of interventions. **Nursing priorities are directed toward (1) preparing the patient psychologically and physically for the procedure, (2) obtaining informed consent, (3) monitoring the patient's physiologic responses, and (4) assessing the patient after the procedure.**

Table 11-7

Cardiovascular Diagnostic Procedures

PROCEDURE	EVALUATION	COMMENTS
Aortography	Aortic valve insufficiency Aneurysms or dissection of ascending aorta Coarctation of aorta Injuries to aorta and major branches	Contrast medium used: check for allergy to iodine, shellfish, and dye; ensure hydration after procedure. Monitor for clinical indications of anaphylaxis (flushing, urticaria, stridor). Monitor puncture site.
Cardiac biopsy	Effect of cardiotoxic drugs Evidence of cardiac transplant rejection Inflammatory heart disease Tumors Cardiomyopathy	Observe closely for signs of cardiac perforation and cardiac tamponade.
Cardiac catheterization and coronary angiography	Severity of coronary artery stenosis Cardiac muscle function Pressures within heart Cardiac output, ejection fraction Arterial blood gas analysis within chambers Allows angioplasty, atherectomy, intracoronary stents, or lasers to reduce coronary artery obstruction	*Before test,* check for allergy to iodine, shellfish, and dye (contrast medium used). *After test:* Ensure hydration (contrast medium used). Keep affected extremity immobilized in a straight position for 6-12 hours. Monitor arterial puncture point for hemorrhage or hematoma. Monitor neurovascular status of affected limb. Note complaints of back pain and vital sign changes (may indicate retroperitoneal hemorrhage).
Chest radiography	Cardiac size and shape Pulmonary congestion or pleural effusion Thoracic aneurysm or aortic calcification Position of pulmonary artery and cardiac catheter, pacemaker, wires	Inquire about possibility of pregnancy.

Table 11-7

Cardiovascular Diagnostic Procedures—*cont'd*

PROCEDURE	EVALUATION	COMMENTS
Computed tomography (CT)	Left ventricular wall motion Cardiac tumors MI Pericardial effusion Aortic aneurysm/dissection	May be done with or without contrast medium. If contrast medium used, check for allergy to iodine, shellfish, and dye; ensure hydration after procedure.
Digital subtraction angiography	Vascular disease Degree of occlusion	Contrast medium used: check for allergy to iodine, shellfish, and dye; ensure hydration after procedure. Monitor for clinical indications of anaphylaxis (flushing, urticaria, stridor). Monitor puncture site.
Doppler ultrasonography	Vascular disease Degree of occlusion	TEE is better choice if patient is obese or has COPD, chest wall deformity, chest trauma, or thick chest dressings.
Echocardiography • *M mode:* Single ultrasound beam • *2D:* Planar ultrasound beam; wider view of heart, structures • *Doppler:* Flow of blood through heart • *Color flow:* Doppler image superimposed on 2D image • *Stress:* Images before, during, and after exercise or pharmacologic stress • *TEE:* Transducer placed in esophagus	Chamber size and wall thickness Valve functioning Papillary muscle functioning Prosthetic valve functioning Ventricular wall motion abnormalities Intracardiac masses Pericardial fluid Intracardiac pressures (Doppler) Ejection fraction, cardiac output (Doppler) Valve gradients (Doppler) Intracardiac shunts (Doppler) Thoracic aneurysm (TEE)	
Electrocardiography (ECG)	Dysrhythmias Conduction defects, including intraventricular blocks Electrolyte imbalance Drug toxicity MI, myocardial ischemia/injury Chamber hypertrophy	List drugs the patient is receiving on ECG request. Be alert to electrical safety hazards.
Electrophysiologic studies (EPS)	Dysrhythmias under controlled circumstances Best therapy for control of dysrhythmia: drug/dosage, pacemaker, catheter ablation	Patient may have near-death experience during EPS; encourage expression of fears, concerns, and anxieties. Monitor puncture site.
Holter monitoring	Suspected dysrhythmias over 24-hour period Pacemaker function Silent ischemia	Instruct patient on importance of keeping diary.
Intravascular ultrasound (IVUS)	Coronary artery size/patency Vessel wall structure Coronary stent position/patency Aorta; aneurysms, aneurysm dissections	As for cardiac catheterization.
Magnetic resonance imaging (MRI)	Three-dimensional view of heart Anatomy/structure of heart and great vessels, including cardiomyopathy, congenital defect, masses, and aneurysms Changes in chemistry of tissues before structural changes occur	Does not involve radiation or dyes. Cannot be used in patients with any implanted metallic device, including pacemakers, defibrillators, metallic heart valves, and intracranial aneurysm clips.
Multiple-gated acquisition (MUGA) scan (radionuclide angiography)	Ventricular size/wall motion Cardiac output, cardiac index, end-systolic volume, end-diastolic volume, ejection fraction Intracardiac shunts	Assure patient that amount of radioactive material is minimal.

Continued

Table 11-7
Cardiovascular Diagnostic Procedures—*cont'd*

PROCEDURE	EVALUATION	COMMENTS
Pericardiocentesis and pericardial fluid analysis	Blood, pus, pathogens, malignancy Emergency relief of cardiac tamponade	Observe closely for signs of cardiac tamponade.
Peripheral angiography	Atherosclerotic plaque Occlusion Aneurysm Traumatic injury	*Before test,* check for allergy to iodine, shellfish, and dye (contrast medium used). *After test:* Ensure hydration (contrast medium used). Keep affected extremity immobilized in a straight position for 6-12 hours. Monitor arterial puncture point for hemorrhage or hematoma. Monitor neurovascular status of affected limb. Monitor for indications of systemic emboli.
Phonocardiography	Extra heart sounds and murmurs in relation to cardiac cycle and ECG	Rarely used at present.
Positron emission tomography (cardiac PET scan)	Severity of coronary artery stenosis Collateral circulation Patency of bypass grafts Size/location of infracted tissue	Assure patient that amount of radioactive material is minimal.
Stress electrocardiography	High-risk patients, patients with known CAD, or postsurgical patients for ischemia with exercise or pharmacologic agents (e.g., adenosine, dipyridamole, dobutamine) Exercise-induced dysrhythmias	≥1 mm of transient ST-segment depression 80 msec after J point suggests CAD. Monitor closely for exercise-induced hypotension and ventricular dysrhythmias.
Technetium-99 pyrophosphate scan	Size and location of acute MI; infracted areas show increased uptake of radioactivity (hot spots) 1-7 days after MI	Assure patient that amount of radioactive material is minimal. Peak accuracy at 12-48 hours after initial symptoms.
Thallium stress electrocardiography	Myocardial ischemia during exercise; ischemic areas show decreased uptake of radioactivity (cold spots).	Assure patient that amount of radioactive material is minimal.
Thallium-201 scan	Myocardial ischemia; ischemic areas show decreased uptake of radioactivity (cold spots).	Assure patient that amount of radioactive material is minimal.
Vectorcardiography	Chamber hypertrophy Bundle branch blocks/hemiblocks Myocardial ischemia or infarction	
Venography (ascending contrast phlebography)	Deep leg veins, DVT Competence of deep vein valves Location of suitable vein for arterial bypass graft	Contrast medium used: check for allergy to iodine, shellfish, and dye; ensure hydration after procedure. Monitor for clinical indications of anaphylaxis (flushing, urticaria, stridor). Monitor puncture site.
Ventriculography	Ventricular wall motion/thickness Ventricular aneurysm Mitral valve motion Left ventricular end-diastolic volume, end-systolic volume, stroke volume, ejection fraction Intracardiac shunt	Contrast medium used: check for allergy to iodine, shellfish, and dye; ensure hydration after procedure. Monitor for clinical indications of anaphylaxis (flushing, urticaria, stridor). Monitor puncture site.

From Dennison RD: *Pass CCRN!*, ed 2, St Louis, 2000, Mosby.
MI, Myocardial infarction; *2D,* two-dimensional; *TEE,* transesophageal echocardiography; *COPD,* chronic obstructive pulmonary disease; *CAD,* coronary artery disease; *DVT,* deep vein thrombosis.

Preparing the patient includes teaching about the procedure, answering questions, and ensuring that the patient is informed about the diagnostic procedure. If the procedure is invasive, the clinician that will perform the procedure must discuss risks, benefits, and potential complications with the patient to ensure that informed consent is obtained. Monitoring the patient's responses during diagnostic procedures includes observing for signs of pain, anxiety, and hemorrhage and monitoring vital signs. Assessing the patient

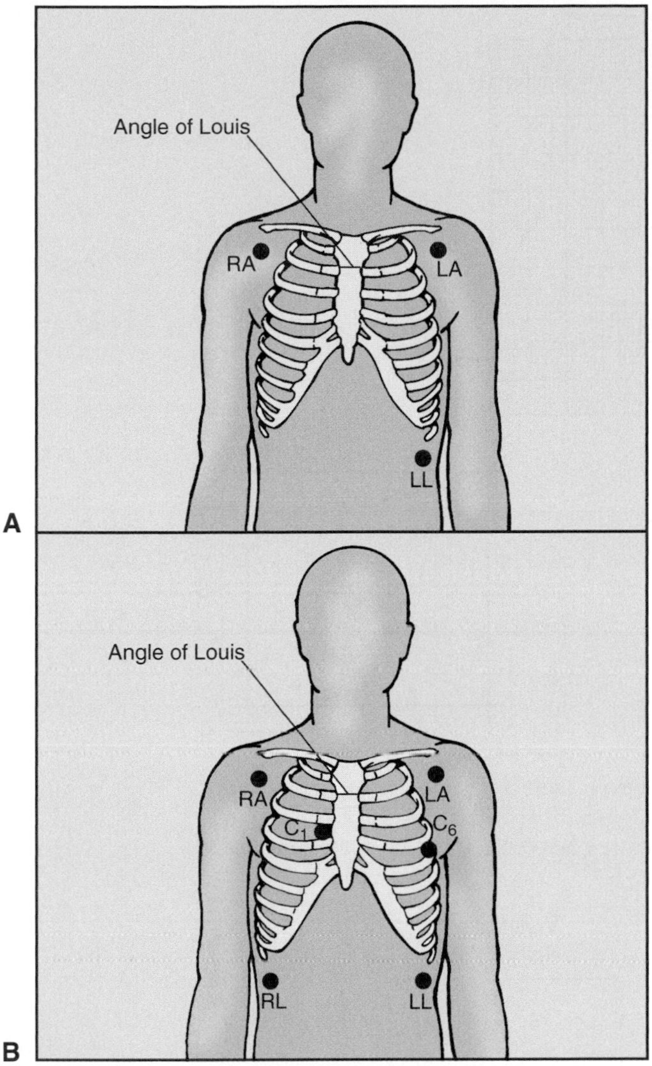

FIGURE 11-6. A, Three electrodes and lead-wire cables allow monitoring of three of the limb leads (I, II, and III) and can also be rearranged to monitor MCL_1 and MCL_6. **B,** Multilead monitoring system: five electrodes and lead-wire cables allow monitoring of any of the six standard limb leads (I, II, III, aV_R, aV_L, or aV_F) and any one precordial lead, either V_1 or V_6. C_1 indicates the proper position of the chest electrode for monitoring lead V_1, and C_6 indicates the proper position of the chest electrode for monitoring V_6. The cable attachments are color coded for quick identification and placement. Accurate electrode placement is essential.

after the procedure includes monitoring for complications and medicating the patient for any postprocedural anxiety, pain, or discomfort. Evidence of bleeding or chest pain should be immediately reported to the physician and emergency measures undertaken to maintain circulation and increase myocardial oxygen supply.

ELECTROCARDIOGRAPHY

ECG Leads

The basic ECG lead system consists of three electrodes: positive electrode, negative electrode, and ground electrode (Figure 11-6, *A*). A system of five electrodes is typically used in critical care (Figure 11-6, *B*). The function of the ground electrode is to prevent the display of background electrical interference on the ECG tracing. Leads do not transmit any electricity to the patient; leads only sense and record electrical impulses. During continuous cardiac monitoring, adhesive pregelled electrodes are placed on the patient to obtain the ECG tracing for a visual display of one, two, or more leads simultaneously.[34]

ECG Analysis

Specialized ECG Paper

ECG paper records the speed and magnitude of electrical impulses on a grid composed of small and large boxes (Figure 11-7). Every large box has five small boxes in it. On the horizontal axis one small box (1 mm) is equivalent to 0.04 second, and one large box (5 mm) represents 0.20 second at a standard paper speed of 25 millimeters per second (mm/sec). Distances along the horizontal axis represent time and are stated in seconds. The vertical axis represents the magnitude, or force, of the electrical signal. The vertical scale is also standardized to a specific calibration. One small box equals 0.1 mm on the vertical scale. The standard ECG calibration is 1 millivolt (mV) is equal to 10 mm (or 10 small boxes) on the vertical ECG scale.[34]

Interpreting ECG Waveforms

Analysis of waveforms and intervals provides the basis for ECG interpretation (Figure 11-8).

P Wave. The P wave represents atrial depolarization. Mechanical contraction will follow electrical depolarization.

QRS Complex. The QRS complex represents ventricular depolarization. It is referred to as a complex because it consists of several different waves. The letter *Q* is used to describe an initial negative deflection; in other words, only if the first deflection from the baseline is negative will the wave be labeled a Q wave. The letter *R* applies to any positive deflection. A second positive deflection within the same complex is termed R prime (R′). The letter *S* refers to any subsequent negative deflection. Any combination of these deflections can occur and is collectively called the QRS complex (see Figure 11-8). The QRS duration is normally less than 0.10 second (2.5 small boxes on the horizontal scale).

T Wave. The T wave represents ventricular repolarization. The onset of the QRS to approximately the midpoint or peak of the T wave represents an absolute refractory period, during which the heart muscle cannot respond to another stimulus regardless of the strength of that stimulus (Figure 11-9). From the midpoint to the end of the T wave, the heart muscle is in the relative refractory period. The heart muscle has not yet fully recovered, but it could be depolarized again if a sufficiently strong stimulus were received.

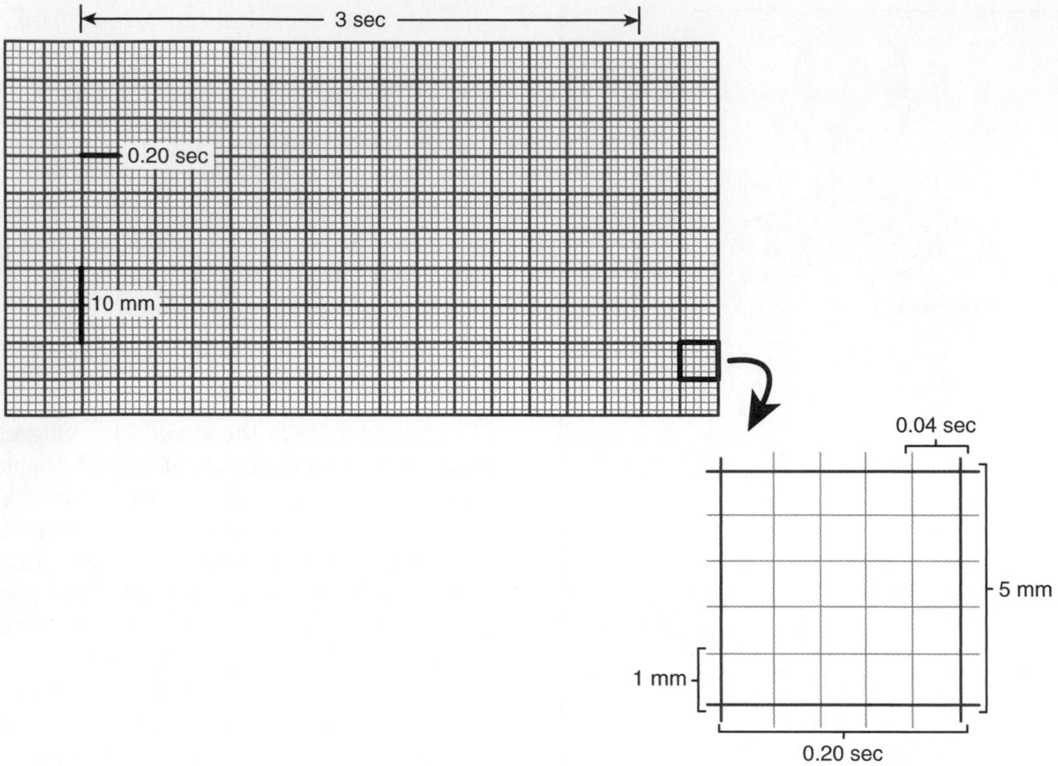

FIGURE 11-7. ECG graph paper. The horizontal axis represents time, and the vertical axis represents magnitude of voltage. Horizontally, each small box is 0.04 second and each large box is 0.20 second. Vertically, each large box is 5 mm. Markings are present every 3 seconds at the top of the paper for ease in calculating heart rate.

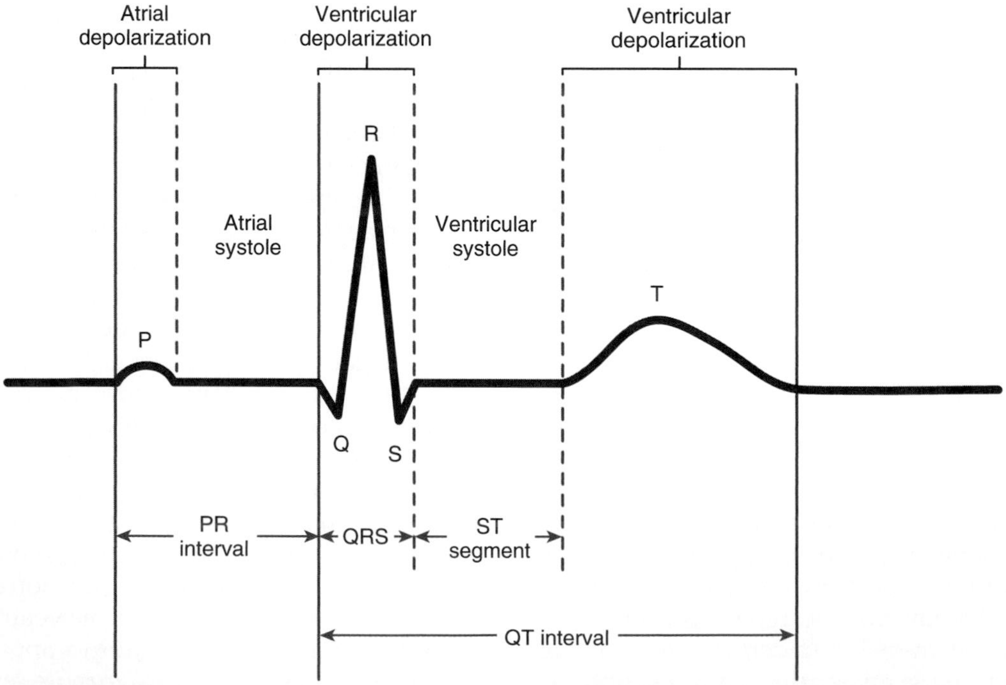

FIGURE 11-8. Normal ECG waveforms, intervals, and correlation with events of the cardiac cycle. The *P wave* represents atrial depolarization, followed immediately by atrial systole. The *QRS* represents ventricular depolarization, followed immediately by ventricular systole. The *ST segment* corresponds to phase 2 of the action potential, during which time the heart muscle is completely depolarized and contraction normally occurs. The *T wave* represents ventricular repolarization. The *PR interval,* measured from the beginning of the P wave to the beginning of the QRS, corresponds to atrial depolarization and impulse delay in the AV node. The *QT interval,* measured from the beginning of the QRS complex to the end of the T wave, represents the time from initial depolarization of the ventricles to the end of ventricular repolarization.

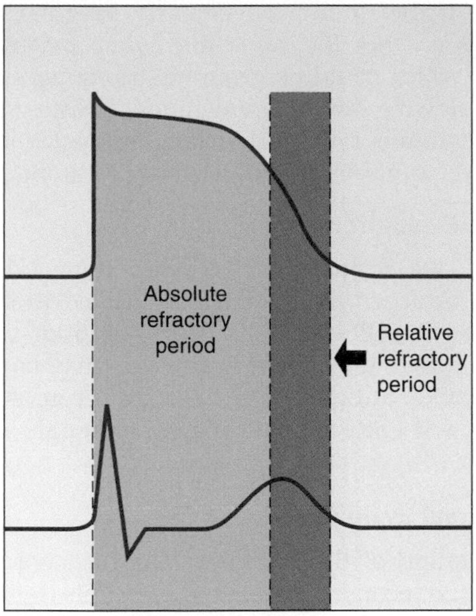

FIGURE 11-9. Absolute and relative refractory periods correlated with the cardiac muscle's action potential and with an ECG tracing.

Intervals Between Waveforms

The intervals between ECG waveforms are also evaluated (see Figure 11-8).

PR Interval. The PR interval is measured from the beginning of the P wave to the beginning of the QRS complex. Normally the PR interval is 0.12 to 0.20 second in length and represents the time between sinus node discharge and the beginning of ventricular depolarization. Because most of this period results from delay of the impulse in the AV node, the PR interval is an indicator of AV nodal function.

ST Segment. The ST segment is the portion of the wave that extends from the end of the QRS to the beginning of the T wave. Its duration is not measured. Instead, its shape and location are evaluated.[34] The ST segment is normally flat and at the same level as the isoelectric baseline. Any change from baseline is expressed in millimeters and may indicate myocardial ischemia (one small box equals 1 mm on the vertical scale). ST-segment elevation (increase greater than 1 mm) is associated with acute myocardial injury. ST-segment depression (decrease from baseline of more than 1 mm) is associated with myocardial ischemia. The measurement of ST elevation or depression is made using the J point in relation to the baseline isoelectric line (Figure 11-10).

QT Interval. The QT interval is measured from the beginning of the QRS complex to the end of the T wave and indicates the total time from the onset of depolarization to the completion of repolarization.[35] The QT length is affected by the heart rate (HR). A faster heart rate shortens the QT interval, a slower heart rate lengthens the QT interval. Thus, the QT is corrected for heart rate. A normal corrected QT (QTc) interval is less than 0.46 second in women and less than 0.45 in men.[34] A prolonged QT interval is significant because it can predispose the patient to the development of polymorphic VT, known also as torsades de pointes.[34] A long QT interval can occur secondary to electrolyte imbalance and antidysrhythmic drug therapy and also some non-antidysrhythmic medications.[34]

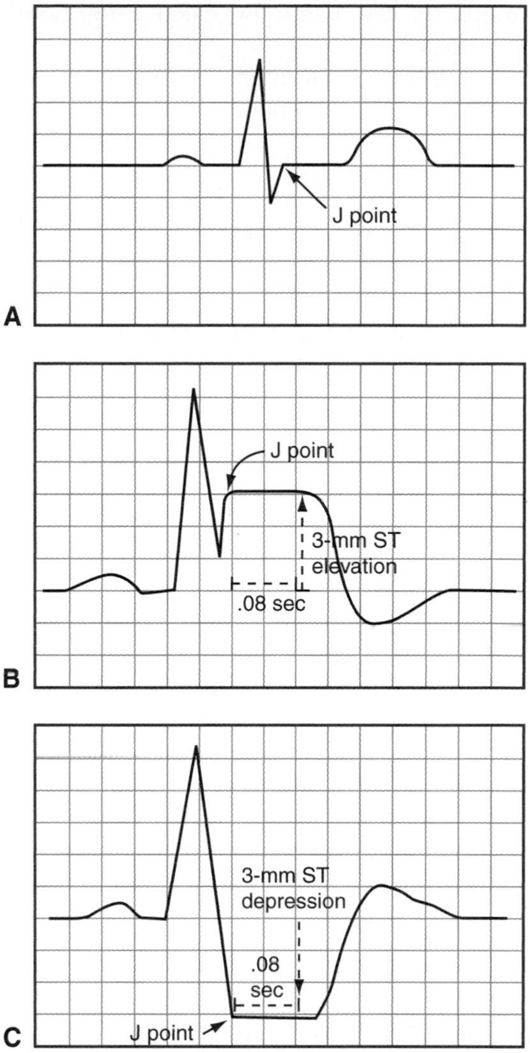

FIGURE 11-10. **A,** Normal position of the J point. **B,** 3-mm ST elevation. **C,** 3-mm ST depression. ST changes are measured 60 to 80 msec (0.06-0.08 sec) after the J point.

HEART RATE DETERMINATION

The first element to assess when evaluating a rhythm strip is the ventricular rate. Regardless of the dysrhythmia involved, the ventricular rate holds the key to whether the patient can tolerate the dysrhythmia (i.e., maintain adequate blood pressure, CO, and mentation). If the ventricular rate is consistently greater than 200 or less than 30 beats/min, emergency measures must be started to correct the rate. A detailed analysis of the underlying rhythm disturbance can proceed later when the immediate crisis is over. The following three methods are used for calculating heart rate (Figure 11-11):

Method 1: Number of RR intervals (in 6 seconds) multiplied by 10. ECG paper is usually marked at the top in 3-second increments, making a 6-second interval easy to identify.

Method 2: Number of large boxes between QRS complexes divided into 300.

Method 3: Number of small boxes between QRS complexes divided into 1500.

In the healthy heart, the atrial rate and the ventricular rate are the same. In many dysrhythmias, however, the atrial and ventricular rates are different, and therefore both must be calculated. To find the atrial rate, the PP interval, instead of the RR interval, is used in one of the three methods.

Rhythm Determination

The term *rhythm* refers to the regularity with which the P waves or R waves occur. Calipers assist in accurately measuring the rhythm. One point of the calipers is placed on the beginning of one R wave while the other point is placed on the next R wave. Leaving the calipers "set" at this interval, each succeeding RR interval is checked to ensure it is the same width.

In describing the rhythm, three terms are used. If the rhythm is regular, the RR intervals are the same (±10%). If the rhythm is regularly irregular, the RR intervals are not the same, but some pattern is involved, which could be grouping, rhythmic speeding up and slowing down, or any other consistent pattern. If the rhythm is irregularly irregular, the RR intervals are not the same, and no pattern can be found.

P-Wave Evaluation

The P wave is analyzed by determining (1) if it is present or absent and (2) if it is related to the QRS complex. One P wave should be in front of every QRS, and two, three, or four P waves may be in front of every QRS at times. If this pattern is consistent, the P wave and QRS are still related, although not on a 1:1 basis.

PR-Interval Evaluation

The duration of the PR interval, which normally is 0.12 to 0.20 second, is measured first. This is measured from the start of a visible P wave to the beginning of the following QRS. Next, all PR intervals on the strip are verified to ensure they have the same duration as the original interval.

QRS-Complex Evaluation

The entire ECG strip must be evaluated to ascertain that the QRS complexes are consistently the same shape and width. The normal QRS duration is 0.06

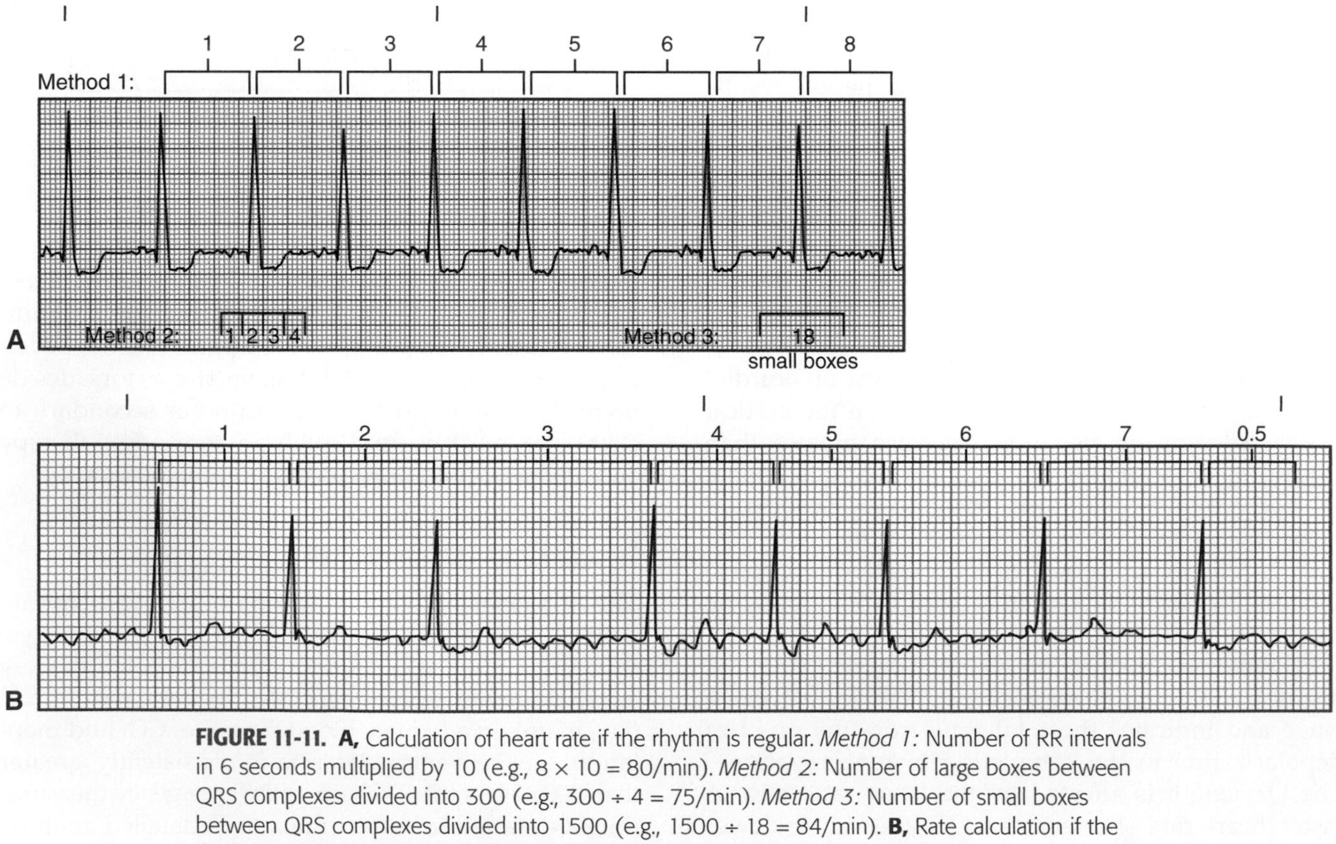

FIGURE 11-11. A, Calculation of heart rate if the rhythm is regular. *Method 1:* Number of RR intervals in 6 seconds multiplied by 10 (e.g., 8 × 10 = 80/min). *Method 2:* Number of large boxes between QRS complexes divided into 300 (e.g., 300 ÷ 4 = 75/min). *Method 3:* Number of small boxes between QRS complexes divided into 1500 (e.g., 1500 ÷ 18 = 84/min). **B,** Rate calculation if the rhythm is irregular. Only method 1 can be used (e.g., 7.5 intervals × 10 = 75/min).

to 0.10 second. If more than one QRS shape is on the strip, each QRS must be measured. The QRS is measured from where it leaves the baseline to where it returns to the baseline.

Dysrhythmia Interpretation

In clinical practice the terms *dysrhythmia* and *arrhythmia* often are used interchangeably. Both are correct, and either may be used in practice; this text favors *dysrhythmia.* A dysrhythmia is any disturbance in the normal cardiac conduction pathway. For this reason, patients in a critical care unit are monitored continuously, using a single or multilead system, and rhythm strips are recorded routinely as well as any time the patient's rhythm changes.

Sinus Rhythms

Normal Sinus Rhythm (Figure 11-12)

RATE: 60 to 100 beats/min.
RHYTHM: Regular (±10%).
P WAVE: Present, all the same shape, with only one preceding each QRS complex.
PR INTERVAL: 0.12 to 0.20 second.
QRS DURATION: 0.06 to 0.10 second.
QRS COMPLEX: Shape and whether deflection is positive or negative vary depending on lead placement and do not provide any key diagnostic information.
ETIOLOGY: Normal conduction.
TREATMENT: None required.

Sinus Bradycardia

Sinus bradycardia meets all of the criteria for normal sinus rhythm, except that the heart rate is less than 60 beats/min. Sinus bradycardia is not treated unless the patient displays signs of hypoperfusion such as hypotension, dizziness, or angina.

Sinus Tachycardia

Sinus tachycardia meets all of the criteria for normal sinus rhythm, except that the heart rate is greater than 100 beats/min. In the critical care setting, it is wise to be skeptical of any "sinus tachycardia" with a rate greater than 150 and to search for a triggering focus other than the sinus node. Sinus tachycardia can be caused by a wide variety of factors, such as exercise, emotion, pain, fever, hemorrhage, shock, heart failure, and thyrotoxicosis.[36] Illegal stimulant drugs such as cocaine, "ecstasy," and amphetamines can raise the resting heart rate significantly.[36] Many drugs used in critical care can also cause sinus tachycardia; common culprits are aminophylline, dopamine, hydralazine, atropine, and catecholamines such as epinephrine. Tachycardia is detrimental to anyone with ischemic heart disease because it decreases the time for ventricular filling, decreases stroke volume, and thus compromises CO. In addition, tachycardia increases heart work and myocardial oxygen demand, while decreasing oxygen supply by decreasing coronary artery filling time. When the cause of the tachycardia can be determined (e.g., fever, pain), the cause is treated rather than trying to treat the heart rate directly.[36]

Sinus Dysrhythmia

Sinus dysrhythmia, commonly called *sinus arrhythmia* in clinical practice, meets all of the criteria for normal sinus rhythm (NSR) except that the rhythm is irregular. This irregularity coincides with the respiratory pattern; heart rate increases with inhalation and decreases with exhalation[37] (Figure 11-13). Sinus dysrhythmia often occurs in children and young adults,

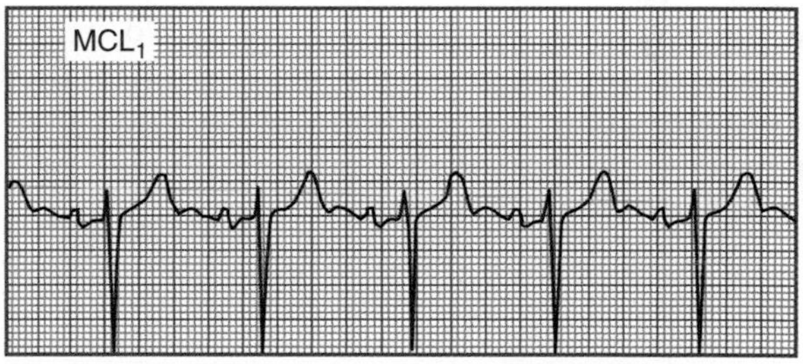

FIGURE 11-12. Normal sinus rhythm. The rate is 70; the rhythm is regular. One P wave is present before each QRS complex. The PR interval is 0.18 second and does not vary throughout the strip. The QRS duration is 0.08 second. All evaluation criteria are within normal limits.

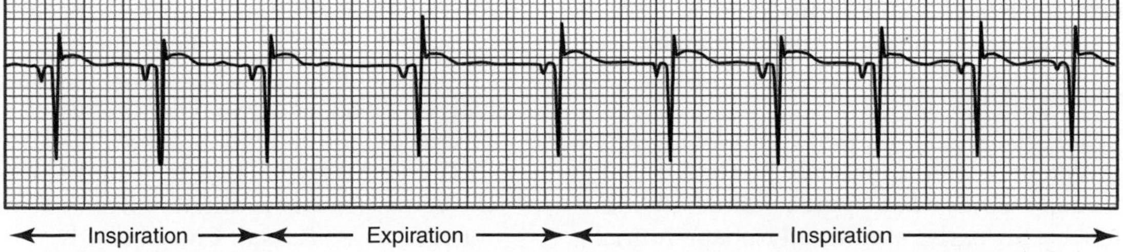

FIGURE 11-13. Sinus dysrhythmia. Note the increase in heart rate during inspiration and decrease in heart rate during expiration.

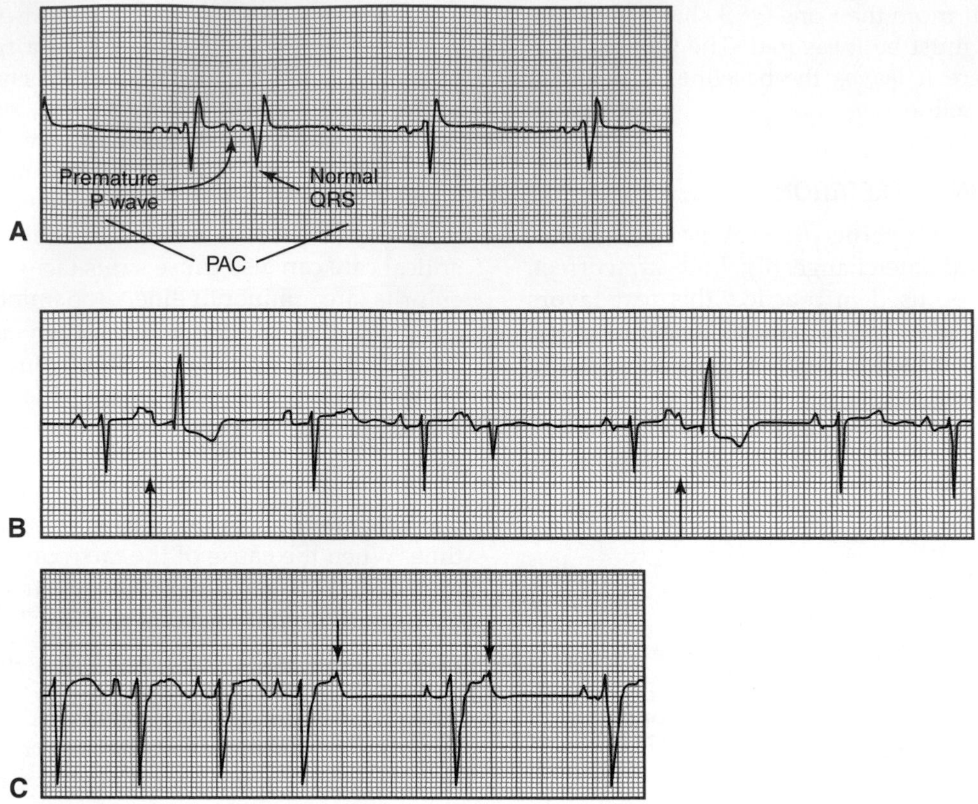

FIGURE 11-14. Premature atrial contractions (PACs). **A,** Normally conducted PAC. The early P wave is indicated by the arrow, and the QRS that follows is of normal shape and duration. **B,** Nonconducted (blocked) PACs. The early P waves are indicated by arrows. Note how they distort the T waves, making them appear peaked, compared with the normal T waves seen after the third and fourth QRS complexes. **C,** Right bundle branch block aberration after a PAC.

and the incidence decreases with age. No treatment is required. To avoid being misled by other rhythm disturbances, one must examine all P waves closely to verify that they are all the same shape and that the PR intervals are all constant.

Atrial Dysrhythmias

Atrial dysrhythmias originate from an ectopic focus in the atria, somewhere other than the sinus node. The ectopic impulse occurs before the normal sinus impulse is due to occur. The premature atrial depolarization may initiate a normal QRS complex, an abnormal or aberrant complex, or initiate a supraventricular tachycardia, clinically described as SVT. In recent years, huge advances have been made in understanding the pathogenesis and management of atrial dysrhythmias.

Premature Atrial Contractions

Premature atrial contractions (PACs) are isolated, early beats from an ectopic focus in the atria. The underlying rhythm is usually sinus. The regular sinus rhythm is interrupted by an early, abnormally shaped atrial P wave. The early atrial wave usually looks different than the sinus P wave and may be inverted. The PR interval may be longer, shorter, or the same as the PR interval of a sinus impulse. The QRS that follows the ectopic atrial P wave can vary in shape depending on the degree of refractoriness of the AV node.

1. *PAC with narrow QRS:* If the atrial impulse arrives in the AV node after the AV node is fully repolarized, the impulse is conducted to the ventricles as a normal QRS. If the ventricles are also fully repolarized, conduction through the bundle branches is expected and a normal QRS is recorded on the ECG (Figure 11-14, *A*).
2. *PAC with wide QRS:* Occasionally, the early ectopic P wave can be conducted through the AV node, but part of the conduction pathway through the ventricular bundle branches is blocked. Because the right bundle branch normally has the longest refractory period, it is usually the right bundle branch that is still blocked when the early impulse arrives. This produces a QRS that is wider than 0.12 second or wider than three small boxes on the ECG paper (Figure 11-14, *C*). Conduction through the ventricles that is different from normal is referred to as *aberrant.* Consequently, these early, abnormally conducted PACs are described as *aberrantly conducted PACs.*

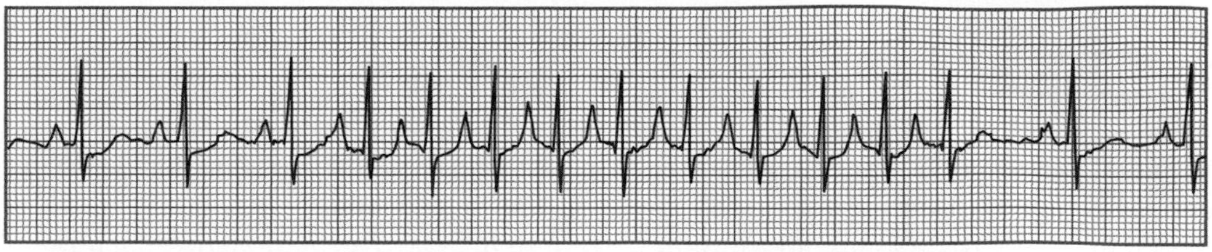

FIGURE 11-15. Paroxysmal supraventricular tachycardia (PSVT). Note that the atrial rate during tachycardia is 158 beats/min. The run starts and stops abruptly.

3. *Nonconducted PAC with pause without QRS:* Sometimes the ectopic P wave arrives so early that the AV node is still in its absolute refractory period. In this case, the wave of depolarization does not move past the AV node and no QRS follows. All that is seen on the ECG is an early, abnormal P wave followed by a pause until the next sinus P wave occurs (Figure 11-14, *B*). This is called a *nonconducted PAC.*

PACs can occur in individuals with normal hearts. PACs are accentuated by emotional upheaval, nicotine, caffeine, and digitalis. Heart failure can cause PACs because of increased pressure within the atria. As atrial pressure begins to rise, the atrial walls are stretched, causing irritability of atrial cells and the occurrence of PACs.

Supraventricular Tachycardia

The term *supraventricular tachycardia* (SVT) is clinically used to describe a varied group of dysrhythmias that originate above the AV node with a heart rate above 150 beats/min. SVT is not a very specific term. SVT includes sinus tachycardia, atrial tachycardia, atrial flutter, atrial fibrillation, and junctional tachycardia. Each of these entities has a distinct pathophysiology, specific therapy, and expected outcome. SVT may also be described as a "narrow-complex tachycardia" defined as a QRS that is less than 0.12 second.[36] Once the specific dysrhythmia is identified, it is generally referred to by a specific name; for example, atrial fibrillation. In other words, the term SVT is used to describe a rapid, sustained atrial or junctional tachycardia when the exact mechanism is not yet known. Women are affected by episodic SVT at about twice the rate of men.[36] SVT is not always benign. About 15% of people with SVT experience syncope (lose consciousness). Medications are used to limit the SVT rate and prevent "blackouts" or syncope.[36] SVT that is persistent for weeks or months may lead to a tachycardia-mediated cardiomyopathy.[36] *Paroxysmal supraventricular tachycardia* (PSVT) is a form of SVT that starts and stops suddenly (Figure 11-15).

Atrial Flutter

Atrial flutter is recognized on the ECG by the *sawtooth* atrial pattern. These sawtooth-shaped atrial wavelets are not P waves; they are more appropriately called *F waves* (flutter waves), as shown in Figure 11-16. Fortunately, the AV node does not allow conduction of all these impulses to the ventricles.

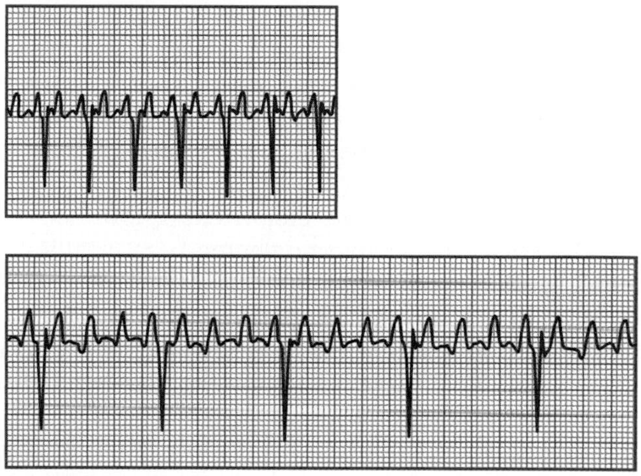

FIGURE 11-16. **A,** Initial strip shows atrial flutter with 2:1 conduction through the AV node. **B,** During carotid sinus massage, the AV conduction rate is decreased, more clearly revealing the flutter waves.

RATE: Atrial rate 250 to 350 beats/min.

RHYTHM: Regular flutter waves. Ventricular response (QRS complexes) may be regular or irregular.

P WAVE: Replaced by flutter (F) waves.

PR INTERVAL: No longer applies; instead a conduction ratio of flutter waves to QRS complexes (e.g., 2:1, 3:1, 4:1) is used. When evaluating the rate of atrial flutter, both atrial and ventricular rates must be calculated. The atrial rate is always faster.

QRS COMPLEX: Shape is usually narrow and normal.

PHYSIOLOGY: Atrial flutter can be started by any isolated atrial impulse, but to be maintained the atrial flutter requires a *reentry circular pathway* around macrostructures in the atria. Typical atrial structures are the vena cava and the tricuspid valve. The *reentry loop* may circle counterclockwise around the tricuspid valve,[36] can run clockwise around the inferior vena cava (IVC), or can make a figure-eight loop around the IVC and the tricuspid valve.[38]

TREATMENT: Nonpharmacologic interventions to convert atrial flutter to sinus rhythm are the most effective; these include electrical cardioversion and atrial overdrive pacing. The conversion rate with DC cardioversion is between 95% and 100%.[36] If atrial flutter has been present for more than 48 hours, up to one third of patients will have thrombi in the atria, and *anticoagulation* is mandated before either pharmacologic or electrical cardioversion. The risk of systemic emboli following cardioversion ranges from 2% to 7%.[36] Overdrive atrial pacing is often favored to convert atrial flutter following cardiac surgery. Epicardial wires that are placed at the time of surgery are connected to an external pacemaker. The overall success rate of atrial overdrive pacing is 83% (range 55% to 100%).[36]

Pharmacologic cardioversion using ibutilide (Corvert) is effective at converting hemodynamically stable atrial flutter to sinus rhythm between 38% and 76% of the time.[36] For patients who responded to the ibutilide, the average conversion time after infusion was 30 minutes.[36] One of the complications of ibutilide is known to be polymorphic tachycardia—also known as torsades de pointes—but in studies with atrial flutter patients the rate of torsades de pointes was under 3%.[36]

For patients with atrial flutter unrelated to an acute disease process, permanent termination of the atrial flutter circuit can be achieved by *radiofrequency ablation* (RFA). RFA is a catheter procedure used to create a line of conduction block across one of more sections of the reentry pathway. The most frequent location for RFA is a narrow band of tissue between the inferior vena cava and the tricuspid annulus known as the cavotricuspid isthmus.[36]

Atrial Fibrillation (Figure 11-17)

RATE: Atrial rate 350 to 600 fibrillatory waves per minute. Ventricular rate 60 to 100 (when controlled by medication), greater than 100 (when uncontrolled by medication).
RHYTHM: Irregularly irregular ventricular rhythm.
P WAVE: Replaced by fibrillating baseline or waves.

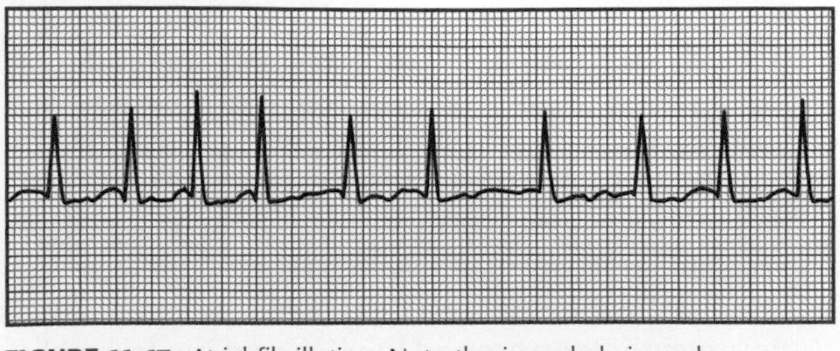

FIGURE 11-17. Atrial fibrillation. Note the irregularly irregular ventricular rhythm.

PR INTERVAL: Absent. Replaced by fibrillating baseline.
QRS DURATION: 0.06 to 0.10 second.
QRS COMPLEX: Usually normal because pathway through ventricles is unchanged once impulse leaves AV node.
ETIOLOGY: The pathogenesis of atrial fibrillation (AF) has traditionally been ascribed to random electrical foci firing in the atria. Recent research using high-density atrial mapping, high-speed video recordings, and ECG analysis has uncovered distinct spatial organization within the atria.[39-41] Atrial fibrillation is now known to involve several reentry circuits within the atria and in some cases to originate at specific anatomic sites. The four pulmonary veins that drain into the left atrium are a trigger site for early atrial foci to both initiate and propagate reentry circuits to maintain atrial fibrillation.[40] The earliest atrial ectopic foci have been electrically mapped 2 to 4 cm within the pulmonary veins.[40] The spread of atrial fibrillation to the rest of the atria is thought to occur via multiple reentry *wavelets* that are maintained in perpetual motion by a "mother rotor," or dominant reentry circuit, that functions at a higher frequency, drives the atrial fibrillation, and originates from the ectopic pulmonary vein tissue.[40]

Risk factors: As more research has focused on the etiology of atrial fibrillation, a clearer picture of incidence and risk factors has emerged. AF is present in 0.4% of the population, although there is a huge variation based on age. It occurs in less than 1% of persons less than 60 years, but the incidence rises to over 6% in those older than 80 years.[39] Men have a higher risk of developing AF than women, and at an earlier age.[39] Average age of onset is 60.5 years for men and 65.5 years for women.[42] The incidence of reported "palpitations" or paroxysmal AF is higher in women.[42] Atrial fibrillation is the most common cardiac dysrhythmia in the United States and responsible for about one third of dysrhythmia-related hospital admissions.[42] According to epidemiologic data from the Framingham study, one in four men and women who are free of AF at age 40 years will develop atrial fibrillation or flutter later in their life.[43] The risk of AF is higher for people with a history of hypertension, heart failure, or myocardial infarction.[43]

TREATMENT: There is currently considerable debate about the most effective approach to treating atrial fibrillation. In the past the gold standard was to convert the patient out of the atrial fibrillation back to normal sinus rhythm. However, recent research has shown that for many patients staying out of atrial fibrillation is an unattainable goal. Furthermore, the long-term clinical outcome for the patient may be similar with either of the two following approaches:

1. Convert the atrial fibrillation back to sinus rhythm using pharmacologic or electrical cardioversion (rhythm control). Anticoagulation is used if the person has been in AF for more than 3 days.
2. Allow the atrial fibrillation to persist and use pharmacologic measures to control the ventricular response rate by antidysrhythmic drugs (rate control).

Rhythm control for atrial fibrillation: For the hospitalized patient with *new-onset* atrial fibrillation with unstable hemodynamics, the focus is generally on rhythm control (conversion to sinus rhythm) using antidysrhythmic drugs or electrical cardioversion. Emergency drugs used to convert atrial fibrillation to sinus rhythm (also known as a chemical cardioversion)[41] flecainide, dofetilide, propafenone, ibutilide and amiodarone. Antidysrhythmic drugs used longterm to maintain the patient in sinus rhythm include amiodarone, disopyramide, flecainide, moricizine, procainamide, propafenone, quinidine, sotalol, and dofetilide or a combination of these medications as needed.[44] Even with drug therapy, recurrence of atrial fibrillation is likely.[44] Electrical cardioversion may be successful in converting the atria to sinus rhythm if attempted within a few days or weeks of the onset of atrial fibrillation. Its success is less likely if the AF has existed for a long time.[41] Without continued antidysrhythmic drug therapy, about 75% of cardioverted patients will be in atrial fibrillation at 1 year.[45] This number changes to about 50% of patients (half in AF, half in sinus rhythm) with continued antidysrhythmic drug therapy.[45] One of the disadvantages to long-term antidysrhythmic drug treatment is drug side-effects and potential "prodysrhythmic" effect of certain medications.[44,46]

Rate control for atrial fibrillation: The most frequently prescribed drugs used to control the ventricular rate in atrial fibrillation include calcium channel blockers, β-blockers, and digoxin. These drugs work to slow conduction through the AV node. They have no impact on the fibrillating atria. In the past it had always been assumed that "rate control" was an inferior strategy, because the patient stayed in atrial fibrillation, lost "atrial kick," and was presumed to have an increased risk of embolic stroke. Two multicenter trials have altered that perception: The *A*trial *F*ibrillation *F*ollow-up: *I*nvestigation of *R*hythm *M*anagement (AFFIRM),[47] and the *RA*te *C*ontrol vs. *E*lectrical Cardioversion for Persistent Atrial Fibrillation (RACE).[48] These two trials found similar morbidity, mortality, and quality of life in patients treated long term with either method: rhythm conversion or rate control.[44,49] For long-term management of atrial fibrillation, rate control is the recommended approach, with mandatory therapeutic anticoagulation to prevent embolic stroke.[41,50]

JUNCTIONAL DYSRHYTHMIAS

Only certain areas of the AV node have the property of automaticity. The area around the AV node is called the *junction;* hence impulses generated there are called *junctional.* When an ectopic impulse arises in the junction, it spreads in two directions at once. One wave of depolarization spreads upward into the atria and depolarizes them, causing the recording of a P wave on the ECG. This is called *retrograde (backward) conduction,* and the P wave is inverted when viewed in an inferior ECG lead such as lead II. At the same time, another wave of depolarization spreads downward into the ventricles through the normal conduction pathway, producing a normal QRS complex. This is termed *antegrade (forward) conduction.* Depending on timing, the P wave (1) may be seen in front of the QRS, with a short PR interval (less than 0.12 second), (2) may be obscured entirely by the QRS, or (3) may immediately follow the QRS.

Premature Junctional Contraction

RATE: Depends on underlying rhythm, usually NSR.
RHYTHM: On ECG, rhythm is regular from sinus node except for early QRS complex (PJC) of normal shape.
P WAVE: May be entirely absent, may be seen in T wave, or may be inverted.
PR INTERVAL: Usually absent. Lack or short PR interval is a defining characteristic of junctional rhythms.
QRS DURATION: 0.06 to 0.10 second.
QRS COMPLEX: Usually narrow and normal.
ETIOLOGY: Premature junctional contraction (PJC) is a single ectopic impulse that originates in AV junctional area.
TREATMENT: Usually none required. PJCs have virtually the same clinical significance as PACs. If the patient is receiving digoxin, however, digitalis toxicity should be considered. Although digoxin slows conduction through AV node, it also increases automaticity in the junction.

Junctional Escape Rhythm (Figure 11-18)

RATE: Intrinsic rate of junction is 40 to 60 beats/min if dominant pacemaker of heart.
RHYTHM: Regular.
P WAVE: Same as for PJC.
PR INTERVAL: Usually absent or very short.
QRS DURATION: 0.06 to 0.10 second.
QRS COMPLEX: Usually narrow and normal because impulse originates above ventricles.

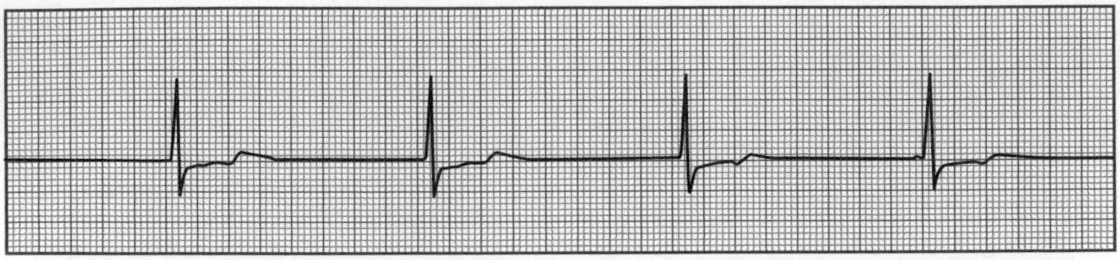

FIGURE 11-18. Junctional escape rhythm. The ventricular rate is 38. P waves are absent, and the QRS is normal width.

ETIOLOGY: Originates in AV junction after failure of sinus node.

PHYSIOLOGY: Under normal conditions, the AV junction is never able to "escape" and depolarize the heart because it is overridden by the faster sinus node. If the sinus node fails, however, AV node junctional impulses can depolarize and pace the heart. This junctional escape rhythm is a protective mechanism to prevent asystole in the event of sinus node failure.

TREATMENT: Generally a junctional escape rhythm is well tolerated hemodynamically, although efforts should be directed toward determining the cause and restoring sinus rhythm. An *accelerated junctional rhythm* has the same characteristics as a junctional escape, except that the rate is faster at 60 to 100 beats/min. Accelerated junctional rhythms are usually well tolerated hemodynamically by patients, because the HR is within normal range. A *junctional tachycardia* also shares the same characteristics but has a rate faster than 100 beats/min.

Ventricular Dysrhythmias

Premature Ventricular Contraction

RATE: Depends on underlying HR, usually NSR.

RHYTHM: Early QRS complexes interrupt underlying rhythm.

PR INTERVAL: Absent or retrograde after PVC.

QRS DURATION: Greater than 0.12 second.

QRS COMPLEX: Wide, with bizarre shape.

Unifocal premature ventricular contractions (PVCs): All ventricular ectopic beats look the same in a particular lead. There are several different names used to describe PVCs:

Unifocal PVCs: Probably all result from the same irritable focus (Figure 11-19, *A*).

Multifocal PVCs: Ventricular ectopic beats have various shapes in the same lead. More serious than unifocal PVCs, multifocal PVCs indicate that a greater area of irritable myocardium is involved. Multifocal PVCs are more likely to deteriorate into ventricular tachycardia/fibrillation (Figure 11-19, *B*).

Ventricular bigeminy: PVC follows each normal beat (Figure 11-19, *C*).

Compensatory pause: There is an apparently long "pause" following a PVC. However, the time interval from the last normal QRS preceding the PVC to the QRS following the PVC is equal to two complete cardiac cycles. The compensatory pause allows the sinus node to resume the normal pattern (Figure 11-19, *D*).

Interpolated PVC: PVC falls between two normal QRS complexes without disturbing the rhythm. RR interval between sinus beats remains the same (Figure 11-19 , *E*).

Couplet: Two consecutive PVCs.

Triplet: Three consecutive PVCs.

R on T: If a PVC occurs on the T wave during the relative refractory period (latter half of T wave) when only part of the muscle is repolarized, individual segments of muscle can depolarize separately from each other, resulting in ventricular fibrillation (Figure 11-19, *F*).

Fusion beats: If a ventricular ectopic impulse and a sinus beat depolarize simultaneously and meet in the middle of a depolarization, a fusion beat results. Fusion beats are narrower than ventricular beats and look like a cross between patient's sinus QRS and ventricular ectopic QRS.

ETIOLOGY: Myocardial ischemia, electrolyte imbalances, hypoxia, acidosis, heart disease (e.g., cardiomyopathy, ventricular aneurysm, previous MI), and prodysrhythmic medications.

PHYSIOLOGY: Ventricular dysrhythmias result from ectopic focus in any portion of ventricular myocardium. Usual conduction pathway through ventricles is not used, and the wave of depolarization spreads from cell to cell.

DOCUMENTATION: Underlying rhythm must always be described first (e.g., sinus bradycardia with frequent unifocal PVCs, atrial fibrillation with occasional multifocal PVCs).

TREATMENT: Not all ventricular ectopy requires treatment. In patients with no significant heart disease, PVCs do not increase the risk for sudden death and are considered benign. If possible, the cause of the PVCs should be treated; for example, PVCs caused by hypokalemia and hypomagnesemia are managed by potassium/magnesium administration. Patients with hypoxia

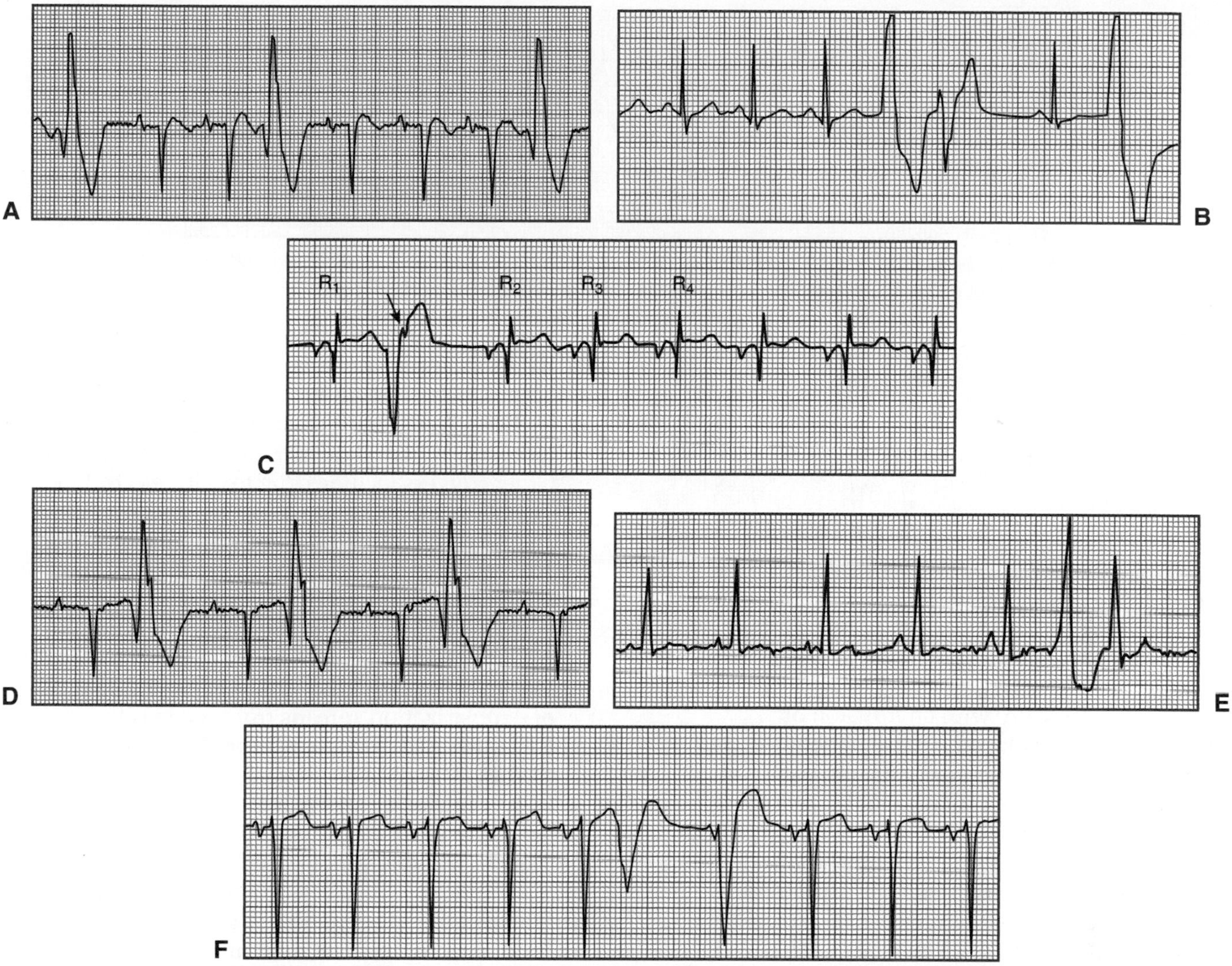

FIGURE 11-19. **A,** Unifocal PVCs. **B,** Multifocal PVCs. **C,** PVC with a fully compensatory pause. The interval between the two sinus beats that surround the PVC (R_1 and R_2) is exactly two times the normal interval between sinus beats (R_3 and R_4). The fully compensatory pause occurs because the sinus node continues to pace despite the PVC. Note the sinus P wave *(arrow)* hidden in the ST segment of the PVC. This P wave did not conduct through to the ventricles because they had just been depolarized and were still in the absolute refractory period. **D,** Ventricular bigeminy. **E,** Interpolated PVC. The PVC falls between two normal QRS complexes without disturbing the rhythm. Note that the RR interval between sinus beats remains the same. **F,** R-on-T phenomenon.

receive oxygen, ventilation if required, and have acidosis corrected.

Idioventricular Rhythms

RATE: 20 to 40 beats/min (escape rhythm). 40 to 100 beats/min (accelerated rhythm) (Figure 11-20).

RHYTHM: Regular.

PR INTERVAL: Absent.

QRS DURATION: Greater than 0.12 second.

P WAVE: Present, but not associated with QRS complex.

QRS COMPLEX: Wide and bizarre because complexes originate in ventricles.

ETIOLOGY: SA and AV nodes may be ischemic, infarcted, or depressed by drug toxicity.

PHYSIOLOGY: At times an ectopic focus in the ventricles can become the dominant pacemaker of the heart. If both SA node and AV junction fail, ventricles will depolarize at their own intrinsic rate of 20 to 40 beats per minute. This is described as an *idioventricular rhythm*. When a ventricular focus assumes control of the heart at a rate greater than 40 beats/min, this is termed an *accelerated idioventricular rhythm*.

TREATMENT: Rather than trying to abolish idioventricular ventricular beats, the aim of treatment is to reestablish a higher pacing site (e.g., SA node, AV junction). As a temporary measure, if the patient is hemodynamically unstable, the heart rate may be increased

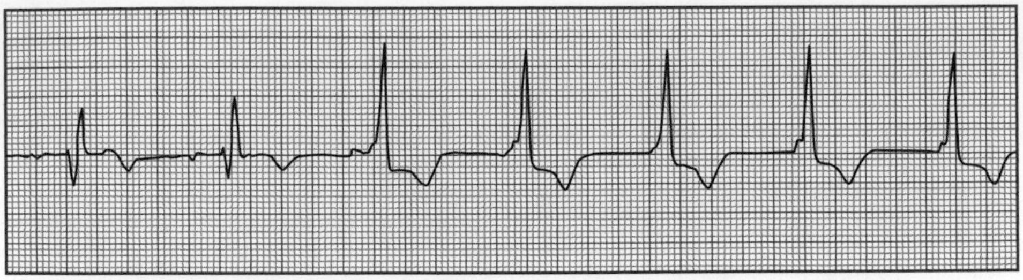

FIGURE 11-20. Accelerated idioventricular rhythm (AIVR). The QRS duration is 0.14 second, and the ventricular rate is 65.

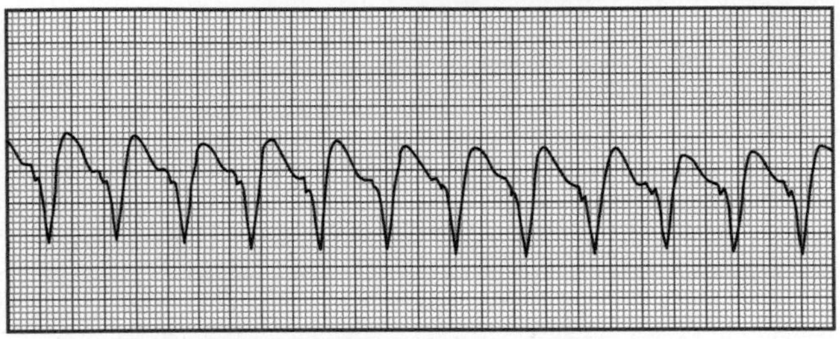

FIGURE 11-21. Ventricular tachycardia.

pharmacologically with an infusion of isoproterenol (Isuprel). Transcutaneous pacing may be used in an emergency. More often, a transvenous temporary pacemaker is inserted and the heart is paced at a faster rate until underlying problems that caused failure of faster pacing sites can be resolved. Drugs such as lidocaine are contraindicated in treatment of idioventricular rhythms because if the ventricular ectopic focus is abolished, the patient could become asystolic.

Ventricular Tachycardia

RATE: Greater than 100 beats/min.

RHYTHM: Mostly regular. May have some irregularities.

P WAVE: Not related to QRS. Sinus node usually is unaffected and will continue to depolarize atria on schedule, so P waves may be seen on ECG and even may conduct a normal impulse to ventricles if timing is right.

PR INTERVAL: Absent.

QRS DURATION: Greater than 0.12 second.

QRS COMPLEX: Wide, with bizarre shape compared with sinus QRS (Figure 11-21).

Nonsustained ventricular tachycardia (VT): Three or more consecutive PVCs, rate greater than 110 beats/min, lasts less than 30 seconds without hemodynamic collapse, and self-terminates.

Torsades de pointes ("twisting of the points"): Specific form of VT that refers to twisting appearance of VT on ECG (Figure 11-22). Torsades may be precipitated by antidysrhythmics that prolong the QT interval

ETIOLOGY: Over 90% of ventricular tachycardia occurs in the presence of structural cardiac disease, such as myocardial ischemia, congenital heart disease, valvular dysfunction, and cardiomyopathy. Other triggers include drug toxicity, electrolyte disturbances, and as an adverse reaction to certain antidysrhythmic drugs (prodysrhythmia). Only 10% of patients experience episodes of VT without known structural heart disease.[51]

PHYSIOLOGY: VT results from repeating ectopic focus in ventricular myocardium. Usual conduction pathway through ventricles is bypassed, and wave of depolarization spreads from cell to cell.

TREATMENT: Pharmacologic, or electrical cardioversion/defibrillation.

How ventricular tachycardia is clinically managed depends on whether the patient is stable or unstable, as well as whether a pulse and adequate blood pressure are present. Pulseless ventricular tachycardia is life-threatening. The patient will lose consciousness and will need immediate defibrillation as described in the American Heart Association (AHA) protocols for Advanced Cardiac Life Support (ACLS).[52] Patients with stable VT who have a heart rate below 150 beats/min, palpable pulse, and stable blood pressure may be treated pharmacologically with amiodarone, β-blockers, lidocaine, procainamide, or overdrive pacing as described in the ACLS protocols.[52]

Once the acute episode is over, patients who have already experienced sustained ventricular tachycardia or cardiac arrest often continue to be at risk for sudden cardiac death (SCD). An extensive clinical evaluation of these patients is warranted, including cardiac catheterization and electrophysiologic testing with programmed ventricular stimulation. Therapy is aimed at preventing a recurrence of sustained VT/VF. It may include treating the underlying cause, administering antidysrhythmic drugs, performing ablation of the reentrant pathway within the ventricle, or inserting an implantable cardioverter-defibrillator (ICD).

Ventricular Fibrillation (Figure 11-23)

RATE: Indeterminable.

RHYTHM: Irregular, wavy baseline without recognizable QRS complexes.

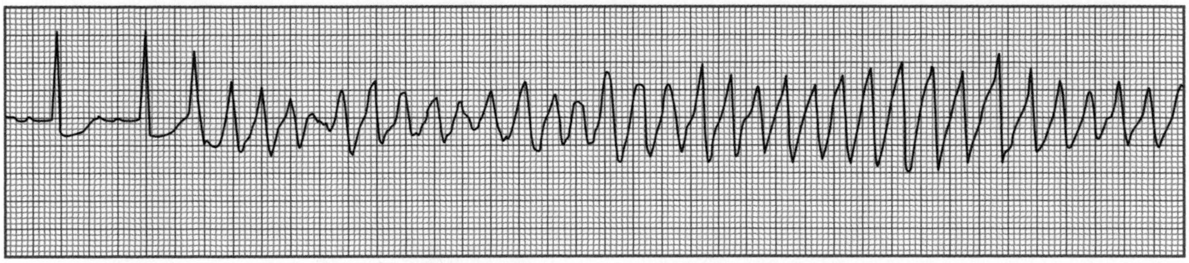

FIGURE 11-22. Torsades de pointes.

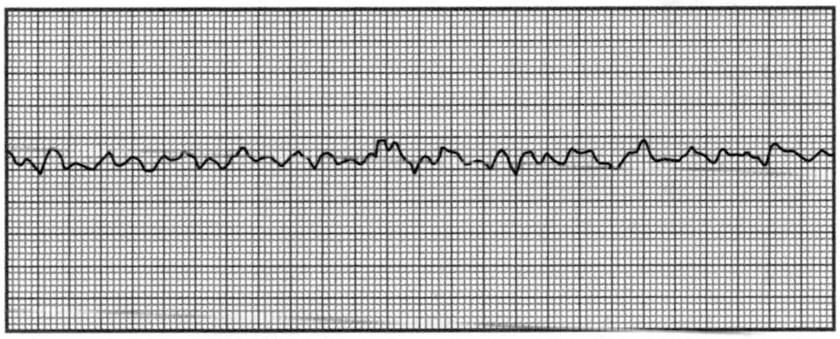

FIGURE 11-23. Ventricular fibrillation.

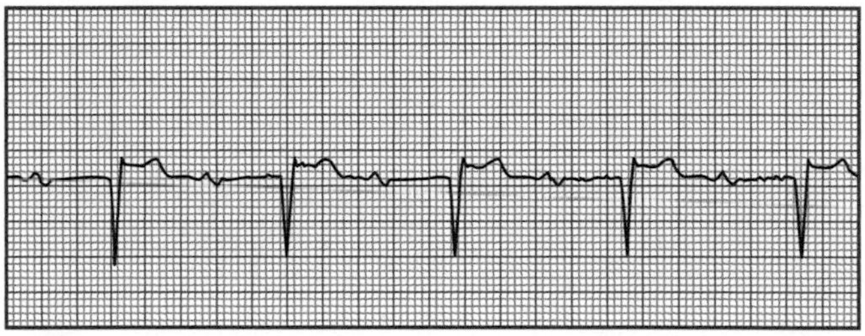

FIGURE 11-24. First-degree AV block. The PR interval is prolonged to 0.44 second.

P WAVE: Absent. Cannot be distinguished from fibrillating ventricular baseline.
PR INTERVAL: Absent.
QRS DURATION: Absent. No QRS complexes present.
QRS COMPLEX: Normal QRS is missing. ECG appears as wavy baseline. This is a life-threatening rhythm. Patients have no pulse or blood pressure, are unconscious, and will not survive without effective resuscitation.
ETIOLOGY: VT is most common precursor of VF. Therefore all the factors that predispose patients to VT apply.
PHYSIOLOGY: VF is a result of electrical impulses from single or multiple ventricular foci that prevent ventricles from contracting. Ventricles merely quiver, with no forward flow of blood.
TREATMENT: Unsynchronized defibrillation is the emergency treatment of choice combined with epinephrine and cardiopulmonary resuscitation (CPR). Supportive measures such as intubation and correction of metabolic abnormalities are performed concurrently following ACLS guidelines.[52]

Heart Blocks

First-Degree Atrioventricular Block (Figure 11-24)

RATE: Depends on underlying rhythm, usually NSR.
RHYTHM: Regular if NSR.
P WAVE: Present, normal shape.
PR INTERVAL: Greater than 0.20 second.
QRS DURATION: 0.06 to 0.10 second.
QRS COMPLEX: Unaffected.
PHYSIOLOGY: All atrial impulses that should be conducted to ventricles are conducted, but PR interval is prolonged.
TREATMENT: None required. Many elderly patients have first-degree AV block as a chronic condition associated with aging of AV junction.
Acute myocardial infarction: Patients with acute MI should be monitored for degeneration into more serious forms of AV block.
Drug side effect: If development of first-degree AV block is new and related to recent antidysrhythmic administration, the medication regimen must be evaluated.

Second-Degree Atrioventricular Block Type I (Figure 11-25)

This is a rhythm known by several different names including: Mobitz I and Wenckebach.

RATE: Atrial rate depends on underlying sinus rate. Ventricular rate depends on P wave/QRS ratio.
RHYTHM: Regular, irregular pattern. P waves regular. As part of Mobitz I pattern, R-to-R intervals become progressively shorter until sinus P wave is not conducted, resulting in a pause. After the pause, the cycle repeats. The PR interval typically lengthens the most with the second beat of the cycle.[53]
P WAVE: Normal shape.
PR INTERVALS: Progressively lengthen until a P wave is not conducted to ventricles and therefore is not followed by QRS complex.
QRS DURATION: 0.06 to 0.10 second.
QRS COMPLEX: Conducted complexes are normal.

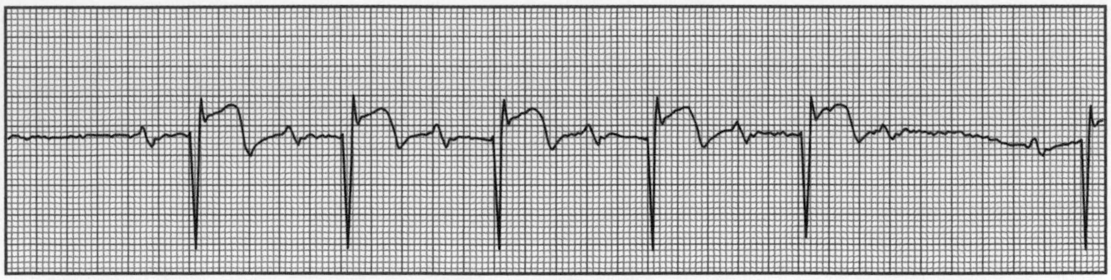

FIGURE 11-25. Mobitz type I (Wenckebach) second-degree AV block. Note that the PR intervals gradually increase from 0.36 to 0.46 second until finally a P wave is not conducted to the ventricles.

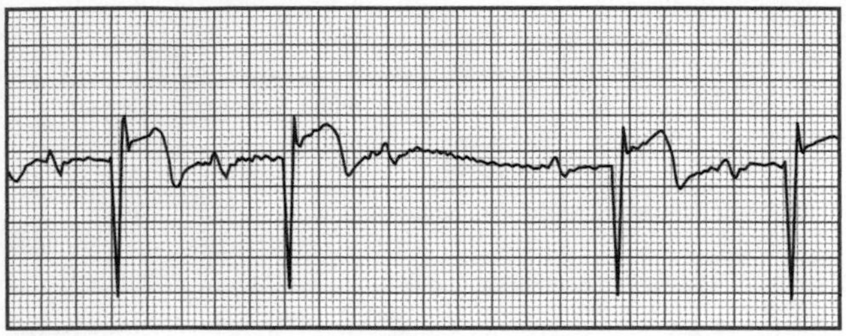

FIGURE 11-26. Mobitz type II second-degree AV block. Note that the PR intervals remain constant.

ETIOLOGY: Anatomic site of block is at level of AV node. If associated with acute inferior wall MI, block is caused by ischemia and is usually transient.
PHYSIOLOGY: AV conduction time lengthens until P wave not conducted to ventricles.
DOCUMENTATION: P wave/QRS complex ratio. For example, if four P waves are conducted to ventricles and fifth wave is not, a 5:4 conduction ratio is present (five P waves to four QRS complexes).
TREATMENT: No treatment required if ventricular rate is sufficient to sustain hemodynamic stability. In certain clinical conditions, such as acute MI, consider the risk of progression to a more serious form of heart block, and if hemodynamic compromise is present or deemed likely, a temporary transvenous pacemaker may be inserted.

Second-Degree Atrioventricular Block Type II (Figure 11-26)

This rhythm is also known as Mobitz II.
RATE: Atrial rate usually 60 to 100 beats/min. Ventricular rate slower and depends on number of conducted P waves.
RHYTHM: Regular if AV node consistently conducts every second or third P wave. Irregular if P waves conducted inconsistently.
P WAVE: Normal in shape. More P waves than QRS complexes.
PR INTERVAL: 0.12 to 0.20 second. Constant interval for P waves that conduct to ventricles. QRS DURATION: 0.06 to 0.10 second. Wider if BBB present.
QRS COMPLEX: May be narrow and normal or widened due to coexisting BBB.
ETIOLOGY: Usually indicates block below level of AV node, either in bundle of His or in both bundle branches. Mobitz II most frequently occurs when one bundle branch is blocked and other is ischemic. Mobitz II is more ominous clinically than Mobitz I block and often progresses to complete AV block.
PHYSIOLOGY: Occurs in presence of long absolute refractory period with virtually no relative refractory period, resulting in an "all or nothing" situation. Sinus P waves may be conducted. When conduction does occur, all PR intervals are the same.
TREATMENT: Mobitz II can be serious and often precedes complete AV block. Use of temporary transvenous pacemaker is usually necessary, but its insertion can be elective if patient remains hemodynamically stable.

Third-Degree Atrioventricular Block (Figure 11-27)

RATE: Depends on underlying rhythm.
RHYTHM: Usually regular.
P WAVE: Normal shape.
PR INTERVAL: P waves are not related to QRS complexes, so PR interval varies widely.
QRS DURATION: Greater than 0.10 second.
QRS COMPLEX: If junctional focus is pacing heart, complex is narrow but is not related to P waves. If ventricular focus is pacing heart, QRS is wide and unrelated to P waves.
ETIOLOGY: Degeneration of AV node caused by underlying heart disease, ischemia, or infarction. Blockage of AV node is a side effect of some antidysrhythmic drugs.
PHYSIOLOGY: In third-degree, or complete, AV block, no atrial impulses can conduct through AV node to cause ventricular depolarization. Opportunity for conduction is optimal but does not occur. Ideally a junctional or ventricular focus depolarizes spontaneously at its intrinsic rate of 20 to 60 beats/min, and ventricular contraction continues. If not, asystole occurs, the pulse stops, and death results if intervention is not immediate.

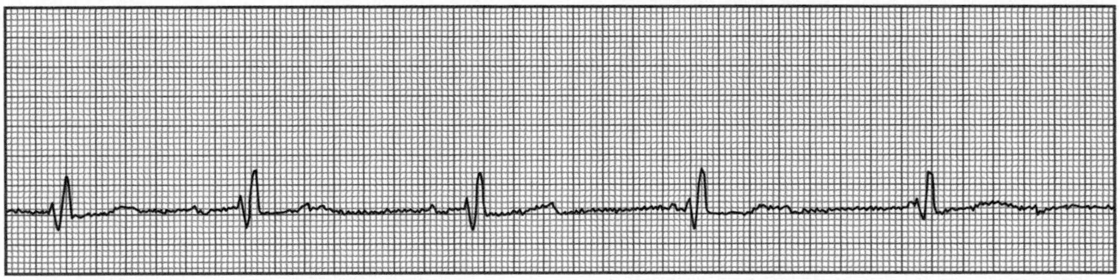

FIGURE 11-27. Third-degree (complete) heart block.

TREATMENT: Almost always requires a pacemaker. If patient is hemodynamically unstable, external pacemaker can be used to maintain an adequate ventricular rate until temporary transvenous pacemaker can be inserted.[52]

Nursing Management

Nursing priorities for the patient with bedside ECG monitoring focus on (1) positioning electrodes correctly to obtain specific lead views, (2) selecting the optimal monitoring lead based on the patient's clinical status, (3) documenting significant changes in the patient's heart rhythm, and (4) initiating emergency measures to treat dysrhythmias when required.

BEDSIDE HEMODYNAMIC MONITORING

Invasive hemodynamic monitoring is one of the major competencies required for the critical care nurse. Using invasive catheters and sophisticated monitors, the nurse evaluates a patient's cardiac function, circulating blood volume, and physiologic response to treatment. Knowledge of the theoretic base that underlies hemodynamic monitoring assists the clinician in developing decision-making skills to interpret and analyze trends and to formulate a nursing management plan appropriate for each individual patient. Research studies have shown that critical care nurses and physicians who frequently manage patients with invasive hemodynamic lines more accurately assess hemodynamic waveforms than clinicians who infrequently work in critical care.

Equipment

A hemodynamic monitoring system has four component parts as shown in Figure 11-28 and described in the following list:

1. An invasive catheter and high-pressure tubing connect the patient to the transducer.
2. The transducer receives the physiologic signal via the catheter and tubing and converts it into electrical energy.
3. The flush system maintains patency of the fluid-filled system and catheter.
4. The bedside monitor contains the amplifier/recorder, which increases the volume of the electrical signal and displays it on an oscilloscope and on a digital scale in millimeters of mercury (mm Hg).

Although many different types of invasive catheters can be inserted to monitor hemodynamic pressures, all such catheters are connected to similar equipment (see Figure 11-28). Even so, there remains considerable variation in the way different hospitals configure their hemodynamic systems. The basic setup consists of the following:

- A bag of 0.9% saline solution as a flush solution. In some hospitals the flush solution will contain 1 unit of heparin (range 0.25 to 2 units) per milliliter of solution; other hospitals do not use heparin in the flush solution because of concern over the development of heparin-induced thrombocytopenia (HIT).[54,55] A pressure infusion cuff covers the bag of flush solution and is inflated to 300 mm Hg.
- IV tubing; three-way stopcocks; and an in-line flow device attached for both continuous fluid infusion and manual flush. High-pressure tubing must be used to connect the invasive catheter to the transducer to prevent damping (flattening) of the waveform.
- A pressure transducer. Transducers are disposable, use a silicon chip, and are highly accurate.

The flush solutions and tubing are usually changed every 96 hours. Some hospitals change flush solutions every 24 hours. For this reason it is essential to be familiar with the specific written procedures that concern hemodynamic monitoring equipment in each critical care unit.

Calibrating Hemodynamic Monitoring Equipment

To ensure accuracy of hemodynamic pressure readings, two baseline measurements are necessary:

1. Calibration of the system to atmospheric pressure, also known as "zeroing" the transducer.
2. Determination of the phlebostatic axis for transducer height placement; this is also termed "leveling" the transducer.[56]

Zeroing the Transducer. To calibrate the equipment to atmospheric pressure, referred to as *zeroing the* *transducer,* the three-way stopcock nearest to the transducer is turned simultaneously to open the transducer to air (atmospheric pressure) and to close it to the patient and the flush system. The monitor is adjusted so that "0" is displayed, which equals atmospheric pressure. Atmospheric pressure is not actually "0"; it is 760 mm Hg at sea level. Using "0" to represent current atmospheric pressure provides a convenient baseline for hemodynamic measurement purposes. Some monitors also require calibration of the upper scale limit while the system remains open to air. At the end of the calibration procedure, the stopcock is returned to the closed position and a closed cap is placed over the open port. At this point the patient's waveform and hemodynamic pressures are displayed. Clinical protocols in most units require the nurse to calibrate the transducer at the beginning of each shift for quality assurance.

Leveling the Transducer. Leveling the transducer is different from zeroing. This process aligns the trans-

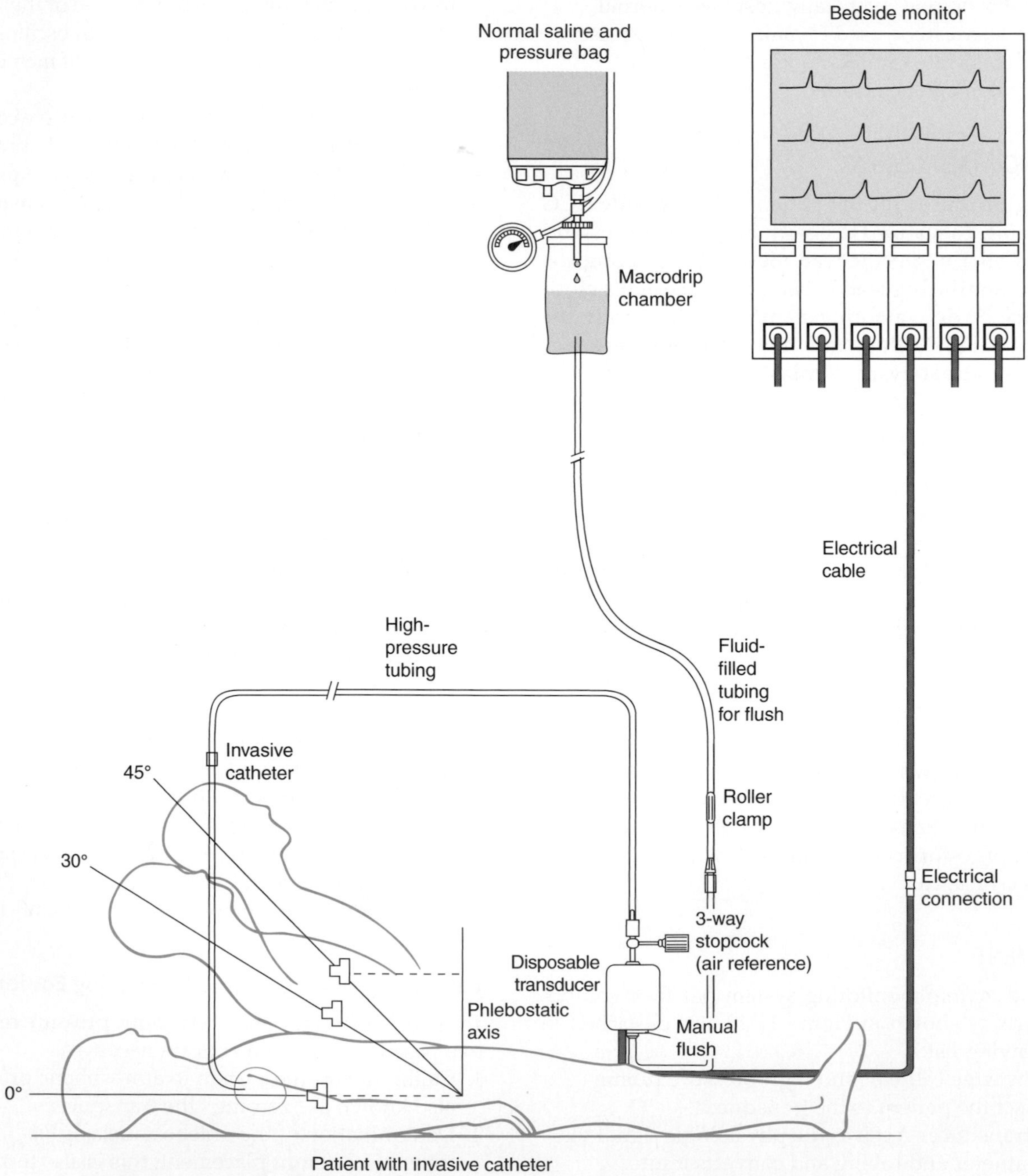

FIGURE 11-28. The four parts of a hemodynamic monitoring system include invasive catheter attached to high-pressure tubing to connect to the transducer; transducer; flush system, including a manual flush; and bedside monitor.

ducer with the level of the left atrium. The purpose is to line up the *air-fluid interface* with the left atrium to correct for changes in *hydrostatic pressure* in blood vessels above and below the level of the heart.[56] The *phlebostatic axis* is a physical reference point on the chest that is used as a baseline for consistent transducer height placement. To obtain the axis, a theoretic line is drawn from the fourth intercostal space (fourth ICP), where it joins the sternum, to a midaxillary line on the side of the chest. The midaxillary line is one half of the anterior-posterior depth of the lateral chest wall.[56] This point approximates the level of the atria, as shown in Figure 11-28. It is used as the reference mark for both central venous and pulmonary artery catheter transducers. The level of the transducer "air reference stopcock" approximates the position of the tip of a central hemodynamic monitoring catheter within the chest.

Recognizing Normal Hemodynamic Values

Once the system is correctly calibrated, the clinical team uses the known normal values as a reference when evaluating clinical patient outcomes and response to interventions (Table 11-8).

Table 11-8

Hemodynamic Pressures and Calculated Hemodynamic Values

HEMODYNAMIC PRESSURE	DEFINITION AND EXPLANATION	NORMAL RANGE
Mean arterial pressure (MAP)	Average perfusion pressure created by arterial blood pressure during the cardiac cycle. The normal cardiac cycle is one third systole and two thirds diastole. These three components are divided by 3 to obtain the average perfusion pressure for the whole cardiac cycle.	70-100 mm Hg
Central venous pressure (CVP)	Pressure created by volume in the right side of the heart. When the tricuspid valve is open, the CVP reflects filling pressures in the right ventricle. Clinically, the CVP is often used as a guide to overall fluid balance.	2-5 mm Hg 3-8 cm water (H_2O)
Left atrial pressure (LAP)	Pressure created by volume in the left side of the heart. When the mitral valve is open, the LAP reflects filling pressures in the left ventricle. Clinically, the LAP is used after cardiac surgery to determine how well the left ventricle is ejecting its volume. In general, the higher the LAP, the lower the ejection fraction from the left ventricle.	5-12 mm Hg
Pulmonary artery pressure (PAP) (systolic, diastolic, mean) PA systolic (PAS) PA diastolic (PAD) PAP mean (PAP_M)	Pulsatile pressure in the pulmonary artery, measured by an indwelling catheter.	PAS 20-30 mm Hg PAD 5-10 mm Hg PAP_M 10-15 mm Hg
Pulmonary artery occlusion pressure (PAOP) (PCW, PCWP, or PAWP)	Pressure created by volume in the left side of the heart. When the mitral valve is open, the PAOP reflects filling pressures in the pulmonary vasculature, and pressures in the left side of the heart are transmitted back to the catheter "wedged" into a small pulmonary arteriole.	5-12 mm Hg
Cardiac output (CO)	The amount of blood pumped out by a ventricle. Clinically, it can be measured using the thermodilution CO method, which calculates CO in liters per minute (L/min).	4-6 L/min (at rest)
Cardiac index (CI)	CO divided by body surface area (BSA), tailoring the CO to individual body size. A BSA conversion chart is necessary to calculate CI, which is considered more accurate than CO because it is individualized to height and weight. CI is measured in liters per minute per square meter BSA (L/min/m^2).	2.5-4.0 L/min/m^2
Stroke volume (SV)	Amount of blood ejected by the ventricle with each heartbeat. Hemodynamic monitoring systems calculate SV by dividing cardiac output (CO in L/min) by the heart rate (HR), then multiplying the answer by 1000 to change liters to milliliters (ml).	60-100 ml
Stroke volume index (SVI)	SV indexed to BSA.	33-47 ml/m^2/beat
Systemic vascular resistance (SVR)	Mean pressure difference across the systemic vascular bed, divided by blood flow. Clinically, SVR represents the resistance against which the left ventricle must pump to eject its volume. This resistance is created by the systemic arteries and arterioles. As SVR increases, CO falls. SVR is measured in either units or dynes/sec/cm^{-5}. If the number of units is multiplied by 80, the valve is converted to dynes/sec/cm^{-5}.	10-18 units or 800-1200 dynes/sec/cm^{-5}

Continued

Table 11-8

Hemodynamic Pressures and Calculated Hemodynamic Values—*cont'd*

HEMODYNAMIC PRESSURE	DEFINITION AND EXPLANATION	NORMAL RANGE
Systemic vascular resistance index (SVRI)	SVR indexed to BSA.	2000-2400 dynes/sec/cm^{-5}
Pulmonary vascular resistance (PVR)	Mean pressure difference across pulmonary vascular bed, divided by blood flow. Clinically, PVR represents the resistance against which the right ventricle must pump to eject its volume. This resistance is created by the pulmonary arteries and arterioles. As PVR increases, the output from the right ventricle decreases. PVR is measured in either units or dynes/sec/cm^{-5}. PVR is normally one sixth of SVR.	1.2-3.0 units or <250 dynes/sec/cm^{-5}
Pulmonary vascular resistance index (PVRI)	PVR indexed to BSA.	225-315 dynes/sec/cm^{-5}/m^2
Left cardiac work index (LCWI)	Amount of work the left ventricle does *each minute* when ejecting blood. The hemodynamic formula represents pressure generated (MAP) multiplied by volume pumped (CO). A conversion factor is used to change mm Hg to kilogram-meter (kg-m). LCWI is always represented as an indexed volume (BSA chart). LCWI increases or decreases because of changes in either pressure (MAP) or volume pumped (CO).	3.4-4.2 kg-m/m^2/beat
Left ventricular stroke work index (LVSWI)	Amount of work the left ventricle performs with *each heartbeat.* The hemodynamic formula represents pressure generated (MAP) multiplied by volume pumped (SV). A conversion factor is used to change ml/mm Hg to gram-meter (g-m). LVSWI is always represented as an indexed volume. LVSWI increases or decreases because of changes in either pressure (MAP) or volume pumped (SV).	50-62 g-m/m^2/beat
Right cardiac work index (RCWI)	Amount of work the right ventricle performs *each minute* when ejecting blood. The hemodynamic formula represents pressure generated (PAP mean) multiplied by volume pumped (CO). A conversion factor is used to change mm Hg to kilogram-meter (kg-m). RCWI is always represented as an indexed value (BSA chart). Similar to LCWI, the RCWI increases or decreases because of changes in either pressure (PAP mean) or volume pumped (CO).	0.54-0.66 kg-m/m^2
Right ventricular stroke work index (RVSWI)	Amount of work the right ventricle does *each heartbeat.* The hemodynamic formula represents pressure generated (PAP mean) multiplied by volume pumped (SV). A conversion factor is used to change mm Hg to gram-meter (g-m). RVSWI is always represented as an indexed value (BSA chart). Similar to LVSWI, the RVSWI increases or decreases because of changes in either pressure (PAP mean) or volume pumped (SV).	7.9-9.7 g-m/m^2/beat

Accommodating Changes in Patient Position

Patient position in the hemodynamically monitored patient would not be an issue if critical care patients always lay flat in the bed. However, lying flat is not always a comfortable position, especially if the patient is alert. Other considerations include elevation of the head of the bed to decrease the work of breathing and to prevent hospital- and ventilator-associated pneumonias.

Head of Bed Position. Nurse researchers have determined that the CVP, pulmonary artery pressure (PAP), and pulmonary artery occlusion pressure (PAOP) (also called *pulmonary artery wedge pressure* [PAWP]) can be reliably measured at head-of-bed positions from 0 (flat) to 60 degrees for most hemodynamically stable patients.[56,57]

Lateral Position. The landmarks for leveling the transducer are different if the patient is turned to the side. Researchers have evaluated hemodynamic pressure measurement readings with the patients in the 30- and 90-degree lateral positions with the head of the bed flat and found the measurements to be reliable.[56] In the 30-degree angle position, the landmark to use for leveling the transducer is half the distance from the surface of the bed to the left sternal border.[56] In the 90-degree right-lateral position the transducer fluid-air interface was positioned at the fourth ICS mid-sternum. In the 90-degree left-lateral position the transducer was positioned at the left parasternal border (beside the sternum).[56] It is important to know that measurements can be recorded in nonsupine positions, because critically ill patients must be turned to prevent development of pressure ulcers and other complications of immobility.

Establishing Safe Monitor Alarm Limits

All bedside hemodynamic monitoring systems have alarm limits that are preset to ensure patient safety. The alarms must be sufficiently distinctive and audible to be heard over the noise of a typical critical care unit. Patient safety guidelines are designed to promote clinical alarm goals. Some clinical situations create special challenges with respect to alarm safety. Nursing care actions that cause the patient to move in the bed will often trigger the alarms. Temporarily silencing the sound for 1 to 3 minutes while continuing to observe the bedside monitor is appropriate. The real challenge occurs when a patient is restless or fidgeting with IV tubing or electrodes, resulting in the alarms being constantly triggered because the monitor is unable to evaluate the ECG rhythms and hemodynamic waveforms effectively. It is tempting to "silence" these "nuisance alarms" permanently. The alarms should not be turned off because the patient is left in a vulnerable position if a dysrhythmia or hemodynamic complication arises. Clinical interventions to ameliorate the root cause of the problem (e.g., restlessness) are more appropriate. The key issues concerning monitor alarms are presented in Patient Safety Priorities: Clinical Alarm Systems.

Troubleshooting Hemodynamic Equipment Problems

Typical problems with bedside monitoring equipment are addressed in Table 11-9.

INTRAARTERIAL BLOOD PRESSURE MONITORING

Indications

Intraarterial blood pressure monitoring is indicated for any major medical or surgical condition that compromises CO, tissue perfusion, or fluid volume status. The system is designed for continuous measurement of three blood pressure parameters—systole, diastole, and mean arterial blood pressure (MAP). In addition, the direct arterial access is helpful in the management of patients with acute respiratory failure who require frequent arterial blood gas (ABG) measurements.

Catheters

The size of the catheter used is proportionate to the diameter of the cannulated artery. The catheter insertion is usually percutaneous, although the technique varies with vessel size. Catheters are most often inserted in the smaller arteries, using a "catheter-over-needle" unit in which the needle is used as a temporary guide for catheter placement. With this method, once the unit has been inserted into the artery, the needle is withdrawn, leaving the supple plastic catheter in place.

Insertion of a catheter into a larger artery usually necessitates the following procedure:
1. Entry into the artery using a needle
2. Passage of a supple guidewire through the needle into the artery
3. Removal of the needle
4. Passage of the catheter over the guidewire
5. Removal of the guidewire, leaving the catheter in the artery

---

PATIENT SAFETY PRIORITIES

Clinical Alarm Systems

Clinical Alarm System Effectiveness
1. Implement regular preventive maintenance and testing of alarm systems.
2. Ensure that alarms are activated with appropriate settings and are sufficiently audible with respect to distances and competing noise within the unit.

Clinical Alarm Safety

Alarm Identification
1. Audible and visual indication should be present for any condition that poses a risk to the patient. Indicator should be visible from at least 10 feet (3 meters).
2. Cause of the alarm must be easily identifiable by health care practitioner.
3. Life-threatening conditions should be clearly differentiated from noncritical alarm situations.
4. High-priority alarms should override low-priority alarms.
5. Alarm must be sufficiently loud or distinctive to be heard over environmental noise of a busy critical care unit.
6. It should never be possible to turn the volume control to "off."

Disabling and Silencing Alarms
1. Alarm silence must have visual indicator to clearly show it is disabled.
2. Critical alarms should not be permanently overridden (turned "off").
3. New, life-threatening alarm conditions should override a silenced alarm.

Power

Battery units should initiate an alarm before a unit stops working effectively.

Alarm Limits
1. Alarm limits can be adjusted to meet clinical needs of patients. The system should default to standard settings between patients.
2. Alarm limits should preferably be displayed on the monitor.

Data from www.jointcomission.org; and Critical alarms and patient safety: ECRI's guide to developing effective alarm strategies and responding to JCAHO's alarm-safety goal, *Health Devices* 31(11):397, 2002.

Table 11-9

Nursing Measures to Ensure Patient Safety and to Troubleshoot Problems With Hemodynamic Monitoring Equipment

PROBLEM	PREVENTION	RATIONALE	TROUBLESHOOTING
Overdamping of waveform	Provide continuous infusion of solution containing heparin through an in-line flush device (1 unit of heparin for each milliliter of flush solution).	To ensure that recorded pressures and waveform are accurate because a damped waveform gives inaccurate readings.	Before insertion, completely flush the line and/or catheter. In a line attached to a patient, back flush through the system to clear bubbles from tubing or transducer.
Underdamping ("overshoot" or "fling")	Use short lengths of noncompliant tubing. Use "fast-flush square waveform" test to demonstrate optimal system damping. Verify arterial waveform accuracy with the cuff blood pressure.	If the monitoring system is underdamped, both the systolic and diastolic values will be overestimated by both the waveform and the digital values. False high systolic values may lead to clinical decisions based on erroneous data.	Perform the "fast-flush square waveform" test to verify optimal function of the monitoring system.
Clot formation at end of catheter	Provide continuous infusion of solution containing heparin through an in-line flush device (1 unit of heparin for each milliliter of flush solution).	Any foreign object placed in the body can cause local activation of the patient's coagulation system as a normal defense mechanism. The clots that are formed may be dangerous if they break off and travel to other parts of the body.	If a clot in the catheter is suspected because of a damped waveform or resistance to forward flush of the system, gently aspirate the line using a small syringe inserted into the proximal stopcock. Then flush the line again once the clot is removed and inspect the waveform. It should return to a normal pattern.
Hemorrhage	Use Luer-Lok (screw) connections in line setup. Close and cap stopcocks when not in use. Ensure that the catheter is either sutured or securely taped in position.	A loose connection or open stopcock creates a low-pressure sump effect, causing blood to back into the line and into the open air. If a catheter is accidentally removed, the vessel can bleed profusely, especially with an arterial line or if the patient has abnormal coagulation factors (resulting from heparin in the line) or has hypertension.	Once a blood leak is recognized, tighten all connections, flush the line, and estimate blood loss. If the catheter has been inadvertently removed, put pressure on the cannulation site. When bleeding has stopped, apply a sterile dressing, estimate blood loss, and inform the physician. If the patient is restless, an armboard may protect lines inserted in the arm.
Air emboli	Ensure that all air bubbles are purged from a new line setup before attachment to an indwelling catheter. Ensure that the drip chamber from the bag of flush solution is more than half full before using the in-line, fast-flush system. Some sources recommend removing all air from the bag of flush solution before assembling the system.	Air can be introduced at several times; including when central venous pressure (CVP) tubing comes apart, when a new line setup is attached, or when a new CVP or pulmonary artery (PA) line is inserted. During insertion of a CVP or PA line, the patient may be asked to hold his or her breath at specific times to prevent drawing air into the chest during inhalation. The in-line, fast-flush devices are designed to permit clearing of blood from the line after withdrawal of blood samples.	Because it is impossible to get the air back once it has been introduced into the blood stream, prevention is the best cure. If any air bubbles are noted, they must be vented through the in-line stopcocks and the drip chamber must be filled. The left atrial pressure (LAP) line setup is the only system that includes an air filter specifically to prevent air emboli.

Table 11-9

Nursing Measures to Ensure Patient Safety and to Troubleshoot Problems With Hemodynamic Monitoring Equipment—*cont'd*

PROBLEM	PREVENTION	RATIONALE	TROUBLESHOOTING
		If the chamber of the IV tubing is too low or empty, the rapid flow of fluid will create turbulence and cause flushing of air bubbles into the system and into the bloodstream.	
Normal waveform with *low* digital pressure	Ensure that the system is calibrated to atmospheric pressure. Ensure that the transducer is placed at the level of the phlebostatic axis.	To provide a 0 baseline relative to atmospheric pressure. If the transducer has been placed *higher* than the phlebostatic level, gravity and the lack of hydrostatic pressure will produce a false *low* reading.	Recalibrate the equipment if transducer drift has occurred. Reposition the transducer at the level of the phlebostatic axis. Misplacement can occur if the patient moves from the bed to the chair or if the bed is placed in a Trendelenburg position.
Normal waveform with *high* digital pressure	Ensure that the system is calibrated to atmospheric pressure. Ensure that the transducer is placed at the level of the phlebostatic axis.	To provide a 0 baseline relative to atmospheric pressure. If the transducer has been placed *lower* than the phlebostatic level, the weight of hydrostatic pressure on the transducer will produce a false *high* reading.	Recalibrate the equipment if transducer drift has occurred. Reposition the transducer at the level of the phlebostatic axis. This situation can occur if the head of the bed was raised and the transducer was not repositioned. Some centers require attachment of the transducer to the patient's chest to avoid this problem.
Loss of waveform	Always have the hemodynamic waveform monitored so that changes or loss can be quickly noted.	The catheter may be kinked, or a stopcock may be turned off.	Check the line setup to ensure that all stopcocks are turned in the correct position and that the tubing is not kinked. Sometimes the catheter migrates against a vessel wall, and having the patient change position restores the waveform.

Insertion. Several major peripheral arteries are suitable for receiving a catheter and for long-term hemodynamic monitoring. The most frequently used site is the radial artery. If this artery is not available, the femoral, dorsalis-pedis, axillary, or brachial arteries may be used.

Allen Test. The major advantage of the radial artery is the supply of collateral circulation to the hand provided by the ulnar artery via the palmar arch in most of the population; thus other avenues of circulation are available if the radial artery becomes blocked after catheter placement. Before radial artery cannulation, collateral circulation is assessed, either by using Doppler flow or by the Allen test. In the Allen test the radial and ulnar arteries are compressed simultaneously. The patient is asked to clench and unclench the hand until it blanches. Pressure is released from one of the arteries and the hand should immediately flush from that side. The same procedure is repeated for the remaining artery.[7]

Nursing Management

Nursing priorities for the patient with intraarterial monitoring focus on (1) assessing arterial perfusion pressures, (2) interpreting the accuracy of the arterial pressure waveform, and (3) troubleshooting hemodynamic monitoring system problems.

Intraarterial blood pressure monitoring is designed for continuous assessment of arterial perfusion to the major organ systems of the body. MAP is the clinical parameter most often used to assess perfusion, because MAP represents perfusion pressure throughout the cardiac cycle. Because one third of the cardiac cycle is spent in systole and two thirds in diastole, the MAP calculation must reflect the greater amount of time spent in diastole. The MAP formula when calculated by hand is:

$$(\text{Diastolic value} \times 2) + (\text{Systolic value} \times 1) \div 3 = \text{MAP}$$

Thus a blood pressure of 120/60 mm Hg produces a MAP of 80 mm Hg. However, the bedside hemodynamic

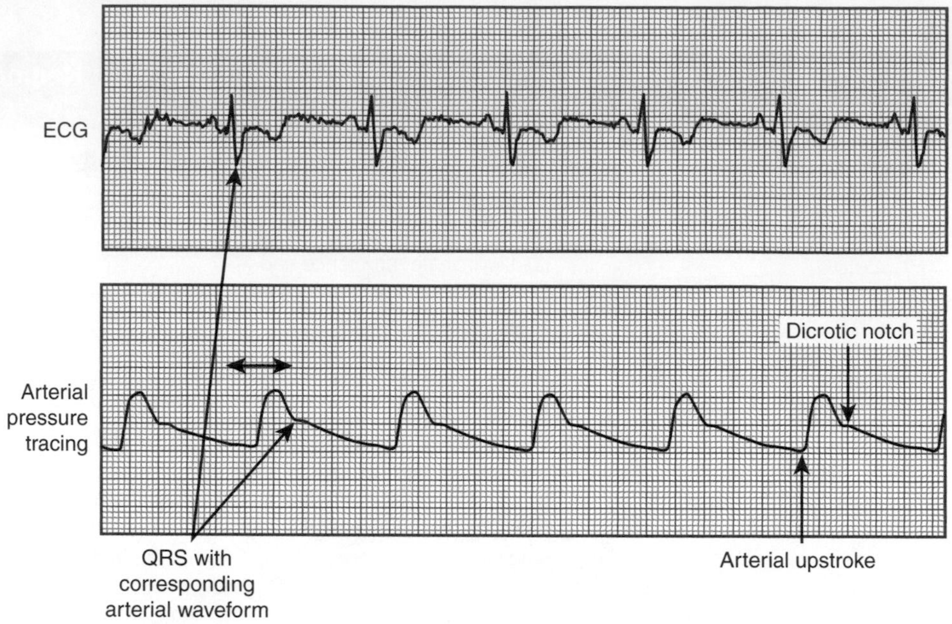

FIGURE 11-29. Simultaneous ECG and normal arterial pressure tracing.

monitor may show a slightly different digital number because most computers calculate the area under the curve of the arterial line tracing.

Assessing Arterial Perfusion Pressures. A MAP greater than 60 mm Hg is necessary to perfuse the coronary arteries. A minimum MAP of 65 mm Hg is suggested as a goal when treating a patient for sepsis. After a carotid endarterectomy or neurosurgery, a MAP of 90 to 110 mm Hg may be more appropriate to increase cerebral perfusion pressure. Systolic and diastolic pressures are monitored in conjunction with the MAP as a further guide to the accuracy of perfusion. Should cardiac output decrease, the body compensates by constricting peripheral vessels to maintain the blood pressure. In this situation the MAP may remain constant but the pulse pressure (difference between systolic and diastolic pressures) narrows. The following examples explain this point:

Mr. A: BP, 90/70 mm Hg; MAP, 76 mm Hg
Mr. B: BP, 150/40 mm Hg; MAP, 76 mm Hg

Both of these patients have a perfusion pressure of 76 mm Hg, but clinically they are very different. Mr. A is peripherally vasoconstricted, as is demonstrated by the narrow pulse pressure (90/70 mm Hg). His skin is cool to touch, and he has weak peripheral pulses. Mr. B has a wide pulse pressure (150/40 mm Hg), warm skin, and normally palpable peripheral pulses. Thus nursing assessment of the patient with an arterial line includes comparison of clinical findings with arterial line readings, including perfusion pressure and MAP.

Interpreting Arterial Pressure Waveforms. As the aortic valve opens, blood is ejected from the left ventricle and is recorded as an increase of pressure in the arterial system. The highest point recorded is called *systole.* After peak ejection (systole), force is decreased and pressure drops. A notch (the dicrotic notch) may be visible on the downstroke of this arterial waveform, representing closure of the aortic valve. The *dicrotic notch* signifies the beginning of diastole. The remainder of the downstroke represents diastolic runoff of blood flow into the arterial tree. The lowest point recorded is called *diastole.* A normal arterial pressure tracing is described in Figure 11-29. Note that electrical stimulation (QRS) is always first and that the arterial pressure tracing follows the initiating QRS. If the arterial line becomes unreliable or dislodged, a cuff pressure can be used as a reserve system. In the normovolemic patient, little difference exists between the cuff blood pressure and arterial pressure. When the arterial catheter is functioning accurately, it is considered the gold standard.[58]

Troubleshooting Monitoring System Problems. Major complications associated with arterial pressure monitoring are rare. The most life-threatening risk is exsanguination if the Luer-Lok connections are not tight or if an in-line stopcock is inadvertently opened to air. Pressure monitor alarms must always be "on" with alarm limits (high and low) set at a safe, audible warning range for each patient. When the arterial monitor displays a low blood pressure digital reading, it is a nursing responsibility to determine whether this is a true patient problem or a problem with the monitoring equipment. A *damped waveform* occurs when communication from the artery to the transducer is interrupted and produces false values on the monitor and oscilloscope. Troubleshooting techniques are used to find the origin of the problem and to remove the cause of damping (see Table 11-9).

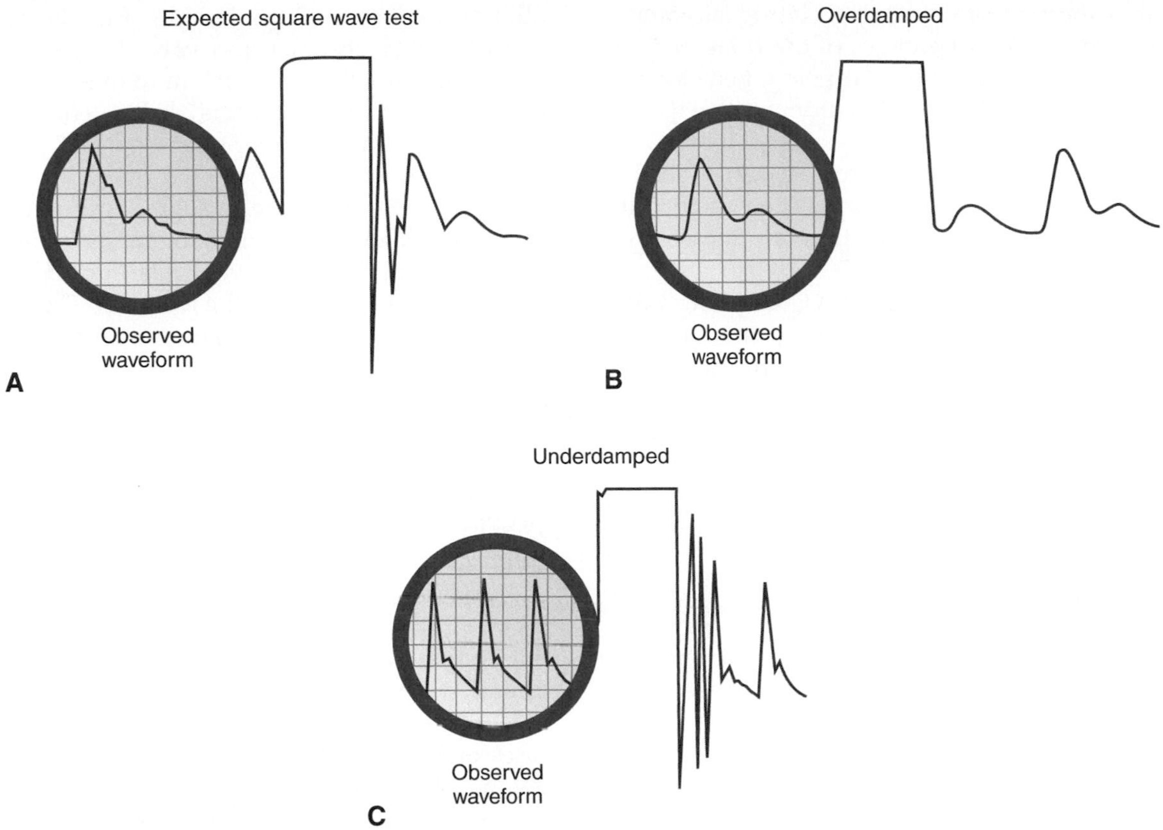

FIGURE 11-30. Square waveform test. **A,** Expected square wave test. **B,** Overdamped. **C,** Underdamped. (From Darovic GO: *Hemodynamic monitoring: invasive and noninvasive clinical application*, ed 3, Philadelphia, 2002, Saunders.)

Fast-Flush Square Waveform Test. The monitoring system can be verified for accuracy at the bedside by the *fast-flush square waveform,* or *dynamic frequency response,* test.[56] The test makes use of the manual flush system on the transducer. Normally the flush device allows only 3 ml of fluid per hour. With the normal waveform displayed, the manual fast-flush is used to generate a rapid increase in pressure, which is displayed on the monitor oscilloscope. If air bubbles, clots, or kinks are in the system, the waveform becomes damped, or flattened, and this will be reflected in the square waveform result as shown in Figure 11-30. This test can be performed with any hemodynamic monitoring system, is easy to do, and should be incorporated into nursing care procedures at the bedside when the hemodynamic system is first set up, at least once a shift, after opening the system for any reason, and whenever there is concern over the accuracy of the waveform.[56] If the pressure waveform is distorted or the digital display is inaccurate, the troubleshooting methods described in Table 11-9 can be implemented.

Central Venous Pressure Monitoring

Indications

CVP monitoring is indicated whenever a patient has significant alteration in fluid volume. The CVP can be used as a guide in fluid volume replacement in hypovolemia and to assess the impact of diuresis after diuretic administration in the case of fluid overload. In addition, when a major IV line is required for volume replacement, a central venous catheter (CVC) is a good choice because large volumes of fluid can easily be delivered.

Central Venous Catheters

A range of CVC options are available as single-, double-, or triple-lumen infusion catheters, depending on the specific needs of the patient. Central venous catheters are made from a variety of materials ranging from polyurethane to silicone; most are soft and flexible.

Insertion. The large veins of the upper thorax—subclavian (SC) and internal jugular (IJ)—are most commonly used for percutaneous CVC line insertion. The femoral vein in the groin is used when the thoracic veins are not accessible. All three major sites have advantages and disadvantages.

Internal Jugular Vein. The IJ is the most frequently used access site for CVC insertion. Compared to the other thoracic veins, it is the easiest to canalize. If the IJ is not available, the external jugular (EJ) may be accessed, although blood flow is significantly higher in the IJ, making it the preferred site. Another advantage of the IJ is that the risk of creating an iatrogenic pneumothorax is small. Disadvantages of the IJ are patient discomfort from the indwelling catheter when moving the head or neck and contamination of the IJ site from oral or tracheal secretions, especially if the patient is intubated or has a tracheostomy. This may be the reason why catheter-related infections are higher in the IJ compared to the SC position for indwelling catheters left in place over 4 days.[59]

Subclavian Vein. If the anticipated CVC dwelling time is prolonged over 5 days, the SC site is preferred. The SC position has the lowest infection rate and produces the least patient discomfort from the catheter. The disadvantages are that the SC vein is more difficult to access and carries a higher risk of iatrogenic pneumothorax or hemothorax, although the risk varies greatly, depending on the experience and skill of the physician inserting the catheter.

Femoral Vein. The femoral vein is considered the easiest cannulation site because there are no curves in the insertion route. The large diameter of the femoral vein carries a high blood flow that is advantageous for specialized procedures such as continuous renal replacement therapy (CRRT) or plasmapheresis. Disadvantages are that the patient cannot bend at the hip, because this interrupts blood flow through the catheter and may lead to thrombus formation; risk of retroperitoneal bleed; and a higher rate of nosocomial infections, probably due to site location near the groin area.[59]

During insertion of the SC or IJ veins, the patient may be placed in a Trendelenburg position. Placing the head in a dependent position causes the IJ veins in the neck to become more prominent, facilitating line placement. To minimize the risk of air embolus during the procedure, the patient may be asked to "take a deep breath and hold it" any time the needle or catheter is open to air. The tip of the catheter is designed to remain in the vena cava and should not migrate into the right atrium.

Because many patients are awake and alert when a CVC is inserted, a brief explanation about the procedure will minimize patient anxiety and result in cooperation during the insertion. This cooperation is important, because CVC insertion is a sterile procedure and because the supine or Trendelenburg position may not be comfortable for many patients.

Nursing Management

Nursing priorities for the patient with CVP monitoring focus on (1) assessing fluid volume status, (2) accommodating changes in patient position, (3) preventing catheter-related complications, and (4) accurately interpreting the CVP waveform and digital pressures.

Assessing Fluid Volume Status. In the critically ill patient the CVC is also used to monitor CVP and waveform. The CVP catheter is used to measure the filling pressures of the right side of the heart. During diastole, when the tricuspid valve is open and blood is flowing from the right atrium to the right ventricle, the CVP accurately reflects right ventricular end-diastolic pressure (RVEDP). The normal CVP is 2 to 5 mm Hg (3 to 8 cm H_2O).

Low Central Venous Pressure. A low CVP often occurs in the hypovolemic patient and suggests that insufficient blood volume is in the ventricle at end-diastole to produce an adequate stroke volume. Thus to maintain normal CO, the heart rate must increase. This increase produces the tachycardia often observed in hypovolemic states and increases myocardial oxygen demand.

The CVP is used in combination with the MAP and other clinical parameters to assess hemodynamic stability. In the hypovolemic patient, the CVP falls before a significant fall in MAP occurs, because peripheral vasoconstriction keeps the MAP normal. Thus the CVP is an excellent early-warning system for the patient who is bleeding, vasodilating, receiving diuretics, or being rewarmed after cardiac surgery.

High Central Venous Pressure. An elevated CVP occurs in cases of fluid overload. To circulate the excess blood volume, the heart must greatly increase its contractile force to move the large volume of blood. This increases the cardiac workload and increases myocardial oxygen consumption. The critical care nurse follows the trend of the CVP measurements to determine subsequent interventions for optimal fluid volume management.

Central Venous Pressure Limitations. The CVP is not a reliable indicator of left ventricular dysfunction. Left ventricular dysfunction, which can occur after an acute MI, increases filling pressures on the left side of the heart. The CVP, because it measures RVEDP, remains normal until the increase in pressure from the left side of the heart is reflected back through the pulmonary vasculature to the right ventricle.

Accommodating Changes in Patient Position. To achieve accurate CVP measurements, the phlebostatic axis is used as a reference point on the body, and the transducer must be level with this point. If the phlebostatic axis is used and the transducer is correctly aligned, any head-of-bed position of up to 60 degrees may be accurately used for CVP readings for most patients.[56] Elevating the head of the bed is especially helpful for the patient with respiratory or cardiac problems who will not tolerate a flat position.

Preventing Catheter-Related Complications. The CVC is an essential tool in care of the critically ill patient, but it is associated with some risks, and for this reason it is the responsibility of all clinicians to be informed of these hazards and to follow hospital procedures to avoid iatrogenic complications. The most frequent CVC complications are air embolus, catheter-associated thrombus formation, and infection.

Air Embolus. The risk of air embolus, although uncommon, is always present for the patient with a central venous line in place. Air can enter during insertion through a disconnected or broken catheter, or air can enter along the path of a removed CVC. This is more likely if the patient is in an upright position, because air can be pulled into the venous system with the increase in negative intrathoracic pressure during inhalation.[60] If a large volume of air is infused rapidly, it may become trapped in the right ventricular outflow tract, stopping blood flow from the right side of the heart to the lungs. If the air embolus is large, the patient will experience respiratory distress and cardiovascular collapse. Two clinical signs are specifically associated with a large venous air embolism: "mill wheel murmur" and "gasp reflex."[61] A mill wheel murmur is a loud, churning sound heard over the middle chest, caused by the obstruction to right ventricular outflow. The gasp reflex is the automatic gasp for air that occurs during hypoxemia. Treatment involves administering 100% oxygen and placing the patient on the left side with the head downward (left lateral Trendelenburg position). This position displaces the air from the right ventricular outflow tract to the apex of the heart, where it can be either resorbed or aspirated. Precautions to prevent an air embolism in a CVP line include using only screw (Luer-Lok) connections, avoiding long loops of IV tubing, and using screw caps on the three-way stopcock.

Thrombus Formation. Clot formation (thrombus) at the CVC site is unfortunately not uncommon. Ultrasound studies have found asymptomatic thrombus formation to be in the range of 33% to 67% when the catheter is in place for over 7 days.[59] Symptomatic thrombi are reported in 0% to 5% of those cases.[59,61] Thrombus formation is not uniform; it may involve development of a *fibrin sleeve* around the catheter, or the thrombus may be attached directly to the vessel wall. Other factors that promote clot formation include rupture of vascular endothelium, interruption of laminar blood flow, and physical presence of the catheter, all of which activate the coagulation cascade. The risk of thrombus formation is higher if insertion was difficult or there were multiple needlesticks.[59] Gradual thrombus formation may lead to "sudden" CVC occlusion. Usually the CVC becomes more difficult to withdraw blood from, or the CVP waveform becomes intermittently damped over a period of hours or even 1 to 2 days and is reported as needing "frequent flushes" to remain patent. This situation is caused by the continued lengthening of a "fibrin sleeve" that extends along the catheter length from the insertion site past the catheter tip.[59,61] Some catheters are heparin-coated to reduce the risk of thrombus formation, although the risk of HIT, reported to be 0.4% with indwelling CVC, does not make this a benign option.[61] Sometimes CVC complications are additive; for example the risk of catheter-related infection is increased in the presence of thrombi. The thrombus likely serves as a culture medium for bacterial growth.[61]

Infection. Infection related to the use of central venous catheters is a major problem. Risk factors for catheter-related infections include extremes of age, impaired host defense mechanisms, severe illness, malnutrition, and presence of other invasive lines. It is estimated that more than 50,000 infections related to CVC use occur annually in the United States, with associated mortality between 10% and 20%.[61]

The incidence of infection is strongly correlated with the length of time the CVC has been left inserted. Catheters that are in place under 3 days almost never lead to infection, providing standard insertion and management procedures are followed. If the CVC remains between 3 and 7 days, the infection rate is 3% to 5%. Catheters remaining in one site over 7 days have an infection rate of 5% to 10%.[61]

CVC-related infection is noted either at the catheter insertion site or as a bloodstream infection (septicemia). Systemic manifestations of infection can be present without inflammation at the catheter site. To determine whether a suspect catheter is contaminated, after removal, the tip is placed in a sterile container and cultured. No decrease in infections was found when catheters were routinely changed to prevent infectious, and this practice is not recommended.[62] A "suspect" CVC changed over guidewire risks a higher rate of infection.[62] Prevention is the best defense against complications resulting from infections. Most infections are transmitted via the skin. Therefore current insertion recommendations state that the physician should use good hand-washing procedures, clean the insertion site with 2% chlorhexidine, utilize sterile technique during catheter insertion, and maintain maximal sterile barrier precautions (see Patient Safety Priorities: Guidelines for Prevention and Management of Central Venous Catheter Infections).[62-65]

To prevent infection all clinicians must use good hand-washing technique and follow aseptic procedures during site care and any time the CVC system is entered to withdraw blood, give medications, or change tubing.[62,65] The infusion of high-dextrose solutions such as TPN may be associated with an increased risk of infection. Methods to lower TPN-related complications include use of a single-lumen CVC that is not accessed for other medications or laboratory samples.[66]

Incidence of infection is higher with use of occlusive dressings that do not allow removal of moisture. Therefore transparent, breathable dressings that allow removal of skin moisture are recommended. Site dressings that have antimicrobial properties are being used to try to lower infection rates. New developments in catheter design may also help to reduce central line infection. Catheters are available that are

PATIENT SAFETY PRIORITIES

Guidelines for Prevention and Management of Central Venous Catheter Infections

1. Use effective hand washing.
2. Educate and train health care providers who insert and maintain central venous catheters (CVCs).
3. Use maximal sterile barrier precautions during CVC insertion.
4. Use 2% chlorhexidine preparation for skin antisepsis.
5. Avoid routine replacement of CVCs as a strategy to prevent infection.
6. Insert antiseptic/antibiotic-impregnated short-term CVCs if rate of infection is high despite adherence to other strategies (education/training, maximal sterile barrier precautions, 2% chlorhexidine).
7. Confirm clinical suspicion of infection by taking cultures of blood and catheter samples.
8. Initially treat intravascular catheter infection with IV antimicrobial therapy, considering severity of patient's acute illness, underlying disease, and potential pathogens. Once the catheter-related pathogen is documented, narrow focus of antimicrobial therapy to treat specific organism(s).
9. Remove CVC if infected.

Data from O'Grady NP et al: *Am J Infect Control* 30:476, 2002; and Boyce JM, Pittet D: *Am J Infect Control* 30(8):S1, 2002.

impregnated with an antimicrobial substance or have a silver-impregnated, tissue-barrier cuff attached to the catheter.[62] These catheters are designed to lower the rate of CVC infection.

Interpreting the CVP Waveform. The normal right atrial (CVP) waveform has three positive deflections—called *a, c,* and *v waves*—that correspond to specific atrial events in the cardiac cycle (Figure 11-31). The *a wave* reflects atrial contraction and follows the P wave seen on the ECG. The downslope of this wave is called the *x descent* and represents atrial relaxation. The *c wave* reflects the bulging of the closed tricuspid valve into the right atrium during ventricular contraction; this wave is small and not always visible, but corresponds to the QRS-T interval on the ECG. The *v wave* represents atrial filling and increased pressure against the closed tricuspid valve in early diastole. The downslope of the v wave is named the *y descent* and represents the fall in pressure as the tricuspid valve opens and blood flows from the right atrium to the right ventricle.

Specialized Catheters. A CVC that incorporates a fiberoptic sensor to measure systemic venous oxygen saturation ($Scvo_2$) can be used as a traditional CVC and also used to follow the trend of venous oxygen saturation.[67] The physiology underlying use of this fiberoptic technology is discussed later in the chapter, in the section on $Scvo_2$ monitoring.

Pulmonary Artery Pressure Monitoring

The pulmonary artery (PA) catheter is the most invasive of the critical care monitoring catheters. It is also known as a *right heart catheter,* or a *Swan-Ganz catheter* (named after the catheter inventors). Routine use of PA catheters has frequently been called into question and is considered controversial.[68] Recent research trials reported no benefit to use of the PA catheter to guide treatment of critically ill patients compared with less-invasive diagnostic methods.[69,70] Other researchers report no additional mortality or morbidity reduction from use of a PA catheter but do report an increase in complications and adverse events.[71,72] The most important clinical advice is not to insert the PA catheter as a routine measure in every patient, but to determine whether the individual's clinical condition and evidence of an effective management strategy warrants this level of monitoring.[68] Approximately 1.5 million PA catheters are used in the United States annually[73]; 30% are used in cardiac surgery units, 30% in cardiac catheterization laboratories and coronary care units, 25% in high-risk surgery and trauma, and 15% in medical intensive care units.[73]

Indications

Traditionally the PA catheter has been used for diagnosis and evaluation of conditions that compromise cardiac or fluid volume status. The PA catheter can simultaneously facilitate assessment of several hemodynamic parameters. These parameters include pulmonary artery systolic and diastolic pressures, pulmonary artery mean pressure, and PAOP. Use of the PA catheter also makes it possible to measure CO and to calculate additional hemodynamic parameters. Currently clinicians are challenged to accurately identify which patients will really benefit from use of a PA catheter.[74]

Pulmonary Artery Catheters

The traditional PA catheter, invented by Swan and Ganz, has four lumens for measurement of right atrial pressure (RAP) or CVP, PA pressures, PAOP (wedge), and cardiac output (Figure 11-32, *A*). Multifunction catheters may have additional lumens, which can be used for IV infusion (Figure 11-32, *B*) and to measure continuous mixed venous oxygen saturation (Svo_2), right ventricular volume, and continuous cardiac output (Figure 11-32, *C*). Other PA catheters include transvenous pacing electrodes to pace the heart if needed.

The PA catheter is 110 cm in length with an indicator marked every 10 cm along the length of the

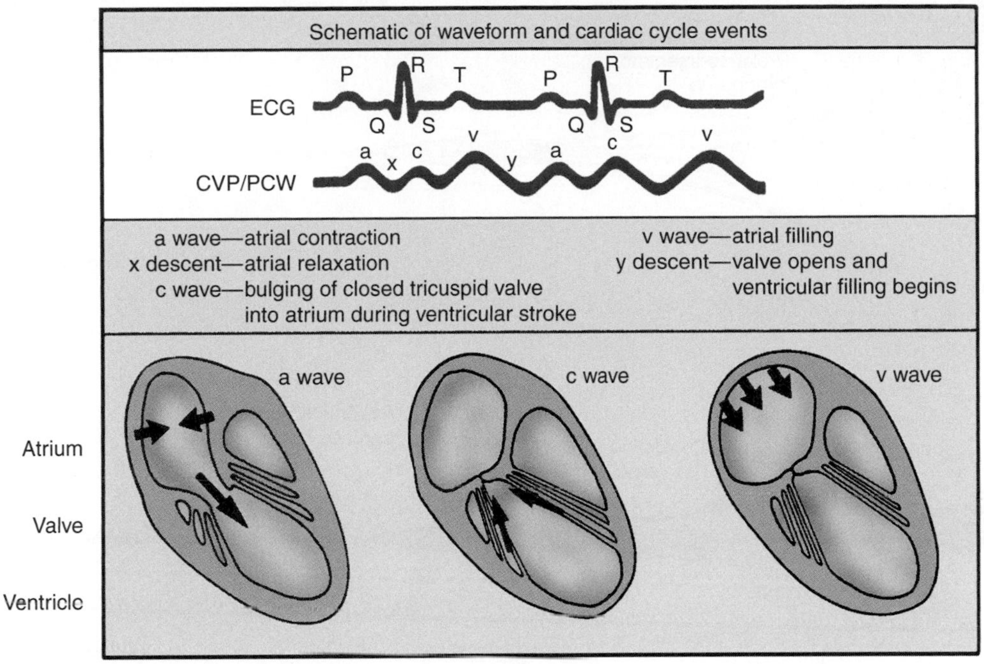

FIGURE 11-31. Cardiac events that produce the CVP waveform with a, c, and v waves. The *a wave* represents atrial contraction. The *x descent* represents atrial relaxation. The *c wave* represents the bulging of the closed tricuspid valve into the right atrium during ventricular systole. The *v wave* represents atrial filling. The *y descent* represents opening of the tricuspid valve and filling of the ventricle.

catheter. The most commonly used size is 7.5 or 8.0 French (Fr), although 5.0 and 7.0 Fr sizes are also available. Each of the four lumens exits into the heart or pulmonary artery at a different point, graduated along the catheter length (see Figure 11-32, *A*).

Right Atrial Lumen. The proximal lumen is situated in the right atrium and is used for IV infusion, CVP measurement, withdrawal of venous blood samples, and injection of fluid for CO determinations. This port is often described as the *right atrial port,* also called the *CVP port.*

Pulmonary Artery Lumen. The distal PA lumen is located at the tip of the PA catheter and is situated in the pulmonary artery. It is used to record PA pressures and can be used for withdrawal of blood samples to measure SvO_2.

Balloon Lumen. The third lumen opens into a balloon at the end of the catheter that can be inflated with 0.8 (7 Fr) to 1.5 (7.5 Fr) ml of air. The balloon is inflated during catheter insertion once the catheter reaches the right atrium to assist in forward flow of the catheter and to minimize right ventricular ectopy from the catheter tip. It is also inflated to obtain the PAOP, or "wedge," measurements when the PA catheter is correctly positioned in the pulmonary artery.

Thermistor Lumen. The fourth lumen is a thermistor (temperature sensor) used to measure changes in blood temperature. It is located 4 cm from the catheter tip and is used to measure thermodilution CO. The connector end of the lumen is attached directly to the CO computer.

Additional Features. If continuous SvO_2 is measured, the catheter has an additional fiberoptic lumen that exits at the tip of the catheter (see Figure 11-32, *C*). If cardiac pacing is used, two PA catheter methods are available. One type of catheter has three atrial (A) and two ventricular (V) pacing electrodes attached to the catheter so that when it is properly positioned, the patient can be connected to a pacemaker and be AV-paced. The other catheter method uses a specific transvenous pacing wire that is passed through an additional catheter lumen and exits into the right ventricle if ventricular pacing is required. In addition, a right ventricular volumetric PA catheter is available that measures stroke volume in the RV.

Insertion

If a PA catheter is to be inserted into a patient who is awake, some brief explanations about the procedure are helpful to ensure that the patient understands what is going to happen. The initial insertion techniques used for placement of a PA catheter are similar to those described in the section on CVC insertion. In addition, because the PA catheter is positioned within the heart chambers and pulmonary artery on the right side of the heart, catheter passage is monitored using either fluoroscopy or waveform analysis on the bedside monitor (Figure 11-33).

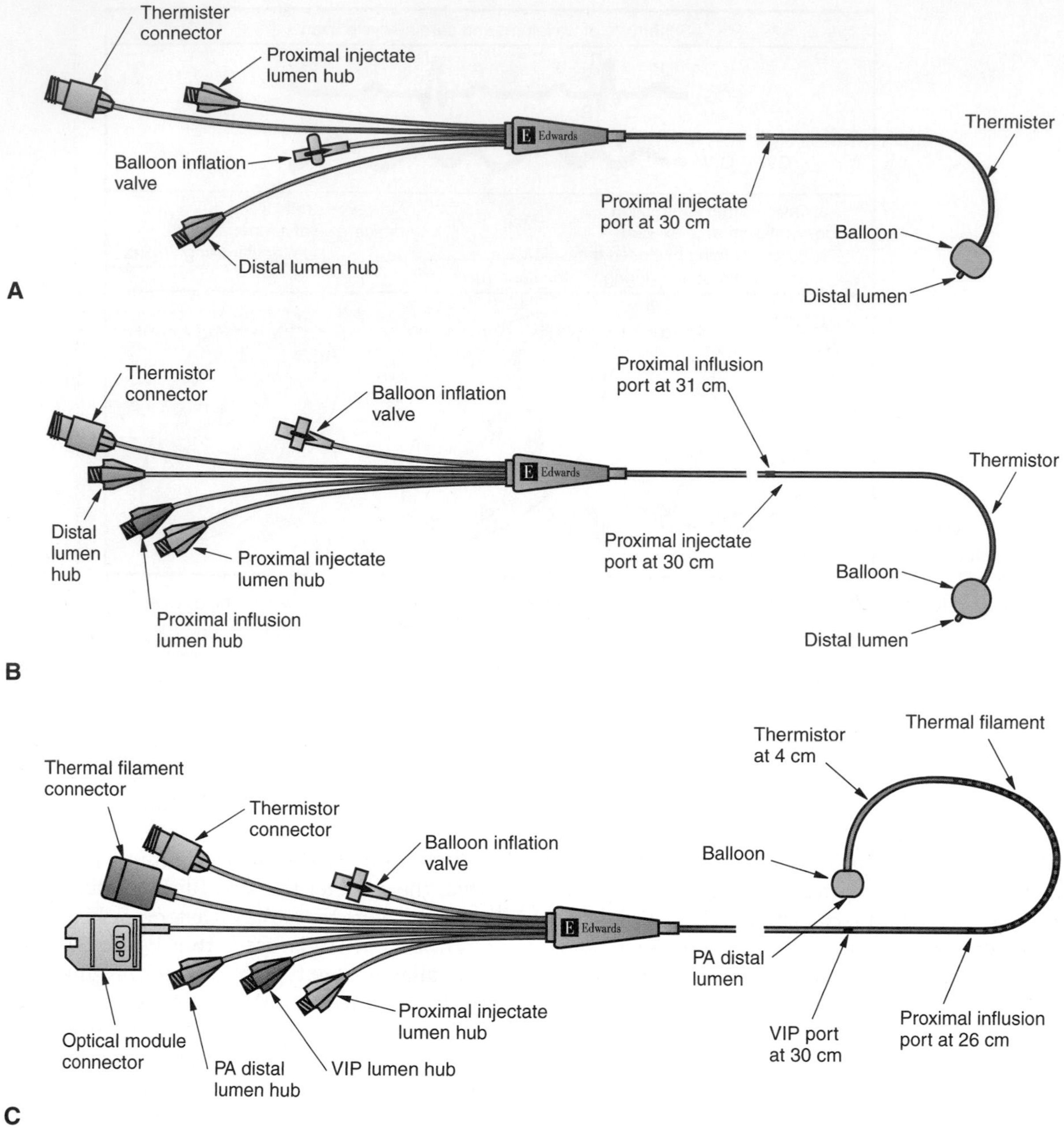

FIGURE 11-32. Types of pulmonary artery catheters. **A,** Four-lumen catheter. **B,** Five-lumen catheter that includes an additional venous infusion port (VIP) into the right atrium. **C,** Seven-lumen catheter that includes a VIP port and two additional lumens for continuous cardiac output (CCO) and thermal filament, and continuous mixed venous oxygen saturation (Svo_2) monitoring (optical module connector). An additional option is to combine use of the CCO filament and the thermistor response time to calculate continuous end-diastolic volume (CEDV). (©2001 Edwards Lifesciences LLC. All rights reserved. Reprinted with permission ©Edwards Lifesciences, Swan-Ganz® is a trademark of Edwards Lifesciences Corporation, registered in the US Patent and Trademark Office.)

Before inserting the catheter into the vein, the physician—using sterile technique—tests the balloon for inflation and flushes the catheter with normal saline solution to remove any air. The PA catheter is then attached to the bedside hemodynamic line setup and monitor so that the waveforms can be visualized while the catheter is advanced through the right side of the heart (see Figure 11-33). A larger introducer sheath (8.5 Fr)—which has the tip positioned in the vena cava and an additional IV side-port lumen—is often used to cannulate the vein first. This introducer sheath is known by several different names in clinical practice, including *sheath, cordis, introducer,* or *side-port*. This introducer sheath remains in place, and the supple PA

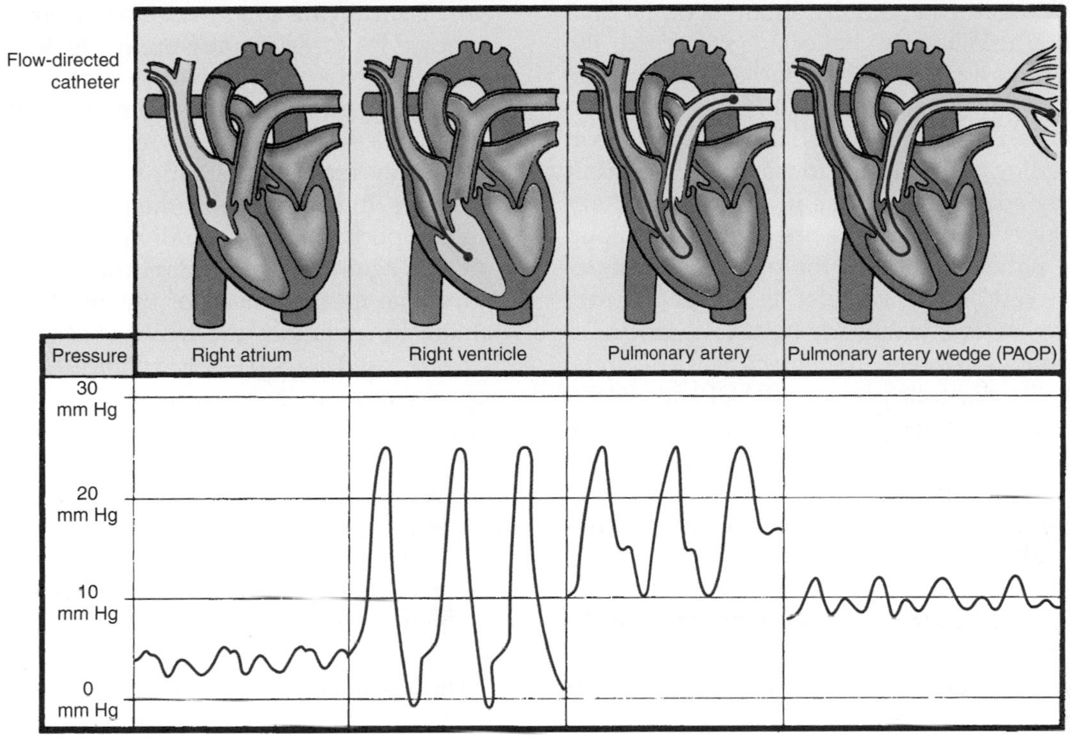

FIGURE 11-33. Pulmonary artery (PA) catheter insertion with corresponding waveforms.

catheter is threaded through it into the vena cava and into the right side of the heart.

Nursing Management

Nursing priorities for the patient with PA catheter monitoring focus on (1) accurately interpreting PA catheter waveforms, (2) accommodating changes in patient position, (3) recognizing the effect of respiratory variation, (4) preventing catheter-related complications, (5) measuring cardiac output, and (6) evaluating hemodynamic performance.

Interpreting Pulmonary Artery Waveforms. Each chamber of the heart has a distinctive waveform with recognizable characteristics. It is the responsibility of the critical care nurse to recognize each waveform displayed on the bedside monitor, both when the catheter enters the corresponding chamber during insertion and also during routine monitoring.

Right Atrial Waveform. As the PA catheter is advanced into the right atrium during insertion, a right atrial waveform must be visible on the monitor, with recognizable a, c, and v waves (see Figure 11-33). The normal mean pressure in the right atrium is 2 to 5 mm Hg. Before passage through the tricuspid valve, the balloon at the tip of the catheter is inflated for two reasons. First, it cushions the pointed tip of the PA catheter so that if the tip comes into contact with the right ventricular wall, it will cause less myocardial irritability and, consequently, fewer ventricular dysrhythmias. Second, inflation of the balloon assists the catheter in floating with the flow of blood from the right ventricle into the pulmonary artery. It is because of these features and the balloon that PA catheters are described as *flow-directional catheters.*

Right Ventricular Waveform. The right ventricular waveform is distinctly pulsatile, with distinct systolic and diastolic pressures. Normal RV pressures are 20 to 30 mm Hg systolic and 0 to 5 mm Hg diastolic. Even with the balloon inflated, it is not uncommon for some ventricular ectopy to occur during passage through the RV. All patients who have a PA catheter inserted must have simultaneous ECG monitoring, with defibrillator and emergency resuscitation equipment nearby.

Pulmonary Artery Waveform. As the catheter enters the pulmonary artery, the waveform again changes. The diastolic pressure rises. Normal PA pressures range from 20 to 30 mm Hg systolic over 10 mm Hg diastolic. A dicrotic notch, visible on the downslope of the waveform, represents closure of the pulmonic valve.

Pulmonary Artery Occlusion Waveform (Wedge). While the balloon remains inflated, the catheter is advanced into the wedge position until the inflated balloon occludes a medium-sized pulmonary artery (1.2 cm diameter).[74] This value is the *pulmonary artery occlusion pressure* (PAOP).[74] In the PAOP (wedge) position, the waveform decreases in size and is nonpulsatile, reflective of a left atrial tracing with a and v wave deflections (see Figure 11-33). The balloon occludes the pulmonary vessel so that the PA lumen is exposed only to left atrial pressure and is protected from the pulsatile influence of the pulmonary artery. When the balloon is deflated, the catheter should spontaneously float back into the PA. When the balloon is reinflated, the wedge tracing should be visible on the bedside monitor. The normal PAOP ranges from 5 to 12 mm Hg.

After insertion, the catheter is sutured to the skin and a chest radiograph is taken to verify placement. If the catheter is advanced too far into the pulmonary bed and produces a PAOP tracing without balloon inflation, the patient is at risk for pulmonary infarction. Alternatively, if the catheter is not sufficiently advanced into the PA, it will not be useful for PAOP (wedge) readings. However, in many critical care units, if the patient's PA diastolic pressure (PADP) and PAOP (wedge) values approximate (within 0 to 3 mm Hg), the PADP is used to follow the trend of left ventricular (LV) filling pressure (preload). This prevents possible trauma from frequent balloon inflation; in such a situation the PA catheter may be consciously pulled back into a nonwedging position in the pulmonary artery.

Accommodating Changes in Patient Position. In the supine position, if the transducer is placed at the level of the phlebostatic axis, a head-of-bed position from flat up to 60 degrees is appropriate for most patients. PA and PAOP measurements in the lateral position may be significantly different from those taken when the patient is lying supine. At this point, if there is concern over the validity of pressure readings in a particular patient, it is more reliable to take measurements with the patient on his or her back, with the head of bed elevated from zero up to 60 degrees. A stabilization period of only 5 minutes is required before taking pressure readings after a patient changes position.[75]

Recognizing the Effect of Respiratory Variation. All PADP and PAOP (wedge) tracings are subject to respiratory interference, especially if the patient is on a positive-pressure, volume-cycled ventilator.[56,74] During inhalation the ventilator "pushes up" the PA tracing, which produces an artificially high reading (Figure 11-34, *A*). During spontaneous respiration, negative intrathoracic pressure "pulls down" the waveform and can produce an erroneously low measurement (Figure 11-34, *B*). To minimize the impact of respiratory variation, the PADP is read at end-expiration, which is the most stable point in the respiratory cycle. If the digital number fluctuates with respiration, a printed readout on paper can be obtained to verify true PADP. In some clinical settings, ECG or airway pressure and flow are recorded simultaneously with the PADP/PAOP tracing to identify end-expiration.[56,74]

Positive End-Expiratory Pressure. Some clinical diagnoses, such as acute respiratory distress syndrome (ARDS), require the use of high levels of positive end-expiratory pressure (PEEP) set with the ventilator to treat refractory hypoxemia. If a PEEP of greater than 10 cm H_2O is used, PAOP (wedge) and PA pressures will be artificially elevated. Because of this impact of PEEP, in the early days of hemodynamic monitoring, patients in some critical care units were taken off the ventilator to record PA pressure measurements. It has since been shown that this practice closes alveoli, decreases the patient's oxygenation level, and may result in persistent hypoxemia. Because patients remain on PEEP for treatment, they remain on it during measurement of PA pressures. In this situation, the trend of PA readings is more important than one individual measurement.

Once again, the most important factor is not one individual measurement, or the absolute number obtained, but whether the trend of the measurements is being used as a basis for clinical interventions to support and improve cardiopulmonary function in the critically ill.

Preventing Catheter-Related Complications. Two randomized controlled trials that involved PA catheters listed the following complications: hematoma at the insertion site (4%),[69] puncture of an artery (3%),[69] catheter-related infection (2.5%),[72] catheter knotting or pulmonary infarction/hemorrhage (1%),[72] and arrhythmias (0.5%).[72]

The PA tracing is continuously monitored. This is to ensure that the catheter does not migrate forward into a spontaneous wedge or PAOP position. A segment of lung can suffer infarction if the wedged catheter occludes an arteriole for a prolonged period. If the catheter is spontaneously "wedged," the critical care nurse can gently pull the catheter back out of the wedge position if the institutional policy allows.[76]

PA Catheter Removal. PA catheters can be safely removed from the patient by critical care nurses competent in this procedure.[56] Removal is not usually associated with major complications. The most common incidents are PVCs in about 2% of patients as the catheter is pulled through the RV.[56,77]

Measuring Cardiac Output. The PA catheter is used to measure CO using either an intermittent (bolus) *or* a continuous CO method.

Thermodilution Cardiac Output Method. The bolus thermodilution method is performed at the bedside and results in CO calculated in liters per minute. Generally, three cardiac outputs that are within a 10% mean range are obtained at one time and then are averaged to calculate CO. A known amount (5-ml or 10-ml bolus) of iced or, more typically, room-temperature normal saline solution is injected into the proximal lumen of the catheter. The injectate exits into the right atrium and travels with the flow of blood past the thermistor (temperature sensor) located at the distal end of the catheter in the pulmonary artery. The injectate can be delivered by hand injection, using individual syringes of saline. Frequently a closed in-line system attached to a 500-ml bag of normal saline is used as a reservoir to deliver the individual injections.[78]

Sometimes the right atrial (proximal) port is clotted off and not usable. If another right atrial port is available, this can be substituted. However, if a usable port

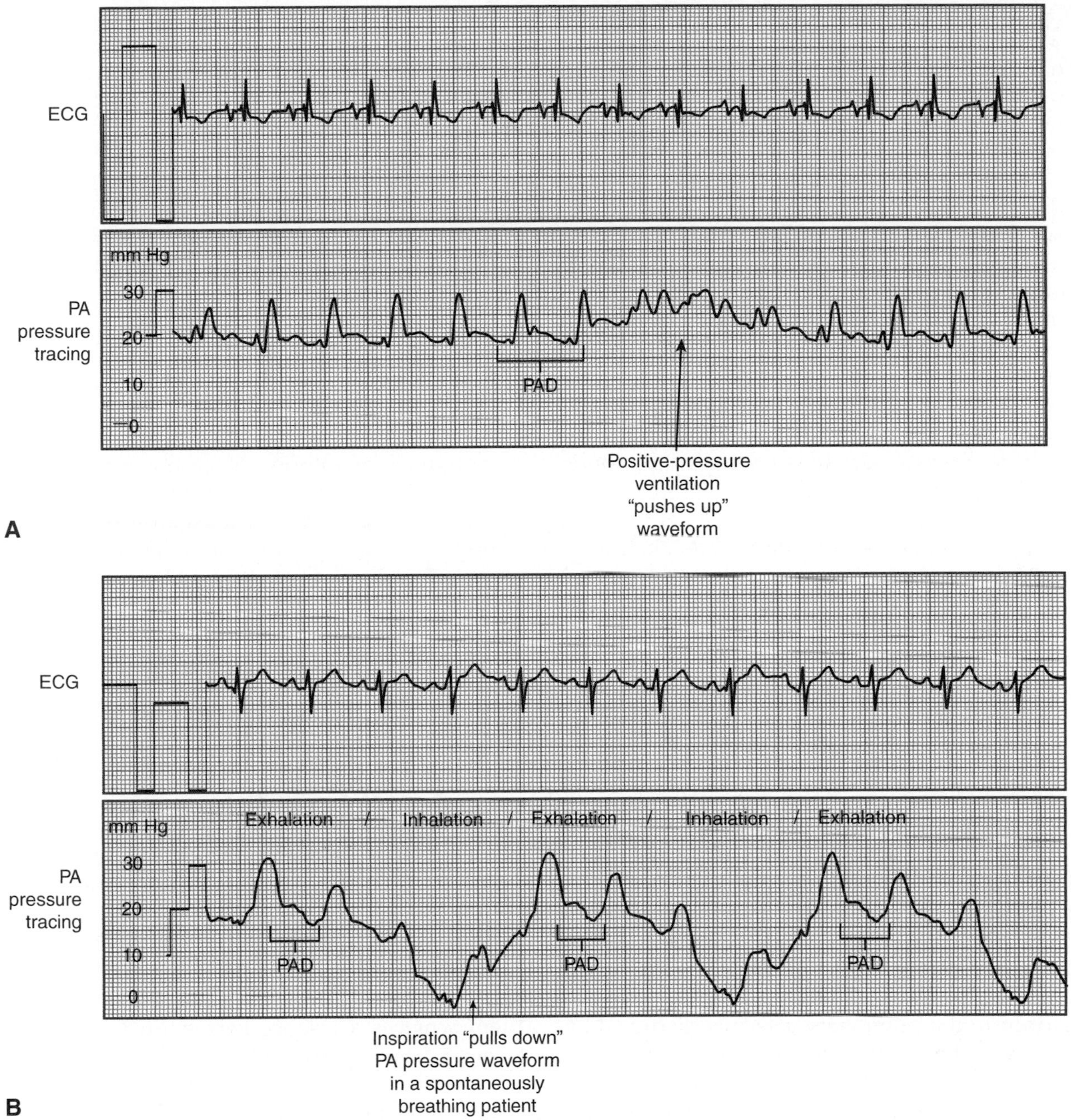

FIGURE 11-34. Pulmonary artery (PA) waveforms that demonstrate the impact of ventilation of PA pressure readings. For accuracy, PA pressures are read at end-exhalation. **A,** Positive-pressure ventilation: the increase in intrathoracic pressure during inhalation "pushes up" the PA pressure waveform, creating a false high reading. **B,** Spontaneous breathing: the decrease in intrathoracic pressure during normal inhalation "pulls down" the PA waveform, creating a false low reading.

is not available, to ensure accurate cardiac output data, a new pulmonary artery catheter is inserted.

Cardiac Output Curve. The thermodilution CO method uses the indicator-dilution principle, in which a known temperature is the indicator. It is based on the principle that the change in temperature over time is inversely proportional to blood flow. Blood flow can be diagrammatically represented as a cardiac output curve on which temperature is plotted against time (Figure 11-35). Most hemodynamic monitors display

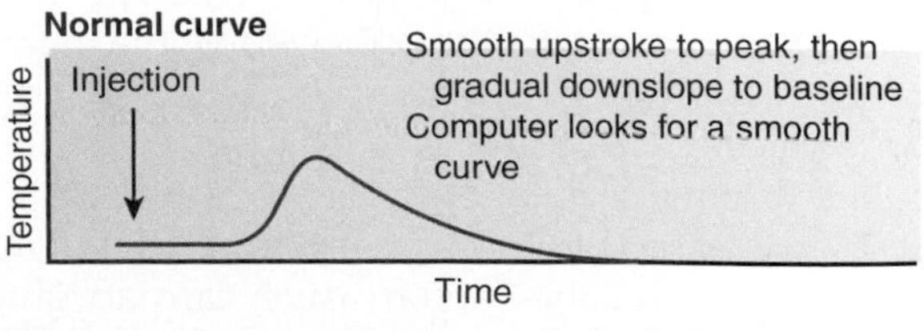

FIGURE 11-35. Normal cardiac thermodilution bolus output curve.

this CO curve, which must then be interpreted to determine whether the CO injection is valid. The normal curve has a smooth upstroke, with a rounded peak and a gradually tapering downslope. If the curve has an uneven pattern, it may indicate faulty injection technique and the CO measurement must be repeated. Patient movement or coughing also alters the CO measurement.

Injectate Temperature. If the CO is within the normal range, it is equally accurate whether iced or room temperature injectate is used. However, if the COs are extremely high or very low, iced injectate may be more accurate. To ensure accurate readings, the difference between injectate temperature and body temperature must be at least 10° C, and the injectate must be delivered within 4 seconds, with minimal handling of the syringe to prevent warming of the solution. This is particularly important if iced injectate is used. With all delivery systems, the injectate is delivered at the same point in the respiratory cycle, usually end-exhalation.

Patient Position and Cardiac Output. In the normovolemic, stable patient, reliable CO measurements can be obtained in a supine position (patient lying on his or her back) with the head of the bed elevated up to 45 degrees.[79] If the patient is hypovolemic or unstable, leaving the head of the bed in a flat position, or only slightly elevated, is the most clinically appropriate choice. CO measurements performed when the patient is turned to the side are not considered as accurate as those performed with the patient in the supine position.

Clinical Conditions That Alter Cardiac Output. Two clinical conditions produce errors in the thermodilution CO measurement: tricuspid valve regurgitation and ventricular septal rupture. If the patient has tricuspid valve regurgitation, the expected flow of blood from the right atrium to the pulmonary artery is disrupted by backflow from the right ventricle to the right atrium. This creates a lower CO measurement than the patient's actual output. If the person has an intracardiac left-to-right shunt, such as occurs following ventricular septal rupture, the thermodilution CO measures the large pulmonary volume and records a higher CO than the patient's true systemic output.

Continuous Invasive Cardiac Output Measurement. The bolus thermodilution method is reliable but performed intermittently. Continuous CO monitoring using a PA catheter is also used in clinical practice.[79] One method employs a thermal filament on the PA catheter to emit small energy signals (the indicator) into the bloodstream. These signals are then detected by the thermistor near the tip of the PA catheter, and the equivalent of an indicator curve is created and a CO value is calculated from this data.

Noninvasive Cardiac Output Measurement. There is a tremendous need for reliable noninvasive cardiac output technologies in critical care. Two methods that show promise are esophageal Doppler flowmetry and pulse contour analysis.[74]

Evaluating the Hemodynamic Profile. For the patient with a thermodilution PA catheter in place, additional hemodynamic information can be calculated using values derived from the PA catheter, BP, CO, and body surface area (BSA). These measurements are calculated using specific formulas that are indexed to a patient's body size, using a body area surface area computer calculation incorporated into the bedside monitor.[74,75]

CONTINUOUS MONITORING OF CENTRAL OR MIXED VENOUS OXYGEN SATURATION

Indications

Continuous monitoring of venous oxygen saturation is indicated for the critically ill patient who has the potential to develop an imbalance between oxygen supply and metabolic tissue demand. This includes the patient in severe sepsis or shock, following high-risk surgery, and the patient with severe respiratory compromise.

Continuous venous oxygen monitoring permits a calculation of the balance achieved between arterial oxygen supply (SaO_2) and oxygen demand at the tissue level by sampling desaturated venous blood from the pulmonary artery catheter distal tip. This sample is termed *mixed venous blood* saturation (SvO_2) because it is a mixture of all of the venous blood drained from many body tissues. Recently the same fiberoptic technology has been used in combination with a fiberoptic triple-lumen CVC. In this situation the venous blood is sampled from the superior vena cava, just above the right atrium, and is abbreviated $ScvO_2$.[80,81]

Under normal conditions the cardiopulmonary system achieves a balance between oxygen supply and demand. Four factors contribute to this balance:

1. Cardiac output (CO)
2. Hemoglobin (Hgb)
3. Arterial oxygen saturation (SaO_2)
4. Tissue metabolism (VO_2)

Three of these factors (CO, Hgb, and SaO_2) contribute to the supply of oxygen to the tissues. Tissue metabolism (VO_2) determines oxygen consumption or the quantity of oxygen extracted at tissue level that creates the demand for oxygen. The relationship of all these factors is illustrated in Figure 11-36.

Catheters

There are two different catheter choices available: a PA catheter with a fiberoptic lumen and a CVC with fiberoptic lumen. The technology used to measure the venous saturation is identical in both catheters. The fiberoptics are attached to an optical module that is integrated into the bedside monitor. The optical module transmits a narrow band of light down one optical

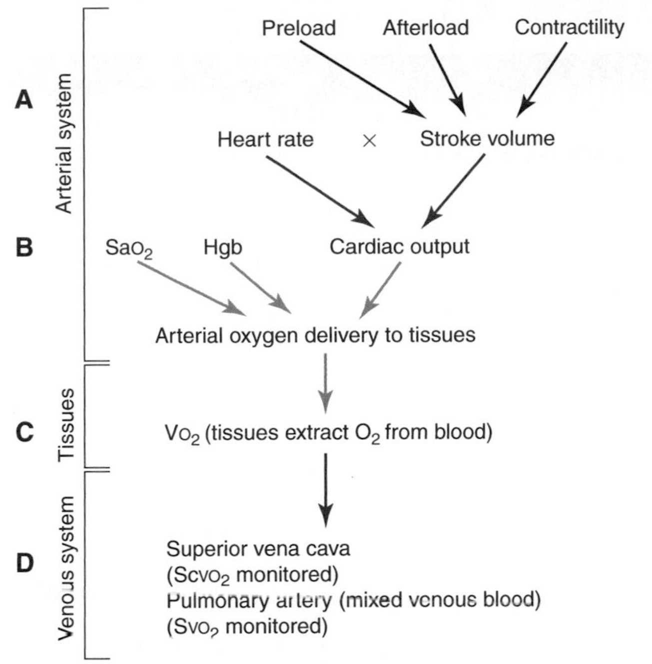

FIGURE 11-36. The factors that contribute to the Svo_2 value. **A,** Cardiac output (CO) is determined by heart rate ($Scvo_2$ HR) × stroke volume (SV). **B,** The Sao_2, Hgb, and CO all contribute to arterial oxygen delivery at the tissue level. **C,** Tissues extract and use the oxygen carried in the blood. This process of cellular oxygen consumption is termed *Vo_2*. **D,** Blood returns to the superior vena cava (recorded as $Scvo_2$) and then to the pulmonary artery, where the mixed venous blood is recorded as Svo_2.

fiber. This light is reflected off the hemoglobin in the blood and returns to the optical module through the receiving fiberoptic. The fiberoptic signal is recorded on a bedside continuous display.[80,81]

***Svo_2* Catheter.** The pulmonary arterial catheter contains the traditional four lumens plus a lumen containing two or three optical fibers. The fiberoptic lumen is located in the pulmonary artery and measures the oxygen concentration (Svo_2) in the pulmonary artery.

***$Scvo_2$* Catheter.** The central venous catheter incorporates the fiberoptic lumen into a multilumen CVC. The fiberoptic catheter tip is positioned in a central vein such as the superior vena cava to measure venous oxygen saturation ($Scvo_2$).

The $Scvo_2$ catheter has been successfully used to guide hemodynamic fluid resuscitation in septic patients in the emergency department and the critical care unit.[82-84] $Scvo_2$ monitoring has also been successfully used for high-risk surgical patients.[85] The relationship between the values obtained from the traditional pulmonary artery (Svo_2) catheter and the central venous ($Scvo_2$) catheter are very similar, although the $Scvo_2$ values are slightly higher. The trend of parallel measurements (up or down as patient condition changes) is in the same direction about 90% of the time.[67]

***Svo_2/$Scvo_2$* Calibration.** The catheter is calibrated before insertion into the patient through a standardized color reference system, which is part of the catheter package. Insertion technique and sites are identical to those used for placement of conventional PA or CVC catheters. Waveform analysis and/or venous saturation measurement can be used for accurate placement. Once the catheter is inserted, recalibration is unnecessary unless the catheter becomes disconnected from the optical module.

To recalibrate the fiberoptic module to verify accuracy when the catheter is already inserted in a patient, a mixed venous blood sample (Svo_2) or central venous sample ($Scvo_2$) must be withdrawn from the appropriate catheter tip and sent to the laboratory for oxygen saturation analysis. In many critical care units, this is a standard daily procedure to ensure that readings used to guide patient care remain accurate.[80]

Nursing Management

Nursing priorities for the patient with a catheter that monitors Svo_2/$Scvo_2$ are to incorporate the Svo_2/$Scvo_2$ values into the overall hemodynamic assessment for each patient.

Svo_2 monitoring provides a continuous assessment of the balance of oxygen supply and demand for an individual patient. Nursing assessment includes evaluation of the Svo_2/$Scvo_2$ value and evaluation of the four factors (Sao_2, CO, Hgb, and Vo_2) that maintain the oxygen supply-demand balance.

Normal Svo_2 Values. Normal Svo_2 is approximately 75% in the healthy individual (range 60% to 80%). In critically ill patients, a venous oxygen saturation between 60% and 80% is evidence of adequate balance between oxygen supply and demand.

Normal $Scvo_2$ Values. The normal values for the $Scvo_2$ catheter are about 5% higher.[67] This is because the reading is taken in the vena cava before the blood enters the right heart chambers, where the *cardiac sinus* (vein) delivers venous blood drained from the myocardium into the right atrium. The heavily desaturated myocardial blood will decrease the oxygen saturation slightly. For this reason, $Scvo_2$ values are always slightly higher than Svo_2 readings in the same patient.[67]

If the Svo_2/$Scvo_2$ value is within the normal range of 60% to 80% and the patient is not clinically compromised, one can assume that oxygen supply and demand are balanced for that individual.

Sepsis and $Scvo_2$. For patients who are septic the $Scvo_2$ central venous catheter is recommended to guide therapy to achieve an $Scvo_2$ above 70%.[82-84]

Low Svo_2/$Scvo_2$. If the Svo_2/$Scvo_2$ value decreases by more than 10% and this change is maintained for more than 10 minutes, the clinician must determine which of the four factors is affecting Svo_2.[83] Specifically, if the Svo_2/$Scvo_2$ falls below 60% and is sustained, the

Table 11-10
Svo_2 Measurements

Svo_2 MEASUREMENT	PHYSIOLOGIC BASIS FOR CHANGE IN $Svo_2/Scvo_2$	CLINICAL DIAGNOSIS AND RATIONALE
High $Svo_2/Scvo_2$ (80%-95%)	Increased oxygen supply Decreased oxygen demand	Patient receiving more oxygen than required by clinical condition Anesthesia, which causes sedation and decreased muscle movement Hypothermia, which lowers metabolic demand (e.g., with cardiopulmonary bypass) Sepsis caused by decreased ability of tissues to use oxygen at a cellular level False high positive because PA catheter is wedged in a pulmonary arteriole (Svo_2 only)
Normal $Svo_2/Scvo_2$ (60% to 80%)	Normal oxygen supply and metabolic demand	Balanced oxygen supply and demand Anemia or bleeding with compromised cardiopulmonary system
Low $Svo_2/Scvo_2$ (less than 60%)	Decreased oxygen supply caused by: Low hemoglobin (Hgb) Low arterial saturation (Sao_2) Low cardiac output (CO) Increased oxygen consumption (Vo_2)	Hypoxemia resulting from decreased oxygen supply or lung disease Cardiogenic shock caused by left ventricular pump failure Metabolic demand exceeds oxygen supply in conditions that increase muscle movement and increase metabolic rate, including physiologic states such as shivering, seizures, and hyperthermia and nursing interventions such as being weighed on a bed scale and turning

Svo_2, Mixed venous oxygen saturation; *$Scvo_2$*, superior vena cava oxygen saturation.

clinician must assume that oxygen supply is not equal to demand and investigate the cause (Table 11-10).

Assessment of $Svo_2/Scvo_2$ Values. It is helpful to assess the cause of decreased $Svo_2/Scvo_2$ in a logical sequence that reflects knowledge of the meaning of the venous saturation value. The following is one such assessment sequence:

1. Clinically assess the patient.
2. Assess whether the decreased $Svo_2/Scvo_2$ is caused by low oxygen supply. Verify the effectiveness of the ventilator or oxygen mask, or check Sao_2 from arterial blood gas values.
3. Assess cardiac function by performing a CO measurement.
4. Assess Hgb value by checking recent laboratory results or by withdrawing a blood sample for laboratory analysis.
5. Assess whether the decreased $Svo_2/Scvo_2$ is the result of a recent patient movement or nursing action that may have temporarily increased Vo_2.

If $Svo_2/Scvo_2$ falls below 40%, the balance of oxygen supply and demand may not be adequate to meet tissue needs at the cellular level. At some point the cells change from an aerobic to anaerobic mode of metabolism, which results in the production of lactic acid and is representative of a shock state in which cellular injury or cell death may result. At this point every attempt must be made to determine the cause of the low $Svo_2/Scvo_2$ and to correct the oxygen supply-demand imbalance. To avoid the risk of lactic acidosis it is helpful to watch the trend of the $Svo_2/Scvo_2$ and to intervene early with a goal of maintaining the venous oxygen saturation above 70%.[80-85]

SUMMARY

The range of diagnostic tools available to the bedside critical care nurse will continue to expand. As critical care patient needs become more complex and nursing responsibilities augment, incorporation of appropriate diagnostic information into the nursing management plan will only increase in importance.

evolve To test your mastery of this chapter, try the Open-Book Quiz at http://evolve.elsevier.com/Urden/priorities/

REFERENCES

1. Gibbons RJ et al: ACC/AHA 2002 guideline update for the management of patients with chronic stable angina—summary article: a report of the American College of Cardiology/American Heart Association Task Force on Practice Guidelines (Committee on the Management of Patients With Chronic Stable Angina), *Circulation* 107(1):149, 2003.
2. Wong WM, Fass R: Noncardiac chest pain, *Curr Treat Options Gastroenterol* 7(4):273, 2004.
3. Faybush EM, Fass R: Gastroesophageal reflux disease in noncardiac chest pain, *Gastroenterol Clin North Am* 33(1):41, 2004.
4. Chun AA, McGee SR: Bedside diagnosis of coronary artery disease: a systematic review, *Am J Med* 117(5):334, 2004.
5. Drazner MH et al: Prognostic importance of elevated jugular venous pressure and a third heart sound in patients with heart failure, *N Engl J Med* 345(8):574, 2001.
6. Drazner MH, Rame JE, Dries DL: Third heart sound and elevated jugular venous pressure as markers of the subsequent development of heart failure in patients with asymptomatic left ventricular dysfunction, *Am J Med* 114(6):431, 2003.

7. Barone JE, Mullinger RV: Should an Allen test be performed before radial cannulation? *J Trauma* 61:468, 2006.
8. Perloff D et al: *Human blood pressure determination by sphygmomanometry,* Dallas, 2001, American Heart Association.
9. Chobanian AV et al: Seventh report of the Joint National Committee on Prevention, Detection, Evaluation, and Treatment of High Blood Pressure, *Hypertension* 42(6): 1206, 2003.
10. Fields LE et al: The burden of adult hypertension in the United States 1999 to 2000: a rising tide, *Hypertension* 44(4):398, 2004.
11. Barrett MJ et al: Mastering cardiac murmurs: the power of repetition, *Chest* 126(2):470, 2004.
12. Criddle LM: Rhabdomyolysis: pathophysiology, recognition, and management, *Crit Care Nurse* 23(6):14, 2003.
13. Malinoski DJ, Slater MS, Mullins RJ: Crush injury and rhabdomyolysis, *Crit Care Clin* 20(1):171, 2004.
14. Davidson MB et al: Pathophysiology, clinical consequences, and treatment of tumor lysis syndrome, *Am J Med* 116(8):546, 2004.
15. Gennari FJ, Segal AS: Hyperkalemia: an adaptive response in chronic renal insufficiency, *Kidney Int* 62(1):1, 2002.
16. Palmer BF: Managing hyperkalemia caused by inhibitors of the renin-angiotensin-aldosterone system, *N Engl J Med* 351(6):585, 2004.
17. Diercks DB et al: Electrocardiographic manifestations: electrolyte abnormalities, *J Emerg Med* 27(2):153, 2004.
18. Ariyan CE, Sosa JA: Assessment and management of patients with abnormal calcium, *Crit Care Med* 32(4 suppl): S146, 2004.
19. Dickerson RN et al: Accuracy of methods to estimate ionized and "corrected" serum calcium concentrations in critically ill multiple trauma patients receiving specialized nutrition support, *JPEN J Parenter Enteral Nutr* 28(3):133, 2004.
20. Ma G et al: Electrocardiographic manifestations: digitalis toxicity, *J Emerg Med* 20(2):145, 2001.
21. Zivin JR et al: Hypocalcemia: a pervasive metabolic abnormality in the critically ill, *Am J Kidney Dis* 37(4):689, 2001.
22. Noronha JL, Matuschak GM: Magnesium in critical illness: metabolism, assessment, and treatment, *Intensive Care Med* 28(6):667, 2002.
23. Braunwald E et al: ACC/AHA guideline update for the management of patients with unstable angina and non-ST-segment elevation myocardial infarction—2002: summary article: a report of the American College of Cardiology/American Heart Association Task Force on Practice Guidelines (Committee on the Management of Patients With Unstable Angina), *Circulation* 106(14):1893, 2002, http://www.ahajournals.org.
24. Antman EM et al: ACC/AHA guidelines for the management of patients with ST-elevation myocardial infarction—executive summary: a report of the American College of Cardiology/American Heart Association Task Force on Practice Guidelines (Writing Committee to Revise the 1999 Guidelines for the Management of Patients With Acute Myocardial Infarction), *Circulation* 110:588, 2004, http://www.ahajournals.org.
25. Novis DA et al: Biochemical markers of myocardial injury test turnaround time: a College of American Pathologists Q-Probes study of 7020 troponin and 4368 creatine kinase-MB determinations in 159 institutions, *Arch Pathol Lab Med* 128(2):158, 2004.
26. Hirsh J, Raschke R: Heparin and low-molecular-weight heparin: the Seventh ACCP Conference on Antithrombotic and Thrombolytic Therapy, *Chest* 126(3 suppl):188S, 2004.
27. Ansell J et al: The pharmacology and management of the vitamin K antagonists: the Seventh ACCP Conference on Antithrombotic and Thrombolytic Therapy, *Chest* 126(3 suppl):204S, 2004.
28. Patrono C et al: Platelet-active drugs: the relationships among dose, effectiveness, and side effects: the Seventh ACCP Conference on Antithrombotic and Thrombolytic Therapy, *Chest* 126(3 suppl):234S, 2004.
29. Hirsh J, Heddle N, Kelton JG: Treatment of heparin-induced thrombocytopenia: a critical review, *Arch Intern Med* 164(4):361, 2004.
30. Hirsh J et al: American Heart Association/American College of Cardiology Foundation guide to warfarin therapy, *Circulation* 107(12):1692, 2003.
31. Executive summary of the Third Report of the National Cholesterol Education Program (NCEP) Expert Panel on Detection, Evaluation, and Treatment of High Blood Cholesterol in Adults (Adult Treatment Panel III), *JAMA* 285(19):2486, 2001, www.ahajournals.org.
32. Grundy SM et al: Implications of recent clinical trials for the National Cholesterol Education Program Adult Treatment Panel III guidelines, *Circulation* 110(2):227, 2004.
33. Grundy SM et al: Clinical management of metabolic syndrome: report of the American Heart Association/National Heart Lung, and Blood Institute/American Diabetes Association Conference on Scientific Issues Related to Management, *Circulation* 10(4):551, 2004, http://www.ahajournals.org.
34. Drew BJ et al: Practice standards for electrocardiographic monitoring in hospital settings, *Circulation* 110(17):2721, 2004, www.ahajournals. org.
35. Roden DM: Drug-induced prolongation of the QT interval, *N Engl J Med* 350(10):1013, 2004.
36. Blomstrom-Lundqvist C et al: ACC/AHA/ESC guidelines for the management of patients with supraventricular arrhythmias—executive summary: a report of the American College of Cardiology/American Heart Association Task Force on Practice Guidelines and the European Society of Cardiology Committee for Practice Guidelines (Writing Committee to Develop Guidelines for the Management of Patients With Supraventricular Arrhythmias) developed in collaboration with NASPE-Heart Rhythm Society, *J Am Coll Cardiol* 42(8):1493, 2003, www.jacc.org.
37. Yasuma F, Hayano J: Respiratory sinus arrhythmia: why does the heartbeat synchronize with respiratory rhythm? *Chest* 125(2):683, 2004.
38. Zhang S et al: Lower loop reentry as a mechanism of clockwise right atrial flutter, *Circulation* 109(13):1630, 2004.
39. Fuster V et al: ACC/AHA/ESC guidelines for the management of patients with atrial fibrillation: a report

of the American College of Cardiology/American Heart Association Task Force on Practice Guidelines and the European Society of Cardiology Committee for Practice Guidelines and Policy Conferences (Committee to Develop Guidelines for the Management of Patients With Atrial Fibrillation) developed in collaboration with the North American Society of Pacing and Electrophysiology, *Circulation* 104(17):2118, 2001, http://www.ahajournals.org
40. Everett TH, Olgin JE: Basic mechanisms of atrial fibrillation, *Cardiol Clin* 22(1):9, 2004.
41. Ufberg JW, Clark JS: Bradydysrhythmias and atrioventricular conduction blocks, *Emerg Clin North Am* 24(1):1-9, 2000.
42. Crystal E, Connolly SJ: Atrial fibrillation: guiding lessons from epidemiology, *Cardiol Clin* 22(1):1, 2004.
43. Lloyd-Jones DM et al: Lifetime risk for development of atrial fibrillation: the Framingham Heart Study, *Circulation* 110(9):1042, 2004.
44. Kellen JC: Implications for nursing care of patients with atrial fibrillation: lessons learned from the AFFIRM and RACE studies, *J Cardiovasc Nurs* 19(2):128, 2004.
45. Weiss EM, Buescher T: Atrial fibrillation: treatment options and caveats, *AACN Clin Issues* 15(3):362, 2004.
46. Corley SD et al: Relationships between sinus rhythm, treatment, and survival in the Atrial Fibrillation Follow-Up Investigation of Rhythm Management (AFFIRM) Study, *Circulation* 109(12):1509, 2004.
47. Wyse DG et al: A comparison of rate control and rhythm control in patients with atrial fibrillation, *N Engl J Med* 347(23):1825, 2002.
48. Van Gelder IC et al: A comparison of rate control and rhythm control in patients with recurrent persistent atrial fibrillation, *N Engl J Med* 347(23):1834, 2002.
49. Jenkins LS et al: Quality of life in atrial fibrillation: the Atrial Fibrillation Follow-up Investigation of Rhythm Management (AFFIRM) study, *Am Heart J* 149(1):112.
50. Snow V et al: Management of newly detected atrial fibrillation: a clinical practice guideline from the American Academy of Family Physicians and the American College of Physicians, *Ann Intern Med* 139(12):1009, 2003.
51. Chiu C, Sequeira IB: Diagnosis and treatment of idiopathic ventricular tachycardia, *AACN Clin Issues* 15(3): 449, 2004.
52. Field JM Hazinski MF, Gilmore D,: *Handbook of emergency cardiovascular care for healthcare providers,* Dallas, Tex, 2006, American Heart Association.
53. Fuster V et al: ACC/AHAESC guidelines for the management of patients with atrial fibrillation: a report of the American College of Cardiology/American Heart Association Task Force on Practice Guidelines and the European Society of Cardiology Committee for Practice Guidelines (Writing Committee to Revise the 2001 guidelines for the management of atrial fibrillation—developed in collaboration with the European Heart Rhythm Association and the Heart Rhythm Society, *Circulation* 114:e257-e354, 2006, http://www.ahajournals.org.
54. Warkentin TE, Greinacher A: Heparin-induced thrombocytopenia: recognition, treatment, and prevention: the Seventh ACCP Conference on Antithrombotic and Thrombolytic Therapy, *Chest* 126(3 Suppl):311S, http://www.accp.org.
55. Cooney MF: Heparin-induced thrombocytopenia, *Crit Care Nurse* 26(6):30, 2006.
56. AACN: *Pulmonary artery pressure monitoring: AACN practice alert,* 2004, American Association of Critical Care Nurses, http://www.aacn.org.
57. Grap MJ et al: Effect of backrest elevation on the development of ventilator-associated pneumonia, *Am J Crit Care* 14(4):325, 2005.
58. Perloff D et al: *Human blood pressure determination by sphygmomanometry,* ed 6, Dallas, 2001, American Heart Association.
59. Polderman KH, Girbes AR: Central venous catheter use. I. Mechanical complications, *Intensive Care Med* 28(1):1, 2002.
60. Dumont CP: Procedures nurses use to remove central venous catheters and complications they observe: a pilot study, *Am J Crit Care* 10(3):151, 2001.
61. Polderman KH, Girbes AR: Central venous catheter use. II. Infectious complications, *Intensive Care Med* 28(1):18, 2002.
62. O'Grady NP et al: Guidelines for the prevention of intravascular catheter-related infections, *Infect Control Hosp Epidemiol* 23(12):759, 2002.
63. Chaiyakunapruk N et al: Chlorhexidine compared with povidone-iodine solution for vascular catheter-site care: a meta-analysis, *Ann Intern Med* 136(11):792, 2002.
64. Hu KK et al: Using maximal sterile barriers to prevent central venous catheter–related infection: a systematic evidence-based review, *Am J Infect Control* 32(3):142, 2004.
65. Boyce JM, Pittet D: Guideline for hand hygiene in health-care settings: recommendations of the Healthcare Infection Control Practices Advisory Committee and the HIPAC/SHEA/APIC/IDSA Hand Hygiene Task Force, *Am J Infect Control* 30(8):S1, 2002.
66. Dimick JB et al: Risk of colonization of central venous catheters: catheters for total parenteral nutrition vs. other catheters, *Am J Crit Care* 12(4):328, 2003.
67. Reinhart K et al: Continuous central venous and pulmonary artery oxygen saturation monitoring in the critically ill, *Intensive Care Med* 30(8):1572, 2004.
68. Hadian M, Pinsky MR: Evidence-based review of the use of the pulmonary artery catheter: impact data and complications. *Crit Care* 10(suppl 3):S8, 2006.
69. Harvey S et al: Pulmonary artery catheters for adult patients in intensive care (review), The Cochrane Library, issue 4, 2006, John Wiley & Sons, http://www.thecochranelibrary.com.
70. Shah MR et al: Impact of the pulmonary artery catheter in critically ill patients, meta-analysis of randomized controlled trials, *JAMA* 294(13):1664, 2005.
71. ARDS Clinical Trials Network: Pulmonary artery versus central venous catheter to guide treatment of acute lung injury, *N Engl J Med* 354(21):2213, 2006.
72. The ESCAPE Investigators and ESCAPE Study Coordinators: Evaluation study of congestive heart failure and pulmonary artery catheter effectiveness, *JAMA* 294(13):1625, 2005.
73. Bernard GR et al: Pulmonary artery catheterization and clinical outcomes: National Heart, Lung, and Blood Institute and Food and Drug Administration Workshop Report: consensus statement, *JAMA* 283(19):2568, 2000.

74. Polanco PM, Pinsky MR: Practical issues of hemodynamic monitoring at the bedside, *Surg Clin North Am*, 86:1431, 2006.
75. Bridges EJ: Monitoring pulmonary artery pressures: just the facts, *Crit Care Nurse* 20(6):59, 2000.
76. Antle DE: Ensuring competency in nurse repositioning of the pulmonary artery catheter, *Dimens Crit Care Nurs* 19(2):44, 2000.
77. Baldwin IC, Heland M: Incidence of cardiac dysrhythmias in patients during pulmonary artery catheter removal after cardiac surgery, *Heart Lung* 29(3):155, 2000.
78. Gawlinski A: Measuring cardiac output: intermittent bolus thermodilution method, *Crit Care Nurse* 20(2):118, 2000.
79. Giuliano KK et al: Backrest angle and cardiac output measurement in critically ill patients, *Nurs Res* 52(4):242, 2003.
80. Jesurum J: Protocols for Practice—Svo_2 Monitoring, *Crit Care Nurse* 24(4):73, 2004.
81. Goodrich C: Continuous central venous oximetry monitoring, *Crit Care Nurs Clin North Am* 18:203, 2006
82. Rivers E et al: Early goal-directed therapy in the treatment of severe sepsis and septic shock, *N Engl J Med* 345(19):1368, 2001.
83. Dellinger RP et al: Surviving sepsis campaign guidelines for management of severe sepsis and septic shock, *Crit Care Med*, 32(3):858, 2004.
84. Picard KM et al: Development and implementation of a multidisciplinary sepsis protocol, *Crit Care Nurse* 26(3):43, 2006.
85. Collaborative Study Group on Perioperative $Scvo_2$ Monitoring: Multicentre study on peri- and postoperative central venous oxygen saturation in high-risk surgical patients, *Crit Care* 10(6), R158,2006, http://ceforum.com.

CHAPTER 12

Cardiovascular Disorders

MARY E. LOUGH

OBJECTIVES

- Describe the etiology and pathophysiology of atherosclerotic coronary artery disease.
- Identify the pathophysiology and clinical manifestations of acute heart failure.
- Explain the treatment of selected cardiovascular disorders: coronary artery disease, cardiomyopathy, and valvular disease.
- Discuss the nursing priorities for managing a patient with an acute cardiovascular disorder.

Cardiovascular disease remains the leading cause of mortality in the United States. There are 2,400,000 deaths from cardiovascular causes in the United States each year, or 60% of "total mortality."[1] The estimated direct and indirect national cost is $133.2 billion.[1] Cardiovascular diseases are the leading cause of death for both women and men.[1] An understanding of the pathology of cardiovascular disease processes and current clinical management allows the critical care nurse to accurately anticipate and plan interventions. This chapter focuses on cardiac disorders commonly seen in the critical care environment.

CORONARY ARTERY DISEASE

DESCRIPTION AND ETIOLOGY

Atherosclerosis is a progressive disease that affects arteries throughout the body. In the heart, atherosclerotic changes are clinically known as *coronary artery disease* (CAD). This disease process is also known by the term *coronary heart disease* (CHD) because ultimately other heart structures will become involved in the disease process. Research and epidemiologic data collected during the past 50 years have demonstrated a strong association between specific risk factors and the development of CAD.[1] These risk factors are further delineated into nonmodifiable and modifiable coronary risk factors (Box 12-1).

RISK FACTORS FOR CORONARY ARTERY DISEASE

Age, Gender, and Race

The severe effects of CAD occur as a person ages. In general, CAD symptoms are seen in middle and old age.[1] Traditionally CAD has been regarded as a male disease, but it is increasingly obvious that in modern society it affects both genders.[1] The average age for a person having a first heart attack is 68.8 years for men and 70.4 years for women.[1] Starting at age 75 the prevalence of cardiovascular disease is higher in women than in men.[3] In fact, CAD rates in postmenopausal women are two to three times higher than those of women the same age before menopause.[1] Nonwhite populations of both genders have higher CAD mortality rates than do white populations of similar socioeconomic status.[1,2]

Family History

A positive family history is one in which a close blood relative has had a myocardial infarction or stroke before the age of 60. This family history suggests a genetic or lifestyle predisposition to the development of coronary artery disease.

Box 12-1

Coronary Artery Disease Risk Factors

Nonmodifiable
Age
Gender
Family history
Race

Modifiable
Elevated serum lipids
Diet high in saturated fat, cholesterol, and calories
Hypertension
Cigarette smoking
Chronic kidney disease
Prediabetes or diabetes mellitus
Obesity
Physical inactivity
Metabolic syndrome
Elevated homocysteine level
Postmenopause (modification is controversial)

Hyperlipidemia

Hyperlipidemia is a leading factor responsible for severe atherosclerosis and the development of CAD. Determining total serum cholesterol and triglyceride levels represents a helpful start in the evaluation process.[3,4] A lipid panel blood test will measure the following values:

- High-density lipoprotein (HDL) cholesterol
- Low-density lipoprotein (LDL) cholesterol
- Very-low-density lipoprotein (VLDL) cholesterol
- Triglycerides

Treatment of hyperlipidemia has advanced beyond the concept of lowering total cholesterol to treatment of specific lipoprotein abnormalities.[3-6] The current target levels for specific serum lipids are listed in Table 12-1.

Total Cholesterol. The total cholesterol is the sum of the HDL, LDL, and VLDL cholesterol in the bloodstream. It is used as a starting point for lipid testing. If the total cholesterol is over 200 mg/dl, that is an indication to investigate the lipid profile and other risk factors for development of CAD.

HDL Cholesterol. HDL cholesterol is frequently described as the "good" cholesterol because higher serum levels exert a protective effect against acute atherosclerotic events. All the reasons are not completely understood, but one recognized physiologic effect is the ability of HDL to promote the efflux of cholesterol from cells. This process may minimize the accumulation of foam cells in the artery wall and thus decrease the risk of developing atherosclerosis.[7] High HDL levels confer both antiinflammatory and antioxidant benefits on the arterial wall.[7] In contrast, a low HDL level is an independent risk factor for the development of CAD and other atherosclerotic conditions. HDL cholesterol is generally higher in women and is raised by physical exercise and by stopping smoking. When lifestyle changes are ineffective in patients with low HDL cholesterol, the HDL level can be raised by drugs such as extended-release nicotinic acid (niacin) and fibrates.

LDL Cholesterol. LDL cholesterol is usually described as the "bad" cholesterol because high levels are associated with an increased risk of acute coronary syndrome, stroke, and peripheral arterial disease. High LDL levels initiate the atherosclerotic process by infiltrating the vessel wall and binding to the matrix of cells beneath the endothelial layer.[7] An individual's target LDL cholesterol level is determined according to his or her risk profile as described in Table 12-1. Some cardiologists advocate a reduction of the LDL goal to a range of 50 to 70 mg/dl for everyone, not only those with a known cardiovascular disease.[8]

Triglycerides. Triglycerides are serum lipids that constitute an additional and separate atherogenic risk factor. An optimal triglyceride level is below 150 mg/dl, and the more elevated the triglyceride serum level the higher the risk of developing coronary artery disease. A value from 150 to 199 mg/dl is borderline high; from 200 to 500 mg/dl is high; and a value above 500 mg/dl signals a high risk of atherogenic complications and a strong risk for the presence or development of type 2 diabetes.

Table 12-1

Lipid Guidelines and Coronary Artery Disease Risk

LIPID	TARGET VALUE*
Total cholesterol	Below 200 mg/dl
HDL cholesterol	Above 40 mg/dl for men Above 50 mg/dl for women
LDL cholesterol	Below 70 mg/dl if very high risk Below 100 mg/dl if high risk Below 130 mg/dl if low risk
VLDL cholesterol	Below 30 mg/dl
Triglycerides	Below 150 mg/dl

*Values outside the target range increase coronary artery disease risk.

HDL, High-density lipoprotein; *LDL*, low-density lipoprotein; *VLDL*, very-low-density lipoprotein.

High-Fat Diet

A diet rich in saturated fats will lead to elevated cholesterol levels in the blood. The first line of treatment to lower elevated serum cholesterol is a low-fat, high-fiber diet and increased physical exercise.[5,6] If these measures are not effective, lipid-lowering drugs are indicated.[1] This sounds simple in theory, but less than half of the people who qualify for lipid reduction therapy are actually taking their medications, only a third of treated patients reach their LDL target, and half of patients prescribed a lipid-lowering drug have stopped taking it 6 months later.[1] Although the drugs are very helpful for some, they are clearly not a panacea for everyone. A collaborative team approach to manage the interaction of diet, abnormal blood lipid levels, and use of medications is recommended.[9]

Obesity

Obesity is a disease of modern times. It is often associated with a sedentary lifestyle. It also increases susceptibility to the development of other risk factors, such as hypertension, decreased insulin sensitivity, and hyperlipidemia, with increased LDL and low HDL cholesterol levels.[10] In the United States, 122 million adults are overweight or obese.[11] Body weight is defined using the body mass index.

Body mass index (BMI) is a mathematic formula used to assess body weight relative to height. BMI is used to evaluate the threat of excess pounds as a risk factor for coronary artery disease and permits comparisons

Box 12-2

How to Calculate and Interpret Body Mass Index (BMI)

Use a Calculator

Metric

Divide body weight in kilograms by height in meters; divide the result again by height in meters.

Formula:

BMI = Weight in kilograms/(Height in meters) × (Height in meters)

Example: A person weighs 100 kg and is 1.91 m tall

BMI = 100 kg/(1.91 m) × (1.91 m) = 27.7

Pounds/Inches

Multiply weight in pounds by 703; divide the result by height in inches, then divide again by height in inches.

Formula:

BMI = Weight in pounds/(Height in inches) × (Height in inches) × 703

Example: A person weighs 222 pounds and is 6 feet 3 inches (75 inches) tall

BMI = 222 pounds/(75 inches) × (75 inches) × 703 = 27.7

How to Interpret the Body Mass Index Result

BMI (kg/m^2)	WEIGHT STATUS
Under 18.5	Underweight
18.5 to 24.9	Normal weight
25 to 29.5	Overweight
Over 30	Obese

of people of different gender, age, height, and body type.[1] BMI is calculated as the weight in kilograms divided by the square of the height in meters (kg/m^2). The BMI calculation in both metric and pounds/inches is shown in Box 12-2. A normal BMI is between 18.5 and 25 kg/m^2. A BMI between 25 and 30 kg/m^2 indicates the person is overweight. A BMI greater than 30 kg/m^2 is the definition of obesity.[4] A waist size greater than 40 inches in men and 35 inches in women increases CAD risk.[1]

Physical Inactivity

Regular vigorous physical activity using large muscle groups promotes physiologic adaptation to aerobic exercise that can prevent the development of coronary artery disease and reduce symptoms in patients with established cardiovascular disease.[12] Exercise will also reduce the incidence of many other diseases, including type 2 diabetes, osteoporosis, obesity, depression, and cancers of the colon and breast.[12] Multiple research trials have demonstrated the positive effects of physical activity on the other major cardiac risk factors.[12] Exercise alters the lipid profile by decreasing LDL cholesterol and triglycerides and increasing HDL cholesterol.[12] Exercise reduces insulin resistance at the cellular level, thus lowering the risk of developing type 2 diabetes, especially if combined with a weight-loss program.[12] Epidemiologic studies indicate that physical athletics as a young person do not confer protection in later years. Lifelong physical activity is necessary to prevent atherosclerotic coronary artery disease and stroke.[12]

Hypertension

Normal blood pressure is described as a systolic blood pressure (SBP) below 120 mm Hg and a diastolic blood pressure (DBP) below 80 mm Hg. *Hypertension* is defined as the elevation of either SBP greater than 140 mm Hg or DBP higher than 90 mm Hg. *Controlled hypertension* describes a situation in which administration of antihypertensive medications maintains the patient's blood pressure (BP) within the normal range. According to recent guidelines, the goal of treatment for the hypertensive person without other risk factors is to achieve a BP below 140/80 mm Hg. For the hypertensive person who already has diabetes or kidney disease, the target BP is lower, below 130/80 mm Hg. A normal BP is below 120/80 mm Hg.[11]

Prehypertension reflects an untreated systolic pressure of 120 to 139 mm Hg or an untreated diastolic pressure between 85 and 90 mm Hg.[11] In the United States this affects a huge number of people: one in five adults is prehypertensive.

Cigarette Smoking

The greater the number of cigarettes smoked per day, the greater the risk of developing CAD, acute myocardial infarction (MI), and stroke.[1,13,14] Cigarette smoking unfavorably alters serum lipid levels, decreases HDL cholesterol level, and increases LDL cholesterol and triglyceride levels. In the United States, smoking remains commonplace; 25% of men and 20% of women over 18 years of age smoke cigarettes. Passive, secondhand smoke exposure also increases cardiovascular risk, and 34.7% of nonsmoking adults are exposed to environmental tobacco smoke at home or at work.[1,13-15]

Diabetes Mellitus

Individuals with diabetes mellitus (types 1 and 2) have a higher incidence of coronary heart disease than the general population. Elevated blood glucose level is a known risk factor for development of vascular inflammation associated with atherosclerosis. The target range for normoglycemia is 70 to 110 mg/dl. It is recommended that patients in the intensive care unit (ICU) have blood glucose maintained within the normal range to decrease complications.[16]

Prediabetes. A fasting blood glucose between 110 and 125 mg/dl represents a prediabetic state and is a risk factor for the development of diabetes and CAD. The upper limit for normal fasting plasma glucose is 126 mg/dl. Patients with diabetes have an increased risk of developing coronary artery disease and have worse clinical outcomes following acute coronary syndrome events.[17] In a recent multinational study of patients who were seen at hospitals with symptoms of acute coronary syndrome, almost one in four had a known history of diabetes.[18]

Chronic Kidney Disease

Chronic kidney disease is considered a "risk equivalent" for coronary artery disease.[3,19] This means patients with chronic kidney disease have as much risk of experiencing a coronary event as if they already had CAD.[3,20] The risk of death for the patient with acute myocardial infarction rises as the serum creatinine level rises.[20] In one study the in-hospital mortality rates for patients with an acute MI was 2% for patients with normal kidney function, 6% for those with mild kidney failure, 14% for those with moderate kidney failure, 21% for those with severe kidney failure, and 30% for patients with end-stage kidney disease.[20]

Metabolic Syndrome

The metabolic syndrome is a combination of several key risk factors that unite to greatly increase the risk of developing CAD and type 2 diabetes. An estimated 47 million adults in the United States (23.7%) manifest measurable signs of metabolic syndrome.[1,5] The following are risk factors, and metabolic syndrome is diagnosed if three of the five are present:

1. Waist circumference is greater than 40 inches (102 cm) in men and greater than 35 inches (88 cm) in women.[21]
2. Serum triglyceride level is greater than 150 mg/dl (>1.7 mmol/L).[21]
3. HDL cholesterol level is less than 40 mg/dl (<1.04 mmol/L) in men, less than 50 mg/dl (<1.29 mmol/L) in women.[21]
4. BP is 130/85 mm Hg or higher. A BP of 130/85 mm Hg is diagnostic for prehypertension; A BP above 140/90 mm Hg is diagnostic for hypertension.[21]
5. Fasting glucose level is greater than 100 mg/dl. A fasting blood glucose between 100 and 110 mg/dl is diagnostic for prediabetes. A fasting blood glucose level greater than 126 mg/dl is diagnostic for diabetes.[21]

In the Framingham epidemiologic study, presence of the factors associated with metabolic syndrome predicted 25% of all new-onset CAD and almost 50% of new-onset diabetes.[21]

Women and Heart Disease—Premenopause and Postmenopause

Serious CAD symptoms occur approximately 5 years later in women than in men.[22] The average age for the first acute MI in men is 65.8 years and in women 70.4 years.[1] Incidence of coronary artery disease in women is two to three times higher in postmenopausal women compared with women who are premenopausal.[1] Thus in the past it had seemed logical to prescribe hormone replacement therapy (HRT) for postmenopausal women. However, well-designed research trials discovered an increase in cardiovascular events in the first year of HRT (estrogen plus progestin) replacement therapy, although cardiac events declined after the first year.[22,23] Subsequent studies have confirmed this result.[22] In 2004 the estrogen-only HRT trial was stopped by the National Institutes of Health (NIH) because of an increased risk of stroke in the women taking estrogen. For these reasons, HRT is no longer recommended for prevention of atherosclerotic cardiovascular disease.[24]

Cardiovascular disease kills more than half a million women annually in the United States. To emphasize the magnitude of the problem, this represents more deaths than the next seven fatal diseases for women combined and also exceeds the number of cardiovascular-related deaths in men each year.[25] Mortality rates for women after an acute MI are also higher than for men: 38% to 25%, respectively. Some of the reasons for the higher mortality are that women wait longer before seeking medical help, have smaller coronary arteries, are older when symptoms occur, and experience very different symptoms than men of the same age.[26]

Risk Equivalents

Certain medical conditions are considered "risk equivalents" of CAD. A *risk equivalent* means the person has the same risk of having an acute MI as if they actually had coronary heart disease already.[3] Two noncardiac medical conditions are considered risk equivalents for CAD: diabetes mellitus and chronic kidney disease. Peripheral arterial disease (PAD) and cerebral vascular disease are atherosclerotic conditions that are also considered CAD risk equivalents.

Multifactorial Risk

The major risk factors for developing CAD have been extensively documented in large epidemiologic studies: smoking, family history, adverse lipid profile, and elevated blood pressure.[3] Coronary artery disease has multifactorial causation; the greater the number of risk factors, the greater the risk of developing CAD.[1,3,21] The best time for an individual to make lifestyle changes is before symptoms of coronary artery disease occur. Patients with two or more risk factors or one or more of the "CAD risk equivalent diseases" have the greatest potential to benefit from risk factor reduction and lifestyle change.[3]

Primary Versus Secondary Prevention

If a person has symptoms of CAD or has previously had an acute coronary syndrome event, the goal of any lifestyle change or medication is termed *secondary prevention,* or preventing another heart attack.[27] If an individual matches the risk profile described in the previous pages, but does *not* have symptoms of CAD or has *not* had an acute MI, the treatment plan is described as *primary prevention.* The constellation of cardiac risk factors is now well established and is predictive for development of CAD for most populations in the developed industrial world.

Genetics

The role of genetic susceptibility to development of atherosclerotic disease in being actively investigated.[28] Most researchers are searching for genetic variants associated with the known risk factors described above. Some individuals may have a higher genetic predisposition than others, but the role of environmental risk factors remains very strong.

PATHOPHYSIOLOGY

Coronary heart disease is a progressive atherosclerotic disorder of the coronary arteries that results in narrowing or complete occlusion. *Atherosclerosis* affects the medium-size arteries that perfuse the heart and other major organs. Normal arterial walls are composed of three layers: the *intima* (inner lining), the *media* (middle muscular layer), and the *adventitia* (outer coat).

Development of Atherosclerosis

It is now well understood that atherosclerosis is a chronic inflammatory disorder that is characterized by an accumulation of macrophages and T lymphocytes in the arterial intimal wall. High LDL is one of the triggers of vascular inflammation. The inflammation injures the wall, allowing the LDL cholesterol to move into the vessel wall below the endothelial surface.[7] In addition, blood monocytes adhere to endothelial cells and migrate into the vessel wall. Within the artery wall, some monocytes differentiate into macrophages that unite with, and then internalize, LDL cholesterol. The *foam cells* that result are the marker cells of atherosclerosis.[7]

Elevated LDL cholesterol levels promote low-level endothelial inflammation that allows lipoproteins to infiltrate the intimal vessel wall. Once infiltrated under the endothelium, the LDL tends to stay within the vessel wall rather than return to the circulation.[7] This is in contrast to the actions of HDL cholesterol. HDL enters the vessel wall, helps efflux cholesterol from cells, and then returns to the circulation.[7] The actions of HDL may help minimize the number of foam cells in the artery wall.[7]

Atherosclerotic Plaque Rupture

When "mature" atherosclerotic plaque develops, it is not uniform in composition. It has a lipid liquid center filled with procoagulant factors. A connective tissue *fibrous cap* covers the top of the fluid lipid center.[3,29-31] The abrupt rupture of this cap allows procoagulant lipids to flood into the vessel lumen and rapidly form a coronary thrombosis as shown in Table 12-2. As the enlarging clot blocks blood flow through the coronary artery, a "heart attack" will occur unless there is adequate collateral circulation from other coronary vessels. Symptoms and suggested cardiac interventions at appropriate stages in development of CAD are listed in Table 12-2.

Plaque Regression

A reduction in blood cholesterol level decreases atherosclerotic plaque size by decreasing the amount of liquid cholesterol within the plaque core.[5] Lowering cholesterol levels will not change the dimensions of the fibrous or calcified portions of the plaque. However, lower cholesterol levels reduce vascular inflammation and make vulnerable plaque less likely to rupture.[3]

ACUTE CORONARY SYNDROMES

The term *acute coronary syndrome* (ACS) is used to describe the array of clinical presentations of coronary artery disease that range from unstable angina to acute MI, as shown in Table 12-2.[1,3,29] It is important to recognize that the general public and media describe an acute myocardial infarction as a "heart attack." The following section will initially discuss stable manifestations of CAD (stable angina) followed by a description of the acute manifestations (unstable angina and acute MI).

Angina

Angina pectoris, or chest pain, caused by myocardial ischemia is not a separate disease, but rather a symptom of CAD. It is caused by a blockage or spasm of a coronary artery, leading to diminished myocardial blood supply. The lack of oxygen causes myocardial ischemia, which is felt as chest pain. Angina may occur anywhere in the chest, neck, arms, or back, but the most commonly described location is pain or pressure behind the sternum. The pain often radiates to the left arm but can also radiate down both arms and to the back, the shoulder, the jaw, and/or the neck (Figure 12-1). Angina symptoms are not the same for all individuals. The presenting characteristics can be highly individualized, as described in Box 12-3. It is essential that patients and families are taught that angina does not always present in the dramatic "Hollywood heart attack" scenario seen on television and in movies, where the person clutches the throat or chest and exhibits extreme distress.[3]

Women and Angina. Many women experience a variety of different symptoms both before an acute MI and during the acute event as shown in Box 12-4.[30] The recognition and publicity about the fact that many

Table 12-2

Timeline of Atherogenesis From a Normal Artery Through Acute Myocardial Infarction Depicted by Longitudinal Section of an Artery, Plus Associated Symptoms and Interventions

ATHEROGENESIS-THROMBOGENESIS	ASSOCIATED SYMPTOMS	CARDIAC INTERVENTION
A. Normal artery, normal vessel wall.	A. No symptoms	A-C. Primary prevention of CAD recommended: low-fat diet, take regular physical exercise, avoid smoking, and achieve normal BMI
B. Lipids in bloodstream.	B. No symptoms	
C. Extracellular lipid accumulates in the intima of the artery (atheroma).	C. No symptoms	
D. Evolves to become a fatty-fibrous (atherosclerotic) lesion. Some lesions will contain a lipid interior covered by a fibrous cap.	D. May experience chest pain symptoms with exercise that are relieved by rest or NTG (stable angina); may have no symptoms at all until the lesion fills over 75% of the vessel lumen	D. PCI if stable angina present and CAD diagnosed by cardiac catheterization
E. Rupture of the cap allows the lipid in the center to be released into the bloodstream, stimulating clot formation (thrombogenesis).	E. Chest pain not relieved by rest, or NTG (ACS—unstable angina)	E. Call 911—immediate transport to a hospital, preferably one with experience treating ACS
F. Fresh clot blocks the vessel. Spasm of the artery may also occur near the thrombus.	F. Chest pain unrelieved by rest or NTG—severity, location of angina and associated symptoms vary greatly between individuals (ACS—acute MI)	F. Emergency intervention to open the artery: fibrinolytic or catheter-based procedure (PCI)
G. Vessel is open, but the atherosclerotic lesion remains.	G. No symptoms	G. Secondary prevention of CAD to prevent repeat MI; β-blockers to prevent arrhythmias; ACE-inhibitor drugs to prevent ventricular remodeling and heart failure; elective PCI

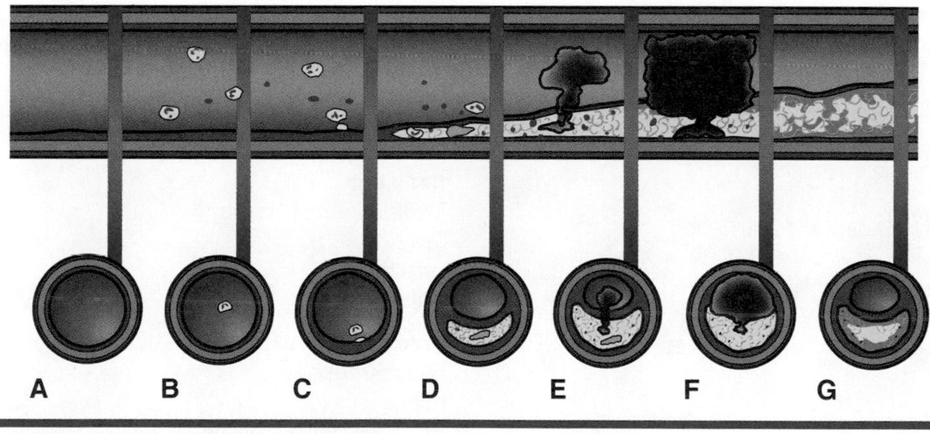

CAD, Coronary artery disease; *BMI,* body mass index; *NTG,* nitroglycerin; *PCI,* percutaneous coronary intervention; *ACS,* acute coronary syndrome; *MI,* myocardial infarction; *ACE,* Angiotensin-converting enzyme.
Figure modified from Antman EM et al: *Circulation* 110:588, 2004.

women do not experience "crushing chest pain" is important if women's symptoms are not to be trivialized by clinicians.[31] Ultimately, it is important that all patients are made aware of *angina symptom equivalents* such as unexpected shortness of breath, breaking out in a cold sweat, or sudden fatigue, nausea, or lightheadedness.[3]

Stable Angina. *Stable angina* is predictable and caused by similar precipitating factors each time; typically it is exercise induced. Patients become used to the pattern of this type of angina and may describe it as "my usual chest pain." Pain control is achieved by rest and by sublingual nitroglycerin within 5 minutes. Stable angina is the result of fixed lesions (blockages) of more than 75% of the coronary artery lumen. Ischemia and chest pain occur when myocardial demand from exertion exceeds the fixed blood oxygen supply.[4]

Unstable Angina. *Unstable angina* is defined as a change in a previously established stable pattern of angina. It is part of the continuum of ACS. Unstable angina usually is more intense than stable angina, may awaken the person from sleep, or may necessitate

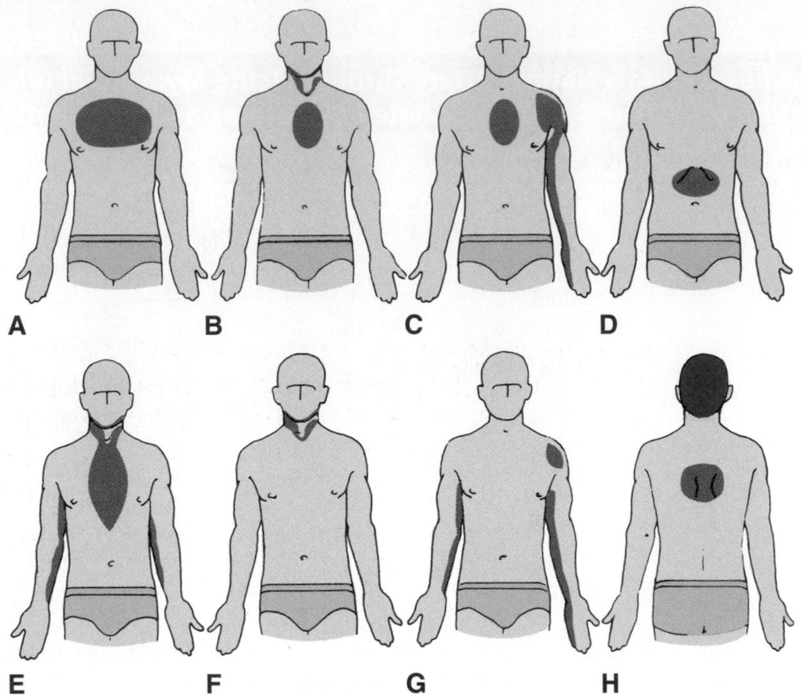

FIGURE 12-1. Common sites for anginal pain. **A,** Upper part of chest. **B,** Beneath sternum, radiating to neck and jaw. **C,** Beneath sternum, radiating down left arm. **D,** Epigastric. **E,** Epigastric, radiating to neck, jaw, and arms. **F,** Neck and jaw. **G,** Left shoulder; inner aspect of both arms. **H,** Intrascapular.

Box 12-3

Characteristics of Angina Pectoris

Location

Beneath sternum, radiating to neck and jaw
Upper chest
Beneath sternum, radiating down left arm
Epigastric
Epigastric, radiating to neck, jaw, and arms
Neck and jaw
Left shoulder, inner aspect of both arms
Intrascapular

Duration

Less than 5 minutes
Less than 5 minutes (stable)
Longer than 5 minutes or worsening symptoms without relief from rest or medication indicates unstable or preinfarction symptoms (unstable)

Quality

Sensation of pressure or heavy weight on the chest
Feeling of tightness, like a vise
Visceral quality (deep, heavy, squeezing, aching)
Burning sensation
Shortness of breath, with feeling of suffocation
Most severe pain ever experienced

Radiation

Medial aspect of left arm
Jaw
Left shoulder
Right arm

Precipitating Factors

Exertion/exercise
Cold weather
Exercising after a large, heavy meal
Walking against the wind
Emotional upset
Fright, anger
Coitus

Medication Relief

Usually within 45 seconds to 5 minutes of sublingual nitroglycerin administration

more than nitrates for pain relief. A change in the level or frequency of symptoms requires immediate medical evaluation. Severe angina that persists for more than 5 minutes, is worsening in intensity, and is not relieved by one nitroglycerin tablet is a medical emergency and the patient or a family member must call 911 immediately.[3] The 911 (emergency medical services [EMS]) system is available to 90% of the population of the United States.[3] In a recent study, patients with an acute MI who used 911 and were transported to the hospital by ambulance had significantly faster receipt of initial reperfusion therapies.[32] Family and friends are dis-

Box 12-4

Cardiovascular Symptoms Experienced by Women Before Acute Myocardial Infarction

SYMPTOMS 1 MONTH BEFORE ACUTE MI	SYMPTOMS DURING ACUTE MI
Unusual fatigue (71%)	Shortness of breath (58%)
Sleep disturbance (48%)	Weakness (55%)
Shortness of breath (42%)	Unusual fatigue (43%)
Indigestion (39%)	Cold sweat (39%)
Anxiety (36%)	Dizziness (39%)
Heart racing (27%)	Nausea (36%)
Arms weak/heavy (25%)	Arm heaviness or weakness (35%)
Changes in thinking or memory (24%)	Ache in arms (32%)
	Heat/flushing (32%)
Vision change (23%)	Indigestion (31%)
Loss of appetite (22%)	Pain centered high in chest (31%)
Hands/arms tingling (22%)	Heart racing (23%)
Difficulty breathing at night (19%)	

From McSweeney JC et al: *Circulation* 108(21):2619, 2003.
MI, Myocardial infarction.

couraged from driving a person experiencing unstable angina to the hospital and instead are encouraged to call 911. Patients should be instructed never to drive themselves but to call EMS via 911.

Unstable angina is an indication of atherosclerotic plaque instability. It can signal atherosclerotic plaque rupture and thrombus formation that can lead to myocardial infarction. The patient who comes to the emergency department with recent onset of unstable angina but who has nonspecific or nonelevated ST-segment changes on the 12-lead electrocardiogram (ECG) should be evaluated according to the latest clinical guidelines, because not all patients who experience an acute MI have ST elevation on the 12-lead ECG.[29]

Medical Management

Accurate assessment of chest pain symptoms is essential if unstable angina is to be recognized and treated effectively. An important reason to ask questions about the chest pain is to differentiate between stable and unstable angina. The change from stable to unstable angina is potentially life-threatening for the patient. If the ST segments are elevated or there is a newly documented left bundle branch block on the 12-lead ECG, the patient will be treated for acute MI.[3] However, if these classic ECG signs are missing and the chest pain continues, the current pharmacologic treatments of choice are aspirin, vasodilation by nitroglycerin, intravenous (IV) antiplatelet agents such as the glycoprotein (GP) IIb/IIIa-inhibitors, and IV unfractionated heparin (UFH).[29] Low-molecular-weight heparin (LMWH) combined with fibrinolysis is an alternative to heparin-fibrinolysis for patients under 75 years of age with a serum creatinine level below 2.5 mg/dl for men and below 2 mg/dl for women.[3]

Another option is to take the patient directly to the cardiac catheterization laboratory for direct visualization of the coronary arteries by the cardiologist. Recanalization of the coronary arteries is recommended, provided the institution performs more than 200 procedures annually or the individual physician performs more than 75 interventional procedures annually.[3,29]

Box 12-5

NURSING DIAGNOSIS PRIORITIES

Coronary Artery Disease and Angina

- Acute Pain related to transmission and perception of cutaneous, visceral, muscular, or ischemic impulses, p. A-7
- Ineffective Cardiopulmonary Tissue Perfusion related to decreased myocardial oxygen supply and/or increased myocardial oxygen demand, p. A-35
- Activity Intolerance related to cardiopulmonary dysfunction, p. A-2
- Powerlessness related to lack of control over current situation, p. A-44
- Anxiety related to threat to biologic, psychologic, and/or social integrity, p. A-9
- Deficient Knowledge: Discharge Regimen related to lack of previous exposure to information, p. A-18
- Readiness for Enhanced Therapeutic Regimen Management

Nursing Management

Nursing management of the patient with CAD and angina incorporates a variety of nursing diagnoses (Box 12-5)**. Nursing priorities focus on (1) identifying myocardial ischemia, (2) relieving chest pain, (3) maintaining a calm environment, and (4) providing patient education.**

Identifying Myocardial Ischemia

Complaints of chest discomfort (angina) must be evaluated quickly, because angina is an indicator of myocardial ischemia (see Box 12-3). The patient is asked to rate the intensity of the chest discomfort on a scale of 0 to 10. The words "chest pain" are not to be used exclusively, because some patients describe their angina as "pressure" or "heaviness." It is important to document the characteristics of the pain and the patient's heart rate and rhythm, blood pressure, respirations, temperature, skin color, peripheral pulses, urine output, mentation, and overall tissue perfusion. A 12-lead ECG is used to identify the area of ischemic myocardium. The major concern is that the chest pain may represent preinfarction angina, and early identification is essential so that the patient can be immediately treated. This may include transfer to the cardiac catheterization laboratory for a coronary arteriogram and opening of a blocked artery. Or, if the hospital does not have a cardiac catheterization laboratory, GP IIb/IIIa receptor–blockers may be infused to prevent the evolution of the acute MI before transfer.[3,29]

Relieving Chest Pain

In the critical care unit, control of angina is achieved by a combination of supplemental oxygen, nitrates, analgesia, and surveillance of the angina and of the effects of pharmacologic therapy.

1. *Oxygen:* All patients with acute ischemic pain are administered supplemental oxygen to increase myocardial oxygenation. Use of pulse oximetry is recommended to guide therapy and maintain oxygen saturation above 90%.[3] Those patients who develop symptoms of acute heart failure may require emergency intubation and mechanical ventilation to correct significant hypoxemia.[3,29]
2. *Nitrates:* A combination of intravenous and sublingual nitroglycerin is used to vasodilate the coronary arteries and decrease pain. After nitrate administration, the critical care nurse closely observes the patient for relief of chest pain, for return of the ST segment to baseline, and for the potential development of unwanted side effects such as hypotension and headache. Avoid administration of a nitrate if the SBP is below 90 mm Hg or if a male patient has recently taken a phosphodiesterase-inhibitor drug (e.g., Viagra).[3,29]
3. *Analgesia:* Morphine 2 to 4 mg IV is the analgesic opiate of choice for preinfarction angina. It both relieves pain and decreases fear and anxiety. After administration, the critical care nurse assesses the patient for pain relief and the development of unwanted side effects such as hypotension and respiratory depression.[3,29]
4. *Aspirin:* Chewing an oral non–enteric-coated aspirin (162 to 325 mg) at the beginning of chest pain has been shown to reduce mortality. The nonenteric formulation is preferred because it increases absorption in the mouth when chewed, not swallowed.[3,29]

Maintaining a Calm Environment

Patients admitted to a critical care unit with unstable angina experience extreme anxiety and fear of death. The critical care nurse is faced with the challenge of ensuring that the elements of a calm environment that will alleviate the patient's fear and anxiety are maintained, while being ready at all times to respond to an acute emergency, such as a cardiac arrest, or to assist with emergency intubation or insertion of hemodynamic monitoring catheters.

Providing Patient Education

In the critical care unit, the patient's ability to retain educational information is severely affected by stress and pain. It is essential to teach avoidance of the *Valsalva maneuver,* which is defined as forced expiration against a closed glottis. This can be explained to the patient as "bearing down" when going to the bathroom or breath holding when repositioning in bed. The Valsalva maneuver causes an increase in intrathoracic pressure that decreases venous return to the right side of the heart and is associated with low blood pressure and symptomatic bradycardia.

Once the anginal pain is controlled, longer-term patient and family education can begin. Points to cover include risk factor modification, signs and symptoms of angina, when to call the physician, medications, and dealing with emotions and stress. However, because the acute hospital length of stay for uncomplicated angina is usually less than 3 days, referral to a cardiac rehabilitation program for a controlled exercise program and risk factor modification after discharge is perhaps the most helpful teaching intervention a critical care nurse can provide. Clinical practice guidelines for the management of coronary artery disease and stable angina are listed in Evidence-Based Collaborative Management: Coronary Artery Disease and Stable Angina.

MYOCARDIAL INFARCTION

Description and Etiology

Myocardial infarction (MI) is the term used to describe irreversible myocardial necrosis (cell death) that results from an abrupt decrease or total cessation of coronary blood flow to a specific area of the myocardium.[1] In the hospital this is often referred to as an "acute MI," indicating both the sudden onset and the life-threatening nature of the event. Increasingly, an acute MI is described in relation to whether there was ST elevation on the diagnostic 12-lead ECG. Thus it may be labeled an acute *non–ST-elevation MI* (NSTEMI)[33] or an acute *ST-elevation MI* (STEMI).[3]

The three mechanisms that block the coronary artery and are responsible for the acute reduction in oxygen delivery to the myocardium are the following:

1. Plaque rupture
2. New coronary artery thrombosis
3. Coronary artery spasm close to the ruptured plaque

Myocardial tissue can best be salvaged within the first 2 hours (120 minutes) after the onset of anginal symptoms as illustrated in Figure 12-2.[3] The earlier the myocardium is revascularized, the better the survival.[33] Unfortunately, many persons do not seek treatment until the acute phase has passed.[3]

Pathophysiology

Ischemia

The outer region of the infarcted myocardial area is the *zone of ischemia,* as illustrated in Figure 12-3. It

EVIDENCE-BASED COLLABORATIVE MANAGEMENT

Coronary Artery Disease and Stable Angina

Summary of Evidence-Based Recommendations for Management of Coronary Artery Disease and Stable Angina

Strong Evidence the Following Lifestyle Interventions Are Helpful to Prevent CAD:

- Diet
  - Low-salt, high-fiber, fruit, vegetables, grains
  - All dietary fat less than 30% of total calories
  - Multivitamin if homocysteine level elevated
  - Limit sugary foods
  - Limit calories if overweight
  - Omega-3 fatty acids included in diet
- Exercise
  - Start by walking more, and increase physical exercise from there
  - Refer to cardiac rehabilitation program
- Obesity
  - Achieve healthy body weight
- Addiction
  - Stop cigarette smoking
  - Limit alcohol intake

Strong Evidence the Following Diagnostic Procedures Are Helpful for the Patient With Angina:

- When a patient is first seen with chest pain, quickly obtaining a detailed history of symptoms, focused physical examination, and risk factor assessment can help determine whether the probability of coronary artery disease (CAD) is low, intermediate, or high.
- Initial laboratory tests include hemoglobin, fasting blood glucose, lipid panel.
- Baseline 12-lead ECG at rest, even if chest pain not present.
- Obtain 12-lead ECG during any episode of chest pain.
- Chest x-ray if symptoms of heart failure are present.
- Exercise 12-lead ECG if condition stable and symptoms suggestive of CAD; or if condition stable with complete right bundle branch block or complete left bundle branch block that makes the ECG difficult to interpret for ischemia.
- Cardiac echocardiography for patients with a systolic murmur suggestive of aortic stenosis.
- Cardiac echocardiography to determine extent of left ventricular (LV) hypertrophy or dysfunction.
- Stress cardiac echocardiography recommended for patient with greater than 1 mm ST-segment depression at rest (stress may be by physical exercise or by pharmacologic stimulation).
- Coronary angiography (typically as part of a cardiac catheterization procedure) is recommended for patients at high risk of adverse coronary events.

Initial Pharmacologic and Lifestyle Treatment Recommendations

- The goal of treatment is to eliminate chest pain.
- The ten most important elements of CAD and stable angina management can be remembered using the A-to-E mnemonic:

  A Aspirin and anti-anginals
  B β-Blocker and blood pressure
  C Cholesterol and cigarettes
  D Diet and diabetes
  E Education and exercise

  The above translates to the following: daily (low-dose) 75-325 mg aspirin; oral nitrates, sublingual nitroglycerin for episodes of angina; β-blockers to decrease LV workload and decrease blood pressure to less than 130/80 mm Hg; and diet or lipid reduction drug therapy (statin) to lower low-density lipoprotein cholesterol (LDL-C) to below 100 mg/dl (LDL-C to below 70 mg/dl if patient at very high risk), increase HDL-C above 40 mg/dl for men, and above 50 mg/dl for women, and reduce triglycerides below 150 mg/dl. Always ask about tobacco use, recommend strongly stopping smoking, encourage nicotine replacement therapy (nicotine patches or gum) as needed; low fat, calorie appropriate diet, nutritional consult as needed; fasting blood glucose 70-100 mg/dl; hemoglobin $A1_C$ below 7%; education about risk factor modification and the CAD disease process; recommend daily exercise for 30-60 minutes (ideal) or at least 3-4 times a week; achieve a BMI between 18.5-24.9 kg/m^2, waist less than 40 inches for men and 35 inches for women. Treat depression if present, hormone replacement therapy is not recommended as a treatment for symptoms of coronary heart disease.

Interventional vs. Surgical Recommendations for Stable High-Risk Patients

Patients are "risk stratified" according to their symptoms and the results of cardiac diagnostic tests.

- Percutaneous catheter interventions (PCI)
  - Angioplasty, atherectomy, stent
  - PCI is more frequently performed than open heart surgery for relief of anginal symptoms
- Coronary artery bypass surgery
  - For patients with left main occlusion or multivessel disease
  - For patients with two-vessel disease with significant proximal LAD stenosis and LV ejection fraction below 50%

Data from Gibbons RJ et al: *Circulation* 107(1):149, 2003; and Mosca L et al: *Circulation* 109(5):672, 2004.
ECG, Electrocardiogram; *BMI,* body mass index; *LAD,* left anterior descending; *PCI,* percutaneous coronary artery.

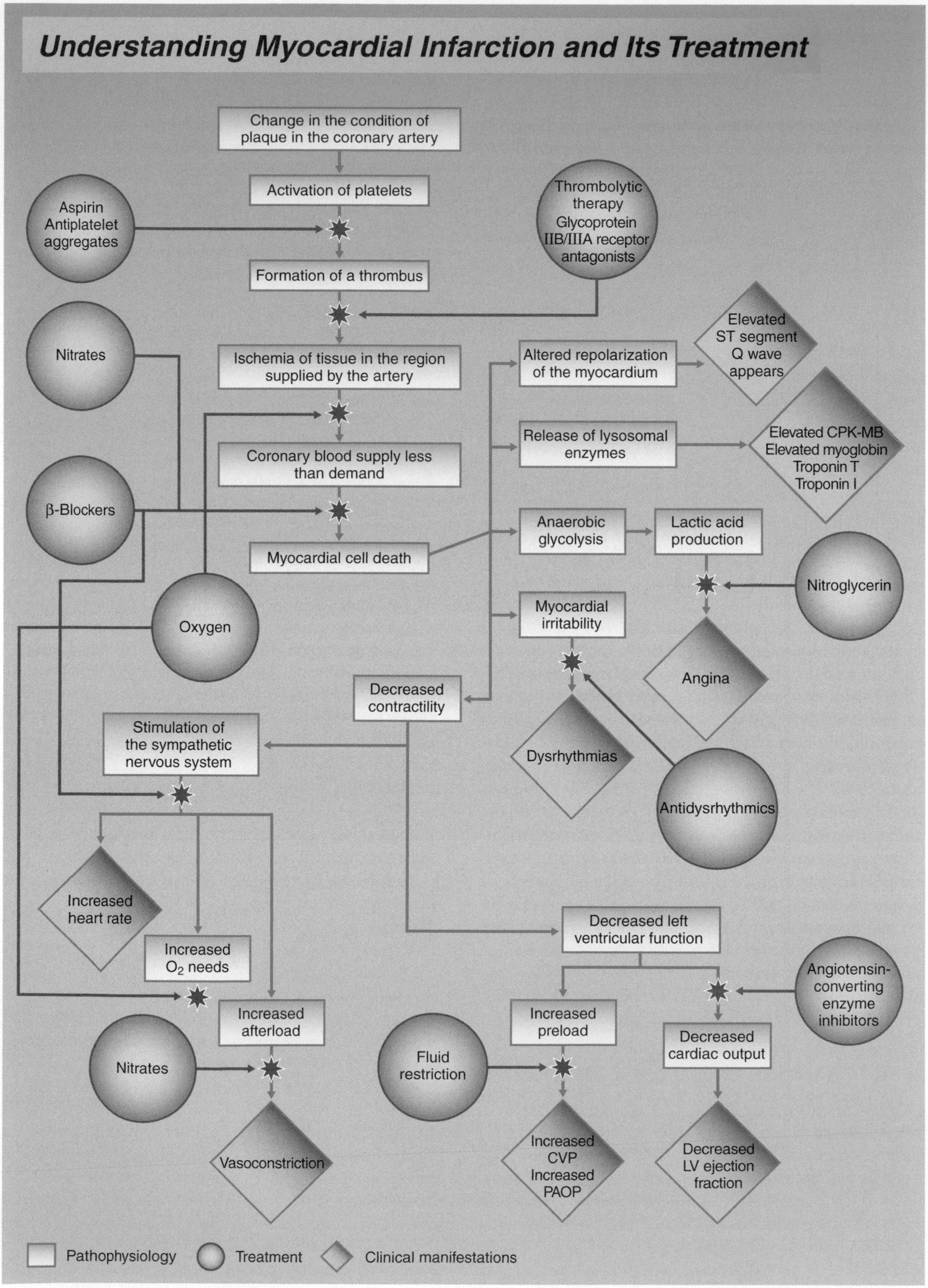
Understanding Myocardial Infarction and Its Treatment
Change in the condition of plaque in the coronary artery
Activation of platelets
Aspirin Antiplatelet aggregates
Thrombolytic therapy Glycoprotein IIB/IIIA receptor antagonists
Formation of a thrombus
Nitrates
Ischemia of tissue in the region supplied by the artery
Altered repolarization of the myocardium
Elevated ST segment Q wave appears
Release of lysosomal enzymes
Elevated CPK-MB Elevated myoglobin Troponin T Troponin I
Coronary blood supply less than demand
β-Blockers
Anaerobic glycolysis
Lactic acid production
Myocardial cell death
Nitroglycerin
Oxygen
Myocardial irritability
Angina
Decreased contractility
Stimulation of the sympathetic nervous system
Dysrhythmias
Antidysrhythmics
Increased heart rate
Increased O2 needs
Decreased left ventricular function
Angiotensin-converting enzyme inhibitors
Increased afterload
Nitrates
Fluid restriction
Increased preload
Decreased cardiac output
Vasoconstriction
Increased CVP Increased PAOP
Decreased LV ejection fraction
Pathophysiology
Treatment
Clinical manifestations

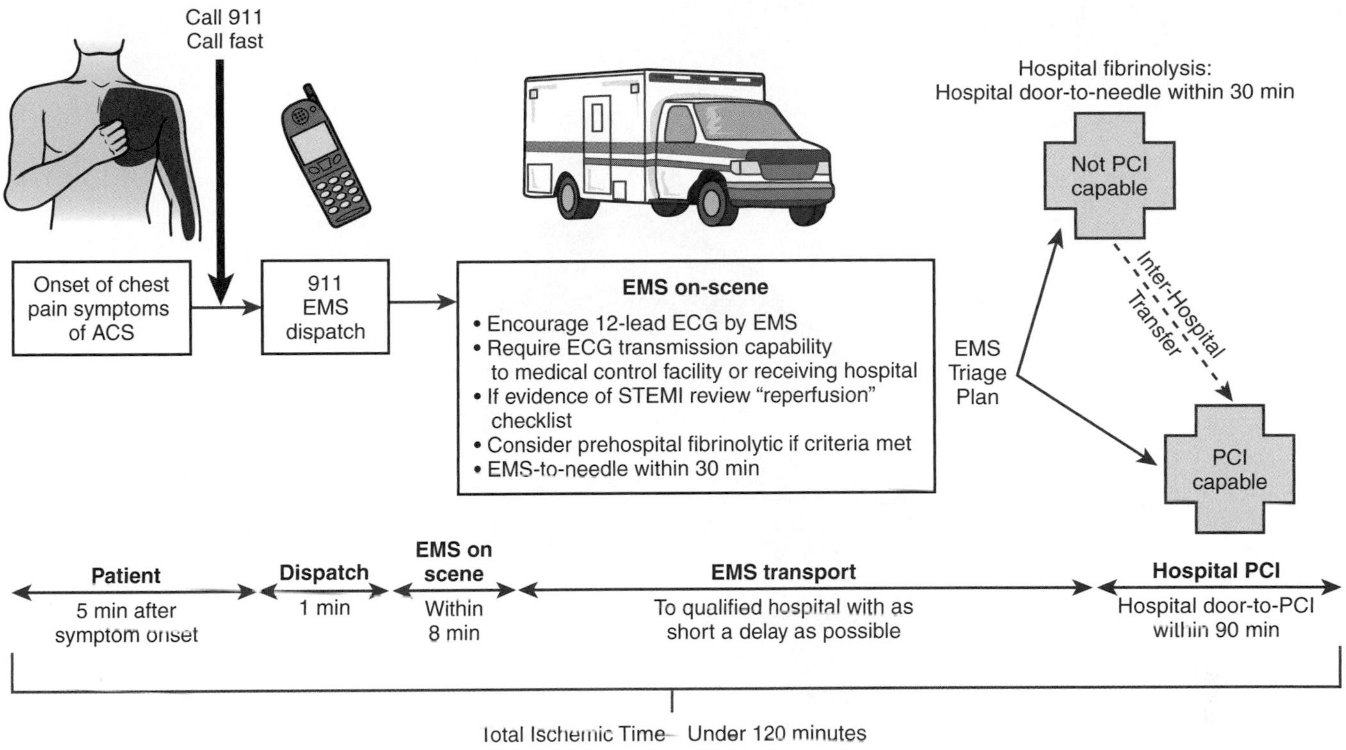

FIGURE 12-2. Prehospital chest pain/ACS evaluation and treatment options. *ACS,* Acute coronary syndrome; *EMS,* emergency medical services; *ECG,* electrocardiogram; *STEMI,* ST-elevation myocardial infarction; *PCI,* percutaneous coronary intervention. (Modified from Antman EM et al: *Circulation* 110[5]:588, 2004.)

is composed of viable cells. Priority interventions are targeted to save this viable muscle. Repolarization in this zone is temporarily impaired but eventually will be restored to normal. Repolarization of the cells in this area manifests as T-wave inversion (Figure 12-4, *B*).

Injury

The infarcted zone is surrounded by injured but still potentially viable tissue in an area known as the *zone of injury* (see Figure 12-3). Cells in this area do not fully repolarize because of the deficient blood supply. This is recorded on the ECG as elevation of the ST segment (Figure 12-4, *C*).

Infarction

The area of dead muscle (necrosis) in the myocardium is known as the *zone of infarction* (see Figure 12-3). On the ECG, evidence of this zone is seen by new pathologic Q waves, which reflect a lack of depolarization from the cardiac surface involved in the MI (Figure 12-4, *D*). As healing takes place, the cells in this area are replaced by scar tissue.

Transmural MI or Q-Wave MI

Myocardial infarctions are classified according to their location on the myocardial surface and the muscle layers affected. Not all infarctions cause necrosis in all layers, as shown in Figure 12-5. A transmural MI involves all three cardiac layers—the *endocardium,* the *myocardium,* and the *epicardium.* A transmural (full-thickness) MI usually provokes significant ECG changes, as shown in Figure 12-4. This is also described as a *Q-wave MI.* It is important to be aware that not every acute MI produces a recognizable series of Q waves on the 12-lead ECG. In addition, some patients who had a demonstrated Q wave on a 12-lead ECG as a result of an acute MI lose the Q wave months or years later. The reasons for this are not yet known, but it may represent the development of collateral circulation.

12-Lead Electrocardiographic Changes

The ECG changes produced by a transmural infarction demonstrate alteration in both myocardial depolarization (QRS complex) and repolarization (ST segment). The changes in repolarization are seen by the presence of new Q waves. These new, pathologic Q waves are deeper and wider than tiny Q waves found on the normal 12-lead ECG.[3]

Location

The location of infarction is determined by correlating the ECG leads with Q waves and the ST-segment T-wave abnormalities (Table 12-3). Infarction most commonly affects the left ventricle and the interventricular septum; however, the right ventricle can also

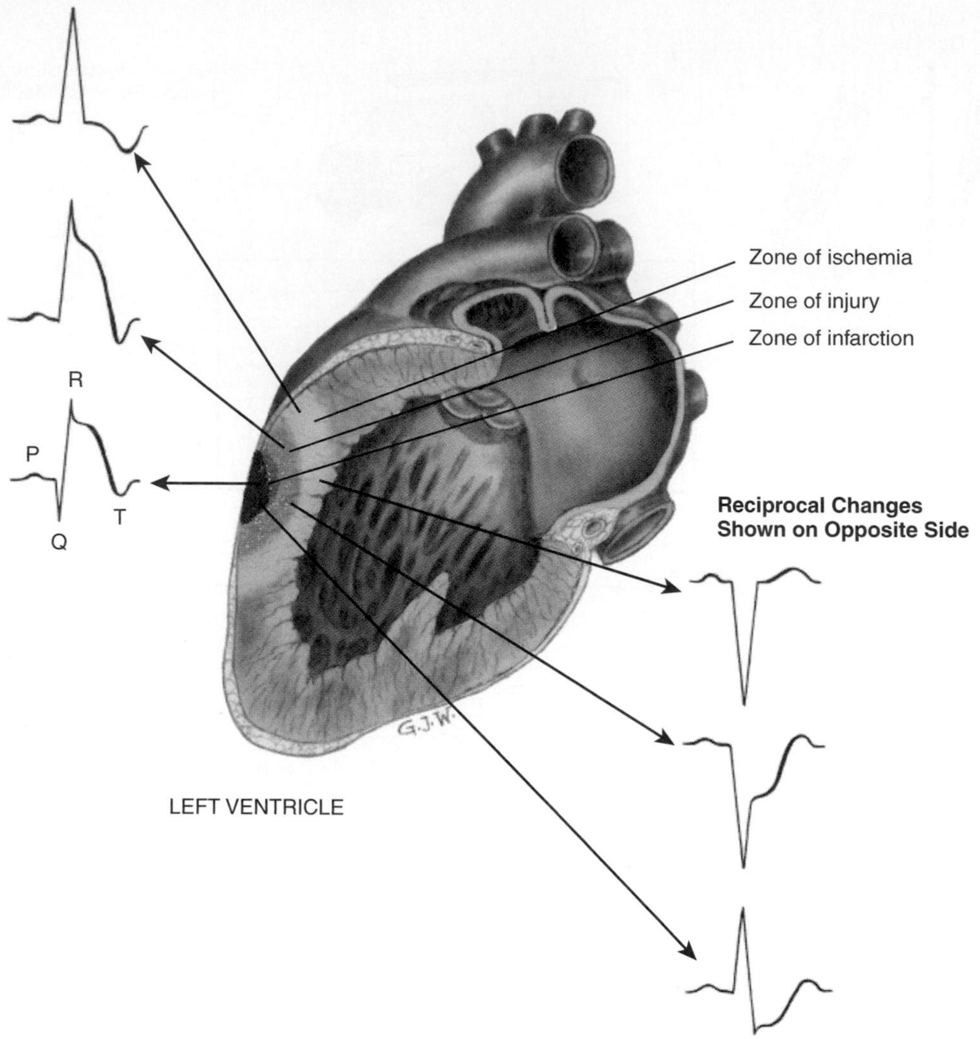

FIGURE 12-3. Zone of ischemia, zone of injury, and zone of infarction, shown through electrocardiogram waveforms and reciprocal waveforms corresponding to each zone.

Table 12-3

Correlations Among Ventricular Surfaces, Electrocardiographic Leads, and Coronary Arteries

SURFACE OF LEFT VENTRICLE	ELECTROCARDIOGRAPHIC LEADS	CORONARY ARTERY USUALLY INVOLVED
Inferior	II, III, aV_F	Right coronary artery
Lateral	V_5-V_6, I, aV_L	Left circumflex
Anterior	V_2-V_4	Left anterior descending
Anterior lateral	V_1-V_6, I, aV_L	Left main coronary artery
Septal	V_1-V_2	Left anterior descending
Posterior	V_1-V_2	Left circumflex or right coronary artery (reciprocal changes)
	V_7-V_9 (direct)	

be infracted and many patients who sustain an inferior MI have some right ventricular damage. The ECG manifestations that are used to diagnose an MI and pinpoint the area of damaged ventricle include inverted T waves, ST-segment elevation, and pathologic Q waves in specific lead groupings as described below.

Anterior Wall Infarction. Anterior wall infarction results from occlusion of the proximal left anterior descending (LAD) artery (see Table 12-3). ST-segment elevation is expected in leads V_1 through V_4 on the 12-lead ECG as shown in Figure 12-6. If the left main coronary artery is occluded, the ECG manifestations will involve almost all of the precordial leads V_1 to V_6 and leads I and aV_L (see Table 12-3). These specific groups of ECG changes that help to locate the part of the heart that is infarcting are termed *indicative changes.* A large anterior wall MI may be associated with left ventricular (LV) pump failure, cardiogenic shock, or death.[3]

Left Lateral Wall Infarction. Left lateral wall infarction occurs as a result of occlusion of the circumflex

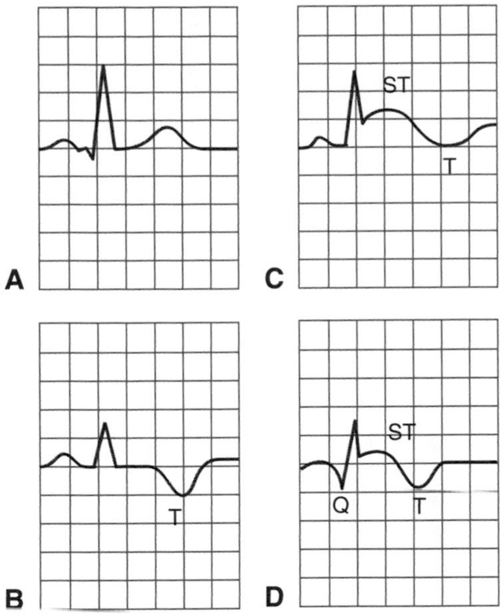

FIGURE 12-4. Electrocardiogram (ECG) changes indicative of ischemia, injury, and infarction (necrosis) of the myocardium. **A,** Normal ECG. **B,** Ischemia indicated by inversion of the T wave. **C,** Ischemia and current of injury indicated by T-wave inversion and ST-segment elevation. The ST segment may be elevated above or depressed below the baseline, depending on whether the tracing is from a lead facing toward or away from the infarcted area and depending on whether epicardial or endocardial injury occurs. Epicardial injury causes ST elevation in leads facing the epicardium. **D,** Ischemia, injury, and myocardial necrosis. The Q wave indicates necrosis of the myocardium.

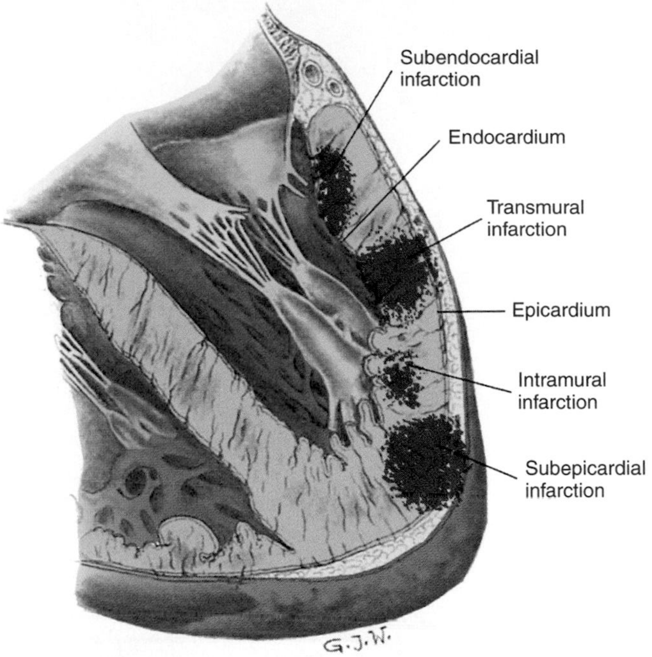

FIGURE 12-5. Location of infarctions in myocardium.

coronary artery. On a 12-lead ECG, new Q waves and ST-segment T-wave changes are seen in leads I, aV_L, V_5, and V_6 as shown in Figure 12-7. In reality, few patients present with only lateral wall ECG changes, and some anterior wall leads (V_3 and V_4) may also show evidence of injury or infarction.

Inferior Wall Infarction. Inferior wall infarction occurs with occlusion of the right coronary artery (RCA). This infarction is manifested by ECG changes in leads II, III, and aV_F as shown in Figure 12-8. Conduction disturbances are expected with an inferior wall MI and are related to the anatomy of the coronary arterial supply. Because the RCA perfuses the sinoatrial (SA) node in just over half of the population and also supplies the proximal bundle of His and atrioventricular (AV) node in over 90% of individuals, heart block and other conduction disturbances should be anticipated. Inferior wall MI carries a mortality of about 6%. If the right ventricle is involved, mortality rises to 25% to 30%.[3]

Right Ventricular Infarction. Infarction of the right ventricle (RV) occurs when there is a blockage in a proximal section of the right coronary artery. This places all of the right ventricle and the inferior wall at risk. RV ischemia can be demonstrated in up to half of inferior wall STEMIs, although only 10% to 15% show the hemodynamic abnormalities associated with classic RV infarction.[3] If massive RV infarction occurs, the patient can suffer cardiogenic shock, which carries over 50% mortality in this population.[33]

Posterior Wall Infarction. Infarction in the posterior wall can occur because of a blockage either in the right coronary artery or in the circumflex artery. This is because both arteries supply this section of the heart, although the RCA is generally the dominant vessel. A posterior wall MI is difficult to detect but may be identified by either specific leads placed in the left scapular area or by very tall R waves in leads V_1 and V_2.

Non–ST-Segment Elevation MI

The 12-lead ECG is a highly useful diagnostic tool. For many years it was considered the "gold standard" when diagnosing an acute MI. Now it is known that the *ST segment* is not elevated in every acute MI. One reason for the lack of ST-segment elevation may be that the infarction and subsequent necrosis are not full thickness. Because some of the muscle in the area can still be depolarized, ST elevation may not occur. This type of MI is also less likely to develop Q waves on a subsequent 12-lead ECG once the acute phase has passed. This situation is diagnostically known as a *non–ST-segment elevation MI* (NSTEMI).[29] This condition has previously been described by several names, including *nontransmural MI; non–Q-wave MI,* or *subendocardial MI.* Because patients who sustain an NSTEMI do have CAD, it is important that they be treated aggressively to minimize the size of the infarcted area.[29] Without the visual clue of the ST-segment elevation on the 12-lead ECG, the patients cannot receive imme-

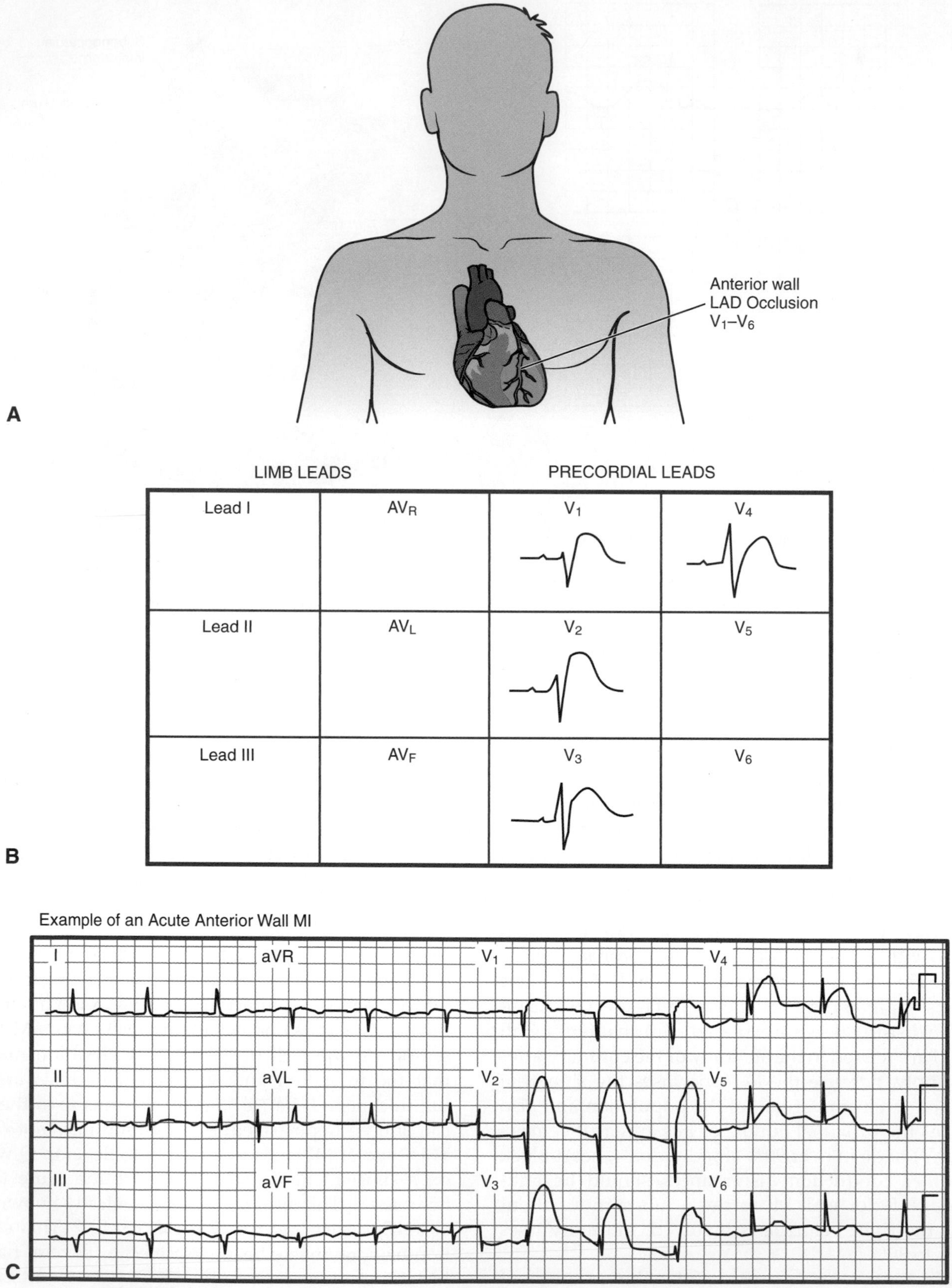

FIGURE 12-6. Twelve-lead electrocardiogram (ECG)—changes with anterior wall ST-elevation myocardial infarction (STEMI). **A,** Myocardial infarction (MI) location on cardiac wall. **B,** ECG leads with expected ST-segment elevation. **C,** Twelve-lead ECG from patient experiencing left anterior wall STEMI.

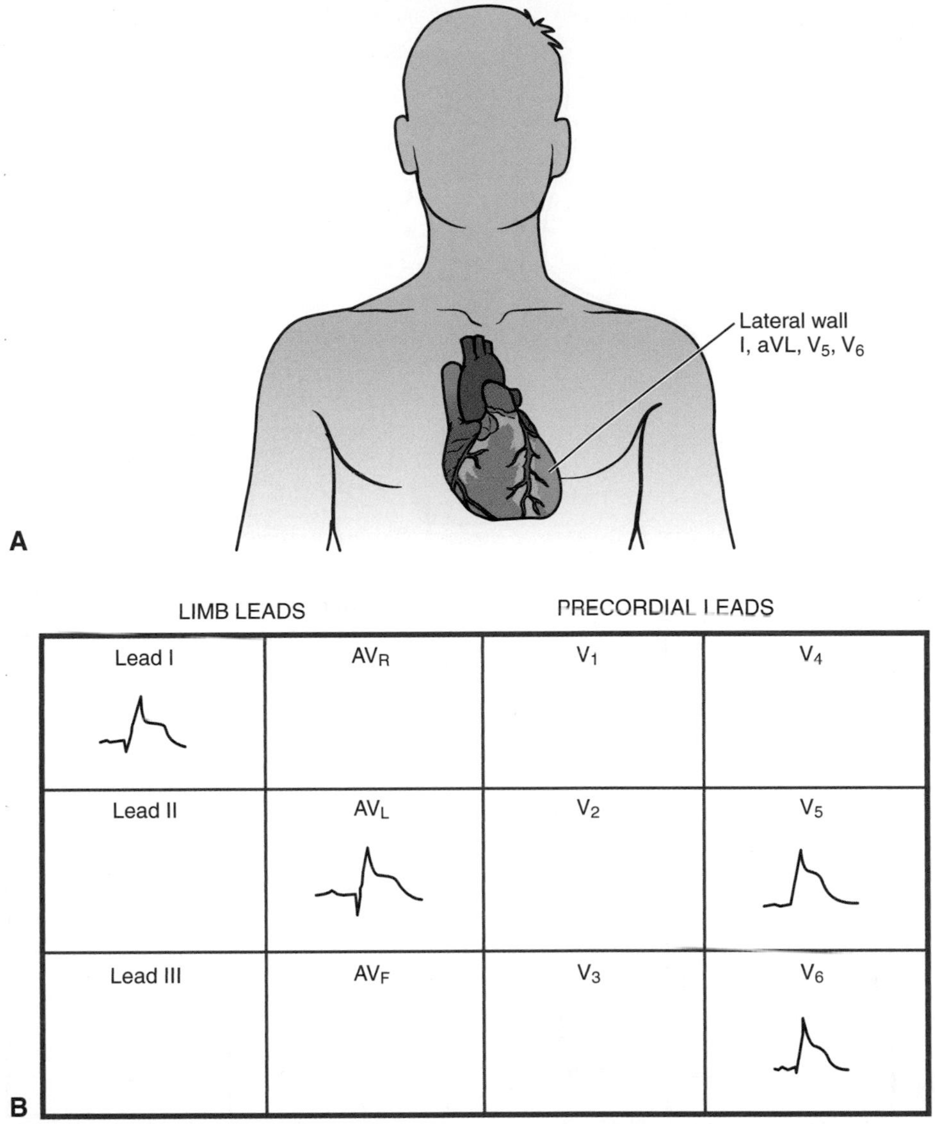

FIGURE 12-7. Twelve-lead electrocardiogram (ECG)—changes with lateral wall ST-elevation myocardial infarction (STEMI). **A,** Myocardial infarction (MI) location on cardiac wall. **B,** ECG leads with expected ST-segment elevation.

diate IV fibrinolytic agents, but they can be appropriately managed in an interventional catheterization laboratory and receive GP IIb/IIIa-inhibitor therapy as illustrated in the timeline in Figure 12-2. The 12-lead ECG plays a vital role in identifying the treatment plan for an acute coronary syndrome. ST elevation is helpful when present, but it would be a mistake to believe that if the ST is not elevated the patient is not in danger of myocardial infarction.

Cardiac Biomarkers During MI

In the presence of damaged or necrosed myocardial muscle cells, cardiac biomarkers are released. These biomarkers were previously called "cardiac enzymes." To confirm the diagnosis of acute MI, the serum biomarkers CK-MB and either troponin I or troponin T are measured. If the coronary artery is opened by fibrinolytic therapy or a percutaneous coronary intervention (PCI) the biomarkers exhibit a more rapid rise and dramatic fall as shown in Figure 12-9.

Complications With Acute MI

Many patients experience complications occurring either early or late in the postinfarction course. These complications may result from electrical dysfunction or from a pump problem. Electrical dysfunctions include bradycardia, bundle branch blocks, and varying degrees of heart block. Pumping complications cause heart failure, pulmonary edema, and cardiogenic shock.[3]

Sinus Bradycardia. Sinus bradycardia (heart rate less than 60 beats/min) occurs in 30% to 40% of patients who sustain an acute MI.[3] It is more prevalent with an inferior wall infarction in the first hour following

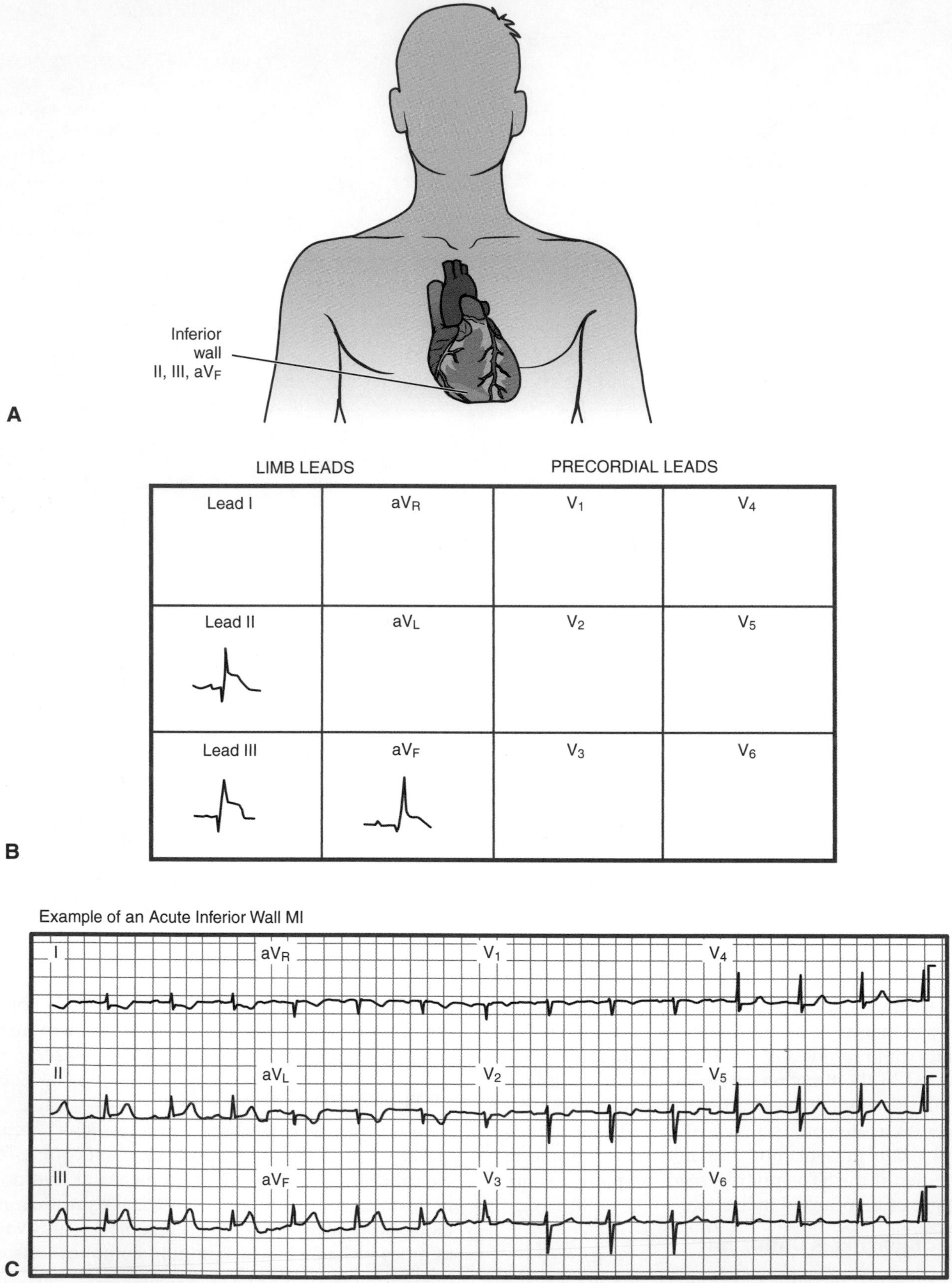

FIGURE 12-8. Twelve-lead electrocardiogram (ECG)—changes with inferior wall ST-elevation myocardial infarction (STEMI). **A,** Myocardial infarction (MI) location on cardiac wall. **B,** ECG leads with expected ST-segment elevation. **C,** Twelve-lead ECG from patient experiencing inferior wall STEMI.

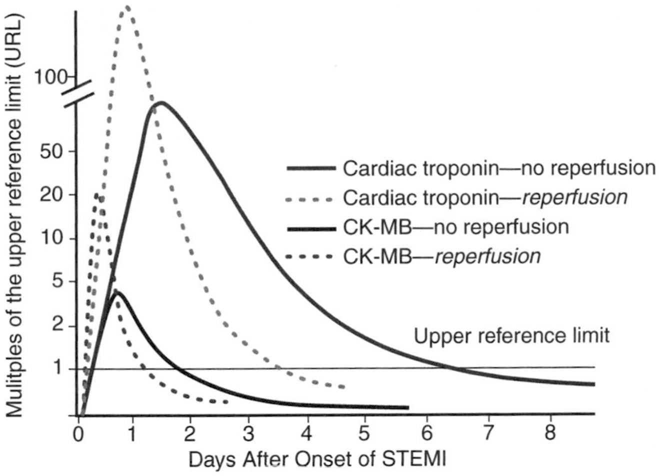

FIGURE 12-9. Cardiac biomarkers during myocardial infarction (MI). *STEMI*, ST-elevation myocardial infarction. (From ACC/AHA guidelines for the management of patients with ST-elevation myocardial infarction—executive summary: a report of the American College of Cardiology/American Heart Association Task Force on Practice Guidelines [Writing Committee to Revise the 1999 Guidelines for the Management of Patients With Acute Myocardial Infarction], *Circulation* 110[9]:e82, 2004).

STEMI.[3] Symptomatic bradycardia with hypotension and low cardiac output is treated with atropine 0.6 to 1.0 mg IV push, repeated every 5 minutes to a maximum dose of 0.04 mg/kg (e.g., 2 mg for a person who weighs 50 kg).[3]

Sinus Tachycardia. Sinus tachycardia (heart rate more than 100 beats/min) most often occurs with an anterior wall MI. Anterior infarctions impair left ventricular pumping ability, thereby reducing the ejection fraction and the stroke volume. In an attempt to maintain cardiac output, the heart rate increases. Sinus tachycardia must be corrected, because it greatly increases myocardial oxygen consumption, leading to further ischemia.

Atrial Dysrhythmias. Premature atrial contractions (PACs) occur frequently in patients who sustain an acute myocardial infarction. Atrial fibrillation is also common and may occur spontaneously or be preceded by PACs. With onset of atrial fibrillation the loss of organized atrial contraction decreases cardiac output by up to 20%. A global registry of patients with ACS found that almost 8% of ACS patients have preexisting atrial fibrillation, whereas just over 6% develop new-onset atrial fibrillation during their hospitalization for ACS.[34] Patients with atrial fibrillation—both new-onset and preexisting—have higher morbidity than patients without atrial fibrillation during an acute coronary syndrome. Specifically, ACS patients with new-onset atrial fibrillation experience a greater number of in-hospital adverse events such as reinfarction, shock, pulmonary edema, bleeding, and stroke.[34] Atrial fibrillation during the hospitalization significantly affects risk of death in the setting of an acute MI; it increases in-hospital mortality by 20% and long-term mortality by 34%.[3]

Ventricular Dysrhythmias. Premature ventricular contractions (PVCs) are seen in almost all patients within the first few hours after a myocardial infarction. They are initially controlled by administering oxygen to reduce myocardial hypoxia and by correcting acid-base or electrolyte imbalances. In the setting of an acute MI, PVCs are pharmacologically treated if they have the following characteristics: frequent (more than 6 per minute), closely coupled (R-on-T phenomenon), multiform in shape, and occur in bursts of three or more, increasing the risk of sustained ventricular tachycardia (VT). Ventricular fibrillation (VF) is a life-threatening dysrhythmia associated with high mortality in acute MI. Increasingly, β-blockers are prescribed after an acute MI to decrease mortality from ventricular dysrhythmias.[3]

Atrioventricular Heart Block During MI. Heart block occurs in 6% to 14% of patients with STEMI, and those patients have increased mortality.[3] In STEMI, AV block most often occurs after an inferior wall infarction. Because the right coronary artery supplies the AV node in 90% of the population, RCA occlusion leads to ischemia and infarction of the AV node cells. The development of sudden heart block is much less common now that most patients receive fibrinolysis or PCI to open the occluded vessel. In the majority of cases, transcutaneous pacing is the primary intervention; transvenous pacemakers are used less frequently.[3]

Ventricular Aneurysm After MI. A ventricular aneurysm (Figure 12-10) is a noncontractile, thinned left ventricular wall, which results from an acute transmural infarction. It most often occurs in the setting of an acute LAD artery occlusion with a wide area of infarcted myocardium.[3] The most effective prevention is early reperfusion of the myocardium, accomplished by opening the thrombosed coronary artery. In one study the rate of ventricular aneurysm was reduced from 18% in untreated patients to 7% when the coronary artery was opened by fibrinolysis.[3] The most common complications of a ventricular aneurysm are acute heart failure, systemic emboli, angina, and VT. Treatment is directed toward management of these complications and surgical repair by left ventricular aneurysmectomy. The affected area may be described as hypokinetic (contracts poorly), *akinetic* (noncontractile scar tissue), or *dyskinetic* (scar tissue that moves in the opposite direction to the normal contractile myocardium). The prognosis depends on the size of the aneurysm, the level of overall left ventricular dysfunction, and the severity of coexisting CAD.

Ventricular Septal Rupture After MI. Postinfarction rupture of the ventricular septal wall is a rare but potentially lethal complication of an acute anterior wall MI. (Figure 12-11). *Ventricular septal rupture,* also known as *acquired ventricular septal defect* (VSD) is an abnormal communication between the right and left ventricle. This complication occurs in less than 1% of all myocardial infarctions, and the incidence has declined, because most STEMI patients have the blocked coronary artery opened.[3] Nevertheless, rupture of the ventricular septum carries an extremely high mortality.[35] Reports of 35% to 73% mortality are typical.[35] Most patients with septal rupture also have signs and symptoms of cardiogenic shock. Ventricular septal rupture manifests as severe chest pain, syncope, hypotension, and sudden hemodynamic deterioration caused by shunting of blood from the high-pressure left ven-

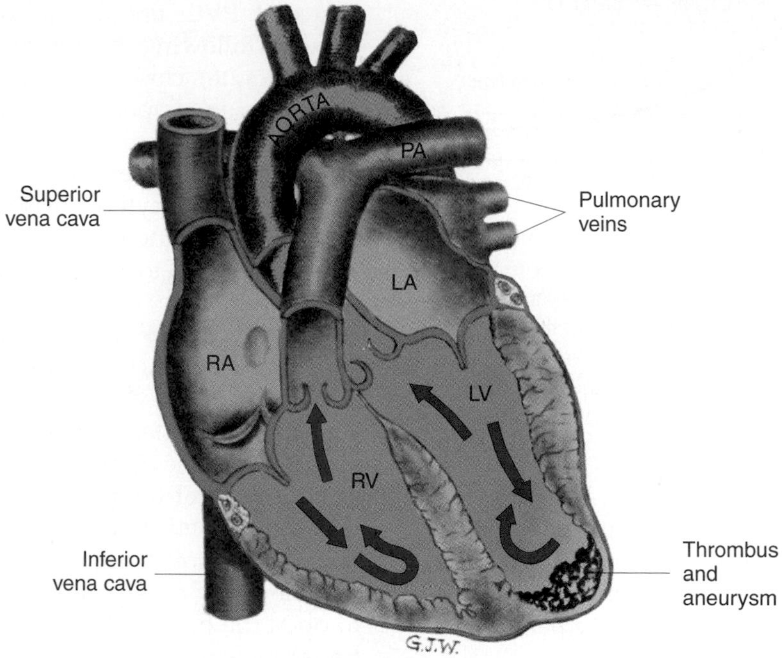

FIGURE 12-10. Ventricular aneurysm after acute myocardial infarction (MI). *PA,* Pulmonary artery; *LA,* left atrium; *RA,* right atrium; *LV,* left ventricle; *RV,* right ventricle.

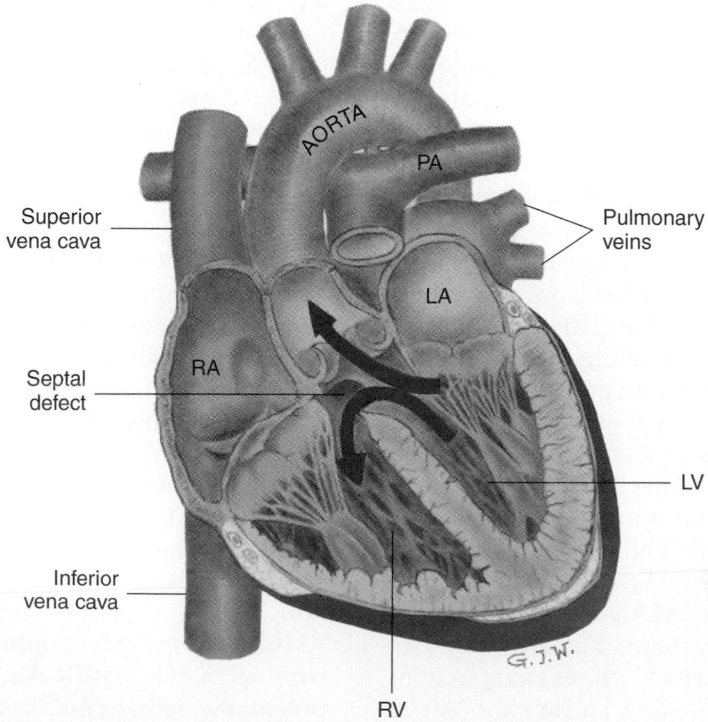

FIGURE 12-11. Ventricular septal rupture after acute myocardial infarction (MI). *PA,* Pulmonary artery; *LA,* left atrium; *RA,* right atrium; *LV,* left ventricle; *RV,* right ventricle.

tricle into the low-pressure right ventricle through the new septal opening. A holosystolic murmur (often accompanied by a thrill) can be auscultated and is best heard along the left sternal border. A diagnosis of postinfarction ventricular septal rupture can be made at the bedside with use of oxygen saturation assessment via a pulmonary artery catheter or by transesophageal echocardiography (TEE). Rupture of the septum is a medical and surgical emergency. The patient's condition is stabilized with vasodilators and an intraaortic balloon pump (IABP) to decrease afterload. The goal of afterload reduction in this patient population is to decrease the amount of blood being shunted to the right side of the heart and consequently to increase the flow of blood to the systemic circulation. If the new septal opening is very small, and the patient's condition is sufficiently stable to wait for scar tissue to form before surgical repair, survival improves. Unfortunately, when the septal opening is large, the massive left-to-right shunt across the septum makes the chances of survival dismal with or without surgery.[35]

Papillary Muscle Rupture After MI. Papillary muscle rupture can occur when the infarct involves the area around one of the papillary muscles that support the mitral valve. Infarction of the papillary muscles results in ineffective mitral valve closure, and blood is forced back into the low-pressure left atrium during ventricular systole. The rupture may be partial or complete. Complete rupture is catastrophic and precipitates severe acute mitral regurgitation, cardiogenic shock, and high risk of death.

Partial rupture (Figure 12-12) also results in mitral regurgitation, but the condition can be stabilized with aggressive medical management using the IABP and vasodilators. Urgent surgical intervention is required to replace the mitral valve.[36] As with other structural complications during acute MI, the incidence is decreased in patients who have their myocardium reperfused early.[3] Of the patients with acute MI who are admitted to the critical care unit in cardiogenic shock, 10% have papillary muscle rupture with acute mitral regurgitation. Mortality is 71% with medical treatment, and 40% with surgical intervention to replace or repair the mitral valve.[3]

Cardiac Wall Rupture After MI. Of the deaths that occur after myocardial infarction, 1% to 6% can be attributed to cardiac rupture.[3] Cardiac wall rupture has two peak times of incidence. The first occurs within the first 24 hours and the second between the third and fifth postinfarction day, when leukocyte scavenger cells are removing necrotic debris, thus thinning the myocardial wall.[3] The onset is sudden and usually catastrophic. Bleeding into the pericardial sac results in cardiac tamponade, cardiogenic shock, pulseless electrical activity (PEA), and death. Survival is rare. If rupture occurs in the hospital, emergency pericardiocentesis is required to relieve the tamponade until a surgical repair can be attempted. The best prevention is early reperfusion of the myocardium.[3]

Pericarditis After MI. Pericarditis is inflammation of the pericardial sac. It can occur during a transmural MI or after an acute MI. Pericarditis may occur in 5%

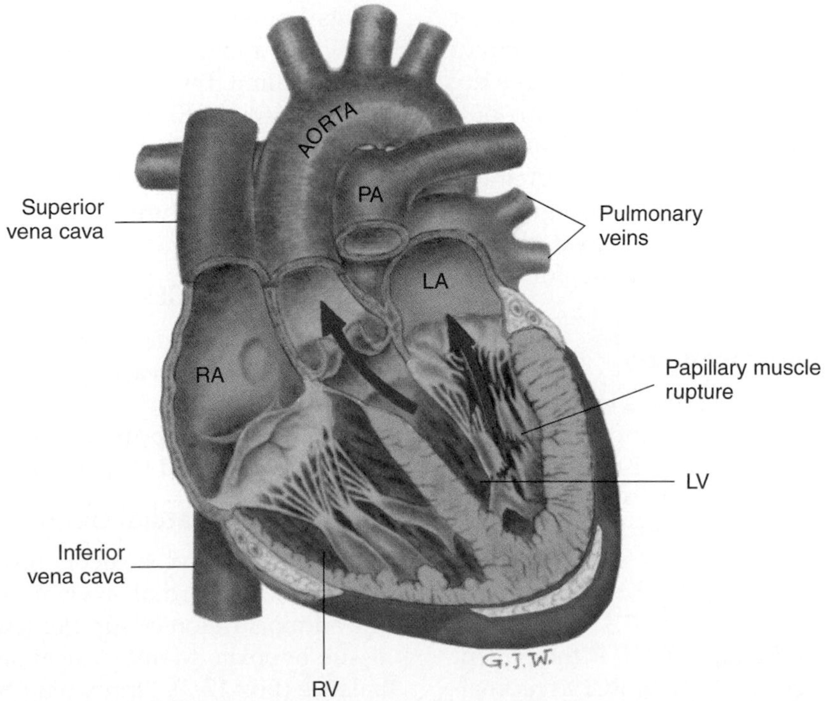

FIGURE 12-12. Papillary muscle rupture after acute myocardial infarction (MI). *PA,* Pulmonary artery; *LA,* left atrium; *RA,* right atrium; *LV,* left ventricle; *RV,* right ventricle.

to 20% of transmural infarctions but is treated only if it is clinically significant.[37] The damaged epicardium becomes rough and inflamed and irritates the pericardium lying adjacent to it, precipitating pericarditis. Pain is the most common symptom of pericarditis, and a pericardial friction rub is the most common initial sign. The friction rub is best auscultated with a stethoscope at the sternal border and is described as a grating, scraping, or leathery scratching. Pericarditis frequently produces a pericardial effusion.[37] Once the effusion (fluid) occurs, the friction rub may disappear. On the 12-lead ECG, pericarditis may manifest as elevation of the ST segment in all of the typically upright leads.[38] Pericarditis is treated with nonsteroidal anti-inflammatory drugs (NSAIDs).

Heart Failure and Acute MI. Almost 20% of patients with acute STEMI also have acute heart failure on admission to the hospital. These patients have often waited longer to come to the hospital and are older and more likely to be female. Compared with acute MI patients without heart failure, these patients have a higher risk of adverse in-hospital events and have longer lengths of stay and higher in-hospital mortality.[39]

MEDICAL MANAGEMENT

Quality outcomes research shows that compliance with the recent research guidelines developed by the American College of Cardiology and the American Heart Association (ACC/AHA) decreases in-hospital mortality following acute MI.[40,41] Patients admitted to hospitals that adhere to the AHA/ACC guidelines for treatment of either STEMI or NSTEMI have 8.3% in-hospital mortality compared with 15.3% mortality for patients managed at hospitals where the most recent guidelines are not fully used.[40,41] The guidelines are research based and are designed to improve the outcome of patients admitted to the hospital with an acute MI. Clinical guidelines address the issues of interventions to open the coronary artery, anticoagulation, prevention of dysrhythmias, tight glucose control, and prevention of ventricular remodeling following STEMI.[3]

Recanalization of the Coronary Artery

The essential immediate intervention is either fibrinolytic therapy or PCI to open the occluded artery for the patient with an acute STEMI.[3] All clinical guidelines emphasize the need for patients with symptoms of acute coronary syndrome to be rapidly triaged and treated.[3]

Anticoagulation

In the acute phase following an STEMI, if the patient has not received fibrinolytic therapy or PCI to recanalize (open) the coronary artery, anticoagulation with heparin is required.[3] It is also prudent to administer IV UFH or subcutaneous (Sub-Q) LMWH if the person is at risk for thrombus development.[3] Patients at risk for thrombotic emboli include those with an anterior wall infarction, atrial fibrillation, previous embolus, cardiomyopathy, or cardiogenic shock. An initial heparin bolus of 60 units/kg IV followed by a continuous heparin drip at 12 units/kg/hr to maintain an activated partial thromboplastin time (aPTT) between 50 and 70 seconds (1.5 to 2.0 times control) is recommended. Alternatively, LMWH may be used at doses that will provide full anticoagulation.[3] When the risk of systemic embolic complications remains high, especially in atrial fibrillation, the patient should be anticoagulated with warfarin (Coumadin).[3]

Dysrhythmia Prevention

The antidysrhythmic with the best safety record following STEMI is amiodarone. The reduction in death related to decreased dysrhythmias after MI is 13%.[3] β-Blockers are another class of antidysrhythmics that are recommended for all patients following STEMI. β-Blockers prevent ventricular dysrhythmias, lower blood pressure, and prevent reinfarction, especially in patients with left ventricular dysfunction.[3]

Tight Glucose Control

Achievement of normal serum blood glucose levels both during the acute phase and after MI improves survival.[3]

Prevention of Ventricular Remodeling

Many patients are at risk for development of heart failure following STEMI. The category of vasodilating drugs known as *angiotensin-converting enzyme (ACE) inhibitors* or angiotensin receptor–blockers (ARBs) can stop or limit the ventricular remodeling that leads to heart failure. Either an ACE inhibitor or, if this not tolerated, an ARB medication is indicated for all patients following STEMI.[3] Information about the clinical effects of heart failure is covered later in this chapter.

NURSING MANAGEMENT

Nursing management of the patient with an acute MI incorporates a variety of nursing diagnoses (Box 12-6**). Nursing priorities focus on (1) balancing myocardial oxygen supply and demand, (2) preventing complications, and (3) providing patient education.**

Balancing Myocardial Oxygen Supply and Demand

In the acute period, if severe heart muscle damage has occurred, myocardial oxygen supply is increased by the administration of supplemental oxygen to prevent tissue hypoxia. Many clinical signs manifest this imbalance (Box 12-7). Drugs play an increasingly important role in balancing supply and demand, and it is the critical care nurse who both administers and monitors

Box 12-6

NURSING DIAGNOSIS PRIORITIES

Myocardial Infarction

- Acute Pain related to transmission and perception of cutaneous, visceral, muscular, or ischemic impulses, p. A-7
- Decreased Cardiac Output related to alterations in preload, p. A-12
- Decreased Cardiac Output related to alterations in afterload, p. A-12
- Decreased Cardiac Output related to alterations in contractility, p. A-13
- Decreased Cardiac Output related to alterations in heart rate or rhythm, p. A-2
- Activity Intolerance related to cardiopulmonary dysfunction
- Ineffective Cardiopulmonary Tissue Perfusion related to decreased myocardial oxygen supply and/or increased myocardial oxygen demand, p. A-35
- Insomnia related to fragmented sleep, p. A-43
- Anxiety related to threat to biologic, psychologic, and/or social integrity, p. A-9
- Ineffective Coping related to situational crisis and personal vulnerability, p. A-38
- Powerlessness related to lack of control over current situation or disease progression, p. A-44
- Deficient Knowledge: Discharge Regimen related to lack of previous exposure to information, p. A-18
- Readiness for Enhanced Therapeutic Regimen Management

Box 12-7

CLINICAL MANIFESTATIONS OF ACUTE MYOCARDIAL INFARCTION

- Tachycardia with or without ectopy
- Bradycardia
- Normotension or hypotension
- Tachypnea
- Diminished heart sounds, especially S_1
- If left ventricular dysfunction present, may have S_3 and/or S_4
- Systolic murmur
- Pulmonary crackles
- Pulmonary edema
- Air hunger
- Orthopnea
- Frothy sputum
- Decreased cardiac output
- Decreased urine output
- Decreased peripheral pulses
- Slow capillary refill
- Restlessness
- Confusion
- Anxiety
- Agitation
- Denial
- Anger

the effectiveness of these agents. For the patient with a low cardiac output, positive inotropic drugs such as dobutamine, dopamine, and milrinone are prescribed. These inotropic agents are used to increase cardiac contractility in the healthy areas of the heart (thus increasing oxygen supply), while avoiding damage to the recently infarcted areas. Myocardial oxygen supply can be further enhanced by the use of coronary artery vasodilators. Nitroglycerin is recommended for the first 48 hours to increase vasodilation and prevent myocardial ischemia.[3] Research evidence supports the administration of early β-blockade therapy to decrease myocardial workload and to prevent dysrhythmias. Administration of β-blockade reduces mortality by 14% in the first 7 days after an MI, and by 23% longterm.[3] However, if the patient is in cardiogenic shock, β-blockers are withheld until the cardiac output has improved.[3] Other interventions to decrease cardiac work and myocardial oxygen consumption include bed rest with bedside commode privileges when the patient is clinically stable.

Preventing Complications

A thorough grasp of the range of potential complications that can occur following STEMI is essential. Cardiac monitoring for early detection of ventricular dysrhythmias is ongoing. Assessment for signs of continued ischemic pain is important, because angina is a warning sign of myocardium at risk. In response to angina, a 12-lead ECG is taken to determine if there is an extension of the infarct, nitroglycerin is administered, and the physician is notified immediately so that interventions may be initiated to limit the size of the MI. Heart failure is a serious complication following STEMI. Therefore whenever the patient's blood pressure is stable, treatment with an ACE inhibitor is initiated. These vasodilators are used to prevent the left ventricular remodeling and dilation that occur in many patients after an acute MI. Hypotension is a potential complication of an ACE inhibitor, especially with the first dose. It is an important nursing responsibility to monitor blood pressure and patient symptoms after taking this medication. Surveillance to detect both obvious and subtle signs of bleeding is also a priority because so many acute MI patients receive antiplatelet, anticoagulant, and fibrinolytic medications.[3]

In the first 24 hours, the stable patient with acute MI may be given only a light diet, because appetite is often poor in such patients. It is no longer considered necessary to restrict iced fluids or caffeine. While the patient is in bed, an upright position is preferred to foster better lung expansion. Deep breathing decreases the risk of atelectasis. An upright position also decreases venous return, lowers preload, and decreases cardiac work. The patient is taught to avoid increasing intraabdominal pressure (Valsalva maneuver). Stool softeners are given to lessen the risk of constipation from analgesics and bed rest and also to decrease the risk of straining. The nurse controls the critical care unit environment by decreasing noise, diminishing sensory overload, and allowing adequate rest periods.

Providing Patient Education

Once the acute phase has passed, education for the patient and family is focused on risk factor reduction, manifestations of angina, when to call a physician or emergency services, medications, and resumption of physical and sexual activity. If possible, a referral is made to a cardiac rehabilitation program so that this education can be reinforced outside the acute care hospital environment.[42] **Clinical practice guidelines for multidisciplinary care of the patient with an acute myocardial infarction are listed in Evidence-Based Collaborative Practice: Acute Coronary Syndrome and Acute Myocardial Infarction (Non-STEMI and STEMI).**

EVIDENCE-BASED COLLABORATIVE PRACTICE

Acute Coronary Syndrome and Acute Myocardial Infarction (NSTEMI and STEMI)

Prevention of Acute Coronary Syndrome

The term ACS is used to define the life-threatening consequences of CAD, notably unstable angina, NSTEMI and STEMI:

- Unstable angina is a term that denotes chest pain that is not relieved by SL nitroglycerin or rest within 5 minutes.
- NSTEMI is an acute MI ***without*** ST elevation on the 12-lead ECG.
- STEMI is an acute MI ***with*** ST elevation on the 12-lead ECG.

All of the recommendations are "class I," meaning there is strong research evidence to support these recommendations.

Recommendations That Decrease the Risk of Developing NSTEMI and STEMI

- Primary care providers should evaluate CAD risk factors for all patients every 3 to 5 years.
- The 10-year risk of ACS and acute MI should be assessed for all patients who have more than two major risk factors.
- An intensive risk factor modification program is recommended for patients with established CAD, or high-risk equivalents such as diabetes or chronic kidney disease.

Recommendations That Patients Be Educated About Emergency ACS Symptoms

- Patients who have previously diagnosed CAD should take one SL nitroglycerin, and patient (if alone) or friends or relatives should call 911 if chest pain/discomfort is unrelieved or worsening in 5 minutes.
- The same recommendation applies to patients without known CAD. If pain is unrelieved with rest or worsening at 5 minutes, patient (if alone) or friends or relatives should call 911.
- Patients with chest discomfort should be transported to the hospital via ambulance rather than be driven by friends or relatives.
- Family members should be advised to take a CPR course before an ACS emergency. This will teach CPR skills, demonstrate use of an AED, and educate participants about the "chain of survival" concept.

Recommendations for Prehospital EMS-Paramedic First Responders

- First responders such as EMS-paramedics can provide early defibrillation and ACLS for patients in cardiac arrest.
- EMS personnel should administer 162 to 325 mg nonenteric aspirin (chewed, not swallowed) to patients with chest pain suspected of having an STEMI.
- A prehospital fibrinolysis protocol is reasonable for patients with STEMI when there are physicians in the ambulance, or when there is a well-organized EMS service with full-time paramedics plus 12-lead ECG transmission capability and online medical direction.
- Patients over 75 years of age or those with cardiogenic shock should be transported to a hospital with the ability to provide fibrinolytics, emergency PCI, or emergency CABG. PCI or CABG, when needed, should be provided within 18 hours of the onset of cardiogenic shock.
- Patients with STEMI who have a contraindication to fibrinolytic therapy should be brought to a hospital capable of emergency PCI or CABG. At the scene the **door-to-departure time should be less than 30 minutes.** PCI should be initiated **within 90 minutes** from initial medical contact.

Data from Braunwald E et al: *J Am Coll Cardiol* 40(7):1366, 2002; and Antman EM et al: *Circulation* 110:588, 2004.

ACS, Acute coronary syndrome; *CAD,* coronary artery disease; *non-STEMI,* non–ST-elevation myocardial infarction; *STEMI,* ST-elevation myocardial infarction; *SL,* sublingual; *ECG,* electrocardiogram; *MI,* myocardial infarction; *CPR,* cardiopulmonary resuscitation; *AED,* automated external defibrillator; *EMS,* emergency medical services; *ACLS,* advanced cardiac life support; *PCI,* percutaneous coronary intervention; *CABG,* coronary artery bypass graft surgery; *ED,* emergency department; *HR,* heart rate; *BP,* blood pressure, *RR,* respiratory rate; Spo_2, oxygen saturation from external pulse oximeter; *RV,* right ventricle; *TTE,* transthoracic echocardiogram; *TEE,* transesophageal echocardiogram; *MRI,* magnetic resonance imaging; Sao_2, arterial oxygen saturation; *IV,* intravenous; *LBBB,* left bundle branch block; *ACE,* angiotensin-converting enzyme; *LDL,* low-density lipoprotein cholesterol; *VSR,* ventricular septal rupture; *IABP,* intraaortic balloon pump; *SBP,* systolic blood pressure; *VF,* ventricular fibrillation; *VT,* ventricular tachycardia; *ICD,* implantable cardioverter-defibrillator; *SCD,* sudden cardiac death; *EF,* ejection fraction; *AV,* atrioventricular; *HRT,* hormone replacement therapy, *STEMI,* S-T elevation myocardial infarction; *NSTEMI,* non-STEMI.

EVIDENCE-BASED COLLABORATIVE PRACTICE

Acute Coronary Syndrome and Acute Myocardial Infarction (NSTEMI and STEMI)—*cont'd*

Recommendations for Initial Emergency Clinical Management

- Hospitals should establish multidisciplinary teams to facilitate rapid triage of patients who present to the ED with chest pain.
- Use of written protocols is recommended to standardize care. An immediate cardiology consult is advised if the patient symptoms fall outside the written protocol.

STEMI

- Fibrinolytics for STEMI: Time from coming into contact with the health care system (paramedics or ED) and receiving fibrinolytics should be **less than 30 minutes.** A brief, focused neurologic examination to determine prior stroke or presence of cognitive defects is necessary prior to administration of fibrinolytics.
- PCI for STEMI: Time from coming into contact with the health care system (paramedics or ED) to balloon inflation PCI should be **less than 90 minutes.**

NSTEMI

- If the level of risk for the patient with NSTEMI is not immediately apparent, a "chest pain unit" within the ED permits close surveillance by competent clinicians without immediate hospital admission.
- Glycoprotein IIb/IIIa inhibitors for NSTEMI, in addition to aspirin and heparin, are indicated when cardiac catheterization or PCI are planned.
- PCI may be indicated for NSTEMI.

Recommendations for Initial Emergency Physical Assessment

Vital Signs

- HR, BP, RR, temperature, Spo_2, ECG monitor to detect presence of dysrhythmias

Physical Assessment

- Assess for warm or cool skin, color, capillary refill, peripheral pulses
- Auscultate heart for cardiac murmur or new S_3 or S_4
- Auscultate lungs for air entry plus crackles, wheezes
- Observe for breathlessness, frothy pink sputum (pulmonary edema)
- Ask patient, family, significant others for relevant history

Recommendations for Emergency Diagnostics

12-Lead ECG

- The 12-lead ECG should be shown to the ED physician within 10 minutes of the patient's arrival in the ED for all patients with chest discomfort or angina equivalent symptoms.
- If the first ECG is normal but the patient continues to have symptoms of chest pain/discomfort, the 12-lead ECG should be repeated at 5- to 10-minute intervals, ***or*** continuous 12-lead ECG monitoring can be used.
- In patients with inferior wall infarction, RV infarction must be suspected and right-sided ECG leads then recorded. V_4R is diagnostic lead of choice to diagnose ST elevation in the RV.

Laboratory Studies

- Laboratory tests should be drawn as part of the general management of STEMI but should not delay the administration of reperfusion therapy.

Cardiac Biomarkers

- Cardiac-specific troponins are recommended for patients with coexistent skeletal muscle injury. Clinicians are advised not wait for results of the biomarker assay before initiating reperfusion therapy. Point-of-care (handheld) biomarker assay results are permissible, but subsequent biomarker assays should be via quantitative laboratory analysis.

Imaging Studies

- Portable chest x-ray: obtaining the chest x-ray must not delay reperfusion therapy unless a major complication such as aortic dissection is suspected.
- Portable echocardiography (TTE or TEE) or MRI scan to distinguish aortic dissection from STEMI, for patients in whom the symptoms are not clear

Recommendations for Routine Care

Prevent Hypoxia

- Supplemental oxygen administered to maintain Sao_2 above 90%

Coronary Vasodilation

- Nitroglycerin 0.04 mg SL every 5 minutes for three doses. If chest pain /discomfort is ongoing, start peripheral IV. Administer IV nitroglycerin for relief of chest pain, control of hypertension, or relief of pulmonary congestion.

Pain Control

- Morphine sulphate 2-4 mg IV in 2-mg increments at 5- to 15-minute intervals for STEMI pain control

Aspirin

- Aspirin 162 mg to be chewed for rapid buccal absorption

β-Blockers

- Oral β-blocker therapy administered to STEMI patients without contraindications to β-blockade, irrespective of fibrinolytic or primary PCI reperfusion

Continued

EVIDENCE-BASED COLLABORATIVE PRACTICE

Acute Coronary Syndrome and Acute Myocardial Infarction (NSTEMI and STEMI)—*cont'd*

Recommendations for Emergency Interventions for STEMI

Fibrinolytic Drugs

- Fibrinolytic drugs administered to STEMI patients with ST elevation greater than 0.1 mV (1 mm or one small box) in two contiguous precordial (chest) leads ***or*** two adjacent limb leads, new LBBB or presumed new LBBB, and onset of symptoms less than 12 hours ago
- Before administration of fibrinolytic therapy, rule out neurologic contraindications.
- Rule out facial trauma, uncontrolled hypertension, or ischemic stroke within the last 3 months
- If contraindications to fibrinolysis are present, PCI is the preferred method of reperfusion.

PCI

- Emergency diagnostic coronary angiography to identify blocked coronary artery before PCI
- Emergency PCI is recommended over fibrinolytic therapy if symptom onset was longer ago than 3 hours
- Emergency PCI can be performed within 12 hours of symptom onset for patients with new LBBB, or presumed new LBBB.
- Emergency PCI balloon inflation within 90 minutes of arrival at the hospital
- If cardiogenic shock develops less than 36 hours after MI, in patients younger than 75 years with ST elevation, or patients with new LBBB, "rescue PCI" is recommended within 18 hours of shock onset.

Cardiac Surgery

- Emergency CABG surgery is undertaken for specific indications in STEMI:
  - Failed PCI with persistent pain or hemodynamic instability
  - Recurrent ischemia refractory to medical therapy in patients with suitable anatomy who are not candidates for PCI
  - Post-MI ventricular septal rupture (VSR) or papillary muscle rupture, both of which frequently lead to cardiogenic shock
  - Cardiogenic shock less than 36 hours after MI, in patients younger than 75 years with ST elevation, or patients with new LBBB who have multivessel or left main disease
  - Recurrent ventricular dysrhythmias with 50% or greater left main coronary artery lesion and/or triple vessel disease

Recommendations for Secondary Prevention of Complications

Medications

- ACE Inhibitors—prevent ventricular remodeling
- Beta-blockers—prevent ventricular dysrhythmias
- Diuretics—if heart failure has developed
- Antihyperlipidemics—if total cholesterol, LDL, or triglycerides elevated

Recommendations for Management of Complications Following STEMI

Cardiogenic Shock

- IABP for patients with hypotension (BP 90 mm Hg or SBP 30 mm Hg below baseline)

Ventricular Arrhythmias

- VF or pulseless VT is managed by standard ACLS criteria (unsynchronized monophasic shock of 200 joules; if unsuccessful a second shock of 200-300 joules, if unsuccessful a third shock of 360 joules).
- Patients with hemodynamically significant VT more than 2 days post-STEMI who have ongoing ventricular dysrhythmias are considered for implantation of an ICD.
- Patients with an EF between 30% and 40% at 1 month after STEMI should undergo an electrophysiology study (EPS), and if they are inducible to VT/VF, an ICD is recommended to reduce risk of SCD.
- Patients with an EF below 30% at 1 month after STEMI are at high risk of SCD.

AV block

- Transvenous pacemaker inserted (emergency) or permanent pacemaker (later elective) for symptomatic second- or third-degree AV block
- All patients after STEMI who require permanent pacing should also be evaluated for ICD indications.

Provide Relevant Education

Medications

- Written and verbal instructions about medication dosages, administration, and side effects

Emergency Information

- Give patient and family information about calling 911 if pain/angina equivalent symptoms persist or are worse after 5 minutes.
- Family members of high-risk patients are advised to take a CPR class and learn about AED.

Risk Factors

- Smoking cessation, hypertension control, weight control, normal blood glucose; low-fat diet; normal lipid panel
- Increase physical activity, no new HRT for women

Cardiac Rehabilitation

- Participation in a cardiac rehabilitation program will help the patient continue the process of risk factor and lifestyle modification.

HEART FAILURE

DESCRIPTION AND ETIOLOGY

The number of patients with heart failure (HF) is increasing in the United States. Currently over 2 million Americans have a diagnosis of HF, and about 500,000 new cases are diagnosed each year.[43] Each year, 300,00 patients die of HF and patients spend over 6.5 million days in the hospital.[43] Heart failure is primarily a disease of the elderly. Approximately 6% to 10% of people over 65 years of age have a diagnosis of HF; for patients who are hospitalized with this diagnosis, 80% of them are over 80 years old. The number of patients diagnosed with HF is increasing. The total inpatient and outpatient costs for HF exceed $38 billion each year, a sum that represents over 5% of the total United States health care budget.[43]

PATHOPHYSIOLOGY

Heart failure is a response to cardiac dysfunction, a condition in which the heart cannot pump blood at a volume required to meet the body's needs. Any condition that impairs the ability of the ventricles to fill or eject blood can cause HF. Coronary artery disease with resultant necrotic damage to the left ventricle is the underlying cause of HF in most patients. Other major conditions that lead to HF include valvular dysfunction, infection (myocarditis or endocarditis), cardiomyopathy, and uncontrolled hypertension.[43]

ASSESSMENT AND DIAGNOSIS

Heart failure is typically classified using the New York Heart Association (NYHA) criteria. Patients are assigned into four groups, I through IV, depending on their degree of symptoms and the amount of patient effort required to elicit symptoms (Table 12-4). Research-based clinical guidelines suggest adding a second level of classification that emphasizes the progressive nature of HF through various stages, with increasing symptom distress and intensified clinical interventions (Table 12-5).[43] Heart failure can manifest itself in many different ways depending on how far the ventricular remodeling and dysfunction has advanced. Heart failure may be discovered secondary to a known clinical syndrome such as acute MI or because of decreased exercise tolerance, fluid retention, or admission to the critical care unit for an unrelated condition.[43] For patients with fluid retention, the most reliable clinical sign of fluid volume overload is jugular vein distention (JVD).[43] The assessment procedure used to estimate JVD is described in Chapter 11.

The first step in diagnosis is to determine the underlying structural abnormality creating the ventricular dysfunction and symptoms. Various imaging tests are available to visualize cardiac anatomy, and laboratory tests are used to evaluate the impact of hormonal or electrolyte imbalance. The results of these tests permit the cardiology team to design a treatment plan to control symptoms and possibly correct the underlying cause. All patients do not have the same type of heart failure, as described below.

Left Ventricular Failure

Failure of the left ventricle is defined as a disturbance of the contractile function of the left ventricle, resulting in a low cardiac output state. This leads to vasoconstriction of the arterial bed that raises systemic vascular resistance (SVR), a condition also described as "high afterload," and creates congestion and edema in the pulmonary circulation and alveoli. Clinical manifestations include decreased peripheral perfusion with weak or diminished pulses; cool, pale extremities; and in later stages, peripheral cyanosis (Table 12-6). Over time, with progression of the disease state the fluid accumulation behind the dysfunctional left ventricle elevates pulmonary pressures, contributes to pulmonary congestion and edema, and produces dysfunction of the right ventricle, resulting in failure of the right side of the heart.

Right Ventricular Failure

Failure of the right side of the heart is defined as ineffective right ventricular contractile function. Pure failure of the right ventricle may result from an acute condition such as a pulmonary embolus or a right ventricular infarction, but it is most commonly caused by failure of the left side of the heart (see ealier discussion). The common manifestations of right ventricular failure are the following: jugular vein distention, elevated central venous pressure (CVP), weakness, peripheral or sacral edema, hepatomegaly (enlarged liver), jaundice, and liver tenderness. Gastrointestinal (GI) symptoms include poor appetite, anorexia, nausea, and an uncomfortable feeling of fullness (see Table 12-6).

Table 12-4

New York Heart Association Functional Classification of Heart Failure

CLASS	DEFINITION
I	Normal daily activity does not initiate symptoms.
II	Normal daily activities initiate onset of symptoms, but symptoms subside with rest.
III	Minimal activity initiates symptoms; patients are usually symptom-free at rest.
IV	Any type of activity initiates symptoms, and symptoms are present at rest.

Table 12-5
Progression of Heart Failure

STAGE	STRUCTURAL HEART DISORDER	SYMPTOMS	MANAGEMENT
A	No, but at risk because of: Hypertension CAD Diabetes mellitus	None	Preventive treatment of known risk factors: Hypertension Lipid disorders Cigarette smoking Diabetes mellitus Discourage alcohol and illicit drug use
B	Yes, but without symptoms: Previous MI Family history of CM Asymptomatic valvular disease/CM	None	Treat all risk factors. When indicated, use the following: ACE inhibitors β-Blockers
C	Yes, with prior or current symptoms	Shortness of breath Fatigue Reduced exercise tolerance	Treat all risk factors, plus HF symptoms: Diuretics ACE inhibitors β-Blockers Digitalis Dietary salt restriction
D	Yes, with refractory HF symptoms despite maximal specialized interventions (pharmacologic, medical, nursing) Recurrently hospitalized for HF symptoms	Marked symptoms at rest despite maximal medical therapy	Refractory HF requires interventions from previous stages (A-C), plus the following: Continuous intravenous inotropic support Mechanical assist devices Heart transplantation Hospice care

Modified from Hunt S et al: *Circulation* 112(12):e154, 2005.
CAD, Coronary artery disease; *MI,* myocardial infarction, *CM,* cardiomyopathy; *ACE,* angiotensin-converting enzyme; *HF,* heart failure.

Table 12-6
Clinical Manifestations of Failure of Right and Left Sides of the Heart

LEFT VENTRICULAR FAILURE		RIGHT VENTRICULAR FAILURE	
SIGNS	SYMPTOMS	SIGNS	SYMPTOMS
Tachypnea	Fatigue	Peripheral edema	Weakness
Tachycardia	Dyspnea	Hepatomegaly	Anorexia
Cough	Orthopnea	Splenomegaly	Indigestion
Bibasilar crackles	Paroxysmal nocturnal dyspnea	Hepatojugular reflux	Weight gain
Gallop rhythms (S_3 and S_4)		Ascites	Mental changes
Increased pulmonary artery pressures	Nocturia	Jugular vein distention	
Hemoptysis		Increased central venous pressure	
Cyanosis		Pulmonary hypertension	
Pulmonary edema			

Systolic Heart Failure

Systolic dysfunction describes an abnormality of the heart muscle that markedly decreases contractility during systole (ejection) and thus lessens the quantity of blood that can be pumped out of the heart. Patients with a diagnosis of systolic heart failure have signs and symptoms of HF combined with a below-normal ejection fraction (EF). Left ventricular systolic dysfunction is the classic picture that most clinicians picture when thinking about heart failure. In addition to the signs and symptoms of left heart failure (see above), the patient will have a low EF. There is some debate as to how low the EF has to be to qualify as systolic heart failure but the range is generally below 50%[44]; some clinicians cite numbers below 45% or even below 40%.[45,46] Symptoms of systolic heart failure include dyspnea, exercise intolerance, and fluid volume overload.

CAD and its sequelae represent the underlying cause in two thirds of patients with systolic heart failure.[43] The remaining patients with systolic dysfunction have nonischemic cardiomyopathy (interchangeably described as *dilated cardiomyopathy*),[47] which results from an identifiable cause such as hypertension, thyroid disease, cardiac valvular disease, alcohol use, or myocarditis.[43] If the cause is unknown, systolic dysfunction is described as *idiopathic dilated cardiomyopathy*.[43] The incidence of systolic heart failure in the general population is 3%; it increases with age and is more common in men.[46] Clinical findings that are required to make a diagnosis of systolic heart failure include the following[43]:

- Signs and symptoms of heart failure
- Left ventricular systolic dysfunction with a low ejection fraction

Diastolic Heart Failure

Diastolic dysfunction describes an abnormality of the heart muscle that makes it unable to relax, stretch, or fill during diastole. The ejection fraction can be normal or abnormal (low), and the patient may be symptomatic or symptom-free.[44,48] Between 20% and 40% of patients with HF are believed to have diastolic muscle dysfunction.[43] The principal causes are similar to systolic heart failure (see above): coronary artery disease, myocardial ischemia, atrial fibrillation, uncontrolled hypertension in 75% of cases, and left ventricular hypertrophy (LVH) in about 40%.[48] Some conditions that are known to markedly alter diastolic function include hypertrophic cardiomyopathy (HCM), restrictive cardiomyopathy, and infiltrative diseases such as amyloidosis and neoplastic infiltrate.[43,47] The incidence of diastolic heart failure is highest in patients older than 75 years and disproportionately affects elderly women.[43] It is postulated that the process of ageing negatively impacts diastolic function, imposing stiffness and fibrosis on both the cardiac muscle and cardiovascular vessels.[43]

Clinical findings that are required to make a diagnosis of diastolic heart failure include the following[43-45]:

- Signs and symptoms of heart failure
- Normal or only mildly abnormal left ventricular systolic dysfunction
- Abnormal left ventricular relaxation, filling, diastolic distensibility, or diastolic stiffness

Diastolic heart failure is caused by dysfunction during the diastolic phase of the cardiac cycle. In affected patients, the heart muscle takes longer to relax compared with a normal heart, the ventricular chamber does not distend to accept the fill-volume, and the myocardium remains stiff throughout diastole.[48,49] Normally, diastole is the filling stage of the cardiac cycle when the ventricle relaxes completely. The abnormal hemodynamics of diastolic heart failure can be elicited by diagnostic tests such as cardiac catheterization and a stress echocardiogram.[48]

In diastolic heart failure, the left ventricular end-diastolic pressure (LVEDP) is high, whereas the left ventricular end-diastolic volume (LVEDV) is paradoxically low, when compared to normal hearts.[44] Another diagnostic clue is that many patients with diastolic heart failure have normal intracardiac pressures at rest, but during exercise the LVEDP and pulmonary vascular pressures rise rapidly.[44] This is because the noncompliant, stiff ventricle cannot increase stroke volume during exercise; thus cardiac output remains low even though physical demand is high. Not unexpectedly, patients with diastolic heart failure often experience a sudden rise in blood pressure and sinus tachycardia during exercise; they are exercise intolerant and experience fatigue, dyspnea, pulmonary venous congestion, and even pulmonary edema.[44,45,48]

Systolic Versus Diastolic Heart Failure

It turns out to be impossible to accurately determine whether a patient has systolic or diastolic heart failure from clinical assessment alone.[44] This is because both types of HF produce similar signs and symptoms. The level of symptoms and quality of life are variable between individuals, and between men and women, even when the EF and presumed cardiac dysfunction is the same.[50] This may be because the majority of symptoms come from the neurohormonal compensatory mechanisms (see below) rather than the cardiac output. An elevated brain natriuretic peptide (BNP) level (greater than 100 pg/ml) is very useful to diagnose heart failure in patients with fluid overload and shortness of breath.[51] The BNP value tends to be higher in patients with a diagnosis of systolic heart failure compared with diastolic heart failure, although this differentiation is not reliable enough to be used to differentiate the two types of heart failure in clinical practice.[51] The more severe the heart failure, the higher the BNP level. The primary use of the BNP test is to diagnose if heart failure is present.

The annual mortality rate in diastolic heart failure is 5% to 8%, markedly less than the 10% to 15% annual mortality for patients with systolic heart failure. To put this in perspective, age-matched controls without any heart failure experience an annual mortality rate of just 1%.[44,48]

It is not possible to distinguish whether a patient has systolic or diastolic heart failure simply by looking at the medications they are prescribed. The same drugs are used to treat the two types of HF, although the underlying rationales may be different.[45] For example, β-blockers are used in diastolic heart failure to slow the heart rate, to prolong diastole to give more time for ventricular filling, and to modify the ventricular response to exercise, especially for patients who have a preserved ejection fraction.[45] When β-blockers are prescribed for treatment of systolic heart failure, the intent is to preserve long-term inotropic (contractile) function and prevent ventricular remodeling.[45] Diuretics are used to treat both types of HF, although a smaller dosage is generally needed in diastolic heart failure.[45] ACE inhibitors and ARBs are also used to treat both types of HF. The medications used to treat heart failure are further discussed in Chapter 13.

Acute Versus Chronic Heart Failure

Acute versus chronic heart failure refers to the rapidity with which the syndrome develops, the presence and activation of compensatory mechanisms, and the presence or absence of fluid accumulation in the interstitial space. In clinical practice guidelines, the terms *acute* and *chronic* have replaced the older name, "congestive heart failure" (CHF), because not all heart failure involves pulmonary congestion.[43] However, the description of a patient with CHF remains commonly employed in clinical practice.

Acute heart failure has a sudden onset, with no compensatory mechanisms. The patient may experience acute pulmonary edema, low cardiac output, or even cardiogenic shock. Patients with chronic heart failure are hypervolemic, have sodium and water retention, and have structural heart chamber changes such as dilation or hypertrophy.[43]

Chronic heart failure is ongoing, with symptoms that may be made tolerable by medication, diet, and a reduced activity level. The deterioration into acute heart failure can be precipitated by the onset of dysrhythmias, acute ischemia, sudden illness, or cessation of medications. This may necessitate admission to a critical care unit.

Neurohormonal Compensatory Mechanisms in Heart Failure

When the heart begins to fail and the cardiac output is no longer sufficient to meet the metabolic needs of the tissues, the body activates several major compensatory mechanisms: the sympathetic nervous system, the renin-angiotensin-aldosterone system (RAAS), and, if hypertension is present, the development of ventricular hypertrophy (see Table 12-5). This process ultimately reshapes the ventricle in a process described as *ventricular remodeling.* These pathophysiologic processes and the pharmacologic measures taken to limit ventricular remodeling are described in the following paragraphs.

1. *Sympathetic nervous system:* The sympathetic nervous system compensates for low cardiac output by increasing heart rate (HR) and BP. As a result, levels of circulating catecholamines are increased, resulting in peripheral vasoconstriction. In addition to raising BP and HR, catecholamines cause shunting of blood from nonvital organs, such as the skin, to vital organs, such as the heart and brain. This mechanism, although initially helpful, may become a negative factor if elevation of HR increases myocardial oxygen demand while shortening the amount of time for diastolic filling and coronary artery perfusion.
2. *Renin-angiotensin-aldosterone system:* Activation of RAAS in heart failure promotes fluid retention.[43,52] The RAAS is activated by low cardiac output that causes the hormone *renin* to be secreted by the kidneys. A physiologic chain of events is then set in motion that leads to volume overload. The renin acts on *angiotensinogen* in the bloodstream and converts it to *angiotensin I;* when angiotensin passes through the lung tissues it is activated by an enzyme named *ACE* that converts the angiotensin I to *angiotensin II,* a powerful vasoconstrictor that increases SVR, raises BP, and increases the workload of the left ventricle; the increased SVR further lowers cardiac output. The mineralocorticoid hormone *aldosterone* is released from the adrenal glands and stimulates sodium retention via the distal tubules of the kidney. In addition, in response to the low cardiac output the renal arterioles constrict, decrease glomerular filtration, and increase reabsorption of sodium from the proximal and distal tubules. To break the RAAS cycle of fluid retention in heart failure, two types of drugs are prescribed to interrupt the steps. To inhibit the conversion of angiotensin I to angiotensin II, a drug in the ACE-inhibitor category is prescribed. These agents prevent arterial vasoconstriction, decrease blood pressure and SVR, and decrease the amount of ventricular remodeling that often occurs with HF. Or, a drug that inhibits angiotensin II directly may be prescribed instead. The drugs in this category are termed *angiotensin receptor-blockers* (ARBs).[53] Spirolactone (Aldactone) is a drug from a different category that is also prescribed to break the RAAS cycle. Aldactone is a *mineralocorticoid receptor–antagonist* that will inhibit (block) the retention of sodium from the distal tubules of the kidney.[50,53] Figure 12-13 shows the mechanism of action by which these drugs act on the RAAS.
3. *Ventricular hypertrophy:* Ventricular hypertrophy is the final compensatory mechanism. It is also strongly associated with preexisting hypertension. Because myocardial hypertrophy increases the force of contraction, hypertrophy helps the ventricle overcome an increase in afterload. When this mechanism is no longer efficient for the ventricle, it will remodel by dilation.
4. *Ventricular remodeling:* As a result of the above mechanisms, the shape of the ventricle changes, or is "remodeled," to resemble a round bowl. A dilated ventricle has poor contractility and is enlarged without hypertrophy. Research trial evidence indicates that synergistic use of drugs from different categories—ACE inhibitor or ARB,

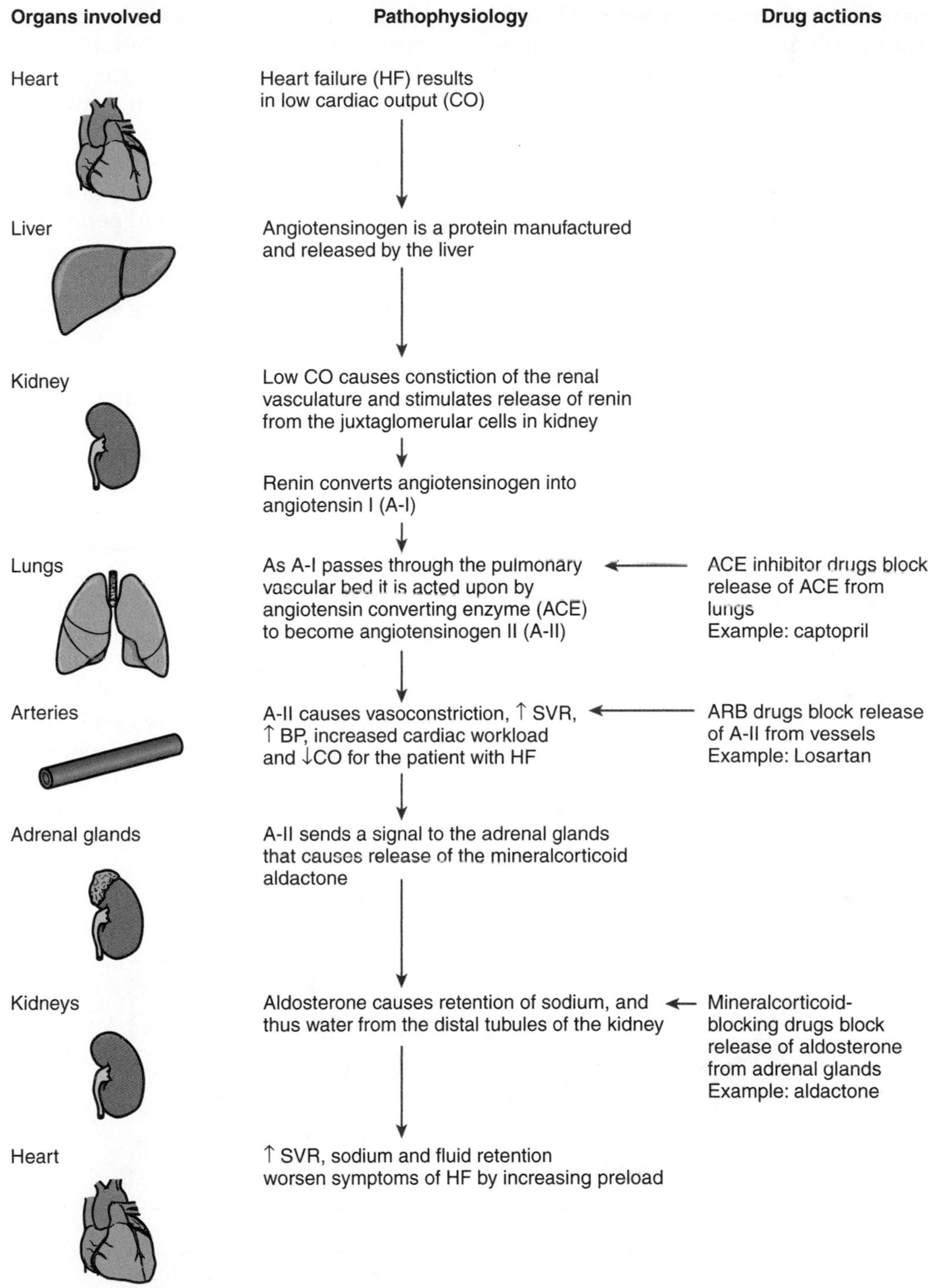
Organs involved
Pathophysiology
Drug actions
Heart
Heart failure (HF) results in low cardiac output (CO)
Liver
Angiotensinogen is a protein manufactured and released by the liver
Kidney
Low CO causes constiction of the renal vasculature and stimulates release of renin from the juxtaglomerular cells in kidney
Renin converts angiotensinogen into angiotensin I (A-I)
Lungs
As A-I passes through the pulmonary vascular bed it is acted upon by angiotensin converting enzyme (ACE) to become angiotensinogen II (A-II)
ACE inhibitor drugs block release of ACE from lungs
Example: captopril
Arteries
A-II causes vasoconstriction, ↑ SVR, ↑ BP, increased cardiac workload and ↓CO for the patient with HF
ARB drugs block release of A-II from vessels
Example: Losartan
Adrenal glands
A-II sends a signal to the adrenal glands that causes release of the mineralcorticoid aldactone
Kidneys
Aldosterone causes retention of sodium, and thus water from the distal tubules of the kidney
Mineralcorticoid-blocking drugs block release of aldosterone from adrenal glands
Example: aldactone
Heart
↑ SVR, sodium and fluid retention worsen symptoms of HF by increasing preload

FIGURE 12-13. Renin-angiotensin-aldosterone system (RAAS), role in heart failure, and interaction of specific drugs. SVR, Systemic vascular resistance; *BP,* blood pressure; *CO,* cardiac output; *ARB,* angiotensin receptor–blocker; *ACE,* angiotensin-converting enzyme.

Aldactone, plus β-blockade—can halt or reduce the progression of heart failure remodeling.[53-56]

Pulmonary Complications of Heart Failure

The clinical manifestations of acute heart failure result from tissue hypoperfusion and organ congestion and are progressive, as described above. The severity of clinical manifestations also progresses as heart failure worsens. Initially manifestations appear only with exertion but eventually occur at rest as well.[43]

Shortness of Breath in Heart Failure

The patient experiences the feeling of shortness of breath first with exertion, but as heart failure worsens, symptoms are also present at rest. Recently a diagnostic blood test has become available to assist clinicians in differentiating whether a patient's shortness of breath is caused by cardiac failure or by pulmonary complications. BNP is released from the cardiac ventricles in response to increased wall tension. Heart failure increases LV wall tension because of the excess preload in the ventricles. When the BNP blood level is greater than 100 pg/ml, the dyspnea is probably related to cardiac rather than pulmonary failure.[57,58] The more severe the heart failure, the higher the BNP test result.[59] If the patient has concomitant kidney disease, the BNP clinical diagnostic point to diagnose heart failure rises to greater than 200 pg/ml.[60] Breathlessness in HF is described by the following terms:

1. *Dyspnea:* the patient's sensation of shortness of breath; it results from pulmonary vascular congestion and decreased lung compliance
2. *Orthopnea:* describes difficulty in breathing when lying flat because of an increase in venous return that occurs in the supine position
3. *Paroxysmal nocturnal dyspnea:* a severe form of orthopnea in which the patient awakens from sleep gasping for air
4. *Cardiac asthma:* dyspnea with wheezing, a nonproductive cough, and pulmonary crackles that progress to the gurgling sounds of pulmonary edema

Pulmonary Edema in Heart Failure

Pulmonary edema, or protein-laden fluid in the alveoli, inhibits gas exchange by impairing the diffusion pathway between the alveolus and the capillary. It is caused by increased left atrial and ventricular pressures and results in an excessive accumulation of serous or serosanguineous fluid in the interstitial spaces and alveoli of the lungs. The formation of pulmonary edema has two stages. The first stage is not as severe and is characterized by interstitial edema, engorgement of the perivascular and peribronchial spaces, and increased lymphatic flow as illustrated in Figure 12-14, *B*. The later stage is characterized by alveolar edema resulting from fluid moving into the alveoli from the interstitium (Figure 12-14, *C*). Eventually, blood plasma moves into the alveoli faster than the lymphatic system can clear it, thereby interfering with diffusion of oxygen, depressing the arterial partial pressure of oxygen ($Pa{O_2}$), and leading to tissue hypoxia (Figure 12-14, *D*).

Heart failure patients in pulmonary edema are extremely breathless and anxious and have a sensation of suffocation. They expectorate pink, frothy liquid and feel as if they are drowning. They may sit bolt upright, gasp for breath, or thrash about. The respiratory rate is elevated, and accessory muscles of ventilation are used, with nasal flaring and bulging neck muscles. Respirations are characterized by loud inspiratory and expiratory gurgling sounds. Diaphoresis is profuse, and the skin may be cold, ashen, and sometimes cyanotic, reflecting low cardiac output, increased sympathetic stimulation, peripheral vasoconstriction, and desaturation of arterial blood.

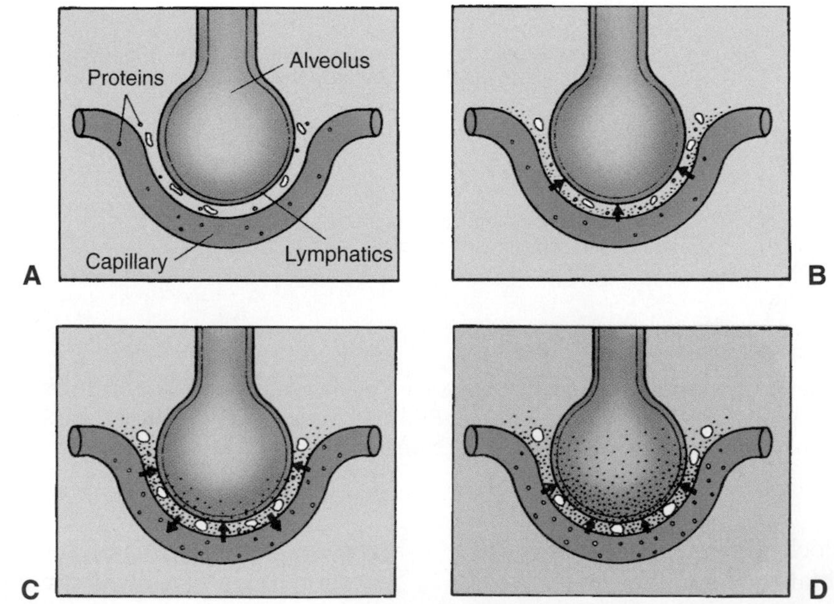

FIGURE 12-14. As pulmonary edema progresses, it inhibits oxygen and carbon dioxide exchange at the alveolar capillary interface. **A,** Normal relationship. **B,** Increased pulmonary capillary hydrostatic pressure causes fluid to move from the vascular space into the pulmonary interstitial space. **C,** Lymphatic flow increases in an attempt to pull fluid back into the vascular or lymphatic space. **D,** Failure of lymphatic flow and worsening of left-sided heart failure results in further movement of fluid into the interstitial space and the alveoli.

Arterial Blood Gases in Pulmonary Edema

Arterial blood gas (ABG) values are variable. In the early stage of pulmonary edema, respiratory alkalosis may be present because of hyperventilation, which eliminates CO_2. As the pulmonary edema progresses and gas exchange becomes impaired, acidosis (pH <7.35) and hypoxemia ensue. A chest x-ray examination usually confirms an enlarged cardiac silhouette, pulmonary venous congestion, and interstitial edema.

Cardiogenic Versus Noncardiogenic Pulmonary Edema

In the critical care unit, when a patient develops pulmonary edema it is often a challenge to determine whether the cause is cardiac, known as *cardiogenic pulmonary edema,* or whether the origin is pulmonary or systemic in origin. The latter is referred to as *noncardiogenic pulmonary edema* or, more commonly, *acute respiratory distress syndrome* (ARDS). Options to determine the

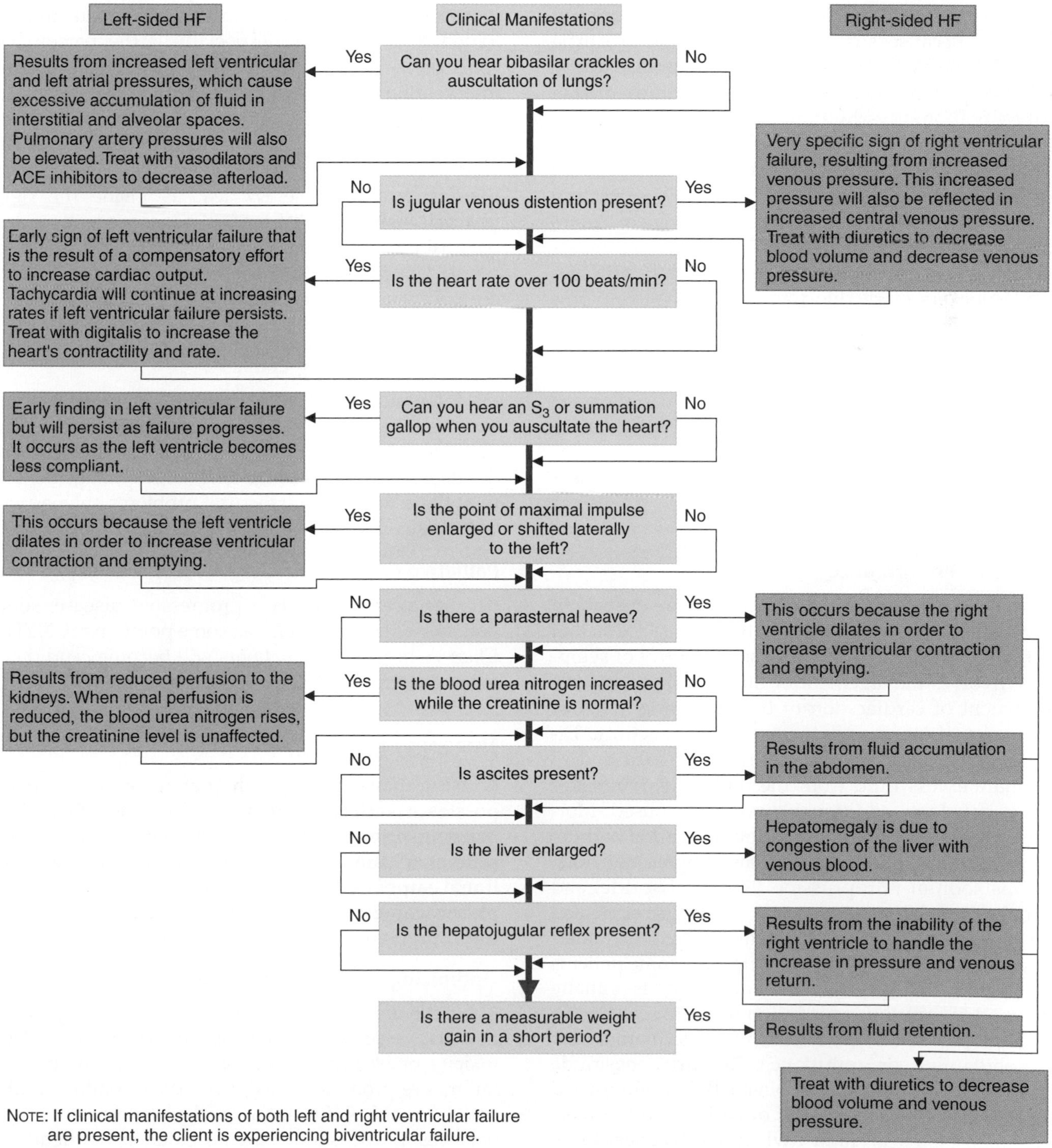

NOTE: If clinical manifestations of both left and right ventricular failure are present, the client is experiencing biventricular failure.

ACE, Angiotensin-converting enzyme; *HF*, heart failure.

cause of the pulmonary edema include use of the serum BNP level[60] or insertion of a pulmonary artery (PA) catheter. The PA catheter is used to determine the patients "wedge" pressure. It is essential to understand the different etiologies because the treatment of each form of pulmonary edema is very specific.

Dysrhythmias and Heart Failure

A ventricular EF below 30% and the presence of NYHA class III or IV heart failure are strongly associated with ventricular dysrhythmias and an increased risk of death.[61,62] Because sustained ventricular tachycardia or fibrillation (VT/VF) initiate sudden cardiac death, high-risk patients with severe heart failure are prescribed both antidysrhythmic drugs and have an implantable cardioverter-defibrillator (ICD) inserted.[62-64]

Many patients with heart failure also have atrial fibrillation. Digoxin is frequently prescribed in atrial fibrillation to control ventricular heart rate. Digoxin does not prolong life but makes patients feel less symptomatic. Digoxin may also work synergistically with specific β-blockers (carvedilol) and make the symptoms more tolerable for patients with severe heart failure.[62,65]

MEDICAL MANAGEMENT

The goals of the medical management of heart failure are to relieve heart failure symptoms, enhance cardiac performance, and correct known precipitating causes of acute heart failure.

Relief of Symptoms and Enhancement of Cardiac Performance

In the acute phase of advanced heart failure the patient may have a pulmonary artery catheter in place so that LV function can be followed closely. Control of symptoms involves management of fluid overload and improvement of cardiac output by decreasing systemic vascular resistance and increasing contractility. Diuretics are administered to decrease preload and to eliminate excess fluid from the body.[54] If pulmonary edema develops, additional diuretics are used. Morphine is given to facilitate peripheral dilation and decrease anxiety. Afterload is decreased by vasodilators, such as sodium nitroprusside (SNP or Nipride) and nitroglycerin. Nitrates are used to decrease preload and vasodilate the coronary arteries if CAD is an underlying cause of the acute heart failure. For some patients an IABP is also required.[66] Contractility is initially increased by continuous infusion of positive inotropic drugs (dopamine) or by combination inodilators such as dobutamine or milrinone. The drug nesiritide (Natrecor) is a human recombinant BNP administered IV. It is indicated for the relief of patients with acutely decompensated heart failure who have dyspnea at rest. Nesiritide lowers pulmonary artery pressures and "wedge" pressure, which decreases symptoms of dyspnea.[67,68]

Once the acute heart failure is controlled, the patient is weaned off IV medications, which are gradually replaced by oral agents. Before the transition out of the critical care unit, the heart failure patient will receive ACE inhibitors to prevent LV chamber remodeling and slow or avoid LV dilation.[43,52,53] If the patient does not tolerate ACE inhibitors, the ARB category of drugs may be substituted.[53] Low dosage β-blockers such as carvedilol may also be prescribed, although strict surveillance is required to anticipate and avoid untoward negative inotropic effects.[62,69] Digoxin may be added to the regimen, especially if the person has concomitant atrial fibrillation.[65] Nonpharmacologic interventions that are increasingly used include pacemaker cardiac resynchronization therapy (CRT).[70] CRT is biventricular pacing where the right and left ventricles each have a pacing lead in contact with the myocardium. The RV lead is inside the right ventricle, while the LV lead is positioned into a left wall tributary of the coronary sinus vein.[71-73] In newer permanent pacemaker models, both RV and LV leads are paced to synchronize the ventricles and improve heart failure symptoms.

Correct Precipitating Causes

Once symptoms of HF are controlled, diagnostic studies such as cardiac catheterization, echocardiogram, and thallium scan are undertaken to uncover the cause of the heart failure and tailor long-term management to treat the cause. Some structural problems such as valvular disease may be amenable to surgical correction.

Palliative Care for End-Stage Heart Failure

Because heart failure is a progressive disease, some patients will not recover.[73] At some point, many NYHA Class IV heart failure patients will become candidates for palliative care.[73]

NURSING MANAGEMENT

Nursing management of the patient with HF incorporates a variety of nursing diagnoses (Box 12-8). Nursing priorities focus on (1) optimizing cardiopulmonary function, (2) promoting comfort and emotional support, (3) monitoring the effectiveness of pharmacologic therapy, (4) providing adequate nutrition, and (5) providing patient education.

Optimizing Cardiopulmonary Function

The patient's ECG is evaluated for any dysrhythmias that may be present or may develop as a result of drug toxicity or electrolyte imbalance. Patients with heart failure are prone to digoxin toxicity secondary to decreased renal perfusion, as well as to electrolyte imbalances. Breath sounds are auscultated frequently to determine adequacy of respiratory effort and to assess for onset or worsening of pulmonary congestion. Oxygen through a nasal cannula is administered to relieve

Box 12-8

NURSING DIAGNOSIS PRIORITIES

Acute Heart Failure

- Impaired Gas Exchange related to ventilation/perfusion mismatching or intrapulmonary shunting, p. A-29
- Decreased Cardiac Output related to alterations in preload, p. A-12
- Decreased Cardiac Output related to alterations in contractility, p. A-12
- Decreased Cardiac Output related to alterations in heart rate or rhythm, p. A-12
- Activity Intolerance related to cardiopulmonary dysfunction, p. A-2
- Anxiety related to threat to biologic, psychologic, and/or social integrity, p. A-9
- Ineffective Coping related to situational crisis and personal vulnerability, p. A-38
- Insomnia related to circadian desynchronization, p. A-43
- Deficient Knowledge: Discharge Regimen related to lack of previous exposure to information, p. A-18
- Readiness for Enhanced Therapeutic Regimen Management

dyspnea. Diuretics or vasodilators are used to decrease excessive preload and afterload.[54,67] If the patient is not hypotensive, morphine may be administered to decrease hyperventilation and anxiety. If the patient's ventilatory status worsens, the nurse must be prepared for endotracheal intubation and mechanical ventilation. Obtaining daily weights is important until the weight stabilizes at a "dry" weight. Generally, the daily weight is used in fluid management, and a weekly weight is optimally used for tracking body weight (muscle, fat).

Promoting Comfort and Emotional Support

During periods of breathlessness, activity must be restricted; bed rest usually is prescribed for the patient, who is positioned with the head of the bed elevated to allow for maximal lung expansion. The arms can be supported on pillows so that no undue stress is placed on the shoulder muscles. The legs may be placed in a dependent position to encourage venous pooling, thereby decreasing venous return. Rest periods must be carefully planned and adhered to, while independence within the patient's activity prescription is fostered. Vital signs are recorded before an activity is begun and after it is completed. Signs of activity intolerance, such as dyspnea, fatigue, sustained increase in pulse, and onset of dysrhythmias, are documented and reported to the physician. Activity is gradually increased according to patient tolerance. Skin breakdown is a risk because of the combination of bed rest, inadequate nutrition, peripheral edema, and decreased perfusion to the skin and subcutaneous tissue. Frequent position changes and mobilization are helpful to provide comfort and prevent this complication.

Monitoring the Effectiveness of Pharmacologic Therapy

Patients experiencing acute heart failure require aggressive pharmacologic therapy.[62,68,74,75] The nurse must know the action, side effects, therapeutic levels, and toxic effects of the diuretics and venodilators used to decrease preload, the positive inotropic agents used to increase ventricular contractility, the vasodilators used to decrease afterload, and any antidysrhythmics used to control heart rate and prevent dysrhythmias. The patient's hemodynamic response to these agents is closely monitored. Fluid intake and output balances are tabulated daily, or even hourly, in the critical care unit.

Providing Adequate Nutrition

Patients experiencing heart failure often experience decreased appetite and nausea; therefore small, frequent meals may be more appropriate than the standard three large meals. Food must be as tasty as possible; favorite foods as well as food from home may be incorporated into the diet as long as the foods are compatible with nutritional restrictions such as low sodium to decrease the risk of fluid retention. Each patient must be assessed for nutritional imbalance individually. Some people with heart failure are well nourished, some are obese, and some are malnourished before they enter the hospital.

Providing Patient Education

The nurse assesses both the patient's and family's understanding of the pathophysiology and individual risk factor profile for heart failure.[76] Primary topics of education include the importance of a low-salt diet, daily weight, fluid restrictions, and written information about the multiple medications used to control the symptoms of heart failure.[43,77] Many patients with a diagnosis of heart failure also require education about lifestyle changes such as smoking cessation, weight loss, energy conservation, and how to incorporate exercise and sodium restriction into their daily life.[55,78,79] Achieving the optimal outcomes for the patient with heart failure requires contributions from a team of educated health care clinicians.[43,55,77,79] **Collaborative multidisciplinary goals, developed from clinical practice guidelines for management of the patient with symptoms of acute heart failure, are listed in Evidence-Based Collaborative Practice: Heart Failure.**

CARDIOMYOPATHY

DESCRIPTION AND ETIOLOGY

Cardiomyopathy is a disease of the heart muscle: *cardio* (heart), *myo* (muscle), and *pathy* (pathology). Cardiomyopathies are classified on the basis of structural abnormalities and, if known, genotype. The classic cardiomyopathic categories are hypertrophic, restrictive, and dilated as illustrated in Figure 12-15. Recently an

EVIDENCE-BASED COLLABORATIVE PRACTICE

Heart Failure

A collaborative heart failure management team provides an integrated approach to care to achieve clinical stability for the patient.

1. **Ensure systematic assessment and management**
   - To achieve an absence of "congestion" and to stabilize patient's condition at the best "stage" possible when in hospital (see Tables 12-4 and 12-5)
   - To maintain same stability once discharged home and to avoid hospital readmission
2. **Counsel and educate patient/family after discharge from hospital. Patients and families should understand the following:**
   - Heart failure disease process.
   - Heart failure medications, dosages, medication schedule, drug side effects.
   - Fluid balance related to salt restriction (2-g sodium diet), daily weight, diuretic regimen.
   - When to call health care provider.
   - Risk of additional complications: sudden cardiac death, progressive heart failure, need for other cardiac procedures (pacemaker; ICD, PCI) or cardiac surgery (bypass graft, valve replacement). Some patients may require a mechanical assist device or heart transplantation.
   - Purpose of "advance directive" for health care decisions.
3. Promote patient compliance with treatment regimen.
   - Patients need support from concerned companions and health care professionals.
   - Patient should remain physically active and involved with life.
4. Facilitate hospital discharge; implement outpatient models of health care delivery.
   - Close communication between inpatient and outpatient health care providers is essential.

Data from Grady KL et al: *Circulation* 102:2443, 2000; and Hunt S et al: *Circulation* 112(12):e154, 2005.
ICD, Implantable cardioverter-defibrillator; *PCI,* percutaneous coronary intervention.

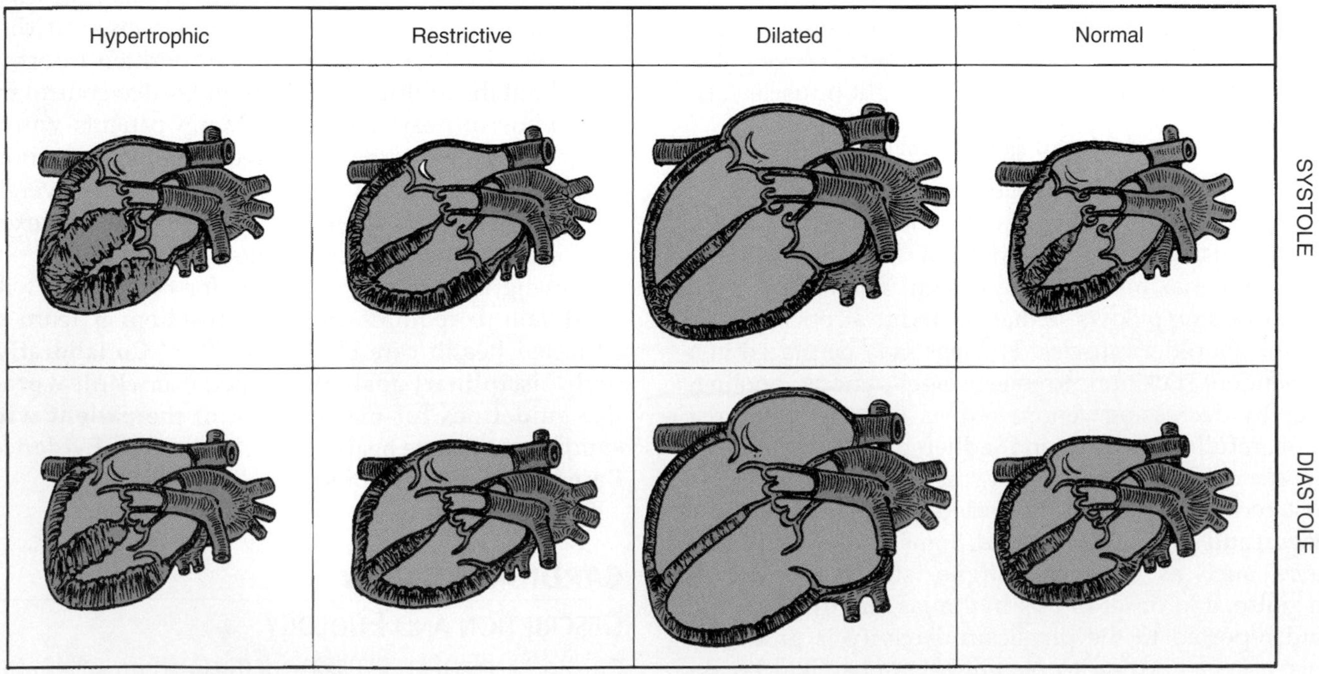

A B C D

FIGURE 12-15. Types of cardiomyopathies and the differences in ventricular diameter during systole and diastole, compared with a normal heart. **A,** Hypertrophic. **B,** Restrictive. **C,** Dilated. **D,** Normal.

additional classification has been proposed with the terms genetic, acquired, and mixed.[80]

Hypertrophic Cardiomyopathy

HCM is a genetically inherited disease that affects the myocardial sarcomere.[81,82] As HCM progresses, the left ventricle becomes stiff, noncompliant, and hypertrophied, sometimes in an asymmetrical fashion.[81] Today it is apparent that HCM occurs in two forms. The most well known, but less frequent, manifestation is a stiff, noncompliant myocardial muscle with LV hypertrophy and bizarre cellular hypertrophy of the upper ventricular septum. This LV septal hypertrophy obstructs outflow through the aortic valve, especially during exercise (see Figure 12-15, *A*). It also pulls the papillary muscle out of alignment, causing mitral regurgitation. This form of HCM used to be known as *idiopathic hypertrophic subaortic stenosis (IHSS)*; however, because IHSS does not describe all patients with hypertrophied hearts, the more general term *HCM* is now used.[81] Other patients with HCM have generalized LV hypertrophy, but the septum is not more enlarged than the rest of the myocardium.[81] HCM causes significant diastolic dysfunction because the muscle-bound, stiff, noncompliant heart muscle cannot fill adequately during diastole.

Symptoms in HCM are similar to those seen with heart failure plus the symptoms of myocardial ischemia, supraventricular tachycardia (SVT), VT syncope, and stroke.[82] Symptoms are generally more intense with physical exercise, especially in the obstructive form of HCM where the aortic outflow tract is obstructed by the enlarged LV septum. There is also a known association between HCM and sudden cardiac death (SCD). For this reason, limitation of physical activity may be recommended. Causes of SCD are thought to stem from ventricular dysrhythmias and also atrial fibrillation.[81] Episodes of paroxysmal atrial fibrillation occur in 20% to 25% of HCM patients.[81] Pharmacologic management includes β-blockers to decrease LV workload, prevention of atrial and ventricular dysrhythmias, anticoagulation if atrial fibrillation or left ventricular thrombi are present, and management of heart failure symptoms. Interventional procedures include insertion of an ICD to decrease the risk of SCD, and percutaneous alcohol ablation of the intraventricular septum to decrease the size of the septal wall.[81,82] Surgical procedures such as septal myectomy and mitral valve replacement are options now used less frequently.[81]

Dilated Cardiomyopathy

Dilated cardiomyopathy is characterized by gross dilation of both ventricles without muscle hypertrophy (see Figure 12-15, *C*). There are several distinct causes of dilated cardiomyopathy, which may be genetic, acquired, or mixed,[80] as discussed below.

Ischemic Dilated Cardiomyopathy. Ischemic dilated cardiomyopathy is caused by repeated myocardial injury or infarction secondary to the sequelae of coronary artery disease. It is the most common cause of acquired dilated cardiomyopathy in the United States. The patient will have signs and symptoms of systolic heart failure and a low EF.[46]

Familial Dilated Cardiomyopathy. When the cause of the dilated cardiomyopathy is unknown, it is termed *idiopathic*. In some, but not all cases, the occurrence is linked to *genetic inheritance*.[84-86] The heritable trait can be expressed as either autosomal-dominant or recessive gene inheritance.[84-86] Preliminary research studies indicate that the genetic picture is highly individual between different family groups, even if the clinical picture appears similar.[84-86]

Acquired Causes of Dilated Cardiomyopathy. There are many acquired causes of dilated cardiomyopathy.[80] Injury can be caused by valvular heart dysfunction that has placed extreme pressure or volume on the chambers; also, viral or bacterial infections such as myocarditis can lead to inflammatory changes that permanently remodel the heart.[80,87] Other noncardiac causes include infiltration by systemic collagens as in amyloidosis or sarcoidosis.[88]

In dilated cardiomyopathy the myocardial muscle fibers contract poorly, resulting in global left ventricular dysfunction, low cardiac output, atrial and ventricular dysrhythmias, blood pooling that leads to ventricular thrombi and embolic episodes, and finally, refractory heart failure and premature death. The goals of the medical management of dilated cardiomyopathy are similar to those for systolic heart failure: improvement of pump function, removal of excess fluid, control of heart failure symptoms, anticipation and management of complications, and prevention of SCD.

Restrictive Cardiomyopathy. Restrictive cardiomyopathy (RCM) is the least commonly encountered cardiomyopathy in industrialized societies (see Figure 12-15, *B*). As with the other cardiomyopathies, this form can have a genetic component or be acquired.[80] RCM results in ventricular wall rigidity as a consequence of myocardial fibrosis. The overall effect is the diastolic inhibition of ventricular filling. Diastolic heart failure, low cardiac output, dyspnea, orthopnea, and liver engorgement are the most common clinical manifestations of restrictive cardiomyopathy. Medical management includes β-blockers to slow the heart rate and allow more time for ventricular filling, diuretics to remove excess fluid, and a low-sodium diet.

Nursing Management

Nursing management of the patient with cardiomyopathy incorporates a variety of nursing diagnoses related to the symptoms of HF (see Box 12-8). **Nursing**

priorities are individualized according to the type of cardiomyopathy and focus on (1) maintaining fluid balance, (2) monitoring effects of pharmacologic therapy, (3) increasing mobility, (4) and providing patient education.

As with HF, a collaborative team of compassionate, knowledgeable professionals is required to provide effective care and education for these challenging patients.[77]

VALVULAR HEART DISEASE

Description and Etiology

Valvular heart disease describes structural and/or functional abnormalities of single or multiple cardiac valves. The result is an alteration in blood flow across the valve. The two types of valvular lesions are stenotic and regurgitant. These are described here with reference to the specific cardiac valves involved.

Usually, if a person is admitted to the critical care unit with valve disease, he or she either is experiencing acute heart failure or is being admitted for cardiac surgical valvular replacement. In the past in the United States, most valvular lesions were rheumatic in origin; that is, damage was a direct result of group A β-hemolytic streptococcal pharyngitis.[89] Today, as a result of aggressive antibiotic treatment of "strep throat," this is rarely a problem, although it has not been completely eliminated as a cause.[89] The elderly person typically presents with symptoms of heart failure and *"degenerative"* valve changes. These may be described as *myxomatous* leaflet degeneration or annular calcification.[90,91]

Pathophysiology

Mitral Valve Stenosis

Mitral stenosis (MS) describes a progressive narrowing of the mitral valve orifice. Symptoms occur when the normal valve size is reduced to 2 cm^2 or less.[91] Symptoms occur at rest when the valve area is reduced below 1 cm.[91] Narrowing is caused by aging valve tissue or by acute rheumatic valvulitis (Table 12-7, *A*). The diffuse valve leaflets fibrose and fuse, reducing mobility and thickening the chordae tendineae. As a result, the mitral valve can no longer open or close passively in response to left atrial and ventricular pressure changes. Thus, blood flow across the valve is impeded. Mitral stenosis increases the risk of developing atrial fibrillation because of the high pressures in the left atrium that will stimulate left atrial remodeling and enlargement. Development of atrial fibrillation will significantly increase symptoms and may increase the need for surgical replacement of the valve.

Table 12-7
Valvular Dysfunction

	PATHOPHYSIOLOGY	CLINICAL MANIFESTATIONS	PHYSICAL SIGNS
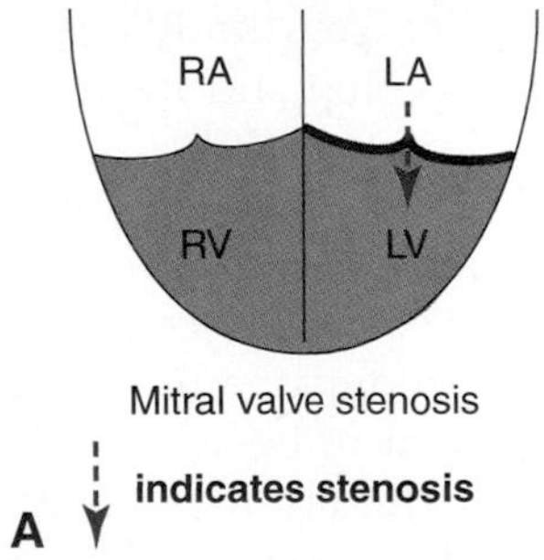	**Mitral Valve Stenosis** Left atrium must generate more pressure to propel blood beyond the lesion Rise in left atrial pressure and volume reflected retrograde into pulmonary vessels Right ventricular hypertrophy Right ventricular failure	Dyspnea on exertion Fatigue and weakness Pronounced respiratory symptoms—orthopnea, paroxysmal nocturnal dyspnea Mild hemoptysis with bronchial capillary rupture Susceptibility to pulmonary infections	Chest radiograph—pulmonary congestion, redistribution of blood flow to upper lobes ECG—atrial fibrillation and other atrial dysrhythmias Auscultation—diastolic murmur, accentuated S_1, opening snap Catheterization—elevated pressure gradient across valve; increased left atrial pressure, pulmonary artery wedge pressure, and pulmonary artery pressure; low cardiac output
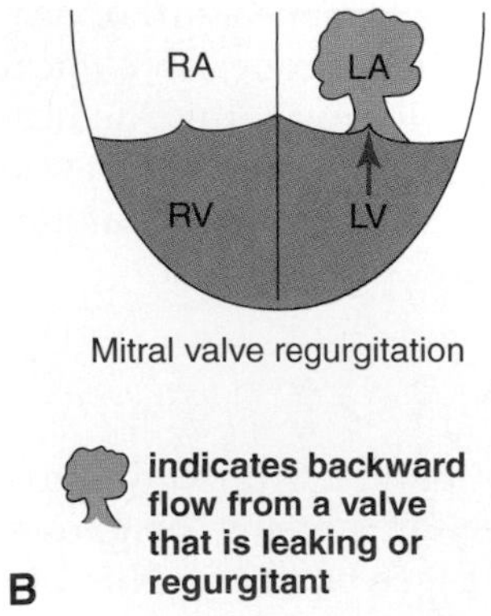	**Mitral Valve Regurgitation** Left ventricular dilation and hypertrophy Left atrial dilation and hypertrophy	Weakness and fatigue Exertional dyspnea Palpitations Severe symptoms precipitated by left ventricular failure, with consequent low output and pulmonary congestion	Chest radiograph—left atrial and left ventricular enlargement, variable pulmonary congestion ECG—P mitrale, left ventricular hypertrophy, atrial fibrillation Auscultation—murmur throughout systole Catheterization—opacification of left atrium during left ventricular injection, v waves, increased left atrial and left ventricular pressures Variable elevations of pulmonary pressures

Table 12-7
Valvular Dysfunction—*cont'd*

	PATHOPHYSIOLOGY	CLINICAL MANIFESTATIONS	PHYSICAL SIGNS
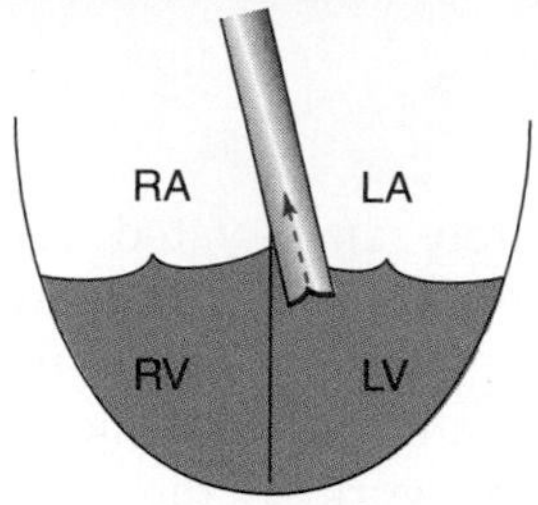 Aortic valve stenosis C ⇡ indicates stenosis	**Aortic Valve Stenosis** Left ventricular hypertrophy Progressive failure of ventricular emptying Pulmonary congestion Failure of right side of heart, with systemic venous congestion Sudden cardiac death	Exertional dyspnea Exercise intolerance Syncope Angina Heart failure (left ventricular failure)	Chest radiograph—poststenotic aortic dilation, calcification ECG—left ventricular hypertrophy Auscultation—systolic ejection murmur Catheterization—significant pressure gradient, increased left ventricular end-diastolic pressure
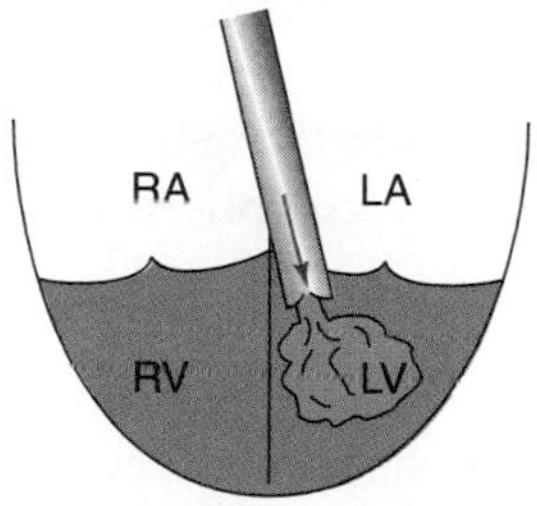 Aortic valve regurgitation D indicates backward flow from a valve that is leaking or regurgitant	**Aortic Valve Regurgitation** Increased volume load imposed on left ventricle Left ventricular dilation and hypertrophy	Fatigue Dyspnea and exertion Palpitations	Chest radiograph—boot-shaped elongation of cardiac apex ECG—left ventricular hypertrophy Auscultation—diastolic murmur Catheterization—opacification of left ventricle during aortic injection Peripheral signs—hyperdynamic myocardial action and low peripheral resistance
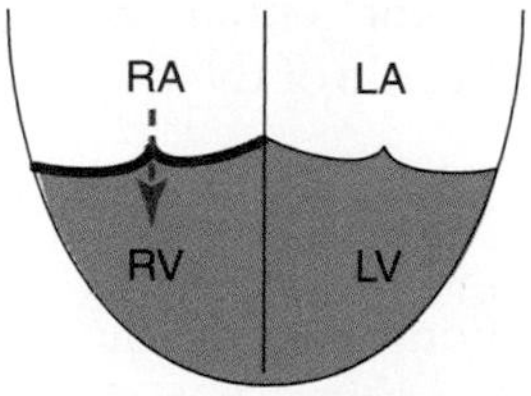 Tricuspid valve stenosis E ⇣ indicates stenosis	**Tricuspid Valve Stenosis** Right atrium must generate higher pressure to eject blood beyond the lesion Right atrial dilation Systemic venous engorgement Increased venous pressure	Venous distention Peripheral edema Ascites Hepatic engorgement Anorexia	Chest radiograph—right atrial enlargement ECG—right atrial enlargement (P pulmonale) Auscultation—diastolic murmur Catheterization—elevated right atrial pressure with large a waves; pressure gradient across the tricuspid valve
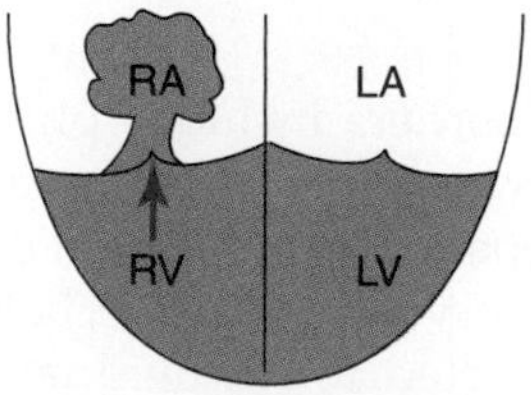 Tricuspid valve regurgitation F indicates backward flow from a valve that is leaking or regurgitant	**Tricuspid Valve Regurgitation** Right ventricular hypertrophy and dilation	Decreased cardiac output Neck vein distention Hepatic engorgement Ascites Edema Pleural effusions	Chest radiograph—right atrial and ventricular enlargement ECG—right ventricular hypertrophy and right atrial enlargement, atrial fibrillation Auscultation—murmur throughout systole Catheterization—elevated right atrial pressure and v waves

RA, Right atrium; *LA,* left atrium; *RV,* right ventricle; *LV,* left ventricle; *ECG,* electrocardiogram.

Mitral Valve Regurgitation

Mitral regurgitation may occur secondary to rheumatic disease, aging of the valve, or it can be caused by endocarditis, or papillary muscle dysfunction (Table 12-7, *B*). In mitral valve regurgitation (MR) the valve annulus, leaflets, chordae tendineae, and papillary muscles may all be dysfunctional, or the dysfunction may be isolated to just one component of the valve. Mitral valve regurgitation results in retrograde flow of blood into the left atrium with each ventricular contraction. MR is always described as either chronic or acute because of the very different impact upon the left-sided chambers.

With *chronic MR,* the left atrium will have dilated to accommodate the additional regurgitant volume, whereas the left ventricle will have hypertrophied (increased muscle) to maintain an adequate stroke volume and cardiac output. By contrast, *acute MR* is precipitated by papillary muscle rupture secondary to an acute MI.[91] This is a medical emergency. This left atrium cannot accommodate the sudden increase in volume and pressure, and use of an IABP and inotropic drug support are often required. Once the patient's condition has stabilized, surgical replacement or repair of the incompetent valve is performed.[92]

Aortic Valve Stenosis

Aortic stenosis (AS) describes a narrowing of the aortic valve area. AS can result from aging, rheumatic valvulitis, or deterioration of a congenital bicuspid valve[93] (Table 12-7, *C*). When the aortic valvular opening is reduced to less than 1.5 cm^2 this is classified as mild AS, and on cardiac catheterization or Doppler echocardiography there will be a *"gradient"* of about 25 mm Hg across the valve.[90] The gradient represents the difference in systolic pressure between the LV and the aorta. A significant pressure difference is a diagnostic hallmark of valvular stenosis.[90] If the valve orifice has narrowed to 1 cm^2 or less, the gradient will be greater than 50 mm Hg and the diagnosis will be upgraded to severe AS.[90] The impedance of LV ejection into the aorta results in increased left ventricular systolic pressure, left ventricular hypertrophy, and eventually left ventricular dilation. When symptoms such as angina, dyspnea, syncope, and other indicators of heart failure develop, it is critical to intervene to prevent further damage to the left ventricle. Aortic valve replacement is usually indicated.

Aortic Valve Regurgitation

Aortic regurgitation (AR), also know as aortic insufficiency (AI) can occur as a result of rheumatic fever, systemic hypertension, Marfan syndrome, syphilis, rheumatoid arthritis, aging valve tissue, or discrete subaortic stenosis (Table 12-7, *D*). Aortic valve incompetence results in a reflux of blood back into the left ventricle during ventricular diastole. To accommodate this extra volume, the left ventricle initially dilates and then hypertrophies in an attempt to empty more completely and to meet the needs of the peripheral circulation. Aortic valve replacement is recommended for symptomatic patients with well-preserved or moderate LV dysfunction.[94]

Tricuspid Valve Stenosis

Tricuspid stenosis (TS) is rarely an isolated lesion (Table 12-7, *E*). TS often occurs in conjunction with mitral or aortic disease. Its origin most often is rheumatic fever or a complication of endocarditis.[89] Tricuspid stenosis increases the pressure work of the usually low-pressure right atrium, resulting in right atrial hypertrophy. In addition, the right atrium dilates in an attempt to accommodate the residual right atrial volume and the incoming venous return. As a result, systemic venous congestion occurs—the consequences of which include jugular venous congestion, liver failure, hepatomegaly, ascites, and peripheral edema.

Tricuspid Valve Regurgitation

Tricuspid regurgitation usually results from advanced failure of the left side of the heart that eventually affects the right side of the heart, severe pulmonary hypertension, or as a complication of infective endocarditis[89] (Table 12-7, *F*).

Pulmonic Valve Disease

Pulmonary valve disease is not a common disorder in adults. It is most often related to congenital anomalies and produces failure of the right side of the heart.

Mixed Valvular Lesions

Many persons have mixed lesions (i.e., an element of both stenosis and regurgitation). Mixed lesions can accentuate the severity of a condition. For example, when combined, aortic stenosis and aortic regurgitation increase left ventricular volume and pressure and thereby multiply the degree of left ventricular work.

Medical Management

Management of valvular disorders includes pharmacologic therapy to control symptoms of heart failure and then cardiac surgical repair or replacement of the affected valve.[90-92] When surgery is not feasible, balloon dilation is a rare option selected for individuals too ill to undergo a major cardiac surgical procedure.

Nursing Management

Nursing management of the patient with valvular disease incorporates a variety of nursing diagnoses (Box 12-9). **Nursing priorities are focused on (1) maintaining adequate cardiac output, (2) optimizing fluid balance, and (3) providing patient education.**

Box 12-9

NURSING DIAGNOSIS PRIORITIES

Valvular Heart Disease

- Decreased Cardiac Output related to alterations in preload, p. A-12
- Decreased Cardiac Output related to alterations in afterload, p. A-12
- Decreased Cardiac Output related to alterations in contractility, p. A-13
- Decreased Cardiac Output related to alterations in heart rate or rhythm, p. A-13
- Activity Intolerance related to cardiopulmonary dysfunction, p. A-18
- Deficient Knowledge: Discharge Regimen related to lack of previous exposure to information, p. A-18
- Readiness for Enhanced Therapeutic Regimen Management

Maintaining Cardiac Output

Low cardiac output is a common finding in patients with valvular heart disease. It can occur because of decreased forward flow through a stenotic valve, because of bidirectional flow across an incompetent valve, or because of associated heart failure. Vital signs and the effect of positive inotropic and afterload-reducing agents are assessed and documented. If the patient has hemodynamic catheters inserted, cardiac output and hemodynamic parameters are measured and evaluated. Patient care activities are carefully planned to provide adequate rest periods to prevent fatigue.

Optimizing Fluid Balance

Fluid status is evaluated by auscultation of breath sounds for crackles, heart sounds for presence of an S_3, daily weight to trend a "sudden weight gain," and presence of peripheral edema. The appearance of pulmonary crackles or an S_3 heart sound confirms volume overload. The jugular vein is assessed for signs of increased distention. Diuretics and vasodilators are administered to counteract excess fluid retention. The patient is weighed daily, and fluid intake and output are monitored and recorded.

Providing Patient Education

Patient education for the patient with acute or chronic heart failure secondary to valvular dysfunction includes (1) information related to diet, (2) fluid restrictions, (3) the actions and side effects of heart failure medications, (4) the need for prophylactic antibiotics before undergoing any invasive procedures such as dental work, and (5) when to call the health care provider to report a negative change in cardiac symptoms. Many patients will also require information about valvular heart surgery. Achieving the optimal outcomes for the patient with valve disease requires contributions from a team of educated health care clinicians. **Collaborative multidisciplinary priorities are listed in** Box 12-10. **See the section on heart valve replacement in Chapter 13 for more information on surgical management.**

Box 12-10

Collaborative Management

Valvular Heart Disease

- **Assess valvular dysfunction**
  - Clinical assessment
  - *Auscultation* for heart murmurs
  - Signs/symptoms of heart failure; dyspnea is usually the earliest symptoms (see Table 12-5)
  - *Echocardiogram:* valve motion, ventricular wall motion
  - *Cardiac catheterization:* valve/ventricular wall motion, ejection fraction
- **Consider valve surgery**
  - If heart failure symptoms appear, surgery is indicated
  - Valve replacement
- **Provide patient/family education**
  - Anticoagulation (if mechanical valve or atrial fibrillation present)
  - Heart failure medications (if heart failure is present)
  - *Infection prevention:* endocarditis prophylaxis

Data from Bonow RO et al: *Circulation* 114(5):e84, 2006.

SUMMARY

The number of patients with cardiovascular disease continues to grow.[1] Fortunately, considerable research and clinical progress has occurred that has clarified the diagnosis and management of many cardiac conditions. To be able to participate fully in the collaborative management of patients with CV disorders, it is essential that the critical care nurse understand the spectrum of interventions from basic nursing care procedures to the most recent advances in therapy.

evolve To test your mastery of this chapter, try the Open-Book Quiz at http://evolve.elsevier.com/Urden/priorities/

REFERENCES

1. American Heart Association: *Heart disease and stroke statistics—2006 update,* Dallas, 2006, The Association.
2. Clark LT: Issues in minority health: atherosclerosis and coronary heart disease in African Americans, *Med Clin North Am* 89(5):977.
3. Antman EM et al: ACC/AHA guidelines for the management of patients with ST-elevation myocardial infarction—executive summary: a report of the American College of Cardiology/American Heart Association Task Force on Practice Guidelines (Writing Committee to Revise the 1999 Guidelines for the Management of Patients With Acute Myocardial Infarction), *Circulation* 110(5):588, 2004.
4. Gibbons RJ et al: ACC/AHA 2002 guideline update for the management of patients with chronic stable angina—summary article: a report of the American College of Cardiology/American Heart Association Task

Force on Practice Guidelines (Committee on the Management of Patients With Chronic Stable Angina), *Circulation* 107(1):149, 2003.

5. Executive summary of the third report of the National Cholesterol Education Program (NCEP) Expert Panel on Detection, Evaluation, and Treatment of High Blood Cholesterol in Adults (Adult Treatment Panel III), *JAMA* 285(19):2486, 2001.
6. Grundy SM et al: Implications of recent clinical trials for the National Cholesterol Education Program Adult Treatment Panel III guidelines, *Circulation* 110(2):227, 2004.
7. Barter PJ et al: Antiinflammatory properties of HDL, *Circ Res* 95(8):764, 2004.
8. O'Keefe JH Jr et al: Optimal low-density lipoprotein is 50 to 70 mg/dl: lower is better and physiologically normal, *J Am Coll Cardiol* 43(11):2142, 2004.
9. Fletcher B et al: Managing abnormal blood lipids: a collaborative approach, *Circulation* 112(20):3184, 2005.
10. Mokdad AH et al: The continuing epidemics of obesity and diabetes in the United States, *JAMA* 286(10):1195, 2001.
11. Chobanian AV et al: Seventh report of the Joint National Committee on Prevention, Detection, Evaluation, and Treatment of High Blood Pressure, *Hypertension* 42(6): 1206, 2003.
12. Thompson PD et al: Exercise and physical activity in the prevention and treatment of atherosclerotic cardiovascular disease: a statement from the Council on Clinical Cardiology (Subcommittee on Exercise, Rehabilitation, and Prevention) and the Council on Nutrition, Physical Activity, and Metabolism (Subcommittee on Physical Activity), *Circulation* 107(24):3109, 2003.
13. Brook RD et al: Air pollution and cardiovascular disease: a statement for healthcare professionals from the Expert Panel on Population and Prevention Science of the American Heart Association, *Circulation* 109(21):2655, 2004.
14. Sargent RP, Shepard RM, Glantz SA: Reduced incidence of admissions for myocardial infarction associated with public smoking ban: before and after study, *BMJ* 328(7446):977, 2004.
15. Houterman S, Verschuren WM, Kromhout D: Smoking, blood pressure and serum cholesterol: effects on 20-year mortality, *Epidemiology* 14(1):24, 2003.
16. Garber AJ et al: American College of Endocrinology position statement on inpatient diabetes and metabolic control, *Endocr Pract* 10(1):77, 2004.
17. McGuire DK et al: Association of diabetes mellitus and glycemic control strategies with clinical outcomes after acute coronary syndromes, *Am Heart J* 147(2):246, 2004.
18. Franklin K et al: Implications of diabetes in patients with acute coronary syndromes: the Global Registry of Acute Coronary Events, *Arch Intern Med* 164(13):1457, 2004.
19. Sarnak MJ et al: Kidney disease as a risk factor for development of cardiovascular disease: a statement from the American Heart Association Councils on Kidney in Cardiovascular Disease, High Blood Pressure Research, Clinical Cardiology, and Epidemiology and Prevention, *Hypertension* 42(5):1050, 2003.
20. Wright RS et al: Acute myocardial infarction and renal dysfunction: a high-risk combination, *Ann Intern Med* 137(7):563, 2002.
21. Grundy SM et al: Clinical management of metabolic syndrome: report of the American Heart Association/National Heart, Lung, and Blood Institute/American Diabetes Association conference on scientific issues related to management, *Circulation* 109(4):551, 2004.
22. Grady D et al: Cardiovascular disease outcomes during 6.8 years of hormone therapy: Heart and Estrogen/progestin Replacement Study follow-up (HERS II), *JAMA* 288(1):49, 2002.
23. Hulley S et al: Randomized trial of estrogen plus progestin for secondary prevention of coronary heart disease in postmenopausal women: Heart and Estrogen/progestin Replacement Study (HERS) Research Group, *JAMA* 280(7):605, 1998.
24. Anderson GL et al: Effects of conjugated equine estrogen in postmenopausal women with hysterectomy: the Women's Health Initiative randomized controlled trial, *JAMA* 291(14):1701, 2004.
25. Mosca L et al: Evidence-based guidelines for cardiovascular disease prevention in women, *Circulation* 109(5): 672, 2004.
26. Lefler LL, Bondy KN: Women's delay in seeking treatment with myocardial infarction: A meta synthesis, *J Cardiovasc Nurs* 19(4):251, 2004.
27. Smith SC et al: AHA/ACC guidelines for secondary prevention for patients with coronary and other atherosclerotic vascular disease: 2006 update—endorsed by the National Heart, Lung, and Blood Institute, *Circulation* 113(19):2363, 2006.
28. Watkins H, Farrall M: Genetic susceptibility to coronary artery disease: from promise to progress, *Nat Rev Genet* 7(3):163, 2006.
29. Pearson TA et al: Markers of inflammation and cardiovascular disease: application to clinical and public health practice—a statement for healthcare professionals from the Centers for Disease Control and Prevention and the American Heart Association, *Circulation* 107(3):499, 2003.
30. Speidl WS et al: High-sensitivity C-reactive protein in the prediction of coronary events in patients with premature coronary artery disease, *Am Heart J* 144(3):449, 2002.
31. Buffon A et al: Widespread coronary inflammation in unstable angina, *N Engl J Med* 347(1):5, 2002.
32. Smith SC Jr et al: ACC/AHA guidelines for percutaneous coronary intervention (revision of the 1993 PTCA guidelines)—executive summary: a report of the American College of Cardiology/American Heart Association task force on practice guidelines (Committee to revise the 1993 Guidelines for Percutaneous Transluminal Coronary Angioplasty) endorsed by the Society for Cardiac Angiography and Interventions, *Circulation* 103(24):3019, 2001.
33. Braunwald E et al: ACC/AHA guideline update for the management of patients with unstable angina and non–ST-segment elevation myocardial infarction—summary article: a report of the American College of Cardiology/American Heart Association Task Force on Practice Guidelines (Committee on the Management of Patients With Unstable Angina), *Circulation* 106(14):1893, 2002.
34. Mehta RH et al: Comparison of outcomes of patients with acute coronary syndromes with and without atrial fibrillation, *Am J Cardiol* 92(9):1031, 2003.
35. Birnbaum Y et al: Ventricular septal rupture after acute myocardial infarction, *N Engl J Med* 347(18):1426, 2002.

36. Birnbaum Y et al: Mitral regurgitation following acute myocardial infarction, *Coron Artery Dis* 13(6):337, 2002.
37. Maisch B et al: Guidelines on the diagnosis and management of pericardial diseases executive summary: the Task Force on the Diagnosis and Management of Pericardial Diseases of the European Society of Cardiology, *Eur Heart J* 25(7):587, 2004.
38. Wang K, Asinger RW, Marriott HJ: ST-segment elevation in conditions other than acute myocardial infarction, *N Engl J Med* 349(22):2128, 2003.
39. Wu AH et al: Hospital outcomes in patients presenting with congestive heart failure complicating acute myocardial infarction: a report from the Second National Registry of Myocardial Infarction (NRMI-2), *J Am Coll Cardiol* 40(8):1389, 2002.
40. Szekendi MK: Compliance with acute MI guidelines lowers inpatient mortality, *J Cardiovasc Nurs* 18(5):356, 2003.
41. Eagle KA et al: Adherence to evidence-based therapies after discharge for acute coronary syndromes: an ongoing prospective, observational study, *Am J Med* 117(2):73, 2004.
42. Balady GJ et al: Core components of cardiac rehabilitation/secondary prevention programs: a statement for healthcare professionals from the American Heart Association and the American Association of Cardiovascular and Pulmonary Rehabilitation Writing Group, *Circulation* 102(9):1069, 2000.
43. Hunt SA et al: ACC/AHA 2005 Guideline Update for the Diagnosis and Management of Chronic Heart Failure in the Adult: a report of the American College of Cardiology/American Heart Association Task Force on Practice Guidelines (Writing Committee to Update the 2001 Guidelines for the Evaluation and Management of Heart Failure)—developed in collaboration with the American College of Chest Physicians and the International Society for Heart and Lung Transplantation: endorsed by the Heart Rhythm Society, *Circulation* 112(12):e154, 2005, http://www.ahajournals.org
44. Zile MR, Brutsaert DL: New concepts in diastolic dysfunction and diastolic heart failure. I. Diagnosis, prognosis, and measurements of diastolic function, *Circulation* 105(11):1387, 2002.
45. Zile MR, Brutsaert DL: New concepts in diastolic dysfunction and diastolic heart failure. II. Causal mechanisms and treatment, *Circulation* 105(12):1503, 2002.
46. Henry LB: Left ventricular systolic dysfunction and ischemic cardiomyopathy, *Crit Care Nurs Q* 26(1):16, 2003.
47. Bolliger K, Sadar AM: Care and management of the patient with right heart failure secondary to diastolic dysfunction: an advanced practice perspective and case review, *Crit Care Nurs Q* 26(1):22, 2003.
48. Aurigemma GP, Gaasch WH: Clinical practice: diastolic heart failure, *N Engl J Med* 351(11):1097, 2004.
49. Zile MR, Baicu CF, Gaasch WH: Diastolic heart failure: abnormalities in active relaxation and passive stiffness of the left ventricle, *N Engl J Med* 350(19):1953, 2004.
50. Riedinger MS et al: Quality of life in patients with heart failure: do gender differences exist? *Heart Lung* 30(2):105, 2001.
51. Maisel AS et al: Bedside B-type natriuretic peptide in the emergency diagnosis of heart failure with reduced or preserved ejection fraction: results from the Breathing Not Properly (BNP) multinational study, *J Am Coll Cardiol* 41(11):2010, 2003.
52. Thohan V, Torre-Amione G, Koerner MM: Aldosterone antagonism and congestive heart failure: a new look at an old therapy, *Curr Opin Cardiol* 19(4):301, 2004.
53. Patten RD, Soman P: Prevention and reversal of LV remodeling with neurohormonal inhibitors, *Curr Treat Options Cardiovasc Med* 6(4):313, 2004.
54. Paul S: Balancing diuretic therapy in heart failure: loop diuretics, thiazides, and aldosterone antagonists, *Congest Heart Fail* 8(6):307, 2002.
55. Paul S: Ventricular remodeling, *Crit Care Nurs Clin North Am* 15(4):407, 2003.
56. Dimopoulos K et al: Meta-analyses of mortality and morbidity effects of an angiotensin receptor blocker in patients with chronic heart failure already receiving an ACE inhibitor (alone or with a beta-blocker), *Int J Cardiol* 93(2-3):105, 2004.
57. McCullough PA, Sandberg KR: B-type natriuretic peptide and renal disease, *Heart Fail Rev* 8(4):355, 2003.
58. Maisel AS et al: Impact of age, race, and sex on the ability of B-type natriuretic peptide to aid in the emergency diagnosis of heart failure: results from the Breathing Not Properly (BNP) multinational study, *Am Heart J* 147(6):1078, 2004.
59. Maisel AS et al: Rapid measurement of B-type natriuretic peptide in the emergency diagnosis of heart failure, *N Engl J Med* 347(3):161, 2002.
60. McCullough PA et al: Uncovering heart failure in patients with a history of pulmonary disease: rationale for the early use of B-type natriuretic peptide in the emergency department, *Acad Emerg Med* 10(3):198, 2003.
61. Buxton AE et al: Relation of ejection fraction and inducible ventricular tachycardia to mode of death in patients with coronary artery disease: an analysis of patients enrolled in the multicenter unsustained tachycardia trial, *Circulation* 106(19):2466, 2002.
62. Stroe AF, Gheorghiade M: Carvedilol: beta-blockade and beyond, *Rev Cardiovasc Med* 5(suppl 1):S18, 2004.
63. Zhang J: Sudden cardiac death: implantable cardioverter defibrillators and pharmacological treatments, *Crit Care Nurs Q* 26(1):45, 2003.
64. Whang W et al: Heart failure and the risk of shocks in patients with implantable cardioverter defibrillators: results from the Triggers of Ventricular Arrhythmias (TOVA) study, *Circulation* 109(11):1386, 2004.
65. Khand AU et al: Carvedilol alone or in combination with digoxin for the management of atrial fibrillation in patients with heart failure? *J Am Coll Cardiol* 42(11):1944, 2003.
66. Chen EW et al: Relation between hospital intra-aortic balloon counterpulsation volume and mortality in acute myocardial infarction complicated by cardiogenic shock, *Circulation* 108(8):951, 2003.
67. Burger AJ et al: Effect of nesiritide (B-type natriuretic peptide) and dobutamine on ventricular arrhythmias in the treatment of patients with acutely decompensated congestive heart failure: the PRECEDENT study, *Am Heart J* 144(6):1102, 2002.
68. Colbert K, Greene MH: Nesiritide (Natrecor): a new treatment for acutely decompensated congestive heart failure, *Crit Care Nurs Q* 26(1):40, 2003.

69. Abraham WT, Iyengar S: Practical considerations for switching beta-blockers in heart failure patients, *Rev Cardiovasc Med* 5(suppl 1):S36, 2004.
70. Albert NM: Cardiac resynchronization therapy through biventricular pacing in patients with heart failure and ventricular dyssynchrony, *Crit Care Nurse* 23(suppl 3):2, 2003.
71. Abraham WT, Hayes DL: Cardiac resynchronization therapy for heart failure, *Circulation* 108(21):2596, 2003.
72. Young JB et al: Combined cardiac resynchronization and implantable cardioversion defibrillation in advanced chronic heart failure: the MIRACLE ICD Trial, *JAMA* 289(20):2685, 2003.
73. Goodlin SJ et al: Consensus statement: palliative and supportive care in advanced heart failure, *J Card Fail* 10(3):200, 2004.
74. Rudisill PT, Kennedy C, Paul S: The use of beta-blockers in the treatment of chronic heart failure, *Crit Care Nurs Clin North Am* 15(4):439, 2003.
75. Fonarow GC et al: Organized Program to Initiate Life-saving Treatment in Hospitalized Patients with Heart Failure (OPTIMIZE-HF): rationale and design, *Am Heart J* 148(1):43, 2004.
76. Callahan HE: Families dealing with advanced heart failure: a challenge and an opportunity, *Crit Care Nurs Q* 26(3):230, 2003.
77. Grady KL et al: Team management of patients with heart failure: a statement for healthcare professionals from the Cardiovascular Nursing Council of the American Heart Association, *Circulation* 102(19):2443, 2000.
78. Coviello JS, Nystrom KV: Obesity and heart failure, *J Cardiovasc Nurs* 18(5):360, 2003.
79. Sneed NV, Paul SC: Readiness for behavioral changes in patients with heart failure, *Am J Crit Care* 12(5):444, 2003.
80. Maron BJ et al: Contemporary definitions and classification of the cardiomyopathies: an American Heart Association scientific statement from the Council on Clinical Cardiology, Heart Failure and Transplantation Committee; Quality of Care and Outcomes Research and Functional Genomics and Translational Biology Interdisciplinary Working Groups; and Council on Epidemiology and Prevention, *Circulation* 113:1807, 2006.
81. Maron BJ et al: American College of Cardiology/European Society of Cardiology clinical expert consensus document on hypertrophic cardiomyopathy: a report of the American College of Cardiology Foundation Task Force on Clinical Expert Consensus Documents and the European Society of Cardiology Committee for Practice Guidelines, *J Am Coll Cardiol* 42(9):1687, 2003.
82. Nishimura RA, Holmes DR Jr: Clinical practice: hypertrophic obstructive cardiomyopathy, *N Engl J Med* 350(13):1320, 2004.
83. Elliott P, McKenna WJ: Hypertrophic cardiomyopathy, *Lancet* 363(9424):1881, 2004.
84. Kamisago M et al: Mutations in sarcomere protein genes as a cause of dilated cardiomyopathy, *N Engl J Med* 343(23):1688, 2000.
85. Li D et al: Novel cardiac troponin T mutation as a cause of familial dilated cardiomyopathy, *Circulation* 104(18): 2188, 2001.
86. Murphy RT et al: Novel mutation in cardiac troponin I in recessive idiopathic dilated cardiomyopathy, *Lancet* 363(9406):371, 2004.
87. Noutsias M et al: Current insights into the pathogenesis, diagnosis and therapy of inflammatory cardiomyopathy, *Heart Fail Monit* 3(4):127, 2003.
88. Syed J, Myers R: Sarcoid heart disease, *Can J Cardiol* 20(1):89, 2004.
89. Bonow RO et al: ACC/AHA 2006 guidelines for the management of patients with valvular heart disease: a report of the American College of Cardiology/American Heart Association Task Force on Practice Guidelines (Writing Committee to Revise the 1998 Guidelines for the Management of Patients With Valvular Heart Disease)—developed in collaboration with the Society of Cardiovascular Anesthesiologists: endorsed by the Society for Cardiovascular Angiography and Interventions and the Society of Thoracic Surgeons, *Circulation* 114(5):e84, 2006.
90. Segal BL: Valvular heart disease. I. Diagnosis and surgical management of aortic valve disease in older adults, *Geriatrics* 58(9):31, 2003.
91. Segal BL: Valvular heart disease. II. Mitral valve disease in older adults, *Geriatrics* 58(10):26, 2003.
92. Wiegand DL: Advances in cardiac surgery: valve repair, *Crit Care Nurse* 23(2):72, 2003.
93. Robicsek F et al: The congenitally bicuspid aortic valve: how does it function? Why does it fail? *Ann Thorac Surg* 77(1):177, 2004.
94. Hicks GL Jr, Massey HT: Update on indications for surgery in aortic insufficiency, *Curr Opin Cardiol* 17(2):172, 2002.

CHAPTER 13

Cardiovascular Therapeutic Management

JONI DIRKS

OBJECTIVES

- Describe the functions of a temporary pacemaker and an implantable cardioverter-defibrillator.
- Identify the signs of reperfusion in a patient undergoing fibrinolytic therapy.
- Outline the nursing management for a patient undergoing cardiac surgery and cardiac interventional procedures.
- List the most important categories of cardiovascular drugs, their intended actions, and major significance.

A wide variety of therapeutic interventions are employed in the management of the patient with cardiovascular dysfunction. This chapter focuses on the priority interventions used to manage acute cardiovascular disorders in the critical care setting.

TEMPORARY PACEMAKERS

Pacemakers are electronic devices that can be used to initiate the heartbeat when the heart's intrinsic electrical system cannot effectively generate a rate adequate to support cardiac output. Pacemakers can be used temporarily, either supportively or prophylactically, until the condition responsible for the rate or conduction disturbance resolves.

Indications

The clinical indications for instituting temporary pacemaker therapy include bradydysrhythmias induced by drug toxicities, electrolyte imbalances, acute coronary syndromes, or as prophylactic support following cardiac surgery.[1] Tachydysrhythmias may also be treated by using a temporary pacing rate set higher than the rate of the dysrythmia.[1]

The Pacemaker System

A pacemaker system is a simple electrical circuit consisting of a pulse generator and a pacing lead (an insulated electrical wire) with one, two, or three electrodes.

Pacing Pulse Generator

The pulse generator is designed to generate an electrical current that travels through the pacing lead and exits through an electrode (exposed portion of the wire) that is in direct contact with the heart. This electrical current initiates a myocardial depolarization. The current then returns to the pulse generator to complete the circuit. The power source for a temporary external pulse generator is a standard 9-volt alkaline battery.

Pacing Lead Systems

The pacing lead used for temporary pacing may be *bipolar* or *unipolar*. In a unipolar system, only one electrode (negative) is in direct contact with the myocardium. In a bipolar system, two electrodes (positive and negative) are located within the heart. The bipolar lead used in transvenous pacing has two electrodes on one catheter (see Figure 13-1, *D*). In both unipolar and bipolar systems, the current flows from the negative terminal of the pulse generator, down the pacing lead to the negative electrode, and into the heart. The current is then picked up by the positive electrode (ground) and flows back up the lead to the positive terminal of the pulse generator. In a bipolar pacing wire, the distal, or negative, electrode is at the tip of the pacing lead and is in direct contact with the heart, usually inside the right atrium or ventricle. Approximately 1 cm from the negative electrode is a positive electrode. The negative electrode is attached to the negative terminal, and the positive electrode is attached to the positive terminal of the pulse generator, either directly or via a bridging cable (Figure 13-1).

Pacing Routes

Several routes are available for temporary cardiac pacing with advantages and disadvantages to each method.

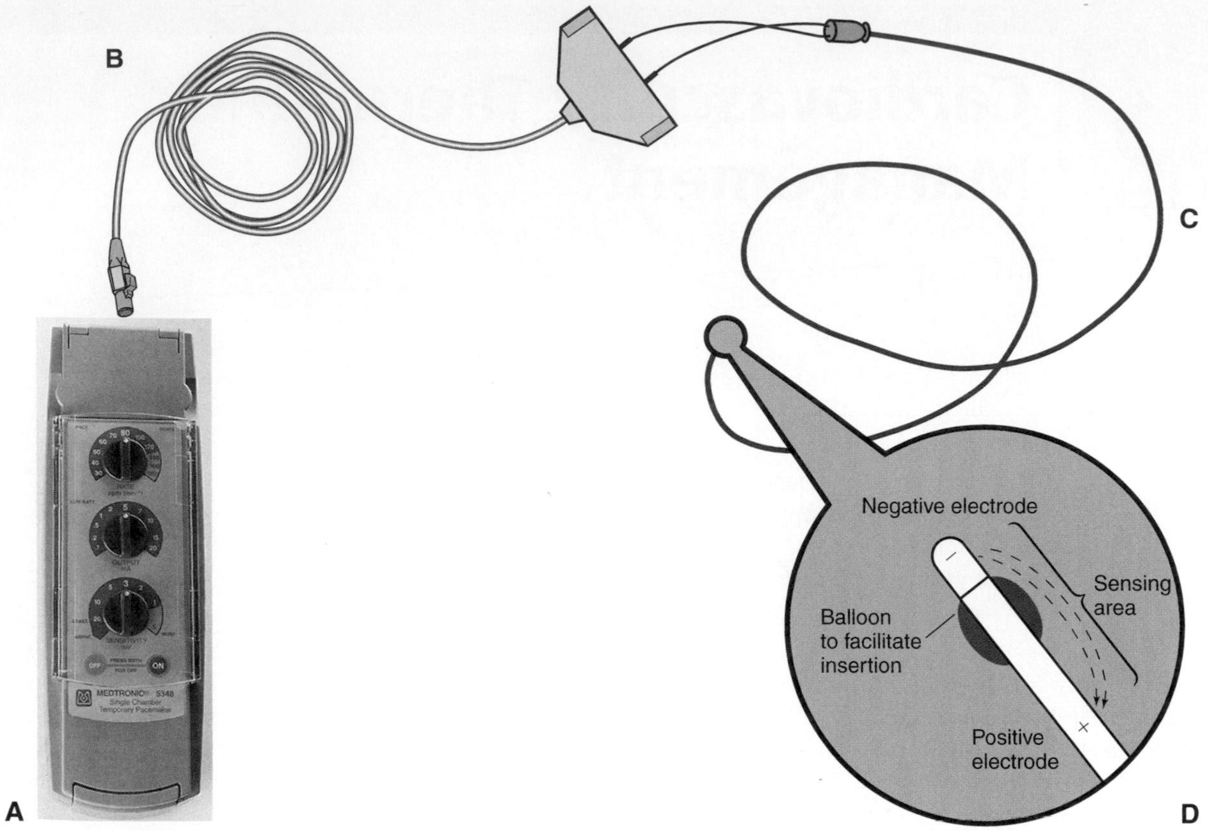

FIGURE 13-1. The components of a temporary bipolar transvenous catheter. **A,** Single-chamber temporary (external) pulse generator. **B,** Bridging cable. **C,** Pacing lead. **D,** Enlarged view of the pacing lead tip. (**A** Courtesy Medtronic Inc, Minneapolis, Minn.)

Transcutaneous Pacing

Transcutaneous cardiac pacing involves the use of two large skin electrodes, one placed anteriorly and the other posteriorly on the chest, connected to an external pulse generator. It is a rapid, noninvasive procedure that nurses can perform in the emergency setting and is recommended as a primary intervention in the advanced cardiac life support (ACLS) algorithm for the treatment of symptomatic bradycardia.[2] Improved technology related to stimulus delivery and the development of large electrode pads that help disperse the energy have helped reduce the pain associated with cutaneous nerve and muscle stimulation. This route is generally used as an emergency short-term therapy until the situation resolves or another route of pacing can be established.

Epicardial Pacing

The insertion of temporary epicardial pacing wires is a routine procedure during most cardiac surgical cases. Ventricular and in many cases atrial pacing wires are loosely sewn to the epicardium. The terminal pins of these wires are pulled through the skin before the chest is closed. The bipolar epicardial lead system often has two separate insulated wires (one negative and one positive electrode) that are loosely secured with sutures to the cardiac chamber to be paced. Both leads are in contact with the myocardial tissue, so either wire may be used as the negative, or pacing, electrode. The remaining wire is then used as the positive, or ground, electrode. If both chambers have pacing wires attached, the atrial wires exit the skin subcostally to the right of the sternum and the ventricular wires exit in the same region but to the left of the sternum. These wires can be removed several days after surgery by gentle traction at the skin surface with minimal risk of bleeding.[3]

Transvenous Pacing

Temporary transvenous endocardial pacing is accomplished by advancing a pacing electrode wire through a vein, often the subclavian or internal jugular, and into the right atrium or right ventricle. Insertion can be facilitated either through direct visualization with fluoroscopy or by the use of the bedside electrocardiogram (ECG).[1] In some cases the pacing wire is inserted through a specialized pulmonary artery catheter via a catheter port that exits in the right atrium or ventricle.

Table 13-1

NASPE/BPEG Generic (NPG) Code

POSITION I CHAMBER(S) PACED	II CHAMBER(S) SENSED	III RESPONSE TO SENSING	IV PROGRAMMABILITY	V ANTITACHYDYSRHYTHMIA FUNCTION(S)
0 = None	0 = None	0 = None	0 = None	0 = None
A = Atrium	A = Atrium	T = Triggered	P = Simple programmability (rate, output, sensitivity)	P = Pacing (antitachydysrhythmia)
V = Ventricle	V = Ventricle	I = Inhibited	M = Multiprogrammability	S = Shock
D = Dual (A + V)	D = Dual (A + V)	D = Dual (T + I)	C = Communicating	D = Dual (P + S)
S* = Single (A or V)	S = Single (A or V)			

Modified from Bernstein AD et al: *Pacing Clin Electrophysiol* 10:794, 1987.
*Used by manufacturer only.
NOTE: Positions I through III are used exclusively for antibradydysrhythmia function.
NASPE, North American Society of Pacing and Electrophysiology; *BPEG,* British Pacing and Electrophysiology Group.

CODES AND MODES

Three-Letter Pacemaker Code

The Inter-Society Commission for Heart Disease (ICHD) has a standardized code for describing the various pacing modes. A three-letter code is used to describe temporary pacing modes. The first letter refers to the cardiac chamber that is paced. The second letter designates which chamber is sensed, and the third letter indicates the pacemaker's response to the sensed event.[4]

Five-Letter Pacemaker Code

The five-letter pacemaker code contains the three-letter code categories plus two sections that list additional programming functions (Table 13-1).[4]

Synchronous Pacing Modes

Synchrony implies that the pacemaker only delivers a stimulus when the heart's intrinsic pacemaker fails to function at a predetermined rate. The most physiologic of the synchronous modes are those in which the normal sequential relationship between atrial and ventricular depolarization and contraction is maintained. Atrioventricular (AV) synchrony increases the volume in the ventricle before contraction and thus improves cardiac output. When atrial-to-ventricular conduction is impaired, as during heart block, AV synchrony can be maintained through dual-chamber (both atrial and ventricular) pacing modes.

DDD Pacing. The most physiologic of the AV pacing modes is the DDD mode.[3] In DDD pacing, atrial and ventricular leads are used for both pacing and sensing (Table 13-2). In response to sensed activity, the pacemaker inhibits the pacing stimulus. Therefore a sensed P wave in the atrium will inhibit the atrial pacing stimulus, whereas a sensed R wave in the ventricle will inhibit the ventricular pacing stimulus. DDD pacing is also described as "universal pacing" or "physiologic pacing" because it most closely resembles the heart's intrinsic conduction system.

Table 13-2

Examples of Temporary Pacing Modes

PACING MODE	DESCRIPTION
Asynchronous	
AOO	Atrial pacing, no sensing
VOO	Ventricular pacing, no sensing
DOO	Atrial and ventricular pacing, no sensing
Synchronous	
AAI	Atrial pacing, atrial sensing, inhibited response to sensed P waves
VVI	Ventricular pacing, ventricular sensing, inhibited response to sensed QRS complexes
DVI	Atrial and ventricular pacing, ventricular sensing; both atrial and ventricular pacing are inhibited if a spontaneous ventricular depolarization is sensed
Universal	
DDD	Both chambers are paced and sensed; inhibited response of the pacing stimuli to sensed events in their respective chamber; triggered response to sensed atrial activity to allow for rate-responsive ventricular pacing

VVI Pacing. The VVI mode is designed to pace the ventricle when the pacemaker does not sense an intrinsic (patient-initiated) ventricular depolarization. Other names that are popularly used for this mode include "backup pacing" or "demand pacing" (see Table 13-2). VVI pacing is necessary in specific circumstances; the classic example is symptomatic bradycardia with atrial fibrillation (AF). Because AF makes it impossible to pace the atria, one effective intervention is to use VVI pacing to maintain ventricular function.

Asynchronous Pacing Modes

Fixed-rate or asynchronous pacing modes ignore the patient's intrinsic heartbeat. These modes are uncommon with the exception of two situations. Emergency DOO or VOO pacing may be used in asystole as a lifesaving measure. These modes are sometimes used in the operating room, where electromagnetic interference (EMI) from electrocautery and other electrical equipment can interfere with normal pacemaker function.[5]

Pacemaker Settings

The controls on all external temporary pulse generators are similar, and their function must be thoroughly understood so that pacing can be initiated quickly in an emergency situation and troubleshooting facilitated should problems with the pacemaker arise.

The *rate control* regulates the number of impulses that can be delivered to the heart per minute. The rate setting depends on the physiologic needs of the patient, but in general it is maintained between 60 and 80 beats/min.

The *output control* regulates the amount of electrical current (measured in milliamperes [mA]) that is delivered to the heart to initiate depolarization. The point at which depolarization occurs is termed *pacing threshold* and is indicated by a myocardial response to the pacing stimulus (capture). The pacing threshold can be determined by gradually decreasing the output setting until 1:1 capture is lost. The output setting is then slowly increased until 1:1 capture is reestablished; this threshold to pace is less than 1 mA with a properly positioned pacing electrode. The output, however, is set two to three times higher than threshold because thresholds tend to fluctuate over time. The procedure for measuring pacing thresholds is described in Box 13-1. Separate output controls for both the atrium and the ventricle are used with a dual-chamber pulse generator.

The *sensitivity control* regulates the ability of the pacemaker to detect the heart's intrinsic electrical activity. Sensitivity is measured in millivolts (mV) and determines the size of the intracardiac signal that the generator will recognize. If the sensitivity is adjusted to its most sensitive setting—a setting of 0.5 to 1.0 mV—the pacemaker can respond even to low-amplitude electrical signals coming from the heart. On the other hand, turning the sensitivity to its least sensitive setting (adjusting the dial to a setting of 20 mV or to the area labeled *async*) will result in the inability of the pacemaker to sense any intrinsic electrical activity and cause the pacemaker to function at a fixed rate. A sense indicator (often a light) on the pulse generator signals each time intrinsic cardiac electrical activity is sensed. A pulse generator may be designed to sense atrial or ventricular activity, or both. The procedure for measuring sensitivity thresholds when a patient is connected to a temporary pacing generator is described in Box 13-2.

The *AV interval control* (available only on dual-chamber generators) regulates the time interval between the atrial and ventricular pacing stimuli. This interval is analogous to the PR interval that occurs in the intrinsic ECG. Proper adjustment of this interval to between 150 and 250 milliseconds (msec) preserves AV synchrony and permits maximal ventricular stroke volume and enhanced cardiac output.

Box 13-1
Temporary Pacemaker Testing for Pacing Thresholds

1. Adjust pacemaker rate setting so that patient is 100% paced. It may be necessary to increase the pacing rate to achieve this setting.
2. Gradually decrease output (milliampere, mA) setting until 1:1 capture is lost. Pacing threshold is located where capture is lost.
3. Slowly increase output setting until 1:1 capture is reestablished. With a properly positioned pacing electrode, the pacing threshold should be less than 1.0 mA.
4. Set output (mA) setting two to three times higher than measured threshold because thresholds tend to fluctuate over time.
5. Evaluate pacing thresholds for both atrial and ventricular leads separately if patient is connected to a dual-chamber pulse generator.

Box 13-2
Temporary Pacemaker Testing for Sensitivity Thresholds

- Set the sensitivity control to its most sensitive setting.
- Adjust the pulse generator rate to 10 beats/min less than the patient's intrinsic rate (the flash indicator should flash regularly).
- Reduce the generator output to the minimal value to prevent the risk of competing with the intrinsic rhythm.
- Gradually increase the sensitivity value until the sense indicator stops flashing and the pace indicator starts flashing.
- Decrease sensitivity until the sense indicator begins to flash again; this is the sensitivity threshold.
- Adjust the sensitivity setting on the generator to half the threshold value; restore generator output and rate to their original values.

Temporary DDD pacemakers have several other digital controls that are unique to this newer type of temporary pulse generator. The *lower rate,* or *base rate,* determines the rate at which the generator will pace when intrinsic activity falls below the set rate of the pacemaker. The *upper rate* determines the fastest ventricular rate the pacemaker will deliver in response to sensed atrial activity. This setting is needed to protect the patient's heart from being paced in response to rapid atrial dysrhythmias. The *pulse width,* which can be adjusted from 0.05 to 2 msec, controls the length of time that the pacing stimulus is delivered to the heart. There also is an *atrial refractory period,* programmable from 150 to 500 msec, which regulates the length of time after either a sensed or paced ventricular event, during which the pacemaker cannot respond to another atrial stimulus. An emergency button is also available on some models to allow for rapid initiation of asynchronous (DOO) pacing during an emergency.

On all newer temporary pacemakers, the on/off switch is coupled with a safety feature that prevents accidental termination of pacing. Also, a "lock" feature is used to prevent unintended changes to the prescribed settings.

Pacing Artifacts

All patients with temporary pacemakers require continuous ECG monitoring. The pacing artifact is the spike that is seen on the ECG tracing as the pacing stimulus is delivered to the heart. A *P wave* is visible after the pacing artifact if the atrium is being paced (Figure 13-2, *A*). Similarly, a *QRS complex* follows a ventricular pacing artifact (Figure 13-2, *B*). With dual-chamber pacing, a pacing artifact precedes both the P wave and the QRS complex (Figure 13-2, *C*).

Pacemaker Malfunctions

Pacing Abnormalities

Most pacemaker malfunctions can be categorized as abnormalities of either pacing or sensing. Immediate and accurate recognition of these malfunctions is critically important in a pacemaker-dependent individual.

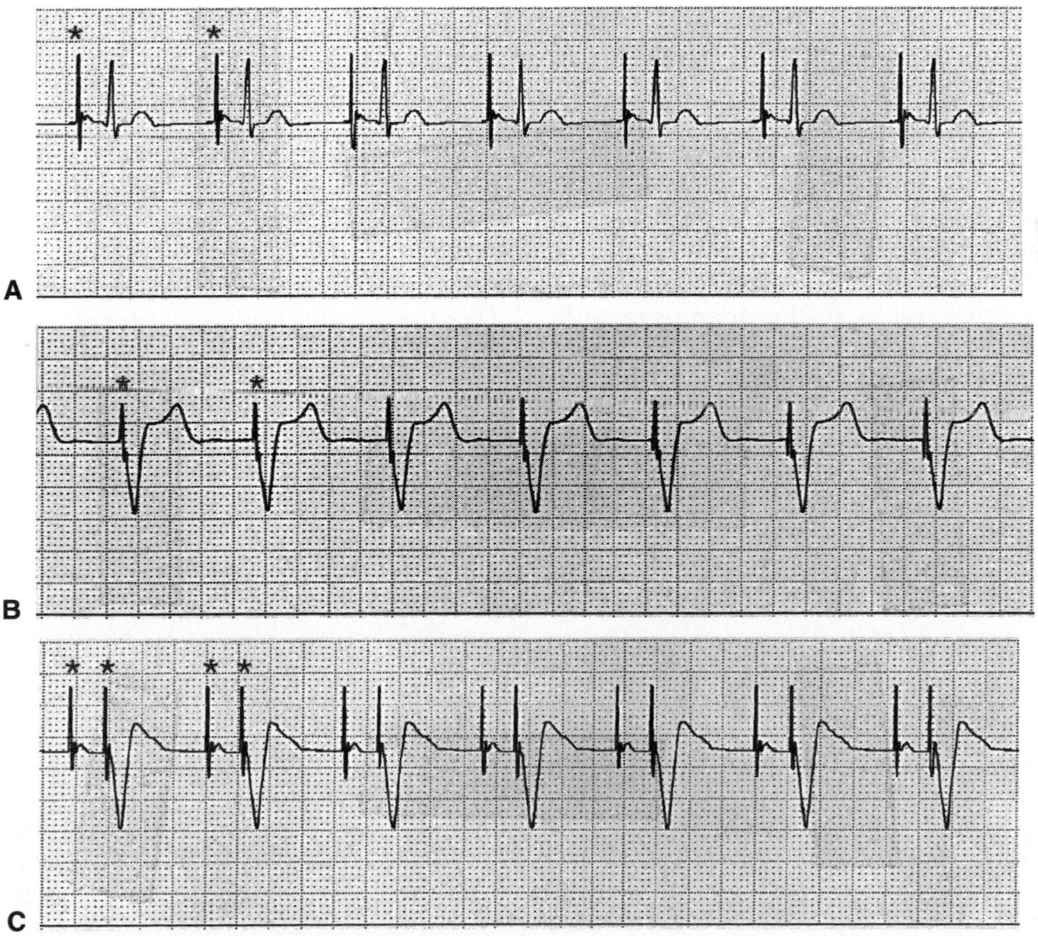

FIGURE 13-2. Pacing examples. **A,** Atrial pacing. **B,** Ventricular pacing. **C,** Dual-chamber pacing. The * represents a pacemaker impulse.

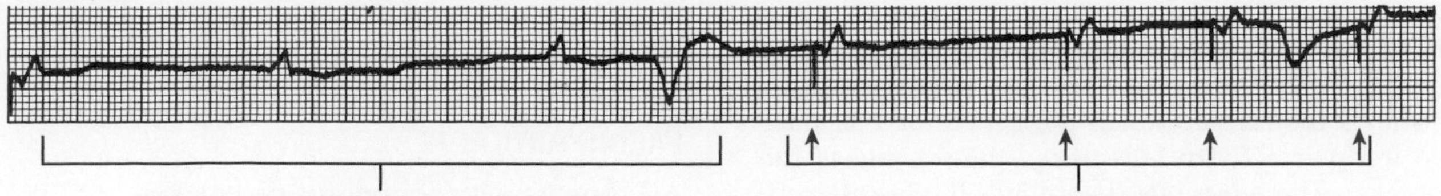

FIGURE 13-3. Pacemaker malfunction: failure to pace. **A,** Patient with a transvenous pacemaker is turned onto the left side. Immediately, there is a failure to pace (loss of pacer artifacts on ECG). The patient's heart rate is extremely low without pacemaker support. **B,** The nurse turns the patient onto the right side, the transvenous electrode floats into contact with the right ventricular wall, and pacing is resumed. (From Kesten KS, Norton CK: *Pacemakers: patient care, troubleshooting, rhythm analysis,* Baltimore, 1985, Resource Applications.)

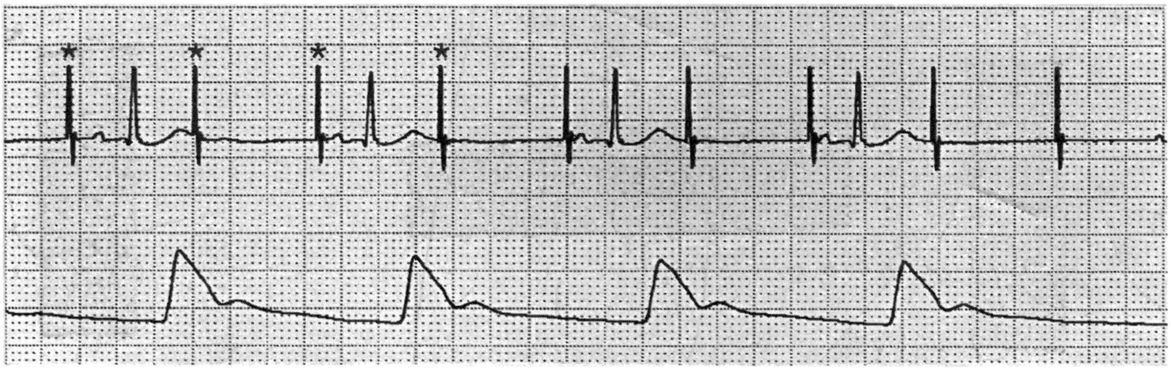

FIGURE 13-4. Pacemaker malfunction: failure to capture. Atrial pacing and capture occur after pacer spike(s) 1, 3, 5, and 7. The remaining pacer spikes fail to capture the tissue, resulting in loss of the P wave, no conduction to the ventricles, and no arterial waveform. The * represents a pacemaker impulse.

Failure to Pace. Failure of the pacemaker to deliver the pacing stimulus results in the disappearance of the pacing artifact on the bedside ECG monitor, even though the patient's intrinsic rate is less than the set rate on the pacemaker (Figure 13-3). This can occur either intermittently or continuously and can be attributed to failure of the pulse generator or its battery, a loose connection between the various components of the pacemaker system, broken lead wires, or stimulus inhibition as a result of EMI. Tightening connections, replacing the batteries or the pulse generator itself, or removing the source of EMI may restore pacemaker function.

Failure to Capture. If the pacing stimulus fires but fails to initiate a myocardial depolarization, a pacing artifact will be present but will not be followed by the expected P wave or QRS complex, depending on the chamber being paced (Figure 13-4). This "loss of capture" most often can be attributed either to displacement of the pacing electrode or to an increase in threshold (electrical stimulus necessary to elicit a myocardial depolarization) as a result of drugs, metabolic disorders, electrolyte imbalances, or fibrosis or myocardial ischemia at the site of electrode placement. In many cases, increasing the output (mA) may elicit capture. For transvenous leads, repositioning the patient to the left side may improve lead contact and restore capture.

Sensing Abnormalities

Sensing abnormalities include both undersensing and oversensing.

Undersensing. When a pacemaker is undersensing, it is unable to sense spontaneous myocardial depolarizations. This results in competition between paced complexes and the heart's intrinsic rhythm. This malfunction can be demonstrated on the ECG by pacing artifacts that occur *after* or are unrelated to spontaneous complexes (Figure 13-5). Undersensing can result in the delivery of pacing stimuli into a relative refractory period of the cardiac depolarization cycle. A ventricular pacing stimulus delivered into the downslope of the T wave (R-on-T phenomenon) is a real danger with this type of pacer aberration, because it may precipitate a lethal dysrhythmia. Quick action is required to determine the cause and initiate appropriate interventions. Often the cause can be attributed to inadequate wave amplitude. If this is the case, the situation can be promptly remedied by increasing the sensitivity

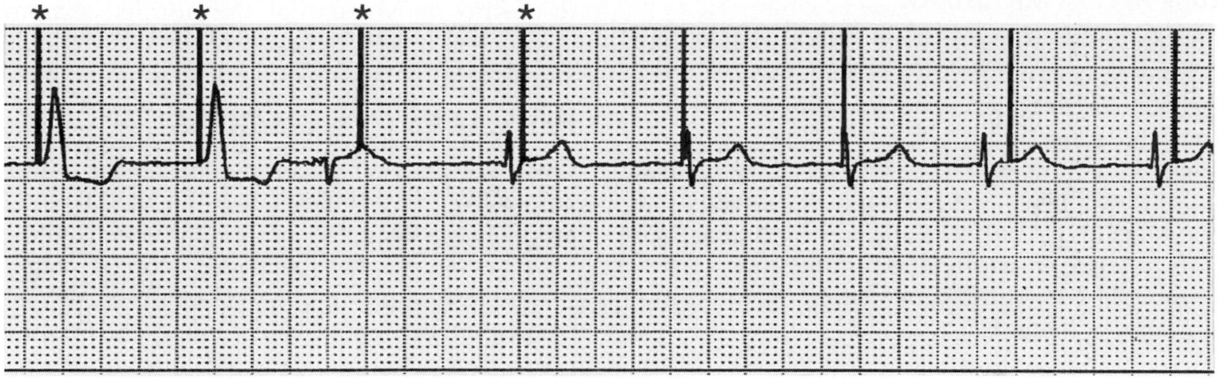

FIGURE 13-5. Pacemaker malfunction: undersensing. Notice that after the first two paced beats, a series of intrinsic beats occur; the pacemaker unit fails to sense these intrinsic QRS complexes. These spikes do not capture the ventricle because they occur during the refractory period of the cardiac cycle. The * represents a pacemaker impulse.

(moving the sensitivity dial toward its lowest setting). Other possible causes include inappropriate (i.e., asynchronous) mode selection, lead displacement or fracture, loose cable connections, and pulse generator failure.

Oversensing. Pacemaker oversensing results from the inappropriate sensing of extraneous electrical signals that can lead to an unnecessary trigger or inhibition of pacemaker output stimuli with abnormal pauses. The source of these electrical signals can range from the presence of tall, peaked T waves to EMI in the critical care environment. Because most temporary pulse generators are programmed in demand (synchronous) modes, oversensing results in unexplained pauses in the ECG tracing as the extraneous signals are sensed and inhibit pacing. Often, simply moving the sensitivity control toward 20 mV stops the pauses.

Medical Management

The physician determines the pacing route based on the patient's clinical situation. Generally, transcutaneous pacing is used in emergent situations until a transvenous lead can be secured. If the patient is undergoing heart surgery, epicardial leads may be electively placed at the end of the operation. The physician places the transvenous or epicardial pacing lead(s), repositioning as needed to obtain adequate pacing and sensing thresholds. Decisions regarding lead placement may later limit the pacing modes available to the clinician. For example, to perform dual-chamber pacing, both atrial and ventricular leads must be placed. In emergent situations, however, interventions are focused on establishing ventricular pacing, and atrial lead placement may not be feasible. After lead placement, the initial settings for output and sensitivity are determined, the pacing rate and mode are selected, and the patient's response to pacing is evaluated.

Nursing Management

Nursing priorities for the patient connected to a temporary pacemaker focus on (1) preventing pacemaker malfunction, (2) protecting against microshock, (3) monitoring for complications, and (4) providing patient education.

Preventing Pacemaker Malfunction

Continuous ECG monitoring is essential to facilitating prompt recognition of and appropriate intervention for pacemaker malfunction. In addition, proper care of the pacing system can do a great deal to prevent pacing abnormalities.

The temporary pacing lead and bridging cable must be properly secured to the body with tape to prevent the accidental displacement of the electrode, which can result in failure to pace or sense. The external pulse generator can be secured to the patient's waist with a strap or placed in a telemetry bag for the mobile patient. For the patient on a regimen of bed rest, the pulse generator can be suspended with twill tape from an intravenous (IV) pole mounted overhead on the ceiling. This not only will prevent tension on the lead while the patient is moved (given adequate length of bridging cable) but also will alleviate the possibility of accidental dropping of the pulse generator.

The nurse inspects for loose connections between the lead(s) and pulse generator on a regular basis. In addition, replacement batteries and pulse generators must always be available on the unit. Although the battery has an anticipated life span of 1 month, it probably is sound practice to change the battery if the pacemaker has been operating continually for several days. Newer generators provide a low-battery signal 24 hours before complete loss of battery function to prevent inadvertent interruptions in pacing. The pulse generator must always be labeled with the date that the battery was replaced.

Protecting Against Microshock

It is important to be aware of all sources of EMI within the critical care environment that could interfere with the pacemaker's function. Sources of EMI in the clinical area include electrocautery, defibrillation current, radiation therapy, magnetic resonance imaging devices, and transcutaneous electrical nerve stimulation (TENS) units. In most cases, if EMI is suspected of precipitating pacemaker malfunction, converting to the asynchronous mode (fixed rate) will maintain pacing until the cause of the EMI is removed.

Because the pacing electrode provides a direct, low-resistance path to the heart, the nurse takes special care while handling the external components of the pacing system to avoid conducting stray electrical current from other equipment. Even a small amount of stray current transmitted via the pacing lead could precipitate a lethal dysrhythmia. The possibility of "microshock" can be minimized by the wearing of rubber gloves when handling the pacing wires and by proper insulation of terminal pins of pacing wires when they are not in use. The latter can be accomplished either by using caps provided by the manufacturer or by improvising with a plastic syringe cover or section of disposable nonlatex glove. The wires are to be taped securely to the patient's chest to prevent accidental electrode displacement. Additional safety measures include using a nonelectric or a properly grounded electric bed, keeping all electrical equipment away from the bed, and permitting the use of only rechargeable electric razors.

Monitoring for Complications

Infection at the lead insertion site is a rare but serious complication associated with temporary pacemakers. The site(s) is carefully inspected for purulent drainage, erythema, and edema, and the patient is observed for signs of systemic infection. Site care is performed according to the institution's policy and procedure. Although most infections remain localized, endocarditis can occur in patients with endocardial pacing leads. A less common complication associated with transvenous pacing is myocardial perforation, which can result in rhythmic hiccoughs or cardiac tamponade. Following insertion a chest x-ray film should be taken to verify the tip of the lead is correctly positioned.[1]

Providing Patient Education

Education of the person with a temporary pacemaker emphasizes prevention of complications. The patient is instructed not to handle any exposed portion of the lead wire and to notify the nurse if the dressing over the insertion site becomes soiled, wet, or dislodged. The patient also is advised not to use any electrical devices brought in from home that could interfere with pacemaker functioning. Furthermore, patients with temporary transvenous pacemakers need to be taught to restrict movement of the affected extremity to prevent lead displacement.

PERMANENT PACEMAKERS

Over 200,000 permanent pacemakers are implanted annually in the United States, and critical care nurses are likely to encounter these devices in their clinical practice.[6] The goal of permanent pacemaker therapy is to simulate, as much as possible, normal physiologic cardiac depolarization and conduction. Sophisticated generators now permit rate-responsive pacing, either in response to sensed atrial activity (DDD) or in response to a variety of physiologic sensors (body motion, QT interval, and minute ventilation). In patients who do not have a functional sinus node that can increase their heart rate, rate-responsive pacemakers have been shown to improve exercise capacity and quality of life.[6] Table 13-3 describes the types of *rate-responsive pacing* modes currently in clinical use.

Cardiac Resynchronization Therapy

About one third of patients with severe heart failure have ventricular conduction delays (prolonged QRS duration or bundle branch block). Such conduction delays create a lack of synchrony between the contraction of the left and right ventricles. The hemodynamic consequences of this dyssynchrony include impaired ventricular filling and decreased ejection fraction, cardiac output, and mean arterial pressure.[7] *Cardiac resynchronization therapy* (CRT) uses atrial pacing, plus it stimulates both the left and right ventricles (*biventricular pacing*), to optimize atrial and ventricular mechanical activity. The CRT device uses three pacing leads, one each in the right atrium and the right ventricle and a specially designed transvenous lead that

Table 13-3
Permanent Pacemaker Rate Response Pacing Modes

PULSE GENERATOR	DESCRIPTION
AAIR	AAI features, plus rate-responsive pacing; used for patients with a symptomatic bradycardia with a paceable atrium and intact atrioventricular (AV) conduction
VVIR	VVI features, plus rate-responsive pacing; used for patients with an atrium that is unpaceable as a result of chronic atrial fibrillation or other atrial dysrhythmia
DDDR	DDD features, plus rate-responsive pacing; used for patients with a symptomatic bradycardia in which the atrium is paceable but AV conduction is, or may become, unreliable

is inserted via the coronary sinus to pace the left ventricle.[8] Because many heart failure patients are also at risk for sudden cardiac death (SCD), biventricular pacing is now available on some implantable cardioverter-defibrillators. A number of clinical trials have shown symptom and structural cardiac improvement with CRT.[9,10]

Permanent Pacemaker Insertion

Permanent pacemakers may be implanted with the patient under local anesthesia in either the operating room or the cardiac catheterization laboratory. Generally, transvenous leads are inserted via the cephalic or subclavian vein and positioned in the right atrium and/or the right ventricle, under fluoroscopy. Satisfactory lead placement is determined by testing stimulation and sensitivity thresholds with a pacing system analyzer. The lead(s) is then attached to the generator, which is inserted into a surgically created "pocket" in the subcutaneous tissue below the clavicle.

IMPLANTABLE CARDIOVERTER-DEFIBRILLATOR

An implantable cardioverter-defibrillator (ICD) is an implantable device capable of identifying and terminating life-threatening ventricular dysrhythmias. Initially an ICD was only recommended for patients who had survived an episode of cardiac arrest caused by ventricular fibrillation (VF) or ventricular tachycardia (VT).[6] A number of clinical trials that compared ICD therapy for such secondary prevention of SCD with antidysrhythmic drug therapy found improved survival with the ICD.[11] Today ICD use has expanded to include primary prevention of SCD in patients with coronary artery disease (CAD), previous myocardial infarction, or left ventricular dysfunction when VT or VF was inducible during an electrophysiology study (EPS). Recent trials have shown improved survival with ICD implantation in high-risk patients (i.e., those with previous myocardial infarction and an ejection fraction <30%) even without evidence of VT/VF on an EPS.[12] These results are likely to further increase the number of patients who receive an ICD.

ICD System

The ICD system contains (1) sensing electrodes to recognize the dysrhythmia and (2) defibrillation electrodes or coils that are in contact with the heart and can deliver a "shock."[13] These electrodes are connected to a generator that is surgically placed in the subcutaneous tissue either in the upper left abdominal quadrant or in the pectoral region (Figure 13-6). The early-model generators could defibrillate or cardiovert only lethal dysrhythmias. Current generation devices deliver a "tiered" therapy with programmable antitachycardia pacing, bradycardia backup pacing, low-energy cardioversion, and high-energy defibrillation options. With tiered therapy, antitachycardia pacing is used as the first line of treatment and will terminate 90% to 96% of spontaneous VT episodes and 81% of fast VT episodes (rate >180 beats/min).[13] If the VT can be pace-terminated successfully, the patient will not receive a "shock" from the generator and may not even realize that the ICD terminated the dysrhythmia. This improves patient comfort and prolongs battery life.[13] If programmed bursts of pacing do not terminate the VT, the ICD will "cardiovert" the rhythm. If the dysrhythmia deteriorates into VF, the ICD is programmed to defibrillate at a higher energy. If the dysrhythmia terminates spontaneously, the device will not discharge (see Figure 13-6). Occasionally, the electrical rhythm may deteriorate to asystole or a slow idioventricular rhythm. In such cases the bradycardia back-up pacing function is activated. Current ICD models retain an electrographic record of such events that can be later interpreted using a computer from the ICD manufacturer.[13]

New product development for ICDs has resulted in dual-chamber devices with leads in both the atria and the ventricles. The introduction of atrial leads allows for dual-chamber pacing to optimize hemodynamic performance, as well as atrial sensing to more accurately discriminate between atrial and ventricular tachycardias and decrease the incidence of inappropriate shocks. Implantable defibrillators with atrial capabilities may also be used to deliver therapies such as cardioversion or antitachycardia pacing to patients with atrial tachydysrhythmias, but research is needed to evaluate the exact role of this therapy.[6]

ICD Insertion

Transvenous electrode leads are inserted into the subclavian vein and advanced into the right side of the heart, where contact with the endocardium is achieved. To improve defibrillation efficacy, an additional subcutaneous patch may be placed with some models. The endocardial leads are used for sensing, pacing, and cardioversion/defibrillation. The leads are tunneled through the subcutaneous tissue.[6] The leads are connected to the ICD generator, which is implanted in a subcutaneous "pocket" in the pectoral position, similar to that used for permanent pacemakers (see Figure 13-6).

Medical Management

Medical management of the ICD patient begins before implantation, with a thorough evaluation of the patient's dysrhythmia and underlying cardiac function. Patients identified at risk for SCD undergo an

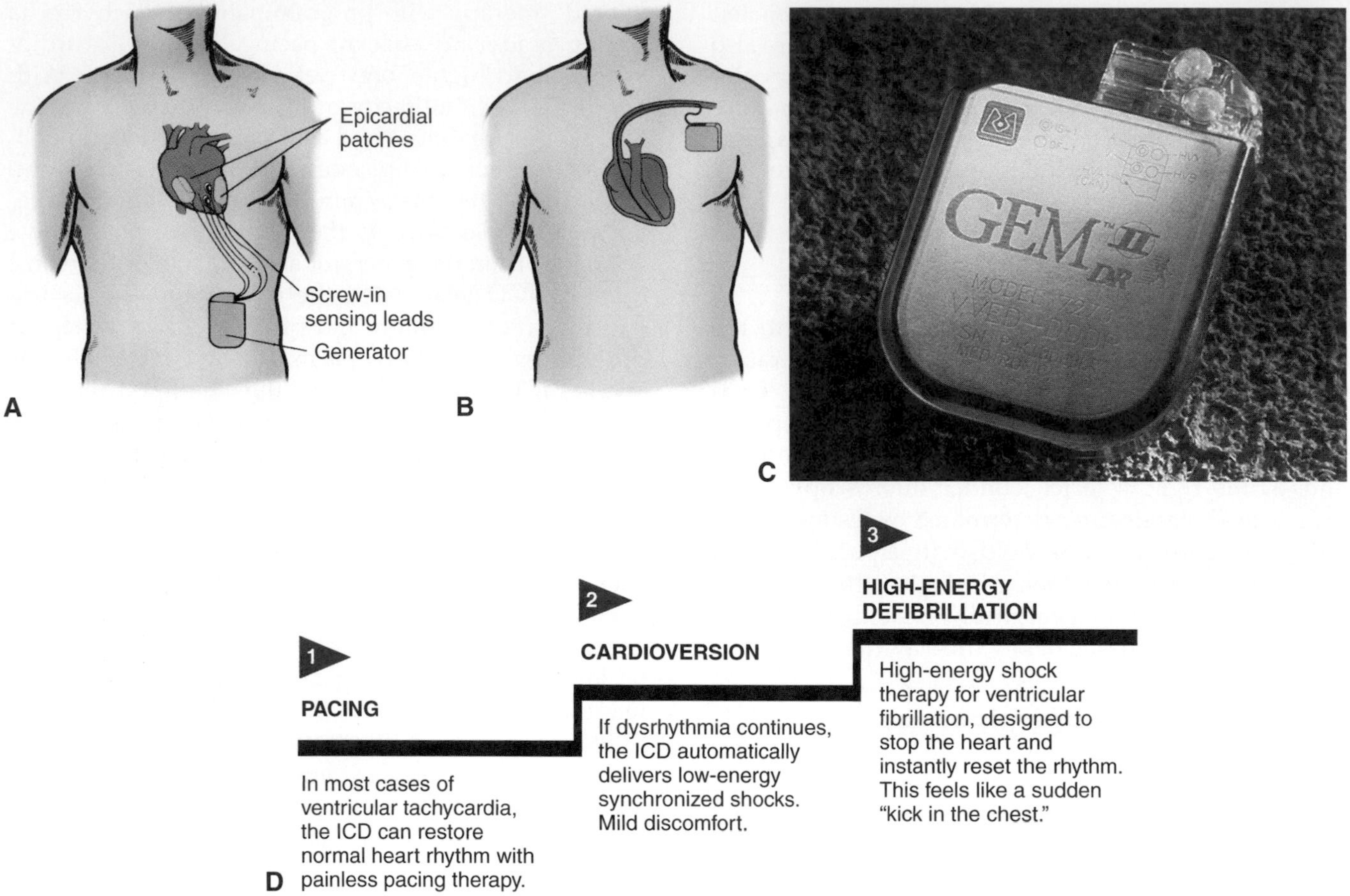

FIGURE 13-6. **A,** Placement of an implantable cardioverter-defibrillator (ICD) and epicardial lead system. The generator is placed in a subcutaneous "pocket" in the left upper abdominal quadrant. The epicardial screw-in sensing leads monitor the heart rhythm and connect to the generator. If a life-threatening dysrhythmia is sensed, the generator can pace-terminate the dysrhythmia or deliver electrical cardioversion or defibrillation through the epicardial patches. With this system, the leads/patches must be placed during open-chest (sternal or thoracotomy) surgery. **B,** In the transvenous lead system, open-chest surgery is not required. The pacing/cardioversion/defibrillation functions are all contained in a lead (or leads) inserted into the right atrium and ventricle. New generators are small enough to place in the pectoral region. **C,** An example of a dual-chamber ICD (Medtronic Gem II DR) with tiered therapy and pacing capabilities. **D,** Tiered therapy is designed to use increasing levels of intensity to terminate ventricular dysrhythmias. (Courtesy Medtronic Inc, Minneapolis, Minn.)

electrophysiology study to identify the origin of the dysrhythmia and to determine the effectiveness of antidysrhythmic agents in suppressing or altering the rate of the dysrhythmia. Further assessment of cardiac status is made to determine whether additional interventions (cardiac surgery, angioplasty) are indicated to improve cardiac function and decrease the risk of ventricular dysrhythmias.

ICD Programming

An electrophysiologist generally performs initial programming of the device at the time of implantation to tailor the ICD algorithm to the specific individual.[13] At implantation, defibrillation threshold measurements are obtained. This involves inducing the dysrhythmia and then evaluating the device's ability to terminate the dysrhythmia. Once it is determined that the ICD functions adequately, further follow-up is conducted on an outpatient basis to monitor the number of discharges and the battery life of the device.

Nursing Management

Nursing priorities for the with an ICD focus on (1) monitoring for ICD-associated complications and (2) providing patient education.

Monitoring for ICD-Associated Complications

In the case of a ventricular dysrhythmia, it is important to know the type of ICD implanted, how the device functions, and whether it is activated (i.e., on). If the patient experiences a shockable rhythm in the critical care unit, the nurse should be prepared to defibrillate in the event that the device fails. When performing external defibrillation, the paddles/patches should not be placed directly over the ICD generator. In addition, standard paddle placement may need to be altered in patients with ICDs to achieve successful defibrillation.[2] Most patients will continue to take some antidysrhythmic medications to decrease the number of "shocks" required and to slow the rate of the tachycardia.[13,14] Complications associated with the ICD include infection from the implanted system, broken leads, and the sensing of supraventricular tachydysrhythmias resulting in unneeded discharges (shocks).

Providing Patient Education

To facilitate a positive psychologic adjustment to the ICD, education of the patient and family about the device is vital. Preoperative teaching for the ICD patient includes information about how the device works and what to expect during the implantation procedure. After implantation, education is focused on aspects of living with an ICD. Patients need information pertaining to scheduled device follow-up and instructions about what to do if they experience a shock or series of shocks. If the shocks are associated with shortness of breath or other symptoms of heart failure, the patient should be taken to a nearby emergency department for monitoring. Many institutions also have successfully used family support groups for this patient population.

FIBRINOLYTIC THERAPY

Fibrinolytic therapy is an important clinical intervention for the patient experiencing acute ST-elevation myocardial infarction (STEMI). Before the introduction of fibrinolytic agents, the medical management of acute myocardial infarction (MI) was focused on decreasing myocardial oxygen demands to minimize myocardial necrosis and thus preserve ventricular function. Today, efforts to limit the size of infarction are directed toward the timely reperfusion of the jeopardized myocardium by restoring blood flow in the culprit vessel. The use of fibrinolytic therapy to accomplish this objective is predicated on the theory that the significant event in an acute coronary syndrome (unstable angina or acute MI) is the rupture of an atherosclerotic plaque with subsequent thrombus formation (Figure 13-7). The thrombus, which is composed of aggregated platelets bound together with fibrin strands, occludes the coronary artery, depriving the myocardium of oxygen previously supplied by that artery. The administration of a fibrinolytic agent results in the lysis of the acute thrombus, thus recanalizing, or opening, the obstructed coronary artery and restoring blood flow to the affected tissue. Once perfusion is restored, adjunctive measures are taken to prevent further clot formation and reocclusion.

Box 13-3

Fibrinolytic Therapy Selection Criteria

- No more than 12 hours from onset of chest pain; less if possible
- ST-segment elevation on electrocardiogram or new-onset left bundle branch block
- Ischemic chest pain of 30 minutes' duration
- Chest pain unresponsive to sublingual nitroglycerin
- No conditions that might cause a predisposition to hemorrhage

Eligibility Criteria

Inclusion Criteria

Criteria have been developed, based on research findings, to determine the patient population that would most likely benefit from the administration of fibrinolytic therapy. In general, patients with recent onset of chest pain (less than 12 hours' duration) and persistent ST elevation (greater than 0.1 mV in two or more contiguous leads) are considered candidates for fibrinolytic therapy.[9] Patients who present with bundle branch blocks that may obscure ST-segment analysis and a history suggestive of an acute MI are also considered candidates for therapy.

Exclusion Criteria

Increased risk of bleeding after use of fibrinolytics constitutes the major exclusion criteria. Patients who have stable clots that might be disrupted by fibrinolytic therapy (those secondary to recent surgery, trauma, or stroke) are generally not considered candidates. Other selection criteria for the use of fibrinolytic therapy are listed in Box 13-3.

Fibrinolytic Agents

Several fibrinolytic agents are currently available for intravenous treatment of acute STEMI.[15] All of these agents stimulate lysis of the clot by converting inactive plasminogen to plasmin, an enzyme responsible for degradation of fibrin (see Figure 13-7). A comparison of current Food and Drug Administration (FDA)-approved fibrinolytic agents is provided in Table 13-4.

Evidence of Reperfusion

In the cardiac catheterization laboratory, the blood flow of a vessel that has been occluded by a thrombus and then opened by fibrinolytic therapy can be observed directly under fluoroscopy. The adequacy of the

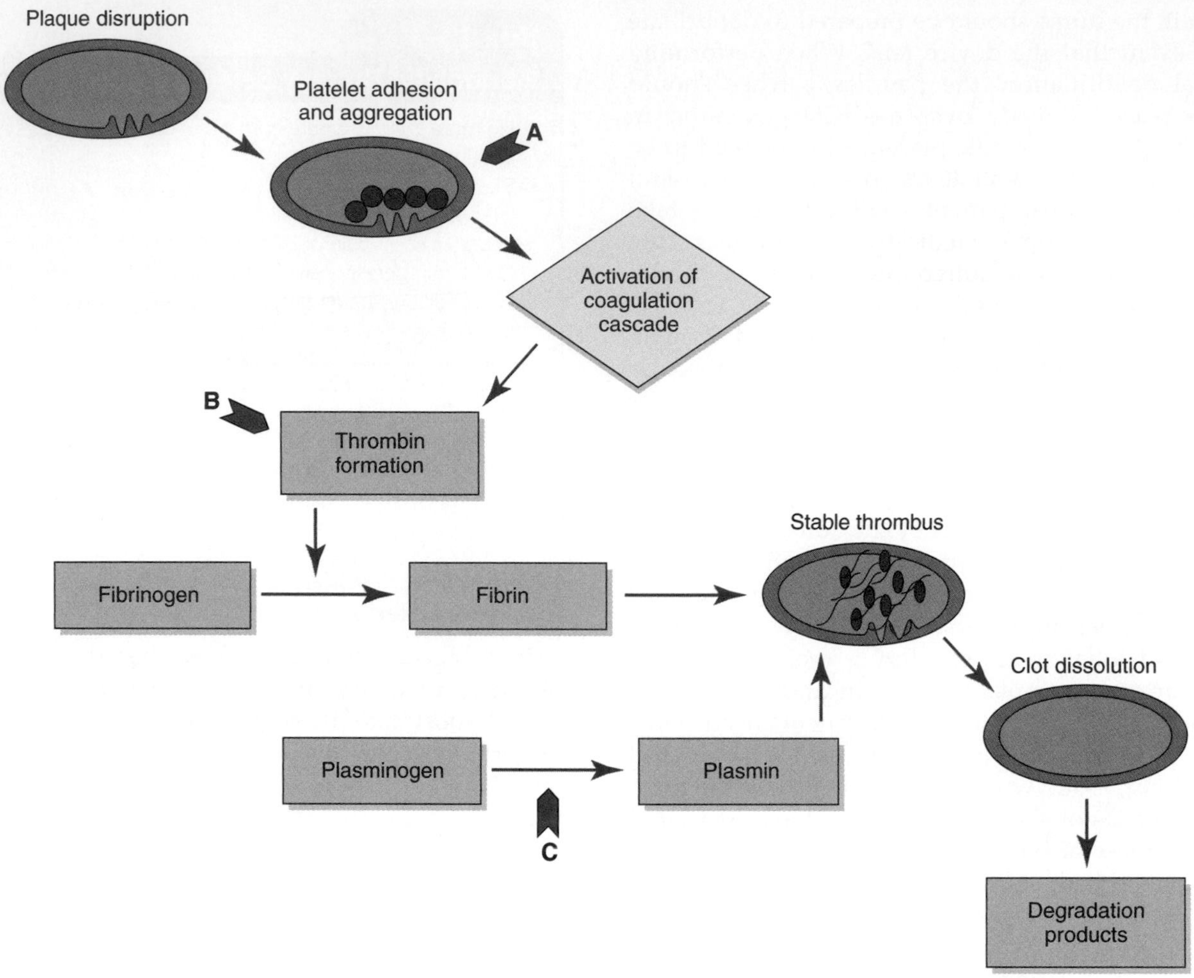

FIGURE 13-7. Thrombus formation and site of action of medications used in the treatment of acute myocardial infarction. **A,** Site of action of antiplatelet agents such as aspirin and glycoprotein IIb/IIIa inhibitors. **B,** Heparin bonds with antithrombin III and thrombin to create an inactive complex. **C,** Fibrinolytic agents convert plasminogen to plasmin, an enzyme responsible for degradation of fibrin clots.

Box 13-4
Flow in the Infarct-Related Artery as Described in the Thrombolysis in Myocardial Infarction (TIMI) Trial

TIMI 3	Normal or brisk flow through the coronary artery
TIMI 2	Partial flow, slower than in normal vessels
TIMI 1	Sluggish flow with incomplete distal filling
TIMI 0	No flow beyond the point of occlusion

flow of blood through the coronary artery is described using the standardized thrombolysis in myocardial infarction (TIMI) scale (Box 13-4).

Nursing Management

Nursing priorities for the patient receiving fibrinolytic therapy focus on (1) identifying candidates for reperfusion therapy, (2) observing for signs of reperfusion, (3) monitoring for signs of bleeding, and (4) providing patient education.

Identifying Candidates for Reperfusion Therapy

Nursing management of the patient undergoing fibrinolytic therapy begins with identifying potential candidates. In many institutions, checklists are used to facilitate rapid identification of patients who are candidates for fibrinolytics. The nurse prepares the patient for fibrinolytic therapy by starting intravenous lines and obtaining baseline laboratory values and vital signs.

Observing for Signs of Reperfusion

Reperfusion of the ischemic myocardium may be observed noninvasively by the following means:

1. Ischemic chest pain ceases abruptly as blood flow is restored.
2. Reperfusion ventricular dysrhythmias may occur; generally these are self-limiting or nonsustained,

Table 13-4

Pharmacologic Management: Fibrinolytic Agents for Use in ST-Elevation Myocardial Infarction (STEMI)

DRUG	DOSAGE	ACTIONS	SPECIAL CONSIDERATIONS
Clot Specific			
t-PA (alteplase)	IV: 100 mg over 90 min with the first 15 mg given as a bolus	Binds to fibrin at the clot and promotes activation of plasminogen to plasmin	Short half-life, so heparin is usually given with the drug as a bolus and then followed with an infusion Aspirin is begun with administration of the drug and continued daily
r-PA (reteplase)	IV: 10 units given as a bolus, repeated in 30 min	Binds to fibrin at the clot and promotes activation of plasminogen to plasmin	Heparin is started with administration of the drug and continued for 24 hours Aspirin is begun with administration of the drug and continued daily
TNKase (tenecteplase)	IV: 30-50 mg based on body weight, given as a single bolus	Binds to fibrin at the clot and promotes activation of plasminogen to plasmin	Heparin is started with administration of the drug Aspirin is begun with administration of the drug and continued daily
Non–Clot Specific			
SK (streptokinase)	IV: 1.5 million units given over 60 min	Catalyzes the conversion of plasminogen to plasmin, which causes lysis of fibrin Has systemic lytic effects	May cause allergic reactions and hypotension Heparin may be administered IV or Sub-Q Aspirin is begun with administration of the drug and continued daily
APSAC (anistreplase)	IV: 30 units via slow bolus over 2-5 min	A molecular combination of streptokinase and plasminogen with actions similar to streptokinase Has systemic lytic effects	May cause allergic reactions and hypotension Long half-life, so heparin is usually started 4-6 hr after APSAC Aspirin is begun with administration of the drug and continued daily

t-PA, Tissue plasminogen activator; *IV*, intravenous; *r-PA*, recombinant plasminogen activator; *Sub Q*, subcutaneous; *APSAC*, anisoylated plasminogen-streptokinase activator complex.

and aggressive antidysrhythmic therapy is not required.

3. Normalization of the previously elevated ST segments occurs. To monitor the ST segment changes a monitoring lead should be chosen that clearly demonstrates the ST elevation before initiation of therapy.[16]
4. The serum concentrations of myocardial biomarkers released by damaged myocardial cells, such as myocardial creatine kinase (CK-MB) or troponin, are monitored. These biomarkers rise rapidly and markedly after reperfusion of the ischemic heart muscle.

Monitoring for Signs of Bleeding

The most common complication related to clot lysis is bleeding, not only as a result of the fibrinolytic therapy but also because the patients routinely receive anticoagulation therapy following fibrinolytic therapy to minimize the possibility of rethrombosis. Mild gingival bleeding and oozing around venipuncture sites is common and not a cause of concern. Should serious bleeding occur, such as intracranial or internal bleeding, all fibrinolytic and heparin therapies are discontinued and volume expanders or coagulation factors, or both, are administered.

Nursing management also includes preventive measures to minimize the potential for bleeding. For example, injections are avoided if at all possible. To ensure hemostasis at venipuncture and arterial puncture sites additional pressure is applied. Intravenous lines are placed before administering fibrinolytic therapy, and a heparin lock may be used for obtaining laboratory specimens during treatment.

Providing Patient Education

Education for the patient receiving fibrinolytic therapy includes information regarding the actions of fibrinolytic drugs, with an emphasis on precautions to minimize bleeding. For example, the patient is cautioned against vigorous toothbrushing and told to refrain from using straight-edge razors. In addition, information is provided regarding ongoing risk factor management in the prevention of atherosclerotic CAD, stroke, and peripheral arterial disease.

CATHETER INTERVENTIONS FOR CORONARY ARTERY DISEASE

During the past three decades, the trend in treatment of CAD is toward percutaneous catheter-based interventions.[17] Today options for percutaneous coronary intervention (PCI) include not only percutaneous transluminal coronary angioplasty (PTCA) but also atherectomy and stent placement, used either alone or in conjunction with angioplasty.

Indications for Catheter-Based Interventions

Indications for catheter-based interventions have been considerably broadened since the initial application of balloon angioplasty. Whereas once only patients with single-vessel CAD were considered for PTCA, now patients with multivessel disease, even those who have previously undergone surgical saphenous vein graft (SVG) and internal mammary artery (IMA) graft or fibrinolytic therapy for acute MI, may be candidates for catheter intervention. Trials comparing fibrinolytics to catheter-based reperfusion in the setting of acute MI have shown an advantage for percutaneous catheter interventions over drug therapy in preventing death, reinfarction, or stroke, even though there may be delays related to transporting patients to facilities with interventional capabilities.[15]

Surgical Backup

Today the majority of coronary arterial dissections are effectively treated with stent placement. As a result, most institutions have evolved to an informal surgical backup plan, such as the first available operating room. Nevertheless, the availability of cardiac surgical services on site is still recommended.[18]

Angioplasty

PTCA, often just called angioplasty, involves the use of a balloon-tipped catheter that, when advanced through an atherosclerotic lesion (atheroma), can be inflated intermittently for the purpose of dilating the stenotic area and improving blood flow through it (Figure 13-8). The high balloon-inflation pressure stretches the vessel wall, fractures the plaque, and enlarges the vessel lumen. A successful angioplasty procedure is one in which the stenosis is reduced to less than 50% of the vessel lumen diameter, although most clinicians aim for less than 20% final diameter stenosis.[18] Procedural success is influenced by patient variables such as age, cardiac function, and comorbidities such as diabetes, as well as by characteristics of the lesion itself. Lesions that are discrete (less than 1 cm in length), concentric, easily accessible, and have little or no calcification are most likely to be treated successfully with angioplasty.

Atherectomy

Atherectomy is the excision and removal of the atherosclerotic plaque by cutting, shaving, or grinding, using specialized coronary catheters. Three atherectomy devices are described in Table 13-5: directional coronary atherectomy (DCA), rotational ablation (Rotablator),

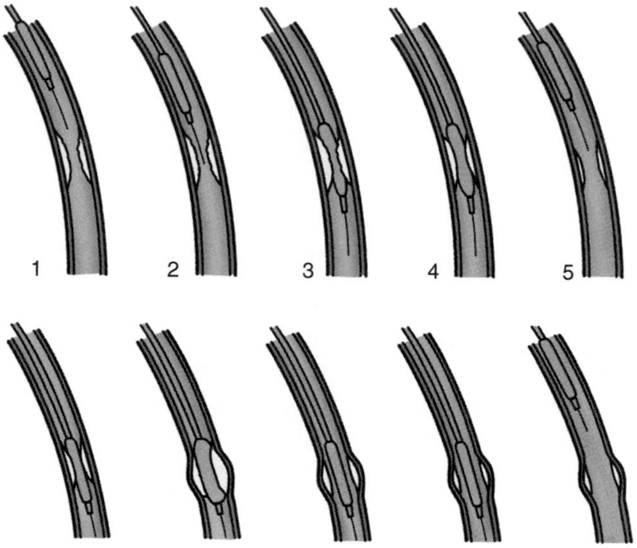

FIGURE 13-8. Percutaneous transluminal coronary angioplasty (PTCA). An angioplasty catheter balloon threaded over a guidewire is used to open a vessel occluded by atherosclerosis.

Table 13-5
Atherectomy Devices

DEVICE	DESIGN	USES
Directional coronary atherectomy	Rotating, cup-shaped cutter within a windowed cylindric housing; plaque that protrudes into window is shaved off and collected within nose cone of cutter housing	Ostial lesions Eccentric lesions in large vessels Proximal, discrete lesions In-stent restenosis
Rotational ablation catheter (Rotablator)	A high-speed, rotating, diamond-studded burr; "sanding effect"; generates microparticles that pass distally into microcirculation	In-stent restenosis Calcified lesions
Transluminal extraction catheter	Motorized cutting head with triangular blades; excised plaque removed by suction	Long, diffuse lesions Occluded saphenous vein graft

and transluminal extraction catheter. All three devices are FDA approved for use in coronary as well as peripheral arteries. Because these devices use different mechanisms, they may offer special advantages for different types of lesions. The current trend is to use a "lesion-specific" approach in the selection of a device for catheter intervention.

CORONARY STENTS

A significant development in interventional cardiology has been the coronary stent prosthesis. Today, stents are used in 80% to 90% of all coronary interventional procedures.[17] The latest development is use of stents coated with drugs that inhibit cell growth to lower restenosis rates. A drug coated with sirolimus (an immunosuppressive drug used to prevent organ transplant rejection) was shown in clinical trials to significantly decrease restenosis when compared with bare metal stents.[19,20] Another stent coated with paclitaxel (an anticancer agent) has also shown promising results.[21]

A stent is introduced into the coronary artery over a guidewire in a region that has been previously dilated with PTCA both to prevent acute closure and restenosis and to obtain a larger lumen diameter as shown in Figure 13-9. Stents are inserted to optimize the results of other treatments (PTCA, atherectomy, fibrinolytics) of acute vessel closure and prevention of restenosis. Also, intravascular ultrasound may be used to evaluate the vessel lumen diameter after stent deployment.[18] Multiple stents may be implanted sequentially within a vessel to fully cover the area of the lesion.

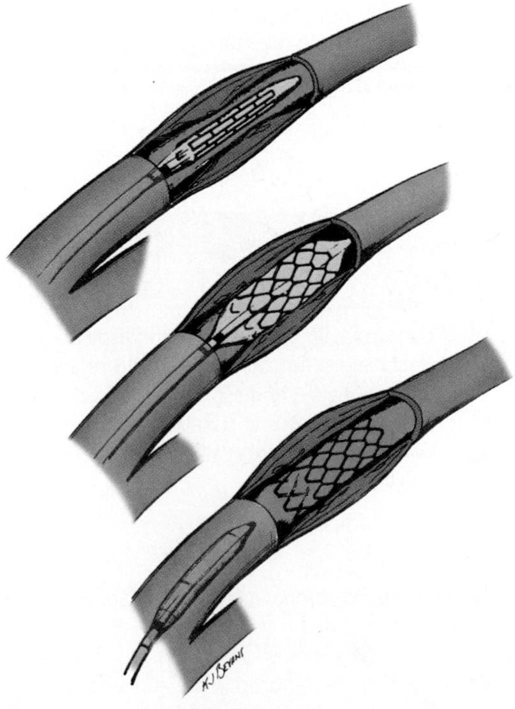

FIGURE 13-9. Intracoronary stent (balloon expandable stent). (From Bevans M, McLimore E: *J Cardiovasc Nurs* 7[1]:34, 1992.)

Procedure

PCI is performed in the cardiac catheterization laboratory under fluoroscopy. Introducer catheters, or "sheaths," are inserted percutaneously into the femoral artery and vein. The venous sheath can be used to perform a right heart catheterization with a pulmonary artery (PA) catheter or to insert a pacing catheter, or both. The patient is systemically heparinized to prevent clots from forming on or in any of the catheters, with dosing adjusted to achieve a target activated clotting time. For patients who cannot tolerate heparin, another anticoagulant may be used.[22] Conventional and newer anticoagulant agents are described in Table 13-6.

A special guiding catheter designed to engage the coronary artery ostia is inserted through the arterial sheath and advanced in a retrograde manner through the aorta. Nitroglycerin or calcium channel blockers may be given at this time to prevent coronary artery spasm and to maximize coronary vasodilation during the procedure. A guidewire is then advanced down the coronary artery and negotiated across the occluding atheroma. The balloon catheter is advanced over this guidewire and positioned across the lesion. The balloon is inflated and deflated repetitively (each inflation not to exceed 90 seconds) until evidence of dilation is demonstrated on an angiogram. In cases that require prolonged balloon inflations, an autoperfusion angioplasty catheter is available with side holes that allow passive blood flow through the central lumen to the distal coronary artery if adequate systemic blood pressure is present.

Platelet Inhibitor Dugs

Recently, potent antiplatelet agents (glycoprotein IIb/IIIa inhibitors) have become available to reduce the formation of intracoronary thrombosis after PCI. Initially used only in patients with high risk for abrupt closure, these agents now have been found to have benefit across the spectrum of interventional procedures, from angioplasty to atherectomy to stenting.[18] Glycoprotein IIb/IIIa inhibitor therapy is usually initiated during the procedure and is continued for 12 to 24 hours, depending on the agent used.[23]

Abciximab (ReoPro) was the first of the glycoprotein IIb/IIIa inhibitors approved by the FDA as an adjunct to PTCA for the prevention of abrupt closure of arteries in high-risk patients. Subsequently, two additional agents, *eptifibatide* (Integrilin) and *tirofiban* (Aggrastat), were also approved. These drugs block the enzyme *glycoprotein IIb/IIIa,* which is essential for platelet aggregation. Indications and dosing of these agents is provided in Table 13-7. The major complication of glycoprotein IIb/IIIa inhibitors is bleeding, and nursing management requires careful assessment of all potential bleeding sites, especially at the femoral sheath site. Extra precautions are used to immobilize the sheath insertion site, either with a sheet tuck to the affected leg or a leg restraint.[24]

Oral antiplatelet therapy is routinely prescribed at discharge and includes agents such as ticlopidine or clopidogrel for 2 to 4 weeks and aspirin indefinitely. Ticlopidine, although proven to be effective, has serious and sometimes fatal side effects, including neutropenia. Clopidogrel, which is similar to ticlopidine but does not cause as much bone marrow suppression, is now used more often.[18]

COMPLICATIONS

Complications that can occur in the period immediately after angioplasty, atherectomy, or stent placement include bleeding and hematoma formation at

Table 13-6

Pharmacologic Management: Anticoagulants

CLASSIFICATION/DRUG	MECHANISM OF ACTION	INDICATIONS	SPECIAL CONSIDERATIONS
Heparin			
Heparin sodium	Enhances activity of antithrombin III, a natural anticoagulant	Prevention of clotting in patients with MI and those undergoing PCI or cardiac surgery	Effectiveness of treatment may be monitored by aPTT or ACT Response is variable due to binding with plasma proteins Effects may be reversed with protamine sulfate Risk of developing HIT
Low-Molecular-Weight Heparin			
Dalteparin (Fragmin) Enoxaparin (Lovenox)	Enhances activity of antithrombin III	Prophylaxis and treatment of thromboembolic complications following surgery Prevention of clots in patients with unstable angina and MI	More predictable response than heparin, because drug is not largely bound to protein aPTT not particularly useful in monitoring treatment
Direct Thrombin Inhibitor			
Lepirudin (Refludan) Bivalirudin (Angiomax)	Directly inhibits thrombin	Prophylaxis and treatment of thrombosis in patients with HIT Prevention of clots in patients with unstable angina or PCI	aPTT may be monitored daily Dose should be adjusted for patients with renal insufficiency No reversal agent available

MI, Myocardial infarction; *PCI,* percutaneous coronary intervention; *aPTT,* activated partial thromboplastin time; *ACT,* activated clotting time; *HIT,* heparin-induced thrombocytopenia.

Table 13-7

Pharmacologic Management: Glycoprotein IIB/IIIA Inhibitors

DRUG	INDICATIONS/DOSE	COMMENTS
Abciximab (ReoPro)	**ACS:** 0.25 mg/kg IVP, then 10 mcg/min until PCI **PCI:** 0.25 mg/kg IVP, then 0.125 mcg/kg/min × 12 hr	Used concomitantly with heparin and aspirin May affect platelet function for up to 48 hr after infusion
Eptifibatide (Integrilin)	**ACS:** IV bolus of 180 mcg/kg followed with an infusion of 2 mcg/kg/min for up to 72 hr; if the patient undergoes PCI, the dose is decreased to 0.5 mcg/kg/min and continued for 24 hr after procedure, for a total of 96 hr **PCI:** 135 mcg/kg IVP, followed by an infusion of 0.5 mcg/kg/min × 24 hr	Concomitant heparin and aspirin may be administered Platelet function returns to baseline within 6-8 hr Contraindicated in patients with significant renal dysfunction
Tirofiban (Aggrastat)	**ACS (with or without PCI):** 0.4 mcg/kg/min for 30 min, then continued at 0.1 mcg/kg/min for 48-108 hr after ACS or for patients undergoing PCI	Administered in combination with heparin for patients undergoing PCI Platelet function returns to baseline within 4-8 hr Dosage should be reduced in patients with severe renal dysfunction

ACS, Acute coronary syndrome; *IVP,* intravenous push; *PCI,* percutaneous coronary intervention; *IV,* intravenous.

the site of vascular cannulation; compromised blood flow to the involved extremity; contrast-induced renal failure; dysrhythmias; and vasovagal response (hypotension, bradycardia, and diaphoresis) during manipulation or removal of introducer sheaths.

Nursing Management

Nursing management of the patient after PCI incorporates a variety of nursing diagnoses (Box 13-5). **Nursing priorities are directed toward (1) monitoring for recurrent angina, (2) managing the femoral access site, (3) assessing for bleeding, (4) palpating peripheral pulses, and (4) providing patient education.**

Monitoring for Recurrent Angina

It is essential that the nurse observe the patient for recurrent angina, a clinical indication of myocardial ischemia. Ischemic chest pain may be accompanied by elevated ST segments on the bedside monitor or the 12-lead ECG. Angina after a coronary procedure may be a result of transient coronary vasospasm, or it may signal a more serious complication. In either case the nurse must act quickly to assess for manifestations of myocardial ischemia and initiate clinical interventions as indicated. IV nitroglycerin is titrated to alleviate chest pain. Continued angina despite maximal vasodilator therapy generally rules out coronary vasospasm as the source of ischemic pain, and a new evaluation in the cardiac catheterization laboratory must be considered to rule out an acute occlusion. The risk is that a clot in the coronary artery, usually occurring at a site where the intimal wall has been dissected, has caused an acute occlusion.

Managing the Femoral Access Site

The patient is transferred to the coronary care or angioplasty unit after the procedure for care and observation. The arterial sheath is attached to a continuous heparinized saline flush, and intravenous fluids must be infused through the venous sheath to maintain luminal patency. Heparin is usually discontinued immediately to facilitate early sheath removal. If the patient's postangioplasty course is uneventful, the sheaths are removed within 2 to 4 hours of the procedure. After sheath removal, the patient may be discharged home 6 to 12 hours later.

Assessing for Bleeding. While the femoral sheath is in place or after its removal, ecchymosis, bleeding, or hematoma at the sheath insertion site may occur from the combined effects of anticoagulation and vessel trauma.[24] The nurse observes the patient's skin for bleeding or swelling at the puncture site and frequently assesses adequacy of circulation to the involved extremity.

The patient is instructed to keep the involved leg straight and not to elevate the head of the bed any more than 30 degrees while the sheath is in place (to prevent dislodgment) and for several hours after its removal (to prevent bleeding). After sheath removal, direct pressure is applied to the puncture site for 15 to 30 minutes; a sandbag may be ordered if direct pressure is inadequate for hemostasis. For stents or atherectomy, which require a larger sheath size, a C-clamp or femoral compression device may be used to apply continued pressure for 1 to 2 hours to ensure adequate hemostasis. Average time to hemostasis in one study was 33 minutes (range 15 to 175 minutes)[24] with femoral site complications more likely to be associated with vascular trauma and antithrombotic drugs, rather than utilization of a specific method of femoral site care.[24]

Hemostatic Devices. Vascular hemostatic devices have been developed to address the problem of achieving hemostasis at the femoral access site after sheath removal. Perclose has marketed a percutaneous vascular surgical device that is inserted into the femoral artery in the same position as a conventional introducer sheath. The device contains needles and sutures that are used to suture the artery closed after the interventional procedure. At the end of the procedure, when the artery is sealed, the needles are removed by the cardiologist and the sutures are knotted firmly. VasoSeal and Angioseal are vascular hemostatic devices that use a collagen plug, injected through a preloaded syringe system into the supraarterial space, to promote hemostasis at the arterial puncture site.[25,26] Gentle pressure is maintained over the puncture site for approximately 5 minutes, until hemostasis is achieved. When devices such as these are used, time to ambulation and discharge can be significantly shortened. The collagen plug is completely absorbed after 90 days, but until that time the site cannot be used for another procedure.

Retroperitoneal Bleeding. Following PCI, the nurse assesses the patient for back pain, which can indicate retroperitoneal bleeding from the internal arterial puncture site.[27] Retroperitoneal hemorrhage occurs in

Box 13-5

NURSING DIAGNOSIS PRIORITIES

Post PTCA, Coronary Atherectomy, and Stent

- Ineffective Cardiopulmonary Tissue Perfusion related to acute myocardial ischemia, p. A-35
- Ineffective Peripheral Tissue Perfusion related to decreased peripheral blood flow, p. A-41
- Acute Pain related to transmission and perception of cutaneous, visceral, muscular, or ischemic impulses, p. A-7
- Anxiety related to threat to biologic, psychologic, and/or social integrity, p. A-9
- Deficient Knowledge: Discharge Regimen related to lack of previous exposure to information, p. A-18

less than 1% of PCI cases but requires prompt volume resuscitation, often requiring blood transfusions to avoid patient demise.[27]

Palpating Peripheral Pulses

Pulses are usually monitored every 15 minutes for the first 1 to 2 hours immediately after the procedure, then hourly with vital signs until the sheaths are removed. After sheath removal, pulses are again monitored at 15-minute intervals for a brief period. If the patient does not have sheaths because a hemostatic device was used at the end of the PCI, the nurse is still responsible for assessing the puncture site, the peripheral distal pulses, and color/warmth of the extremity. Bleeding around the puncture site can decrease blood flow to the extremity. Patients usually are allowed to resume ambulation 6 to 8 hours later, depending on institution protocol.

Providing Patient Education

Typically, patients undergoing elective angioplasty, atherectomy, or stent procedures are hospitalized for under 24 hours. All patients require education about their medication regimen and CAD risk factor modification. Because of the abbreviated hospital stay, the nurse often can do little more than identify the offending risk factors and initiate basic instruction. Patients are referred to a local cardiac rehabilitation center for more extensive teaching and follow-up to facilitate understanding and compliance with risk factor modification.

Another important point of instruction concerns the discharge medications. Patients are discharged home on a regimen of antiplatelet drugs (e.g., clopidogrel, aspirin), as well as a nitrate (e.g., isosorbide) to promote vasodilation. In addition, if the patient has coronary artery vasospasm, calcium channel blockers are prescribed. It is essential that the patient clearly understand the rationale for therapy and potential side effects of each drug. It is essential to provide written information and an emergency telephone number the patient can call if problems occur. In all aspects of patient care management after PCI, health care professionals work as a team with the goal of providing the best possible outcome for each patient as described in Evidence-Based Collaborative Practice: Percutaneous Catheter Intervention: Angioplasty, Atherectomy, Stents.

CARDIAC SURGERY

The nursing management of the patient undergoing cardiac surgery is both demanding and exciting and

EVIDENCE-BASED COLLABORATIVE PRACTICE

Percutaneous Catheter Intervention: Angioplasty, Atherectomy, Stents

Definitions

- Primary percutaneous catheter intervention (PCI): Urgent balloon angioplasty—with or without stent placement—*without* fibrinolytic therapy or platelet glycoprotein IIb/IIIa medications to open the infarct-related artery in STEMI. Successful in over 90% of patients.
- Facilitated PCI: Administration of fibrinolytics or platelet glycoprotein IIb/IIIa medications to open the artery before PCI.
- Elective PCI: Scheduled procedure, nonurgent.

PCI in ST-Elevation Myocardial Infarction

- Primary PCI preferred over fibrinolytic therapy for chest pain up to 12 hours' duration, when PCI performed in hospitals with skillful practitioners, cardiac catheterization facilities, where the "door to balloon" time is under 90 minutes. With cardiac surgery backup.
- Fibrinolytic therapy is utilized when the first medical contact for a patient with ST-elevation myocardial infarction (STEMI) is less than 3 hours after onset of symptoms and PCI is not available.
- See Figure 12-2, p. 185, for more information on PCI emergency management of STEMI.

Stents

- Stents placed in the STEMI-related artery decrease the incidence of abrupt closure to around 1%.
- Stents reduce risk of artery restenosis compared with catheter procedures alone.
- Drug-eluting stents appear to further reduce restenosis risk within the first 12 months after PCI.
- Stent thrombosis in the first 12 months is about 1.5%.

Biomarkers

- For any signs or symptoms suggestive of an MI during or after PCI, measure troponin I or T and CK-MB.
- There is no evidence to support routine measurement without untoward symptoms.

Antiplatelet Therapy for 12 Months

- Dual antiplatelet therapy (oral) with aspirin and a thienopyridine (such as clopidogrel) for 12 months following placement of a drug-eluting stent as recommended. Premature stoppage of one or both the antiplatelet agents increases the risk of acute MI, stent thrombosis, and death.

Data from Smith SC et al: *Circulation* 113:156, 2006; and Keeley EC, Hillis LD: *N Engl J Med* 356(1):47, 2007.

requires the talents of an experienced team of critical care nurses. The following discussion introduces basic cardiac surgical techniques and principles of cardiopulmonary bypass and highlights the key points about postoperative care of the adult patient who requires either valve replacement or coronary artery revascularization.

Coronary Artery Bypass Surgery

The combined results of three major randomized trials support the view that coronary artery bypass grafting (CABG) affords dramatic improvement of symptoms and quality of life. CABG is more effective than medical therapy for improving survival in patients with left main-vessel or triple-vessel disease or with double-vessel disease involving the left anterior descending (LAD) artery, as well as more effective for relieving exercise-induced ischemia or chronic ischemia leading to left ventricular (LV) dysfunction. Medical therapy is recommended when ischemia is prevented by antianginal drugs that are well tolerated by the patient.[18] Surgical revascularization has been shown to be more efficacious than angioplasty in patients with diabetes mellitus.[24] CABG also offers advantages over percutaneous revascularization in patients with multivessel disease. When arterial grafts are used, CABG has superior long-term patency rates, surpassing those of angioplasty or stents.[28] In addition, bypass surgery may allow for more complete revascularization because it can be used on vessels that are not amenable to treatment with a percutaneous approach, such as those with total occlusions or excessive tortuosity. Myocardial revascularization involves the use of a conduit, or channel, designed to bypass an occluded coronary artery. Currently, the two most common conduits are the SVG and the IMA. A comparison of conduits used for myocardial revascularization is provided in Table 13-8.

Saphenous Vein Graft

SVG involves the anastomosis of an excised portion of the saphenous vein proximal to the aorta and distal to the coronary artery below the obstruction (Figure 13-10). Traditionally the SVG was obtained through an open incision as shown in Figure 13-10, but recent technology has allowed for the endoscopic harvesting of this vessel. This minimally invasive technique of graft procurement decreases postoperative pain and reduces both scarring and infection rates.[29]

Internal Mammary Artery Grafts

The IMA, which usually remains attached to its origin at the subclavian artery, is swung down and anastomosed distal to the coronary artery (Figure 13-11). Both the right IMA (RIMA) and the left IMA (LIMA) may be used as conduits. Of note, emergency coronary artery bypass surgery may preclude the use of the IMA because of the extra time required to mobilize the artery, as well as the inability to effect cardioplegia through this conduit. However, the current trend is to use arterial conduits such as the IMA when possible, because their long-term patency rates are superior to those of the SVG.[30]

Radial Artery Grafts

The potential benefit of long-term patency associated with arterial conduits has revived interest in the use of radial artery (RA) grafts. First introduced as a potential conduit for myocardial revascularization in the 1970s, RA grafts were abandoned because of a high incidence of early graft occlusion and vasospasm. Current early patency rates of 90% or better have been attributed to improved harvesting techniques and the

Table 13-8
Conduits Used for Coronary Artery Bypass Grafts

TYPE OF GRAFT	ADVANTAGES	DISADVANTAGES
Saphenous vein	Easily harvested Length allows for multiple grafts No anatomic limitations to graft sites	Long-term patency is not as good as that of arterial grafts Requires at least two anastomosis sites Associated with leg edema postoperatively
Internal mammary artery	Improved patency over venous grafts Only requires one anastomosis	Requires extensive dissection Not accessible for emergency bypass Associated with increased chest-wall discomfort postoperatively Anatomic limitations to bypassing some areas of the heart
Gastroepiploic artery	Improved patency over venous grafts Only requires one anastomosis Associated with increased gastrointestinal complications postoperatively	Technically difficult to harvest Not accessible for emergency bypass Anatomic limitations to bypassing some areas of the heart
Radial artery	Improved patency over venous grafts Easily harvested	Requires adequate collateral flow to hand via ulnar artery May be associated with higher rates of vasospasm Requires two anastomosis sites

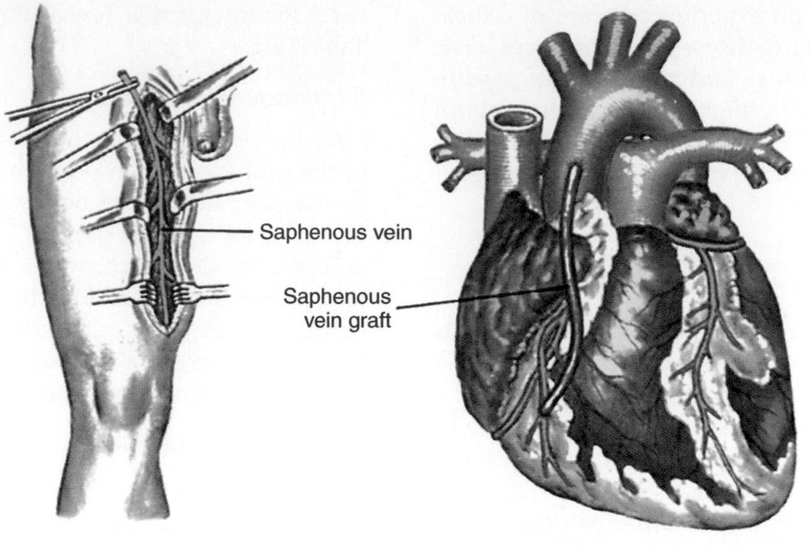

FIGURE 13-10. Saphenous vein graft.

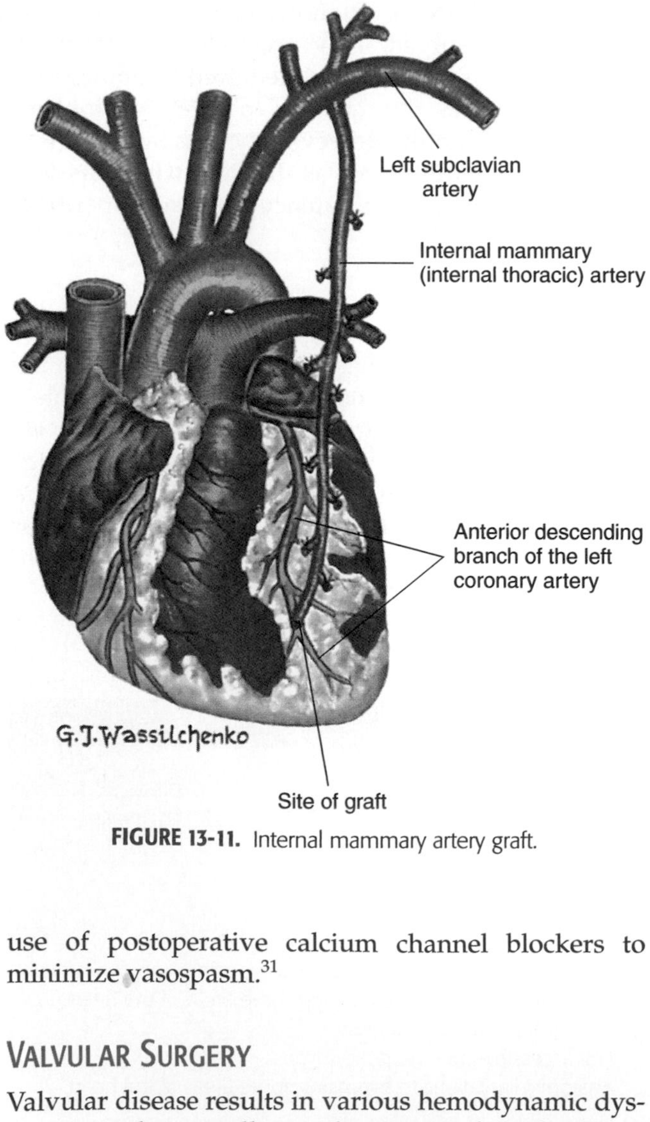

FIGURE 13-11. Internal mammary artery graft.

use of postoperative calcium channel blockers to minimize vasospasm.[31]

Valvular Surgery

Valvular disease results in various hemodynamic dysfunctions that usually can be managed medically as long as the patient remains symptom-free. There is reluctance to intervene surgically early in the course of this disease because of the surgical risks and long-term complications associated with prosthetic valve replacement. These consequences, however, must be weighed against the possibility of irreversible deterioration in left ventricular function that may develop during the compensated asymptomatic phase.

Symptomatic aortic valve disease necessitates replacement of the damaged valve.[32] Symptomatic mitral valve disease may be treated by valve repair or valve replacement depending on the disease process.[32] If reconstruction and repair of the mitral valve is not possible, the valve is replaced with a prosthetic valve. The two categories of prosthetic valves are mechanical valves and biologic valves, or tissue valves. *Mechanical valves* are made from combinations of metal alloys, pyrolite carbon, Dacron, and Teflon and have rigid occluding devices (Figure 13-12). Their construction renders them highly durable, but all patients with mechanical valves require anticoagulation to reduce the incidence of thromboembolism. *Biologic valves* are constructed from animal or human cardiac tissue and have flexible occluding mechanisms. Because of their low thrombogenicity, tissue valves offer the patient freedom from therapeutic anticoagulation. Their durability, however, is limited by their tendency toward early calcification (see Box 13-6 for a description of various prosthetic valves).

Minimally Invasive Cardiac Surgery

Over the past decade, new techniques have been developed to address some of the problems associated with traditional cardiac surgery procedures. Some of these procedures are accomplished without a median sternotomy, using a series of holes or "ports" in the chest and/or small thoracotomy incisions. CABG or valve surgery can then be performed using a thoraco-

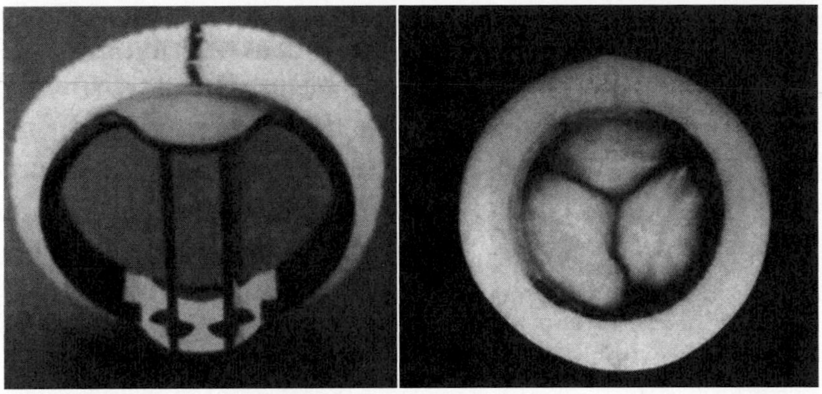

FIGURE 13-12. Prosthetic valves. **A,** The Starr-Edwards caged-ball valve model 4320 with completely covered Stellite cage and hollow Stellite ball, with specific gravity close to that of blood. **B,** The Hancock II porcine aortic valve. The flexible Delrin stent and sewing ring are covered in Dacron cloth. (From Eagle K et al: *The practice of cardiology,* ed 2, Boston, 1989, Little Brown.)

Box 13-6

Classification of Prosthetic Cardiac Valves

Mechanical Valves

Caged-ball: a ball moves freely within a three- or four-sided metallic cage mounted on a circular sewing ring
- Starr-Edwards

Tilting-disk: a free-floating, lens-shaped disk mounted on a circular sewing ring
- Björk-Shiley (discontinued)
- Medtronic Hall
- Omniscience
- Monostrut

Bi-leaflet: two semicircular leaflets, mounted on a circular sewing ring that opens centrally
- St. Jude Medical
- Duromedics
- CarboMedics
- On-X ATS

Biologic (Tissue) Valves (Bioprostheses)

Porcine heterograft: a porcine aortic valve mounted on a semiflexible stent and preserved in glutaraldehyde
- Hancock
- Carpentier-Edwards
- Toronto Stentless (St. Jude)
- Free Style Stentless (Medtronic)

Homograft: a human heart valve (aortic or pulmonic) harvested from a donated heart and cryopreserved; may or may not be mounted on a support ring

scope for visualization and specially designed instruments.[33] Off-pump coronary artery bypass (OPCAB) is increasingly used to avoid the complications of cardiopulmonary bypass. Or, surgeons use a less invasive, catheter-based system of cardiopulmonary bypass with access via the femoral artery and vein.[34]

A variety of incisional approaches can be used for "beating heart" surgery. In minimally invasive direct coronary artery bypass graft (MIDCABG) surgery, a small left anterior thoracotomy incision is used to directly harvest the LIMA, which is then anastomosed to the left anterior descending artery. Alternative approaches may use a segment of saphenous vein or radial artery, one end of which is attached to the LIMA and the other to accessible coronary arteries.[34] Studies comparing off-pump surgery with conventional surgery have shown comparable graft patency and similar or less surgical morbidity with off-pump procedures.[35]

Heart Transplant

Heart transplant is performed for end-stage heart failure with a life expectancy of only 6 to 12 months. A median incision and sternotomy is for visualization of the thorax. All of the diseased heart is removed except the posterior walls of the atria that contain the openings of the pulmonary veins and the vena cava. Four major anastomoses are performed to connect the donor heart to the remaining atrial wall. The right atria, left atria, aorta, and pulmonary artery are connected in that order (Figure 13-13). Immediate postoperative management is similar to other cardiac surgical procedures. The recipient must take lifelong immunosuppressive drugs to prevent rejection of the new heart. Surveillance for rejection, prevention of infection, and comprehensive education about transplant self-care are essential to ensuring a long-term success.

Cardiopulmonary Bypass

Cardiopulmonary bypass (CPB) is a mechanical means of circulating and oxygenating a patient's blood while diverting most of the circulation from the heart and lungs during cardiac surgical procedures. Numerous clinical sequelae can result from CPB (Table 13-9). Knowledge of these physiologic effects allows the nurse to anticipate problems and intervene effectively.

NURSING MANAGEMENT

Nursing management of the patient after cardiac surgery incorporates a variety of nursing diagnoses (Box 13-7). **Nursing priorities are directed toward (1) normalizing cardiac output, (2) rewarming after hypothermia, (3) controlling bleeding complications, (4) maintaining chest tube patency, (5) recognizing cardiac tamponade, (6) promoting early extubation, (7) assessing for neurologic complications, (8) preventing infection, (9) preserving kidney function, and (10) providing patient education.**

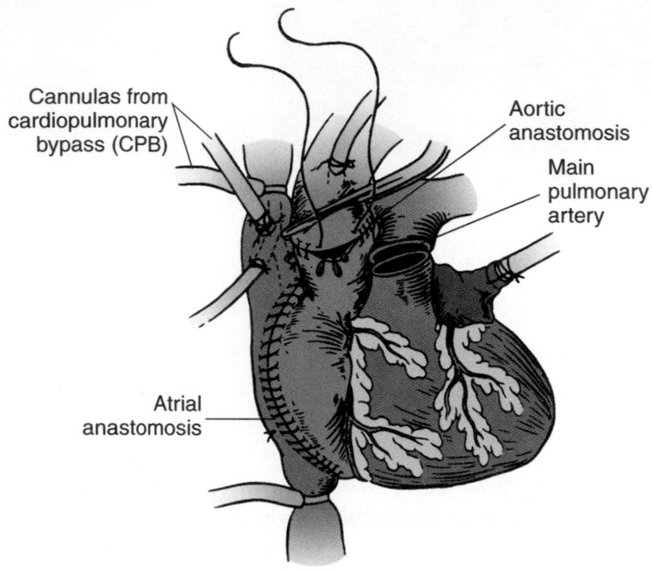

FIGURE 13-13. Heart transplantation: surgical procedure. (Modified from Hurst JW et al: *The heart,* ed 7, New York, 1990, McGraw-Hill.)

Normalizing Cardiac Output

Using standardized protocols, the nurse actively intervenes to normalize cardiac output (CO) by optimizing the patient's heart rate, preload, afterload, and contractility.

Heart Rate. In the presence of low cardiac output, the heart rate can be appropriately regulated by means of temporary pacing or drug therapy. Temporary epicardial pacing usually is instituted when the heart rate of the adult patient who has had cardiac surgery drops to less than 80 beats/min. In the case of tachycardia, intravenous β-blockers (esmolol) or calcium channel blockers (diltiazem) may be used in the acute postoperative period to slow supraventricular rhythms with a ventricular response that exceeds 110 beats/min. Because ventricular ectopy can result from hypokalemia, serum potassium levels are maintained in the high-normal range (4.5 to 5 mEq/L) to provide some margin for error. Maintaining serum magnesium in a therapeutic range (2 mEq/L) has also been shown to reduce the incidence of dysrhythmias in the postoperative period.[36]

Table 13-9

Physiologic Effects of Cardiopulmonary Bypass (CPB)

EFFECTS	CAUSES
Intravascular fluid deficit (hypotension)	Third spacing Postoperative diuresis Sudden vasodilation (drugs, rewarming)
Third spacing (weight gain, edema)	Decreased plasma protein concentration Increased capillary permeability
Myocardial depression (decreased cardiac output)	Hypothermia Increased systemic vascular resistance Prolonged CPB pump run Preexisting heart disease Inadequate myocardial protection
Coagulopathy (bleeding)	Systemic heparinization Mechanical trauma to platelets Depressed release of clotting factors from liver as a result of hypothermia
Pulmonary dysfunction (decreased lung mechanics and impaired gas exchange)	Decreased surfactant production Pulmonary microemboli Interstitial fluid accumulation in lungs
Hemolysis (hemoglobinuria)	Red blood cells damaged in pump circuit
Hyperglycemia (rise in serum glucose)	Decreased insulin release Stimulation of glycogenolysis
Hypokalemia (low serum potassium)	Intracellular shifts during bypass and postoperative diuresis
Hypomagnesemia (low serum magnesium)	Postoperative diuresis secondary to hemodilution
Neurologic dysfunction (decreased level of consciousness, motor/sensory deficits)	Inadequate cerebral perfusion Microemboli to brain (air, plaque fragments, fat globules)
Hypertension (transient rise in blood pressure)	Catecholamine release and systemic hypothermia causing vasoconstriction

Atrial fibrillation occurs in a third of patients after cardiac surgery, with a peak occurrence in the first 2 to 3 days after surgery.[36,37] The incidence of atrial fibrillation is lower in patients who had off-pump cardiac surgery.[38] This rhythm induces hemodynamic compromise, prolongs hospitalization, and increase the patient's risk of stroke. Prophylactic administration of antidysrhythmic agents such as β-blockers or amiodarone has been shown to decrease the incidence of atrial fibrillation and its clinical sequelae.[36,37]

Preload. In most patients, reduced preload is the cause of low postoperative cardiac output. If a pulmonary artery catheter has been inserted during surgery, monitoring pulmonary artery occlusion pressure (PAOP), also known as the "wedge pressure," can provide a more convenient and accurate guide to left ventricular preload than can monitoring central venous pressure (CVP) alone. To enhance preload, volume may be administered in the form of crystalloid, colloid, or packed red cells. It is not uncommon to achieve the greatest hemodynamic stability in cardiac surgery patients when filling pressures (pulmonary artery diastolic pressure [PADP] or PAOP) are in the range of 18 to 20 mm Hg (normal values range from 5 to 12 mm Hg).

Afterload. Partly as a result of the peripheral vasoconstrictive effects of hypothermia, many patients who have had cardiac surgery demonstrate postoperative hypertension and elevated systemic vascular resistance (SVR). Although transient, postoperative hypertension can precipitate or exacerbate bleeding from the mediastinal chest tubes. In addition, the high SVR (afterload) can increase left ventricular workload. Therefore vasodilator therapy with intravenous sodium nitroprusside (Nipride) often is used to reduce afterload, control hypertension, and improve CO.

Contractility. If these adjustments in heart rate, preload, and afterload fail to produce significant improvement in CO, contractility can be enhanced with positive inotropic drug support to augment cardiac output.[39]

Rewarming After Hypothermia

Hypothermia can contribute to depressed myocardial contractility in the patient who has had cardiac surgery. In addition, hypothermia may contribute to postoperative bleeding, because functioning of clotting factors is depressed during hypothermia. After surgery, patients may be rewarmed using warmed air or water blankets. To prevent subsequent excessive temperature elevations, care must be taken to remove the blankets promptly when the body temperature reaches 98.6° F (37° C).

Controlling Bleeding Complications

Postoperative bleeding from the mediastinal chest tubes can be caused by inadequate hemostasis, disruption of suture lines, or coagulopathy associated with CPB or hypothermia. Bleeding is more likely to occur with IMA grafts as a result of the extensive chest-wall dissection required to free the IMA. If bleeding in excess of 150 ml/hr occurs early in the postoperative period, clotting factors (fresh-frozen plasma, fibrinogen, and platelets) and additional protamine (used to reverse the effects of heparin) may be administered, along with prompt blood replacement. Other medications used in the treatment of postoperative bleeding are described in Table 13-10.

In some institutions, autotransfusion devices, which facilitate the collection and reinfusion of shed mediastinal blood, may be used to replace red blood cell loss.[40] A number of chest drainage systems are configured for either intermittent or continuous autotransfusion. These systems contain a special reservoir section where blood is collected directly from the chest tubes. The accumulated blood is then passed through a microaggregate filter before reinfusion into the patient. Once bleeding slows and autotransfusion is no longer required, the chest tubes are connected directly to the chest tube drainage system.

The use of prophylactic positive end-expiratory pressure (PEEP) in conjunction with mechanical ventilation has been used to increase intoracic pressure to effect tamponade of oozing mediastinal blood vessels. However, although 10 cm H_2O PEEP is safe, it does not lessen postoperative blood loss via chest tubes.[41] Rewarming the patient reverses the depressed manufacture and release of clotting factors that result from hypothermia. However, persistent mediastinal bleeding—usually in excess of 500 ml in 1 hour or

Box 13-7

NURSING DIAGNOSIS PRIORITIES

Post Cardiac Surgery

- Decreased Cardiac Output related to alterations in preload, p. A-12
- Decreased Cardiac Output related to alterations in afterload, p. A-12
- Decreased Cardiac Output related to alterations in contractility, p. A-13
- Decreased Cardiac Output related to alterations in heart rate or rhythm, p. A-13
- Impaired Gas Exchange related to ventilation/perfusion mismatching or intrapulmonary shunting, p. A-29
- Ineffective Airway Clearance related to excessive secretions or abnormal viscosity of mucus, p. A-33
- Activity Intolerance related to cardiopulmonary dysfunction, p. A-2
- Deficient Fluid Volume related to absolute loss, p. A-16
- Risk for Infection: invasive procedures, p. A-46
- Acute Pain related to transmission and perception of cutaneous, visceral, muscular, or ischemic impulses, p. A-7
- Anxiety related to threat to biologic, psychologic, and/or social integrity, p. A-9
- Insomnia related to fragmented sleep, p. A-43
- Deficient Knowledge: Discharge Regimen related to lack of previous exposure to information, p. A-18

Table 13-10

Pharmacologic Management: Postoperative Bleeding

DRUG	DOSE	ACTION/SIDE EFFECTS
Aminocaproic acid (Amicar)	Loading dose: 5 g over 1 hr, followed by a continuous infusion of 1 g/hr for 8 hr or until bleeding is controlled	Inhibits conversion of plasminogen to plasmin to prevent fibrinolysis, helping to stabilize clots
Desmopressin acetate (DDAVP)	0.3 mg/kg IV over 20-30 min	Improves platelet function by increasing levels of factor VIII Side effects include facial flushing, tachycardia, headache, and hypotension
Protamine sulfate	25-50 mg IV slowly over 10 min	Neutralizes the anticoagulant effect of heparin Can cause hypotension, bradycardia, and allergic reactions

IV, Intravenous.

300 ml/hr for 2 consecutive hours despite normalization of clotting studies—is an indication for reexploration of the surgical site.

Maintaining Chest Tube Patency

Chest tube stripping to maintain patency of the tubes is controversial because of the high negative pressure generated by routine methods of stripping. It is believed to result in tissue damage that can actually contribute to bleeding. This risk, however, must be carefully weighed against the very real danger of cardiac tamponade if blood is not effectively drained from around the heart. Therefore chest tube stripping often is advocated in instances of excessive postoperative bleeding. However, the technique of "milking" the chest tubes is advisable for routine postoperative care, because this technique generates less negative pressure and decreases the risk of bleeding.

Recognizing Cardiac Tamponade

Cardiac tamponade may occur after surgery if blood accumulates in the mediastinal space, impairing the heart's ability to pump. Signs of tamponade include elevated and equalized filling pressures (CVP, PADP, PAOP), decreased cardiac output, decreased blood pressure, jugular venous distention, pulsus paradoxus, muffled heart sounds, sudden cessation of chest tube drainage, and a widened cardiac silhouette on chest x-ray film. Interventions for tamponade may include emergency sternotomy in the intensive care unit or a return to the operating room for surgical evacuation of the clot.

Promoting Early Extubation

Protocols that facilitate early extubation (within the first 4 to 8 hours) have now been implemented in most institutions.[42] Early extubation requires a multidisciplinary approach that incorporates anesthesiologists, surgeons, nurses, and respiratory therapists. Potential candidates must be identified before surgery so that the anesthetic regimen can be modified to support early extubation. One approach is to use short-acting anesthetic agents such as propofol at the end of the surgery and minimize the use of opioids. Another option is to administer neostigmine and glycopyrrolate at the end of the surgery to reverse the neuromuscular blockade used during the procedure.

Assessing for Neurologic Complications

Neurologic complications may range from mild disorientation to stroke. The transient neurologic dysfunction often seen in patients who have had cardiac surgery probably can be attributed to decreased cerebral perfusion and to cerebral microemboli, both related to the CPB pump run. Off-pump CABG surgery is associated with a lower incidence of stroke.[43]

The term *postcardiotomy delirium* has been used to describe a postoperative syndrome that initially may be seen as only a mild impairment of orientation but that may progress to agitation, hallucinations, and delusions. Environmental factors, such as sensory deprivation and sensory overload associated with being in a critical care unit, may contribute to this condition. Treatment of delirium may require the use of medications such as benzodiazepines or haloperidol (Haldol). Environmental modifications such as noise reduction, restoring normal day/night lighting patterns, and placing familiar objects at the bedside may help to calm and reorient the patient. Liberalizing visitation policies to allow family members a prolonged presence at the bedside is also highly desirable. Nursing management is organized to maximize optimal sleep patterns whenever possible.

Preventing Infection

Postoperative fever is fairly common after CPB. However, persistent temperature elevation to more than 101° F (38.3° C) must be investigated. Sternal wound infections and infective endocarditis are the most devastating infectious complications, but leg wound infection, pneumonia, and urinary tract infection also can occur. Surgical site infection rates are greater in

Box 13-8

Indications for the Use of Intraaortic Balloon Pump

- Left ventricular failure after cardiac surgery
- Unstable angina refractory to medications
- Recurrent angina after acute MI
- Complications of acute MI
  - Cardiogenic shock
  - Papillary muscle dysfunction/rupture with mitral regurgitation
  - Ventricular septal rupture

Refractory ventricular dysrhythmias

MI, Myocardial infarction.

diabetic patients.[44] Recent studies have shown that maintaining blood glucose between 80 and 110 mg/dl in the perioperative period through a continuous insulin infusion decreases the risk of infection in this population.[45]

Preserving Kidney Function

Hemolysis caused by trauma to the red blood cells in the extracorporeal circuit results in hemoglobinuria, which can damage kidney tubules. Administration of adequate fluid volume, judicious use of diuretics, and prompt attention to a decreased urine output can help conserve kidney function.

Providing Patient Education

Patient education includes information related to the surgical procedure, as well as content related to risk factor management for the prevention of atherosclerosis. Patients who have undergone valve surgery may also require information regarding the need for antibiotic prophylaxis before invasive procedures and specifics pertaining to their anticoagulation regimen.

Collaborative Management

Care of the patient following cardiac surgery is complex and requires a collaborative team approach to ensure optimal outcomes. Evidence-Based Practice: Coronary Artery Bypass Graft Surgery reviews guidelines for collaborative management of the patient who requires CABG surgery.

INTRAAORTIC BALLOON PUMP

The intraaortic balloon pump (IABP) is the most widely used temporary mechanical circulatory assist device for supporting failing circulation (Box 13-8). Its therapeutic effects are based on the hemodynamic principles of diastolic augmentation and afterload reduction.

The most commonly used intraaortic balloon (IAB) catheter consists of a single, sausage-shaped polyurethane balloon that is wrapped around the distal end of a vascular catheter and positioned in the descending thoracic aorta just distal to the takeoff of the left subclavian artery. The newest generation of IAB catheters are very flexible, can be wrapped to a smaller diameter, and can be inserted into the femoral artery percutaneously rather than surgically. When attached to a bedside pumping console and properly synchronized to the patient's cardiac cycle, the intraaortic balloon inflates during diastole and deflates just before systole.

Initially, as the balloon is inflated in diastole concurrent with aortic valve closure, the blood in the aortic arch above the level of the balloon is displaced retrograde (backward) toward the aortic root, augmenting diastolic coronary arterial blood flow and increasing myocardial oxygen supply (Figure 13-14, *A*). The blood volume in the aorta below the level of the balloon is propelled forward toward the peripheral vascular system, which may enhance renal perfusion. Subsequently, the deflation of the balloon just before the opening of the aortic valve creates a potential space or vacuum in the aorta, toward which blood flows unimpeded during ventricular ejection (Figure 13-14, *B*). This decreased resistance to left ventricular ejection, or decreased afterload, facilitates ventricular emptying and reduces myocardial oxygen demands. The overall physiologic effect of IABP therapy is an improvement in the balance between myocardial oxygen supply and demand. Contraindications to balloon pumping include aortic aneurysm, aortic valve insufficiency, and severe peripheral vascular disease.[46]

IABP Insertion

The intraaortic balloon may be inserted in the operating room, the cardiac catheterization laboratory, or the critical care unit. The IAB catheter is usually inserted percutaneously through the femoral artery and advanced to the correct position in the descending thoracic aorta. The physician may insert the balloon through an introducer sheath or perform a sheathless insertion to minimize the degree of vessel occlusion created by the catheter. After insertion, the balloon is attached to the console and filled with the prescribed volume of helium, and pumping is initiated. If the balloon fails to unwrap completely during filling, the physician may rapidly inflate and deflate the balloon manually, using a syringe.

Nursing Management

The management of the pumping console and its timing functions may be performed by the nurse caring for the patient or delegated to specially trained personnel on the unit. In either situation, several important nursing diagnoses and management responsibilities

EVIDENCE-BASED COLLABORATIVE PRACTICE

Coronary Artery Bypass Graft Surgery

Strong Evidence to Support the Following:

Coronary Artery Bypass Graft (CABG) Criteria for Stable and Unstable Angina

- CABG should be performed in patients who have significant left main coronary artery stenosis.
- CABG should be performed in patients who have left main stenosis greater than or equal to 70% stenosis of the proximal left anterior descending (LAD) artery and proximal left circumflex artery.
- CABG is useful in patients who have three-vessel disease. Survival benefit is greater in patients with abnormal left ventricular (LV) function, such as when LV ejection fraction (LVEF) is less than 0.50 (50%) and/or there are large areas of demonstrable myocardial ischemia.
- CABG is beneficial for patients with one- or two-vessel disease plus extensive ischemia and LVEF less than 0.50 (50%).
- CABG is beneficial for patients with disabling or unstable angina despite maximal noninvasive therapy, when surgery can be performed with acceptable risk. If the angina is not typical, objective evidence of ischemia should be obtained.
- CABG is recommended for unstable angina/non–ST-elevation myocardial infarction (NSTEMI) in patients in whom emergency percutaneous coronary intervention (PCI) revascularization is not optimal or possible and who have ongoing ischemia not responsive to maximal nonsurgical therapy.

CABG Criteria During ST-Elevation Myocardial Infarction

- Emergency or urgent CABG in patients with ST-elevation myocardial infarction (STEMI) should be undertaken in the following circumstances:
  1. Failed angioplasty with persistent pain or hemodynamic instability in patients with coronary anatomy suitable for surgery
  2. Persistent or recurrent ischemia refractory to medical therapy in patients who have coronary anatomy suitable for surgery, who have a significant area of myocardium at risk, and who are not candidates for PCI
  3. At the time of surgical repair of postinfarction ventricular septal rupture or mitral valve insufficiency
  4. Cardiogenic shock in patients less than 75 years old with ST-segment elevation or left bundle branch block or posterior myocardial infarction (MI) who develop shock within 36 hours of MI and are suitable for revascularization that can be performed within 18 hours of shock, unless further support is futile because of the patient's wishes or contraindications/unsuitability for further invasive care

CABG Criteria With Life-Threatening Ventricular Dysrhythmias

- Life-threatening ventricular dysrhythmias in the presence of greater than or equal to 50% left main stenosis and/or three-vessel coronary disease

CABG Plus Valve Surgery Criteria

- Patients undergoing CABG who also have severe aortic stenosis (AS) should undergo aortic valve replacement (AVR). Severe AS is measured by a mean gradient greater than or equal to 50 mm Hg or Doppler velocity greater than or equal to 4 m/sec.

Reduction in Intraoperative Complications

- Significant atherosclerosis of the ascending aorta mandates a surgical approach that will minimize the possibility of arteriosclerotic emboli and stroke.
- Blood cardioplegia should be considered in patients undergoing cardiopulmonary bypass (CPB) accompanying CABG surgery for acute MI or unstable angina.
- In every patient undergoing CABG, the left internal mammary artery (IMA) should be given primary consideration for revascularization of the LAD artery.

Reduction in Risk of Infection

- Preoperative antibiotic administration should be used in all patients to reduce the risk of postoperative infection.
- A deep sternal wound infection should be treated with aggressive surgical debridement and early revascularized muscle flap coverage, unless there are complicating circumstances.

Prevention of Postoperative Dysrhythmias

- Preoperative or early postoperative administration of β-blockers in patients without contraindications should be used as the standard therapy to reduce the incidence and/or clinical sequelae of atrial fibrillation after CABG surgery.

Antiplatelet Therapy

- Aspirin is the drug of choice for prophylaxis against early saphenous vein graft (SVG) closure.
- If clinical circumstances permit, clopidogrel should be withheld for 5 days before the performance of CABG surgery.

Pharmacologic Management of Hyperlipidemia

- All CABG surgery patients should receive statin therapy unless otherwise contraindicated.

Smoking Cessation Is Important

- All smokers should receive educational counseling and be offered smoking cessation therapy after CABG surgery.
- Pharmacologic therapy including nicotine replacement and bupropion (in select patients) should be offered to patients indicating a willingness to quit.

Cardiac Rehabilitation Is Beneficial

- Cardiac rehabilitation should be offered to all eligible patients after CABG.

Data from Eagle A et al: *Circulation* 110(14:):e340, 2004.

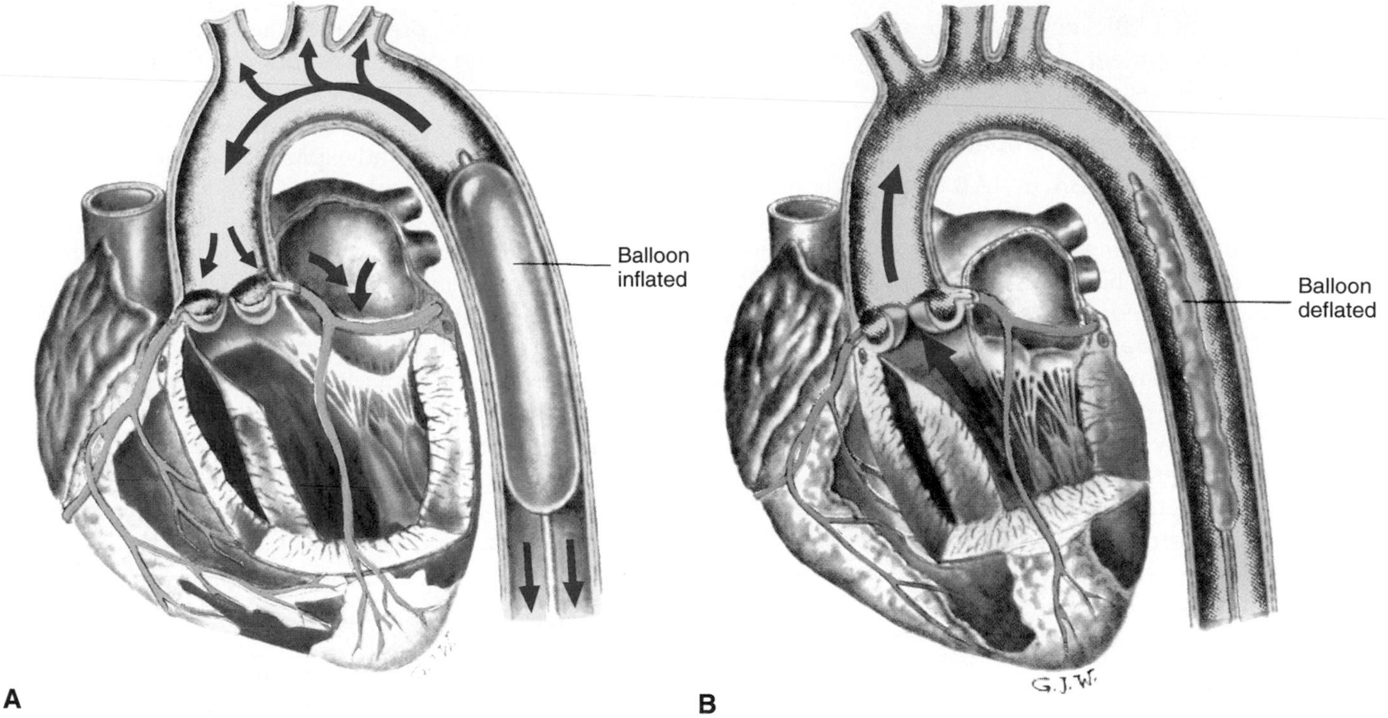

FIGURE 13-14. Mechanisms of action of the intraaortic balloon pump. **A,** Diastolic balloon inflation augments coronary blood flow. **B,** Systolic balloon deflation decreases afterload.

Box 13-9
NURSING DIAGNOSIS PRIORITIES

Intraaortic Balloon Pump

- Decreased Cardiac Output related to alterations in preload, p. A-12
- Decreased Cardiac Output related to alterations in afterload, p. A-12
- Decreased Cardiac Output related to alterations in contractility, p. A-13
- Decreased Cardiac Output related to alterations in heart rate or rhythm, p. A-13
- Activity Intolerance related to cardiopulmonary dysfunction, p. A-2
- Ineffective Cardiopulmonary Tissue Perfusion related to acute myocardial ischemia, p. A-35
- Ineffective Peripheral Tissue Perfusion related to decreased peripheral blood flow, p. A-41
- Risk for Infection: invasive procedures, p. A-46
- Insomnia related to circadian desynchronization, p. A-43
- Disturbed Body Image related to functional dependence on life-sustaining technology, p. A-20
- Deficient Knowledge: Discharge Regimen related to lack of previous exposure to information, p. A-18

relate to the management of the patient receiving IABP therapy (Box 13-9).

Preventing Dysrhythmias

The ECG and arterial pressure tracing are constantly monitored to verify the timing and effect of balloon counterpulsations. For counterpulsation to occur, the pump must receive a trigger signal to identify the beginning of a new cardiac cycle. The trigger can be the R wave of the ECG, the upstroke of the arterial pressure waveform, or a pacemaker spike. Dysrhythmias can adversely affect the timing of balloon inflation and deflation; thus rhythm disturbances must be detected and treated promptly. Current balloon pumps have automatic timing features that use internal algorithms to adjust inflation and deflation in response to changes in the patient's heart rate or rhythm. Mean arterial pressure is ideally maintained at about 80 mm Hg with adequate pumping.

Preventing Peripheral Ischemia

The most common complication of IABP support is lower extremity ischemia secondary to occlusion of the femoral artery, either by the catheter itself or by emboli from thrombus formation on the balloon.[47] Although ischemic complications have decreased with sheathless insertion techniques and the introduction of smaller balloon catheters (8.0 Fr versus 9.5 Fr), evaluation of peripheral circulation remains an important nursing assessment.[48] Consequently, the presence and quality of peripheral pulses distal to the catheter insertion site are assessed frequently, along with color, temperature, and capillary refill of the involved extremity. Doppler localization of peripheral pulses may be required if pulses are difficult to palpate on the cannulated extremity. Signs of diminished perfusion must be reported immediately. Anticoagulation such as a heparin infusion may be prescribed to decrease the incidence of thrombosis. Other vascular complications associated with IABP include acute aortic dissection and the development of pseudoaneurysms at the catheter insertion site.

Monitoring for Balloon Complications

A potential complication of IAB therapy is balloon perforation. Perforation occurs secondary to repeated contact of the balloon membrane with calcified plaque in the aorta as the balloon inflates and deflates. The patient is monitored for evidence of a balloon leak, such as a gas leak alarm from the pump console and the presence of blood in the IAB tubing. If a balloon leak is detected, pumping is stopped and the physician immediately notified so that the balloon can be removed. If the balloon is not promptly removed or pumping is attempted after the perforation, the IAB may become entrapped as the blood hardens within the catheter, creating a mass. If this occurs, the balloon must be surgically removed.

Monitoring Balloon Catheter Position

The balloon catheter must be maintained in proper position to optimize its effectiveness and minimize complications. The balloon may migrate proximally and occlude the left subclavian artery, or it may move distally, compromising renal circulation. Therefore careful assessment of the left radial pulse and urinary output is essential. Measures to prevent accidental displacement of the balloon catheter include ensuring that the patient observes complete bed rest, with the head of the bed elevated no more than 30 degrees, and avoids any flexion of the involved hip. Logrolling, in which the patient is moved from side to side every 2 hours, is used to maintain skin integrity and to prevent pulmonary atelectasis.

Weaning the IABP

Weaning from the balloon pump is considered when hemodynamic stability has been achieved with no, or only minimal, pharmacologic support. One weaning procedure consists of slowly decreasing the pumping frequency from every beat to every second, third, or eighth beat, as tolerated.[47] To prevent thrombus formation on the balloon surface, the IABP must remain at a minimal pumping ratio (or volume) until its removal.

Providing Patient Education

Patient education for the patient with an IAB is focused on the reasons for use of the balloon pump and any movement restrictions. Many of the IABP manufacturers provide helpful educational booklets designed for patients and families.

EFFECTS OF CARDIOVASCULAR DRUGS

Multiple medications are used in the treatment of critically ill cardiovascular patients. The critical care nurse is responsible for preparation and administration of these drugs and often is required to titrate the dose on the basis of the patient's hemodynamic response. The medications used to treat cardiovascular disease are rapidly changing and expanding as more is learned about the pathophysiology of cardiac disease and as improved formulas are developed by pharmaceutical companies. The critical care nurse who has an understanding of the mechanisms of action of the various drug classifications can readily apply this knowledge to new drugs within the same classification. The following discussion provides a concise review of drugs commonly administered to support cardiovascular function in the critical care setting. The emphasis is on intravenously administered medications that are used for the acute rather than the chronic management of cardiovascular conditions.

ANTIDYSRHYTHMIC DRUGS

Antidysrhythmic drugs constitute a diverse category of pharmacologic agents used to terminate or prevent an array of abnormal cardiac rhythms. These drugs commonly are classified according to their primary effect on the action potential of cardiac cells. The classification scheme shown in Table 13-11 is the most commonly used system. Classification of newer agents is more difficult, because some of these agents have characteristics of more than one class and others have no characteristics of the current system.

Table 13-11

Classification of Antidysrhythmic Agents

CLASS	ACTION	DRUGS
I	Blocks sodium channels ("stabilizes" cell membrane)	
IA	Blocks sodium channels and delays repolarization, thus lengthening the duration of the action potential	Quinidine Procainamide Disopyramide
IB	Blocks sodium channels and accelerates repolarization, thus shortening the duration of the action potential	Lidocaine Mexiletine Tocainide
IC	Blocks sodium channels and slows conduction through the His-Purkinje system, thus prolonging the QRS duration	Flecainide Encainide Propafenone
II	Blocks β-receptors	Esmolol Metoprolol Propranolol
III	Slows repolarization and prolongs the duration of the action potential	Amiodarone Ibutilide Sotalol Dofetilide
IV	Blocks calcium channels	Diltiazem Verapamil

CLASS I DRUGS

Class I agents are sodium channel blockers that decrease the influx of sodium ions through "fast" channels during phase 0 depolarization. This prolongs the absolute (effective) refractory period, thus decreasing the risk of premature impulses from ectopic foci. In addition, these drugs depress automaticity by slowing the rate of spontaneous depolarizations of pacemaker cells during the resting phase (phase 4).

CLASS II DRUGS

Class II drugs are β-adrenergic blockers (beta-blockers). These agents inhibit dysrhythmias mediated by the sympathetic nervous system by competing with endogenous catecholamines for available receptor sites. As a result, spontaneous depolarization during the resting phase (phase 4) is depressed and atrioventricular conduction is slowed. Drugs in this class can be further subdivided into cardioselective (those that block only β_1 cardiac receptors) and noncardioselective (those that block both the β_1 and β_2 receptors). Knowledge of the effects of adrenergic-receptor stimulation allows for anticipation of not only the therapeutic responses brought about by β-blockade but also the potential adverse effects such as bronchospasm (Table 13-12). Although numerous β-blockers are available, only *esmolol, metoprolol,* and *propranolol* are available as intravenous agents for the treatment of acute dysrhythmias. Of these, esmolol (Brevibloc) offers significant advantages for the critically ill patient because of its short half-life (approximately 9 minutes). It is used in the treatment of supraventricular tachycardias, such as atrial fibrillation and atrial flutter.

CLASS III DRUGS

Class III agents include *amiodarone, dofetilide, ibutilide,* and *sotalol.* These agents markedly slow the rate of phase 3 repolarization, increasing the effective refractory period and the action potential duration. Although their effect on the action potential is similar, these drugs differ greatly in their mechanism of action and their side effects. At this time, sotalol is approved only for oral use. Intravenous amiodarone was originally approved for treatment of serious ventricular dysrhythmias that were refractory to other medications. Because of its effectiveness, it is now used for both atrial and ventricular dysrhythmias.[2] Dofetilide (Tikosyn) is a new class III antidysrhythmic agent used for the conversion to and maintenance of normal sinus rhythm in patients with highly symptomatic atrial fibrillation/flutter. Because dofetilide prolongs the refractoriness of both atrial and ventricular tissue, prolongation of the QT interval can occur, which is associated with an increased risk of torsades de pointes.[49] Therapy with dofetilide is initiated in a hospital setting under close monitoring. Ibutilide (Corvert) is a short-term antidysrhythmic agent used for the rapid conversion of acute atrial fibrillation or atrial flutter to sinus rhythm. The drug is administered as a 10-minute infusion in a carefully monitored clinical setting. The most serious side effect of ibutilide is its potential for inducing life-threatening dysrhythmias, especially torsades de pointes.[50]

Table 13-12

Actions of Adrenergic Receptors

RECEPTOR	LOCATION	RESPONSE TO STIMULATION
α	Vessels of skin, muscles, kidneys, and intestines	Vasoconstriction of peripheral arterioles
β_1	Cardiac tissue	Increased heart rate Increased conduction Increased contractility
β_2	Vascular and bronchial smooth muscle	Vasodilation of peripheral arterioles Bronchodilation

CLASS IV DRUGS

Class IV agents are calcium channel blockers that inhibit the influx of calcium through slow calcium channels during the plateau phase (phase 2). This effect occurs primarily in tissue in which slow calcium channels predominate, primarily in the sinus and AV nodes and the atrial tissue. *Verapamil* was the first drug in this category available as an intravenous antidysrhythmic. It depresses sinus and AV node conduction and is effective in terminating supraventricular tachycardias caused by AV nodal reentry. *Diltiazem* (Cardizem) in IV form is also effective in treating supraventricular dysrhythmias, with fewer hypotensive side effects.

UNCLASSIFIED ANTIDYSRHYTHMICS

Adenosine (Adenocard) is an antidysrhythmic agent that remains unclassified under the current system. Adenosine occurs endogenously in the body as a building block of adenosine triphosphate (ATP). Given in intravenous boluses, adenosine slows conduction through the AV node, causing transient AV block. It is used clinically to convert supraventricular tachycardias and to facilitate differential diagnosis of rapid dysrhythmias. Because of its short half-life, the drug is administered intravenously as a rapid bolus, followed by a saline flush. The bolus is delivered as centrally as possible so that the drug reaches the heart before it is metabolized.[2] Side effects are transient because the drug is rapidly taken up by the cells and is cleared from the body within 10 seconds.

Magnesium is also unclassified under the present system. Although its action as an antidysrhythmic agent is not entirely understood, clinical studies suggest that it may reduce the incidence of both ventricular and supraventricular dysrhythmias in selected patient populations. It is considered the treatment of choice in patients with torsades de pointes. For acute treatment, 1 to 2 g of magnesium is administered over 1 to 2 minutes. In patients with confirmed hypomagnesemia, this bolus may be followed with a 24-hour infusion.[2]

Side Effects

Antidysrhythmic drugs carry the risk of serious side effects, some of which may be life-threatening. The major side effects of the intravenous antidysrhythmic agents are listed in the Table 13-13. The most severe complication is the potential for a "prodysrhythmic" effect. This may result in a worsening of the underlying dysrhythmia, the occurrence of a new dysrhythmia, or the development of a bradydysrhythmia. For example, torsades de pointes is a prodysrhythmia caused by a number of drugs. The development of a prodysrhythmia is unpredictable; thus the nurse plays an important role in evaluating ECG changes, monitoring drug levels, and assessing patient symptoms. Antidysrhythmic agents may also alter the amount of energy required for defibrillation and pacing. For example, increases in an antidysrhythmic drug dose may increase the amount of output (mA) required to depolarize the myocardium. Table 13-13 contains information about frequently prescribed antidysrhythmic agents.

Inotropic Drugs

Critically ill patients with compromised cardiac function often require the use of medications to enhance

Table 13-13

Pharmacologic Management: Selected Antidysrhythmic Agents

DRUG/SITE OF ACTION	INDICATIONS	DOSAGE	MAJOR SIDE EFFECTS
Sinus Node, Atria, or AV Node			
Adenosine	SVT, PSVT	6 mg IV rapid push; if unsuccessful, repeat with 12 mg over 1-2 sec; follow with IV fluid 10 ml flush (NS or D5W)	Transient; flushing, dyspnea, hypotension
Digoxin	AFib, AF, PSVT	0.5-1 mg loading dose in divided doses; maintenance dose of 0.125-0.375 mg daily	Bradycardia, heart block Toxicity: CNS and GI symptoms
Diltiazem	SVT, AFib, AF	Bolus dose of 0.25 mg/kg IV over 2 min, followed by an infusion of 5-15 mg/hr	Bradycardia, hypotension, AV block
Esmolol	ST, SVT	Loading dose of 500 mcg/kg/min over 1 min, followed by an infusion of 50 mcg/kg/min for 4 min; repeat procedure every 5 min, increasing infusion by 25-50 mcg/kg/min to maximum of 300 mcg/kg/min	Hypotension, bradycardia, heart failure
Ibutilide	AFib, AF	0.010-0.025 mg/kg infused over 10 min (may repeat once) or 1 mg diluted in 50 ml infused over 10 min (may repeat once)	Minimal side effects except for rare polymorphic VT (torsades de pointes)
Propranolol	SVT	1-3 mg IV every 5 min not to exceed 0.1 mg/kg	Bradycardia, heart block, heart failure
Verapamil	AF, PSVT	5-10 mg IV; may repeat in 15-30 min	Hypotension, bradycardia, heart failure
Ventricle			
Lidocaine	PVCs, VT, VF	1-1.5 mg/kg bolus, followed by continuous infusion of 1-4 mg/min	CNS toxicity, nausea, vomiting with repeated doses
Atria and Ventricle			
Amiodarone	VT/VT arrest Stable, VT, AFib, AF	300 mg IV push; may repeat with 150 mg in 3-5 min (maximum dose of 2.2 g/24 hr) 150 mg IV over 10 min, followed by 360 mg over 6 hr (1 mg/min); maintenance infusion of 0.5 mg/min	Hypotension, abnormal liver function tests
Procainamide	AF, SVT, PVCs, VT	Loading dose of 12-17 mg/kg at a rate of 20 mg/min, followed by infusion of 1-4 mg/min	Hypotension, GI effects Widening of QRS and QT lengthening

AV, Atrioventricular; *SVT,* supraventricular tachycardia; *PSVT,* paroxysmal supraventricular tachycardia; *IV,* intravenous; *NS,* normal saline; *D5W,* dextrose 5% in water; *AFib,* atrial fibrillation; *AF,* atrial flutter; *CNS,* central nervous system; *GI,* gastrointestinal; *ST,* sinus tachycardia; *VT,* ventricular tachycardia; *PVCs,* premature ventricular contractions; *VF,* ventricular fibrillation.

myocardial contractility (positive inotropes). Clinically available inotropes include cardiac glycosides, sympathomimetics, and phosphodiesterase inhibitors. These agents increase myocardial contractility, resulting in improved cardiac output, more complete emptying of the ventricles, and decreased filling pressures.

Cardiac Glycosides

Cardiac glycosides include digitalis and its derivatives. Although these drugs have been used for centuries, their slow onset of action and risk of toxicity make them more appropriate for the management of chronic heart failure. Because digoxin also causes slowing of the sinus rate and a decrease in AV conduction, it may be administered intravenously in the acute care setting to control supraventricular dysrhythmias.

Sympathomimetics

Sympathomimetic agents stimulate adrenergic receptors, thereby simulating the effects of sympathetic nerve stimulation. Included in this category are naturally occurring catecholamines (epinephrine, dopamine, and norepinephrine), as well as synthetic catecholamines (dobutamine and isoproterenol). The cardiovascular effects of these drugs, which vary according to their selectivity for specific receptor sites, are often dose dependent as well. Table 13-14 describes the cardiovascular effects of sympathomimetic drugs at various dosages.

Dopamine

Dopamine (Intropin) is one of the most widely used drugs in the critical care setting. It is a chemical precursor of norepinephrine, which, in addition to both α- and β-receptor stimulation, can activate dopaminergic receptors in the renal and mesenteric blood vessels. The actions of this drug are entirely dose-related.[51] At low dosages of 1 to 2 mcg/kg/min, dopamine stimulates dopaminergic receptors, causing renal and mesenteric vasodilation. However, it is now clear that this increase in urine output does not confer protection against development of acute renal failure. The resultant increase in renal perfusion increases urinary output. Moderate dosages result in stimulation of β_1-receptors to increase myocardial contractility and improve cardiac output. At dosages greater than 10 mcg/kg/min, dopamine predominantly stimulates α-receptors, resulting in vasoconstriction that often negates both the β-adrenergic and dopaminergic effects.

Dobutamine

Dobutamine (Dobutrex) is a synthetic catecholamine with predominantly β_1-effects. It also produces some β_2-stimulation, resulting in a mild systemic vasodilation. Dobutamine is as effective as dopamine in increasing myocardial contractility and is useful in the treatment of heart failure, especially in hypotensive patients who cannot tolerate vasodilator therapy. The usual dosage range is 2.5 to 20 mcg/kg/min, titrated on the basis of hemodynamic parameters.

Epinephrine

Epinephrine (Adrenalin) is produced by the adrenal gland as part of the body's response to stress. This agent has the ability to stimulate both α- and β-receptors,

Table 13-14

Physiologic Effects of Sympathomimetic Agents

		RECEPTOR ACTIVATED*			CARDIOVASCULAR EFFECTS			
DRUG	DOSAGE	α	β_1	β_2	DOPA	CO	HR	SVR
Dobutamine	<5 mcg/kg/min	0	↑↑↑	↑	0	↑↑	↑	0/↓
	5-20 mcg/kg/min	0	↑↑↑	↑↑	0	↑↑↑	↑↑	↓
	>20 mcg/kg/min	0	↑↑↑	↑↑	0	↑↑↑	↑↑↑	↓↓
Dopamine	<3 mcg/kg/min	0	↑	↑	↑↑↑	0/↑	0/↑	0
	3-10 mcg/kg/min	↑	↑↑↑	↑	↑↑↑	↑↑↑	↑	↑
	11-20 mcg/kg/min	↑↑↑	↑↑↑	↑	↑↑	↑↑	↑↑	↑↑↑
	>20 mcg/kg/min	↑↑↑↑	↑↑	0	0	↑	↑	↑↑↑
Epinephrine	<2 mcg/min	0	↑	↑↑	0	0/↑	0/↑	↓
	2-8 mcg/min	↑↑	↑↑↑	↑↑	0	↑↑↑	↑	↑
	9-20 mcg/min	↑↑↑	↑↑	↑↑	0	↑↑	↑↑	↑↑
Isoproterenol	1-7 mcg/min	0	↑↑↑	↑↑↑	0	↑↑↑	↑↑↑	↓↓↓
Norepinephrine	<2 mcg/min	↑↑↑	↑↑	0	0	↑	0/↑	↑↑↑
	2-16 mcg/min	↑↑↑↑	↑↑	0	0	↓	↑	↑↑↑↑
Phenylephrine	10-100 mcg/min	↑↑↑↑	0	0	0	0	↓	↑↑↑

*Refer to Table 13-12 for actions of receptors.

Dopa, Dopaminergic; *CO,* cardiac output; *HR,* heart rate; *SVR,* systemic vascular resistance; 0, no effect; ↑, increased; ↓, decreased (the number of arrows indicates the degree of effect [e.g., ↑, mild and ↑↑↑, strong effect]).

depending on the dose administered (see Table 13-14). At doses of 1 to 2 mcg/min, epinephrine binds with β_1-receptors to increase heart rate, cardiac conduction, contractility, and vasodilation, thereby increasing cardiac output. As the dosage is increased, peripheral α-receptors are stimulated, resulting in increased vascular resistance and blood pressure. At these doses, epinephrine's impact on cardiac output depends on the heart's ability to pump against the increased afterload. Epinephrine accelerates the sinus rate and may precipitate ventricular dysrhythmias in the ischemic heart. Other side effects include restlessness, angina, and headache.

Norepinephrine

Norepinephrine (Levophed) used at low infusion activates β_1-receptors to produce increased contractility and thus augment cardiac output. At higher doses the inotropic effects are limited by marked vasoconstriction mediated by α-receptors. Clinically norepinephrine is used most often as a vasopressor to elevate blood pressure in shock states.

Phosphodiesterase Inhibitors

Phosphodiesterase inhibitors are inotropic agents that also are potent vasodilators (inodilators). Drugs in this classification inhibit the enzyme *phosphodiesterase,* resulting in increased levels of cyclic adenosine monophosphate (AMP) and intracellular calcium. Amrinone (Inocor) and milrinone (Primacor) were the first of these agents approved for use in the United States. Increases in cardiac output occur as a result of increased contractility (inotropic effects) and decreased afterload (vasodilative effects). Filling pressures tend to decrease, whereas the heart rate and blood pressure remain fairly constant. Amrinone may cause thrombocytopenia, so platelet counts are monitored and patients observed for hemorrhagic complications. Milrinone is associated with a lower rate of thrombocytopenia but can induce ventricular dysrhythmias (premature ventricular complexes, ventricular tachycardia) in a significant number of patients.[52]

VASODILATOR DRUGS

Vasodilators are pharmacologic agents that improve cardiac performance by various degrees of arterial or venous dilation, or both. The goal of vasodilator therapy may be a reduction of preload or afterload, or both. Afterload reduction is accomplished by vasodilation of arterial vessels. This results in decreased resistance to left ventricular ejection and may improve cardiac output without increasing myocardial oxygen demands. Reduction of preload is accomplished by dilating venous vessels to increase capacitance. This results in decreased filling pressures. These drugs may be classified into four groups on the basis of mechanism of action. Table 13-15 shows characteristics of selected vasodilators.

Direct Smooth Muscle Relaxants

Direct-acting vasodilators include *sodium nitroprusside* (Nipride), *nitroglycerin* (Tridil), and *hydralazine* (Apresoline). These drugs produce relaxation of vascular smooth muscle via the activation of nitric oxide, resulting in decreased peripheral vascular resistance.

Table 13-15
Pharmacologic Management: Characteristics of Selected Vasodilators

DRUG CLASSIFICATION	DOSAGE	PRELOAD	AFTERLOAD	SIDE EFFECTS
Direct Smooth Muscle Relaxants				
Sodium nitroprusside (Nipride)	0.25-6 mcg/kg/min IV infusion	Moderate	Strong	Hypotension, thiocyanate toxicity, reflex tachycardia
Nitroglycerin (Tridil)	5-300 mcg/min IV infusion	Strong	Mild	Headache, reflex tachycardia, hypotension
Calcium Channel Blockers				
Nicardipine (Cardene)	5 mg/hr IV, titrated to 15 mg/hr	None	Strong	Hypotension, headache, reflex tachycardia
Nifedipine (Procardia)	10-30 mg PO	None	Strong	Hypotension, headache, reflex tachycardia
ACE Inhibitors				
Captopril (Capoten)	6.25-100 mg PO every 8-12 hr	Moderate	Moderate	Hypotension, chronic cough, neutropenia
Enalapril (Vasotec)	0.625 mg IV over 5 min, then every 6 hr	Moderate	Moderate	Hypotension, elevation of liver enzymes
α-Adrenergic Blockers				
Labetalol (Normodyne)	20-80 mg IV bolus every 10 min, then 1-2 mg/min infusion	Moderate	Moderate	Orthostatic hypotension, bronchospasm, AV block
Phentolamine (Regitine)	1-2 mg/min infusion	Moderate	Moderate	Hypotension, tachycardia

IV, Intravenous; *PO,* by mouth; *ACE,* angiotensin-converting enzyme; *AV,* atrioventricular.

Hypotension may occur as a result of peripheral vasodilation, and headaches may be caused by cerebral vasodilation. Compensatory mechanisms can occur in response to the drop in blood pressure. These include baroreceptor activation that causes reflex tachycardia and activation of the renin-angiotensin-aldosterone system (RAAS), with resultant sodium and water retention.

Sodium Nitroprusside. *Sodium nitroprusside* (Nipride) is a potent, rapidly acting venous and arterial vasodilator, particularly suitable for rapid reduction of blood pressure in hypertensive emergencies and perioperatively. It also is effective for afterload reduction in the setting of severe heart failure. The drug is administered by continuous intravenous infusion, with the dosage titrated to maintain the desired blood pressure and SVR. This drug is covered from direct light during IV administration. Prolonged administration can result in thiocyanate toxicity, manifested by nausea, confusion, and tinnitus.[53]

Nitroglycerin. *Intravenous nitroglycerin* (Tridil) causes both arterial and venous vasodilation, but its venous effect is more pronounced. It is used in the critical care setting for the treatment of acute heart failure (HF) because it reduces cardiac filling pressures, relieves pulmonary congestion, and decreases cardiac workload and oxygen consumption. In addition, nitroglycerin dilates the coronary arteries and is a useful adjunct in the treatment of unstable angina and acute MI. The initial dosage is 10 mcg/min, and the infusion is titrated upward to achieve the desired clinical effect: a reduction or elimination of chest pain, decreased PAOP (wedge pressure), or a decrease in blood pressure. Nitroglycerin also is administered prophylactically to prevent coronary vasospasm after coronary angioplasty, atherectomy, stent insertion, or fibrinolytic therapy. The most common side effects of this drug include hypotension, flushing, and headache. It is dispensed in a glass bottle to prevent loss of drug potency when in contact with plastic.

Calcium Channel Blockers

Calcium channel blockers are a chemically diverse group of drugs with differing pharmacologic effects.

Nifedipine (Procardia) and *nicardipine* (Cardene) are *dihydropyridines*. Drugs in this group of calcium channel blockers (with the suffix "pine") are used primarily as arterial vasodilators. These drugs reduce the influx of calcium in the arterial resistance vessels. Both coronary and peripheral arteries are affected. They are used in the critical care setting to treat hypertension. Nifedipine is available in an oral form only but in the past was prescribed sublingually during hypertensive emergencies. Reports of adverse events associated with sublingual nifedipine have prompted the FDA to discourage its use.[54] Nicardipine is now available as an intravenous calcium channel blocker, and as such it offers more accurate titration for effective control of hypertension. Side effects of nifedipine and nicardipine are related to vasodilation and include hypotension, reflex tachycardia, flushing, headache, and ankle edema.

Diltiazem (Cardizem) is from the *benzothiazine* group of calcium channel blockers. Verapamil (Calan, Isoptin) is part of the *phenylalkylamine* group. The different classifications account for the variety of action between these calcium channel blockers. These drugs dilate coronary arteries but have little effect on the peripheral vasculature. They are used in the treatment of angina, especially that which has a vasospastic component, and as antidysrhythmics in the treatment of supraventricular tachycardias.

Angiotensin-Converting Enzyme Inhibitors

Angiotensin-converting enzyme (ACE) inhibitors produce vasodilation by blocking the conversion of angiotensin I to angiotensin II. Because angiotensin is a potent vasoconstrictor, limiting its production decreases peripheral vascular resistance. In contrast to the direct vasodilators and nifedipine, ACE inhibitors do not cause reflex tachycardia or induce sodium and water retention. However, these drugs may cause a profound fall in blood pressure, especially in patients who are volume depleted. Blood pressure must be monitored carefully, especially during initiation of therapy.

Captopril (Capoten) and enalapril (Vasotec) are used in patients with heart failure to decrease SVR (afterload) and PAOP (preload). Captopril is available in an oral form only but has a relatively rapid onset of action (approximately 1 hour). Enalapril is available in an intravenous form and may be used to decrease afterload in more emergent situations.

B-Type Natriuretic Peptide

Nesiritide (Natrecor) is a new vasodilator used in the treatment of acute heart failure. This agent is a recombinant form of human brain natriuretic peptide (BNP), the hormone released by cardiac cells in response to ventricular distention. The primary effects of nesiritide include decreasing filling pressures (PAOP, CVP), reducing vascular resistance (SVR, pulmonary vascular resistance [PVR]), and increasing urine output. Although nesiritide has proven to be as effective as traditional vasodilator therapy for managing acute heart failure, further analysis has raised concerns that the drug may be associated with decreased renal function and increased mortality after discharge.[55] The recommended dose is an IV bolus of 2 mcg/kg, followed by a continuous infusion of 0.01 mcg/kg/min. The primary side effect is hypotension. If this occurs, nesiritide may need to be discontinued for a time and then restarted at a lower dose after the patient's condition has stabilized.[56]

α-Adrenergic Blockers

Peripheral adrenergic blockers block α-receptors in arteries and veins, resulting in vasodilation. Orthostatic hypotension is a common side effect and may result in syncope. Long-term therapy also may be complicated by fluid and water retention.

Labetalol (Normodyne), a combined peripheral α-blocker and cardioselective β-blocker, is used in the treatment of acute stroke and hypertensive emergencies. Because the blockade of β_1-receptors permits the decrease of blood pressure without the risk of reflexive tachycardia and increased cardiac output, this drug also is useful in the treatment of acute aortic dissection.[57]

Phentolamine (Regitine) is a peripheral α-blocker that causes decreased afterload via arterial vasodilation. It is given as a continuous infusion at a rate of 1 to 2 mg/min and is titrated to achieve the required reduction in blood pressure and SVR. Phentolamine is the drug of choice in the treatment of pheochromocytoma.[53] This drug also is used to treat the extravasation of dopamine. If this occurs, 5 to 10 mg is diluted in 10 ml normal saline and administered intradermally into the infiltrated area.

Dopamine A-1-Receptor Agonists

Fenoldopam (Corlopam) is the first of a new class of vasodilators called *dopamine A-1-receptor agonists.* The drug is a potent vasodilator that affects peripheral, renal, and mesenteric arteries. It is administered via continuous IV infusion beginning at 0.1 mcg/kg/min and titrated up to the desired blood pressure effect with a maximum recommended dose of 0.5 mcg/kg/min. It can be administered as an alternative to sodium nitroprusside or other antihypertensives in the treatment of hypertensive emergencies.[53] Fenoldopam can reduce the risk of kidney injury in critically ill patients.[58]

VASOPRESSORS

Vasopressors are sympathomimetic agents that mediate peripheral vasoconstriction through stimulation of α-receptors (see Table 13-14). This results in increased systemic vascular resistance and thus elevates blood pressure. Some of these drugs (epinephrine and norepinephrine) also have the ability to stimulate α-receptors. Vasopressors are not widely used in the

Table 13-16

Pharmacologic Management: Atrial Fibrillation

TREATMENT GOAL	CLASSIFICATION/DRUG	SPECIAL CONSIDERATIONS
Conversion/maintenance of sinus rhythm	***Class IA*** Quinidine Procainamide (Pronestyl) Disopyramide (Norpace)	Class IA drugs prolong QT intervals and may cause torsades de pointes. Rate control should be achieved before initiation of therapy.
	Class IC Flecainide (Tambocor) Propafenone (Rythmol)	Class IC drugs are prodysrhythmic in patients with CAD or previous MI and should be avoided in these patients.
	Class III Amiodarone (Cordarone) Dofetilide (Tikosyn) Ibutilide (Corvert) Sotalol (Betapace)	Amiodarone and sotalol also have β-blocking properties and may help with rate control. Treatment with dofetilide requires careful monitoring for prodysrhythmic effects. Ibutilide is an intravenous agent and is used for conversion only.
Control of ventricular rate	***β-Blockers*** Esmolol (Brevibloc) Metoprolol (Lopressor) Propranolol (Inderal)	Intravenous esmolol or may be used in acute settings to control ventricular rate. Oral agents are used for maintenance therapy. β-Blockers provide good rate control during exercise.
	Calcium Channel Blockers Diltiazem (Cardizem) Verapamil (Isoptin)	Intravenous calcium channel blockers may be used in emergency situations, followed by oral agents for maintenance therapy.
	Digitalis Compounds Digoxin (Lanoxin)	Digoxin does not effectively control rate with exercise, so it may be used in combination with other drugs.
Prevention of thromboembolism	***Anticoagulants*** Heparin Warfarin (Coumadin)	Heparin may be used in emergency situations, before cardioversion. Warfarin is used long term, with monitoring to achieve an INR of 2.0-3.0.
	Antiplatelet Agents Aspirin	May be used in patients with contraindications to warfarin or low-risk patients under age 65.

CAD, Coronary artery disease; *MI,* myocardial infarction; *INR,* international normalized ratio.

treatment of cardiac patients, because the dramatic increase in afterload is taxing to a damaged heart.

Vasopressin

Vasopressin, also known as antidiuretic hormone (ADH) has recently become popular in the critical care setting for its vasoconstrictive effects. At higher doses, vasopressin directly stimulates contraction of vascular smooth muscle, resulting in vasoconstriction of capillaries and small arterioles. A one-time dose of 40 units intravenously is recommended in the ACLS guidelines as first-line drug therapy for any pulseless arrest. This includes VF or pulseless VT that is refractory to initial defibrillation, as well as asystole and pulseless electrical activity (PEA).[59] Continuous infusions of 0.02 units/min up to 0.1 units/min have been used in the treatment of vasodilatory shock in patients with refractory hypotension following CPB.[60] Patients must be monitored for side effects such as heart failure (due to the antidiuretic effects) and myocardial ischemia. Vasopressin should be infused through a central line to avoid the risk of peripheral extravasation and resultant tissue necrosis.[60]

Medications for Specific Conditions

Atrial Fibrillation

The goals of treatment for atrial fibrillation include reestablishing and maintaining sinus rhythm, decreasing the rapid ventricular response during episodes of atrial fibrillation, and preventing the risk of thromboembolism. More information about atrial fibrillation is available in Chapter 11. Table 13-16 lists current drugs used in the treatment of atrial fibrillation.

Heart Failure

The goals of treatment in heart failure include alleviating symptoms, slowing the progression of the disease, and improving survival. Results from a number of randomly controlled clinical trials have resulted in guidelines for the pharmacologic treatment of heart failure. More information about heart failure is available in Chapter 12. Table 13-17 lists the drugs currently recommended for the treatment of heart failure.

evolve To test your mastery of this chapter, try the Open-Book Quiz at http://evolve.elsevier.com/Urden/priorities/

Table 13-17
Pharmacologic Management: Heart Failure

CLASSIFICATION/ DRUG	MECHANISM OF ACTION	EFFECTS	SPECIAL CONSIDERATIONS
ACE Inhibitors Captopril (Capoten) Enalapril (Vasotec) Lisinopril (Prinivil)	Interferes with the renin-angiotensin-aldosterone system by preventing conversion of angiotensin I to angiotensin II	Decreases afterload Decreases preload Reverses ventricular remodeling	Agents appear equivalent in treatment of heart failure Monitor closely for hypotension when initiating therapy May be contraindicated in patients with renal insufficiency
Angiotensin Receptor Blockers Losartan (Cozaar) Valsartan (Diovan)	Interferes with the renin-angiotensin-aldosterone system by blocking the effect of angiotensin II at the angiotensin II receptor site	Decreases afterload Decreases preload Reverses ventricular remodeling	Reserved for patients who cannot tolerate ACE inhibitors due to side effects such as severe cough or angioedema
β-Blockers Metoprolol (Lopressor) Carvedilol (Coreg)	Counteracts the SNS response activated in heart failure by blocking receptor sites Metoprolol is a cardioselective β-blocker, while carvedilol blocks both α- and β-receptor sites	Slows heart rate Prevents dysrhythmias Decreases blood pressure Reverses ventricular remodeling	Not initiated during decompensated stage of heart failure Use cautiously in patients with reactive airway disease, poorly controlled diabetes, bradydysrhythmias, or heart block Carvedilol dose is increased slowly, while monitoring for symptoms secondary to vasodilation, such as dizziness or hypotension
Aldosterone Antagonist Spironolactone (Aldactone)	Counteracts the effects of aldosterone, which include sodium and water retention	Decreases preload Decreases myocardial hypertrophy	May increase serum potassium
Inotropes Digoxin (Lanoxin)	Affects the Na^+/K^+-ATPase pump in myocardial cells to increase the strength of contraction	Increases contractility Increases cardiac output Prevents atrial dysrhythmias	Risk of toxicity is increased with hypokalemia

ACE, Angiotensin-converting enzyme; *SNS*, sympathetic nervous system; *Na^+/K^+-ATPase*, sodium, potassium, adenosine triphosphatase.

REFERENCES

1. Timothy PR, Rodeman BJ: Temporary pacemakers in critically ill patients: assessment and management strategies, *AACN Clin Issues* 15(3):305, 2004.
2. American Heart Association: ECC guidelines. V. Electrical therapies: automated external defibrillators, defibrillation, cardioversion and pacing, *Circulation* 112(24): IV-35, 2005.
3. Boyle J, Rost MK: Present status of cardiac pacing: a nursing perspective, *Crit Care Nurs Q* 23(1):1, 2000.
4. Bernstein AD et al: The NASPE/BPEG generic pacemaker code for antibradycardia and adaptive rate pacing and antitachyarrhythmia devices, *Pacing Clin Electrophysiol* 10:794, 1987.
5. Stone KR, McPherson CA: Assessment and management of patients with pacemakers and implantable cardioverter defibrillators, *Crit Care Med* 32(4):S155, 2004.
6. Gregoratos G et al: ACC/AHA/NASPE 2002 guideline update for implantation of cardiac pacemakers and antiarrhythmia devices: summary article, *Circulation* 106:2145, 2002.
7. Albert NM: Cardiac resynchronization therapy through biventricular pacing in patients with heart failure and ventricular dyssynchrony, *Crit Care Nurse Suppl* 23(3):2, 2003.
8. Flanagan J et al: Heart failure patients with ventricular dysynchrony: management with a cardiac resynchronization therapy device, *Prog Cardiovasc Nurs* 18:184, 2003.
9. Abraham WT et al: Cardiac resynchronization in chronic heart failure, *N Engl J Med* 344:1845, 2002.
10. Bradley DJ et al: Cardiac resynchronization and death from progressive heart failure: a meta-analysis of randomized controlled trials, *JAMA* 289:730, 2003.
11. Zipes DP et al: ACC/AHA/ESC 2006 guidelines for management of patients with ventricular arrhythmias and the prevention of sudden cardiac death—executive summary: a report of the ACC/AHA task force on practice guidelines, *Circulation* 114(10):1088, 2006.
12. Moss AJ et al for the MADIT II Investigators: Prophylactic implantation of a defibrillator in patients with myocardial infarction and reduced ejection fraction, *N Engl J Med* 346:877, 2002.
13. Gheri AK et al: Evaluation and management of patients after implantable cardioverter-defibrillator, *JAMA* 296(23):2839, 2006.
14. Bollmann A et al: Antiarrhythmic drugs in patients with implantable cardioverter-defibrillators, *Am J Cardiovasc Drugs* 5(6):371, 2005.
15. Topol EJ: Current status and future prospects for acute myocardial infarction therapy, *Circulation* 108(suppl III): III-6, 2003.
16. Leeper B: Continuous ST segment monitoring, *AACN Clin Issues* 14(2):145, 2003.
17. Arjomand H et al: Percutaneous coronary intervention: historical perspectives, current status and future directions, *Am Heart J* 146(5):787, 2003.
18. Smith SC et al: ACC/AHA/SCAI 2005 guideline update for percutaneous coronary intervention: summary article—a report of the ACC/AHA task force on practice guidelines, *Circulation* 113(1):156, 2006.
19. Morice MC et al: A randomized comparison of a sirolimus-eluting stent with a standard stent for coronary revascularization, *N Engl J Med* 347:561, 2003.
20. Sousa JE et al: New frontiers in cardiology: drug-eluting stents, part I, *Circulation* 107:2274, 2003.
21. Park SJ et al: A paclitaxel-eluting stent for the prevention of coronary restenosis, *N Engl J Med* 348:1537, 2003.
22. Hilt T, Bayat M: Drugs used to limit blood surface interactions, *Crit Care Nurs Clin North Am* 14(1):7, 2002.
23. Mixon TA, Dehmer GJ: Patient care before and after percutaneous coronary interventions, *Am J Med* 115:642, 2003.
24. Chian LL et al: Effects of three groin compression methods on patient discomfort, distress, and vascular complications following a percutaneous coronary intervention procedure, *Nurs Res* 54(6):391, 2005.
25. Schickel SI et al: Achieving femoral artery hemostasis after cardiac catheterization: a comparison of methods, *Am J Crit Care* 8(6):406, 1999.
26. Hamner JB et al: Predictors of complications associated with closure devices after transfemoral percutaneous coronary procedures, *Crit Care Nurse* 25(3):30, 2005.
27. Ellis SG et al: Correlates and outcomes of retroperitoneal hemorrhage complicating percutaneous coronary intervention, *Catheter Cardiovasc Interv* 67(4):541, 2006.
28. Eagle KA et al: ACC/AHA 2004 guideline update for coronary artery bypass graft surgery, *Circulation* 110(14): e340, 2004.
29. Bitondo JM et al: Endoscopic versus open saphenous vein harvest: a comparison of postoperative wound infections, *Ann Thorac Surg* 73:523, 2002.
30. Mack MJ: Advances in the treatment of coronary artery disease, *Ann Thorac Surg* 76:S2240, 2003.
31. Verma S et al: Should radial arteries be used routinely for coronary artery bypass grafting? *Circulation* 110:e40, 2004.
32. Bonow RO et al: ACC/AHA 2006 guidelines for the management of patients with valvular heart disease, *Circulation* 114(5):e84, 2006.
33. Wegund DL: Advances in cardiac surgery: valve repair, *Crit Care Nurs* 23(2):72, 2003.
34. Chen-Scarabelli C: Beating heart coronary artery bypass surgery, *Crit Care Nurse* 22(5):44, 2002.
35. Puskas JD et al: Off-pump vs conventional coronary artery bypass grafting: early and 1-year graft patency, cost, and quality of life outcomes: a randomized trial, *JAMA* 291(15):1841, 2004.
36. Kern LS: Postoperative atrial fibrillation: new directions in prevention and treatment, *J Cardiovasc Nurs* 19(2):103, 2004.
37. Brantman L, Howie, J: Use of amiodarone to prevent atrial fibrillation after cardiac surgery, *Crit Care Nurse* 26(1):48, 2006.
38. Wijevsundera DN et al: Off-pump coronary artery surgery for reducing mortality and morbidity: meta-analysis of randomized and observational studies, *J Am Coll Cardiol* 46(5):872, 2005.
39. Gillies M et al: Bench to bedside review: Inotropic drug therapy after adult cardiac surgery—a systematic literature review, *Crit Care* 9(3):241, 2005.

40. Reger TB, Roditski D: Bloodless medicine and surgery for patients having cardiac surgery, *Crit Care Nurs* 21(4):35, 2001.
41. Collier B et al: Prophylactic positive end-expiratory pressure and reduction of postoperative blood loss in open heart surgery, *Ann Thorac Surg* 74(4):1194.
42. Meade MO et al: Trials comparing early vs. late extubation following cardiovascular surgery, *Chest* 120:445S, 2001.
43. Sedrakyan A et al: Off pump surgery is associated with reduced occurrence of stroke and other morbidity as compared with traditional coronary artery bypass grafting: a meta-analysis of systematically reviewed trials, *Stroke* 27(11):2759, 2006.
44. Streeler NB: Considerations in prevention of surgical site infections following cardiac surgery: when your patient is diabetic, *J Cardiovasc Nurs* 21(3)E14, 2006
45. Furnary AP et al: Continuous insulin infusion reduces mortality in patient with diabetes undergoing coronary artery bypass grafting, *J Thorac Cardiovasc Surg* 125:1007, 2003.
46. Trost JC, Hillis LD: Intra-aortic balloon counterpulsation, *Am J Cardiol* 97(9):1391, 2006
47. Metules T: IABP therapy: getting patients treatment fast, *RN* 66(5):56, 2003.
48. Meco M et al: Mortality and morbidity from intra-aortic balloon pumps: risk analysis, *J Cardiovasc Surg* 43(1):12, 2002.
49. Diaz AL, Clifton GD: Dofetilide: a new class III antiarrhythmic for the management of atrial fibrillation, *Prog Cardiovasc Nurs* 16:126, 2001.
50. Haugh KH: Antidysrhythmic agents at the turn of the 21st century, *Crit Care Nurs Clin North Am* 14(1):53, 2002.
51. Kee VR: Hemodynamic pharmacology of intravenous vasopressors, *Crit Care Nurse* 23(4):79, 2003.
52. Branum K: Decompensated heart failure, *AACN Clin Issues* 14(4):498, 2003.
53. Devlin JW et al: Fenoldopam versus nitroprusside for the treatment of hypertensive emergency, *Ann Pharmacother* 38:755, 2004.
54. Cohen MR: Medication errors, *Nursing* 34(11):20, 2004.
55. Fontana D: Nesiritide: The latest drug for treating heart failure, *Crit Care Nurse* 26(1):39, 2006.
56. Prahash A, Lynch T: B-type natriuretic peptide: a diagnostic, prognostic, and therapeutic tool in heart failure, *Am J Crit Care* 13(1):46, 2004.
57. Harrington C: Managing hypertension in patients with stroke: are you prepared for labetalol infusion? *Crit Care Nurse* 23(3):30, 2003.
58. Landoni G et al. Beneficial impact of fenoldopam in critically ill patients with or at risk for acute renal failure: a meta analysis of randomized controlled clinical trials, *Am J Kidney Dis* 49(1):56, 2007.
59. American Heart Association: ECC guidelines. Part 7.2. Management of cardiac arrest, *Circulation* 112(24): IV-58, 2005.
60. Albright TN et al: Vasopressin in the cardiac surgery intensive care unit, *Am J Crit Care* 11(4):326, 2002.

CHAPTER 14

Pulmonary Assessment and Diagnostic Procedures

KATHLEEN M. STACY ■ JEANNE M. MAIDEN

OBJECTIVES

- Identify the components of a pulmonary history.
- Describe inspection, palpation, percussion, and auscultation of the patient with pulmonary dysfunction.
- Outline the steps in analyzing an arterial blood gas.
- Identify key diagnostic procedures used in assessment of the patient with pulmonary dysfunction.
- Discuss the nursing management of a patient undergoing a pulmonary diagnostic procedure.
- Delineate the use of pulse oximetry for bedside monitoring.

Assessment of the patient with pulmonary dysfunction is a systematic process that incorporates both a history and a physical examination. The purpose of the assessment is twofold: (1) to recognize changes in the patient's pulmonary status that would necessitate nursing or medical intervention and (2) to determine the ways in which the patient's pulmonary dysfunction is interfering with self-care activities. To complete the assessment, the patient's laboratory studies and diagnostic tests must be reviewed. This chapter focuses on priority clinical assessments, laboratory studies, and diagnostic tests for the critically ill patient with pulmonary dysfunction.

HISTORY

The initial presentation of the patient determines the rapidity and direction of the interview. For a patient in acute distress, the history is curtailed to just a few questions about the patient's chief complaint and precipitating events. For a patient in no obvious distress, the history focuses on four different areas: (1) review of the patient's present illness, (2) overview of the patient's general respiratory status, (3) examination of the patient's general health status, and (4) survey of the patient's lifestyle.[1] Questions to be included in the interview are outlined in Box 14-1.

A description of the patient's current symptoms is also obtained. Symptoms that are common in the pulmonary patient include dyspnea, cough, wheezing, edema, palpitations, fatigue, chest pain, hemoptysis, and sputum. Information is elicited regarding the location, onset and duration, characteristics, setting, aggravating and alleviating factors, associated symptoms, and efforts to treat the symptoms. If the cough is productive, the patient is asked questions about the color, amount, odor, and consistency of the sputum.[2-5]

CLINICAL ASSESSMENT

INSPECTION

Inspection of the patient focuses on three priorities: (1) observation of the tongue and sublingual area, (2) assessment of chest wall configuration, and (3) evaluation of respiratory effort. If possible, the patient is positioned upright, with the arms resting at the sides.[3]

Observation of the Tongue and Sublingual Area

The patient's tongue and sublingual area are observed for a blue, gray, or dark purple tint or discoloration, indicating the presence of central cyanosis. Central cyanosis is a sign of hypoxemia, or inadequate oxygenation of the blood, and is considered to be life threatening. The fingers and toes may also appear discolored, an indication of the presence of peripheral cyanosis.[6]

Assessment of Chest Wall Configuration

The size and shape of the patient's chest wall are assessed for an increase in the anteroposterior (AP) diameter and for structural deviations. Normally the ratio of AP diameter to lateral diameter ranges from 1:2 to 5:7.[2,4,5] An increase in the AP diameter is suggestive of chronic obstructive pulmonary disease (COPD).[2,4,5] The shape of the chest is inspected for any structural deviations. Some of the more commonly seen abnormalities are pectus excavatum, pectus carinatum,

Box 14-1

Pulmonary History Questions

Present Illness

What brought you to the hospital?
What were the precipitating events?
When did the problem start?

Respiratory Status

Do you currently have a chronic lung disease, such as asthma, bronchitis, or emphysema?
Do you have a history of any lung disease, such as chronic respiratory infections or tuberculosis?
Have you had any chest surgery?

General Health Status

Do you have any other chronic disease or illness?
Do you have a history of any other disease, illness, or surgery?
Are you currently taking any medications, prescription or nonprescription?

Lifestyle

Do you smoke, or have you smoked in the past?
Have you been exposed to secondhand smoke?
Have you ever been exposed to lung irritants or cancer-causing agents, such as asbestos, chemicals, fumes, beryllium, coal or stone quarry dust, or Agent Orange?

barrel chest, and spinal deformities. In pectus excavatum (funnel chest), the sternum and lower ribs are displaced posteriorly, creating a funnel or pit-shaped depression in the chest. This causes a decrease in the AP diameter of the chest and may interfere with respiratory function. In pectus carinatum (pigeon breast), the sternum projects forward, causing an increase in the AP diameter of the chest. A barrel chest also results in an increase in AP diameter of the chest and is characterized by displacement of the sternum forward and the ribs outward. Spinal deformities such as kyphosis, lordosis, and scoliosis may also be present and can interfere with respiratory function.[7]

Evaluation of Respiratory Effort

The patient's respiratory effort is evaluated for rate, rhythm, symmetry, and quality of ventilatory movements.[2] Normal breathing at rest is effortless and regular and occurs at a rate of 12 to 20 breaths per minute.[3] Some of the more commonly seen patterns in patients with pulmonary dysfunction are tachypnea, hyperventilation, and air trapping. Tachypnea is manifested by an increase in the rate and decrease in the depth of ventilation. Hyperventilation is manifested by an increase in both the rate and depth of ventilation. Patients with COPD often experience obstructive breathing, or air trapping. As the patient breathes, air becomes trapped in the lungs and ventilations become progressively shallower until the patient actively and forcefully exhales.[8]

Additional Assessment Areas

Other areas assessed are patient position, use of accessory muscles, presence of intercostal retractions, unequal movement of the chest wall, flaring of nares, and pausing midsentence to take a breath.[2,4,5] The presence of other iatrogenic features, such as chest tubes, central venous lines, artificial airways, and nasogastric tubes, should be noted as they may affect assessment findings.

PALPATION

Palpation of the patient focuses on three priorities: (1) confirmation of tracheal position, (2) assessment of respiratory excursion, and (3) evaluation of fremitus. In addition, the thorax is assessed for any areas of tenderness, lumps, or bony deformities. The anterior, posterior, and lateral areas of the chest are evaluated in a systematic fashion.[2]

Confirmation of Tracheal Position

The patient's tracheal position is confirmed at midline. It is assessed by placing the fingers in the suprasternal notch and moving upward.[8] Deviation of the trachea to either side can indicate pneumothorax, unilateral pneumonia, diffuse pulmonary fibrosis, a large pleural effusion, or severe atelectasis. With atelectasis, the trachea shifts to the same side as the problem, and with pneumothorax the trachea shifts to the opposite side of the problem.[7]

Assessment of Respiratory Excursion

The patient's respiratory excursion is assessed for the degree and symmetry of movement. It is evaluated by placing the hands on the anterolateral chest with the thumbs extended along the costal margin, pointing to the xiphoid process, or by placing the hands on the posterolateral chest with the thumbs on either side of the spine at the level of the tenth rib. The patient is instructed to take a few normal breaths, then a few deep breaths. Chest movement is assessed for equality, which signifies symmetry of thoracic expansion.[3,7,8] Asymmetry is an abnormal finding that can occur with pneumothorax, pneumonia, or other disorders that interfere with lung inflation. The degree of chest movement is felt to ascertain the extent of lung expansion. The thumbs should separate 3 to 5 cm during deep inspiration.[5,8] Lung expansion of a hyperinflated chest is less than that of a normal one.[5,8]

Evaluation of Tactile Fremitus

Assessment of tactile fremitus is performed to identify, describe, and localize any areas of increased or decreased fremitus. Fremitus refers to the palpable vibrations felt through the chest wall when the patient speaks. It is assessed by placing the palmar surface of the hands against opposite sides of the chest wall

Table 14-1

Percussion Tones: Description and Associated Conditions

TONE	INTENSITY	PITCH	DURATION	QUALITY	CONDITIONS
Resonance	Loud	Low	Long	Hollow	Normal lung Bronchitis
Hyperresonance	Very loud	Very low	Long	Booming	Asthma Emphysema Pneumothorax
Tympany	Loud	Musical	Medium	Drumlike	Large pneumothorax Emphysematous blebs
Dullness	Medium	Medium to high	Medium	Thudlike	Atelectasis Pleural effusion Pulmonary edema Pneumonia Lung mass
Flatness	Soft	High	Short	Extremely dull	Massive atelectasis Pneumonectomy

and having the patient repeat the word "ninety-nine." The hands are moved systematically around the thorax until the anterior, posterior, and both lateral areas have been assessed.[7,8] Fremitus varies from patient to patient and depends on the pitch and intensity of the voice. Fremitus is described as normal, decreased, or increased. With normal fremitus, vibrations can be felt over the trachea but are barely palpable over the periphery.[2] With decreased fremitus, there is interference with the transmission of vibrations. Examples of disorders that decrease fremitus include pleural effusion, pneumothorax, bronchial obstruction, pleural thickening, and emphysema. With increased fremitus, there is an increase in the transmission of vibrations. Examples of disorders that increase fremitus include pneumonia, lung cancer, and pulmonary fibrosis.[5]

PERCUSSION

Percussion of the patient focuses on two priorities: (1) evaluation of the underlying lung structure and (2) assessment of diaphragmatic excursion. Although not often used, percussion is useful for confirming suspected abnormalities.

Evaluation of Underlying Lung Structure

The patient's underlying lung structure is evaluated to estimate the amounts of air, liquid, or solid material present. It is performed by placing the middle finger of the nondominant hand on the chest wall. The distal portion, between the last joint and the nailbed, is then struck with the middle finger of the dominant hand. The hands are moved side to side systematically around the thorax to compare similar areas until the anterior, posterior, and both lateral areas have been assessed. Five different tones can be elicited: resonance, hyperresonance, tympany, dullness, and flatness. These tones are distinguished by differences in intensity, pitch, duration, and quality. Table 14-1 describes the different percussion tones and their associated conditions.[3,7]

Assessment of Diaphragmatic Excursion

Diaphragmatic excursion is assessed by measuring the difference in the level of the diaphragm on inspiration and expiration. It is performed by instructing the patient to inhale and hold the breath. The posterior chest is percussed downward, over the intercostal spaces, until the dull sound produced by the diaphragm is heard. The spot is marked. The patient is then instructed to take a few breaths in and out, exhale completely, and then hold his or her breath. The posterior chest is percussed again, and the new area of dullness over the diaphragm is then located and marked. The difference between the two spots is noted and measured. Normal diaphragmatic excursion is 3 to 5 cm.[8] It is decreased in disorders or conditions such as ascites, pregnancy, hepatomegaly, and emphysema. It is increased in pleural effusion or disorders that elevate the diaphragm, such as atelectasis or paralysis.[7]

AUSCULTATION

Auscultation of the patient focuses on three priorities: (1) evaluation of normal breath sounds, (2) identification of abnormal breath sounds, and (3) assessment of voice sounds. Auscultation requires a quiet environment, proper positioning of the patient, and a bare chest.[9] Breath sounds are best heard with the patient in the upright position.[5]

Evaluation of Normal Breath Sounds

The patient's breath sounds are auscultated to evaluate the quality of air movement through the pulmonary system and to identify the presence of abnormal

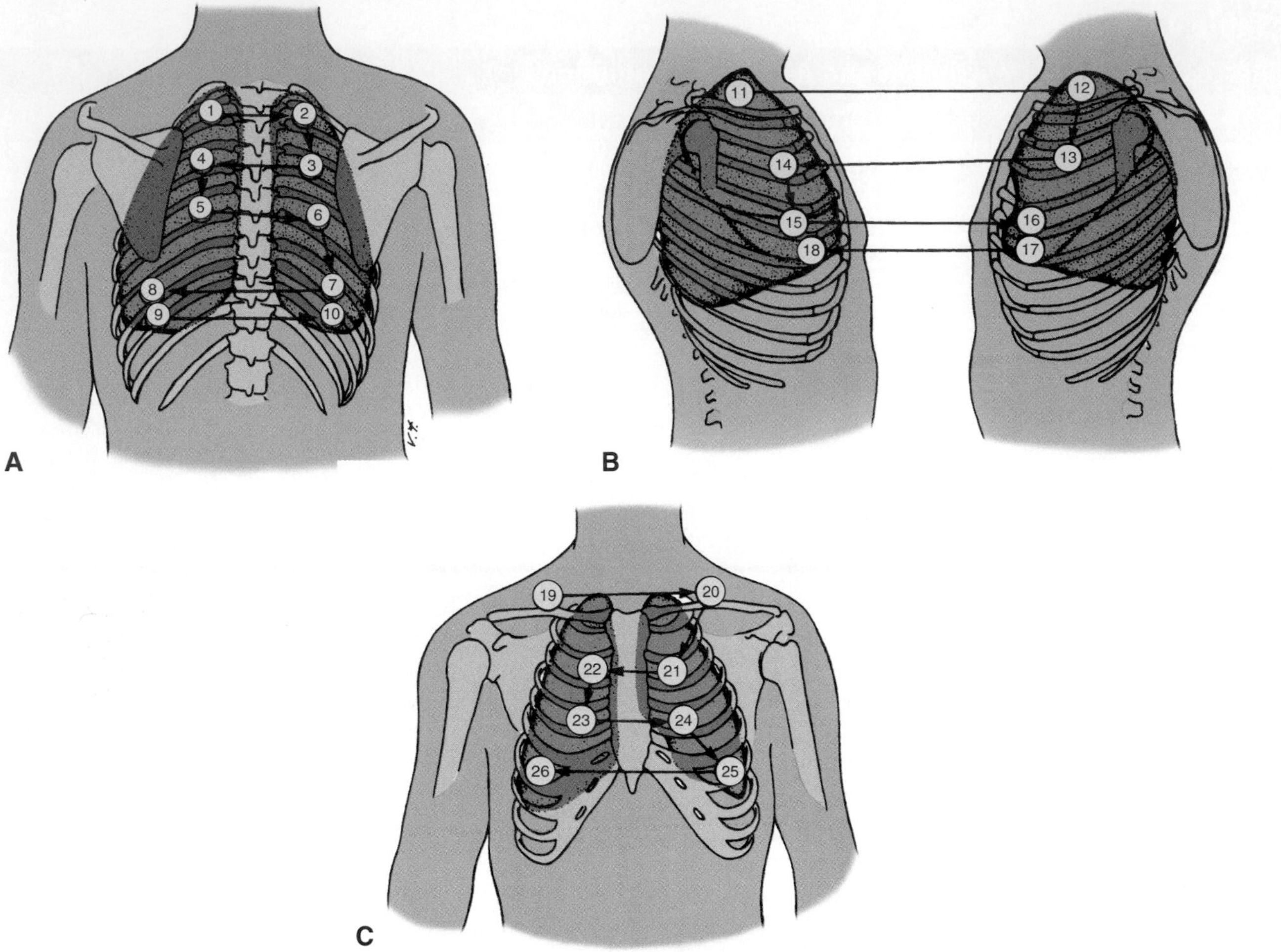

FIGURE 14-1. Auscultation sequence. **A,** Posterior. **B,** Lateral. **C,** Anterior. (From Perry AG, Potter PA: *Clinical nursing skills and techniques,* ed 5, St Louis, 2002, Mosby.)

sounds. It is performed by placing the diaphragm of the stethoscope against the chest wall and instructing the patient to breathe in and out slowly with his or her mouth open.[2] Both the inspiratory and expiratory phases are assessed. Auscultation is done in a systematic sequence—side to side, top to bottom, posteriorly, laterally, and anteriorly[5] (Figure 14-1).

Normal breath sounds are different, depending on their location. They are classified into three categories: bronchial, bronchovesicular, and vesicular. Table 14-2 describes the characteristics of normal breath sounds.[2,5,9]

Identification of Abnormal Breath Sounds

Abnormal breath sounds are identified once the normal breath sounds have been clearly delineated. There are three categories of abnormal breath sounds: absent or diminished breath sounds, displaced bronchial breath sounds, and adventitious breath sounds. Table 14-3 describes the various abnormal breath sounds and their associated conditions.[2,5,9]

An absent or diminished breath sound indicates that there is little or no airflow to a particular portion of the lung (either a small segment or an entire lobe).[9]

Table 14-2
Characteristics of Normal Breath Sounds

SOUND	CHARACTERISTICS
Vesicular	Heard over most of lung field; low pitch; soft, short exhalation and long inhalation
Bronchovesicular	Heard over main bronchus area and upper right posterior lung field; medium pitch; exhalation equals inhalation
Bronchial	Heard only over trachea; high pitch; loud and long exhalation

Modified from Thompson JM et al: *Mosby's clinical nursing,* ed 5, St Louis, 2002, Mosby.

Displaced bronchial breath sounds are normal bronchial sounds heard in the peripheral lung fields instead of over the trachea. This condition is usually indicative of fluid or exudate present in the alveoli.[9]

Adventitious breath sounds are extra or added sounds heard in addition to the other sounds already discussed. They are classified as crackles, rhonchi,

Table 14-3
Abnormal Breath Sounds and Associated Conditions

SOUND	DESCRIPTION	CONDITIONS
Absent breath sounds	No airflow to particular portion of lung	Pneumothorax Pneumonectomy Emphysematous blebs Pleural effusion Lung mass Massive atelectasis Complete airway obstruction
Diminished breath sounds	Little airflow to particular portion of lung	Emphysema Pleural effusion Pleurisy Atelectasis Pulmonary fibrosis
Displaced bronchial sounds	Bronchial sounds heard in peripheral lung fields	Atelectasis with secretions Lung mass with exudate Pneumonia Pleural effusion Pulmonary edema
Crackles (rales)	Short, discrete, popping or crackling sounds	Pulmonary edema Pneumonia Pulmonary fibrosis Atelectasis Bronchiectasis
Rhonchi	Coarse, rumbling, low-pitched sounds	Pneumonia Asthma Bronchitis Bronchospasm
Wheezes	High-pitched, squeaking, whistling sounds	Asthma Bronchospasm
Pleural friction rubs	Creaking, leathery, loud, dry, coarse sounds	Pleural effusion Pleurisy

wheezes, and friction rubs. Crackles (also referred to as rales) are short, discrete, popping or crackling sounds produced by fluid in the smaller airways or alveoli or by the snapping open of collapsed airways during inspiration. They are mainly heard on inspiration and are not cleared by coughing.[8] Crackles can be further classified as fine, medium or coarse, depending on pitch.[9] Rhonchi are coarse, rumbling, low-pitched sounds produced by airflow over secretions in the larger airways or by narrowing of the larger airways. They are mainly heard on expiration and may be cleared with coughing.[8] Rhonchi can further be classified as bubbling, gurgling, or sonorous, depending on the characteristics of the sound.[9] Wheezes are high-pitched, squeaking, whistling sounds produced by airflow through narrowed smaller airways. They are mainly heard on expiration but may be heard throughout the ventilatory cycle.[8] Depending on their severity, wheezes can be further classified as mild, moderate, or severe.[9] Pleural friction rubs are creaking, leathery, loud, dry, coarse sounds produced by irritated pleural surfaces rubbing together. They are usually heard best in the lower anterolateral chest area during the latter portion of inspiration and the beginning of expiration. Pleural friction rubs are caused by inflammation of the pleura.[3,8,9]

Assessment of Voice Sounds

Assessment of the patient's voice sounds is particularly useful in detecting lung consolidation or lung compression. Three abnormal types of voice sounds are bronchophony, whispering pectoriloquy, and egophony. Bronchophony describes a condition in which the spoken voice is heard on auscultation with higher intensity and clarity than usual. Normally the spoken word is muffled when heard through the stethoscope. It is assessed by placing the diaphragm of the stethoscope against the posterior side of the patient's chest and instructing the patient to say "ninety-nine." Bronchophony is present when the sound heard is clear, distinct, and loud. Whispering pectoriloquy describes a condition of unusually clear transmission of the whispered voice on auscultation. Normally the whispered word is unintelligible when heard through the stethoscope. It is assessed by placing the stethoscope against the posterior side of the patient's chest and instructing the patient to whisper "One, two, three." Whispering pectoriloquy is present when the sound heard is clear and distinct. Egophony describes a condition in which the voice sounds increase in intensity and develop a nasal bleating quality on auscultation. It is assessed by placing the stethoscope against the posterior side of the patient's chest and instructing the patient to say "e-e-e." Egophony is present when the "e" sound changes to an "a" sound.[2,4,9]

LABORATORY STUDIES

ARTERIAL BLOOD GASES

Interpretation of arterial blood gas (ABG) levels can be difficult, especially if one is under pressure to do it quickly and accurately. One method that can help ensure accuracy when analyzing arterial blood gas levels is to follow the same steps of interpretation each time. A specific method to be used each time that blood gas values must be interpreted is presented in brief in Box 14-2.

Step 1: Look at the PaO_2 Level and Answer the Quesion, "Does the PaO_2 Level Show Hypoxemia?" The PaO_2 is a measure of the partial pressure of oxygen dissolved in arterial blood plasma, with *P* standing for *partial pressure* and *a* standing for *arterial*. It is reported in millimeters of mercury (mm Hg). PaO_2 reflects 3% of total oxygen in the blood.[10]

Box 14-2

Steps for Interpretation of Arterial Blood Gas Values

Step 1
Look at arterial oxygen tension (PaO_2) and answer the following:
- Does the PaO_2 show hypoxemia?

Step 2
Look at the pH and answer the following:
- Is the pH on the acid or alkaline side of 7.40?

Step 3
Look at arterial carbon dioxide tension (PaCO_2) and answer the following:
- Does the PaCO_2 show respiratory acidosis, respiratory alkalosis, or normalcy?

Step 4
Look at bicarbonate (HCO_3^-) and answer the following:
- Does the HCO_3^- show metabolic acidosis, alkalosis, or normalcy?

Step 5
Look back at the pH and answer the following:
- Does the pH show a compensated or an uncompensated condition?

The normal range in PaO_2 for persons breathing room air at sea level is 80 to 100 mm Hg. However, the normal range is age dependent in two groups: infants and persons 60 years and older. The normal level for infants breathing room air is 40 to 70 mm Hg.[10] The normal level for persons 60 years and older decreases with age as changes occur in the ventilation/perfusion (V/Q) matching in the aging lung.[11] The correct PaO_2 for older persons can be ascertained as follows: 80 mm Hg (the lowest normal value) minus 1 mm Hg for every year that a person is over the age of 60. Using this formula, a 65-year-old individual can have a PaO_2 as low as 75 mm Hg and still be within the normal range (formula for 5 years over 60 years of age: 80 mm Hg − 5 mm Hg = 75 mm Hg). An acceptable range for an 80-year-old person is 60 mm Hg (formula for 20 years over the age of 60: 80 mm Hg − 20 mm Hg = 60 mm Hg). At any age, a PaO_2 lower than 40 mm Hg represents a life-threatening situation that requires immediate action.[10,12] In addition, a PaO_2 less than the predicted lowest value indicates hypoxemia, which means that a lower-than-normal amount of oxygen is dissolved in plasma.[10]

Step 2: Look at the pH Level and Answer the Question, "Is the pH on the Acid or Alkaline Side of 7.40?" The pH is the hydrogen ion (H^+) concentration of plasma. Calculation of pH is accomplished by using the partial pressure of carbon dioxide (PaCO_2) and the plasma bicarbonate level (HCO_3^-).[13,14]

The normal pH of arterial blood is 7.35 to 7.45, with the mean being 7.40. If the pH level is less than 7.40, it is on the acid side of the mean. A pH level less than 7.35 is known as *acidemia,* and the overall condition is called *acidosis.* If the pH level is greater than 7.40, it is on the alkaline side of the mean. A pH level greater than 7.45 is known as *alkalemia,* and the overall condition is called *alkalosis.*[13,14]

Step 3: Look at the PaCO_2 Level and Answer the Question, "Does the PaCO_2 Show Respiratory Acidosis, Alkalosis, or Normalcy?" The PaCO_2 is a measure of the partial pressure of carbon dioxide dissolved in arterial blood plasma and is reported in mm Hg. It is the acid-base component that reflects the effectiveness of ventilation in relation to the metabolic rate.[13,14] In other words, the PaCO_2 value indicates whether the patient can ventilate well enough to rid the body of the carbon dioxide produced as a consequence of metabolism.

The normal range for PaCO_2 is 35 to 45 mm Hg. This range does not change as a person ages. A PaCO_2 value of greater than 45 mm Hg defines *respiratory acidosis,* which is caused by alveolar hypoventilation. Hypoventilation can result from COPD, oversedation, head trauma, anesthesia, drug overdose, neuromuscular disease, or inadequate ventilation with mechanical ventilation.[13,14] A PaCO_2 value that is less than 35 mm Hg defines *respiratory alkalosis*, which is caused by alveolar hyperventilation. Hyperventilation can result from hypoxia, anxiety, pulmonary embolism, pregnancy, and over ventilation with mechanical ventilation or as a compensatory mechanism to metabolic acidosis.[11,13,14]

Step 4: Look at the HCO_3^- Level and Answer the Question, "Does the HCO_3^- Show Metabolic Acidosis, Alkalosis, or Normalcy?" The bicarbonate (HCO_3^-) is the acid-base component that reflects kidney function. The bicarbonate is reduced or increased in the plasma by renal mechanisms. The normal range is 22 to 26 mEq/L.[11,13,14] A bicarbonate level of less than 22 mEq/L defines *metabolic acidosis*, which can result from ketoacidosis, lactic acidosis, renal failure, or diarrhea. The cumulative effect is a gain of acids or a loss of base. A bicarbonate level that is greater than 26 mEq/L defines *metabolic alkalosis*, which can result from fluid loss from the upper gastrointestinal tract (vomiting or nasogastric suction), diuretic therapy, severe hypokalemia, alkali administration, or steroid therapy.[11,13,14]

Step 5: Look Back at the pH level and Answer the Question, "Does the pH Show a Compensated or an Uncompensated Condition?" If the pH level is abnormal (<7.35 or >7.45), the $Paco_2$ value or the HCO_3^- level, or both, will also be abnormal. This is an uncompensated condition because there has not been enough time for the body to return the pH to its normal range (Box 14-3).[13,14] If the pH level is within normal limits and both the $Paco_2$ value and the HCO_3^- level are abnormal, the condition is compensated because there has been enough time for the body to restore the pH to within its normal range.[13,14] Differentiating the primary disorder from the compensatory response can be difficult. The primary disorder is the abnormality that caused the pH level to shift initially; thus, on whichever side of 7.40 the pH level occurs is considered the primary disorder (Box 14-4).[13,14] Partial compensation may also be present and is evidenced by abnormal pH, $Paco_2$, and HCO_3^- levels, indications that the body is attempting to return the pH to its normal range.[13,14]

Table 14-4 summarizes the changes in the acid-base components that accompany various acid-base disorders.[13,14] In addition to the parameters previously discussed, other factors must be considered when reviewing a patient's ABGs, including oxygen saturation, oxygen content, expected Pao_2, and base excess and deficit.

Oxygen Saturation

Oxygen saturation is a measure of the amount of oxygen bound to hemoglobin, compared with hemoglobin's maximal capability for binding oxygen. It can be assessed as a component of the ABG (Sao_2) or can be measured noninvasively using a pulse oximeter (Spo_2).[10,15] Oxygen saturation is reported as a percentage or as a decimal, with normal being greater than 95% on room air. Normally, the saturation level cannot reach 100% (on room air) because of the physiologic shunting.[10,11] However, when supplemental oxygen is administered, oxygen saturation may approach 100% so closely that it is reported as 100%.

Proper evaluation of the oxygen saturation level is vital. For example, an Sao_2 of 97% means that 97% of the available hemoglobin is bound with oxygen. The word "available" is essential to evaluating the Sao_2 level, because the hemoglobin level is not always within normal limits and oxygen can bind only with what is available. A 97% saturation level associated with 10 g of hemoglobin does not deliver as much oxygen to the tissues as does a 97% saturation associated

Box 14-3

Arterial Blood Gas Values: Uncompensated Conditions

Example 1

Pao_2	90 mm Hg
pH	7.25
$Paco_2$	50 mm Hg
HCO_3^-	22 mEq/L

Interpretation: Uncompensated respiratory acidosis

Example 2

Pao_2	90 mm Hg
pH	7.25
$Paco_2$	40 mm Hg
HCO_3^-	17 mEq/L

Interpretation: Uncompensated metabolic acidosis

Box 14-4

Arterial Blood Gas Values: Compensated Conditions

Example 1

Pao_2	90 mm Hg
pH	7.37
$Paco_2$	60 mm Hg
HCO_3^-	38 mEq/L

Interpretation: Compensated respiratory acidosis with metabolic alkalosis. (The acidosis is considered the main disorder, and the alkalosis the compensatory response because the pH is on the acid side of 7.40.)

Example 2

Pao_2	90 mm Hg
pH	7.42
$Paco_2$	48 mm Hg
HCO_3^-	35 mEq/L

Interpretation: Compensated metabolic alkalosis with respiratory acidosis. (The alkalosis is considered the main disorder, and the acidosis the compensatory response because the pH is on the alkaline side of 7.40.)

Table 14-4

Arterial Blood Gas Values in Respiratory/Metabolic Disorders

DISORDER	PH	$Paco_2$ (mm Hg)	HCO_3^- (mEq/L)
Respiratory Acidosis			
Uncompensated	<7.35	>45	22-26
Partially compensated	<7.35	>45	>26
Compensated	7.35-7.39	>45	>26
Respiratory Alkalosis			
Uncompensated	>7.45	<35	22-26
Partially compensated	>7.45	<35	<22
Compensated	7.41-7.45	<35	<22
Metabolic Acidosis			
Uncompensated	<7.35	35-45	<22
Partially compensated	<7.35	<35	<22
Compensated	7.35-7.39	<35	<22
Metabolic Alkalosis			
Uncompensated	>7.45	35-45	>26
Partially compensated	>7.45	>45	>26
Compensated	7.41-7.45	>45	>26
Combined Respiratory/Metabolic Acidosis	<7.35	>45	<22
Combined Respiratory/Metabolic Alkalosis	>7.45	<35	>26

$Paco_2$ Arterial carbon dioxide partial pressure (tension); *HCO_3^-*, bicarbonate.

Table 14-5

Guideline Values for Estimating Fio_2 With Low-Flow O_2 Devices*

100% O_2 FLOW RATE (L/MIN)	Fio_2 (%)
Nasal Cannula or Catheter	
1	24
2	28
3	32
4	36
5	40
6	44
Oxygen Mask	
5-6	40
6-7	50
7-8	60
Mask With Reservoir Bag	
6	60
7	70
8	80
9	90
10	99+

From Scanlon CL, Wilkins RL, Stoller JK: *Egan's fundamentals of respiratory care,* ed 7, St Louis, 1999, Mosby.

*Normal ventilatory pattern assumed.

Fio_2, Fraction of inspired oxygen.

with 15 g of hemoglobin. Thus assessing only the Sao_2 level and finding it within normal limits must not lead one to believe that the patient's oxygenation status is normal. The hemoglobin level must also be evaluated before a decision on oxygenation status can be made.[10,16]

Oxygen Content

Oxygen content (Cao_2) is a measure of the total amount of oxygen carried in the blood, including the amount dissolved in plasma (measured by the Pao_2) and the amount bound to the hemoglobin molecule (measured by the Sao_2). Cao_2 is reported in milliliters (ml) of oxygen carried per 100 ml of blood. The normal value is 20 ml of oxygen per 100 ml of blood. To calculate the oxygen content, the Pao_2, the Sao_2, and the hemoglobin level are used (see Appendix B). A change in any one of these parameters will affect the Cao_2.[10,15,16]

Expected Pao_2

When a patient receives supplemental oxygen, the Pao_2 level is expected to rise. Knowing the level to which the Pao_2 should rise in normal subjects on a given Fio_2 and comparing that with the level to which the Pao_2 actually does rise in patients with pulmonary disease has value because it illustrates how well the lung is functioning. Calculating the expected Pao_2 is accomplished by multiplying the Fio_2 value by 5.[17] Thus the expected Pao_2 on an Fio_2 of 30% is at least 150 mm Hg (30×5), whereas the expected Pao_2 on an Fio_2 of 50% is 250 mm Hg (50×5). These expected Pao_2 values represent the oxygen level achievable with healthy lungs. Pulmonary disease can radically decrease the expected Pao_2 level. It is impossible to apply the "Fio_2 value $\times$ 5" rule to achieve the expected Pao_2 value when the patient is on a system that delivers oxygen by liters per minute.[17] For these situations, Table 14-5 shows the Fio_2 levels that correspond to various oxygen delivery systems.

Classic Shunt Equation and Oxygen Tension Indices

Measuring the degree of intrapulmonary shunting that occurs in a patient at any one time, using the classic shunt equation and oxygen tension indices, can assess the efficiency of oxygenation. *Intrapulmonary shunting* (QS/QT [the portion of cardiac output not exchanging with alveolar blood divided by the total cardiac output]) refers to venous blood that flows to the lungs without being oxygenated because of nonfunctioning alveoli.[15] Other names for this condition include shunt effect, low V/Q, wasted blood flow, and venous admixture.[11] Direct determination of intrapulmonary shunting requires the use of the classic shunt equation, which is both invasive and cumbersome. A shunt of 5% to 15% is considered mild, of 15% to 30% is considered major, and a shunt greater than 30% is a serious and potentially life-threatening condition.[15]

Oftentimes, intrapulmonary shunting is estimated by using the oxygen tension indices. One advantage to these methods is the ease of performance, though they have been found to be unreliable in critically ill patients.[10] An estimate of intrapulmonary shunting can be determined by computing the difference between the alveolar and arterial oxygen concentrations. Normally, alveolar and arterial PO_2 values are approximately equal.[15] When they are not, it indicates that venous blood is passing malfunctioning alveoli and returning unoxygenated to the left side of the heart.[10,15] The most common oxygen tension indices used to estimate intrapulmonary shunting are the PaO_2/FIO_2 ratio, the PaO_2/PAO_2 ratio, and the alveolar-arterial (A-a) gradient (see Appendix B for formulas).[15]

PaO_2/FIO_2 Ratio

The PaO_2/FIO_2 ratio is clinically the easiest formula to calculate because it does not call for the computation of the alveolar PO_2. Normally, the PaO_2/FIO_2 ratio is greater than 300,[15] with the lower the value the worse the lung function.[15]

PaO_2/PAO_2 Ratio

The PaO_2/PAO_2 ratio (arterial/alveolar O_2 ratio) is normally greater than 75%.[15] The disadvantage to using this formula is that it calls for the computation of the alveolar PO_2, but the advantage is that it is unaffected by changes in the FIO_2 as long as the underlying lung condition is stable.[10,15]

Alveolar-Arterial Gradient

The A-a gradient ($P[A\text{-}a]O_2$) is normally less than 15 mm Hg on room air.[15] This estimate of intrapulmonary shunting is the least reliable clinically but is frequently used in clinical decision making. One of the major disadvantages to using this formula is that it is greatly influenced by the amount of oxygen the patient is receiving.[10,15]

Dead Space/Tidal Volume Ratio

The efficiency of ventilation can be measured using the dead space/tidal volume (Vd/Vt) equation (see Appendix B). The formula measures the fraction of tidal volume not participating in gas exchange. Dead space greater than 0.4[18] indicates a dead space–producing disorder and is considered abnormal. The major limitations to using this formula are that it requires the measurement of exhaled carbon dioxide to complete and that the work of breathing by patients must remain stable during the collection.[18]

Box 14-5

Procedure for Collection of Tracheal/Endotracheal Specimen

1. Clear the endotracheal or tracheostomy tube of all local secretions, avoiding deep airway penetration.
2. Attach a sputum trap to a sterile suction catheter, and advance the catheter into the trachea while trying to avoid contact with the endotracheal tube or tracheostomy tube.
3. After the catheter is fully advanced, apply suction until secretions return to the sputum trap. When enough secretions are collected, discontinue suctioning and remove the catheter.
4. Do not apply suction while the catheter is being withdrawn because this can contaminate the sample with sputum from the upper airway. Do not flush the catheter with sterile water because this dilutes the sample.
5. If the catheter becomes plugged with secretions, place it in a sterile container and send it to the laboratory. The specimen must be transported immediately.

Sputum Studies

Careful analysis of sputum specimens is crucial for the rapid identification and treatment of pulmonary infections. The most difficult aspect of sputum examination is proper collection of the specimen. In general, collection of a good sputum sample requires a conscious, cooperative, sufficiently hydrated patient. When the patient has difficulty producing sputum, heated, nebulized saline may help to loosen secretions for expectoration. Chest physiotherapy combined with nebulization can improve the success rate. Collection of a sputum specimen is best done in the morning because there is a greater volume of secretions as a result of nighttime pooling.[19]

Many critically ill patients cannot cough effectively, and thus sputum collection by other means is required. These methods include tracheobronchial aspiration, transtracheal aspiration, and the use of a fiberoptic bronchoscopy with a protected brush catheter. Because each method has its own benefits and risks, the patient's clinical condition determines the appropriate technique.[20]

Many critically ill patients have endotracheal or tracheostomy tubes already in place. Collecting sputum specimens from these patients requires special attention to technique (Box 14-5). Deep specimens are obtained to avoid collecting specimens that contain resident upper airway flora that may have migrated down the tube. Colonization of the lower airways with upper airway flora can occur within 48 hours of intubation.[20]

Once a sputum specimen is obtained, it is examined for volume, physical properties, mucopurulence, and color. Next, a microscopic examination is done to identify the source of the specimen. If a bacterial infection is suspected, a Gram stain followed by a culture and sensitivity (C&S) is performed.[21]

DIAGNOSTIC PROCEDURES

Table 14-6 presents an overview of the various diagnostic procedures used to evaluate the patient with pulmonary dysfunction.

NURSING MANAGEMENT

The nursing management of a patient undergoing a diagnostic procedure involves a variety of interventions. **Priorities are directed toward preparing the patient psychologically and physically for the procedure, monitoring the patient's responses to the procedure, and assessing the patient after the procedure.** Preparing the patient includes teaching the patient about the procedure, answering any questions, and transporting and/or positioning the patient for the procedure. Monitoring the patient's responses to the procedure includes observing the patient for signs of pain, anxiety, or respiratory decompensation (Box 14-6) and monitoring vital signs. Assessing the patient after the procedure includes observing for complications of the procedure and medicating the patient for any postprocedure discomfort. **Any evidence of respiratory distress should be immediately reported to the physician, and emergency measures to maintain breathing must be initiated.**

Box 14-6

Clinical Manifestations of Respiratory Decompensation

Inadequate Airway
Stridor
Noisy respirations
Supraclavicular and intercostal retractions
Flaring of nares
Labored breathing with use of accessory muscles

Inadequate Ventilation
Absence of air exchange at nose and mouth (breathlessness)
Minimal/absent chest wall motion
Manifestations of obstructed airway
Central cyanosis
Decreased or absent breath sounds (bilateral, unilateral)
Restlessness, anxiety, confusion
Paradoxical motion involving significant portion of chest wall
Decreased Pa_{O_2}, increased Pa_{CO_2}, decreased pH

Inadequate Gas Exchange
Tachypnea
Decreased Pa_{O_2}
Increased dead space
Central cyanosis
Chest infiltrates on radiographic evaluation

BEDSIDE MONITORING

PULSE OXIMETRY

Pulse oximetry is a noninvasive method for monitoring oxygen saturation (Sp_{O_2}). It is indicated in any situation in which the patient's oxygenation status requires continuous observation. It consists of a microprocessor and a probe that attaches to the patient (finger, ear, toe, or nose). The probe consists of two light-emitting diodes and a photodetector. The diodes transmit red and infrared light wavelengths through the pulsating vascular bed to the photodetector on the other side. The photodetector converts the light signals into an electric signal, which is then sent to the microprocessor, which converts it to a digital reading. The pulse oximeter is considered very accurate, within ±2% at a saturation greater than 70%.[22,23]

Nursing priorities are directed toward minimizing the physiologic and technical factors that can limit the monitoring system.

Physiologic Limitations

Physiologic limitations include elevated levels of abnormal hemoglobins, presence of vascular dyes, and poor tissue perfusion. The pulse oximeter cannot differentiate between normal and abnormal hemoglobin. Elevated levels of abnormal hemoglobin falsely elevate the Sp_{O_2}. Vascular dyes, such as methylene blue, indigo carmine, indocyanine green, and fluorescein, also interfere with pulse oximetry and can lead to falsely low readings. Poor tissue perfusion to the area with the probe leads to loss of pulsatile flow and signal failure.[22,23]

Technical Limitations

Technical limitations include bright lights, excessive motion, and incorrect placement of the probe. Bright lights may interfere with the photodetector and cause inaccurate results. The probe must be covered to limit optical interference. Excessive motion can mimic arterial pulsations and can lead to false readings. Incorrect placement of the probe can lead to inaccurate results because part of the light can reach the photodetector without having passed through blood (optical shunting). Interventions to limit these problems include using the proper probe in the appropriate spot (e.g., not using a finger probe on the ear), applying the probe according to the directions, and ensuring that the area being monitored has adequate perfusion.[22,23]

CAPNOGRAPHY

Capnography is the measurement of exhaled carbon dioxide (CO_2) gas and is also known as *end-tidal* CO_2 monitoring. Normally, alveolar and arterial CO_2 concentrations are equal in the presence of normal ventilation/perfusion relationships. In a patient who is

Table 14-6
Pulmonary Diagnostic Procedures

PROCEDURE	EVALUATION	COMMENTS
Bronchography	Detects obstruction or malformation of tracheobronchial tree.	Patient ingests radiopaque substance, then radiographs are taken. Inquire about possibility of pregnancy.
Chest radiography	Detects lung pathology (e.g., pneumonia, pulmonary edema, atelectasis, tuberculosis). Determines size and location of lung lesions and tumors. Verifies placement of endotracheal tube, central venous catheters, and chest tubes.	Noninvasive test with minimal radiation exposure. Inquire about possibility of pregnancy. PA and lateral films most common, but in critical care areas, AP portable films often necessary because patient cannot be transported. Lateral decubitus films aid in identification of pleural effusion.
Exercise testing	Identify early disability. Differentiate between cardiac and pulmonary disease.	Monitor for changes in Spo_2 during exercise. Monitor closely for exercise-induced hypotension and ventricular dysrhythmias.
Laryngoscopy, bronchoscopy, mediastinoscopy	Obtain cytology specimen or biopsy. Identify tumors, obstructions, secretions, and foreign bodies in tracheobronchial tree. Locate a bleeding site. May be used therapeutically to remove secretions, foreign bodies, other contaminants.	Patient is sedated before procedure, usually with a benzodiazepine (e.g., diazepam, midazolam). Monitor patient for subcutaneous emphysema after study; indicates tracheal or bronchial tear. Monitor for hemoptysis; some blood in sputum is normal after biopsy, but frank hemoptysis requires immediate attention.
Lung biopsy	Obtain specimen for cytologic evaluation.	Transthoracic needle biopsy performed under fluoroscopy; inquire about possibility of pregnancy. Open lung biopsy requires thoracotomy.
Magnetic resonance imaging (MRI)	Distinguishes tumors from other structures (e.g., tumor, pleural thickening, fibrosis).	Noninvasive test. Contraindicated for patients with pacemakers or implanted metallic devices.
Pulmonary angiography	Detects changes in lung tissue (e.g., masses). Diagnoses abnormalities in pulmonary vasculature, including thrombi and emboli. Identifies congenital abnormalities of circulation.	Invasive test. Inquire about possibility of pregnancy. Contrast media injected into pulmonary artery; ensure adequate hydration after study. Monitor arterial puncture point for hematoma and hemorrhage.
Pulmonary function tests (PFTs) • Spirometry • Ventilatory mechanics • Flow-volume loop • Diffusing capacity	Measure lung volumes, capacities, and flow rates. RV, FRC, and TLC require nitrogen washout technique. Identify features of restrictive or obstructive lung disease. Evaluate responsiveness to bronchodilator. Aids in evaluation of surgical risk. Documents a disability or cause of dyspnea.	Noninvasive studies. Frequently repeated after bronchodilator therapy
Sleep studies	Diagnose and differentiate between obstructive, central, and cardiac sleep apnea.	Restrict caffeine before testing. Usually done during normal sleep hours.
Thoracentesis (may include pleural biopsy)	Obtain pleural fluid/tissue specimen. May be used therapeutically to remove pleural fluid.	Monitor patient for indications of pneumothorax. Monitor for leakage from puncture point.
Thoracic computed tomography (CT)	Defines lesions, masses, cavities, or shadows seen on normal chest radiograph. Evaluates tracheal and bronchial narrowing. Aids in planning radiation therapy.	X-ray films are taken at different angles.
Ultrasonography	Evaluates pleural disease. Visualizes diaphragm and detects disease around diaphragm (e.g., subphrenic hematoma, abscess).	Noninvasive test.
Ventilation scan Lung perfusion scan V/Q scan	Diagnoses ventilation and perfusion abnormalities (e.g., emphysema, pulmonary emboli).	Invasive test: radioisotope ingested and injected intravascularly. Inquire about possibility of pregnancy. Assure patient that amount of radioactive material is minimal.

PA, Posteroanterior; *AP,* anteroposterior; *Spo_2,* oxygen saturation; *V/Q,* ventilation/perfusion ratio.

Table 14-6

Pulmonary Diagnostic Procedures—*cont'd*

VOLUME	DEFINITION	NORMAL VALUE
Lung Volumes and Capacities		
Tidal volume (Vt, VT, VT)	Volume of air moved in/out of lungs with each normal breath.	7 ml/kg (≈500 ml)
Inspiratory reserve volume (IRV)	Volume of air that can be maximally inspired above normal inspiratory level.	3000 ml
Expiratory reserve volume (ERV)	Volume of air that can be maximally exhaled beyond normal expiratory level.	1000 ml
Residual volume (RV)	Volume of air remaining in lungs at end of a maximal expiration.	1000 ml
Inspiratory capacity (IC)	Vt + IRC; volume of air that can be maximally inspired from a normal expiratory level.	3500 ml
Functional residual capacity (FRC)	RV + ERV; volume of air remaining in lungs at end of a normal expiration.	2000 ml
Vital capacity (VC)	Vt + IRC + ERV; volume of air that can be maximally expired after a maximal inspiration.	4500 ml
Total lung capacity (TLC)	Vt + IRC + ERV + RV; volume of air that lungs can hold with maximal inspiration.	5500-6000 ml
Respiratory rate or frequency (f)	Number of breaths per minute.	12-20
Minute ventilation (VE)	Vt ∞ f; volume of air expired per minute.	5-10 L
Dead space (Vd)	$Vd/Vt = Paco_2 - Petco_2/Paco_2$*	<0.4
Alveolar ventilation (VA)	Vt – Vd; volume of tidal air involved in alveolar gas exchange.	350 ml
Forced vital capacity (FVC)	Volume of air in a forceful maximal expiration.	Same as VC: 4500 ml
Forced expiratory volume (FEV)	Volume of air exhaled in prescribed period. FEV_1: in 1 second; FEV_3: in 3 seconds.	FEV_1: >75% VC FEV_3: >95% VC

From Dennison RD: *Pass CCRN!,* ed 2, St. Louis, 2000, Mosby.

*See Appendix B; volume or percentage of Vt that does not participate in gas exchange; includes volume of air in conducting pathways (anatomic dead space) plus volume of alveolar air not involved in gas exchange due to pathology (alveolar dead space); Vd/Vt >0.6 is usually an indication for mechanical ventilation.

hemodynamically stable, the end-tidal CO_2 ($Petco_2$) can be used to estimate the $Paco_2$, with the $Petco_2$ levels 1 to 5 mm Hg less than $Paco_2$ levels. The practitioner must determine first that a normal V/Q relationship exists before correlation of the $Petco_2$ and the $Paco_2$ can be assumed.[24-26] Causes of increased $Petco_2$ include situations in which CO_2 production is increased, such as hyperthermia, sepsis, and seizures, or in which alveolar ventilation is decreased such as respiratory depression. Causes of decreased $Petco_2$ include situations in which CO_2 production is decreased, such as hypothermia, cardiac arrest, and pulmonary embolism, or in which alveolar ventilation is increased such as hyperventilation.[24]

In the critical care area continuous capnography is used for assessment and monitoring of the patient's ventilatory status in a variety of situations, including weaning from mechanical ventilation and undergoing procedural sedation. In addition, capnography can be used to confirm proper placement of an endotracheal tube. Assessment of changes in physiologic dead space can be carried out with end-tidal CO_2 monitoring, based on the degree of difference between the $Paco_2$ and the $Petco_2$. As the severity of pulmonary impairment increases, so does the disparity between the $Paco_2$ and the $Petco_2$, as indicated by an increased gradient. A gradient of greater than 5 mm Hg can be seen with underperfused alveolar-capillary units (dead space–producing situations) and nonperfused alveolar-capillary units (alveolar dead space). Increased dead space ventilation is a result of decreased pulmonary blood flow/cardiac output and lung disease. This leads to an abnormality in the transfer of CO_2 from the blood to the lung. The result is a $Petco_2$ level that is lower than the $Paco_2$ because of the mixing of carbon dioxide between perfused and nonperfused units. The end result is an increased or widened $Paco_2$-to-$Petco_2$ gradient.[25,26]

Currently there are three forms of capnography: mainstream, sidestream, and microstream. All forms can be used in intubated patients, but sidestream and microstream can also be used in nonintubated patients, thus broadening the application of end-tidal CO_2 monitoring. Mainstream capnography measures the CO_2 level directed via a sensor in the exhalation port of the ventilator tubing. During exhalation gas passes over the sensor and the information is transferred via an electrical cable to the display unit. The display unit produces a waveform, called a *capnogram* (Figure 14-2) and a numerical recording ($Petco_2$). Disadvantages to this form of capnography include the weight of the sensor on the ventilator tubing and possible obstruction of the sensor by secretions and condensation. In sidestream capnography the CO_2 gas is continuously aspirated via a side port in the ventilator tubing or nasal cannula and is measured and analyzed by a side unit. Disadvantages to this form of capnography include obstruction of the sampling tube with secretions and slow response time. Microstream capnography is a newer and improved version of sidestream capnography that minimizes the disadvantages.[26]

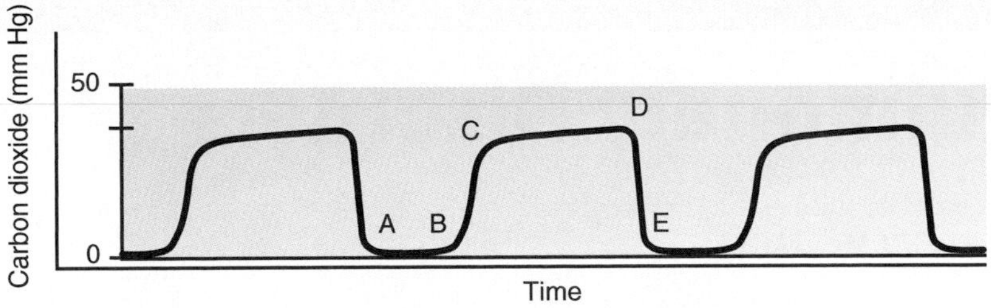

FIGURE 14-2. Normal findings on a capnogram. A→B, indicates the baseline; B→C, expiratory upstroke; C→D, alveolar plateau; D, partial pressure of end-tidal carbon dioxide ($Petco_2$); D→E, inspiratory downstroke. (From Frakes M: Measuring end-tidal carbon dioxide: clinical applications and usefulness, *Crit Care Nurse* 21[5]:23, 2001.)

Nursing priorities are directed toward monitoring the capnogram for changes. Any change in the waveform can indicate a change in the patient's pulmonary status and warrants further evaluation. Loss of the waveform may signal loss of effective respirations.[24]

evolve To test your mastery of this chapter, try the Open-Book Quiz at http://evolve.elsevier.com/Urden/priorities/

REFERENCES

1. Gehring PE: Physical assessment begins with a history, *RN* 54(11):26, 1991.
2. O'Hanlon-Nichols T: Basic assessment series: the adult pulmonary system, *Am J Nurs* 98(2):39, 1998.
3. Brenner M, Welliver J: Pulmonary and acid-base assessment, *Nurs Clin North Am* 25:761, 1990.
4. Finesivler C: Pulmonary assessment: what you need to know, *Prog Cardiovasc Nurs* 18:83, 2003.
5. Wilkins RL: Bedside assessment of the patient. In Wilkins RL, Stoller JK, Scanlan CL, editors: *Egan's fundamentals of respiratory care,* ed 8, St Louis, 2003, Mosby.
6. Carpenter KD: A comprehensive review of cyanosis, *Crit Care Nurs* 13(4):66, 1993.
7. Barkauskas V et al: *Health and physical assessment,* ed 3, St Louis, 2002, Mosby.
8. Seidel HM et al: *Mosby's guide to physical examination,* ed 5, St Louis, 2003, Mosby.
9. Boyda EK et al: *Pulmonary auscultation,* St Paul, 1987, 3M Health Care Group.
10. Scanlan CL, Wilkins RL: Gas exchange and transport. In Wilkins RL, Stoller JK, Scanlan CL, editors: *Egan's fundamentals of respiratory care,* ed 8, St Louis, 2003, Mosby.
11. Michota FA: *Diagnostic procedures handbook,* ed 2, Hudson, Ohio, 2001, Lexi-comp.
12. Hardie JA et al: Reference for arterial blood gases in the elderly, *Chest* 125:2053, 2004.
13. Beachey W: Acid-base balance. In Wilkins RL, Stoller JK, Scanlan CL, editors: *Egan's fundamentals of respiratory care,* ed 8, St Louis, 2003, Mosby.
14. Whittier WL, Rutecki GW: Primer on clinical acid-base problem solving, *Dis Mon* 50:122, 2004.
15. Johnson KL: Diagnostic measures to evaluate oxygenation in critically ill adults: implications and limitations, *AACN Clin Issues* 15:506, 2004.
16. Berry B, Pinard A: Assessing tissue oxygenation, *Crit Care Nur* 22(3):22, 2002.
17. Schallorn L, Ahrens T: Clinical application: using oxygenation profiles to manage patients, *Crit Care Nurs Clin North Am* 11:437, 1999.
18. Ruppel GL: Ventilation. In Wilkins RL, Stoller JK, Scanlan CL, editors: *Egan's fundamentals of respiratory care,* ed 8, St Louis, 2003, Mosby.
19. Fink J: Humidity and bland aerosol therapy. In Wilkins RL, Stoller JK, Scanlan CL, editors: *Egan's fundamentals of respiratory care,* ed 8, St Louis, 2003, Mosby.
20. Albert RK, Spiro SG, Jett JR: *Clinical respiratory medicine,* ed 3, St Louis, 2004, Mosby.
21. Wilkins RL: Electrocardiogram and laboratory test assessment. In Wilkins RL, Stoller JK, Scanlan CL, editors: *Egan's fundamentals of respiratory care,* ed 8, St Louis, 2003, Mosby.
22. Scanlan CL, Wilkins RL: Analysis and monitoring of gas exchange. In Wilkins RL, Stoller JK, Scanlan CL, editors: *Egan's fundamentals of respiratory care,* ed 8, St Louis, 2003, Mosby.
23. Soubani AO: Noninvasive monitoring of oxygen and carbon dioxide, *Am J Emerg Med* 19:141, 2001.
24. Ahrens T, Sona C: Capnography application in acute and critical care, *AACN Clin Issues* 14:123, 2003.
25. Ahrens T: Monitoring carbon dioxide in critical care: the newest vital sign? *Crit Care Nurs Clin N Am* 16:445, 2004.
26. Zwernemann K: End-tidal carbon dioxide monitoring: A VITAL sign worth watching, *Crit Care Nurs Clin N Am* 18:217, 2006.

CHAPTER

15 Pulmonary Disorders

KATHLEEN M. STACY

OBJECTIVES

- Describe the etiology and pathophysiology of selected pulmonary disorders.
- Identify the clinical manifestations of selected pulmonary disorders.
- Explain the treatment of selected pulmonary disorders.
- Discuss the nursing priorities for managing the patient with selected pulmonary disorders.

Understanding the pathology of a disease, the areas of assessment on which to focus, and the usual medical management allows the critical care nurse to more accurately anticipate and plan nursing interventions. This chapter focuses on pulmonary disorders commonly seen in the critical care environment.

ACUTE RESPIRATORY FAILURE

Acute respiratory failure (ARF) is a clinical condition in which the pulmonary system fails to maintain adequate gas exchange.[1] It is the most common organ failure seen in the intensive care unit today,[2,3] with a mortality rate of 22% to 75%.[2] Mortality varies directly with the number of additional organ failures.[2] Additional risk factors for mortality include history of liver, renal, or hematological dysfunction; presence of shock, and age greater than 55 years.[3]

ARF results from a deficiency in the performance of the pulmonary system.[1,4] It usually occurs secondary to another disorder that has altered the normal function of the pulmonary system in such a way as to decrease the ventilatory drive, decrease muscle strength, decrease chest wall elasticity, decrease the lung's capacity for gas exchange, increase airway resistance, or increase metabolic oxygen requirements.[5]

ARF can be classified as hypoxemic normocapnic respiratory failure (type I) or hypoxemic hypercapnic respiratory failure (type II), depending on the patient's arterial blood gas (ABG) levels. In type I respiratory failure the patient presents with a low $Pa{O_2}$ and a normal $Pa{CO_2}$, whereas in type II respiratory failure $Pa{O_2}$ is low and $Pa{CO_2}$ is high.[4]

ETIOLOGY

The etiologies of ARF may be classified as *extrapulmonary* or *intrapulmonary*, depending on the component of the respiratory system that is affected. Extrapulmonary causes include disorders that affect the brain, spinal cord, neuromuscular system, thorax, pleura, and upper airways. Intrapulmonary causes include disorders that affect the lower airways and alveoli, pulmonary circulation, and alveolar-capillary membrane.[6] Table 15-1 lists the different etiologies of ARF and their associated disorders.

PATHOPHYSIOLOGY

Hypoxemia is the result of impaired gas exchange and is the hallmark of acute respiratory failure. Hypercapnia may be present, depending on the underlying cause of the problem. The mains causes of hypoxemia are alveolar hypoventilation, ventilation/perfusion (V/Q) mismatching, and intrapulmonary shunting.[7] Type I respiratory failure usually results from V/Q mismatching and intrapulmonary shunting, whereas type II respiratory failure usually results from alveolar hypoventilation, which may or may not be accompanied by V/Q mismatching and intrapulmonary shunting.[1]

Alveolar Hypoventilation

Alveolar hypoventilation occurs when the amount of oxygen being brought into the alveoli is insufficient to meet the metabolic needs of the body.[6] This can be the result of increasing metabolic oxygen needs or decreasing ventilation.[5] Hypoxemia caused by alveolar hypoventilation is associated with hypercapnia and commonly results from extrapulmonary disorders.[1,7]

Ventilation/Perfusion Mismatching

V/Q mismatching occurs when ventilation and blood flow are mismatched in various regions of the lung in excess of what is normal. Blood passes through alveoli that are underventilated for the given amount of perfusion, leaving these areas with a lower-than-

Table 15-1

Etiologies of Acute Respiratory Failure

AFFECTED AREA	DISORDERS*
Extrapulmonary	
Brain	Drug overdose Central alveolar hypoventilation syndrome Brain trauma or lesion Postoperative anesthesia depression
Spinal cord	Guillain-Barré syndrome Poliomyelitis Amyotrophic lateral sclerosis Spinal cord trauma or lesion
Neuromuscular system	Myasthenia gravis Multiple sclerosis Neuromuscular-blocking antibiotics Organophosphate poisoning Muscular dystrophy
Thorax	Massive obesity Chest trauma
Pleura	Pleural effusion Pneumothorax
Upper airways	Sleep apnea Tracheal obstruction Epiglottitis
Intrapulmonary	
Lower airways and alveoli	Chronic obstructive pulmonary disease Asthma Bronchiolitis Cystic fibrosis Pneumonia
Pulmonary circulation	Pulmonary emboli
Alveolar-capillary membrane	Acute lung injury Inhalation of toxic gases Near-drowning

*Not an inclusive list.

normal amount of oxygen. V/Q mismatching is the most common cause of hypoxemia and is usually the result of alveoli that are partially collapsed or partially filled with fluid.[6-8]

Intrapulmonary Shunting

The extreme form of V/Q mismatching, intrapulmonary shunting, occurs when blood reaches the arterial system without participating in gas exchange. The mixing of unoxygenated (shunted) blood and oxygenated blood lowers the average level of oxygen present in the blood. Intrapulmonary shunting occurs when blood passes through a portion of a lung that is not ventilated. This may be the result of (1) alveolar collapse secondary to atelectasis or (2) alveolar flooding with pus, blood, or fluid.[6,7]

If allowed to progress, hypoxemia can result in a deficit of oxygen at the cellular level. As the tissue demands for oxygen continue and the supply diminishes, an oxygen supply/demand imbalance occurs and tissue hypoxia develops. Decreased oxygen to the cells contributes to impaired tissue perfusion and the development of lactic acidosis and multiple organ dysfunction syndrome.[8]

Assessment and Diagnosis

The patient with ARF may experience a variety of clinical manifestations, depending on the underlying cause and the extent of tissue hypoxia. The clinical manifestations commonly seen in the patient with ARF are usually related to the development of hypoxemia, hypercapnia, and acidosis.[9] Because the clinical symptoms are so varied, they are not considered reliable in predicting the degree of hypoxemia or hypercapnia[8] or the severity of ARF.[3]

Diagnosing and following the course of respiratory failure are best accomplished by ABG analysis. ABG analysis confirms the level of $Paco_2$, Pao_2, and blood pH. ARF is generally accepted as being present when the Pao_2 is less than 60 mm Hg and the $Paco_2$ is greater than 45 mm Hg (type II). In patients with chronically elevated $Paco_2$ levels, these criteria must be broadened to include a pH less than 7.35.[9]

A variety of additional tests are performed depending on the patient's underlying condition. These include bronchoscopy for airway surveillance or specimen retrieval, chest radiography, thoracic ultrasound, thoracic computed tomography (CT) and selected lung function studies.[10]

Medical Management

Medical management of the patient with ARF is aimed at treating the underlying cause, promoting adequate gas exchange, correcting acidosis, initiating nutrition support, and preventing complications. Medical interventions to promote gas exchange are aimed at improving oxygenation and ventilation.

Oxygenation

Actions to improve oxygenation include supplemental oxygen administration and the use of positive airway pressure. The purpose of oxygen therapy is to correct hypoxemia, and although the absolute level of hypoxemia varies in each patient, most treatment approaches aim to keep the arterial hemoglobin oxygen saturation greater than 90%.[9] The goal is to keep the tissues' needs satisfied but not produce hypercapnia or oxygen toxicity.[9] Supplemental oxygen administration is effective in treating hypoxemia related to alveolar hypoventilation and V/Q mismatching. When intrapulmonary shunting exists, supplemental oxygen alone is ineffective.[11] In this situation, positive pressure is necessary to open collapsed alveoli and facilitate

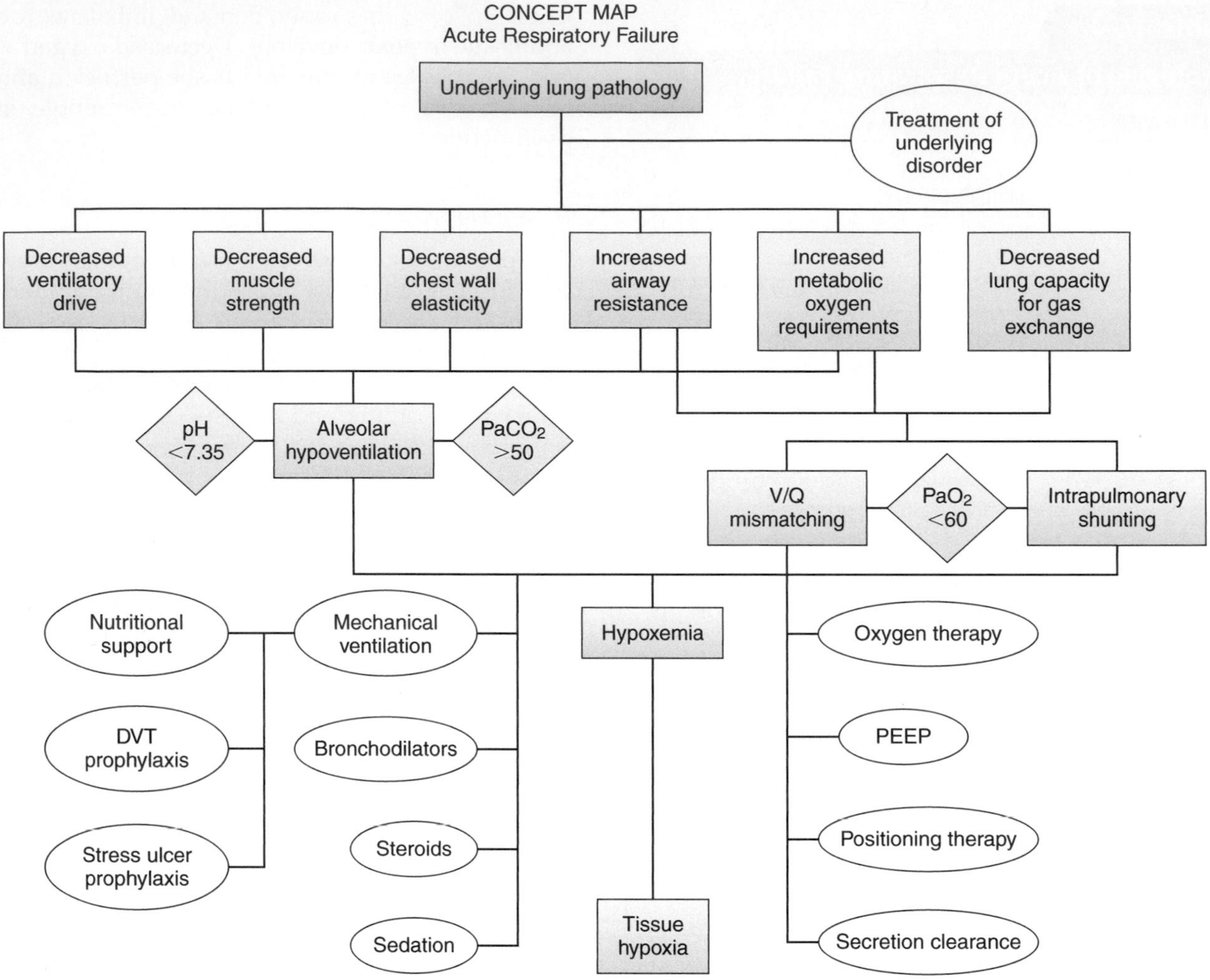

their participation in gas exchange. To avoid intubtion, positive pressure can be delivered noninvasively via a nasal or oronasal mask.[12] One recent study found that an oronasal mask is better tolerated than a nasal mask.[13] For further information on noninvasive ventilation see Chapter 16.

Ventilation

Interventions to improve ventilation include the use of noninvasive and invasive mechanical ventilation. Depending on the underlying cause and the severity of the ARF, the patient may be initially treated with noninvasive ventilation.[12] One study found, however, that those patients with a pH of less than 7.25 at initial presentation had an increased likelihood of the need for invasive mechanical ventilation.[14] The selection of ventilatory mode and settings depends on the patient's underlying condition, severity of respiratory failure, and body size. Initially the patient is started on volume ventilation in the assist/control mode. In the patient with chronic hypercapnia, the settings should be adjusted to keep the arterial blood gas values within the parameters expected to be maintained by the patient after extubation.[15] For further information on mechanical ventilation see Chapter 16.

Pharmacology

Medications to facilitate dilatation of the airways may also be of benefit in the treatment of the patient with ARF. Bronchodilators, such as β_2-agonists and anti cholinergic agents, aid in smooth muscle relaxation and are of particular benefit to patients with airflow limitations. Methylxanthines, such as aminophylline, are no longer recommended because of their negative side effects. Steroids also are often administered to decrease airway inflammation and enhance the effects of the β_2-agonists. Mucolytics and expectorates are also no longer used as they have been found to be of no benefit in this patient population.[16]

Sedation is necessary in many patients to assist with maintaining adequate ventilation. It can be used to comfort the patient and decrease the work of breathing, particularly if the patient is fighting the ventilator. Analgesics should be administered for pain control.[17] In some patients, sedation does not decrease spontaneous respiratory efforts enough to allow adequate ventilation. Neuromuscular paralysis may be necessary to facilitate optimal ventilation. Paralysis also may be necessary to decrease oxygen consumption in the severely compromised patient.[18]

Acidosis

Acidosis may occur in the patient for a number of reasons. Hypoxemia causes impaired tissue perfusion, which leads to the production of lactic acid and the development of metabolic acidosis. Impaired ventilation leads to the accumulation of carbon dioxide and the development of respiratory acidosis. Once the patient is adequately oxygenated and ventilated, the acidosis should correct itself. The use of sodium bicarbonate to correct the acidosis has been shown to be of minimal benefit to the patient and thus is no longer recommended even in the presence of severe acidosis ($pH<7.2$).[19]

Nutrition Support

The initiation of nutrition support is of utmost importance in the management of the patient with ARF. The goals of nutrition support are to meet the overall nutritional needs of the patient, while avoiding overfeeding, to prevent nutrition delivery–related complications and to improve patient outcomes.[20] Failure to provide the patient with adequate nutrition support results in the development of malnutrition. Both malnutrition and overfeeding can interfere with the performance of the pulmonary system, thus further perpetuating ARF. Malnutrition decreases the patient's ventilatory drive and muscle strength, whereas overfeeding increases carbon dioxide production, which then increases the patient's ventilatory demand, resulting in respiratory muscle fatigue.[21]

The enteral route is the preferred method of nutrition administration. If the patient cannot tolerate enteral feedings or cannot receive enough nutrients enterally, he or she will be started on parenteral nutrition. Because the parenteral route is associated with a higher rate of complications, the goal is to switch to enteral feedings as soon as the patient can tolerate them.[20,21] Nutrition support should be initiated before the third day of mechanical ventilation for the well-nourished patient and within 24 hours for the malnourished patient.[20,21]

Complications

The patient with acute respiratory failure may experience a number of complications, including ischemic-anoxic encephalophathy,[22] cardiac dysrhythmias,[23] venous thromboembolism,[24] and gastrointestina bleeding.[25] Ischemic-anoxic encephalopathy results from hypoxemia, hypercapnia, and acidosis.[22] Dysrhythmias are precipitated by hypoxemia, acidosis, electrolyte imbalances, and the administration of β_2-agonists.[23] Maintaining oxygenation, normalizing electrolytes, and monitoring drug levels will facilitate the prevention and treatment of encephalopathy and dysrhythmias.[22,23] Venous thromboembolism is precipitated by venous stasis resulting from immobility and can be prevented through the use of pneumatic compression stockings and low-dose unfractionated heparin or low-molecular-weight heparin.[24] Gastrointestinal bleeding can be prevented through the use of histamine$_2$-antagonists, cytoprotective agents, or gastric proton pump inhibitors.[25] In addition, the patient is at risk for the complications associated with an artificial airway, mechanical ventilation, enteral and parenteral nutrition, and peripheral arterial cannulation.

Box 15-1

NURSING DIAGNOSIS PRIORITIES

Acute Respiratory Failure

- Impaired Gas Exchange related to alveolar hypoventilation
- Impaired Gas Exchange related to ventilation/perfusion mismatching or intrapulmonary shunting, p. A-29
- Ineffective Breathing Pattern related to musculoskeletal fatigue or neuromuscular impairment, p. A-34
- Imbalanced Nutrition: Less Than Body Requirements related to lack of exogenous nutrients or increased metabolic demand, p. A-28
- Acute Confusion related to sensory overload, sensory deprivation, and sleep pattern disturbance, p. A-3
- Deficient Knowledge: Discharge Regimen related to lack of previous exposure to information (see Patient Education: Acute Respiratory Failure), p. A-18

NURSING MANAGEMENT

Nursing management of the patient with acute respiratory failure incorporates a variety of nursing diagnoses (Box 15-1). Nursing care is directed by the specific etiology of the respiratory failure, although some common interventions are used. **Nursing priorities are directed toward (1) optimizing oxygenation and ventilation, (2) providing comfort and emotional support, (3) maintaining surveillance for complications, and (4) providing patient education.**

Optimizing Oxygenation and Ventilation

Nursing interventions to optimize oxygenation and ventilation include positioning, preventing desaturation, and promoting secretion clearance.

Positioning. Positioning of the patient with ARF depends on the type of lung injury and the underlying cause of hypoxemia. For those patients with V/Q mismatching, positioning is used to facilitate better matching of ventilation with perfusion to optimize gas exchange.[26] Because gravity normally facilitates preferential ventilation and perfusion to the dependent areas of the lungs, the best gas exchange would take

PATIENT EDUCATION

Acute Respiratory Failure

- Pathophysiology of disease
- Specific etiology
- Precipitating factor modification
- Importance of taking medications
- Breathing techniques (e.g., pursed-lip breathing, diaphragmatic breathing)
- Energy conservation techniques
- Measures to prevent pulmonary infections (e.g., proper nutrition, hand washing, immunization against *Streptococcus pneumoniae* and influenza viruses)
- Signs and symptoms of pulmonary infections (e.g., sputum color change, shortness of breath, fever)
- Cough enhancement techniques (e.g., cascade cough, huff cough, end-expiratory cough, augmented cough)

place in the dependent areas of the lungs.[11] Thus the goal of positioning is to place the least affected area of the patient's lung in the most dependent position. Patients with unilateral lung disease should be positioned with the healthy lung in a dependent position.[26,27] Patients with diffuse lung disease may benefit from being positioned with the right lung down, because it is larger and more vascular than the left lung.[27,28] For those patients with alveolar hypoventilation, the goal of positioning is to facilitate ventilation. These patients benefit from nonrecumbent positions, such as sitting or a semierect position.[29] In addition, semirecumbency has been shown to decrease the risk of aspiration and inhibit the development of hospital-associated pneumonia.[30] Frequent repositioning (at least every 2 hours) is beneficial in optimizing the patient's ventilatory pattern and V/Q matching.[31]

Preventing Desaturation. A number of activities can prevent desaturation from occurring. These include performing procedures only as needed, hyperoxygenating the patient before suctioning, providing adequate rest and recovery time between various procedures, and minimizing oxygen consumption. Interventions to minimize oxygen consumption include limiting the patient's physical activity, administering sedation to control anxiety, and providing measures to control fever.[29] The patient should be continuously monitored with a pulse oximeter to warn of signs of desaturation.

Promoting Secretion Clearance. Interventions to promote secretion clearance include providing adequate systemic hydration, humidifying supplemental oxygen, coughing, and suctioning. Postural drainage and chest percussion and vibration have been found to be of little benefit in the critically ill patient[32,33] and thus are not discussed here.

To facilitate deep breathing, the patient's thorax should be maintained in alignment and the head of the bed elevated 30 to 45 degrees. This position best accommodates diaphragmatic descent and intercostal muscle action.

Once the patient is extubated, deep breathing and incentive spirometry should be started as soon as possible. Deep breathing involves having the patient take a deep breath and hold it for approximately 3 seconds or longer. Incentive spirometry involves having the patient take at least 10 deep, effective breaths per hour using an incentive spirometer. These actions help prevent atelectasis and reexpand any collapsed lung tissue. The chest should be auscultated during inflation to ensure that all dependent parts of the lung are well ventilated and to help the patient understand the depth of breath necessary for optimal effect. Coughing should be avoided unless secretions are present because it promotes collapse of the smaller airways.

Patient Education

Early in the patient's hospital stay, the patient and family should be taught about acute respiratory failure, its etiologies, and its treatment. As the patient moves toward discharge, teaching should focus on the interventions necessary for preventing the reoccurrence of the precipitating disorder. If the patient smokes, he or she should be encouraged to stop smoking and be referred to a smoking cessation program (see Evidence-Based Collaborative Practice: Smoking Cessation Guidelines). In addition, the importance of participating in a pulmonary rehabilitation program should be stressed. Additional information for the patient can be found at the American Lung Association website (http://www.lungusa.org).

Collaborative management of the patient with acute respiratory failure is outlined in Box 15-2.

ACUTE LUNG INJURY

Acute lung injury (ALI) is a systemic process that is considered to be the pulmonary manifestation of multiple organ dysfunction syndrome.[34] It is characterized by noncardiac pulmonary edema and disruption of the alveolar-capillary membrane as a result of injury to either the pulmonary vasculature or airways.[35]

Many different diagnostic criteria have been used to identify ALI, which has led to confusion, particularly among researchers. In an attempt to standardize the identification of this disorder, the American-European Consensus Committee on ARDS recommended the following criteria be used to diagnose ALI:

- Acute in onset
- Ratio of partial pressure of oxygen (PaO_2) to fraction of inspired oxygen (FIO_2) less than or equal to 300 mm Hg (regardless of positive end-expiratory pressure [PEEP] level)

EVIDENCE-BASED COLLABORATIVE PRACTICE

Smoking Cessation Guidelines

The following are the key recommendations of the updated guideline, *Treating Tobacco Use and Dependence,* based on the literature review and expert panel opinion:

1. Tobacco dependence is a chronic condition that often requires repeated intervention. However, effective treatments exist that can produce long-term or even permanent abstinence.
2. Because effective tobacco dependence treatments are available, every patient who uses tobacco should be offered at least one of these treatments:
   - Patients *willing* to try to quit tobacco use should be provided treatments identified as effective in this guideline.
   - Patients *unwilling* to try to quit tobacco use should be provided a brief intervention designed to increase their motivation to quit.
3. It is essential that clinicians and health care delivery systems (including administrators, insurers, and purchasers) institutionalize the consistent identification, documentation, and treatment of every tobacco user seen in a health care setting.
4. Brief tobacco dependence treatment is effective, and every patient who uses tobacco should be offered at least brief treatment.
5. There is a strong dose-response relation between the intensity of tobacco dependence counseling and its effectiveness. Treatments involving person-to-person contact (via individual, group, or proactive telephone counseling) are consistently effective, and their effectiveness increases with treatment intensity (e.g., minutes of contact).
6. Three types of counseling and behavioral therapies were found to be especially effective and should be used with all patients attempting tobacco cessation:
   - Provision of practical counseling (problem solving/skills training)
   - Provision of social support as part of treatment (intratreatment social support)
   - Help in securing social support outside of treatment (extratreatment social support)
7. Numerous effective pharmacotherapies for smoking cessation now exist. Except in the presence of contraindications, these should be used with all patients attempting to quit smoking.
   - Five *first-line* pharmacotherapies were identified that reliably increase long-term smoking abstinence rates:
     - Bupropion SR
     - Nicotine gum
     - Nicotine inhaler
     - Nicotine nasal spray
     - Nicotine patch
   - Two *second-line* pharmacotherapies were identified as efficacious and may be considered by clinicians if first-line pharmacotherapies are not effective:
     - Clonidine
     - Nortriptyline
   - Over-the-counter nicotine patches are effective relative to placebo, and their use should be encouraged.
8. Tobacco dependence treatments are both clinically effective and cost-effective relative to other medical and disease prevention interventions. As such, insurers and purchasers should ensure that the following occurs:
   - All insurance plans include as a reimbursed benefit the counseling and pharmacotherapeutic treatments identified as effective in this guideline
   - Clinicians are reimbursed for providing tobacco dependence treatment just as they are reimbursed for treating other chronic conditions

From Fiore MC et al: *Treating tobacco use and dependence* (Clinical Practice Guideline), Rockville, MD, June 2000, U.S. Department of Health and Human Services, Public Health Service.

Box 15-2

Collaborative Management

Acute Respiratory Failure

- Identify and treat underlying cause
- Administer oxygen therapy
- Intubate patient
- Initiate mechanical ventilation
- Administer medications
  - Bronchodilators
  - Steroids
  - Sedatives
  - Analgesics
- Position patient to optimize ventilation/perfusion matching
- Suction as needed
- Provide adequate rest and recovery time between various procedures
- Correct acidosis
- Initiate nutritional support
- Maintain surveillance for complications
  - Encephalopathy
  - Cardiac dysrhythmias
  - Venous thromboembolism
  - Gastrointestinal bleeding
- Provide comfort and emotional support

Box 15-3

Risk Factors for Acute Lung Injury

Direct Injury
Aspiration
Near-drowning
Toxic inhalation
Pulmonary contusion
Pneumonia
Oxygen toxicity
Transthoracic radiation

Indirect Injury
Sepsis
Nonthoracic trauma
Hypertransfusion
Cardiopulmonary bypass
Severe pancreatitis
Embolism—air, fat, amniotic fluid
Disseminated intravascular coagulation (DIC)
Shock states

- Bilateral infiltrates on chest radiography
- Pulmonary artery occlusion pressure (PAOP) less than or equal to 18 mm Hg or no clinical evidence of left atrial hypertension.[36,37]

The severest form of ALI is called acute (formerly called "adult") respiratory distress syndrome (ARDS).[36] ARDS is identified by the same diagnostic criteria as ALI except that the ratio of PaO_2 to FIO_2 is less than or equal to 200 mm Hg. Because the etiology, pathophysiology, and treatment of ALI are the same as for ARDS, the discussion will use the broader term of ALI.[37]

ETIOLOGY

A wide variety of clinical conditions are associated with the development of ALI. These are categorized as *direct* or *indirect*, depending on the primary site of injury (Box 15-3).[35,38] Direct injuries are those in which the lung epithelium sustains a direct insult. Indirect injuries are those in which the insult occurs elsewhere in the body and mediators are transmitted via the bloodstream to the lungs. Sepsis, aspiration of gastric contents, diffuse pneumonia, and trauma are major risk factors for the development of ALI.[37]

The mortality rate for ALI is estimated to be 30% to 40%.[37]

PATHOPHYSIOLOGY

The progression of ALI can be described in three phases: exudative, fibroproliferative, and resolution. ALI is initiated with stimulation of the inflammatory-immune system as a result of a direct or indirect injury (Figure 15-1). Inflammatory mediators are released from the site of injury, resulting in the activation and accumulation of the neutrophils, macrophages, and platelets in the pulmonary capillaries. These cellular mediators initiate the release of humoral mediators that cause damage to the alveolar-capillary membrane.[38]

Exudative Phase

Within the first 72 hours after the initial insult, the exudative phase or acute phase ensues. Once released, the mediators cause injury to the pulmonary capillaries, resulting in increased capillary membrane permeability, leading to the leakage of fluid filled with protein, blood cells, fibrin, and activated cellular and humoral mediators into the pulmonary interstitium. Damage to the pulmonary capillaries also causes the development of microthrombi and elevation of pulmonary artery pressures. As fluid enters the pulmonary interstitium, the lymphatics are overwhelmed and unable to drain all the accumulating fluid, resulting in the development of interstitial edema. Fluid is then forced from the interstitial space into the alveoli, resulting in alveolar edema. Pulmonary interstitial edema also causes compression of the alveoli and small airways. Alveolar edema causes swelling of the type I alveolar epithelial cells and flooding of the alveoli. Protein and fibrin in the edema fluid precipitate the formation of hyaline membranes over the alveoli. Eventually, the type II alveolar epithelial cells are also damaged, leading to impaired surfactant production. Injury to the alveolar epithelial cells and the loss of surfactant lead to further alveolar collapse.[38,39]

Hypoxemia occurs as a result of intrapulmonary shunting and V/Q mismatching secondary to compression, collapse, and flooding of the alveoli and small airways. Increased work of breathing occurs as a result of increased airway resistance, decreased functional residual capacity (FRC), and decreased lung compliance secondary to atelectasis and compression of the small airways. Hypoxemia and the increased work of breathing lead to patient fatigue and the development of alveolar hypoventilation. Pulmonary hypertension occurs as a result of damage to the pulmonary capillaries, microthrombi, and hypoxic vasoconstriction, leading to the development of increased alveolar dead space and right ventricular afterload. Hypoxemia worsens as a result of alveolar hypoventilation and increased alveolar dead space. Right ventricular afterload increases and leads to right ventricular dysfunction and a decrease in cardiac output.[38]

Fibroproliferative Phase

This phase begins as disordered healing starts in the lungs. Cellular granulation and collagen deposition occur within the alveolar-capillary membrane. The alveoli become enlarged and irregularly shaped (fibrotic), and the pulmonary capillaries become scarred and

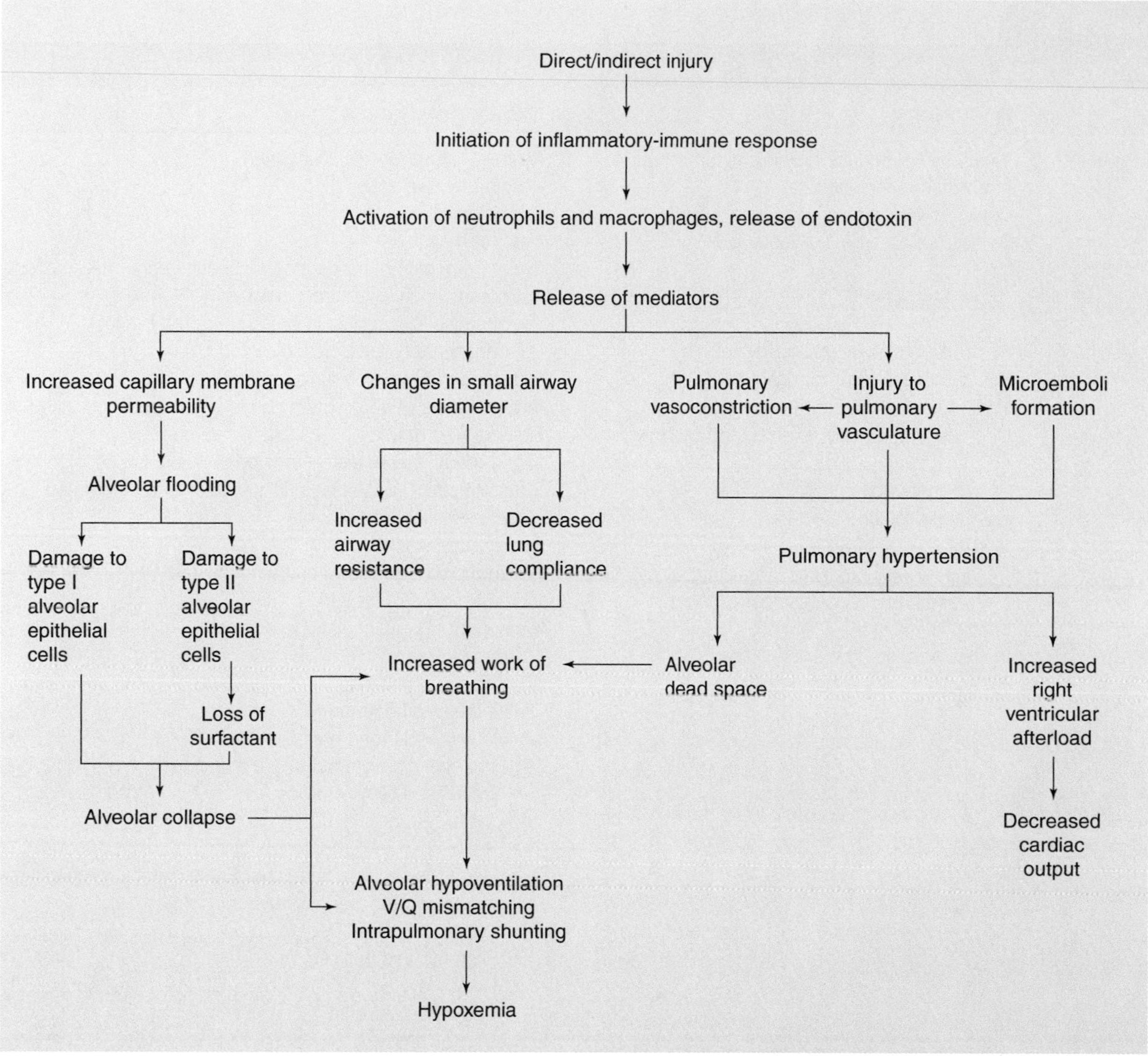

FIGURE 15-1. Pathophysiology of acute lung injury.

obliterated. This leads to further stiffening of the lungs, increasing pulmonary hypertension, and continued hypoxemia.[38,39]

Resolution Phase

Recovery occurs over several weeks as structural and vascular remodeling take place to reestablish the alveolar-capillary membrane. The hyaline membranes are cleared, and intraalveolar fluid is transported out of the alveolus into the interstitium. The type II alveolar epithelial cells multiply, some of which differentiate to type I alveolar epithelial cells, facilitating the restoration of the alveolus. Alveolar macrophages remove cellular debris.[38,39]

Assessment and Diagnosis

Initially the patient with ALI may present with a variety of clinical manifestations, depending on the precipitating event. As the disorder progresses, the patient's signs and symptoms can be associated with the phase of ALI that he or she is experiencing (Table 15-2). During the exudative phase, the patient presents with tachypnea, restlessness, apprehension, and moderate increase in accessory muscle use. During the fibroproliferative phase, the patient's signs and symptoms progress to agitation, dyspnea, fatigue, excessive accessory muscle use, and fine crackles as respiratory failure develops.[40,41]

Arterial blood gas analysis reveals a low $Pa{O_2}$, despite increases in supplemental oxygen administration (refractory hypoxemia).[40] Initially the $Pa{CO_2}$ is low as a result of hyperventilation, but eventually the $Pa{CO_2}$ increases as the patient fatigues. The pH is high initially but decreases as respiratory acidosis develops.[40,41]

Initially the chest x-ray film may be normal, because changes in the lungs do not become evident for up to

Table 15-2

Physiology and Associated Physical Examination of Patient With Acute Lung Injury

PHASE	PHYSIOLOGY	PHYSICAL EXAMINATION
Exudative phase	Parenchymal surface hemorrhage Interstitial or alveolar edema Compression of terminal bronchioles Destruction of type 1 alveolar cells	Restless, apprehensive, tachypneic Respiratory alkalosis Pao_2 normal CXR: normal Chest examination: moderate use of accessory muscles, lungs clear Pulmonary artery pressures: elevated Pulmonary artery occlusion pressure: normal or low
Fibroproliferative phase	Destruction of type 2 alveolar cells Gas exchange compromised Increased peak inspiratory pressure Decreased compliance (static and dynamic) Refractory hypoxemia: • Intraalveolar atelectasis • Increased shunt fraction • Decreased diffusion Decreased functional residual capacity Interstitial fibrosis Increased dead space ventilation	Pulmonary artery pressures: elevated Increased workload on right ventricle Increased use of accessory muscles Fine crackles or rales Increasing agitation related to hypoxia CXR: interstitial or alveolar infiltrates; elevated diaphragm Hyperventilation; hypercarbia Decreased Svo_2 Widening alveolar-arterial gradient Increased work of breathing Worsening hypercarbia and hypoxemia Lactic acidosis (related to aerobic metabolism) Alteration in perfusion: • Increased heart rate • Decreased blood pressure • Change in skin temperature and color • Decreased capillary filling End-organ dysfunction: • Brain: change in mentation, agitation, hallucinations • Heart: decreased cardiac output→angina, CHF, papillary muscle dysfunction, dysrhythmias, MI • Renal: decreased urinary output or GFR • Skin: mottled, ischemic • Liver: elevated SGOT, bilirubin, alkaline phosphatase, PT/PTT; decreased albumin

Modified from Phillips JK: *Crit Care Clin North Am* 11:233, 1999.

Pao_2, Arterial oxygen pressure; *CXR,* chest radiograph; *Svo_2,* venous oxygen saturation; *CHF,* congestive heart failure; *MI,* myocardial infarction; *GFR,* glomerular filtration rate; *SGOT,* serum glutamate oxaloacetate transaminase; *PT,* prothrombin time; *PTT,* partial thromboplastin time.

24 hours. As the pulmonary edema becomes apparent, diffuse, patchy interstitial and alveolar infiltrates appear. This progresses to multifocal consolidation of the lungs, which appears as a "white out" on the chest x-ray film.[40]

Medical Management

Medical management of the patient with ALI involves a multifaceted approach. This strategy includes treating the underlying cause, promoting gas exchange, supporting tissue oxygenation, and preventing complications. Given the severity of hypoxemia, the patient is intubated and mechanically ventilated to facilitate adequate gas exchange.[42]

Ventilation

Traditionally, the patient with ALI was ventilated with a mode of volume ventilation, such as assist/control ventilation (A/CV) or synchronized intermittent mandatory ventilation (SIMV), with tidal volumes adjusted to deliver 10 to 15 ml/kg. Current research now indicates that this approach may have actually led to further lung injury. It is now known that repeated opening and closing of the alveoli cause injury to the lung units (atelectrauma), resulting in inhibited surfactant production, and increased inflammation (biotrauma), resulting in the release of mediators and an increase in pulmonary capillary membrane permeability. In addition, excessive pressure in the alveoli (barotrauma) or excessive volume in the alveoli (volutrauma) leads to excessive alveolar wall stress and damage to the alveolar-capillary membrane, resulting in air escaping into the surrounding spaces.[42] Thus several different approaches have been developed to facilitate the mechanical ventilation of the patient with ALI.

Low Tidal Volume. Low tidal volume ventilation uses smaller tidal volumes (6 to 10 ml/kg) to ventilate the patient, in an attempt to limit the effects of barotrauma and volutrauma. The goal is to provide the maximum tidal volume possible while maintaining an airway pressure less than 30 cm H_2O. To allow for adequate carbon dioxide elimination the respiratory rate is increased to 20 to 30 breaths/min.[42,43]

Permissive Hypercapnia. Permissive hypercapnia uses low tidal volume ventilation in conjunction with normal respiratory rates in an attempt to limit the effects of atelectrauma and biotrauma. Normally the patient's respiratory rate would have to be increased to compensate for the small tidal volume to maintain normocapnia. In ALI though, increasing the respiratory rate can lead to worsening alveolar damage. Thus the patient's carbon dioxide level is allowed to rise, and the patient becomes hypercapnic. As a general rule, the patient's $Paco_2$ should not rise faster than 10 mm Hg per hour and overall should not exceed 80 to 100 mg Hg. Because of the negative cardiopulmonary effects of severe acidosis, the arterial pH is generally maintained at 7.20 or greater. To maintain the pH, the patient is given intravenous sodium bicarbonate or the respiratory rate and/or tidal volume are increased. Permissive hypercapnia is contraindicated in patients with increased intracranial pressure, pulmonary hypertension, seizures, and cardiac failure.[44]

Pressure Control Ventilation. In pressure control ventilation (PCV) mode, each breath is delivered or augmented with a preset amount of inspiratory pressure as opposed to tidal volume, which is used in volume ventilation. Thus the actual tidal volume the patient receives varies from breath to breath. PCV is used to limit and control the amount of pressure in the lungs and decrease the incidence of volutrauma. The goal is to keep the patient's plateau pressure (end-inspiratory static pressure) less than 30 cm H_2O. A known problem with this mode of ventilation is that as the patient's lungs get stiffer, it becomes harder and harder to maintain an adequate tidal volume and severe hypercapnia can occur.[42,43]

Inverse Ratio Ventilation. Another alternative ventilatory mode that is used in managing the patient with ALI is inverse ratio ventilation (IRV), either pressure-controlled or volume-controlled. IRV prolongs the inspiratory (I) time and shortens the expiratory (E) time, thus reversing the normal I:E ratio. The goal of IRV is to maintain a more constant mean airway pressure throughout the ventilatory cycle, which helps keep alveoli open and participating in gas exchange. It also increases FRC and decreases the work of breathing. In addition, because the breath is delivered over a longer period of time, the peak inspiratory pressure in the lungs is decreased. A major disadvantage to IRV is the development of auto-PEEP. Because the expiratory phase of ventilation is shortened, air can become trapped in the lower airways, creating unintentional PEEP (also known as auto-PEEP), which can cause hemodynamic compromise and worsening gas exchange. Patients on IRV usually require heavy sedation with neuromuscular blockade to prevent them from fighting the ventilator.[42,43]

Oxygen Therapy. Oxygen is administered at the lowest level possible to support tissue oxygenation. Continued exposure to high levels of oxygen can lead to oxygen toxicity, which further perpetuates the entire process. The goal of oxygen therapy is to maintain an arterial hemoglobin oxygen saturation of 90% or greater using the lowest level of oxygen—preferably less than 0.50.[35]

Positive End-Expiratory Pressure. Because the hypoxemia that develops with ALI is often refractory or unresponsive to oxygen therapy, it is necessary to facilitate oxygenation with PEEP. The purpose of using PEEP in the patient with ALI is to improve oxygenation while reducing Fio_2 to less toxic levels. PEEP has several positive effects on the lungs, including opening collapsed alveoli, stabilizing flooded alveoli, and increasing FRC. Thus PEEP decreases intrapulmonary shunting and increases compliance. PEEP also has several negative effects, including (1) decreasing cardiac output (CO) as a result of decreasing venous return secondary to increased intrathoracic pressure and (2) barotrauma, as a result of gas escaping into the surrounding spaces secondary to alveolar rupture. The amount of PEEP a patient requires is determined by evaluating both arterial hemoglobin oxygen saturation and cardiac output. In most cases a PEEP of 10 to 15 cm H_2O is adequate. If PEEP is too high, it can result in overdistention of the alveoli, which can impede pulmonary capillary blood flow, decrease surfactant production, and worsen intrapulmonary shunting. If PEEP is too low, it allows the alveoli to collapse during expiration, which can result in more damage to alveoli.[42]

Tissue Perfusion. Adequate tissue perfusion depends on an adequate supply of oxygen being transported to the tissues. An adequate CO and hemoglobin level is critical to oxygen transport. CO depends on heart rate, preload, afterload, and contractility. A variety of fluids and medications are used to manipulate this parameter. Newer approaches to fluid management include maintaining a very low intravascular volume (pulmonary artery occlusion pressure of 5 to

Box 15-4

NURSING DIAGNOSIS PRIORITIES

Acute Lung Injury (ALI)

- Impaired Gas Exchange related to ventilation/perfusion mismatching or intrapulmonary shunting, p. A-29
- Decreased Cardiac Output related to alterations in preload, p. A-12
- Imbalanced Nutrition: Less Than Body Requirements related to lack of exogenous nutrients or increased metabolic demand, p. A-28
- Anxiety related to threat to biologic, psychologic, and/or social integrity, p. A-9
- Compromised Family Coping related to critically ill family member, p. A-11

8 mm Hg) with fluid restriction and diuretics while supporting the CO with vasoactive and inotropic medications. The goal is to decrease the amount of fluid leakage into the lungs.[45]

Nursing Management

Nursing management of the patient with ALI incorporates a variety of nursing diagnoses (Box 15-4). **Nursing priorities are directed toward (1) optimizing oxygenation and ventilation, (2) providing comfort and emotional support, and (3) maintaining surveillance for complications.**

Optimizing Oxygenation and Ventilation

Nursing interventions to optimize oxygenation and ventilation include positioning, preventing desaturation, and promoting secretion clearance (see Nursing Management of ARF). One additional nursing intervention that can be used to improve the oxygenation and ventilation of the patient with ALI is prone positioning.

Prone Positioning. A number of studies have shown that prone positioning the patient with ALI results in an improvement in oxygenation. Although a number of theories propose how prone positioning improves oxygenation, the discovery that ALI causes greater damage to the dependent areas of the lungs probably provides the best explanation. It was originally thought that ALI was a diffuse homogenous disease that affected all areas of the lungs equally. It is now known that the dependent lung areas are more heavily damaged than the nondependent lung areas. Turning the patient prone improves perfusion to less damaged parts of lungs and improves V/Q matching and decreases intrapulmonary shunting. Prone positioning appears to be more effective when initiated during the early phases of ALI.[46] For more information on prone positioning, see Chapter 16.

Box 15-5

Collaborative Management

Acute Lung Injury

- Administer oxygen therapy
- Intubate patient
- Initiate mechanical ventilation
  - Permissive hypercapnia
  - Pressure control ventilation
  - Inverse ratio ventilation
- Use PEEP
- Administer medications
  - Bronchodilators
  - Sedatives
  - Analgesics
  - Neuromuscular blocking agents
- Maximize cardiac output
  - Preload
  - Afterload
  - Contractility
- Turn patient to prone position
- Suction as needed
- Provide adequate rest and recovery time between various procedures
- Initiate nutritional support
- Maintain surveillance for complications
  - Encephalopathy
  - Cardiac dysrhythmias
  - Venous thromboembolism
  - Gastrointestinal bleeding
  - Atelectrauma
  - Biotrauma
  - Volutrauma
  - Barotrauma
  - Oxygen toxicity
- Provide comfort and emotional support

PEEP, Positive end-expiratory pressure.

Collaborative management of the patient with ALI is outlined in Box 15-5.

PNEUMONIA

Pneumonia is an acute inflammation of the lung parenchyma that is caused by an infectious agent that can lead to alveolar consolidation. Pneumonia can be classified as community-acquired (CAP) or hospital-associated (HAP). Community-acquired pneumonia is acquired outside of the hospital.[47] Severe CAP requires admission to the intensive care unit and accounts for about 10% of all patients with pneumonia. The mortality for this patient group is in excess of 50%.[48] Hospital-associated pneumonia is acquired while in the hospital for at least 48 hours.[49] Ventilator-associated pneumonia (VAP) is a subgroup of HAP that refers to development of pneumonia after the insertion of an artificial airway. VAP represents 80% of all HAP cases.[49]

Etiology

The spectra of etiologic pathogens of pneumonia vary with the type of pneumonia as do the risk factors for the disease.

Severe Community-Acquired Pneumonia

Pathogens that can cause severe CAP include *Streptococcus pneumoniae, Legionella* species, *Haemophilus influenzae, Staphylococcus aureus, Mycoplasma pneumoniae,* respiratory viruses, *Chlamydia pneumoniae,* and *Pseudomonas aeruginosa.*[50] A number of factors increase the risk for developing CAP, including alcoholism, chronic obstructive pulmonary disease (COPD), and comorbid conditions such as diabetes, malignancy, and coronary artery disease.[47] Impaired swallowing and altered mental status also contribute to the development of CAP because they result in an increased exposure to the various pathogens due to chronic aspiration of oropharyngeal secretions.[47]

Hospital-Associated Pneumonia

Pathogens that can cause HAP include *Staphylococcus aureus, Streptococcus pneumoniae, Pseudomonas aeruginosa, Acinetobacter baumannii, Klebsiella* species, *Proteus* species, *Serratia* species, fungi, and respiratory viruses.[49] Two of the pathogens most frequently associated with VAP are Staphylococcus aureus and Pseudomonas aeruginosa.[51] Risk factors for these conditions are host-related, device-related, and personnel/procedure-related. Host-related factors include age greater than 65 years, underlying illness (e.g., COPD, immunosuppression, diabetes), alcoholism, smoking, depressed consciousness and malnutrition, and thoracic or abdominal surgery. Device-related factors include endotracheal intubation, mechanical ventilation, and gastric intubation with enteral feedings. Personnel/procedure-related factors include cross contamination by hands, infected personnel, antibiotic therapy, and histamine blockers and antacid therapy. Histamine blockers, antacid therapy, and enteral feedings elevate the pH of the stomach and promote bacterial overgrowth. The nasogastric tube acts as a wick, facilitating the movement of bacteria to the oropharynx, where it can be aspirated.[52]

Pathophysiology

Development of acute pneumonia implies a defect in host defenses, a particularly virulent organism, or an overwhelming inoculation event. Bacterial invasion of the lower respiratory tract can occur by inhalation of aerosolized infectious particles, aspiration of organisms colonizing the oropharynx, migration of organisms from adjacent sites or colonization, direct inoculation of organisms into the lower airway, spread of infection to the lungs from adjacent structures, spread of infection to the lung through the blood, and reactivation of latent infection (usually in the setting of immunosuppression). The most common mechanism appears to be aspiration of oropharyngeal organisms.[53] Table 15-3 lists the precipitating conditions that can facilitate the development of pneumonia.

Table 15-3
Precipitating Conditions of Pneumonia

CONDITION	ETIOLOGIES
Depressed epiglottal and cough reflexes	Unconsciousness, neurologic disease, endotracheal or tracheal tubes, anesthesia, aging
Decreased cilia activity	Smoke inhalation, smoking history, oxygen toxicity, hypoventilation, intubation, viral infections, aging, COPD
Increased secretions	COPD, viral infections, bronchiectasis, general anesthesia, endotracheal intubation, smoking
Atelectasis	Trauma, foreign body obstruction, tumor, splinting, shallow ventilations, general anesthesia
Decreased lymphatic flow	Heart failure, tumor
Fluid in alveoli	Heart failure, aspiration, trauma
Abnormal phagocytosis and humoral activity	Neutropenia, immunocompetent disorders, patients receiving chemotherapy
Impaired alveolar macrophages	Hypoxemia, metabolic acidosis, cigarette smoking history, hypoxia, alcohol use, viral infections, aging

COPD, Chronic obstructive pulmonary disease.

Figure 15-2 depicts the pathophysiology of HAP. Colonization of the patient's oropharynx with infectious organisms is a major contributor to the development of HAP. Normally, the oropharynx has a stable population of resident flora that may be anaerobic or aerobic. When stress occurs, such as with illness, surgery, or infection, pathogenic organisms replace normal resident flora. Previous antibiotic therapy also affects the resident flora population, making replacement by pathologic organisms more likely. The pathogens are then able to invade the sterile lower respiratory tract.[51]

Disruption of the gag and cough reflexes, altered consciousness, abnormal swallowing, and artificial airways all predispose the patient to aspiration and colonization of the lungs and subsequent infection. Histamine blockers, antacids, and enteral feedings also contribute to this problem because they raise the pH of the stomach and promote bacterial overgrowth. The nasogastric tube then acts as a wick, facilitating the movement of bacteria from the stomach to the pharynx, where the bacteria can be aspirated.[47]

Infection results in pulmonary inflammation with or without significant exudates. Increased capillary

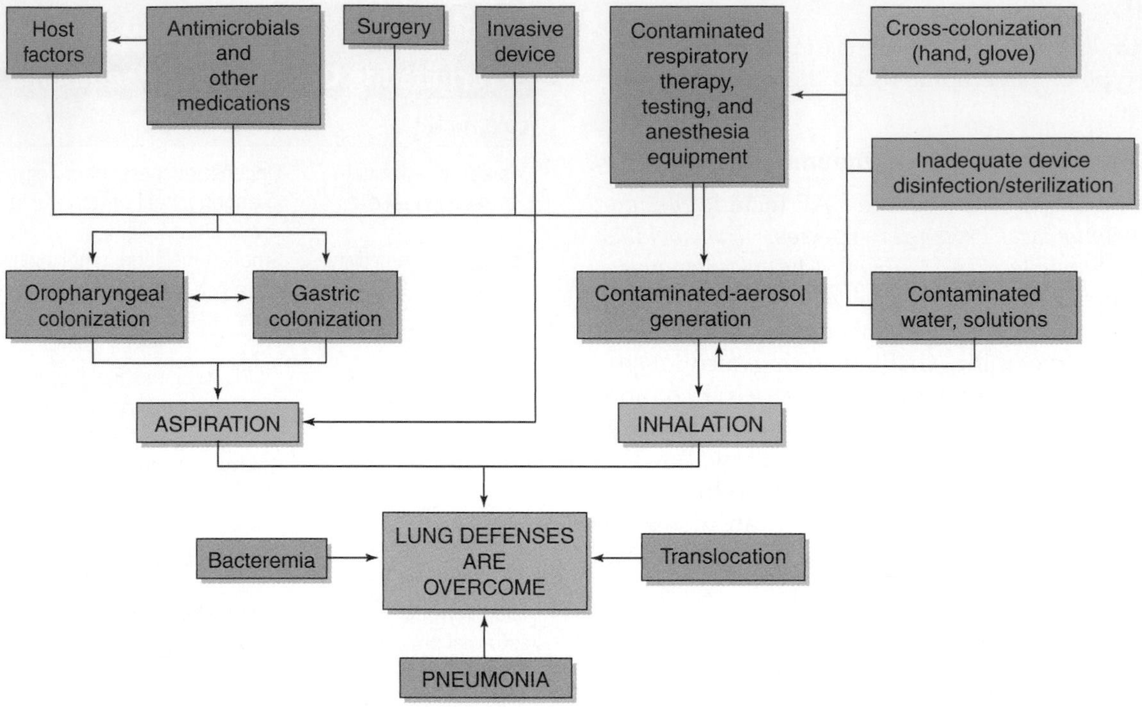

FIGURE 15-2. Pathophysiology of pneumonia. (From Tablan OC et al: *Am J Infect Control* 22:247, 1994.)

permeability occurs with increased interstitial and alveolar fluid. V/Q mismatching and intrapulmonary shunting occurs, resulting in hypoxemia as lung consolidation progresses. Untreated pneumonia can result in ARF and initiation of the inflammatory-immune response. In addition, the patient may develop a pleural effusion. This is the result of the vascular response to inflammation, whereby capillary permeability is increased and fluid from the pulmonary capillaries diffuses into the pleural space.[47,53]

Prevention of VAP is discussed under the mechanical ventilation section of Chapter 16.

Assessment and Diagnosis

The clinical manifestations of pneumonia will vary with the offending pathogen. The patient may present with a variety of signs and symptoms, including dyspnea, fever, and cough (productive or nonproductive).[54] Coarse crackles on auscultation and dullness to percussion may also be present.[54]

Chest radiography is used to evaluate the patient with suspected pneumonia. The diagnosis is established by the presence of a new pulmonary infiltrate. The radiographic pattern of the infiltrates will vary with the organism.[54] A sputum Gram stain and culture are done to facilitate the identification of the infectious pathogen. In 50% of cases, though, a causative agent is not identified.[47] A diagnostic bronchoscopy may be needed, particularly if the diagnosis is unclear or current therapy is not working.[48] In addition, a complete blood count with differential, chemistry panel, blood cultures, and arterial blood gas levels are obtained.[50]

Medical Management

Medical management of the patient with pneumonia should include antibiotic therapy, oxygen therapy for hypoxemia, mechanical ventilation if acute respiratory failure develops, fluid management for hydration, nutritional support, and treatment of associated medical problems and complications. For patients having difficulty mobilizing secretions, a therapeutic bronchoscopy may be necessary.[48,49]

Antibiotic Therapy

Although bacteria-specific antibiotic therapy is the goal, this may not always be possible because of difficulties in identifying the organism and the seriousness of the patient's condition. The time involved obtaining cultures should be balanced against the need to begin some treatment based on patient condition. Empirical therapy has become a generally acceptable approach. In this approach, choice of antibiotic treatment is based on the most likely etiologic organism while avoiding toxicity, superinfection, and unnecessary cost. If available, Gram stain results should be used to guide choices of antibiotics. Antibiotics should be chosen that offer broad coverage of the usual pathogens in the hospital or community. Failure to respond to such therapy may indicate that the chosen antibiotic regi-

Box 15-6

NURSING DIAGNOSIS PRIORITIES

Pneumonia

- Ineffective Airway Clearance related to excessive secretions or abnormal viscosity of mucus, p. A-33
- Impaired Gas Exchange related to ventilation/perfusion mismatching or intrapulmonary shunting, p. A-29
- Risk for Infection Risk Factor: invasive monitoring devices, p. A-46
- Powerlessness related to lack of control over current situation or disease progression, p. A-44

men does not appropriately cover all of the etiologic pathogens or that a new source of infection has developed.[49,50]

Independent Lung Ventilation

In patients with unilateral pneumonia or severely asymmetric pneumonia, this alternative mode of mechanical ventilation may be necessary to facilitate oxygenation. As the alveoli in the affected lung become flooded with pus, the lung becomes less compliant and difficult to ventilate. This results in a shifting of ventilation to the good lung without a concomitant shift in perfusion and thus an increase in V/Q mismatching. Independent lung ventilation (ILV) allows each lung to be ventilated separately, thus controlling the amount of flow, volume, and pressure each lung receives. A double-lumen endotracheal tube is inserted, and each lumen is usually attached to a separate mechanical ventilator. The ventilator settings are then customized to the needs of each lung to facilitate optimal oxygenation and ventilation.[55]

Nursing Management

Nursing management of the patient with pneumonia incorporates a variety of nursing diagnoses (Box 15-6). **Nursing priorities are directed toward (1) optimizing oxygenation and ventilation, (2) preventing the spread of infection, (3) providing comfort and emotional support, and (4) maintaining surveillance for complications.** In addition, the patient's response to the antibiotic therapy should be monitored for adverse effects.

Optimizing Oxygenation and Ventilation

Nursing interventions to optimize oxygenation and ventilation include positioning, preventing desaturation, and promoting secretion clearance. For further discussion on these interventions, see Nursing Management of ARF.

Preventing the Spread of Infection. Prevention should be directed at eradicating pathogens from the environment and interrupting the spread of organisms from person to person. Significant progress has been made in removing contaminants from the patient environment through proper disinfection of respiratory equipment and increased use of disposable supplies. Other possible environmental sources of pathogens include suctioning equipment and indwelling lines. These invasive tools must be given proper aseptic care.[51]

Proper hand hygiene is the single most important measure available to prevent the spread of bacteria from person to person (see Evidence-Based Collaborative Practice: Hand Hygiene Guidelines). In addition, meticulous oral care, including suctioning of the secretions pooling above the cuff of the artificial airway,

EVIDENCE-BASED COLLABORATIVE PRACTICE

Hand Hygiene Guidelines

- Wash hands with soap and water when visibly dirty or contaminated with blood and other body fluids.
- When washing hands with soap and water, wet hands first with water, apply an amount of product recommended by the manufacturer to hands, and rub hands together vigorously for at least 15 seconds, covering all surfaces of the hands and fingers. Rinse hands with water and dry thoroughly with a disposable towel. Use towel to turn off the faucet. Avoid using hot water, because repeated exposure to hot water may increase the risk of dermatitis.
- If hands are not visibly soiled, use an alcohol-based hand rub for routinely decontaminating hands.
- When decontaminating hands with an alcohol-based hand rub, apply product to palm of one hand and rub hands together, covering all surfaces of hands and fingers, until hands are dry (follow the manufacturer's recommendations regarding the volume of product to use).
- Decontaminate hands before and after having direct contact with patients.
- Decontaminate hands before and after donning gloves.
- Wear gloves when contact with blood or other potentially infectious materials, mucous membranes, or nonintact skin could occur.
- Change gloves during patient care if moving from a contaminated body site to a clean body site.
- Remove gloves after caring for a patient. Do not wear the same pair of gloves for the care of more than one patient, and do not wash gloves between uses with different patients.
- Decontaminate hands after contact with inanimate objects (including medical equipment).
- Do not wear artificial fingernails or extenders when having direct contact with patients at high risk (e.g., those in critical care units or operating rooms).
- Keep natural nails tips less than 1/4-inch long.

From Advisory Committee and the HICPAC/SHEA/APIC/IDSA Hand Hygiene Task Force: *MMWR* 51(RR16):1, 2002.

Box 15-7

Collaborative Management

Pneumonia

- Administer oxygen therapy
- Initiate mechanical ventilation as required
- Administer medications
  - Antibiotics
  - Bronchodilators
- Position patient to optimize ventilation/perfusion matching
- Suction as needed
- Provide adequate rest and recovery time between various procedures
- Maintain surveillance for complications
  - Acute respiratory failure
- Provide comfort and emotional support

is critical to decreasing the bacterial colonization of the oropharynx.[30]

Collaborative management of the patient with pneumonia is outlined in Box 15-7.

ASPIRATION PNEUMONITIS

The presence of abnormal substances in the airways and alveoli as a result of aspiration is misleadingly called *aspiration pneumonia.* This term is misleading because the aspiration of toxic substances into the lung may or may not involve an infection. *Aspiration pneumonitis* is a more accurate title, because injury to the lung can result from the chemical, mechanical, and/or bacterial characteristics of the aspirate.

ETIOLOGY

A number of factors have been identified that place the patient at risk for aspiration (Table 15-4). Gastric

Table 15-4

Risk Factors for Aspiration/Aspiration-Related Pneumonia

RISK FACTOR	RATIONALE
Decreased LOC, either because of CNS problems or use of sedatives	Decreased ability to protect airway from oropharyngeal secretions and regurgitated gastric contents Cough and gag reflexes diminish as LOC diminishes, whether from CNS disorder or sedation Slowed gastric emptying Decreased tone of lower esophageal sphincter
Supine position	Increases probability of gastroesophageal reflux
Presence of a nasogastric tube	Interferes with closure of lower esophageal sphincter Biofilm on tube predisposes to aspiration of pathogenic organisms
Vomiting	Sudden and forceful entry of gastric contents into oropharynx predisposes to aspiration Predisposes to displacement of feeding tube ports into esophagus
Feeding tube ports positioned in esophagus	Infused feedings reflux into oropharynx
Tracheal intubation	Reduction in upper airway defense related to ineffective cough, desensitization of the oropharynx and larynx, disuse atrophy of laryngeal muscles, and esophageal compression by an inflated cuff
Mechanical ventilation	Positive abdominal pressure predisposes to aspiration of gastric contents, probably by increasing gastroesophageal reflux
Accumulation of subglottic secretions above endotracheal cuff	Subglottic secretions can leak around cuff into the lower respiratory tract, especially when cuff is deflated.
Inadequate cuff inflation of tracheal devices	Persistent low cuff pressure (e.g., 20 cm H_2O) predisposes to aspiration of oropharyngeal secretions and refluxed gastric contents
Gastric feeding site when gastric emptying significantly impaired	Accumulation of formula and gastrointestinal secretions predisposes to gastroesophageal reflux and aspiration
High GRVs	High GRVs predispose to gastroesophageal reflux and aspiration
Bolus feedings	Volume of infused formula may exceed the tolerance of patients who have poor cough and gag reflexes
Poor oral health	Colonized oropharyngeal secretions may be aspirated into respiratory tract
Advanced age	Older patients tend to have a reduced swallowing ability and are more likely to have neurologic disorders that increase aspiration risk Strong association between advanced age and probability of developing pneumonia once aspiration has occurred
Hyperglycemia	Even mild hyperglycemia can cause delayed gastric emptying by disrupting postprandial antral contractions

CNS, Central nervous system; *GRVs,* gastric residual volumes; *LOC,* level of consciousness.

From Metheny NA: *Respir Care Clin* 12:603, 2006.

contents and oropharyngeal bacteria (see Pneumonia) are the most common aspirates of the critically ill patient.[56,57] The effects of gastric contents on the lungs will vary based on the pH of the liquid. If the pH is less than 2.5, the patient will develop a severe chemical pneumonitis resulting in hypoxemia. If the pH is greater than 2.5, the immediate damage to the lungs will be lessened but the elevated pH may have promoted bacterial overgrowth of the stomach.[56,57] Once the bacteria-laden gastric contents are aspirated into the lungs, overwhelming bacterial pneumonia can develop.[57]

PATHOPHYSIOLOGY

The type of lung injury that develops after aspiration is determined by a number of factors, including the quality of the aspirate and the status of the patient's respiratory defense mechanisms.

Acid Liquid

The aspiration of acid (pH <2.5) liquid gastric contents results in the development of bronchospasm and atelectasis almost immediately. Over the next 4 hours, tracheal damage, bronchitis, bronchiolitis, alveolar-capillary breakdown, interstitial edema, and alveolar congestion and hemorrhage occur.[58] Severe hypoxemia develops as a result of intrapulmonary shunting and V/Q mismatching. As the disorder progresses, necrotic debris and fibrin fill the alveoli, hyaline membranes form, and hypoxic vasoconstriction occurs, resulting in elevated pulmonary artery pressures.[57,58] The clinical course will follow one of three patterns: (1) rapid improvement in 1 week, (2) initial improvement followed by deterioration and development of ALI or pneumonia, or (3) rapid death from progressive ARF.[58]

Acid Food Particles

The aspiration of acid (pH <2.5) nonobstructing food particles can produce the most severe pulmonary reaction because of extensive pulmonary damage.[58] Severe hypoxemia, hypercapnia, and acidosis occur.[57,58]

Nonacid Liquid

The aspiration of nonacid (pH >2.5) liquid gastric contents is similar to acid liquid aspiration initially but with minimal structural damage occurring.[58] Intrapulmonary shunting and V/Q mismatching usually start to reverse within 4 hours, and hypoxemia clears within 24 hours.[57,58]

Nonacid Food Particles

The aspiration of nonacid (pH >2.5) nonobstructing food particles is similar to acid aspiration initially, with significant edema and hemorrhage occurring within 6 hours. After the initial reaction, the response changes to a foreign body type of reaction with granuloma formation occurring around the food particles within 1 to 5 days.[58] In addition to hypoxemia, hypercapnia and acidosis occur as a result of hypoventilation.[57,58]

ASSESSMENT AND DIAGNOSIS

Clinically, the patient presents with signs of acute respiratory distress, and gastric contents may be present in the oropharynx. The patient will have shortness of breath, coughing, wheezing, cyanosis, and signs of hypoxemia. Tachypnea, tachycardia, hypotension, fever, and crackles also are present. Copious amounts of sputum are produced as alveolar edema develops.[56,57]

ABG levels reflect severe hypoxemia. Chest x-ray film changes appear 12 to 24 hours after the initial aspiration, with no one pattern being diagnostic of the event. Infiltrates will appear in a variety of distribution patterns depending on the position of the patient during aspiration and the volume of the aspirate. If bacterial infection becomes established, leukocytosis and positive sputum cultures occur.[57]

MEDICAL MANAGEMENT

Management of the patient with aspiration lung disorder includes both emergency and follow-up treatment. When aspiration is witnessed, emergency treatment should be instituted to secure the airway and minimize pulmonary damage. The upper airway should be immediately suctioned to remove the gastric contents.[56,57] Direct visualization by bronchoscopy is indicated to remove large particulate aspirate[56] or to confirm an unwitnessed aspiration event.[58] Bronchoalveolar lavage is not recommended because this practice disseminates the aspirate in lungs and increases damage. Prophylactic antibiotics are also not recommended.[58]

After airway clearance, attention should be given to supporting oxygenation and hemodynamics. Hypoxemia should be corrected with supplemental oxygen or mechanical ventilation with PEEP, if necessary.[56-58] Hemodynamic changes result from fluid shifts into the lungs that can occur after massive aspirations. Monitoring intravascular volume is essential, and judicious amounts of replacement fluids should be instituted to maintain adequate urinary output and vital signs.[58]

Initially antibiotic therapy is not indicated. If symptoms fail to resolve within 48 hours, empiric antibiotic therapy should be initiated. Corticosteroids have not demonstrated to be of any benefit in the treatment of aspiration pneumonitis and thus are not recommended.[57]

NURSING MANAGEMENT

Nursing management of the patient with aspiration lung disorder incorporates a variety of nursing diagnoses

Box 15-8

NURSING DIAGNOSIS PRIORITIES

Aspiration Lung Disorder

- Impaired Gas Exchange related to ventilation/perfusion mismatching or intrapulmonary shunting, p. A-29
- Ineffective Airway Clearance related to excessive secretions or abnormal viscosity of mucus, p. A-33
- Risk for Aspiration, p. A-45
- Risk for Infection, p. A-46
- Ineffective Coping related to situational crisis and personal vulnerability, p. A-39

Box 15-9

Collaborative Management

Aspiration Pneumonitis

- Administer oxygen therapy
- Secure patient's airway
- Place patient in slight Trendelenburg position
- Turn patient to right lateral decubitus position
- Suction patient's oropharyngeal area
- Initiate mechanical ventilation as required
- Maintain surveillance for complications
  - Pneumonia
  - Acute respiratory failure
  - Acute lung injury
- Provide comfort and emotional support

(Box 15-8). **Nursing priorities are directed toward (1) optimizing oxygenation and ventilation, (2) preventing further aspiration events, (3) providing comfort and emotional support, and (4) maintaining surveillance for complications.**

Optimizing Oxygenation and Ventilation

Nursing interventions to optimize oxygenation and ventilation include positioning, preventing desaturation, and promoting secretion clearance. For further discussion on these interventions, see Nursing Management of ARF.

Preventing Aspiration

One of the most important interventions for preventing aspiration is identifying the patient at risk for aspiration. Actions to prevent aspiration include confirming feeding tube placement, checking for signs and symptoms of feeding intolerance, elevating the head of the bed at least 30 degrees, feeding the patient via a small-bore feeding tube or gastrostomy tube, avoiding the use of a large-bore nasogastric tube, ensuring proper inflation of artificial airway cuffs, and frequent suctioning of the oropharynx of an intubated patient to prevent secretions from pooling above the cuff of the tube. For patients at risk for aspiration or intolerant of gastric feedings, the feeding tube should be placed in the small bowel.[59]

Collaborative management of the patient with aspiration pneumonitis is outlined in Box 15-9.

PULMONARY EMBOLISM

DESCRIPTION

A pulmonary embolism (PE) occurs when a clot (thrombotic emboli) or other matter (nonthrombotic emboli) lodges in the pulmonary arterial system, disrupting the blood flow to a region of the lungs. The majority of thrombotic emboli arise from the deep leg veins, particularly the iliac, femoral, and popliteal veins.[60] Other sources include the right ventricle, the upper extremities, and the pelvic veins. Nonthrombotic emboli arise from fat, tumors, amniotic fluid, air, and foreign bodies. This section of the chapter focuses on thrombotic emboli.

ETIOLOGY

A number of predisposing factors and precipitating conditions put a patient at risk for developing a PE (Box 15-10). Of the three predisposing factors (i.e., hypercoagulability, injury to vascular endothelium, and venous stasis [Virchow's triad]), endothelial injury appears to be the most significant.[60]

PATHOPHYSIOLOGY

A massive PE occurs with the blockage of a lobar or larger artery, resulting in occlusion of more than 40% of the pulmonary vascular bed. Blockage of the pulmonary arterial system has both pulmonary and hemodynamic consequences. The effects on the pulmonary system are increased alveolar dead space, bronchoconstriction, and compensatory shunting. The hemodynamic effects include an increase in pulmonary vascular resistance and right ventricular workload.[61]

Increased Dead Space

An increase in alveolar dead space occurs because an area of the lung is receiving ventilation without being perfused. The ventilation to this area is known as *wasted ventilation,* because it does not participate in gas exchange. This effect leads to alveolar dead space ventilation and an increase in the work of breathing. To limit the amount of dead space ventilation, localized bronchoconstriction occurs.[61]

Bronchoconstriction

Bronchoconstriction develops as a result of alveolar hypocarbia, hypoxia, and the release of mediators. Alveolar hypocarbia occurs as a consequence of decreased carbon dioxide in the affected area and leads

Box 15-10

Risk Factors for Pulmonary Thromboembolism

Predisposing Factors

- Venous stasis
  - Atrial fibrillation
  - Decreased cardiac output (CO)
  - Immobility
- Injury to vascular endothelium
  - Local vessel injury
  - Infection
  - Incision
  - Atherosclerosis
- Hypercoagulability
  - Polycythemia

Precipitating Conditions

- Previous pulmonary embolus
- Cardiovascular disease
  - Heart failure
  - Right ventricular infarction
  - Cardiomyopathy
  - Cor pulmonale
- Surgery
  - Orthopedic
  - Vascular
  - Abdominal
- Cancer
  - Ovarian
  - Pancreatic
  - Stomach
  - Extrahepatic bile duct system
- Trauma (injury or burns)
  - Lower extremities
  - Pelvis
  - Hips
- Gynecologic status
  - Pregnancy
  - Postpartum
  - Birth control pills
  - Estrogen replacement therapy

to constriction of the local airways, increased airway resistance, and redistribution of ventilation to perfused areas of the lungs. A variety of mediators are released from the site of the injury, either from the clot or the surrounding lung tissue, which further causes constriction of the airways. Bronchoconstriction promotes the development of atelectasis.[61]

Compensatory Shunting

Compensatory shunting occurs because the unaffected areas of the lungs have to accommodate the entire cardiac output. This creates a situation in which perfusion exceeds ventilation and blood is returned to the left side of the heart without participating in gas exchange. This leads to the development of hypoxemia.[61]

Hemodynamic Consequences

The major hemodynamic consequence of a PE is the development of pulmonary hypertension, which is part of the effect of a mechanical obstruction when more than 50% of the vascular bed is occluded. In addition, the mediators released at the injury site and the development of hypoxia cause pulmonary vasoconstriction, which further exacerbates pulmonary hypertension. As the pulmonary vascular resistance increases, so does the workload of the right ventricle as reflected by a rise in pulmonary artery (PA) pressures. Consequently, right ventricular failure occurs, which can lead to a decrease in left ventricular preload, decrease in CO, decrease in blood pressure, and shock.[61]

Assessment and Diagnosis

The patient with a pulmonary embolism may have any number of presenting signs and symptoms, with the most common being tachycardia and tachypnea. Additional signs and symptoms that may be present include dyspnea, apprehension, increased pulmonic component of the second heart sound (P_1), fever, rales, pleuritic chest pain, cough, evidence of a deep vein thrombosis (DVT), and hemoptysis.[61] Syncope and hemodynamic instability can occur as a result of right ventricular failure.[60]

Initial laboratory studies and diagnostic procedures that may be done are ABG analysis, d-dimer, electrocardiogram (ECG), chest radiography, and echocardiography (ECHO). ABG analysis may show a low Pao_2, indicating hypoxemia; a low $Paco_2$, indicating hypocarbia; and a high pH, indicating a respiratory alkalosis. The hypocarbia with resulting respiratory alkalosis is caused by tachypnea.[60] The D-dimer is used to rule out PE as a diagnosis. An elevated D-dimer will occur with a PE and a number of other disorders. A normal D-dimer will not occur with a PE and thus can be used to rule a PE out as the diagnosis.[62] The most frequent ECG finding seen in the patient with a PE is sinus tachycardia[60] The classic ECG pattern often associated with a PE, S wave in lead I and Q wave with inverted T wave in lead III, is seen in fewer than 20% of the patients.[60] Other ECG findings associated with a PE include right bundle branch block, new-onset atrial fibrillation, T-wave inversion in the anterior or inferior leads,[60] and ST-segment changes.[61] Chest x-ray examination findings vary from normal to abnormal and are of little value in confirming the presence of a PE. Abnormal findings include cardiomegaly, pleural effusion, elevated hemidiaphragm, enlargement of the right descending pulmonary artery (Palla sign), a wedge-shaped density above the diaphragm (Hampton hump), and the presence of atelectasis.[60]An ECHO, either transthoracic or transesophageal, is also useful in the identification of a PE because it can provide visualization of any emboli in the central pulmonary arteries. In addition, it can be used for assessing the hemodynamic consequences of the PE on the right side of the heart.[62]

Differentiating a PE from other illnesses can be difficult because many of its clinical manifestations are found in a variety of other disorders.[60] Thus a variety of other tests may be necessary, including a V/Q scintigraphy, pulmonary angiogram, and DVT studies.[60-62] Given the advent of more sophisticated CT scanners, the spiral CT is also being used to diagnose a PE.[62,63] A definitive diagnosis of a PE requires confirmation by a high-probability V/Q scan, positive pulmonary angiogram, positive CT, or strong clinical suspicion coupled with abnormal findings on lower extremity DVT studies.[62]

Box 15-11

NURSING DIAGNOSIS PRIORITIES

Pulmonary Embolus

- Impaired Gas Exchange related to ventilation/ perfusion mismatching or intrapulmonary shunting, p. A-29
- Acute Pain related to transmission and perception of cutaneous, visceral, muscular, or ischemic impulses, p. A-7
- Powerlessness related to lack of control over current situation or disease progression, p. A-44
- Deficient Knowledge: Discharge Regimen related to lack of previous exposure to information (see Patient Education: Pulmonary Embolus), p. A-18

Medical Management

Medical management of the patient with a pulmonary embolism involves both prevention and treatment strategies. Prevention strategies include the use of prophylactic anticoagulation with low-dose or adjusted-dose heparin, low-molecular-weight heparin, or oral anticoagulants. The use of graduated compression stockings and intermittent pneumatic leg compression have also been demonstrated as effective methods of prophylaxis in low-risk patients.[64]

Treatment strategies include preventing the recurrence of a PE, facilitating clot dissolution, reversing the effects of pulmonary hypertension, promoting gas exchange, and preventing complications. Medical interventions to promote gas exchange include supplemental oxygen administration, intubation, and mechanical ventilation.[61]

Prevention of Recurrence

Interventions to prevent the recurrence of a PE include the administration of unfractionated or low-molecular-weight heparin and warfarin (Coumadin).[64] Heparin is administered to prevent further clots from forming and has no effect on the existing clot. The heparin should be adjusted to maintain the activated partial thromboplastin time (aPTT) in the range of 1.5 to 2.3 times control.[64] Warfarin should be started at the same time, and when the international normalized ratio (INR) reaches 3.0, the heparin should be discontinued. The INR should be maintained between 2.0 and 3.0. The patient should remain on warfarin for 3 to 12 months depending on the patient's risk for thromboembolic disease.[64]

Interruption of the inferior vena cava is reserved for patients in whom anticoagulation is contraindicated. The procedure involves placement of a percutaneous venous filter (e.g., Greenfield filter) into the vena cava, usually below the renal arteries. The filter prevents further thrombotic emboli from migrating into the lungs.[64]

Clot Dissolution

The administration of thrombolytic agents in the treatment of PE has had limited success. Currently, thrombolytic therapy is reserved for the patient with a massive PE and concomitant hemodynamic instability. Either recombinant tissue-type plasminogen activator (rt-PA) or streptokinase may be used. The therapeutic window for using thrombolytic therapy is 14 days.[65]

Though often considered as a last resort, a pulmonary embolectomy may be performed to surgically remove the clot. Generally it is performed as an open procedure while the patient is on cardiopulmonary bypass.[66]

Reversal of Pulmonary Hypertension

To reverse the hemodynamic effects of pulmonary hypertension, additional measures may be taken. These include the administration of inotropic agents and fluid. Fluids should be administered to increase right ventricular preload, which would stretch the right ventricle and increase contractility, thus overcoming the elevated pulmonary arterial pressures. Inotropic agents also can be used to increase contractility to facilitate an increase in CO.[61]

Nursing Management

Prevention of pulmonary embolism should be a major nursing focus, because the majority of critically ill patients are at risk for this disorder. Nursing actions are aimed at preventing the development of DVT, which is a major complication of immobility and a leading cause of PE. These measures include the use of antiembolic stockings and/or pneumatic compression stockings, elevation of the legs, active/passive range-of-motion exercises, adequate hydration, and progressive ambulation.

Nursing management of the patient with a PE incorporates a variety of nursing diagnoses (Box 15-11).

PATIENT EDUCATION

Pulmonary Embolus

- Pathophysiology of disease
- Specific etiology
- Precipitating factor modification
- Measures to prevent deep vein thrombosis (e.g., avoid tight-fitting clothes, crossing legs, and prolonged sitting or standing; elevate legs when sitting; exercise)
- Signs and symptoms of deep vein thrombosis (e.g., redness, swelling, sharp or deep leg pain)
- Importance of taking medications
- Signs and symptoms of anticoagulant complications (e.g., excessive bruising, discoloration of the skin, changes in color of urine or stools)
- Measures to prevent bleeding (e.g., use soft-bristle toothbrush, caution when shaving)

Box 15-12

Collaborative Management

Pulmonary Embolus

- Administer oxygen therapy
- Intubate patient
- Initiate mechanical ventilation
- Administer medications
  - Thrombolytic therapy
  - Anticoagulants
  - Bronchodilators
  - Inotropic agents
  - Sedatives
  - Analgesics
- Administer fluids
- Position patient to optimize ventilation/perfusion matching
- Maintain surveillance for complications
  - Bleeding
  - Acute lung injury
- Provide comfort and emotional support

Nursing priorities are directed toward (1) optimizing oxygenation and ventilation, (2) monitoring for bleeding, (3) providing comfort and emotional support, and (4) maintaining surveillance for complications.

Optimizing Oxygenation and Ventilation

Nursing interventions to optimize oxygenation and ventilation include positioning, preventing desaturation, and promoting secretion clearance. For further discussion on these interventions, see Nursing Management of ARF.

Monitoring for Bleeding

The patient receiving anticoagulant or thrombolytic therapy should be observed for signs of bleeding. The patient's gums, skin, urine, stool, and emesis should be screened for signs of overt or covert bleeding. In addition, monitoring the patient's INR or aPTT is critical to managing the anticoagulation therapy.

Patient Education

Early in the patient's hospital stay, the patient and family should be taught about pulmonary embolus, its etiologies, and its treatment. As the patient moves toward discharge, teaching should focus on the interventions necessary for preventing the reoccurrence of deep vein thrombosis and subsequent emboli, signs and symptoms of deep vein thrombosis and anticoagulant complications, and measures to prevent bleeding. If the patient smokes, he or she should be encouraged to stop smoking and be referred to a smoking cessation program.

Collaborative management of the patient with a pulmonary embolus is outlined in Box 15-12.

STATUS ASTHMATICUS

Description

Asthma is a chronic obstructive pulmonary disease that is characterized by partially reversible airflow obstruction, airway inflammation, and hyperresponsiveness to a variety of stimuli.[67] Status asthmaticus is a severe asthma attack that fails to respond to conventional therapy with bronchodilators, which may result in acute respiratory failure.[68]

Etiology

The precipitating cause of the attack is usually an upper respiratory infection, allergen exposure, or a decrease in antiinflammatory medications. Other factors that have been implicated include overreliance on bronchodilators, environmental pollutants, lack of access to health care, failure to identify worsening airflow obstruction, and noncompliance with the health care regimen.[67]

Pathophysiology

An asthma attack is initiated when exposure to an irritant or trigger occurs, resulting in the initiation of the inflammatory-immune response in the airways. Bronchospasm occurs along with increased vascular permeability and increased mucus production. Mucosal edema and thick, tenacious mucus further increase airway responsiveness. The combination of bronchospasm, airway inflammation, and hyperresponsiveness results in narrowing of the airways and airflow obstruction. These changes have significant effects on the pulmonary and cardiovascular systems.[67]

Pulmonary Effects

As the diameter of the airways decreases, airway resistance increases, resulting in increased residual volume, hyperinflation of the lungs, increased work of breathing, and abnormal distribution of ventilation. V/Q mismatching occurs, which results in hypoxemia. Alveolar dead space also increases as hypoxic vasoconstriction occurs, resulting in hypercapnia.[67]

Cardiovascular Effects

Inspiratory muscle force also increases in an attempt to ventilate the hyperinflated lungs. This results in a significant increase in negative intrapleural pressure, leading to an increase in venous return and pooling of blood in the right ventricle. The stretched right ventricle causes the intraventricular septum to shift, thereby impinging on the left ventricle. In addition, the left ventricle has to work harder to pump blood from the markedly negative pressure in the thorax to elevated pressure in systemic circulation. This leads to a decrease in cardiac output and a fall in systolic blood pressure on inspiration (pulsus paradoxus).[67]

Assessment and Diagnosis

Initially the patient may present with a cough, wheezing, and dyspnea. As the attack continues, the patient develops tachypnea, tachycardia, diaphoresis, increased accessory muscle use, and pulsus paradoxus greater than 25 mm Hg. Decreased level of consciousness, inability to speak, significantly diminished or absent breath sounds, and inability to lie supine herald the onset of acute respiratory failure.[68-70]

Initial ABG levels indicate hypocapnia and respiratory alkalosis caused by hyperventilation. As the attack continues and the patient starts to fatigue, hypoxemia and hypercapnia develop.[68] Lactic acidosis also may occur as a result of lactate overproduction by the respiratory muscles. The end result is the development of respiratory and metabolic acidosis.[69]

Deterioration of pulmonary function tests despite aggressive bronchodilator therapy is diagnostic of status asthmaticus and indicates the potential need for intubation. A peak expiratory flow rate (PEFR) less than 40% of predicted or an FEV_1 (maximum volume of gas that the patient can exhale in 1 second [forced expiratory volume in 1 second]) less than 20% of predicted indicates severe airflow obstruction, and the need for intubation with mechanical ventilation may be imminent.[70]

Medical Management

Medical management of the patient with status asthmaticus is directed toward supporting oxygenation and ventilation. Bronchodilators, corticosteroids, oxygen therapy, and intubation and mechanical ventilation are the mainstays of therapy.[68]

Bronchodilators

Inhaled β_2-agonists and anticholinergics are the bronchodilators of choice for status asthmaticus. β_2-Agonists promote bronchodilation and can be administered by nebulizer or metered-dose inhaler (MDI). Usually larger and more frequent doses are given, and the drug is titrated to the patient's response. Anticholinergics that inhibit bronchoconstriction are not very effective by themselves, but in conjunction with β_2-agonists they have a synergistic effect and produce a greater improvement in airflow. The routine use of xanthines is not recommended in the treatment of status asthmaticus because they have been shown to have no therapeutic benefit.[67-70]

A number of studies have focused on the bronchodilator abilities of magnesium. Although it has been demonstrated that magnesium is inferior to β_2-agonists as a bronchodilator, in patients who are refractory to conventional treatment, magnesium may be beneficial. A bolus of 1 to 4 g of intravenous magnesium given over 10 to 40 minutes has been reported to produce desirable effects.[67,68,70]

A number of studies of other studies are evaluating the effects of leukotriene inhibitors, such as zafirlukast, montelukast, and zileuton, in the treatment of status asthmaticus. Leukotrienes are inflammatory mediators known to cause bronchoconstriction and airway inflammation. Research suggests that these agents may be beneficial as bronchodilators in those patients who are refractory to β_2-agonists.[70]

Systemic Corticosteroids

Intravenous or oral corticosteroids also are used in the treatment of status asthmaticus. Their antiinflammatory effects limit mucosal edema, decrease mucus production, and potentiate β_2-agonists. It usually takes 6 to 8 hours for the effects of the corticosteroids to become evident.[68] The use of inhaled corticosteroids for the treatment of status asthmaticus remains undecided at this time.[67,70] Initial studies indicate they may be beneficial in certain patient populations.[70]

Oxygen Therapy

Initial treatment of hypoxemia is with supplemental oxygen. High-flow oxygen therapy is administered to keep the patient's SpO_2 greater than 92%.[67]

Another therapy currently under investigation is heliox. A mixture of helium and oxygen, heliox has a lower density and higher viscosity than an oxygen and air mixture. Heliox is believed to reduce the work of breathing and improve gas exchange because it flows more easily through constricted areas. Studies have shown that it reduces air trapping and carbon dioxide and helps relieve respiratory acidosis.[67]

Intubation and Mechanical Ventilation

Indications for mechanical ventilation include cardiac or respiratory arrest, disorientation, failure to respond to bronchodilator therapy, and exhaustion.[67,69,70] A large endotracheal tube (8 mm) should be used to decrease airway resistance and to facilitate suctioning of secretions. Ventilating the patient with status asthmaticus can be very difficult. High inflation pressures should be avoided because they can result in barotrauma. The use of PEEP should be monitored closely because the patient is prone to developing air trapping. Patient-ventilator asynchrony also can be a major problem. Sedation and neuromuscular paralysis may be necessary to allow for adequate ventilation of the patient.[67,69]

Nursing Management

Nursing management of the patient with status asthmaticus incorporates a variety of nursing diagnoses (Box 15-13). **Nursing priorities are directed toward (1) optimizing oxygenation and ventilation, (2) providing comfort and emotional support, and (3) maintaining surveillance for complications.**

Optimizing Oxygenation and Ventilation

Nursing interventions to optimize oxygenation and ventilation include positioning, preventing desaturation, and promoting secretion clearance. For further discussion on these interventions, see Nursing Management of ARF.

Patient Education

Early in the patient's hospital stay, the patient and family should be taught about asthma, its triggers, and its treatment. As the patient moves toward discharge, teaching should focus on the interventions necessary for preventing the recurrence of status asthmaticus, early warning signs of worsening airflow obstruction, correct use of an inhaler and a peak flow meter, measures to prevent pulmonary infections, and signs and symptoms of a pulmonary infection. If the patient smokes, he or she should be encouraged to stop smoking and be referred to a smoking cessation program. In addition, the importance of participating in a pulmonary rehabilitation program should be stressed.

Collaborative management of the patient with status asthmaticus is outlined in Box 15-14.

Box 15-13

NURSING DIAGNOSIS PRIORITIES

Status Asthmaticus

- Impaired Gas Exchange related to alveolar hypoventilation, p. A-29
- Ineffective Breathing Pattern related to musculoskeletal fatigue or neuromuscular impairment, p. A-34
- Ineffective Airway Clearance related to excessive secretions or abnormal viscosity of mucus, p. A-33
- Anxiety related to threat to biologic, psychologic, and/or social integrity, p. A-9
- Deficient Knowledge: Discharge Regimen related to lack of previous exposure to information (see Patient Education: Status Asthmaticus), p. A-18

LONG-TERM MECHANICAL VENTILATION DEPENDENCE

Description

Long-term mechanical ventilation dependence (LTMVD) is a secondary disorder that occurs when a patient

PATIENT EDUCATION

Status Asthmaticus

- Pathophysiology of disease
- Specific etiology
- Early warning signs of worsening airflow obstruction (20% drop in peak expiratory flow rate [PEFR] below predicted or personal best, increase in cough, shortness of breath, chest tightness, wheezing)
- Treatment of attacks
- Importance of taking prescribed medications and avoidance of over-the-counter asthma medications
- Correct use of an inhaler (with and without spacer device)
- Correct use of a peak flow meter
- Removal or avoidance of environmental triggers (e.g., pollen; dust; mold spores; cat and dog dander; cold, dry air; strong odors; household aerosols; tobacco smoke; air pollution)
- Measures to prevent pulmonary infections (e.g., proper nutrition and hand washing, immunization against *Streptococcus pneumoniae* and influenza viruses)
- Signs and symptoms of pulmonary infection (e.g., sputum color change, shortness of breath, fever)
- Importance of participating in pulmonary rehabilitation program

Box 15-14

Collaborative Management

Status Asthmaticus

- Administer oxygen therapy
- Intubate patient
- Initiate mechanical ventilation
- Administer medications
  - Bronchodilators
  - Corticosteroids
  - Sedatives
- Maintain surveillance for complications
  - Acute respiratory failure
- Provide comfort and emotional support

Box 15-15

Physiologic Factors Contributing to LTMVD

- Decreased gas exchange
  - Ventilation/perfusion mismatching
  - Intrapulmonary shunting
  - Alveolar hypoventilation
  - Anemia
  - Acute heart failure
- Increased ventilatory workload
  - Decreased lung compliance
  - Increased airway resistance
  - Small endotracheal tube
  - Decreased ventilatory sensitivity
  - Improper positioning
  - Abdominal distention
  - Dyspnea
- Increased ventilatory demand
  - Increased pulmonary dead space
  - Increased metabolic demands
  - Improper ventilator mode/settings
  - Metabolic acidosis
  - Overfeeding
- Decreased ventilatory drive
  - Respiratory alkalosis
  - Metabolic alkalosis
  - Hypothyroidism
  - Sedatives
  - Malnutrition
- Increased respiratory muscle fatigue
  - Increased ventilatory workload
  - Increased ventilatory demand
  - Malnutrition
  - Hypokalemia
  - Hypomagnesemia
  - Hypophosphatemia
  - Hypothyroidism
  - Critical illness polyneuropathy
  - Inadequate muscle rest

LTMVD, Long-term mechanical ventilation dependence.

requires assisted ventilation longer than expected given the patient's underlying condition[71] and has usually failed at least one weaning attempt.[72] It is the result of complex medical problems that do not allow the normal weaning process to take place in a timely manner.

Etiology and Pathophysiology

A wide variety of physiologic and psychologic factors contribute to the development of LTMVD. Physiologic factors include those conditions that result in decreased gas exchange, increased ventilatory workload, increased ventilatory demand, decreased ventilatory drive, and increased respiratory muscle fatigue (Box 15-15).[73] Psychologic factors include those conditions that result in loss of breathing pattern control, lack of motivation and confidence, and delirium (Box 15-16).

Box 15-16

Psychologic Factors Contributing to LTMVD

- Loss of breathing pattern control
  - Anxiety
  - Fear
  - Dyspnea
  - Pain
  - Ventilator asynchrony
  - Lack of confidence in ability to breathe
- Lack of motivation and confidence
  - Inadequate trust in staff
  - Depersonalization
  - Hopelessness
  - Powerlessness
  - Depression
  - Inadequate communication
- Delirium
  - Sensory overload
  - Sensory deprivation
  - Sleep deprivation
  - Pain
  - Medications

LTMVD, Long-term mechanical ventilation dependence.

The development of LTMVD also is affected by the severity and duration of the patient's current illness and any underlying chronic health problems.[74]

Medical and Nursing Management

The goal of medical and nursing management of the patient with LTMVD is successful weaning. The Third National Study Group on Weaning From Mechanical Ventilation, sponsored by the American Association of Critical-Care Nurses, proposed the Weaning Continuum Model that divides weaning into three stages: preweaning, weaning process, and weaning outcome.[75] It is within this framework that the management of the long-term ventilator-dependent patient is described. In addition, the common nursing diagnoses for this patient population are listed in Box 15-17.

Preweaning Stage

For the long-term ventilator-dependent patient, the preweaning phase consists of resolving the precipitating event that necessitated ventilatory assistance and preventing the physiologic and psychologic factors that can interfere with weaning. Before any attempts at weaning, the patient should be assessed for weaning readiness, an approach should be determined, and a method should be selected.[76]

Weaning Preparedness. The patient should be physiologically and psychologically prepared to initiate the weaning process by addressing those factors that can interfere with weaning. Aggressive medical management to prevent and treat ventilation/perfusion

Box 15-17

NURSING DIAGNOSIS PRIORITIES

Long-Term Mechanical Ventilation Dependence

- Impaired Spontaneous Ventilation related to respiratory muscle fatigue or neuromuscular impairment, p. A-30
- Dysfunctional Ventilatory Weaning Response related to physical, psychosocial, or situational factors, p. A-22
- Risk for Aspiration, p. A-45
- Imbalanced Nutrition: Less Than Body Requirements related to lack of exogenous nutrients or increased metabolic demand, p. A-28
- Risk for Infection, p. A-46
- Acute Confusion related to sensory overload, sensory deprivation, and sleep pattern disturbance, p. A-3
- Anxiety related to threat to biologic, psychologic, and/or social integrity, p. A-9
- Powerlessness related to lack of control over current situation or disease progression, p. A-44

mismatching, intrapulmonary shunting, anemia, cardiac failure, decreased lung compliance, increased airway resistance, acid-base disturbances, hypothyroidism, abdominal distention, and electrolyte imbalances should be initiated. In addition, interventions to decrease the work of breathing should be implemented, such as replacing a small endotracheal tube with a larger tube or a tracheostomy, suctioning airway secretions, administering bronchodilators, optimizing the ventilator settings and trigger sensitivity, and positioning the patient in straight alignment with the head of the bed elevated at least 30 degrees. Enteral or parenteral nutrition should be started and the patient's nutritional state optimized. Physical therapy should be initiated for the patient with critical illness polyneuropathy because increased mobility facilitates weaning. A means of communication should be established with the patient. Sedatives can be administered to provide anxiety control, but the avoidance of respiratory depression is critical.[77]

Weaning Readiness. Although a variety of different methods for assessing weaning readiness have been developed, none of them have proven to be very accurate in predicting weaning success in the patient with LTMVD. One study did indicate that the presence of left ventricular dysfunction, fluid imbalance, and nutritional deficiency did increase the duration of mechanical ventilation. Another study suggested that the upward trending of the albumin level may be predictive of weaning success. Because so many variables can affect the patient's ability to wean, any assessment of weaning readiness should incorporate these variables. Cardiac function, gas exchange, pulmonary mechanics, nutritional status, electrolyte and fluid balance, and motivation should all be considered when making the decision to wean. This assessment should be ongoing to reflect the dynamic nature of the process.[78]

Weaning Approach. Although weaning the patient requiring short-term mechanical ventilation is a relatively simple process that can usually be accomplished with a nurse and respiratory therapist, weaning the patient with LTMVD is a much more complex process that usually requires a multidisciplinary team approach. Multidisciplinary weaning teams that use a coordinated and collaborative approach to weaning have demonstrated improved patient outcomes and decreased weaning times. The team should consist of a physician, nurse, respiratory therapist, dietitian, physical therapist, and a case manager, clinical outcomes manager, or clinical nurse specialist. Additional members, if possible, should include an occupational therapist, speech therapist, discharge planner, and social worker. Working together, the team members should develop a comprehensive plan of care for the patient that is efficient, consistent, progressive, and cost-effective.[79] Several studies have demonstrated successful weaning through the use of nurse and respiratory therapist–managed protocols.[80]

Weaning Method. A variety of weaning methods are available, but no one method has consistently proven to be superior to the others. These methods include T-tube (T-piece), continuous positive airway pressure (CPAP), pressure support ventilation (PSV), and SIMV. One recent multicenter study lends evidence to support the use of PSV for weaning over T-tube or SIMV weaning. Often these weaning methods are used in combination with each other, such as SIMV with PSV, CPAP with PSV, or SIMV with CPAP.[72]

Weaning Process Stage

For the long-term ventilator patient, the weaning process phase consists of initiating the weaning method selected and minimizing the physiologic and psychologic factors that can interfere with weaning.[75] It is imperative that the patient not become exhausted during this phase, because this can result in a setback in the weaning process.[77] During this phase the patient is assessed for weaning progress and signs of weaning intolerance.[72]

Weaning Initiation. Weaning should be initiated in the morning while the patient is rested. Before starting the weaning process, the patient is provided with an explanation of how the process works, a description of the sensations to expect, and reassurances that he or she will be closely monitored and returned to the original ventilator mode and settings if any difficulty occurs.[72] This information should be reinforced with each weaning attempt.

T-tube and CPAP weaning are accomplished by removing the patient from the ventilator and then placing the patient on a T-tube or by placing the patient on CPAP mode for a specified duration of time, known as a weaning trial, for a specified number of times per day. When the weaning trial is over, the patient is placed on the assist-control mode (continuous mandatory ventilation mode on the Puritan-Bennett 7200 ventilator) of the ventilator and allowed to rest to prevent respiratory muscle fatigue. Gradually the duration of time spent weaning is increased, as is the frequency, until the patient is able to breathe spontaneously for 24 hours. If PSV is used in conjunction with CPAP, the PSV is initially set to provide the patient with an assisted tidal volume of 10 to 12 ml/kg, and this is gradually weaned until a level of 6 to 8 cm H_2O of pressure support is achieved. SIMV and PSV weaning

Table 15-5

Weaning Intolerance Indications and Interventions

INDICATOR	ETIOLOGY	INTERVENTION
Pulmonary Signs (Emotional)		
Altered breathing pattern	Inadequate understanding of weaning process	Build trust in staff; consistent care providers
Dyspnea intensity		Encouragement; concrete goals for extubation
Change in facial expression	Inability to control breathing pattern	Involve patient in process and planning daily activities
		Efficient communication established
	Environmental factors	Organize care; avoid interruptions during weaning
		Adequate sleep
		Calm, caring presence of nurse; nonsedating anxiolytics
		Measure dyspnea
		Fan; music
		Biofeedback; relaxation; breathing control
		Family involvement; normalizing daily activities
Pulmonary Signs (Physiologic)		
Accessory muscle use	Airway obstruction	Suction/air-mask bag unit ventilation; manually ventilate patient
Prolonged expiration	Secretions/atelectasis	
Asynchronous movements of chest and abdomen	Bronchospasm	Bronchodilators
	Patient position/kinked	Sitting upright in bed or chair or per patient preference
Retractions	ET tube	
Facial expression changes	Increased workload or muscle	
Dyspnea	Fatigue	
Shortened inspiratory time	Caloric intake	Dietary assessment
Increased breathing	Electrolyte imbalances	Assess electrolytes; give replacements as necessary
frequency, decreased V_T	Inadequate rest	Rest between weaning trials (i.e., SIMV frequency rate >5)
	Patient/ventilator interactions	Assess ventilator settings (i.e., flow rate, trigger sensitivity)
	Increased V_E requirement	Muscle training if appropriate
	Infection	Check for infection (treat if indicated)
	Overfeeding	Appropriate caloric intake
	Respiratory alkalosis	Baseline ABGs achieved (ventilate according to pH)
	Anxiety	Coaching to regularize breathing pattern; give nonsedating anxiolytics
	Pain	Judicious use of analgesics
CNS Changes		
Restless/irritable	Hypoxemia/hypercarbia	Increase FIO_2
Decreased responsiveness		Return to mechanical ventilation
		Discern etiology and treat
CV Deterioration		
Excessive change in BP or HR	Heart failure	Diuretics as ordered
	Increase venous return	β-blockers
Dysrhythmias	Ischemia	Increase FIO_2
Angina		Return to mechanical ventilation
Dyspnea		Discern etiology and treat

Modified from Knebel AR: *Am J Crit Care* 1(3):19, 1992.

ET, Endotracheal; V_T, tidal volume; *SIMV,* synchronized intermittent mandatory ventilation; V_E, respiratory minute volume; *ABGs,* arterial blood gases; *CNS,* central nervous system; FiO_2, fraction of inspired oxygen; *CV,* cardiovascular; *BP,* blood pressure; *HR,* heart rate.

are accomplished by gradually decreasing the number of breaths or the amount of pressure support the patient receives by a specified amount until the patient is able to breathe spontaneously for 24 hours.[72]

Weaning Progress. Weaning progress can be evaluated using various methods. Evaluation of weaning progress when using a weaning method that gradually withdraws ventilatory support, such as SIMV or PSV, can be accomplished by measuring the percentage of the minute ventilation requirement that is provided by the ventilator. If the percentage steadily decreases, weaning is progressing. Evaluation of weaning progress when using a weaning method that removes ventilatory support, such as T-tube or CPAP, can be accomplished by measuring the amount of time the patient remains free from support. If the time steadily increases, weaning is progressing.[72]

Weaning Intolerance. Once the weaning process has begun, the patient should be continuously assessed for signs of intolerance. When present, these signs indicate when to place the patient back on the ventilator or to return the patient to the previous ventilator settings. Commonly used indicators include dyspnea; accessory muscle use; restlessness; anxiety; change in facial expression; changes in heart rate and blood pressure; rapid, shallow breathing; and discomfort.[78] Table 15-5 lists the different weaning intolerance indicators and actions that can be taken to control or prevent them.

Facilitative Therapies. Additional therapies may be needed to facilitate weaning in the patient who is having difficulty making weaning progress. These therapies include ventilatory muscle training and biofeedback. Inspiratory muscle training is used to enhance the strength and endurance of the respiratory muscles. Biofeedback can be used to promote relaxation and assist in the management of dyspnea and anxiety.[72]

Weaning Outcome Stage

Two outcomes are possible for a patient with LTMVD: weaning completed and incomplete weaning.[71]

Weaning Completed. Weaning is deemed successful when a patient is able to breathe spontaneously for 24 hours without ventilatory support. Once this occurs, the patient may be extubated or decannulated at any time, though this is not necessary for weaning to be considered successful.[71]

Incomplete Weaning. Weaning is deemed incomplete when a patient has reached a plateau (5 days at the same ventilatory support level without any changes) in the weaning process despite managing the physiologic and psychologic factors that impede weaning. Thus the patient is unable to breathe spontaneously for 24 hours without full or partial ventilatory support. Once this occurs, the patient should be placed in a subacute ventilator facility or discharged home on a ventilator with home health care nursing follow-up.[71]

evolve To test your mastery of this chapter, try the Open-Book Quiz at http://evolve.elsevier.com/Urden/priorities/

REFERENCES

1. Christie HA, Goldstein LS: Respiratory failure and the need for ventilatory support. In Wilkins RL, Stoller JK, Scanlan CL, editors: *Egan's fundamentals of respiratory care,* ed 8, St Louis, 2003, Mosby.
2. Flaatten H et al: Outcome after acute respiratory failure is more dependent on dysfunction in other vital organs than on severity of the respiratory failure, *Crit Care* 7:R72, 2003.
3. Vincent JL et al: The epidemiology of acute respiratory failure in critically ill patient, *Chest* 121:1602, 2002.
4. Balk R, Bone RC: Classification of acute respiratory failure, *Med Clin North Am* 67:551, 1983.
5. Curtis JR, Hudson LD: Emergent assessment and management of acute respiratory failure in COPD, *Clin Chest Med* 15:481, 1994.
6. Raju P, Manthous CA: The pathogenesis of respiratory failure, *Respir Care Clin N Am* 6:195, 2000.
7. Wagner PD, West JB: Ventilation, blood flow and gas exchange. In Mason RJ et al, editors: *Murray and Nadel's textbook of respiratory medicine,* ed 4, Philadelphia, 2005, Saunders.
8. Levy MM: Pathophysiology of oxygen delivery in repiratory failure, *Chest* 28(5 Suppl 2): 547S, 2005.
9. Sigillito RJ, DeBlieux PM: Evaluation and initial management of the patient in respiratory distress, *Emerg Med Clin North Am* 21:239, 2003.
10. Dakin J, Griffiths M: The pulmonary physician in critical care 1: pulmonary investigations for acute respiratory failure, *Thorax* 57:79, 2002.
11. Misasi RS, Keyes JL: Matching and mismatching ventilation and perfusion in the lung, *Crit Care Nurse* 16(3):23, 1996.
12. Keenan SP et al: Does noninvasive positive pressure ventilation improve outcome in acute hypoxemic respiratory failure? A systematic review, *Crit Care Med* 32:2516, 2004.
13. Kwok H et al: Controlled trial of oronasal versus nasal mask ventilation in the treatment of acute respiratory failure, *Crit Care Med* 31:468, 2003.
14. Soo Hoo GW, Hakimian N, Santiago SM: Hypercapnic respiratory failure in COPD patients: response to therapy, *Chest* 117:169, 2000.
15. Gali B, Goyal DG: Positive pressure mechanical ventilation, *Emerg Med Clin North Am* 21:453, 2003.
16. Rodríguez-Roisin R: COPD exacerbations. V. Management, *Thorax* 61:535, 2006.
17. Jacobi J et al: Clinical practice guidelines for the sustained use of sedatives and analgesics in the critically ill adult, *Crit Care Med* 30:119, 2002.
18. Murray MJ et al: Clinical practice guidelines for sustained neuromuscular blockade in the adult critically ill patient, *Crit Care Med* 30:142, 2002.
19. Holmes CL: The evaluation and management of shock, *Clin Chest Med* 24:775, 2003.
20. Parrish CR, Krenitsk J, Willcutts K: Nutritional support for mechanically ventilated patients. In Burns SM, editor:

AACN protocols for practice: care of mechanically ventilated patients, ed 2, Sudbury, Mass, 2007, Jones & Bartlett.
21. Sloan DS: Nutritional support of the critically ill and injured patient, *Crit Care Clin* 20:135, 2004.
22. Misra S, Ganzini L: Delirium, depression, and anxiety, *Crit Care Clin* 19:771, 2003.
23. Seidlitz M: Cardiac problems in the post acute ventilated patient, *Clin Chest Med* 22:175, 2001.
24. Kehl-Pruett W: Deep vein thrombosis in hospitalized patients: a review of evidence-based guidelines for prevention, *Dimens Crit Care Nurs* 25:53, 2006.
25. Cash BD: Evidence-based medicine as it applies to acid suppression in the hospitalized patient, *Crit Care Med* 30:S373, 2002.
26. Wong WP: Use of body positioning in the mechanically ventilated patient with acute respiratory failure: application of Sackett's rules of evidence, *Physiother Theory Pract* 15(1):25, 1999.
27. Force TR et al: Patient position and motion strategies, *Respir Care Clin N Am* 4:665, 1998.
28. Lasater-Erhand M: The effect of patient position on arterial saturation, *Crit Care Nurse* 15(5):31, 1995.
29. Cosenza JJ, Norton LC: Secretion clearance: state-of-the-art from a nursing perspective, *Crit Care Nurse* 6(4):23, 1986.
30. Collar HR et al: Prevention of ventilator-associated pneumonia: an evidence-based systematic review, *Ann Intern Med* 138:494, 2003.
31. Krishnagopalan S et al: Body positioning of intensive care patients: clinical practice versus standards, *Crit Care Med* 30:2588, 2002.
32. Stiller K: Physiotherapy in intensive care: towards an evidence-based practice, *Chest* 118:1801, 2000.
33. Jones A, Rowe BH: Bronchopulmonary hygiene physical therapy in bronchiectasis and chronic obstructive pulmonary disease: a systematic review, *Heart Lung* 29:125, 2000.
34. Khadaroo RG, Marshall JC: ARDS and the multiple organ dysfunction syndrome: common mechanisms of a common systemic process, *Crit Care Clin* 18:127, 2002.
35. Michaels AJ: Management of post traumatic respiratory failure, *Crit Care Clin* 20:83, 2004.
36. Bernard GR et al: The American-European consensus conference on ARDS: definitions, mechanisms, relevant outcomes, and clinical trial coordination, *Am J Respir Crit Care Med* 149:818, 1994.
37. Neff MJ: The epidemiology and definition of the acute respiratory distress syndrome, *Respir Care Clin N Am* 9:273, 2003.
38. Piantadosi CA et al: The acute respiratory distress syndrome, *Ann Intern Med* 141: 460, 2004.
39. Suratt Bt, Parsons PE: Mechanisms of acute injury lacute respiratory distress syndrome, *Clin Chest Med* 27:579, 2006.
40. Taylor MM: ARDS diagnosis and management: implications for the critical care nurse, *Dimens Crit Care Nurse* 24:197, 2005.
41. Perina DG: Noncardiogenic pulmonary edema, *Emerg Med Clin North Am* 21:385, 2003.
42. Hass CF: Lung protective mechanical ventilation in acute respiratory distress syndrome, *Respir Care Clin N Am* 9:363, 2003.
43. Rouby JJ et al: Mechanical ventilation in patients with acute respiratory distress syndrome, *Anesthesiology* 101:228, 2004.
44. Hickling KG: Permissive hypercapnia, *Respir Care Clin North Am* 8:155, 2002.
45. Roseberg AL: Fluid management in patients with acute respiratory distress syndrome, *Resp Care Clin N Am* 9:481, 2003.
46. Vollman KM: Prone positioning in the patient who has acute respiratory distress syndrome: the art and science, *Crit Care Nurs Clin North Am* 16:319, 2004.
47. Pimentel L, McPherson SJ: Community-acquired pneumonia in the emergency department: a practical approach to diagnosis and management, *Emerg Med Clin North Am* 21:395, 2003.
48. Baudouin SV: The pulmonary physician in critical care. III. Critical care management of community acquired pneumonia, *Thorax* 57:267, 2002.
49. Rello J, Diaz E, Rodríguez A: Etiology of ventilator-associated pneumonia, *Clin Chest Med* 26:87, 2005.
50. Apisarnthanarak A, Mundy LM: Etiology of community-acquired pneumonia, *Clin Chest Med* 26:47, 2005.
51. Flanders SC, Collard HR, Saint S: Nosocomial pneumonia: state of the science, *Am J Infect Control* 34:84, 2006.
52. Craven DE: Preventing ventilator-associated pneumonia in adults: sowing seeds of change, *Chest* 130:251, 2006.
53. Alcón A, Fàbregas N, Torres A: Pathophysiology of pneumonia, *Clin Chest Med* 26:39, 2005.
54. Mabie M, Wunderink RG: Use and limitation of clinical and radiologic diagnosis of pneumonia, *Semin Respir Infect* 18:72, 2003.
55. Thomas AR, Bryce TL: Ventilation in the patient with unilateral lung disease, *Crit Care Clin* 14:743, 1998.
56. Johnson JL, Hirsch CS: Aspiration pneumonia, *Postgrad Med* 113(3):99, 2003.
57. Marik PE: Aspiration pneumonitis and aspiration pneumonia, *N Engl J Med* 344:665, 2001.
58. Tietjen PA, Kaner RJ, Quinn CE: Aspiration emergencies, *Clin Chest Med* 15:117, 1994.
59. Metheny NA: Strategies to prevent aspiration-related pneumonia in tube-fed patients, *Respir Care Clin* 12:603, 2006.
60. Sadosty AT, Boie ET, Stead LG: Pulmonary embolism, *Emerg Med Clin North Am* 21:363, 2003.
61. Wood KE: Major pulmonary embolism: review of a pathophysiologic approach to the golden hour of hemodynamically significant pulmonary embolism, *Chest* 121:877, 2002.
62. Kearon C: Diagnosis of pulmonary embolism, *CMAJ* 168:183, 2003.
63. Trowbridge RL et al: The effects of helical computed tomography on diagnostic and treatment strategies in patients with suspected pulmonary complications, *Am J Med* 116:84, 2004.
64. Piazza G, Goldhaber SZ: Acute pulmonary embolism. II. Treatment and prophylaxis, *Circulation* 114:e42, 2006.
65. Agnelli G, Becattini C, Kirschstein T: Thrombolysis vs heparin in the treatment of pulmonary embolism: a clinical outcome-based meta-analysis, *Arch Intern Med* 162:2537, 2002.
66. Yalamanchili K et al: Open pulmonary embolectomy for treatment of major pulmonary embolism, *Ann Thorac Surg* 77:819, 2004.

67. Rodrigo GJ, Rodrigo C, Hall JB: Acute asthma in adults: a review, *Chest* 125:1081, 2004.
68. Higgins JC: The 'crashing asthmatic,' *Am Fam Physician* 67:997, 2003.
69. Phipps P, Garrard CS: The pulmonary physician in critical care. XII. Acute severe asthma in the intensive care unit, *Thorax* 58:81, 2003.
70. Siwik JP, Nowak RM, Zoratti EM: The evaluation and management of acute, severe asthma, *Med Clin North Am* 5:1049, 2002.
71. Knebel AR et al: Weaning from mechanical ventilation: concept development, *Am J Crit Care Nurs* 3:416, 1994.
72. Burns SM: Weaning from mechanical ventilation. In Burns SM, editor: *AACN protocols for practice: care of mechanically ventilated patients*, ed 2, Boston, 2007, Jones & Bartlett.
73. Rossi A, Poggi R, Roca J: Physiologic factors predisposing to chronic respiratory failure, *Respir Care Clin N Am* 8:379, 2002.
74. MacIntyre NR: Psychological factors in weaning from mechanical ventilatory support, *Respir Care* 40:277, 1995.
75. Knebel AR et al: Weaning from mechanical ventilatory support: refinement of a model, *Am J Crit Care Nurs* 7:149, 1998.
76. Chatila WM, Criner GJ: Complications of long-term mechanical ventilation, *Respir Care Clin N Am* 8:419, 2002.
77. Goldstone J: The pulmonary physician in critical care. X. Difficult weaning, *Thorax* 57:986, 2002.
78. Scheinhorn DJ, Chao DC, Stearn-Hassenpflug M: Liberation from prolonged mechanical ventilation, *Crit Care Clin* 18:569, 2002.
79. Grap MJ et al: Collaborative practice: development, implementation, and evaluation of a weaning protocol for patients receiving mechanical ventilation, *Am J Crit Care* 12:454, 2003.
80. Tietsort J, McPeck M, Rinaldo-Gallo S: Respiratory care protocol development and impact, *Respir Care Clin N Am* 10:223, 2004.

CHAPTER

16 Pulmonary Therapeutic Management

KATHLEEN M. STACY

OBJECTIVES

- Describe nursing management of a patient receiving oxygen therapy.
- List the indications and complications of the different artificial airways.
- Outline the principles of airway management.
- Discuss the various modes of invasive and noninvasive mechanical ventilation.
- Describe the management of a patient on mechanical ventilation.
- Delineate the care of the postoperative thoracic surgery patient.

OXYGEN THERAPY

Normal cellular function depends on an adequate supply of oxygen being delivered to the cells to meet their metabolic needs. The goal of oxygen therapy is to provide a sufficient concentration of inspired oxygen to permit full use of the oxygen-carrying capacity of the arterial blood, thus ensuring adequate cellular oxygenation given an adequate cardiac output (CO) and hemoglobin (Hgb) concentration.[1,2]

PRINCIPLES OF THERAPY

Oxygen is an atmospheric gas that must also be considered a drug, because—like most other drugs—oxygen has both detrimental and beneficial effects. Oxygen is one of the most commonly used and misused drugs. As a drug, it must be administered for good reason and in a proper, safe manner. Oxygen is generally ordered in liters per minute (L/min); as a concentration of oxygen expressed as a percentage, such as 40%; or as a fraction of inspired oxygen (F_{IO_2}), such as 0.4.

The primary indication for oxygen therapy is hypoxemia.[3] The amount of oxygen administered depends on the pathophysiologic mechanisms affecting the patient's oxygenation status. In most cases the amount required should provide an arterial partial pressure of oxygen (Pa_{O_2}) of greater than 60 mm Hg or an arterial hemoglobin saturation (Sa_{O_2}) of greater than 90% during both rest and exercise.[2] The concentration of oxygen given to an individual patient is a clinical judgment based on the many factors that influence oxygen transport, such as Hgb concentration, CO, and the arterial oxygen tension.[1,2]

Once oxygen therapy has begun, the patient is continuously assessed for level of oxygenation and the factors affecting it. The patient's oxygenation status is evaluated several times daily until the desired oxygen level is reached and has stabilized. If the desired response to the amount of oxygen delivered is not achieved, the oxygen supplementation is adjusted and the patient's condition reevaluated. It is important to use this dose-response method so that the lowest possible level of oxygen is administered that will still achieve a satisfactory Pa_{O_2} or Sa_{O_2}.[2,3]

METHODS OF DELIVERY

Oxygen therapy can be delivered by many different devices (Table 16-1). Common problems with these devices include system leaks and obstructions, device displacement, and skin irritation. These devices are classified as low-flow, reservoir, or high-flow systems.[3]

Low-flow Systems

A low-flow oxygen delivery system provides supplemental oxygen directly into the patient's airway at flows of less than or equal to 8 L/min. Because this flow is insufficient to meet the patient's inspiratory volume requirements, it results in a variable F_{IO_2} as the inspired oxygen is mixed with room air. The patient's ventilatory pattern will also affect the F_{IO_2} of a low-flow system. As the patient's ventilatory pattern changes, the inspired oxygen concentration varies

Table 16-1

Oxygen Therapy Systems

CATEGORY	DEVICE	FLOW	F_{IO_2} RANGE (%)	F_{IO_2} STABILITY	ADVANTAGES	DISADVANTAGES	BEST USE
Low-flow	Nasal cannula	1/4-8 L/min (adults) ≤2 L/min (infants)	22-45	Variable	Use on adults, children, infants; easy to apply; disposable, low cost; well tolerated	Unstable, easily dislodged; high flows uncomfortable; can cause dryness/bleeding; polyps, deviated septum may block flow	Stable patient needing low F_{IO_2}; home care patient requiring long- term therapy
	Nasal catheter	1/4-8 L/min	22-45	Variable	Use on adults, children, infants; good stability; disposable, low cost	Difficult to insert; high flows increase back pressure; needs regular changing; polyps, deviated septum may block insertion; may provoke gagging, air swallowing, aspiration	Procedures where cannula difficult to use (bronchoscopy); long-term care for infants
	Transtracheal catheter	1/4-4 L/min	22-35	Variable	Lower O_2 usage/cost; eliminates nasal/skin irritation; improved compliance; increased exercise tolerance; increased mobility; enhanced image	High cost; surgical complications; infection; mucus plugging; lost tract	Home care or ambulatory patients who need increased mobility or who do not accept nasal oxygen
Reservoir	Reservoir cannula	1/4-4 L/min	22-35	Variable	Lower O_2 usage/cost; increased mobility; less discomfort because of lower flows	Unattractive, cumbersome; poor compliance; must be regularly replaced; breathing pattern affects performance	Home care or ambulatory patients who need increased mobility
	Simple mask	5-12 L/min	35-50	Variable	Use on adults, children, infants; quick, easy to apply; disposable, inexpensive	Uncomfortable; must be removed for eating; prevents radiant heat loss; blocks vomitus in unconscious patients	Emergencies, short-term therapy requiring moderate F_{IO_2}
	Partial rebreathing mask	6-10 L/min (prevent bag collapse on inspiration)	35-60	Variable	Same as simple mask; moderate to high F_{IO_2}	Same as simple mask; potential suffocation hazard	Emergencies, short-term therapy requiring moderate to high F_{IO_2}
	Nonrebreathing mask	10-15 L/min (prevent bag collapse on inspiration)	55-70	Variable	Same as simple mask; high F_{IO_2}	Same as simple mask; potential suffocation hazard	Emergencies, short-term therapy requiring high F_{IO_2}
	Nonrebreathing circuit (closed)	3 × V_E (prevent bag collapse on inspiration)	21-100	Fixed	Full range of F_{IO_2}	Potential suffocation hazard; requires 50 psi air/O_2; blender failure common	Patients requiring precise F_{IO_2} at any level (21%-100%)
High-flow	Air-entrainment mask (AEM)	Varies; should provide output flow >60 L/min	24-50	Fixed	Easy to apply; disposable, inexpensive; stable, precise F_{IO_2}	Limited to adult use; uncomfortable, noisy; must be removed for eating; F_{IO_2} >0.40 not ensured; F_{IO_2} varies with back pressure	Unstable patients requiring precise low F_{IO_2}
	Air-entrainment nebulizer	10-15 L/min input; should provide output flow of at least 60 L/min	28-100	Fixed	Provides temperature control and extra humidification	F_{IO_2} <28% or >0.40 not ensured; F_{IO_2} varies with back pressure; high infection risk	Patients with artificial airways requiring low to moderate F_{IO_2}

Modified from Wilkins RL, Stoller JK, Scanlan CL, editors: *Egan's fundamentals of respiratory care,* ed 8, St Louis, 2003, Mosby.

F_{IO_2}, Fraction of inspired oxygen; *V_E*, minute volume.

because of differing amounts of room air gas mixing with the constant flow of oxygen. A nasal cannula is an example of a low-flow device.[3]

Reservoir Systems

A reservoir system incorporates some type of device to collect and store oxygen between breaths. When the patient's inspiratory flow exceeds the oxygen flow of the oxygen delivery system, the patient is able to draw from the reservoir of oxygen to meet his or her inspiratory volume needs. Thus there is less mixing of the inspired oxygen with room air. A reservoir oxygen delivery system can deliver a higher FIO_2 than a low-flow system. Examples of reservoir systems are simple face masks, partial rebreathing masks, and nonrebreathing masks.[3]

High-Flow Systems

With a high-flow system, the oxygen flows out of the device into the patient's airways in amounts sufficient to meet all inspiratory volume requirements. This type of system is not affected by the patient's ventilatory pattern. An air-entrainment mask is an example of a high-flow system.[1,3]

COMPLICATIONS OF OXYGEN THERAPY

Oxygen, like most drugs, has adverse effects and complications resulting from its use. The old adage "if a little is good, a lot is better" does not apply to oxygen. The lung is designed to handle a concentration of 21% oxygen, with some adaptability to higher concentrations, but adverse effects and oxygen toxicity can result if a high concentration is administered for too long.[4]

Oxygen Toxicity

The most detrimental effect of breathing a high concentration of oxygen is the development of oxygen toxicity. It can occur in any patient breathing oxygen concentrations of greater than 50% for more than 24 hours. Patients most likely to develop oxygen toxicity are those who require intubation, mechanical ventilation, and high oxygen concentrations for extended periods.[1,3]

Hyperoxia, or the administration of higher-than-normal oxygen concentrations, produces an overabundance of oxygen free radicals. These radicals are responsible for the initial damage to the alveolar-capillary membrane. Oxygen free radicals are toxic metabolites of oxygen metabolism. Normally, enzymes neutralize the radicals, which prevents any damage from occurring. During the administration of high levels of oxygen, the large number of oxygen free radicals produced exhausts the supply of neutralizing enzymes. Thus damage to the lung parenchyma and vasculature occurs, resulting in the initiation of acute lung injury (ALI).[1,4]

A number of clinical manifestations are associated with oxygen toxicity. The first symptom is substernal chest pain that is exacerbated by deep breathing. A dry cough and tracheal irritation follow. Eventually, definite pleuritic pain occurs on inhalation, followed by dyspnea. Upper airway changes may include a sensation of nasal stuffiness, sore throat, and eye and ear discomforts. Chest radiographs and pulmonary function tests show no abnormalities until symptoms are severe. Complete, rapid reversal of these symptoms occurs as soon as normal oxygen concentrations return.[4]

Carbon Dioxide Retention

In patients with severe chronic obstructive pulmonary disease (COPD), carbon dioxide (CO_2) retention may occur as a result of administering oxygen in higher concentrations. A number of possible theories have been proposed for this phenomenon. One theory states that in patients with COPD the normal stimulus to breathe (increasing CO_2 levels) is muted and decreasing oxygen levels become the stimulus to breathe. When oxygen is administered and hypoxemia corrected, the stimulus to breathe is abolished and hypoventilation develops, resulting in a further increase in the arterial partial pressure of carbon dioxide ($PaCO_2$).[3] Another theory is that the administration of oxygen abolishes the compensatory response of hypoxic pulmonary vasoconstriction. This results in an increase in perfusion of underventilated alveoli and the development of dead space, producing ventilation/perfusion mismatching. As alveolar dead space increases, so does the retention of CO_2.[3,5] One further theory states that the rise in CO_2 is related to the proportion of deoxygenated hemoglobin to oxygenated hemoglobin (Haldane effect). Because deoxygenated hemoglobin carries more CO_2 than oxygenated hemoglobin, when oxygen is administered it increases the amount of oxygenated hemoglobin, which results in an increase in the release of CO_2 at the lung level.[5] Because of the risk of CO_2 accumulation, all chronically hypercapnic patients require careful low-flow oxygen administration.[3]

Absorption Atelectasis

Another adverse effect of high concentrations of oxygen is absorption atelectasis. Breathing high concentrations of oxygen washes out the nitrogen that normally fills the alveoli and helps hold them open (residual volume). As oxygen replaces the nitrogen in the alveoli, the alveoli start to shrink and collapse because oxygen is absorbed into the bloodstream faster than it can be replaced in the alveoli, particularly in areas of the lungs that are minimally ventilated.[1,3]

NURSING MANAGEMENT

Nursing priorities for the patient receiving oxygen focus on (1) ensuring the oxygen is being adminis-

tered as ordered and (2) observing for complications of the therapy. Confirming that the O_2 therapy device is properly positioned and replacing it after removal is important. During meals an oxygen mask should be changed to a nasal cannula if the patient can tolerate one. The patient receiving O_2 therapy should also be transported with the oxygen. In addition, Spo_2 should be periodically monitored using a pulse oximeter.

ARTIFICIAL AIRWAYS

PHARYNGEAL AIRWAYS

Pharyngeal airways are used to maintain airway patency by keeping the tongue from obstructing the upper airway. The two types of pharyngeal airways are *oropharyngeal* and *nasopharyngeal*. Complications of these airways include trauma to the oral or nasal cavity, obstruction of the airway, laryngospasm, gagging, and vomiting.[6,7]

Oropharyngeal Airway

An oropharyngeal airway is made of plastic and is available in a variety of sizes. The proper size is selected by holding the airway against the side of the patient's face and ensuring that it extends from the corner of the mouth to the angle of the jaw. If the airway is improperly sized, it will occlude the airway.[6,7] An oral airway is placed by inserting a tongue depressor into the patient's mouth to displace the tongue downward and then passing the airway into the patient's mouth, slipping it over the patient's tongue.[7] When properly placed, the tip of the airway lies above the epiglottis at the base of the tongue. It should be used only in an unconscious patient who has an absent or diminished gag reflex.[6,7]

Nasopharyngeal Airway

A nasopharyngeal airway is usually made of plastic or rubber and is available in a variety of sizes. The proper size is selected by holding the airway against the side of the patient's face and ensuring that it extends from the tip of the nose to the earlobe.[6,7] A nasal airway is placed by lubricating the tube and inserting it midline along the floor of the naris into the posterior pharynx.[7] When properly placed, the tip of the airway lies above the epiglottis at the base of the tongue.[6,7]

ENDOTRACHEAL TUBES

An endotracheal tube (ETT) is the most commonly used artificial airway for providing short-term airway management. Indications for endotracheal intubation include maintenance of airway patency, protection of the airway from aspiration, application of positive-pressure ventilation, facilitation of pulmonary toilet, and use of high oxygen concentrations.[8] An ETT may be placed through the orotracheal or nasotracheal route.[9,10] In most situations involving emergency placement, the orotracheal route is used because the approach is simpler and affords use of a larger-diameter endotracheal tube.[10,11] Nasotracheal intubation provides greater patient comfort over time and is preferred in situations in which the patient has a jaw fracture.[9,11,12] The advantages of orotracheal intubation and nasotracheal intubation are presented in Table 16-2.

ETTs are available in a variety of sizes, sized according to the inner diameter of the tube, and have a radiopaque marker that runs the length of the tube. On one end of the tube is a cuff that is inflated using the pilot balloon. Because of the high incidence of cuff-related problems, low-pressure, high-volume cuffs are preferred. On the other end of the tube is a 15-mm adaptor that facilitates the connection of the tube to a manual resuscitation bag (MRB), T-tube, or ventilator (Figure 16-1).[13]

Intubation

Before intubation, the necessary equipment is gathered and organized to facilitate the procedure. Readily available equipment should include a suction system with catheters and tonsil suction, an MRB with a mask connected to 100% oxygen, a laryngoscope

Table 16-2
Advantages of Orotracheal, Nasotracheal, and Tracheostomy Tubes

OROTRACHEAL TUBES	NASOTRACHEAL TUBES	TRACHEOSTOMY TUBES
Easier access	Easily secured and stabilized	Easily secured and stabilized
Avoid nasal and sinus complications	Reduced risk of unintentional extubation	Reduced risk of unintentional decannulation
Allow for larger diameter tube, which facilitates:	Well tolerated by patient	Well tolerated by patient
• Work of breathing	Enable swallowing and oral hygiene	Enable swallowing, speech, and oral hygiene
• Suctioning	Facilitate communication	Avoid upper airway complications
• Fiberoptic bronchoscopy	Avoid need for bite block	Allow for larger diameter tube, which facilitates:
		• Work of breathing
		• Suctioning
		• Fiberoptic bronchoscopy

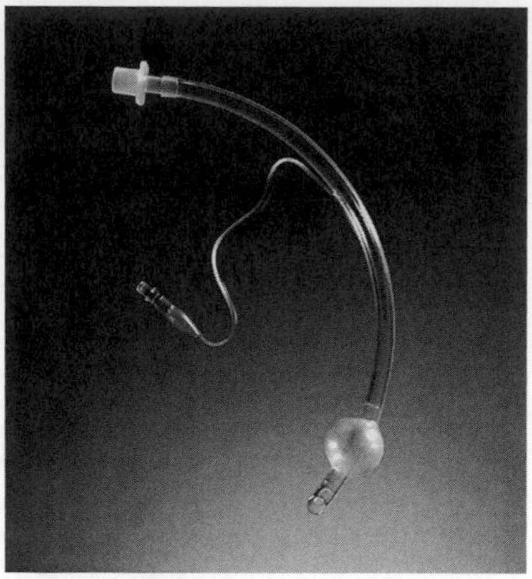

FIGURE 16-1. Endotracheal tube. (Courtesy Nellcor Puritan Bennett, Pleasanton, Calif.)

handle with assorted blades, a variety of sizes of ETTs, and a stylet. Before the procedure is initiated, all equipment is inspected to ensure it is in working order. The patient should be prepared for the procedure, if possible, with an intravenous catheter in place, and should be monitored with a pulse oximeter. The patient is sedated before the procedure (as clinical condition allows), and a topical anesthetic is applied to facilitate placement of the tube. In some cases a paralytic agent may be necessary if the patient is extremely agitated.[8,11]

The procedure is initiated by positioning the patient with the neck flexed and head slightly extended in the "sniff" position. The oral cavity and pharynx are suctioned, and any dental devices are removed. The patient is preoxygenated and ventilated using the MRB and mask with 100% oxygen. Each intubation attempt is limited to 30 seconds. Once the ETT is inserted, the patient is assessed for bilateral breath sounds and chest movement. Absence of breath sounds is indicative of an esophageal intubation, whereas breath sounds heard over only one side is indicative of a mainstem intubation. A disposable end-tidal CO_2 detector is used to initially verify correct airway placement, after which the cuff of the tube is inflated and the tube is secured. Finally, a chest radiograph is obtained to confirm placement.[8,10,11] The tip of the endotracheal tube should be approximately 3 to 4 cm above the carina when the patient's head is in the neutral position.[10] Once final adjustment of the position is complete, the level of insertion (marked in centimeters on the side of the tube) at the teeth is noted.[8,10] A number of complications can occur during the intubation procedure, including nasal and oral trauma, pharyngeal and hypopharyngeal trauma, vomiting with aspiration, and cardiac arrest.[14,15] Hypoxemia and hypercapnia can also occur, resulting in bradycardia, tachycardia, dysrhythmias, hypertension, and hypotension.[8,12]

Complications

A number of complications can occur while the ETT is in place, including nasal and oral inflammation and ulceration, sinusitis and otitis, laryngeal and tracheal injuries, and tube obstruction and displacement. A number of complications can occur days to weeks after the ETT is removed, including laryngeal and tracheal stenosis and a cricoid abscess (Table 16-3). Delayed complications usually require some form of surgical intervention to correct.[14,15]

TRACHEOSTOMY TUBES

A tracheostomy tube is the preferred method of airway maintenance in the patient requiring long-term intubation. Although no ideal time to perform the procedure has been identified, it is commonly accepted that if the patient has been intubated or is anticipated to be intubated for more than 2 to 3 weeks, a tracheotomy should be performed.[16] A tracheotomy is also indicated in several other situations, including upper airway obstruction or trauma and in patients with neuromuscular diseases.[16]

A tracheostomy tube provides the best route for long-term airway maintenance because it avoids the oral, nasal, pharyngeal, and laryngeal complications associated with an ETT. The tube is shorter, of wider diameter, and less curved than an ETT; thus the resistance to airflow is less, and breathing is easier. Additional advantages of a tracheostomy tube include easier secretion removal, increased patient acceptance and comfort, the possibility of the patient being able to eat and talk, and the facilitation of ventilator weaning.[11,16] Table 16-2 presents a list of the advantages of a tracheostomy tube.

Tracheostomy tubes are made of plastic or metal and may be single lumen or double lumen. Single-lumen tubes consist of the tube and a built-in cuff, which is connected to a pilot balloon for inflation purposes, and an obturator, which is used during tube insertion. The double-lumen tubes consist of the tube with the attached cuff, the obturator, and an inner cannula that can be removed for cleaning and then reinserted or, if disposable, replaced by a new sterile inner cannula. The inner cannula can quickly be removed if it becomes obstructed, making the system safer for patients with significant secretion problems. Single-lumen tubes provide a larger internal diameter for airflow than do double-lumen tubes, thus reducing airflow resistance and allowing the patient to ventilate through the tube with greater ease. Plastic tracheostomy tubes also have a 15-mm adaptor on the end (Figure 16-2).[17]

Tracheotomy

A tracheostomy tube is inserted via either an open procedure or a percutaneous procedure. An open

Table 16-3

Endotracheal Tubes: Complications, Causes, and Treatment

COMPLICATION	CAUSES	PREVENTION/TREATMENT
Tube obstruction	Patient biting tube Tube kinking during repositioning Cuff herniation Dried secretions, blood, or lubricant Tissue from tumor Trauma Foreign body	*Prevention:* Place bite block Sedate patient PRN Suction PRN Humidify inspired gases *Treatment:* Replace tube
Tube displacement	Movement of patient's head Movement of tube by patient's tongue Traction on tube from ventilator tubing Self-extubation	*Prevention:* Secure tube to upper lip Restrain patient's hands as needed Sedate patient PRN Ensure that only 2 inches of tube extends beyond lip Support ventilatory tubing *Treatment:* Replace tube
Sinusitis and nasal injury	Obstruction of the paranasal sinus drainage Pressure necrosis of nares	*Prevention:* Avoid nasal intubations Cushion nares from tube and tape/ties *Treatment:* Remove all tubes from nasal passages Administer antibiotics
Tracheoesophageal fistula	Pressure necrosis of posterior tracheal wall, resulting from overinflated cuff and rigid nasogastric tube	*Prevention:* Inflate cuff with minimal amount of air necessary Monitor cuff pressures every 8 hours *Treatment:* Position cuff of tube distal to fistula Place gastrostomy tube for enteral feedings Place esophageal tube for secretion clearance proximal to fistula
Mucosal lesions	Pressure at tube and mucosal interface	*Prevention:* Inflate cuff with minimal amount of air necessary Monitor cuff pressures every 8 hours Use appropriate-size tube *Treatment:* May resolve spontaneously Perform surgical intervention
Laryngeal or tracheal stenosis	Injury to area from end of tube or cuff, resulting in scar tissue formation and narrowing of airway	*Prevention:* Inflate cuff with minimal amount of air necessary Monitor cuff pressures every 8 hours Suction area above cuff frequently *Treatment:* Perform tracheostomy Place laryngeal stent Perform surgical repair
Cricoid abscess	Mucosal injury with bacterial invasion	*Prevention:* Inflate cuff with minimal amount of air necessary Monitor cuff pressures every 8 hours Suction area above cuff frequently *Treatment:* Perform incision and drainage of area Administer antibiotics

PRN, As needed.

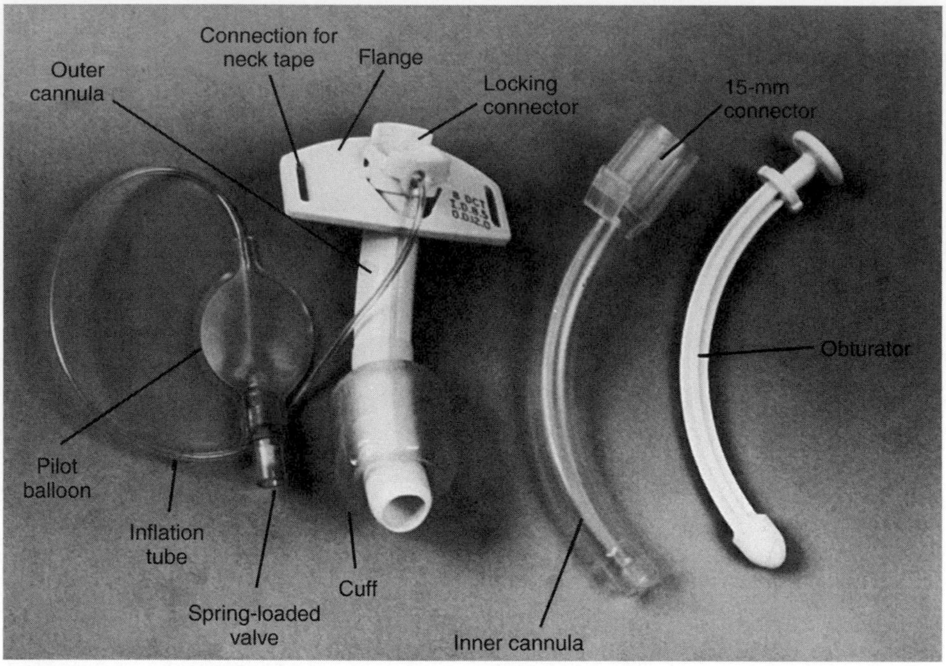

FIGURE 16-2. Tracheostomy tube. (From Scanlan CL: Airway management. In Wilkins RL, Stoller JK, Scanlan CL, editors: *Egan's fundamentals of respiratory care,* ed 8, St Louis, 2003, Mosby.)

procedure is usually performed in the operating room, whereas a percutaneous procedure can be done at the patient's bedside.[16] A number of complications can occur during the tracheotomy procedure, including misplacement of the tracheal tube, hemorrhage, laryngeal nerve injury, pneumothorax, pneumomediastinum, and cardiac arrest.[15]

Complications

A number of complications can occur while the tracheostomy tube is in place, including stomal infection, hemorrhage, tracheomalacia, tracheoesophageal fistula, tracheoinnominate artery fistula, and tube obstruction and displacement. A number of complications can occur days to weeks after the tracheostomy tube is removed; these include tracheal stenosis and a tracheocutaneous fistula (Table 16-4). Delayed complications usually require some form of surgical intervention to correct.[18,19]

NURSING MANAGEMENT

The patient with an endotracheal or tracheostomy tube requires some additional measures to address the effects associated with tube placement on the respiratory and other body systems. **Nursing priorities in the management of the patient with an artificial airway include (1) humidification, (2) cuff management, (3) suctioning, and (4) communication.** Because the tube bypasses the upper airway system, warming and humidifying of air must be performed by external means. Because the cuff of the tube can cause damage to the walls of the trachea, proper cuff inflation and management is imperative. In addition, the normal defense mechanisms are impaired and secretions may accumulate; thus suctioning may be needed to promote secretion clearance. Because the tube does not allow airflow over the vocal cords, developing a method of communication is also very important. Last, observing the patient to ensure proper placement of the tube and patency of the airway is essential. Patient safety issues are addressed in Patient Safety Priorities: Artificial Airways.

PATIENT SAFETY PRIORITIES

Artificial Airways

In the event of unintentional extubation or decannulation, the patient's airway should be opened with the head tilt–chin lift maneuver and maintained with an oropharyngeal or nasopharyngeal airway. If the patient is not breathing, he or she should be manually ventilated with a manual resuscitation bag and face mask with 100% oxygen. In the case of a tracheostomy, the stoma should be covered to prevent air from escaping through it.

Humidification

Humidification of air normally is performed by the mucosal layer of the upper respiratory tract. When this area is bypassed, such as occurs with both endotracheal

Table 16-4
Tracheostomy Tubes: Complications, Causes, and Treatment

COMPLICATION	CAUSES	PREVENTION/TREATMENT
Hemorrhage	Vessel opening after surgery Vessel erosion caused by tube	*Prevention:* Use appropriate-size tube Treat local infection Suction gently Humidify inspired gases Position tracheal window not lower than third tracheal ring *Treatment:* Pack lightly Perform surgical intervention
Wound infection	Colonization of stoma with hospital flora	*Prevention:* Perform routine stoma care *Treatment:* Remove tube, if necessary Perform aggressive wound care and debridement Administer antibiotics
Subcutaneous emphysema	Positive-pressure ventilation Coughing against a tight, occlusive dressing or sutured or packed wound	*Prevention:* Avoid suturing or packing wound closed around tube *Treatment:* Remove any sutures or packing if present
Tube obstruction	Dried blood or secretions False passage into soft tissues Opening of cannula positioned against tracheal wall Foreign body Tissue from tumor	*Prevention:* Suction PRN Humidify inspired gases Use double-lumen tube Position tube so that opening does not press against tracheal wall *Treatment:* Remove/replace inner cannula Replace tube
Tube displacement	Patient movement Coughing Traction on ventilatory tubing	*Prevention:* Use commercial tube holder Suture tube in place Use tubes with adjustable neck plates for patients with short necks Support ventilatory tubing Sedate patient PRN Restrain patient as needed *Treatment:* Cover stoma and manually ventilate patient via mouth Replace tube
Tracheal stenosis	Injury to area from end of tube or cuff, resulting in scar tissue formation and narrowing of airway	*Prevention:* Inflate cuff with minimal amount of air necessary Monitor cuff pressures every 8 hours *Treatment:* Perform surgical repair
Tracheoesophageal fistula	Pressure necrosis of posterior tracheal wall, resulting from overinflated cuff and rigid nasogastric tube	*Prevention:* Inflate cuff with minimal amount of air necessary Monitor cuff pressures every 8 hours *Treatment:* Perform surgical repair
Tracheoinnominate artery fistula	Direct pressure from the elbow of the cannula against the innominate artery Placement of tracheal stoma below fourth tracheal ring Downward migration of the tracheal stoma, resulting from traction on tube High-lying innominate artery	*Prevention:* Position tracheal window not lower than third tracheal ring *Treatment:* Hyperinflate cuff to control bleeding Remove tube and replace with endotracheal tube and apply digital pressure through stoma against the sternum Perform surgical repair
Tracheocutaneous fistula	Failure of stoma to close after removal of tube	*Treatment:* Perform surgical repair

PRN, As needed.

and tracheostomy tubes, or when supplemental oxygen is used, humidification by external means is necessary. Various humidification devices add water to inhaled gas to prevent drying and irritation of the respiratory tract, to prevent undue loss of body water, and to facilitate secretion removal.[20,21] The humidification device should provide inspired gas conditioned (heated) to body temperature and saturated with water vapor.[22]

Cuff Management

Because the cuff of the endotracheal or tracheostomy tube is a major source of the complications associated with artificial airways, proper cuff management is essential. To prevent the complications associated with cuff design, only low-pressure, high-volume cuffed tubes are used in clinical practice.[13,23] Even with these tubes, cuff pressures can be generated that are high enough to lead to tracheal ischemia and injury. Both cuff inflation techniques and cuff pressure monitoring are critical components of the care of the patient with an artificial airway.[10,23]

Cuff Inflation Techniques. Two different cuff inflation techniques currently are being used: the minimal leak (ML) technique and the minimal occlusion volume (MOV) technique. The ML technique consists of injecting air into the cuff until no leak is heard and then withdrawing the air until a small leak is heard on inspiration. Problems with this technique include difficulty maintaining positive end-expiratory pressure (PEEP) and aspiration around the cuff. The MOV technique consists of injecting air into the cuff until no leak is heard at peak inspiration. The problem with this technique is that it generates higher cuff pressures than does the ML technique. The selection of one technique over the other is determined by individual patient needs. If the patient needs a seal to provide adequate ventilation and/or is at high risk for aspiration, the MOV technique is used. If these are not concerns, usually the ML technique is used.[10-11,22,23]

Cuff Pressure Monitoring. Cuff pressures are monitored at least every shift with a cuff pressure manometer. Cuff pressures should be maintained at 20 to 25 mm Hg (24 to 30 cm H_2O), because greater pressures decrease blood flow to the capillaries in the tracheal wall and lesser pressures increase the risk of aspiration. Pressures in excess of 22 mm Hg (30 cm H_2O) should be reported to the physician. In addition, cuffs are not routinely deflated, because this increases the risk of aspiration.[10,22,23]

Foam Cuff Tracheostomy Tubes. One tracheostomy tube on the market has a cuff made of foam that is self-inflating. It is deflated during insertion; afterwards the pilot port is opened to atmospheric pressure (room air), and the cuff self-inflates. Once inflated, the foam cuff conforms to the size and shape of the patient's trachea, thereby reducing the pressure against the tracheal wall. The pilot port is either left open to atmospheric pressure or attached to the mechanical ventilator tubing, thus allowing the cuff to inflate and deflate with the cycling of the ventilator. Routine maintenance of a foam cuff tracheostomy tube includes aspirating the pilot port every 8 hours to measure cuff volume, to remove any condensation from the cuff area, and to assess the integrity of the cuff. Removal is accomplished by deflating the cuff; this can be complicated if the plastic sheath covering the foam is perforated. When perforation occurs, the foam may not be deflatable because the air cannot be totally aspirated.[24]

Suctioning

Suctioning is often required to maintain a patent airway in the patient with an endotracheal or tracheostomy tube. Suctioning is a sterile procedure that is performed only when the patient needs it and not on a routine schedule.[10,22] Indications for suctioning include coughing, secretions in the airway, respiratory distress, presence of rhonchi on auscultation, increased peak airway pressures on the ventilator, and decreasing SpO_2 or PaO_2.[11] A number of complications are associated with suctioning, including hypoxemia, atelectasis, bronchospasms, dysrhythmias, increased intracranial pressure, and airway trauma.[11]

Complications. Hypoxemia can result from disconnecting the oxygen source from the patient and/or removing the oxygen from the patient's airways when the suction is applied. Atelectasis is thought to occur when the suction catheter is larger than half the diameter of the ETT. Excessive negative pressure occurs when suction is applied, promoting collapse of the distal airways. Bronchospasms are the result of the stimulation of the airways with the suction catheter. Cardiac dysrhythmias, particularly bradycardias, are attributed to vagal stimulation. Airway trauma occurs with impaction of the catheter in the airways and excessive negative pressure applied to the catheter.[10,11]

Suctioning Protocol. A number of protocols regarding suctioning have been developed. Several different practices have been found helpful in limiting the complications of suctioning. Hypoxemia can be minimized by giving the patient three hyperoxygenation breaths (breaths at 100% FIO_2) with the ventilator before the procedure and again after each pass of the suction catheter.[10,25] If the patient exhibits signs of desaturation, hyperinflation (breaths at 150% tidal volume) should be added to the procedure.[10] Atelectasis can be avoided by using a suction catheter with an external diameter less than one half of the internal diameter of the ETT. Using no greater than 120 mm Hg of suction will decrease the chances of hypoxemia, atelectasis, and airway trauma.[10] Limiting the duration of each suction pass to 10 to 15 seconds[10] and the number of passes to three or less also will help minimize hypoxemia, airway trauma, and cardiac dysrhythmias.[26] The process of applying intermittent (instead of continuous) suction has been shown to be of no benefit.[27] In addition, the instillation of normal saline to help remove secretions has not proven to be of any benefit[28] and may actually contribute to the development of hypoxemia[10,29] and lower airway colonization, resulting in hospital-acquired pneumonia.[10,30]

Closed Tracheal Suction System. One device to facilitate suctioning a patient on the ventilator is the closed tracheal suction system (CTSS) (Figure 16-3). This device consists of a suction catheter in a plastic sleeve that attaches directly to the ventilator tubing. It allows the patient to be suctioned while remaining on the ventilator. Advantages of the CTSS include the maintenance of oxygenation and PEEP during suctioning, the reduction of hypoxemia-related complications, and the protection of staff members from the patient's secretions. The CTSS is convenient to use, requiring only one person to perform the procedure.

Concerns related to the CTSS include autocontamination, inadequate removal of secretions, and increased risk of unintentional extubation resulting from the extra weight of the system on the ventilator tubing. Autocontamination has been shown not to be an issue if the catheter is cleaned properly after every use. Inadequate removal of secretions may or may not be a problem, and further investigation is required to settle this issue.[11] Though recommendations for changing the catheter vary, one study indicated that the catheter could be changed on an as-needed basis without increasing the incidence of hospital-acquired pneumonia.[31]

Communication

One of the major stressors for the patient with an artificial airway is impaired communication. This is related to the inability to speak, insufficient explanations from staff members, inadequate understanding, fear of being unable to communicate, and difficulty with communication methods.[32] A number of interventions can facilitate communication in the patient with an endotracheal or tracheostomy tube. These include performing a complete assessment of the patient's ability to communicate, teaching the patient how to communicate, using a variety of methods to communicate, and facilitating the patient's ability to communicate by providing the patient with his or her eyeglasses or hearing aid.[33]

A number of methods are available to facilitate communication in this patient population. These include the use of verbal and nonverbal language and a variety of devices to assist the short-term and long-term ventilator-assisted patient. Nonverbal communication may include the use of sign language, gestures, lip-reading, pointing, facial expressions, or eye blinking.

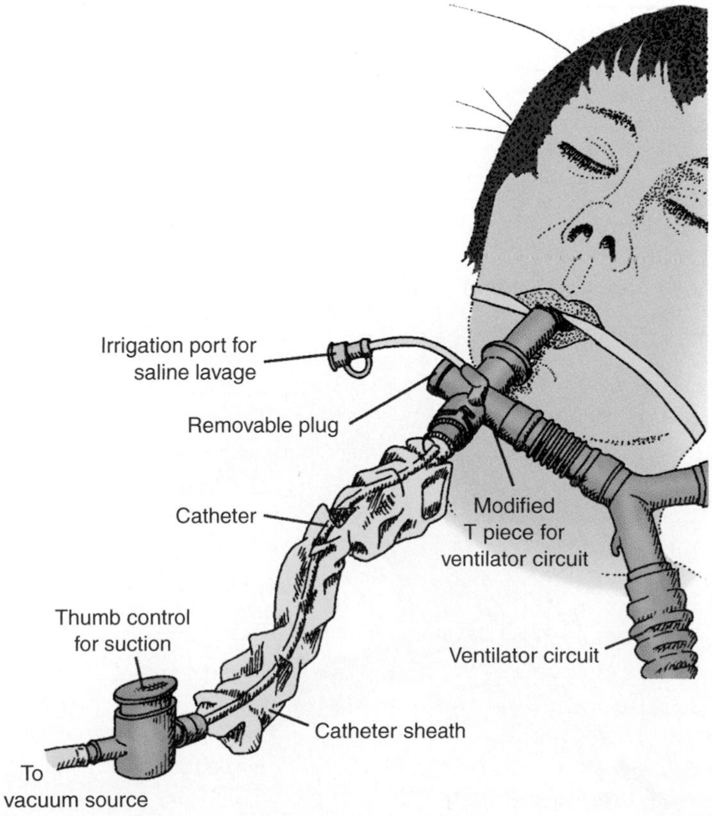

FIGURE 16-3. Closed tracheal suction system. (From Sills JR: Entry-level respiratory therapist exam guide, St Louis, 2000, Mosby.)

Simple devices available include pencil and paper; Magic Slates; magnetic boards with plastic letters; picture, alphabet, or symbol boards; and flash cards. More sophisticated devices include typewriters, computers, talking tracheostomy and endotracheal tubes, and external handheld vibrators. Regardless of the method selected, the patient must be taught how to use the device.[10,33]

Passy-Muir Valve. One of the best devices used to assist the mechanically ventilated patient with a tracheostomy to speak is the Passy-Muir valve. This one-way valve opens on inhalation, allowing air to enter the lungs through the tracheostomy tube, and closes on exhalation, forcing air over the vocal cords and out the mouth, thus permitting the patient to speak (Figure 16-4). Before placing the valve on a tracheostomy tube, the cuff must be deflated to allow air to pass around the tube, and the tidal volume of the ventilator has to be increased to compensate for the air leak. In addition to assisting the patient with communicating, the Passy-Muir valve can assist the ventilator-dependent patient with relearning normal breathing patterns. The valve is contraindicated in patients with laryngeal and pharyngeal dysfunction, excessive secretions, and poor lung compliance.[34]

Oral Hygiene

Patients with artificial airways are extremely susceptible to developing hospital-acquired pneumonia due to microaspiration of subglottic secretions. Subglottic secretions are fluids from the oropharyngeal area that pool above the inflated cuff of the endotracheal tube or tracheostomy tube. These secretions are full of microorganisms from the patient's mouth. Because the cuff of the artificial airway does not create a tight seal in the patient's airway, these secretions seep around the cuff and into the patient's lungs, thus promoting the development of hospital-acquired pneumonia.[35] Though bacteria are normally present in a patient's mouth, in the critically ill patient there are increased amounts of bacteria and more resistant bacteria. Decreased salivary flow, poor mucosal status,[36] and dental plaque all contribute to this problem.[37]

Proper oral hygiene has the potential to decrease the incidence of hospital-acquired pneumonia.[38,39] However, recent studies have shown that routine oral care is not a priority intervention for many nurses.[38,39] Currently there is no evidence-based protocol for oral care. Research studies are lacking, particularly with regard to frequency and effectiveness of different procedures.[40] Most experts agree, though, that oral care should consist of brushing the patient's teeth with a soft toothbrush to reduce plaque, brushing the patient's tongue and gums with a foam swab to stimulate the tissue, and performing deep oropharyngeal suction to remove any secretions that have pooled above the patient's cuff.[38,39]

Extubation/Decannulation

Once the airway is no longer needed, it is removed. Extubation is the process of removing an ETT. It is a simple procedure that can be accomplished at the bedside.[10,11] Before deflating the cuff of an endotracheal or tracheostomy tube in preparation for removal, it is

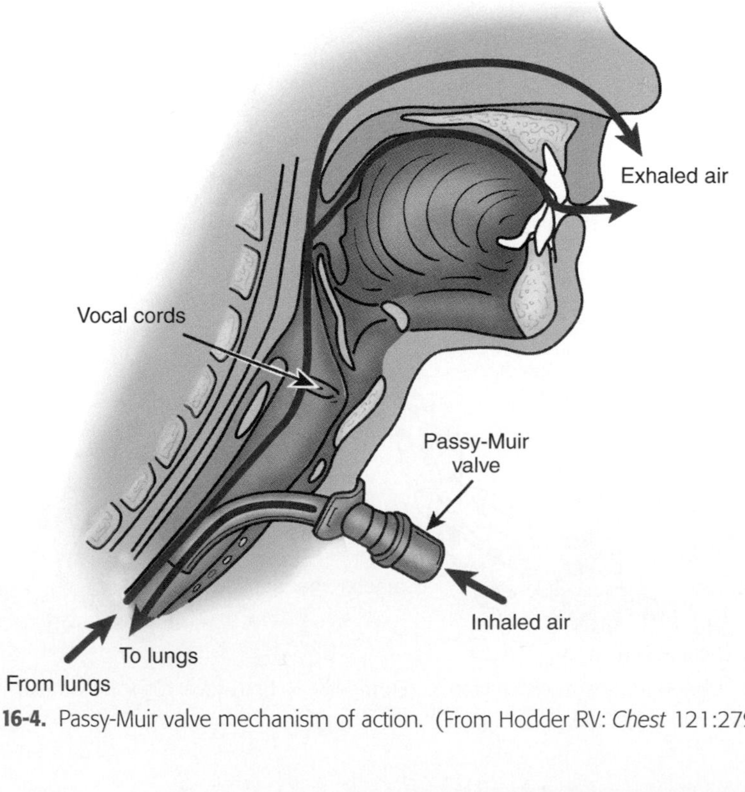

FIGURE 16-4. Passy-Muir valve mechanism of action. (From Hodder RV: *Chest* 121:279, 2002.)

very important to ensure that secretions are cleared from above the tube cuff. Complications of extubation include sore throat, stridor, hoarseness, odynophagia, vocal cord immobility, pulmonary aspiration, and cough.[15] Decannulation is the process of removing a tracheostomy tube. It is also a simple process that can be performed at the bedside. After the removal of the tracheostomy tube, the stoma is usually covered with a dry dressing, with the expectation that the stoma will close within several days.[10,11] Difficulty removing the tracheostomy tube as a result of a tight stoma is usually the only complication associated with decannulation.[15]

INVASIVE MECHANICAL VENTILATION

INDICATIONS

Mechanical ventilation is indicated for a variety of physiologic and clinical reasons. Physiologic objectives include supporting cardiopulmonary gas exchange (alveolar ventilation and arterial oxygenation), increasing lung volume (end-expiratory lung inflation and functional residual capacity), and reducing the work of breathing. Clinical objectives include reversing hypoxemia and acute respiratory acidosis, relieving respiratory distress, preventing or reversing atelectasis and respiratory muscle fatigue, permitting sedation and/or neuromuscular blockade, decreasing oxygen consumption, reducing intracranial pressure, and stabilizing the chest wall.[41]

TYPES OF VENTILATORS

The two main types of ventilators currently available are positive-pressure ventilators and negative-pressure ventilators. Negative-pressure ventilators are applied externally to the patient and decrease the atmospheric pressure surrounding the thorax to initiate inspiration. They generally are not used in the critical care environment. Positive-pressure ventilators use a mechanical drive mechanism to force air into the patient's lungs through an endotracheal or tracheostomy tube.[42]

Ventilator Mechanics

The ventilator must complete four phases of ventilation to properly ventilate the patient: (1) change from exhalation to inspiration, (2) inspiration, (3) change from inspiration to exhalation, and (4) exhalation. The ventilator uses four different variables to begin, sustain, and terminate each of these phases. These variables are described in terms of *volume, pressure, flow,* and *time.*[43]

Trigger. The phase variable that initiates the change from exhalation to inspiration is called the *trigger.* Breaths may be pressure-triggered or flow-triggered, based on the sensitivity setting of the ventilator and the patient's inspiratory effort, or time-triggered, based on the rate setting of the ventilator. A breath that is initiated by the patient is known as a *patient-triggered* or *patient-assisted* breath, whereas a breath that is initiated by the ventilator is known as a *machine-triggered* or *machine-controlled* breath. A *time-triggered breath* is a machine-controlled breath in which the ventilator initiates a breath after a preset amount of time has elapsed. It is controlled by the rate setting on the ventilator (thus a rate of 10 breaths/min yields one breath every 6 seconds). *Flow-triggered* and *pressure-triggered* breaths are patient-assisted breaths in which the patient initiates the breath by decreasing the flow or pressure (respectively) within the breathing circuit. Flow-triggering (also known as *flow-by*) is controlled by adjusting the flow-sensitivity setting of the ventilator, whereas pressure triggering is controlled by adjusting the pressure-sensitivity setting. Many ventilators offer the different types of triggers in combination with each other. Thus a breath may be both time-triggered and flow-triggered, depending on the patient's ability to interact with the ventilator and initiate a breath.[42,43]

Limit. The variable that maintains inspiration is called the *limit* or *target.* Inspiration can be pressure-limited, flow-limited, or volume-limited. A pressure-limited breath is one in which a preset pressure is attained and maintained during inspiration. A flow-limited breath is one in which a preset flow is reached before the end of inspiration. A volume-limited breath is one in which a preset volume is delivered during the inspiration. However, the limit variable does not end inspiration; it only sustains it.[42,43]

Cycle. The variable that ends inspiration is called the *cycle.* The four classifications of positive-pressure ventilators are based on the cycle variable: volume-cycled, pressure-cycled, flow-cycled, and time-cycled. *Volume-cycled ventilators* are designed to deliver a breath until a preset volume is delivered. *Pressure-cycled ventilators* deliver a breath until a preset pressure is reached within the patient's airways. *Flow-cycled ventilators* deliver a breath until a preset inspiratory flow rate is achieved. *Time-cycled ventilators* deliver a breath over a preset time interval.[42,43]

Baseline. The variable that is controlled during exhalation is called the *baseline.* Pressure is almost always used to adjust this variable. The patient exhales to a certain baseline pressure that is set on the ventilator. It may be set at zero, which is atmospheric pressure, or above atmospheric pressure, which is known as *positive end-expiratory pressure (PEEP).*[42,43]

MODES OF VENTILATION

The term *ventilator mode* refers to how the machine will ventilate the patient. In other words, selection of a particular mode of ventilation determines how much the patient will participate in his or her own ventilatory pattern. The choice depends on the patient's situation and the goals of treatment. The mode is determined by the combination of phase variables selected. A large variety of modes are available (Table 16-5).[42-44] Many of these modes may be used in conjunction with each other. Because brands of ventilators vary in their ability to perform certain functions, not all modes are available on all ventilators.[43]

VENTILATOR SETTINGS

A variety of settings on the ventilator allow the ventilator parameters to be individualized to the patient and also allow selection of the desired ventilation mode (Table 16-6). In addition, each ventilator has a patient-

Table 16-5
Modes of Mechanical Ventilation

MODE OF VENTILATION	CLINICAL APPLICATION	NURSING IMPLICATIONS
Continuous mandatory (volume or pressure) ventilation (CMV) also known as assist-control (A/C) ventilation: Delivers gas at preset tidal volume or pressure (depending on selected cycling variable) in response to patient's inspiratory efforts and will initiate breath if patient fails to do so within preset time	Volume controlled CMV (VC-CMV) is used as the primary mode of ventilation in spontaneously breathing patients with weak respiratory muscles Pressure controlled CMV (PC-CMV) is used in patients with decreased lung compliance or increased airway resistance particularly when the patient is at risk for volutrauma	Hyperventilation can occur in patients with increased respiratory rates Sedation may be necessary to limit the number of spontaneous breaths Patient on VC-CMV should be monitored for volutrauma Patient on PC-CMV should be monitored for hypercapnia
Pressure-regulated volume control ventilation (PRVCV): A variation of CMV that combines both volume and pressure features; delivers a preset tidal volume using the lowest possible airway pressure; airway pressure will not exceed preset maximum pressure limit	PRVCV is used in patients with rapidly changing pulmonary mechanics (airway resistance and lung compliance), thus limiting potential complications	
Pressure-controlled inverse ratio ventilation (PC-IRV): PC-CMV mode in which the inspiratory-to-expiratory (I/E) time ratio is greater than 1:1	PC-IRV is used in patients with hypoxemia refractory to PEEP; the longer inspiratory time increases functional residual capacity and improves oxygenation by opening collapsed alveoli, and the shorter expiratory time induces auto-PEEP that prevents alveoli from recollapsing	Requires sedation and/or pharmacologic paralysis because of discomfort Increased intrathoracic pressure can result in excessive air trapping and decreased cardiac output
Intermittent mandatory (volume or pressure) ventilation (IMV) also known as synchronous intermittent mandatory ventilation (SIMV): Delivers gas at preset tidal volume or pressure (depending on selected cycling variable) and rate while allowing patient to breathe spontaneously; ventilator breaths are synchronized to patient's respiratory effort	Volume controlled IMV (VC-IMV) is used both as a primary mode of ventilation in a wide variety of clinical situations and as a weaning mode Pressure controlled IMV (PC-IMV) is used in patients with decreased lung compliance or increased airway resistance when the need to preserve the patient's spontaneous effects is important	May increase the work of breathing and promote respiratory muscle fatigue Patient should be monitored for hypercapnia, particularly with PC-IMV
Adaptive support ventilation (ASV): Ventilator automatically adjusts settings to maintain100 ml/min/kg of minute ventilation; pressure support	ASV is a computerized mode of ventilation that increases or decreases ventilatory support based on patient needs; can be used with any patient requiring volume controlled ventilation	Not intended as a weaning mode Adapts to changes in patient position
Constant positive airway pressure (CPAP): Positive pressure applied during spontaneous breaths; patient controls rate, inspiratory flow, and tidal volume	CPAP is a spontaneous breathing mode used in patients to increase functional residual capacity and improve oxygenation by opening collapsed alveoli at end expiration; it is also used for weaning	Side effects include decreased cardiac output, volutrauma, and increased intracranial pressure No ventilator breaths are delivered in PEEP and CPAP mode unless used with CMV or IMV
Airway pressure release ventilation (APRV): Two different levels of CPAP (inspiratory and expiratory) are applied for set periods of time, allowing spontaneous breathing to occur at both levels	APRV is a spontaneous breathing mode used in patients to maintain alveolar recruitment without imposing additional peak inspiratory pressures that could lead to barotraumas	Patient needs to be monitored for hypercapnia

Table 16-5
Modes of Mechanical Ventilation—*cont'd*

MODE OF VENTILATION	CLINICAL APPLICATION	NURSING IMPLICATIONS
Pressure support ventilation (PSV): Preset positive pressure used to augment patient's inspiratory efforts; patient controls rate, inspiratory flow, and tidal volume	PSV is a spontaneous breathing mode used as the primary mode of ventilation in patients with stable respiratory drive to overcome any imposed mechanical resistance (e.g., artificial airway) PSV can also be used with IMV to support spontaneous breaths	Patient should be monitored for hypercapnia Advantages include reduced patient work of breathing and improved patient-ventilator synchrony
Volume-assured pressure support ventilation (VAPSV) also known as pressure augmentation (PA): A variation of PSV with a set tidal volume to ensure that patient receives minimum tidal volume with each pressure support breath	VAPSV is a spontaneous breathing mode used to treat acute respiratory illness and to facilitate weaning	Advantages include increased patient comfort, decreased work of breathing and decreased respiratory muscle fatigue, and promotion of respiratory muscle conditioning
Independent lung ventilation (ILV): Each lung is ventilated separately	ILV is used in patients with unilateral lung disease, bronchopleural fistulas, and bilateral asymmetric lung disease	Requires a double-lumen endotracheal tube, two ventilators, sedation, and/or pharmacologic paralysis
High-frequency ventilation (HFV): Delivers a small volume of gas at a rapid rate High-frequency positive-pressure ventilation (HFPPV): Delivers 60-100 breaths/min High-frequency jet ventilation (HFJV): Delivers 100-600 cycles/min High-frequency oscillation (HFO): Delivers 900-3000 cycles/min	HFV is used in situations in which conventional mechanical ventilation compromises hemodynamic stability, with bronchopleural fistulas, during short-term procedures, and with diseases that create a risk of volutrauma	Patients require sedation and/or pharmacologic paralysis Inadequate humidification can compromise airway patency Assessment of breath sounds is difficult

PEEP, Positive end-expiratory pressure.

Table 16-6
Ventilator Settings

PARAMETER	DESCRIPTION	TYPICAL SETTINGS
Respiratory rate (f)	Number of breaths the ventilator delivers per minute	6-20 breaths/min
Tidal volume (V_T)	Volume of gas delivered to patient during each ventilator breath	10-12 ml/kg 6-8 ml/kg in acute lung injury (ALI)
Oxygen concentration (FIO_2)	Fraction of inspired oxygen delivered to patient	May be set between 21% and 100%; adjusted to maintain PaO_2 level greater than 60 mm Hg or SpO_2 level greater than 90%
Positive end-expiratory pressure (PEEP)	Positive pressure applied at the end of expiration of ventilator breaths	3-5 cm H_2O
Pressure support (PS)	Positive pressure used to augment patient's inspiratory efforts	5-10 cm H_2O
Inspiratory flow rate and time	Speed with which the tidal volume is delivered	40-80 L/min Time: 0.8-1.2 second
Inspiration/expiration (I/E) ratio	Duration of inspiration to duration of expiration	Rate: 1:2 to 1:1.5 unless inverse ratio ventilation is desired
Sensitivity	Determines the amount of effort the patient must generate to initiate a ventilator breath; it may be set for pressure-triggering or flow-triggering	Pressure trigger: 0.5-1.5 cm H_2O below baseline pressure Flow trigger: 1-3 L/min below baseline flow
High pressure limit	Regulates the maximal pressure the ventilator can generate to deliver the tidal volume; when the pressure limit is reached, the ventilator terminates the breath and spills the undelivered volume into the atmosphere	10-20 cm H_2O above peak inspiratory pressure

PaO_2, Arterial partial pressure of oxygen; *SpO_2,* oxygen saturation.

monitoring system that allows all aspects of the patient's ventilatory pattern to be assessed, monitored, and displayed.[41,42,45]

COMPLICATIONS

Mechanical ventilation is often lifesaving, but similar to other interventions, it is not without complications. Some complications are preventable, whereas others can be minimized but not eradicated. Physiologic complications associated with mechanical ventilation include ventilator-induced lung injury, cardiovascular compromise, gastrointestinal disturbances, patient-ventilator dyssynchrony, and hospital-acquired pneumonia.

Ventilator-Induced Lung Injury

Mechanical ventilation can cause two different types of injury to the lungs: air leaks and biotrauma.[46] Air leaks related to mechanical ventilation are the result of excessive pressure or volume in the alveoli (volutrauma) or shearing due to repeated opening and closing of the alveoli (atelectrauma).[47] Volutrauma and atelectrauma can lead to excessive alveolar wall stress and damage to the alveolar-capillary membrane, resulting in air leaking into the surrounding spaces. Once in the space, the air travels out through the hilum and into the mediastinum (pneumomediastinum), pleural space (pneumothorax), subcutaneous tissues (subcutaneous emphysema), pericardium (pneumopericardium), peritoneum (pneumoperitoneum), and retroperitoneum (pneumoretroperitoneum). The resultant disorders vary from the fairly benign to the potentially lethal—the most lethal of which include a pneumothorax or a pneumopericardium resulting in cardiac tamponade.[48] Volutrauma and atelectrauma can also cause the release of cellular mediators and the initiation of the inflammatory-immune response. This type of ventilator-induced injury is known as biotrauma.[49] Biotrauma can result in the development of acute lung injury.[50] To limit ventilator-induced lung injury, the plateau pressure (pressure needed to inflate the alveoli) should be kept less than 32 cm H_2O, PEEP should be used to avoid end-expiratory collapse and reopening, and the tidal volume should be set at 6 to 10 ml/kg.[46,49]

Cardiovascular Compromise

Positive-pressure ventilation increases intrathoracic pressure, which decreases venous return to the right side of the heart. Impaired venous return decreases preload, which results in a decrease in CO.[48,51] As a secondary consequence, hepatic and renal dysfunction may occur. In addition, positive-pressure ventilation impairs cerebral venous return. In patients with impaired autoregulation, positive-pressure ventilation can result in increased intracranial pressure.[51]

Gastrointestinal Disturbances

A number of gastrointestinal disturbances also can occur as a result of positive-pressure ventilation. Gastric distention occurs when air leaks around the endotracheal or tracheostomy tube cuff and overcomes the resistance of the lower esophageal sphincter.[43,48] Vomiting can occur as a result of pharyngeal stimulation from the artificial airway.[15] These problems can be prevented by inserting a nasogastric tube and ensuring appropriate cuff inflation.[43,48] In addition, hypomotility and constipation may occur as a result of immobility and the administration of paralytic agents, analgesics, and sedatives.[48]

Patient-Ventilator Dyssynchrony

Because the normal ventilatory pattern is usually initiated by the establishment of negative pressure within the chest, the application of positive pressure can lead to patient difficulties in breathing on the ventilator. To achieve optimal ventilatory assistance, the patient should breathe in synchrony with the machine. The selected mode of ventilation, the settings, and the type of ventilatory circuitry used can also increase the work of breathing and lead to the patient breathing out of synchrony with the ventilator. Patient-ventilatory dyssynchrony can result in a decrease in effectiveness of mechanical ventilation, the development of auto-PEEP, and psychologic distress in the patient. Patients who are not breathing in synchrony with the ventilator appear to be fighting or "bucking" the ventilator. To minimize this problem, the ventilator is adjusted to accommodate the patient's spontaneous breathing pattern and to work with the patient. If this is not possible, the patient may need to be sedated and/or pharmacologically paralyzed.[43,52]

Ventilator-Associated Pneumonia

Ventilator-associated pneumonia (VAP) is a subgroup of hospital-acquired pneumonia that refers to development of pneumonia while undergoing mechanical ventilation (see Evidence-Based Collaborative Practice: American Association of Critical-Care Nurses Practice Alert: Ventilator-Associated Pneumonia). There is great potential for the development of pneumonia after the placement of an artificial airway, because the tube bypasses or impairs many of the lung's normal defense mechanisms. Once an artificial airway is placed, contamination of the lower airways follows within 24 hours. This results from a number of factors that directly and indirectly promote airway colonization. The use of respiratory therapy devices (e.g., ventilators, nebulizers, and intermittent positive-pressure breathing machines) also can increase the risk of pneumonia. The severity of the patient's illness, presence of acute lung injury, or malnutrition significantly increases the likelihood that an infection will ensue. In addition, such therapeutic measures as nasogastric tubes, antacids, and histamine$_2$-antagonists facilitate the development of pneumonia. Nasogastric tubes promote aspiration by acting as a wick for stomach contents, whereas antacids and histamine inhibitors increase the pH level of the stomach, thus promoting the growth of bacteria that can then be aspirated.[53] Managing the patient with pneumonia is discussed in Chapter 15.

WEANING

Weaning is the gradual withdrawal of the mechanical ventilator and the reestablishment of spontaneous breathing. Weaning should begin only after the original process requiring ventilator support for the patient has been corrected and patient stability has been achieved.

EVIDENCE-BASED COLLABORATIVE PRACTICE

American Association of Critical-Care Nurses Practice Alert: Ventilator-Associated Pneumonia

Expected Practice

✓ All patients receiving mechanical ventilation, as well as those at high risk for aspiration (e.g., decreased level of consciousness; with enteral tube in place), should have the head of the bed (HOB) elevated at an angle of 30 to 45 degrees unless medically contraindicated.

✓ Use an endotracheal tube (ET) with a dorsal lumen above the endotracheal cuff to allow drainage by continuous suctioning of tracheal secretions that accumulate in the subglottic area.

✓ Do not routinely change, on the basis of duration of use, the patient's ventilator circuit.

Supporting Evidence

- Critically ill patients who are intubated for >24 hours are at 6 to 21 times the risk of developing ventilator-associated pneumonia (VAP),[1-3] and those intubated for <24 hours are at 3 times the risk of VAP.[4] Other risk factors for VAP include decreased level of consciousness, gastric distention, presence of gastric or small intestine tubes, and a trauma or COPD diagnosis. VAP is reported to occur at rates of 10 to 35 cases/1000 ventilator days, depending on the clinical situation.[3]
- Aspiration of oral and/or gastric fluids is presumed to be an essential step in the development of VAP. Pulmonary aspiration is increased by supine positioning and pooling of secretions above the ET tube cuff.[1,5,6]
- Morbidity and mortality associated with the development of VAP is high, with mortality rates ranging from 20% to 41%.[4,7,8] Development of VAP increases ventilator days, critical care lengths of stay (LOS), and hospital LOS by 4, 4, and 9 days, respectively,[2-7] and results in >$40,000 additional costs/VAP case.[2,6]
- Compared to supine positioning, studies have shown that simple positioning of the HOB to 30 degrees or higher significantly reduces gastric reflux and VAP (8% versus 34%, respectively),[4,9-12] yet national surveys and reports in the literature describe poor compliance rates with HOB elevation in critical care units.[4,13-15]
- Studies show that the use of special ET tubes which remove secretions pooled above the cuff with continuous suction decrease VAP by 45% to 50%.[16-19]
- Studies on the frequency of ventilator circuit changes have found no increase in VAP with prolonged use.[20-22]
- National regulatory and expert consensus groups include these interventions as critical to decrease VAP.[1,23-25]

What You Should Do

- Always keep mechanically ventilated patients' HOB elevated to 30 degrees or higher, unless medically contraindicated; use an ET tube with continuous suction above the cuff; do not routinely change ventilator circuits.
- Ensure that your critical care unit has written practice documents such as a policy, procedure, or standard of care that includes these practice alerts.
- Determine your unit's rate of compliance with the HOB elevation directive, and use an ET tube with continuous suction above the cuff.
- If compliance is <90%, develop a plan to improve compliance[13]:
  - → Consider forming a multidisciplinary task force (nurses, physicians, respiratory therapist, clinical pharmacist) or a unit core group of staff to address VAP practice changes.
  - → Educate staff about the significance of nosocomial pneumonias in critically ill patients and how these interventions can reduce VAP.
  - → Incorporate content into orientation programs and initial and annual competency verifications.
  - → Develop a variety of communication strategies to alert and remind staff of the importance of these VAP interventions.
  - → Develop documentation standards for HOB elevation that include rationale for when the HOB is not elevated.
  - → Incorporate HOB elevation to at least 30 degrees in any unit standing orders (include those for monitoring into your critical care scorecard), quality improvement plan, and/or process improvement activities to ensure that practice changes continue.

COPD, Chronic obstructive pulmonary disease.

Continued

Other factors to consider when weaning are length of time on ventilator, sleep deprivation, and nutritional status. Major factors that affect the patient's ability to wean include the ability of the lungs to participate in ventilation and respiration, cardiovascular performance, and psychologic readiness.[54] This discussion focuses on weaning the patient from short-term (3 days or less) mechanical ventilation. Managing the patient requiring long-term mechanical ventilation is discussed in Chapter 15.

EVIDENCE-BASED COLLABORATIVE PRACTICE

American Association of Critical-Care Nurses Practice Alert: Ventilator-Associated Pneumonia—*cont'd*

References

1. Weinstein R et al: Guidelines for prevention of healthcare-associated pneumonia, *MMWR Morb Mortal Wkly Rep,* in press.
2. Rello J et al: Epidemiology and outcomes of ventilator-associated pneumonia in a large US database, *Chest* 122:2115-2121, 2002.
3. Craven D: Epidemiology of ventilator-associated pneumonia, *Chest* 117:186S-187S, 2000.
4. Kollef M: Ventilator-associated pneumonia: a multivariate analysis, *JAMA* 270:1965-1970, 1993.
5. Torres A et al: Pulmonary aspiration of gastric contents in patients receiving mechanical ventilation: the effect of body position, *Ann Intern Med* 116:540-542, 1992.
6. Craven D et al: Nosocomial pneumonia: emerging concepts in diagnosis, management and prophylaxis, *Curr Opin Crit Care* 8:421-429, 2002.
7. Bercault N, Boulain T: Mortality rate attributable to ventilator-associated nosocomial pneumonia in an adult intensive care unit: a prospective case-control study, *Crit Care Med* 29:2303-2309, 2001.
8. Heyland D et al: The attributable morbidity and mortality of ventilator-associated pneumonia in the critically ill patient, *Am J Resp Crit Care Med* 159:1249-1256, 1999.
9. Ibanez J et al: Gastroesophageal reflux in intubated patients receiving enteral nutrition: effect of supine and semi recumbent positions, *JPEN J Parenter Enteral Nutr* 16:419-422, 1992.
10. Orozco-Levi M et al: Semi-recumbent position protects from pulmonary aspiration but not completely from gastroesophageal reflux in mechanically ventilated patients, *Am J Respir Crit Care Med* 152:1387-1390, 1995.
11. Drakulovic M et al: Supine body position as a risk factor for nosocomial pneumonia in mechanically ventilated patients: a randomized trial, *Lancet* 354:1851-1854, 1999.
12. Dotson R, Robinson R, Pingleton S: Gastroesophageal reflux with nasogastric tubes: effect of nasogastric tube size, *Am J Respir Crit Care Med* 149:1659-1662, 1994.
13. Zack J et al: Effect of an educational program aimed at reducing the occurrence of ventilator-associated pneumonia, *Crit Care Med* 30:2407-2412, 2002.
14. Berenholtz S, Pronovost P: Barriers to translating evidence into practice, *Curr Opin Crit Care* 9:321-325, 2003.
15. Grap M et al: Use of backrest elevation in critical care: pilot study, *Am J Crit Care* 8:475-480, 1999.
16. Valles J et al: Continuous aspiration of subglottic secretions in preventing ventilator-associated pneumonia, *Int Care Med* 122:179-186, 1995.
17. Mahul P et al: Prevention of nosocomial pneumonia in intubated patients: respective role of mechanical subglottic secretion drainage and stress ulcer prophylaxis, *Int Care Med* 18:20-25, 1992.
18. Kollef M, Skubas N, Sundt T: A randomized clinical trial of continuous aspiration of subglottic secretions in cardiac surgery patients, *Chest* 116:1339-1346, 1999.
19. Cook D et al: Influence of airway management on ventilator-associated pneumonia: evidence from randomized trials, *JAMA* 279:761-787, 1998.
20. Dreyfuss D et al: Prospective study of nosocomial pneumonia and of patient circuit colonization during mechanical ventilation with circuit changes every 48 hours versus no change, *Am Rev Respir Dis* 143:738-743, 1991.
21. Kotilainen H, Keroack M: Cost analysis and clinical impact of weekly ventilator circuit changes in patients in intensive care unit, *Am J Infect Control* 25:117-120, 1997.
22. Kollef M et al: Mechanical ventilation with or without 7-day circuit changes: a randomized controlled trial, *Ann Intern Med* 123:168-174, 1995.
23. Joint Commission on Accreditation of Healthcare Organizations. ICU Core Measures—draft statement, http://www.jcaho,org/pms/core+measures/candidate+core+measure+set.htm, accessed September 26, 2003.
24. Parrish C, Krenitsky J, McCray C: Nutritional support for the mechanically ventilated patient. In AACN's *Protocols for Practice, Care of the Mechanically Ventilated Patient* series, Aliso Viejo, Calif, 1998, AACN.
25. Collard H, Saint S: Prevention of ventilator-associated pneumonia, Agency for Health Care Policy and Research (AHCPR) website: http://www.ahcpr.gov/clinic/ ptsafety/chap17a.htm.

Other VAP Articles of Interest

Hixon S, Sole M, King T: Nursing strategies to prevent ventilator-associated pneumonia, *AACN Clin Issues* 9:76-90, 1998.

Pfeifer L et al: Preventing ventilator-associated pneumonia, *Am J Nurs* 101:24AA-24GG, 2001.

Readiness to Wean

Once the decision is made to wean the patient, the patient is assessed for readiness to wean. Evaluation of the patient includes the patient's level of consciousness, physiologic and hemodynamic stability, adequacy of oxygenation and ventilation, spontaneous breathing capability, and respiratory rate and pattern. In addition, pulmonary mechanics may be measured. Two strong predictors for weaning readiness are vital capacity (VC)/kg greater than 15 ml and negative inspiratory pressure (NIP) of –30 cm H_2O or less.[55]

Once readiness to wean has been established, the patient is prepared for the weaning trial. The patient is positioned upright to facilitate breathing and suctioned to ensure airway patency. In addition, the process is explained to the patient, and the patient is offered reassurance and diversional activities. The patient is assessed immediately before the start of the trial and frequently during the weaning period for signs of weaning intolerance (Boxes 16-1 and 16-2).[54-56]

Weaning Methods

A number of methods can be used to wean a patient from the ventilator. The method selected depends on the patient, his or her pulmonary status, and the length of time on the ventilator. The three main methods for weaning are (1) T-tube (T-piece) trials, (2) synchronized intermittent mandatory ventilation (SIMV), and (3) pressure support ventilation (PSV).[54-56]

T-Piece. T-piece weaning trials consist of alternating periods of ventilatory support (usually on assist/control [A/C] or continuous mandatory ventilation [CMV]) with periods of spontaneous breathing. The trial is initiated by removing the patient from the ventilator and having the patient breathe spontaneously on a T-piece oxygen delivery system. After a set amount of time, the patient is placed back on the ventilator. The goal is to progressively increase the duration of time spent off the ventilator. During the weaning process, the patient is observed closely for respiratory muscle fatigue.[49-51] Continuous positive airway pressure (CPAP) may be added to prevent atelectasis and improve oxygenation.[56]

Synchronized Intermittent Mandatory Ventilation. The goal of SIMV weaning is the gradual transition from ventilatory support to spontaneous breathing. It is initiated by placing the ventilator in the SIMV mode and slowly decreasing the rate until zero (or close to zero) is reached. The rate is usually decreased one to three breaths at a time, and an arterial blood gas (ABG) sample is usually obtained 30 minutes afterward. This method of weaning can increase the work of breathing, and thus the patient must be closely monitored for signs of respiratory muscle fatigue.[54-56]

Pressure Support Ventilation. PSV weaning consists of placing the patient on the pressure support mode and setting the pressure support at a level that facilitates the patient's achieving a spontaneous tidal volume of 10 to 12 ml/kg. PSV augments the patient's spontaneous breaths with a positive-pressure "boost" during inspiration. During the weaning process, the level of pressure support is gradually decreased in increments of 3 to 6 cm H_2O, while maintaining a tidal volume of 10 to 15 ml/kg, until a level of 5 cm H_2O is achieved. If the patient is able to maintain adequate spontaneous respirations at this level, extubation is considered. PSV also can be used with SIMV weaning to help overcome the resistance in the ventilator system.[54-56]

Box 16-1

Weaning Intolerance Indicators

- Decrease in level of consciousness
- Systolic blood pressure increased or decreased by 20 mm Hg
- Diastolic blood pressure greater than 100 mm Hg
- Heart rate increased by 20 beats/min
- Premature ventricular contractions greater than 6 per minute, couplets, or runs of ventricular tachycardia
- Changes in ST segment (usually elevation)
- Respiratory rate greater than 30 breaths/min or less than 10 breaths/min
- Respiratory rate increased by 10 breaths/min
- Spontaneous tidal volume less than 250 ml
- $Paco_2$ increased by 5 to 8 mm Hg and/or pH less than 7.30
- Spo_2 less than 90%
- Use of accessory muscles of ventilation
- Complaints of dyspnea, fatigue, or pain
- Paradoxic chest wall motion
- Diaphoresis

PATIENT SAFETY PRIORITIES

Invasive Mechanical Ventilation

A number of measures are required to maintain a trouble-free ventilator system. These include maintaining a functional manual resuscitation bag connected to oxygen at the bedside, ensuring that the ventilator tubing is free of water, positioning the ventilator tubing to avoid kinking, maintaining the patency of ventilator tubing and connections, changing ventilator tubing per hospital policy, and monitoring the temperature of the inspired air. In the event that the ventilator malfunctions, the patient is removed from the ventilator and ventilated manually with a manual resuscitation bag (MRB). In addition, alarms should be sufficiently audible with respect to distances and competing noise within the unit.

NURSING MANAGEMENT

Nursing priorities for the patient with invasive mechanical ventilation are directed toward monitoring the patient for both patient-related and ventilator-related complications. Monitoring should include a total patient assessment, with particular emphasis on the pulmonary system, placement of the artificial airway, and observation for subcutaneous emphysema and synchrony with the ventilator. Assessment of the ventilator includes a review of all the ventilator settings and alarms. A clear understanding of the alarms and their related problems is important (Table 16-7). In addition, the peak inspiratory pressure, exhaled tidal volume, and arterial blood gas levels are also monitored. Patient safety issues are addressed in Patient Safety Priorities: Invasive Mechanical Ventilation.

Bedside evaluation of VC, minute ventilation, ABG values, and other pulmonary function tests may be warranted, according to the patient's condition. The use of pulse oximetry can facilitate continuous, noninvasive assessment of oxygenation. Static and dynamic compliance should also be monitored to assess for changes in lung compliance (see Appendix B).

Semirecumbency

Positioning of the patient requiring mechanical ventilation is also important. Semirecumbent positioning (elevation of the head of the bed) may help reduce the incidence of gastroesophageal reflux and lead to a decreased incidence of VAP. Thus the head of the patient's bed should be elevated to 30 to 45 degrees at all times unless contraindicated (e.g., hemodynamic instability).[35,57] However, this intervention does increase the risk of skin sheer on the coccyx, and extra surveillance is mandatory for prevention of pressure ulcers.[57]

NONINVASIVE MECHANICAL VENTILATION

Noninvasive mechanical ventilation is a relatively new method of ventilation that uses a mask instead of an ETT to administer positive-pressure ventilation (Figure 16-5). Advantages of this type of ventilation include decreased frequency of hospital-acquired pneumonia, increased comfort, and the noninvasive nature of the procedure, which allows easy application and removal. It is indicated in both type I and type II acute respiratory failure and when intubation is not an option. Contraindications to noninvasive mechanical ventilation include hemodynamic instability, dysrhythmias, apnea, uncooperativeness, intolerance of the mask, and the inability to maintain a patent airway, clear secretions, and properly fit the mask.[58] One recent study found that a full-face mask is better tolerated than a nasal mask.[59]

Noninvasive mechanical ventilation can be applied using a nasal or facial mask and ventilator or a BiPAP (trademark of Respironics) machine (see Figure 16-5). This mode of therapy uses a combination of PSV (ventilator) or inspiratory positive airway pressure (IPAP) (BiPAP machine) and PEEP (ventilator) or expiratory positive airway pressure (EPAP) (BiPAP machine) to assist the spontaneously breathing patient with ventilation. On inspiration, the patient receives PSV or IPAP to increase tidal volume and minute ventilation, which results in increased alveolar ventilation, a decreased $Paco_2$ level, relief of dyspnea, and reduced accessory muscle use. On expiration, the patient receives PEEP or EPAP to increase functional residual capacity, which results in an increased Pao_2 level. Humidified supplemental oxygen is administered to maintain a clinically acceptable Pao_2 level, and timed breaths may be added if necessary.[60]

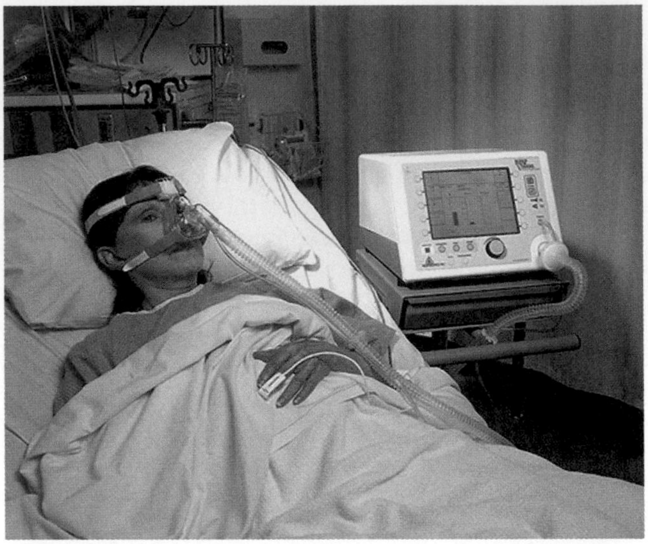

FIGURE 16-5. BiPAP Vision Face Mask in use. (Courtesy Respironics Inc, Murrysville, Pa.).

NURSING MANAGEMENT

Nursing priorities for the patient with noninvasive mechanical ventilation are directed toward monitoring the patient for both patient-related and ventilator-related complications. As with invasive mechanical ventilation, the patient must be closely monitored while receiving noninvasive mechanical ventilation. Respiratory rate, accessory muscle use, and oxygenation status are continually assessed to ensure that the patient is tolerating this method of ventilation. Continued pulse oximetry with a set alarm parameter is initiated.[60]

The key to ensuring adequate ventilatory support is a properly fitted mask. Either a nasal mask or a full-face mask may be used, depending on the patient. A properly fitted mask minimizes air leakage and discomfort for the patient. Transparent dressings placed over the pressure points of the face help minimize

Table 16-7
Troubleshooting Ventilator Alarms

PROBLEM	CAUSES	INTERVENTIONS
Low exhaled V_T	Altered settings; any condition that triggers high- or low-pressure alarm; patient stops spontaneous respirations; leak in system preventing V_T from being delivered; cuff insufficiently inflated; leak through chest tube; airway secretions; decreased lung compliance; spirometer disconnected or malfunctioning	Check settings; evaluate patient, check respiratory rate; check all connections for leaks; suction patient's airway; check cuff pressure; calibrate spirometer
Low inspiratory pressure	Altered settings; unattached tubing or leak around ET tube; ET tube displaced into pharynx or esophagus; poor cuff inflation or leak; tracheosophageal fistula; peak flows that are too low; low V_Ts; decreased airway resistance resulting from decreased secretions or relief of bronchospasm; increased lung compliance resulting from decreased atelectasis; reduction in pulmonary edema; resolution of ALI; change in position	Reset alarm; reconnect tubing; modify cuff pressures; tighten humidifier; check chest tube; adjust peak flow to meet or exceed patient demand and correct for the patient's V_T; reposition or change ET tube
Low exhaled minute volume	Altered settings; leak in system; airway secretions; decreased lung compliance; malfunctioning spirometer; decreased patient-triggered respiratory rate resulting from drugs; sleep; hypocapnia; alkalosis; fatigue; change in neurologic status	Check settings; assess patient's respiratory rate, mental status, and work of breathing; evaluate system for leaks; suction airway; assess patient for changes in disease state; calibrate spirometer
Low PEEP/CPAP pressure	Altered settings; increased patient inspiratory flows; leak; decreased expiratory flows from ventilator	Check settings and correct; observe for leaks in system; if unable to correct problem, increase PEEP settings
High respiratory rate	Increased metabolic demand; drug administration; hypoxia; hypercapnia; acidosis; shock; pain; fear; anxiety	Evaluate ABGs; assess patient; calm and reassure patient
High pressure limit	Improper alarm setting; airway obstruction resulting from patient fighting ventilator (holding breath as ventilator delivers V_T); patient circuit collapse; tubing kinked; ET tube in right mainstem bronchus or against carina; cuff herniation; increased airway resistance resulting from bronchospasm, airway secretions, plugs, and coughing; water from humidifier in ventilator tubing; decreased lung compliance resulting from tension pneumothorax; change in patient position; ALI; pulmonary edema; atelectasis; pneumonia; or abdominal distention	Reset alarms; clear obstruction from tubing; unkink and reposition patient off tubing; empty water from tubing; check breath sounds; reassure patient and sedate if necessary; check ABGs for hypoxemia; observe for abdominal distention that would put pressure on the diaphragm; check cuff pressures; obtain chest x-ray film and evaluate for ET tube position, pneumothorax, and pneumonia; reposition ET tube; give bronchodilator therapy
Low-pressure oxygen inlet	Improper oxygen alarm setting; oxygen not connected to ventilator; dirty oxygen intake filter	Correct alarm setting; reconnect or connect oxygen line to a 50-psi source; clean or replace oxygen filter
I/E ratio	Inspiratory time longer than expiratory time; use of an inspiratory phase that is too long with a fast rate; peak flow setting too low while rate too high; machine too sensitive	Change inspiratory time or adjust peak flow; check inspiratory phase, or hold; check machine sensitivity
Temperature	Sensor malfunction; overheating resulting from too low or no gas flow; sensor picking up outside airflow (from heaters, open doors or windows, air conditioners); improper water levels	Test or replace sensor; check gas flow; protect sensor from outside source that would interfere with readings; check water levels

Modified from Flynn JBM, Bruce NP: *Introduction to critical care nursing skills,* St Louis, 1993, Mosby.
V_T, Tidal volume; *ET,* endotracheal; *ALI,* acute lung injury; *PEEP,* positive end-expiratory pressure; *CPAP,* constant positive airway pressure; *ABGs*, arterial blood gases.

air leakage and prevent facial skin necrosis from the mask. The BiPAP machine is able to compensate for air leaks.[61]

The patient is positioned with the head of the bed elevated at 45 degrees to minimize the risk of aspiration and facilitate breathing. Insufflation of the stomach is a complication of this mode of therapy and places the patient at risk for aspiration. Thus the patient is closely monitored for gastric distention, and a nasogastric tube is placed for decompression as necessary. Often patients are very anxious and have high levels of dyspnea before the initiation of noninvasive mechanical ventilation. Once adequate ventilation has been established, anxiety and dyspnea are usually suffi-

PATIENT SAFETY PRIORITIES

Noninvasive Mechanical Ventilation

The patient requiring noninvasive mechanical ventilation with a full-face mask should never be restrained. The patient has to be able to remove the mask in the event that the mask becomes displaced or the patient vomits. A displaced mask can force the patient's bottom jaw inward and occlude the patient's airway.

ciently relieved. Heavy sedation should be avoided, but if needed, it would constitute the need for intubation and invasive mechanical ventilation. Spending 30 minutes with the patient after the initiation of noninvasive ventilation is important because the patient needs reassurance and must learn how to breathe on the machine.[59,61] Patient safety issues are addressed in Patient Safety Priorities: Noninvasive Mechanical Ventilation.

POSITION THERAPY

Position therapy can help match ventilation and perfusion through the redistribution of oxygen and blood flow in the lungs, which improves gas exchange. Using the concept that there is preferential blood flow to the gravity-dependent areas of the lungs, position therapy is used to place the least damaged portion of the lungs into a dependent position. Thus the least damaged portions of the lungs receive preferential blood flow, resulting in less ventilation/perfusion mismatching.[62] Currently there are two different approaches to position therapy: prone positioning and rotation therapy. Which position works best with each specific pulmonary disorder is still under investigation.

PRONE POSITIONING

Prone positioning is a relatively new therapeutic modality used to improve oxygenation in ALI. It involves turning the patient completely over onto his or her stomach into the facedown position. Although a number of theories have been proposed to explain how prone positioning improves oxygenation, the discovery that ALI causes greater damage to the dependent areas of the lungs probably provides the best explanation. It was originally thought that ALI was a diffuse homogenous disease that affected all areas of the lungs equally. It is now known that the dependent lung areas are more heavily damaged than the nondependent lung areas. Turning the patient prone improves perfusion to less damaged areas of the lungs and improves ventilation/perfusion matching and de-

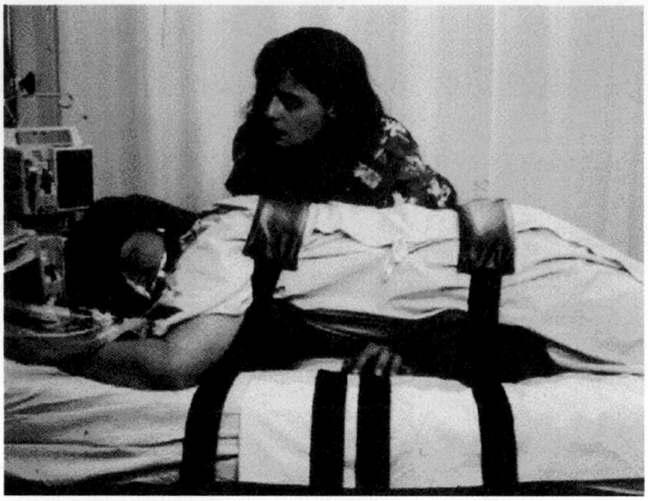

FIGURE 16-6. Patient in prone position. (Courtesy Kathleen Vollman and Hill-Rom Services, Inc, Batesville, Ind.)

creases intrapulmonary shunting.[63] In addition, prone positioning can be used to facilitate the mobilization of secretions and provide pressure relief.[64] Prone positioning is contraindicated in patients with increased intracranial pressure, hemodynamic instability, spinal cord injuries, and abdominal surgery. Patients who are unable to tolerate a facedown position are also not appropriate candidates for this type of therapy.[63]

Currently no standard for the length of time a patient should remain in the prone position has been established. A review of the research on this subject revealed a wide variation, anywhere from 30 minutes to 40 hours.[64] The therapy is considered successful if the patient has an improvement in Pao_2 of greater than 10 mm Hg within 30 minutes of being placed in the prone position.[63,64] Thus the positioning schedule (length of time in prone position and frequency of turning) is usually based on the patient's tolerance of the procedure, the success of the procedure in improving the patient's Pao_2, and whether the patient is able to sustain improvements in Pao_2 when turned back to the supine position.[64] Prone positioning is discontinued when the patient no longer demonstrates a response to the position change.[63]

The biggest limitation to prone positioning is the actual mechanics of turning the patient. A number of procedures have been discussed in the literature that advise using either pillows to support the patient or the Vollman Prone Positioner (Hill-Rom, Inc.).[64] The latter is a steel frame with four cushions to support the patient's forehead, chin, chest, and pelvic area. The device is applied to the patient in the supine position and then used to turn the patient to the prone position (Figure 16-6).[64] Regardless of the method used, the abdomen must be allowed to hang free to facilitate diaphragmatic descent.[63,64]

EVIDENCE-BASED COLLABORATIVE PRACTICE

Summary of Evidence and Evidence-Based Recommendations for Physiotherapy in the Intensive Care Unit

Strong Evidence of the Following:
- Physiotherapy is the treatment of choice for patients with acute lobar atelectasis.
- Prone positioning improves oxygenation for some patients with severe acute respiratory failure or ALI.
- Positioning in side-lying position (affected lung uppermost) improves oxygenation for some patients with unilateral lung disease.
- Hemodynamic status should be monitored during physiotherapy to detect any deleterious side effects of treatment.
- Sedation before physiotherapy will decrease or prevent adverse hemodynamic or metabolic responses.
- Preoxygenation, sedation, and reassurance are necessary before suction to avoid suction-induced hypoxemia.
- Rotation therapy (kinetic therapy) decreases the incidence of pulmonary complications.

Moderate Evidence of the Following:
- Multimodality physiotherapy has a short-lived beneficial effect on respiratory function.
- MH may have a short-lived beneficial effect on respiratory function, but hemodynamic status, airway pressure, or V_T should be monitored to detect any deleterious side effects of treatment.
- ICP and CPP should be monitored on appropriate patients during physiotherapy to detect any deleterious side effects of treatment.

Very Limited or No Evidence of the Following:
- Routine physiotherapy in addition to nursing care prevents pulmonary complications commonly found in ICU patients.
- Physiotherapy is effective in the treatment of pulmonary conditions commonly found in ICU patients (with the exception of acute lobar atelectasis).
- Physiotherapy facilitates weaning, decreases length of stay in the ICU or hospital, and reduces mortality or morbidity.
- Positioning (with the exception of examples cited above), percussion, vibrations, suction, or mobilization are effective components of physiotherapy for ICU patients.
- Limb exercises prevent loss of joint range or soft-tissue length, or improve muscle strength and function, for ICU patients.

From Stiller K: *Chest* 118:1801, 2000.
ICU, Intensive care unit; *ALI,* acute lung injury; *MH,* manual hyperinflation; V_T, tidal volume; *ICP,* intracranial pressure; *CPP,* cerebral perfusion pressure.

Before turning the patient to the prone position, the patient's eyes are lubricated and taped closed, the patient's tubes and drains are secured, and the procedure is explained to the patient and family. A team is organized to implement the turning procedure, and one member is positioned at the head of the bed to maintain the patient's airway. Complications of the procedure include dislodgment or obstruction of tubes and drains, hemodynamic instability, massive facial edema, pressure ulcers, aspiration, and corneal ulcerations.[63]

Rotation Therapy

The use of automated turning beds to provide rotation therapy is often found in the critical care setting. Kinetic therapy (KT) and continuous lateral rotation therapy (CLRT) are two forms of rotation therapy. KT is defined as the continuous turning of a patient from side to side with a 40-degree or greater rotation. CLRT is defined as the continuous turning of a patient from side to side with a less-than-40-degree rotation.[57,65] There are two different types of beds that can perform this type of therapy: an oscillation bed and a kinetic bed. An oscillation bed is one in which the mattress inflates and deflates to provide rotation and a kinetic bed is one which the entire platform of the bed rotates.[57,66]

Rotation therapy is thought to improve oxygenation through better matching of ventilation to perfusion[67] and to prevent pulmonary complications associated with bed rest and mechanical ventilation.[68] Studies have found, however, that to achieve such benefits, rotation must be aggressive and the patient must be at least 40 degrees per side, with a total arc of at least 80 degrees,[69] for at least 18 hours a day.[68] Thus continuous lateral rotation therapy has been shown to be of minimal pulmonary benefit to the critically ill patient. However, kinetic therapy has been shown to decrease the incidence of VAP particularly in neurologic and postoperative patients.[69] One recent study demonstrated that kinetic therapy decreased the incidence of both VAP and lobar atelectasis in a variety of medical, surgical, and trauma patients[68] (see Evidence-Based Collaborative Practice: Recommendations for Physiotherapy in the Intensive Care Unit).

Complications of the procedure include dislodgment or obstruction of tubes, drains, and lines; hemodynamic instability; and pressure ulcers. Lateral rotation does not replace manual repositioning to prevent pressure ulcers.[70] Repositioning changes the relationship of the patient's posterior surface to the mattress. This gives the skin a chance to reperfuse and to ventilate. In addition, repositioning shifts weight-bearing points. To prevent pressure ulcers the patient should be positioned 30 degrees from the surface of the mattress regardless of the degree of rotational turn. One study found that patients receiving rotational therapy actually developed pressure ulcers of the sacrum, occiput, and heels.[71]

THORACIC SURGERY

Types Of Surgery

Thoracic surgery refers to a number of surgical procedures that involve opening the thoracic cavity (thoracotomy) and/or the organs of respiration. Indications for thoracic surgery range from tumors and abscesses to repair of the esophagus and thoracic vessels.[72] Table 16-8 describes a variety of thoracic surgical procedures and their indications. This discussion focuses only on the surgical procedures that involve the removal of lung tissue.

Preoperative Care

Before surgery, a complete evaluation of the patient is needed to determine the appropriateness of surgery as a treatment and to determine whether lung tissue can be removed without jeopardizing respiratory function. This is especially important when a lobectomy or pneumonectomy is being considered. When resection is being undertaken for tumor treatment, preoperative care includes evaluation of the type and extent of the tumor and the physical condition of the patient.[72]

The evaluation of the patient's physical status should focus on the adequacy of cardiopulmonary function. The preoperative evaluation should include pulmonary function tests to determine the patient's ability to manage with less lung tissue. Cardiac function also should be evaluated. Uncontrolled dysrhythmias, acute myocardial infarction, severe chronic heart failure, and unstable angina are all contraindications to surgery.[73]

Surgical Considerations

The type and location of surgery will dictate the type of surgical approach that is used. The most common approach is the posterolateral thoracotomy, which allows for exposure of both the lung and mediastinum. Other approaches that are used include anterolateral thoracotomy and median sternotomy.[72]

Special care is taken to avoid drainage of blood or secretions into the unaffected lung during surgery, because such an occurrence could cause hypoxemia and cardiac dysfunction. A double-lumen endotracheal tube is used during the surgery to protect the unaffected lung from secretions and necrotic tumor fragments. To decrease the incidence of hypoxemia during the procedure, 5 to 10 cm H_2O of PEEP is maintained to the deflated lung. In addition, the deflated lung is intermittently ventilated during the procedure.[74]

Complications and Medical Management

A number of complications are associated with a lung resection. These include acute respiratory failure, bronchopleural fistula, hemorrhage, cardiovascular disturbances, and mediastinal shift.

Acute Respiratory Failure

In the postoperative period, acute respiratory failure may result from atelectasis or pneumonia. Atelectasis can occur as a result of anesthesia, the surgical procedure, immobilization, and pain.[75] Treatment should be aimed at correcting the underlying problems and supporting gas exchange. Supplemental oxygen and mechanical ventilation with PEEP may be necessary.[74] For further discussion on acute respiratory failure see Chapter 15.

Bronchopleural Fistula

Development of a postoperative bronchopleural fistula is a major cause of mortality after a lung resection. A bronchopleural fistula develops when the suture line fails to secure occlusion of the bronchial stump and an opening develops. This can result from an imperfect stump closure, perforation of the stump (e.g., with a suction catheter), high pressure within the airways (e.g., caused by mechanical ventilation),[76] or infection.[77] During surgery, careful attention is given to isolating and closing the bronchus in an attempt to secure a lasting seal with subsequent stump healing.[72] In addition, early extubation is encouraged to eliminate the possibility of perforation of the stump and high airway pressures.[76] Clinical manifestations of a bronchopleural fistula include shortness of breath and coughing up serosanguineous sputum. Immediate surgery is usually necessary to close the stump and prevent flooding of the remaining lung with fluid from the residual space.[77] If this occurs, the patient should be placed with the operative side down (remaining lung up) and a chest tube should be inserted to drain the residual space.[72]

Hemorrhage

Hemorrhage is an early, life-threatening complication that can occur after a lung resection. It can result from bronchial or intercostal artery bleeding or

Table 16-8
Thoracic Surgeries

PROCEDURE	DEFINITION	INDICATIONS
Pneumonectomy 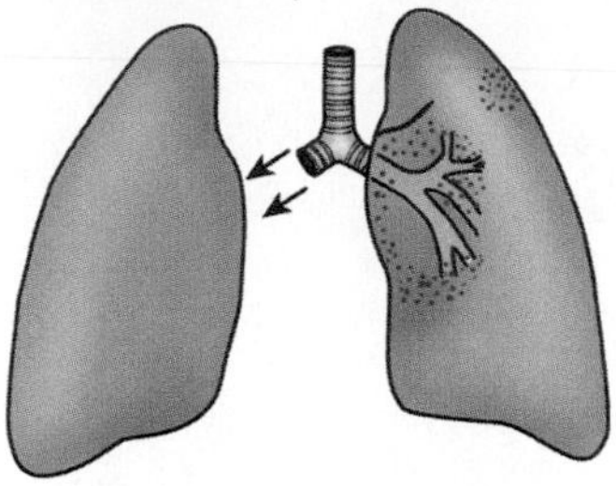	Removal of entire lung with or without resection of the mediastinal lymph nodes	Malignant lesions Unilateral tuberculosis Extensive unilateral bronchiectasis Multiple lung abscesses Massive hemoptysis Bronchopleural fistula
Lobectomy 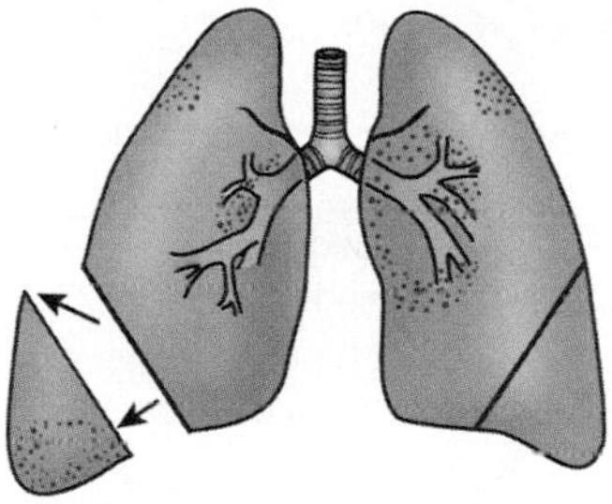	Resection of one or more lobes of lung	Lesions confined to a single lobe Pulmonary tuberculosis Bronchiectasis Lung abscesses or cysts Trauma
Segmental resection 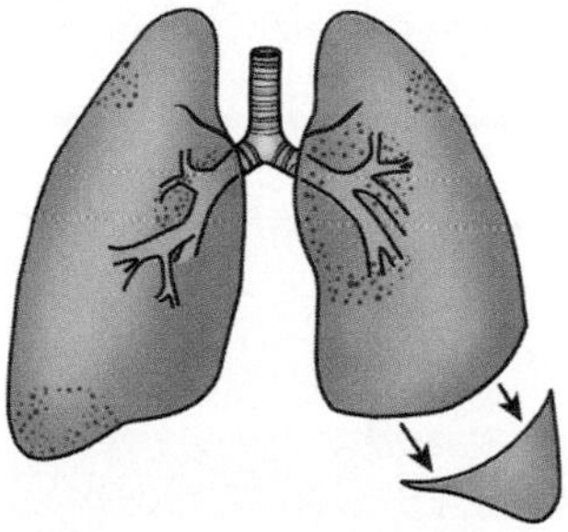	Resection of bronchovascular segment of lung lobe	Small peripheral lesions Bronchiectasis Congenital cysts or blebs
Wedge resection 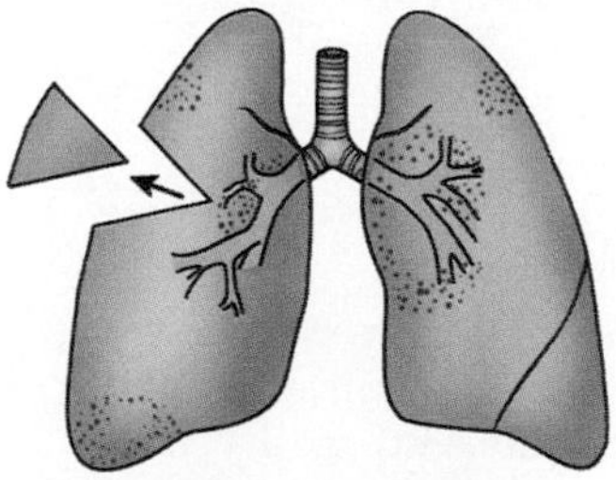	Removal of small wedge-shaped section of lung tissue	Small peripheral lesions (without lymph node involvement) Peripheral granulomas Pulmonary blebs
Bronchoplastic reconstruction (also called sleeve resection) 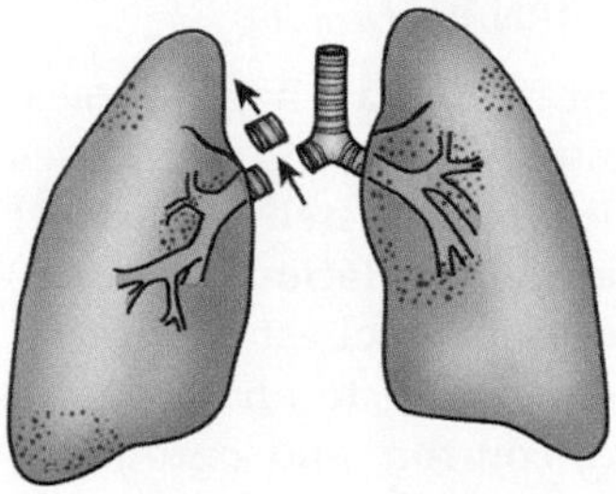	Resection of lung tissue and bronchus with end-to-end reanastomosis of bronchus	Small lesions involving the carina or major bronchus without evidence of metastasis May be combined with lobectomy

Table 16-8

Thoracic Surgeries—*cont'd*

PROCEDURE	DEFINITION	INDICATIONS
Lung volume reduction surgery	Resection of the most damaged portions of lung tissue, allowing more normal chest wall configuration	Severe emphysema
Bullectomy	Resection of a large bulla (an airspace that is greater than 1 cm in diameter that formed as a result of pulmonary tissue destruction)	Severe emphysema with large bullae compressing surrounding tissue
Open lung biopsy	Resection of a small portion of the lung for biopsy	Failure of closed lung biopsy Removal of small lesions
Decortication	Removal of fibrous membrane from pleural surface of lung	Fibrothorax resulting from hemothorax or empyema
Drainage of empyema	Drainage of pus in the pleural space	Acute and chronic infections
Partial rib resection	Removal of one or more ribs to allow healing of underlying lung tissue	Chronic empyemic infections
Video-assisted thoracoscopy (VATS)	Endoscopic procedure performed through small incisions in the chest	Evaluation of pulmonary, pleural, mediastinal, or pericardial conditions Biopsy of lung, pleural, or mediastinal lesions Recurrent spontaneous pneumothorax Evacuation of emphysema, hemothorax, pleural effusion, or pericardial effusion Blebectomy/bullectomy Pleurodesis Sympathectomy Closure of bronchopleural fistula Lysis of adhesions

disruption of a suture or clip around a pulmonary vessel.[76] Excessive chest tube drainage can signal excessive bleeding. During the immediate postoperative period, chest tube drainage should be measured every 15 minutes; this frequency should be decreased as the patient stabilizes. If chest tube loss is greater than 100 ml/hr, fresh blood is noted, or a sudden increase in drainage occurs, hemorrhage should be suspected.

Cardiovascular Disturbances

Cardiovascular complications after thoracic surgery include dysrhythmias and pulmonary edema. Resections of a large lung area or a pneumonectomy may be followed by a rise in central venous pressure. With the loss of one lung, the right ventricle must empty its stroke volume into a vascular bed that has been reduced by 50%. This means a higher pressure system is created, which increases right ventricular workload and precipitates right ventricular failure. Depending on previous heart function, acute decompensation of both ventricles can result. Measures are aimed at supporting cardiac function and avoiding intravascular volume excess. These measures include optimizing preload, afterload, and contractility with vasoactive agents.[76]

Box 16-2

NURSING DIAGNOSIS PRIORITIES

Thoracic Surgery

- Ineffective Breathing Pattern related to decreased lung expansion, p. A-34
- Impaired Gas Exchange related to ventilation/perfusion mismatching or intrapulmonary shunting, p. A-29
- Impaired Gas Exchange related to alveolar hypoventilation, p. A-29
- Acute Pain related to transmission and perception of cutaneous, visceral, muscular, or ischemic impulses, p. A-7
- Disturbed Body Image related to actual change in body structures, function, or appearance, p. A-20

Postoperative Nursing Management

Nursing care of the patient who has had thoracic surgery incorporates a number of nursing diagnoses (Box 16-2). **Nursing priorities are directed toward (1) optimizing oxygenation and ventilation, (2) preventing atelectasis, (3) monitoring chest tubes, (4) assisting the patient with returning to an adequate activity level, (5) providing comfort and emotional support, and (6) maintaining surveillance for complications.**

Optimizing Oxygenation and Ventilation

Nursing interventions to optimize oxygenation and ventilation include positioning, preventing desaturation during procedures, and promoting secretion clearance.

Preventing Atelectasis

Nursing interventions to prevent atelectasis include proper patient positioning and early ambulation, deep-breathing exercises, incentive spirometry (IS), and pain management. The goal is to promote maximal lung ventilation and prevent hypoventilation.

Patient Positioning and Early Ambulation. The nurse should consider the surgical incision site and the type of surgery when positioning the patient. After a lobectomy, the patient should be turned onto the nonoperative side to promote ventilation/perfusion (V/Q) matching. When the good lung is dependent and blood flow is greater to the area with better ventilation, V/Q matching is better. V/Q mismatching results when the affected lung is positioned down because of the increase in blood flow to an area with less ventilation. The patient should be turned frequently to promote secretion removal but should have the affected lung dependent as little as possible. The patient who has had a pneumonectomy should be positioned supine or on the operative side during the initial period. Turning onto the operative side promotes splinting of the incision and facilitates deep-breathing exercises. Tilting the patient slightly toward the unaffected side is possible, but the surgeon should indicate when free side-to-side positioning is safe.[78]

When sitting at the bedside or ambulating, patients must be encouraged to keep the thorax in straight alignment while they breathe deeply. This position best accommodates diaphragmatic descent and intercostal muscle action. The sitting or standing position provides enhanced ventilation to areas of the lung that are dependent in the supine position, thus accommodating maximal inflation and promoting gas exchange. Ambulation is essential in restoring lung function and should be initiated as soon as possible.[79]

Deep Breathing and Incentive Spirometry. Deep breathing and incentive spirometry should be performed regularly by patients who have undergone a thoracotomy. Deep breathing involves having the patient take a deep breath and hold it for approximately 3 seconds or longer. Incentive spirometry involves having the patient take at least 10 deep, effective breaths per hour using an incentive spirometer. These activities help reexpand collapsed lung tissue, thus promoting early resolution of the pneumothorax in patients with partial lung resections. The chest should be auscultated during inflation to ensure that all dependent parts of the lung are well ventilated and to help the patient understand the depth of breath necessary for optimal effect. Coughing, which should be encouraged only when secretions are present, assists in mobilizing secretions for removal.[79]

Pain Management. Pain can be a major problem after thoracic surgery. Pain can increase the workload of the heart, precipitate hypoventilation, and inhibit mobilization of secretions. Clinical manifestations of pain include tachypnea, tachycardia, elevated blood pressure, facial grimacing, splinting of the incision, hypoventilation, moaning, and restlessness. Several alternatives for pain management after thoracic surgery can be used. The two most common methods are systemic narcotic administration and epidural narcotic administration. Systemic narcotics can be administered intravenously or via the patient-controlled analgesia (PCA) method. In addition, the patient should be assisted with splinting the incision with a pillow or blanket when deep breathing and coughing. Splinting stabilizes the area and reduces pain when moving, deep breathing, or coughing.[75]

Maintaining the Chest Tube System

Chest tubes are placed after most thoracic surgery procedures to remove air and fluid. The drainage will initially appear bloody, becoming serosanguineous and then serous over the first 2 to 3 days postoperatively. Approximately 100 to 300 ml of drainage will occur during the first 2 hours postoperatively, which will decrease to less than 50 ml/hr over the next several hours. Routine stripping of chest tubes is not recommended because excessive negative pressure can be generated in the chest. If blood clots are present in the drainage tubing or an obstruction is present, the chest tubes may be carefully milked. The chest tube may be placed to suction or water seal.[80]

During auscultation of the lungs, air leaks should be evaluated. In the early phase, an air leak is commonly heard over the affected area, because the pleura have not yet tightly sealed. As healing occurs, this leak should disappear. An increase in an air leak or the appearance of a new air leak should prompt investigation of the chest drainage system to discover whether air is leaking into the system from outside or whether the leak is originating from the incision. Increased air leaks not related to the thoracic drainage system may indicate disruption of sutures.[76]

Assisting Patient With Returning to Adequate Activity Level

Within a few days after surgery, range-of-motion exercises for the shoulder on the operative side should be performed. The patient frequently splints the operative side and avoids shoulder movement because of pain. If immobility is allowed, stiffening of the shoulder joint can result. This is referred to as *frozen shoulder* and may require physical therapy and rehabilitation to regain satisfactory range of motion of the shoulder joint.[78]

Usually on the day after surgery, the patient is able to sit in a chair. Activity should be systematically increased, with attention to the patient's activity tolerance. With adequate pulmonary function before surgery and a surgical approach designed to preserve respiratory function, full return to previous activity levels is possible. This may take as long as 6 months to 1 year, depending on the tissue resected and the patient's general condition.[72]

SINGLE-LUNG AND DOUBLE-LUNG TRANSPLANTATIONS

Lung transplantation includes the transplantation of one or two lungs depending on the patient's underlying condition. Generally speaking, single-lung transplantation (SLT) is most appropriate for patients with restrictive lung diseases such as idiopathic pulmonary fibrosis (IPF) and sarcoidosis or noninfectious obstructive lung diseases such as emphysema in the absence of significant cardiac dysfunction.[81] Pulmonary diseases that typically are associated with chronic lung infections, such as cystic fibrosis and bronchiectasis, require transplantation of both lungs because of the risk of cross-infection from the native lung into the transplanted lung.[81]

SINGLE-LUNG TRANSPLANT SURGICAL PROCEDURE

Transplantation contralateral (opposite side) to a previous thoracotomy is preferable in order to avoid adhesions that require further surgical dissection. The left lung is sometimes preferred because it is easier to expose and has a longer left main bronchus. The longer bronchus gives the surgeon more flexibility in trimming the suture site as needed for anastomosis (Figure 16-7).[72] If there is a significant disproportion of ventilation and perfusion to one side, transplantation of the worse side may be the preferred option. With SLT the remaining native lung, which has either restrictive or obstructive pathophysiology, will have a higher vascular resistance than the transplanted lung. The blood flow is then automatically directed toward the new lung.[82]

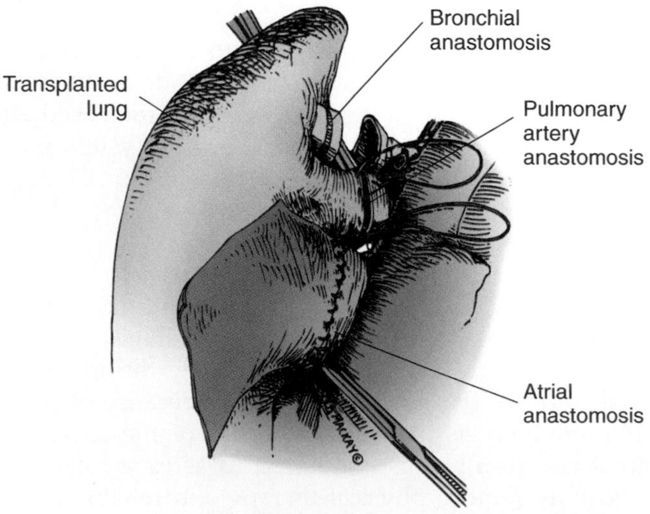

FIGURE 16-7. Single-lung transplant: surgical procedure. (Modified from Baumgartner WA et al: *Heart and heart-lung transplantation,* ed 2, Philadelphia, 2002, Saunders.)

Use of cardiopulmonary bypass (CPB) is becoming less and less common during lung transplantation. However, patients with moderate to severe pulmonary hypertension generally require CPB because clamping of the pulmonary artery necessary for removal of the diseased lung may cause sudden right heart failure. Inability to maintain adequate oxygenation and ventilation with a single lung, sudden increases in pulmonary artery pressure, poor right ventricular function, and hemodynamic compromise indicate the need for CPB.[81]

DOUBLE-LUNG TRANSPLANT SURGICAL PROCEDURE

The surgical procedure for both single- and double-lung transplantation (DLT) is similar, with a few exceptions. In fact, a DLT is performed as a bilateral, sequential SLT. The surgical incision for an SLT can be through either an anterolateral or posterolateral thoracotomy at the level of the fourth or fifth intercostal space. A DLT is performed through bilateral anterior thoracosternotomies extending from the midaxillary line and across the sternum at the fourth intercostal space. This approach is also known as a *clamshell incision.* The clamshell incision is exquisitely painful for the majority of patients, necessitating frequent pain assessment and intervention by the nurse. A median sternotomy or bilateral anterior thoracotomies are alternative surgical approaches.[72,83]

The anastomotic sites for DLT include the back wall of the atria (containing the four pulmonary vein orifices), the bronchus, and the main pulmonary artery as illustrated in Figure 16-8. Donor and recipient arteries are trimmed to suitable lengths, and an end-to-end anastomosis is performed. Bronchial anastomosis is performed with a running suture. After the atrial clamp is slowly removed, the patient is assessed for bleeding. In some transplant centers the omentum is brought through the diaphragm from the abdomen and is wrapped around the bronchus for added stability of the anastomosis and increased vascular supply. Disadvantages of this maneuver include a larger incision and involvement of the abdominal cavity.[72]

LIVING-DONOR LUNG TRANSPLANTATION

Another alternative to traditional lung transplantation is living-donor lung transplantation. In living-donor transplantation the lungs are harvested not from a brain-dead donor but from two living donors who provide either a right or left lower lobe to the recipient.

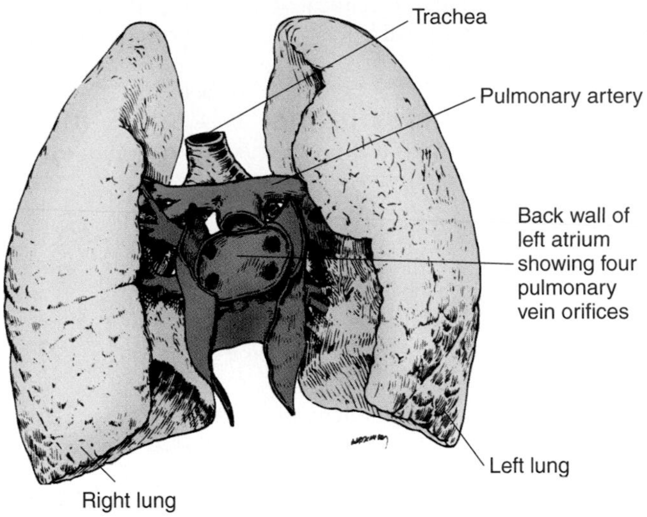

FIGURE 16-8. Double-lung transplant graft before implantation into a recipient. (Modified from Baumgartner WA et al: *Heart and heart-lung transplantation*, ed 2, Philadelphia, 2002, Saunders.)

The two donated lobes essentially function as new lungs. Recipients of this type of transplant tend to be patients with cystic fibrosis or other patients who are smaller in size. Smaller recipients increase the likelihood that two lobes are able to provide adequate pulmonary function. Living-donor lung transplantation is still fairly specialized and is therefore not as commonly practiced as cadaveric lung transplantation.[84]

POSTOPERATIVE MEDICAL AND NURSING MANAGEMENT

Several nursing diagnoses are associated with care of single-lung and double-lung transplant patients (Box 16-3). **Nursing priorities are directed toward (1) optimizing oxygenation and ventilation, (2) providing comfort and emotional support, and (3) maintaining surveillance for complications.** SLT patients generally require mechanical ventilation for a shorter duration. Less bleeding can be anticipated because of the brevity of the surgical procedure. A single pleural chest tube usually is sufficient for drainage. A pulmonary artery catheter may be used to measure right ventricular response when significant V/Q mismatch occurs. In the event of elevated pulmonary artery pressures, pharmacologic vasodilation or afterload reduction can be instituted. Patients with pulmonary hypertension potentially may have a greater V/Q mismatch, resulting in larger alveolar-arterial (A-a) O_2 gradients.

Surveillance of rejection and infection is similar to that in heart lung transplant (HLT). Pulmonary function testing is not initiated until the second or third week postoperatively to allow for surgical recovery. Decreased lung function because of fluid shifts, microatelectasis, and splinting from incisional pain would interfere with accurate testing. In unilateral lung transplantation the transplanted lung functions in parallel with the native lung, which can be expected to retain any pathologic condition. The patient must be measured by a comparison with his or her own baseline and not with normal standards. This concept also can be applied to the immediate postoperative period of intubation during the evaluation of arterial blood gas levels. Oxygenation and ventilation occur in both the diseased and transplanted lungs, and parameters for evaluation need to be adjusted accordingly.[85]

It is important that patient education is provided to cover all aspects of the immunosuppressive medication regimen, signs and symptoms of infection, role of pulmonary function tests, transbronchial biopsy, and clinical signs of pulmonary failure. In addition, a discussion of lifestyle adjustments, long-term considerations, and follow-up visits is included.

Box 16-3

NURSING DIAGNOSIS PRIORITIES

Single-Lung and Double-Lung Transplantation

- Ineffective Airway Clearance related to excessive secretions or abnormal viscosity of mucus, p. A-33
- Impaired Gas Exchange related to ventilation/perfusion mismatching or intrapulmonary shunting, p. A-29
- Risk for Infection , p. A-46
- Disturbed Body Image related to actual change in body structure, function, or appearance, p. A-46
- Anxiety related to threat to biologic, psychologic, and/or social integrity, p. A-20
- Readiness for Enhanced Knowledge: Posttransplant Self-Care Regimen, immunosuppressive drugs, pulmonary drugs, diuretics, and clinical manifestations of infection, p. A-9

evolve To test your mastery of this chapter, try the Open-Book Quiz at http://evolve.elsevier.com/Urden/priorities/

REFERENCES

1. O'Connor BS, Vender JS: Oxygen therapy, *Crit Care Clin* 11:67, 1995.
2. Kruse JA: Oxygen therapy. In Kruse JA, Fink MP, Carlson RW: *Saunders manual of critical care*, Philadelphia, 2003, Saunders.
3. Heuer AJ, Scanlan CL: Medical gas therapy. In Wilkins RL, Stoller JK, Scanlan CL, editors: *Egan's fundamentals of respiratory care*, ed 8, St Louis, 2003, Mosby.
4. White AC: The evaluation and management of hypoxemia in the chronic critically ill patient, *Clin Chest Med* 22:123, 2001.
5. Rossi A, Poggi R, Roca J: Physiologic factors predisposing to chronic respiratory failure, *Respir Care Clin N Am* 8:379, 2002.
6. Marshak AB: Emergency life support. In Wilkins RL, Stoller JK, Scanlan CL, editors: *Egan's fundamentals of respiratory care*, ed 8, St Louis, 2003, Mosby.

7. Greenberg RS: Facemask, nasal, and oral airway devices, *Anesthesiol Clin North Am* 20:833, 2002.
8. Shuster M, Nolan J, Barnes TA: Airway and ventilation management, *Cardiol Clin* 20:23, 2002.
9. Rodricks MB, Deutschman CS: Emergent airway management: indications and methods in the face of confounding conditions, *Crit Care Clin* 16:389, 2000.
10. St John RE, Seckel MA: Airway management. In Burns S, editor: *AACN protocols for practice: care of mechanically ventilated patients,* ed 2, Sudbury, Mass, 2007, Jones & Bartlett.
11. Simmons KF, Scanlan CL: Airway management. In Wilkins RL, Stoller JK, Scanlan CL, editors: *Egan's fundamentals of respiratory care,* ed 8, St Louis, 2003, Mosby.
12. Blanda M, Gallo UE: Emergency airway management, *Emerg Med Clin North Am* 21:1, 2003.
13. Colice GL: Technical standards for tracheal tubes, *Clin Chest Med* 12:433, 1991.
14. Loh KS, Irish JC: Traumatic complications of intubation and other airway management procedures, *Anesthesiol Clin North Am* 20:953, 2002.
15. Feller-Kopman D: Acute complications of artificial airways, *Clin Chest Med* 24:445, 2003.
16. St John RE, Malen JF: Contemporary issues in adult tracheostomy management, *Crit Care Nurs Clin North Am* 16:413, 2004.
17. Walts PA, Murthy SC, DeCamp MM: Techniques of surgical tracheostomy, *Clin Chest Med* 24:413, 2003.
18. Hess DR: Tracheostomy tubes and related appliances, *Respir Care* 50:497, 2005.
19. Sue RD, Susanto I: Long-term complications of artificial airways, *Clin Chest Med* 24:457, 2003.
20. Zuchner K: Humidification: measurement and requirements, *Respir Care Clin N Am* 12:149, 2006.
21. Fink J: Humidity and bland aerosol therapy. In Wilkins RL, Stoller JK, Scanlan CL, editors: *Egan's fundamentals of respiratory care,* ed 8, St Louis, 2003, Mosby.
22. Sottiaux TM: Consequences of under- and over-humidification. *Respir Care Clin N Am* 12:233, 2006.
23. Wright SE, VanDahm K: Long-term care of the tracheostomy patient, *Clin Chest Med* 24:473, 2003.
24. Bivona: *Fome-Cuf users manual,* Gary, Ind, 1991, Bivona.
25. Grap MJ et al: Endotracheal suctioning: ventilator vs. manual delivery of hyperoxygenation breaths, *Am J Crit Care* 5:192, 1996.
26. Stone KS: Ventilator versus manual resuscitation bag as the method of delivering hyperoxygenation before endotracheal suctioning, *AACN Clin Issues Crit Care Nurs* 1:289, 1990.
27. Czarnik RE et al: Differential effects of continuous versus intermittent suction on tracheal tissue, *Heart Lung* 20:144, 1991.
28. Raymond SJ: Normal saline instillation before suctioning: helpful or harmful? A review of the literature, *Am J Crit Care* 4:267, 1995.
29. Kinloch D: Instillation of normal saline during endotracheal suctioning: effects on mixed venous oxygen saturation, *Am J Crit Care* 8:231, 1999.
30. Hagler DA, Traver GA: Endotracheal saline and suction catheters: sources of lower airway contamination, *Am J Crit Care* 3:444, 1994.
31. Kollef MH et al: Mechanical ventilation with or without daily changes of in-line suction catheters, *Am J Respir Crit Care Med* 156:466, 1997.
32. Jablonski RS: The experience of being mechanically ventilated, *Qual Health Res* 4:186, 1994.
33. Williams ML: An algorithm for selecting a communication technique with intubated patients, *Dimens Crit Care Nurs* 11:222, 1992.
34. Hodder RV: A 55-year-old patient with advanced COPD, tracheostomy tube, and sudden respiratory distress, *Chest* 120:279, 2002.
35. Flanders SA, Collard HR, Saint S: Nosocomial pneumonia: state of the science, *Am J Infect Control* 34:84, 2006.
36. Dennesen P et al: Inadequate salivary flow and poor oral mucosal status in intubated intensive care patients, *Crit Care Med* 31:781, 2003.
37. Munro CL et al: Oral health status and development of ventilator-associated pneumonia: a descriptive study, *Am J Crit Care* 15:453, 2006.
38. Binkley et al: Survey of oral care practices in U.S. intensive care units, *Am J Infect Control* 32:161, 2004.
39. Munro CL, Grap MJ: Oral health and care in the intensive care unit: state of the science, *Am J Crit Care* 13:25, 2004.
40. Garcia R: A review of the possible role of oral and dental colonization on the occurrence of health care–associated pneumonia: underappreciated risk and a call for interventions, *Am J Infect Control* 33:527, 2005.
41. Gali B, Goyal DG: Positive-pressure mechanical ventilation, *Emerg Med Clin North Am* 21:453, 2003.
42. Chatburn RL, Volsko TA: Mechanical ventilators. In Wilkins RL, Stoller JK, Scanlan CL, editors: *Egan's fundamentals of respiratory care,* ed 8, St Louis, 2003, Mosby.
43. Pilbeam SP, Cairo JM: *Mechanical ventilation: physiological and clinical applications*, ed 4, St Louis, 2006, Mosby.
44. Pierce LNB: Invasive and noninvasive modes and methods of mechanical ventilation. In Burns S, editor: *AACN protocols for practice: care of mechanically ventilated patients,* ed 2, Sudbury, Mass, 2007, Jones & Bartlett.
45. Shelledy DC, Peters JI: Initiating and adjusting ventilatory support. In Wilkins RL, Stoller JK, Scanlan CL, editors: *Egan's fundamentals of respiratory care,* ed 8, St Louis, 2003, Mosby.
46. Adams AB, Simonson DA, Dries DJ: Ventilator-induced lung injury, *Respir Care Clin N Am* 9:343, 2003.
47. Carney D, DiRocco J, Nieman G: Dynamic alveolar mechanics and ventilator-induced lung injury, *Crit Care Med* 33(3 suppl):S122, 2005.
48. Chatila WM, Criner GJ: Complications of long-term mechanical ventilation, *Respir Care Clin N Am* 8:631, 2002.
49. Ramnath VR, Hess DR, Thompson BT: Conventional mechanical ventilation in acute lung injury and acute respiratory distress syndrome, *Clin Chest Med* 27:601, 2006.
50. dos Santos CC, Slutsky AS: The contribution of biophysical lung injury to the development of biotrauma, *Annu Rev Physiol* 68:585, 2006.
51. Kuiper JW et al: Mechanical ventilation and acute renal failure, *Crit Care Med* 33:1408, 2005.
52. Ramar K, Sassoon CS: Potential advantages of patient-ventilator synchrony, *Respir Care Clin N Am* 11:307, 2005.

53. Craven DE: Preventing ventilator-associated pneumonia in adults: sowing the seeds of change, *Chest* 130: 251, 2006.
54. Shelledy DC: Discontinuing ventilatory support. In Wilkins RL, Stoller JK, Scanlan CL, editors: *Egan's fundamentals of respiratory care,* ed 8, St Louis, 2003, Mosby.
55. Burns SM: Weaning from mechanical ventilation. In Burns S, editor: *AACN protocols for practice: care of mechanically ventilated patients,* ed 2, Sudbury, Mass, 2007, Jones & Bartlett.
56. Hess D: Ventilator modes used in weaning, *Chest* 120 (6 suppl):474S, 2001.
57. Hess D: Patient positioning and ventilator-associated pneumonia, *Respir Care* 50:892, 2005.
58. Hamel DS, Klonin H: The role of noninvasive ventilation for acute respiratory failure, *Respir Care Clin N Am* 12:421, 2006.
59. Kwok H et al: Controlled trial of oronasal versus nasal mask ventilation in the treatment of acute respiratory failure, *Crit Care Med* 31:468, 2003.
60. Calfee CS, Matthay MA: Recent advances in mechanical ventilation, *Am J Med* 118:584, 2005.
61. Vines DL: Noninvasive positive-pressure ventilation. In Wilkins RL, Stoller JK, Scanlan CL, editors: *Egan's fundamentals of respiratory care,* ed 8, St Louis, 2003, Mosby.
62. Misasi RS, Keyes JL: Matching and mismatching ventilation and perfusion in the lung, *Crit Care Nurse* 16(3):23, 1996.
63. Piedalue F, Albert RK: Prone positioning in acute respiratory distress syndrome, *Respir Care Clin N Am* 9:495, 2003.
64. Vollman KM: Prone positioning in the patient who has acute respiratory distress syndrome: the art and science, *Crit Care Nurs Clin North Am* 16:319, 2004.
65. Goldhill DR et al: Rotational bed therapy to prevent and treat respiratory complications: a review and meta-analysis, *Am J Crit Care* 16:50, 2007.
66. Stiller K: Physiotherapy in intensive care: towards an evidence-based practice, *Chest* 118:1801, 2000.
67. McLean B: Rotational kinetic therapy for ventilation/perfusion mismatch, *Crit Care Nurs Eur* 1:113, 2001.
68. Ahrens T et al: Effect of kinetic therapy on pulmonary complications, *Am J Crit Care* 13:376, 2004.
69. Collard HR: Prevention of ventilator-associated pneumonia: an evidence-based systematic review, *Ann Intern Med* 138:494, 2003.
70. Powers J, Daniels D: Turning points: implementing kinetic therapy in the ICU, *Nurs Manage* 35(5):1, 2004.
71. Russell T, Logsdon A: Pressure ulcers and lateral rotation beds: a case study, *J Wound Ostomy Continence Nurs* 30:143, 2003.
72. Dawes BSG: Thoracic surgery. In Rothrock JC, Smith DA, McEwen DR, editors: *Alexander's care of the patient in surgery,* ed 12, St Louis, 2003, Mosby.
73. Tamul PC, Peruzzi WT: Assessment and management of patients with pulmonary disease, *Crit Care Med* 32: S137, 2004.
74. Cohen E: Management of one-lung ventilation, *Anesthesiol Clin North Am* 19:475, 2001.
75. Gottschalk A et al: Preventing and treating pain after thoracic surgery, *Anesthesiology* 104:594, 2006.
76. Kopec SE: The postpneumonectomy state, *Chest* 114: 1158, 1998.
77. Lois M, Noppen M: Bronchopleural fistulas: an overview of the problem with special focus on endoscopic management, *Chest* 128: 3955, 2005.
78. Brenner Z, Addona C: Caring for the pneumonectomy patient: challenges and changes, *Crit Care Nurse* 15(5):65, 1995.
79. Brooks, JA: Postoperative nosocomial pneumonia: nurse-sensitive interventions, *AACN Clin Issues* 12:305, 2001.
80. Cerfolio RJ: Advances in thoracostomy tube management, *Surg Clin North Am* 82:833, 2002.
81. Hartwig MG, Davis RD Surgical considerations in lung transplantation: transplant operation and early post-operative management, *Respir Care Clin N Am* 10:473, 2004.
82. Trindade AJ, Palmer SM: Current concepts and controversies in lung transplantation, *Respir Care Clin N Am* 10:427, 2004.
83. Roselli EE, Smedira NG: Surgical advances in heart and lung transplantation, *Anesthesiol Clin North America* 22:789, 2004.
84. Bowdish ME, Barr ML: Living lobar lung transplantation, *Respir Care Clin N Am* 10:563, 2004.
85. Arcasoy SM: Medical complications and management of lung transplant recipients, *Respir Care Clin N Am* 10:505, 2004.

CHAPTER 17

Neurologic Clinical Assessment and Diagnostic Procedures

KATHLEEN M. STACY

OBJECTIVES

- Identify the components of a neurologic history.
- Describe the five components of the neurologic assessment.
- Discuss the neurologic changes associated with intracranial hypertension.
- Identify key diagnostic procedures used in assessment of the patient with neurologic dysfunction.
- Discuss the nursing management of a patient undergoing a neurologic diagnostic procedure.
- Identify the different types of intracranial pressure monitoring devices.

Assessment of the critically ill patient with neurologic dysfunction includes a review of the patient's health history, a thorough physical examination, and an analysis of the patient's laboratory data. Numerous invasive and noninvasive diagnostic procedures may also be performed to assist in the identification of the patient's disorder. This chapter focuses on clinical assessments, laboratory studies, and diagnostic procedures for the critically ill patient with a neurologic dysfunction.

CLINICAL ASSESSMENT

A thorough clinical assessment of the patient with neurologic dysfunction is imperative for the early identification and treatment of neurologic disorders. Once completed, the assessment serves as the foundation for developing the management plan for the patient. The assessment process can be brief or can involve a detailed history and examination, depending on the nature and immediacy of the patient's situation.

HISTORY

Neurologic assessment encompasses a wide variety of applications and a multitude of techniques. This chapter focuses on the type of assessment performed in a critical care environment. The one factor common to all neurologic assessments is the need to obtain a comprehensive history of events preceding hospitalization. An adequate neurologic history includes information about clinical manifestations, associated complaints, precipitating factors, progression, and familial occurrences. If the patient is incapable of providing this information, family members or significant others should be contacted as soon as possible. When someone other than the patient is the source of the history, it should be an individual who was in contact with the patient on a daily basis. Frequently, valuable information is gained, which directs the caregiver to focus on certain aspects of the patient's clinical assessment.[1]

PHYSICAL EXAMINATION

Five major components make up the neurologic examination of the critically ill patient. **Nursing assessment priorities focus on evaluating (1) level of consciousness, (2) motor function, (3) pupillary function, (4) respiratory function, and (5) vital signs.** Until all five components have been assessed, a complete neurologic examination has not been performed.[1]

LEVEL OF CONSCIOUSNESS

Assessment of the level of consciousness is the most important aspect of the neurologic examination. In most situations, a patient's level of consciousness deteriorates before any other neurologic changes are noted. These deteriorations often are subtle and must be monitored carefully. **Nursing priorities in assessment of level of consciousness focus on (1) evaluating arousal or alertness and (2) appraising consciousness or awareness.**[1] Though universally accepted definitions for various levels of consciousness do not exist, the categories outlined in Box 17-1 are often used to describe the patient's level of consciousness.[1-4]

Evaluating Arousal

Assessment of the arousal component of consciousness is an evaluation of the reticular activating system and its connection with the thalamus and the cerebral cortex. Arousal is the lowest level of consciousness, and observation centers on the patient's ability to respond to verbal or noxious stimuli in an appropriate manner. To stimulate the patient, the nurse should begin with verbal stimuli in a normal tone. If the patient does not respond, the nurse should increase the stimuli by shouting at the patient. If the patient still does not respond, the nurse should further increase the stimuli by shaking the patient. Noxious stimuli should follow if previous attempts to arouse the patient are unsuccessful. To assess arousal, central stimulation should be used (Box 17-2).

Appraising Awareness

Content of consciousness is a higher-level function and is concerned with assessment of the patient's orientation to person, place, and time. Assessment of content of consciousness requires the patient to give appropriate answers to a variety of questions. Changes in the patient's answers that indicate increasing degrees of confusion and disorientation may be the first sign of neurologic deterioration.[1,3,4]

Glasgow Coma Scale

The most widely recognized level of consciousness assessment tool is the Glasgow Coma Scale (GCS).[5] This scored scale is based on evaluation of three categories: eye opening, verbal response, and best motor response (Table 17-1). The best possible score on the

Box 17-1

Categories of Consciousness

Alert	Patient responds immediately to minimal external stimuli.
Confused	Patient is disoriented to time or place but usually oriented to person, with impaired judgment and decision making and decreased attention span.
Delirious	Patient is disoriented to time, place, and person with loss of contact with reality and often has auditory or visual hallucinations.
Lethargic	Patient displays a state of drowsiness or inaction in which the patient needs an increased stimulus to be awakened.
Obtunded	Patient displays dull indifference to external stimuli, and response is minimally maintained. Questions are answered with a minimal response.
Stuporous	Patient can be aroused only by vigorous and continuous external stimuli. Motor response is often withdrawal or localizing to stimulus.
Comatose	Vigorous stimulation fails to produce any voluntary neural response.

From Barker E: *Neuroscience nursing: a spectrum of care,* ed 2, St Louis, 2002, Mosby.

Box 17-2

Stimulation Techniques in Patient Arousal

Central Stimulation

- *Trapezius pinch:* Squeeze trapezius muscle between thumb and first two fingers.
- *Sternal rub:* Apply firm pressure to sternum with knuckles, using a rubbing motion.

Peripheral Stimulation

- *Nail bed pressure:* Apply firm pressure, using object such as a pen, to nail bed.
- *Pinching of inner aspect of arm/leg:* Firmly pinch small portion of patient's tissue on sensitive inner aspect of arm or leg.

Table 17-1

Glasgow Coma Scale

CATEGORY	SCORE	RESPONSE
Eye opening	4	Spontaneous—eyes open spontaneously without stimulation
	3	To speech—eyes open with verbal stimulation but not necessarily to command
	2	To pain—eyes open with noxious stimuli
	1	None—no eye opening regardless of stimulation
Verbal response	5	Oriented—accurate information about person, place, time, reason for hospitalization, and personal data
	4	Confused—answers not appropriate to question, but use of language is correct
	3	Inappropriate words—disorganized, random speech, no sustained conversation
	2	Incomprehensible sounds—moans, groans, and incomprehensible mumbles
	1	None—no verbalization despite stimulation
Best motor response	6	Obeys commands—performs simple tasks on command; able to repeat performance
	5	Localizes to pain—organized attempt to localize and remove painful stimuli
	4	Withdraws from pain—withdraws extremity from source of painful stimuli
	3	Abnormal flexion—decorticate posturing spontaneously or in response to noxious stimuli
	2	Extension—decerebrate posturing spontaneously or in response to noxious stimuli
	1	None—no response to noxious stimuli; flaccid

GCS is 15, and the lowest score is 3. Generally a score of 7 or less on the GCS indicates coma. Originally the scoring system was developed to assist in general communication concerning the severity of neurologic injury. Recent testing of the GCS revealed a moderate to high agreement rating among both physicians and nurses.[6,7] Several points should be kept in mind when the GCS is used for serial assessment. It provides data about level of consciousness only and never should be considered a complete neurologic examination. It is not a sensitive tool for evaluation of an altered sensorium, nor does it account for possible aphasia. The GCS is also a poor indicator of lateralization of neurologic deterioration.[7] Lateralization involves decreasing motor response on one side or unilateral changes in pupillary reaction.

MOTOR FUNCTION

Nursing priorities in assessment of motor function focus on (1) evaluating muscle size and tone and (2) estimating muscle strength. Each side should be assessed individually and then compared together.[1,8]

Evaluating Muscle Size and Tone

Initially the muscles should be inspected for size and shape. The presence of atrophy or hypertrophy is noted. Muscle tone is assessed by evaluating the opposition to passive movement. The patient is instructed to relax the extremity while the nurse performs passive range of motion and evaluates the degree of resistance. Muscle tone is appraised for signs of flaccidity (no resistance), hypotonia (little resistance), hypertonia (increased resistance), spasticity, or rigidity.[8]

Estimating Muscle Strength

Having the patient perform a number of movements against resistance assesses muscle strength. The strength of the movement is then graded on a six-point scale (Box 17-3). Asking the patient to grasp, squeeze, and release the nurse's index and middle fingers tests the upper extremities. If weakness or asymmetry is suspected, the patient is instructed to extend both arms with the palms turned upward and holds that position with the eyes closed. If the patient has a weaker side, the arm will drift downward and pronate. The lower extremities are tested by asking the patient to push and pull the feet against resistance.[9]

Abnormal Motor Responses

If the patient is incapable of comprehending and following a simple command, noxious stimuli is required to determine motor responses. The stimulus is applied to each extremity separately to allow evaluation of individual extremity function. Peripheral stimulation is used to assess motor function.[1,2] Motor responses elicited by noxious stimuli are interpreted differently than those elicited by voluntary demonstration. These responses may be classified into the categories listed in Box 17-4.[8]

Abnormal flexion also is known as *decorticate posturing* (Figure 17-1, *A*). In response to painful stimuli, the upper extremities exhibit flexion of the arm, wrist, and fingers with adduction of the limb. The lower extremity exhibits extension, internal rotation, and plantar flexion. Abnormal flexion occurs with lesions above the midbrain, in the region of the thalamus or cerebral hemispheres. Abnormal extension also is known as *decerebrate rigidity*, or *posturing* (Figure 17-1, *B*). When the patient is stimulated, teeth clench and the arms are stiffly extended, adducted, and hyperpronated. The legs are stiffly extended with plantar flexion of the feet. Abnormal extension occurs with lesions in the area of the brain stem. Because abnormal flexion and extension appear similar in the lower extremities, the upper extremities are used to determine the presence of these abnormal movements. It is possible for the patient to exhibit abnormal flexion on one side of the body and extension on the other (Figure 17-1, *C*).[1-3] Outcome studies indicate that abnormal flexion, or decorticate posturing, has a less serious prognosis than does extension, or decerebrate posturing. Onset of posturing or a change from abnormal

Box 17-3

Muscle Strength Grading Scale

0—No movement or muscle contraction
1—Trace contraction
2—Active movement with gravity eliminated
3—Active movement against gravity
4—Active movement with some resistance
5—Active movement with full resistance

Box 17-4

Classification of Abnormal Motor Function

Spontaneous	Occurs without regard to external stimuli and may not occur by request
Localization	Occurs when the extremity opposite the extremity receiving pain crosses midline of the body in an attempt to remove the noxious stimulus from the affected limb
Withdrawal	Occurs when the extremity receiving the painful stimulus flexes normally in an attempt to avoid the noxious stimulus
Decortication	Abnormal flexion response that may occur spontaneously or in response to noxious stimuli (see Figure 17-1, *A* and *C*)
Decerebration	Abnormal extension response that may occur spontaneously or in response to noxious stimuli (see Figure 17-1, *B* and *C*)
Flaccid	No response to painful stimuli

flexion to abnormal extension requires immediate physician notification.[3]

Pupillary Function

Nursing priorities in assessment of pupillary function focus on (1) estimating pupil size and shape, (2) evaluating pupillary reaction to light, and (3) assessing eye movements.[1]

Pupillary function is an extension of the autonomic nervous system. Parasympathetic control of the pupil occurs through innervation of the oculomotor nerve (CN III), which exits from the brain stem in the midbrain area. When the parasympathetic fibers are stimulated, the pupil constricts. Sympathetic control originates in the hypothalamus and travels down the entire length of the brain stem. When the sympathetic fibers are stimulated, the pupil dilates. Pupillary changes provide a valuable tool to assessment because of pathway location. The oculomotor nerve lies at the junction of the midbrain and the tentorial notch. Any increase of pressure that exerts force down through the tentorial notch compresses the oculomotor nerve. Oculomotor nerve compression results in a dilated, nonreactive pupil. Sympathetic pathway disruption occurs with involvement in the brain stem. Loss of sympathetic control leads to pinpoint, nonreactive pupils. Control of eye movements occurs with interaction of three cranial nerves: oculomotor (CN III), trochlear (CN IV), and abducens (CN VI). The pathways for these cranial nerves provide integrated function through the internuclear pathway of the medial longitudinal fasciculus (MLF) located in the brain stem. The MLF provides coordination of eye movements with the vestibular (CN VIII) nerve and the reticular formation.[3]

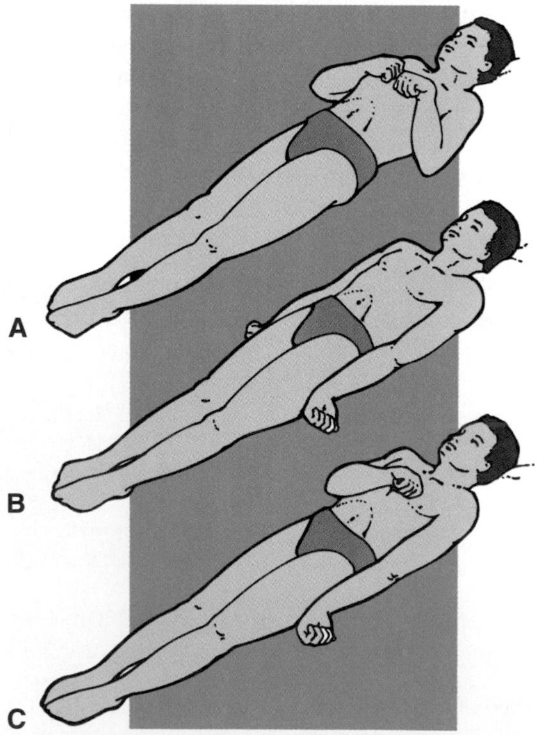

FIGURE 17-1. Abnormal motor responses. **A,** Decorticate posturing. **B,** Decerebrate posturing. **C,** Decorticate posturing on right side and decerebrate posturing on left side of body.

Estimating Pupil Size and Shape

Pupil size should be documented in millimeters with the use of a pupil gauge to reduce the subjectivity of description. Although most people have pupils of equal size, a discrepancy up to 1 mm between the two pupils is normal. Inequality of pupils is known as anisocoria and occurs in 16% to 17% of the human population.[10] Change or inequality in pupil size, especially in patients who previously have not shown this discrepancy, is a significant neurologic sign. It may indicate impending danger of herniation and should be reported immediately. With the location of CN III at the notch of the tentorium, pupil size and reactivity play a key role in the physical assessment of intracranial pressure (ICP) changes and herniation syndromes. In addition to CN III compression, changes in pupil size occur for other reasons. Large pupils can result from the instillation of cycloplegic agents, such as atropine or scopolamine, or can indicate extreme stress. Extremely small pupils can indicate narcotic overdose, lower brain stem compression, or bilateral damage to the pons.[10,11]

Pupil shape also is noted in the assessment of pupils. Although the pupil is normally round, an irregularly shaped or oval pupil may be noted in patients with elevated intracranial pressure. An oval pupil can indicate the initial stages of CN III compression.[1] It has been observed that an oval pupil almost always is associated with an elevated ICP between 18 and 35 mm Hg.[12]

Evaluation of Pupillary Reaction to Light

The pupillary light reflex depends on both optic nerve (CN II) and CN III function (Figure 17-2).[3] The technique for evaluation of the pupillary light response involves use of a narrow-beamed bright light shone into the pupil from the outer canthus of the eye. If the light is shone directly onto the pupil, glare or reflection of the light may prevent the assessor's proper visualization. Pupillary reaction to light is identified as brisk, sluggish, or nonreactive or fixed.[1] Each pupil should be evaluated both for direct light response and for consensual response. The consensual pupillary response is constriction in response to a light shone into the opposite eye. This reflex occurs as a result of crossing of nerve fibers at the optic chiasm.[1] Evaluation of consensual response is necessary to rule out optic nerve dysfunction as a cause for lack of a direct light reflex. Because the optic nerve is the afferent pathway for the light reflex, shining a light into a blind eye will produce neither a direct light response in that eye nor a consensual response in the opposite eye. A consensual response in the blind eye produced by shining a light into the opposite eye demonstrates an intact oculomotor nerve. Oculomotor compression associated with transtentorial herniation will affect both the direct light response and the consensual response in the affected pupil.[1,2,10,11]

Assessment of Eye Movement

In the conscious patient, the function of the three cranial nerves of the eye and their MLF innervation can be assessed by asking the patient to follow a finger through the full range of eye motion. If the eyes move together into all six fields, extraocular movements are intact (Figure 17-3).[1]

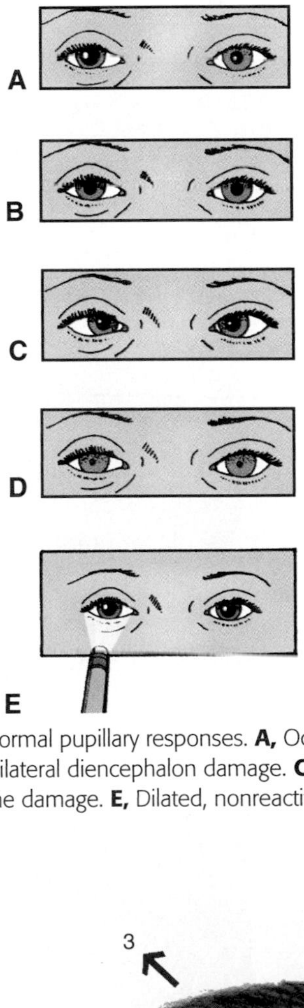

FIGURE 17-2. Abnormal pupillary responses. **A,** Oculomotor nerve compression. **B,** Bilateral diencephalon damage. **C,** Midbrain damage. **D,** Pontine damage. **E,** Dilated, nonreactive pupils.

In the unconscious patient, assessment of ocular function and innervation of the MLF is performed by eliciting the doll's eyes reflex. If the patient is unconscious as a result of trauma, the nurse must ascertain the absence of cervical injury before performing this examination. To assess the oculocephalic reflex, the nurse holds the patient's eyelids open and briskly turns the head to one side while observing the eye movements, then briskly turns the head to the other side and observes. If the eyes deviate to the opposite direction in which the head is turned, doll's eyes are present and the oculocephalic reflex arc is intact (Figure 17-4, *A*). If the oculocephalic reflex arc is not intact, the reflex is absent. This lack of response, in which the eyes remain midline and move with the head, indicates significant brain stem injury (Figure 17-4, *C*). The reflex may also be absent in severe metabolic coma. An abnormal oculocephalic reflex is present when the eyes rove or move in opposite directions from each other (Figure 17-4, *B*). Abnormal oculocephalic reflex indicates some degree of brain stem injury.[1-3]

Evaluation of the oculovestibular reflex is performed by a physician, often as one of the final clinical assessments of brain stem function. Following confirmation that the tympanic membrane is intact, the head is raised to a 30-degree angle. Then 20 to 100 ml of ice water is injected into the external auditory canal. The normal eye movement response is a conjugate, slow, tonic nystagmus deviating toward the irrigated ear and lasting 30 to 120 seconds. This response indicates brain stem integrity. Rapid nystagmus returns the eyes back to the midline only in the conscious patient with cortical functioning (Figure 17-5).[1] An abnormal response is disconjugate eye movement, which indicates a brain stem lesion, or no response, which indicates little to no brain stem function. The oculovestibular reflex may also be temporarily absent in reversible metabolic encephalopathy.[3] This test is an extremely noxious stimulation and may produce a decorticate or decerebrate posturing response in the comatose patient. In the conscious patient, this procedure may produce nausea, vomiting, or dizziness.[1,10,11]

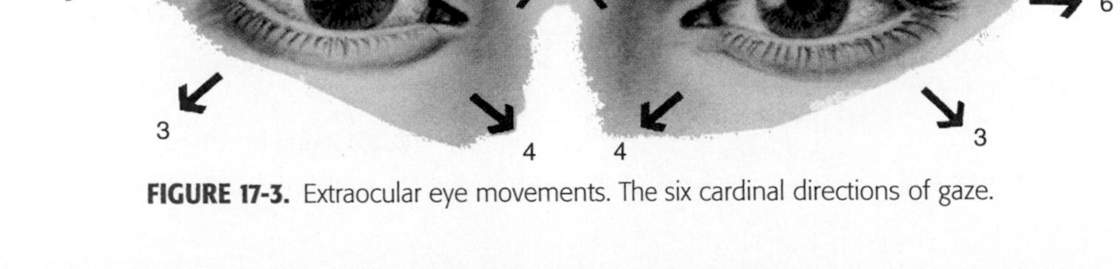

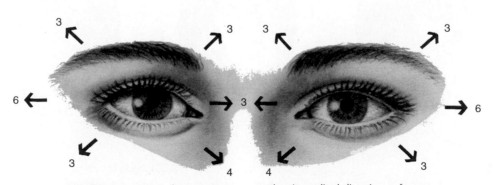

FIGURE 17-3. Extraocular eye movements. The six cardinal directions of gaze.

RESPIRATORY FUNCTION

Nursing priorities in assessment of respiratory function focus on (1) observing respiratory pattern and (2) evaluating airway status.[1]

The activity of respiration is a highly integrated function that receives input from the cerebrum, brain stem, and metabolic mechanisms. A close correlation exists in clinical assessment among altered levels of consciousness, the level of brain or brain stem injury, and the respiratory pattern noted. Under the influence of the cerebral cortex and the diencephalon, three brain stem centers control respirations. The lowest center, the medullary respiratory center, sends impulses through the vagus nerve to innervate muscles of inspiration

A

B

C

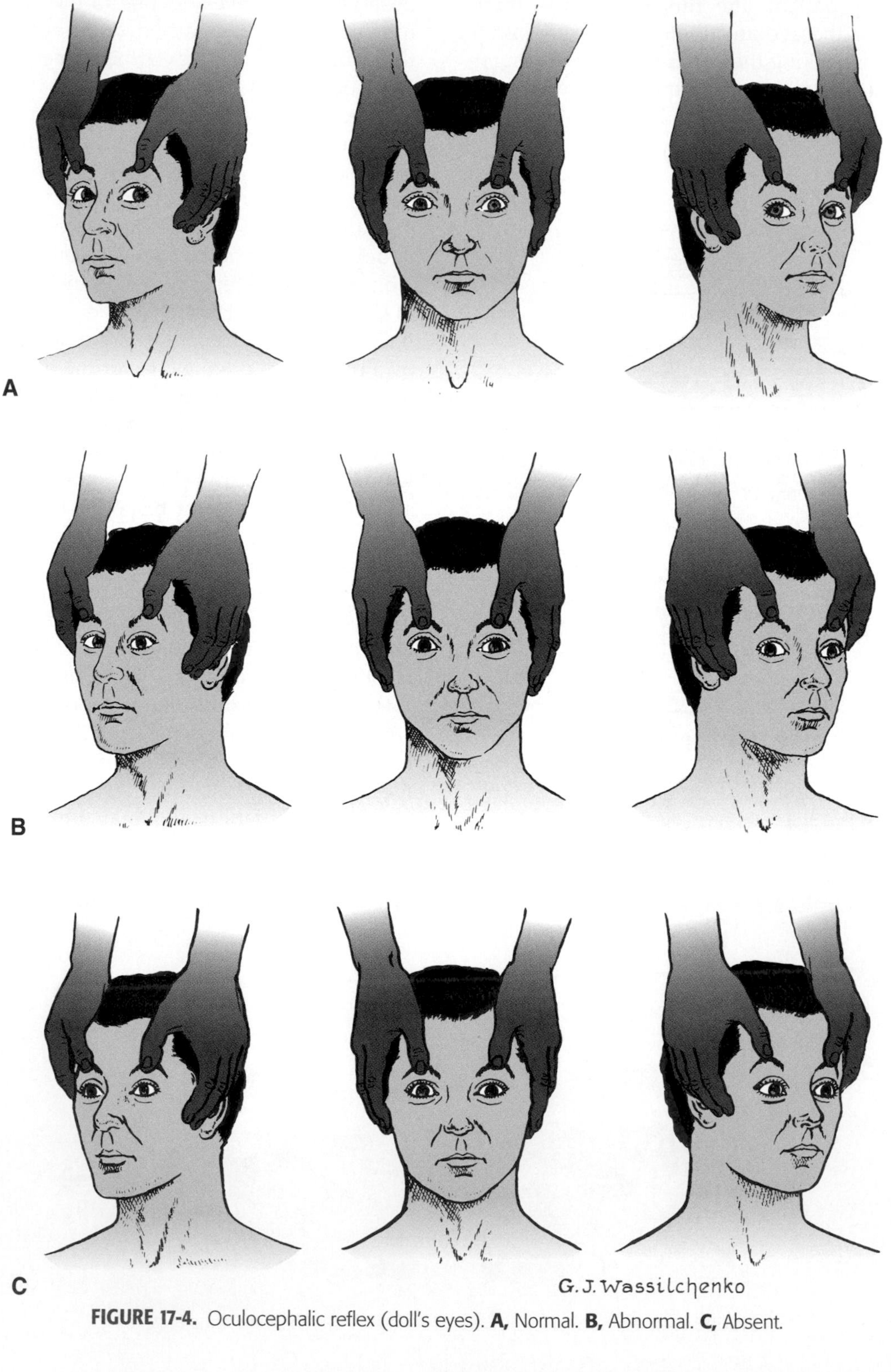

FIGURE 17-4. Oculocephalic reflex (doll's eyes). **A,** Normal. **B,** Abnormal. **C,** Absent.

and expiration. The apneustic and pneumotaxic centers of the pons are responsible for the length of inspiration and expiration and the underlying respiratory rate.[1-3]

Observation of Respiratory Pattern

Changes in respiratory patterns assist in identifying the level of brain stem dysfunction or injury (Table 17-2). Evaluation of respiratory pattern must also include evaluation of the effectiveness of gas exchange in maintaining adequate oxygen and carbon dioxide levels. Hypoventilation is not uncommon in the patient with an altered level of consciousness. Alterations in oxygenation or carbon dioxide levels can result in further neurologic dysfunction. ICP increases with hypoxemia or hypercapnia.[1-3]

Evaluation of Airway Status

Finally, assessment of the respiratory function in a patient with neurologic deficit must include assessment of airway maintenance and secretion control. Cough, gag, and swallow reflexes responsible for protection of the airway may be absent or diminished.[13]

Vital Signs

Nursing priorities in assessment of vital signs focus on (1) evaluating blood pressure and (2) monitoring heart rate and rhythm. As a result of the brain and brain stem influences on cardiac, respiratory, and body temperature functions, changes in vital signs can indicate deterioration in neurologic status.

Evaluation of Blood Pressure

A common manifestation of intracranial injury is systemic hypertension. Cerebral autoregulation, responsible for the control of cerebral blood flow (CBF), frequently is lost with any type of intracranial injury. After cerebral injury, the body often is in a hyperdynamic state (increased heart rate, blood pressure,

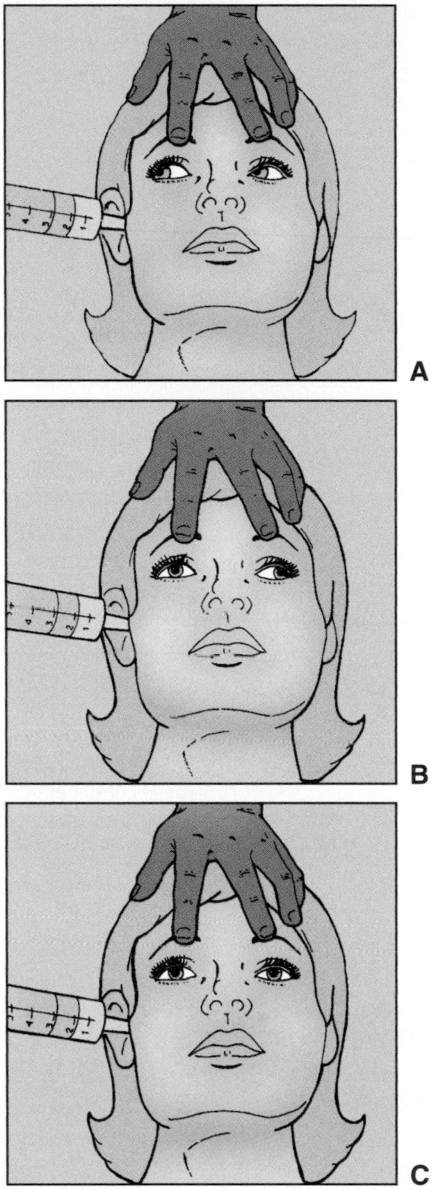

FIGURE 17-5. Oculovestibular reflex (cold caloric test). **A,** Normal. **B,** Abnormal. **C,** Absent.

Table 17-2
Respiratory Patterns

PATTERN	DESCRIPTION	SIGNIFICANCE
Cheyne-Stokes	Rhythmic crescendo and decrescendo of rate and depth of respiration; includes brief periods of apnea	Usually seen with bilateral deep cerebral lesions or some cerebellar lesions
Central neurogenic hyperventilation	Very deep, very rapid respirations with no apneic periods	Usually seen with lesions of the midbrain and upper pons
Apneustic	Prolonged inspiratory and/or expiratory pause of 2-3 sec	Usually seen in lesions of the mid to lower pons
Cluster breathing	Clusters of irregular, gasping respirations separated by long periods of apnea	Usually seen in lesions of the lower pons or upper medulla
Ataxic respirations	Irregular, random pattern of deep and shallow respirations with irregular apneic periods	Usually seen in lesions of the medulla

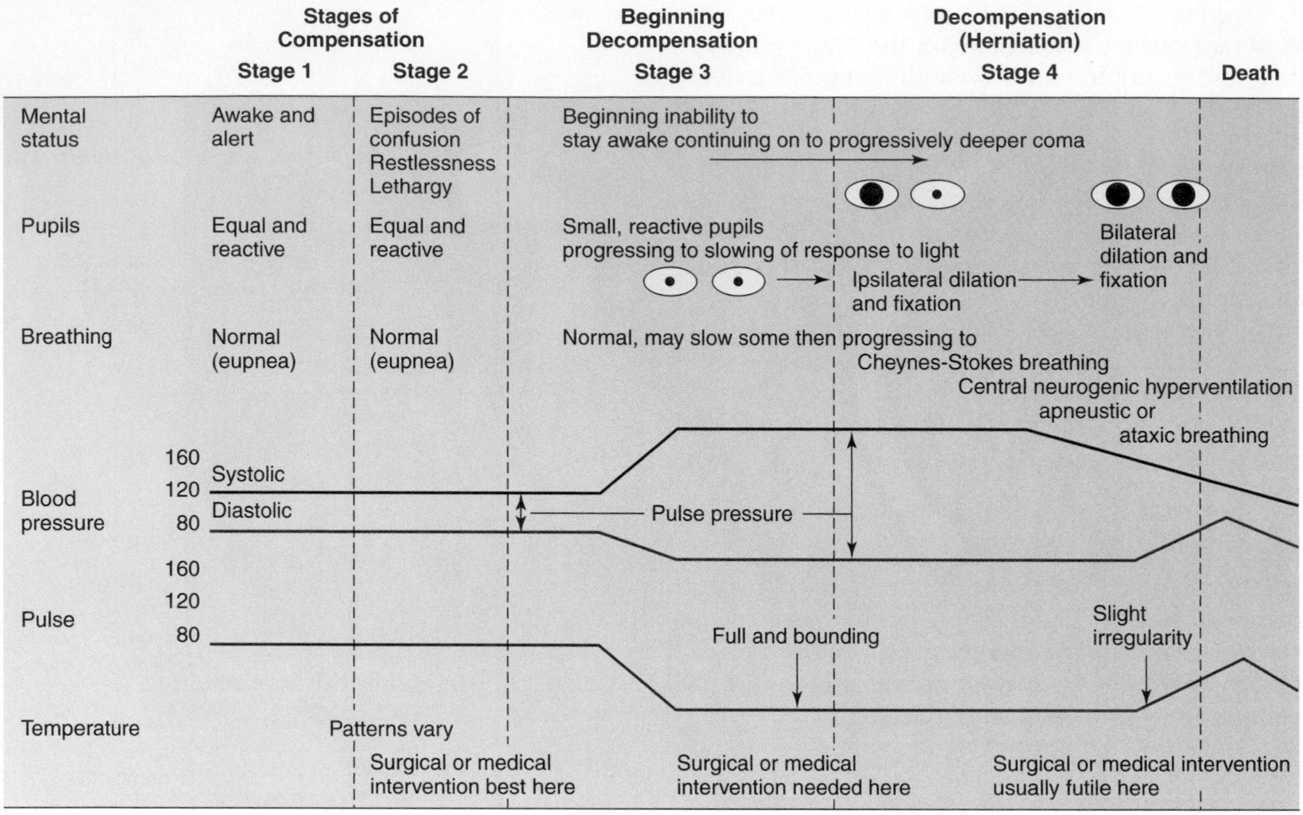

FIGURE 17-6. Clinical correlates of compensated and decompensated phases of intracranial hypertension. (From Beare PG, Myers JL: *Principles and practice of adult health nursing,* ed 3, St Louis, 1998, Mosby.)

and cardiac output) as part of a compensatory response. With the loss of autoregulation as blood pressure increases, cerebral blood flow and cerebral blood volume increase and therefore ICP increases. Control of systemic hypertension is necessary to stop this cycle. However, caution must be exercised. The mean arterial pressure must be maintained at a level sufficient to produce adequate cerebral blood flow in the presence of elevated ICP. Attention must also be paid to the pulse pressure because widening of this value may occur in the late stages of intracranial hypertension.[13]

Observation of Heart Rate and Rhythm

The medulla and the vagus nerve provide parasympathetic control to the heart. When stimulated, this lower brain stem system produces bradycardia. Sympathetic stimulation increases the rate and contractility. Various intracranial pathologic conditions and abrupt ICP changes can produce cardiac dysrhythmias, such as bradycardia, premature ventricular contractions (PVCs), atrioventricular (AV) block, or ventricular fibrillation and myocardial damage.[14]

Cushing's Triad

Cushing's triad is a set of three clinical manifestations (bradycardia, systolic hypertension, and widening pulse pressure) related to pressure on the medullary area of the brain stem. These signs often occur in response to intracranial hypertension or a herniation syndrome. The appearance of Cushing's triad is a late finding that may be absent in neurologic deterioration. Attention should be paid to alteration in each component of the triad and intervention initiated accordingly.[3]

NEUROLOGIC CHANGES ASSOCIATED WITH INTRACRANIAL HYPERTENSION

Assessment of the patient for signs of increasing intracranial pressure is an important responsibility of the critical care nurse. Increasing ICP can be identified by changes in level of consciousness, pupillary reaction, motor response, vital signs, and respiratory patterns (Figure 17-6).

LABORATORY STUDIES

The major laboratory study performed in the patient with neurologic dysfunction is cerebrospinal fluid (CSF) analysis obtained via a lumbar puncture or a ventriculostomy.[1] A complete analysis of CSF is described in Table 17-3.

Table 17-3

Analysis of Cerebrospinal Fluid

CHARACTERISTIC	NORMAL FINDINGS	ABNORMAL FINDINGS	POSSIBLE CAUSES/COMMENTS
Pressure	Less than 200 mm H_2O	<60 mm H_2O	Faulty needle placement Dehydration Spinal block along subarachnoid space Block of foramen magnum Hydrocephalus
		>200 mm H_2O	Muscle tension Abdominal compression Brain tumor Subdural hematoma Brain abscess Brain cyst Cerebral edema (any cause)
Color	Clear, colorless	Cloudy/turbid	Cloudy as a result of microorganisms (e.g., WBCs) Turbid as a result of increased cell count
		Yellow (xanthochromic)	Breakdown of RBCs with RBC pigments, high protein count
		Smoky	RBCs
Blood	None	Red blood cells: blood tinged	Traumatic tap—bloody in first sample
		Grossly bloody	Traumatic tap—bloody in all samples
Volume	150 ml	Increase	Hydrocephalus
Specific gravity	1.007	Increase	Infection, presence of cells or protein
White blood cells (WBCs)	0-5/mm^3	<500/mm^3	Bacterial or viral infections of meninges, neurosyphilis, subarachnoid hemorrhage, infarction, abscess, tuberculous meningitis, metastatic lesions
		>500/mm^3	Purulent infection
Glucose	50-75 mg/dl or 60%-70% of blood glucose	<40 mg/dl	Meningitis: bacterial, tuberculosis, parasitic, fungal carcinomatous, subarachnoid hemorrhage
		>80 mg/dl	May not be of neurologic significance
Chloride	700-750 mg/dl	Decreased (<625 mg/dl)	Meningeal infection, tuberculosis meningitis, hypochloremia
		Increased (>800 mg/dl)	May not be of neurologic significance; correlated with blood levels of chloride and not routine—done only on request
Culture and sensitivity	No organisms present	*Neisseria* or *Streptococcus*	Identify organisms to begin therapy; Gram stain for some cultures may take several weeks
Serology for syphilis	Negative	Positive	Syphilis
Protein (If CSF contains blood, this will raise the protein level)	15-50 mg/dl	Increased (>60 mg/dl)	Bacterial meningitis, brain tumors (both benign and malignant), complete spinal block, ALS, Guillain-Barré syndrome, subarachnoid hemorrhage, infarction, CNS trauma, CNS degenerative diseases, herniated disk, DM with polyneuropathy
		Decreased (<10 mg/dl)	May not be of neurologic significance
Osmolality	295 Osm/L	Increased	Protein, WBCs, microorganisms, RBCs
Lactate	10-20 mg/dl	Increased	Bacterial, seizure activity, fungal meningitis, CNS trauma, coma related to toxic or metabolic causes

From Barker E: *Neuroscience nursing: a spectrum of care,* ed 2, St Louis, 2002, Mosby.
WBC, White blood cell; *RBC,* red blood cell; *CSF,* cerebrospinal fluid; *ALS,* amyotrophic lateral sclerosis; *CNS,* central nervous system; *DM,* diabetes mellitus.

DIAGNOSTIC PROCEDURES

Table 17-4 presents an overview of the various diagnostic procedures used to evaluate the patient with neurologic dysfunction.

Nursing Management

The nursing management of a patient undergoing a diagnostic procedure involves a variety of interventions. **Priorities are directed toward preparing the patient psychologically and physically for the procedure, monitoring the patient's responses to the procedure, and assessing the patient after the procedure.** Preparing the patient includes teaching the patient about the procedure, answering any questions, and transporting and/or positioning the patient for the procedure. Monitoring the patient's responses to the procedure includes observing the patient for signs

Table 17-4
Neurologic Diagnostic Procedures

PROCEDURE	PURPOSES	COMMENTS
Angiography	Visualizes extracranial and intracranial vasculature Identifies aneurysm, AV malformation, vasospasm, vascular tumors	Contraindicated if patient has bleeding disorder or is receiving anticoagulants. May cause local hematoma, vasospasm, vessel occlusion, allergic reaction to contrast media, transient or permanent neurologic dysfunction. ***Before Test:*** • Keep patient NPO for 4 hours and provide sedation before study • Check for allergy to iodine. ***After Test:*** • Ensure hydration (contrast medium used). • Maintain bed rest for 8-12 hours. • Monitor arterial puncture point for hemorrhage or hematoma. • Assess neurovascular status of affected limb. • Monitor for indications of systemic emboli.
Cisternogram	Views CSF flow Identifies hydrocephalus Evaluates CSF leakage through dural tear Evaluates abnormality of structures at base of brain and upper cervical cord region	Contraindicated in intracranial hypertension.
Computed tomography (CT)	Views intracranial structures: size, shape, location, shifts Differentiates among tumors, hemorrhage, and infarction Identifies hydrocephalus, cerebral edema, infectious processes, trauma, aneurysm, hematoma, AV malformation, and cerebral atrophy	Patient must be cooperative. Contrast media may be used. • Check for allergy to iodine or seafood before study. • Patient is NPO for 4-8 hours before study. • Sedation may be given. • Monitor for signs of allergic reaction. • Encourage fluids.
Digital subtraction angiography (DSA): brain, spine	Visualizes vasculature, especially carotid and larger cerebral arteries Evaluates occlusive vascular disease Identifies tumors, aneurysms, AV malformations and vascular abnormalities	May be done intravenously (IV) or intraarterially. • IV: less invasive with fewer complications than cerebral angiography. • Intraarterial: care as for angiography. Contrast media is used. • Check for allergy to iodine or seafood before study. • Patient is NPO for 4-8 hours before study. • Monitor for signs of allergic reaction. • Encourage fluids.
Electroencephalography (EEG)	Differentiates epilepsy from mass lesion Detects focus of seizure activity Evaluates drug intoxication Evaluates cerebral blood flow Localizes tumor, abscess, and other mass lesions May be used in designation of brain death	Stimulants, anticonvulsants, tranquilizers, and antidepressants may be withheld for 24-48 hours before study. Hair is shampooed before and after study.
Electromyography (EMG); nerve conduction velocity studies	Detects muscle disease Identifies peripheral neuropathies and nerve compression Identifies nerve regeneration and muscle recovery	Patient must be cooperative. Contraindicated in patients on anticoagulants, with bleeding disorders, or with skin infection. May be uncomfortable for patient.
Electronystagmography (ENG)	Detects nystagmus, which may aid in identification of cerebellar or vestibular problem	

AV, Arteriovenous; *NPO*, nothing by mouth.

Table 17-4
Neurologic Diagnostic Procedures—*cont'd*

PROCEDURE	PURPOSES	COMMENTS
Evoked-potential studies (EPS)	Evaluate brain's electrical potentials (responses) to external stimuli; evaluate sensory and somatosensory neurologic pathways Identifies neuromuscular disease, cerebrovascular disease, spinal cord injury, head injury, peripheral nerve disease, tumors Determines prognosis in severe head injury Contributes to diagnosis of multiple sclerosis, brain stem injury	Hair is shampooed before and after study.
Isotope ventriculography	Visualizes CSF circulation system	No CSF withdrawn. May cause meningeal irritation and aseptic meningitis.
Lumbar puncture (LP) or cisternal puncture	Obtains CSF for analysis Measures CSF opening pressure (about equivalent to intracranial pressure for most patients if done recumbent and no blockage is present)	Cisternal puncture is higher risk but may be used if there is scar tissue, which prevents LP. Patient must be cooperative. Contraindicated in patients with intracranial hypertension because herniation may occur. Contraindicated in bleeding disorders and in patients receiving anticoagulants. Patient kept flat for 4-8 hours to prevent headache. May cause headache, low back pain, meningitis, abscess, CSF leak, puncture of spinal cord.
Magnetic resonance angiography (MRA)	As for CT except better visualization of vasculature Identifies aneurysms, AV malformations, and vasospasm Identifies large vein patency and venous sinuses	Patient must be cooperative. Cannot be performed in patients receiving mechanical ventilation. Contraindicated in patients with implanted metallic devices, including pacemakers. Tends to overestimate degree of stenosis.
Magnetic resonance imaging (MRI)	As for CT except better visualization of vasculature Identifies vascular lesions, tissue abnormalities, cerebral hemorrhage, cerebral infarction, epileptic foci, and multiple sclerosis Identifies brain stem abnormalities Identifies type, location, and extent of brain injury	More sensitive than CT scan, especially for posterior fossa. Patient must be cooperative. Cannot be performed in patient receiving mechanical ventilation. Contraindicated in patients with implanted metallic devices, including pacemakers.
Myelography	Visualization of spinal subarachnoid space Detects spinal cord lesions and cord/nerve root compression Detects pressure on spinal nerve roots	If done with oil based iophendylate (Pantopaque): • Patient must lie flat for 4-8 hours after study. • May cause headache, nerve root irritation, allergic reaction, and adhesive arachnoiditis. If done with water- soluble metrizamide (Amipaque): • Patient should have head of bed elevated. • May cause headache, nausea, vomiting, back and neck ache, chest pain, seizures, hallucinations, speech disorders, dysrhythmias, and allergic reaction. Encourage fluids with either type of dye.
Nerve conduction velocity studies	Identifies peripheral neuropathies and nerve compression	Needle electrodes are used.
Oculoplethysmography (OPG)	Indirectly measures ocular artery pressure Reflects adequacy of cerebrovascular blood flow in the carotid artery	Contraindicated in patients who have undergone eye surgery within last 6 months, who have had lens implants or cataracts, or who have had retinal detachment. May cause conjunctival hemorrhage, corneal abrasions, and transient photophobia.

CSF, Cerebrospinal fluid.

Continued

Table 17-4

Neurologic Diagnostic Procedures—*cont'd*

PROCEDURE	PURPOSES	COMMENTS
Pneumoencephalography	Visualizes ventricular system and subarachnoid space Identifies intracranial tumors Identifies cerebral atrophy	Care as for LP. Contraindicated in patients with intracranial hypertension. May cause headache, nausea, vomiting, autonomic dysfunction, herniation, subdural hematoma, air embolus, and seizures. Patient kept flat for 12-24 hours after study.
Positron emission tomography (PET) Single-proton emission computed tomography (SPECT)	Evaluates oxygen and glucose metabolism Evaluates cerebral blood flow Identifies cerebral ischemia, injuries, epilepsy, and Alzheimer's disease	Patient must be cooperative. Contraindicated in pregnant patients.
Radioisotope brain scan	Identifies tumors, cerebrovascular disease, cerebral infarction, trauma, infectious processes, and seizures	Generally, has been replaced by CT scan. Reassure patient that amount of radioactive material is minimal. Patient must be cooperative. Contraindicated in pregnant patients.
Regional cerebral blood flow (xenon-133 [^{133}Xe] inhalation)	Evaluates blood flow to the cerebral cortex Identifies cerebrovascular disease Detects regions of increased or decreased perfusion Determines presence of collateral blood flow Evaluates cerebral vasospasm	Reassure patient that amount of radioactive material is minimal. Contraindicated in pregnant patients.
Skull radiography	Detects skull fracture, facial fracture, tumor, bone erosion, cranial anomalies, air-fluid level in sinuses, abnormal intracranial calcification, and radiopaque foreign bodies	Linear and basal fractures are frequently missed by routine x-ray films. Contraindicated in pregnant patients.
Somnography	Records EEG during sleep Evaluates sleep and sleep disorders	
Spinal cord angiography	Differentiates among spinal AV malformation, angioma, tumor, and ischemia	As for angiography. May cause thrombosis of spinal vessels; allergy to contrast agent may occur.
Spinal radiography	Detects vertebral dislocation or fracture, degenerative disease, tumor, bone erosion, and calcification Identifies structural spinal deficits and rules out associated cervical spinal injuries	Care must be taken to prevent fracture displacement and spinal cord injury. C1-C2 view best via open mouth. C6-C7 view best with arms pulled down. Contraindicated in pregnant patients.
Suboccipital puncture	Obtains CSF for analysis Measures CSF pressure Useful when LP contraindicated	May cause trauma to the medulla.
Transcranial Doppler imaging	Measures blood flow velocity through the cerebral arteries Identifies cerebral vasospasm, emboli, vascular stenosis, and brain death	
Ventriculography	Obtains CSF for analysis Measures CSF pressure Used especially when intracranial hypertension contraindicates LP	May cause meningeal irritation, seizures, herniation, and intracerebral/ intraventricular hemorrhage.

From Dennison RD: *Pass CCRN!,* ed 2, St Louis, 2000, Mosby.

of pain, anxiety, or hemorrhage and monitoring vital signs. Assessing the patient after the procedure includes observing for complications of the procedure and medicating the patient for any postprocedure discomfort. Any evidence of increasing intracranial pressure should be immediately reported to the physician, and emergency measures to maintain circulation must be initiated.

BEDSIDE MONITORING

INTRACRANIAL PRESSURE MONITORING

In the patient with suspected intracranial hypertension, a monitoring device may be placed within the cranium to quantify ICP. Under normal physiologic conditions, ICP is maintained below 15 mm Hg mean pressure.[1,15] It is used to monitor serial intracranial pressures and assist with the management of intracranial hypertension. An increase in intracranial pressure can cause a decrease in blood flow to the brain, causing brain damage.[1,15] It can also provide a sterile access for draining excess CSF.[1]

Monitoring Sites

The four sites for monitoring ICP are the intraventricular space, the subarachnoid space, the epidural space, and the parenchyma (Figure 17-7). Each site has advantages and disadvantages for monitoring ICP (Table 17-5). The type of monitor chosen depends on both the suspected pathologic condition and physician's preferences.[16,17] Nursing considerations for each type of device are also discussed in Table 17-5.

Intraventricular Space. ICP monitoring is accomplished by placing a small catheter into the ventricular system; this procedure is known as a *ventriculostomy.* The catheter is inserted through a burr hole with the patient under local anesthesia and usually is placed in the anterior horn of the lateral ventricle. If at all possible, the side chosen for placement of the ventriculostomy is the nondominant hemisphere.[15-17]

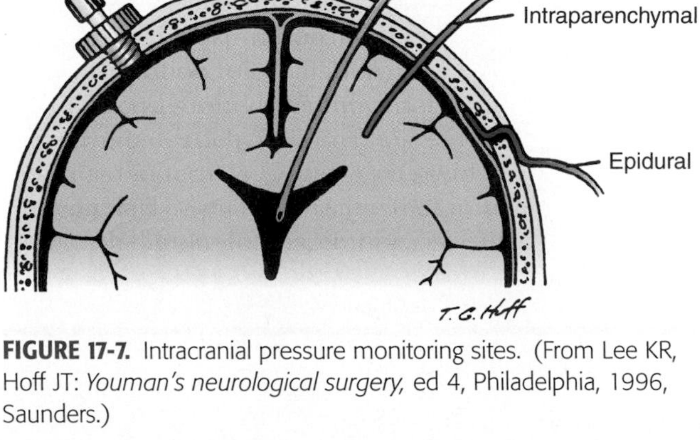

FIGURE 17-7. Intracranial pressure monitoring sites. (From Lee KR, Hoff JT: *Youman's neurological surgery,* ed 4, Philadelphia, 1996, Saunders.)

Subarachnoid Space. ICP monitoring is accomplished by placing a small hollow bolt or screw into the subarachnoid space. It is inserted though a burr hole, usually located in the front of the skull behind the hairline, with the patient under local anesthesia. Inserting this device is easier than inserting the ventriculostomy catheter.[16,17]

Epidural Space. ICP monitoring is accomplished by placing a small fiberoptic sensor into the epidural space. It is also inserted through a burr hole while the patient is under local anesthesia. The physician strips the dura away from the inner table of the skull before inserting the epidural monitor.[16,17]

Intraparenchymal. ICP monitoring is accomplished by placing a small fiberoptic catheter into the parenchymal tissue. After placing a subarachnoid bolt (as just described), a hole is punched in the dura and the catheter is inserted approximately 1 cm into the brain's white matter.[16,17]

Intracranial Pressure Waves

The ICP pulse waveform is observed on a continuous, real-time pressure display and corresponds to each heartbeat. The waveform arises primarily from pulsations of the major intracranial arteries, receiving retrograde venous pulsations as well.[16,17]

Normal ICP Waveform. The normal ICP wave has three or more defined peaks (Figure 17-8). The first peak, or P1, is called the *percussion wave.* Originating from the pulsations of the choroid plexus, it has a sharp peak and is fairly consistent in its amplitude. The second peak, or P2, is called the *tidal wave.* The tidal wave is more variable in shape and amplitude, ending on the dicrotic notch. The P2 portion of the pulse waveform has been most directly linked to the state of decreased compliance. When the P2 component is equal to or higher than P1, decreased compliance occurs (Figure 17-9). Immediately after the dicrotic notch is the third wave, P3, which is called the *dicrotic wave.* After the dicrotic wave, the pressure usually tapers down to the diastolic position, unless retrograde venous pulsations add a few more peaks.[17-19]

A, B, and C pressure waves are not true waveforms (Figure 17-10). Rather, they are the graphically displayed trend data of intracranial pressure over time. These waves reflect spontaneous alterations in ICP associated with respiration, systemic blood pressure, and deteriorating neurologic status.

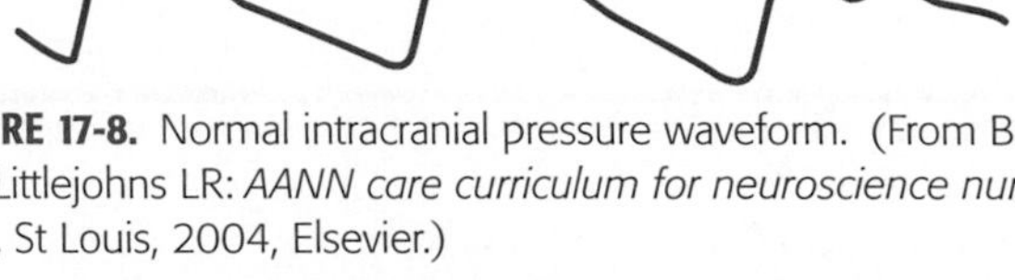

FIGURE 17-8. Normal intracranial pressure waveform. (From Bader MK, Littlejohns LR: *AANN care curriculum for neuroscience nursing,* ed 4, St Louis, 2004, Elsevier.)

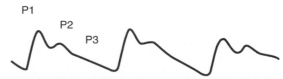

Table 17-5

Advantages, Disadvantages, and Nursing Considerations of Intracranial Pressure Monitoring Techniques

MONITORING DEVICE	ADVANTAGES	DISADVANTAGES	NURSING CONSIDERATIONS
Intraventricular catheter (ventriculostomy)	Allows accurate ICP measurement Provides access to CSF for drainage or sampling Provides access for instillation of contrast media Allows reliable evaluation of intracranial compliances (volume-pressure relationships)	Provides an additional site for infection Is most invasive ICP monitoring technique Requires frequent transducer balancing or recalibration Catheter may become occluded by blood clot or tissue debris Insertion is difficult if ventricles are small, compressed, or displaced Is associated with risk for CSF leakage around insertion site Is associated with increased risk for infection	Provide appropriate sedatives or analgesics during catheter insertion Do baseline and serial neurologic assessments Measure patient's temperature at least every 4 hours Note character, amount, and turbidity of CSF drainage Document ICP/CPP measurements, response to stimulation, nursing care activities per hospital/unit protocol Monitor quality of ICP waveform Monitor system/tubing for air bubbles, and flush or purge system as appropriate Drain CSF as indicated for treatment of ICP elevation Notify physician if CSF drainage is not within prescribed parameters Monitor insertion site for bleeding, drainage, swelling, CSF leakage Zero or calibrate device per hospital/unit protocol Level transducer at the foramen of Monro; external landmarks include the tragus of the patient's ear and the external auditory canal, among others; all ICP measurements should be made with the transducer at a consistent level relative to external landmarks Administer sedatives or analgesics as appropriate to decrease risk of catheter being dislodged by patient's movements Educate patient's family as indicated Notify physician if ICP/CPP not within specified parameters
Subarachnoid bolt or screw	Is associated with lower infection rates than is ventriculostomy Is quickly and easily placed Can be used with small or collapsed ventricles Requires no penetration of brain tissue	Has potential for dampened waveform (cerebral edema, blood or tissue debris) Is less accurate at high ICP elevations Requires frequent balancing/recalibration (and with position changes) Provides no access for CSF sampling	Administer appropriate sedatives or analgesics during insertion Do baseline and serial neurologic assessments Measure patient's temperature at least every 4 hours Monitor insertion site for bleeding, drainage, swelling, CSF leakage Monitor quality of ICP waveform Document ICP/CPP measurements, response to stimulation per hospital/unit protocol Administer sedatives or analgesics as appropriate to decrease risk of catheter being dislodged by patient's movements Zero or calibrate device per hospital/unit protocol

ICP, Intracranial pressure; *CSF,* cerebrospinal fluid; *CPP,* cerebral perfusion pressure.

Table 17-5

Advantages, Disadvantages, and Nursing Considerations of Intracranial Pressure Monitoring Techniques—*cont'd*

MONITORING DEVICE	ADVANTAGES	DISADVANTAGES	NURSING CONSIDERATIONS
Subarachnoid bolt or screw—*cont'd*			Level transducer at the foramen of Monro; external landmarks include the tragus of the patient's ear and the external auditory canal, among others; all ICP measurements should be made with the transducer at a consistent level relative to external landmarks Educate patient's family as indicated Notify physician if ICP/CPP is not within specified parameters
Subdural or epidural catheter or sensor	Is least invasive Is associated with decreased risk of infection Is easily and quickly placed	Increase in baseline drift over time means possible loss of reliability or accuracy Provides no access for CSF drainage/sampling	Administer appropriate sedatives or analgesics during insertion Do baseline and serial neurologic assessments Measure patient's temperature at least every 4 hours Monitor insertion site for bleeding, drainage, swelling Monitor quality of ICP waveform, drift over time Document ICP/CPP measurements, response to stimulation per hospital/unit protocol Administer sedatives or analgesics as appropriate to decrease risk of catheter being dislodged or damaged by patient's movements Educate patient's family as indicated Notify physician if ICP/CPP is not within specified parameters
Fiberoptic transducer-tipped catheter	Can be placed in subdural or subarachnoid space, in a ventricle, or directly within brain tissue Is easily transported Requires zeroing only once (during insertion) Has baseline drift of up to 1 mm Hg per day Is associated with decreased risk for infection when brain tissue is not penetrated Provides good-quality ICP waveforms (less artifact than with other devices) Requires no adjustment in level of transducer with patient's change of position	Provides no access for CSF sampling/drainage Cannot be recalibrated after placement Requires periodic replacement of probe Is easily damaged	Administer appropriate sedatives or analgesics during insertion Do baseline and serial neurologic assessments Measure patient's temperature at least every 4 hours Monitor insertion site for bleeding, drainage, swelling, CSF leakage Monitor quality of ICP waveform, drift over time Document ICP/CPP measurements, response to stimulation per hospital/unit protocol Administer sedatives or analgesics as appropriate to decrease risk of catheter being dislodged or damaged by patient's movements Educate patient's family as indicated Notify physician if ICP/CPP is not within specified parameters

From Arbour R: *Crit Care Nurse* 24(5):19, 2004.

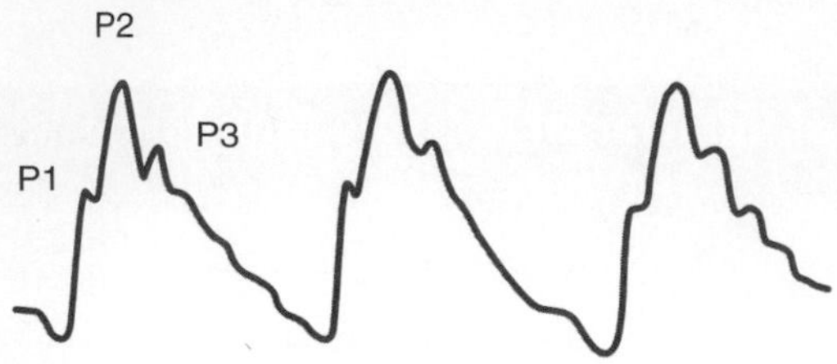

FIGURE 17-9. Abnormal intracranial pressure waveform. ((From Bader MK, Littlejohns LR: *AANN care curriculum for neuroscience nursing*, ed 4, St Louis, 2004, Elsevier.)

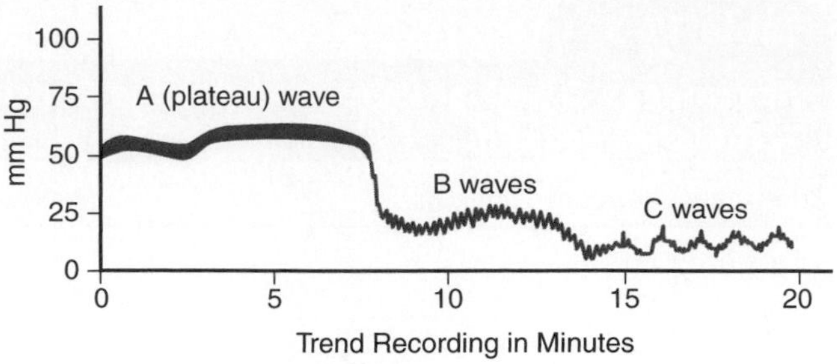

FIGURE 17-10. Intracranial pressure waves. Composite diagram of A (plateau) waves, B (sawtooth) waves, and C (small rhythmic) waves. (From Barker E: *Neuroscience nursing: a spectrum of care*, ed 2, St Louis, 2002, Mosby.)

A Waves. Also called *plateau waves* because of their distinctive shape, A waves are the most clinically significant of the three types. They usually occur in an already elevated baseline ICP (greater than 20 mm Hg) and are characterized by sharp increases in ICP of 30 to 69 mm Hg, which plateau for 2 to 20 minutes and then return to baseline. The actual cause of A waves is unknown, but they may result from vasodilation and increased CBF, decreased venous outflow (and therefore increased cerebral blood volume), fluctuations in $Paco_2$ (and therefore changes in cerebral blood volume), or decreased CSF absorption. B waves often precede A waves. Plateau waves are considered significant because of the reduced cerebral perfusion pressure associated with ICP in the 50 to 100 mm Hg range. Transient signs of intracranial hypertension such as a decreased level of consciousness, bradycardia, pupillary changes, or respiratory changes may accompany these waves. Some research suggests that prolonged increases in ICP associated with plateau waves could result in transient as well as permanent cell damage from ischemia.[2,17]

B Waves. B waves are sharp, rhythmic oscillations with a sawtooth appearance that occur every 30 seconds to 2 minutes and can raise the ICP from 5 to 70 mm Hg. They are a normal physiologic phenomenon that can occur in any patient, but they are amplified in states of low intracranial compliance. B waves appear to reflect fluctuations in cerebral blood volume. Decompensation of normal intracranial volume compensatory capacity is indicated by B waves with a high amplitude (greater than 15 mm Hg pressure change from peak to trough of wave).[2,17]

C Waves. C waves are smaller, rhythmic waves that occur every 4 to 8 minutes and at normal levels of ICP. They are related to normal fluctuations in respiration and systemic arterial pressure. C waves are considered clinically insignificant.[2,17]

Cerebral Perfusion Pressure

Measuring CBF in the clinical setting is difficult, but at the bedside an estimated pressure of cerebral perfusion can be derived. Cerebral perfusion pressure (CPP) is the blood pressure gradient across the brain and is calculated as the difference between the incoming mean arterial pressure (MAP) and the opposing ICP on the arteries:

$$CPP = MAP - ICP$$

The CPP in the average adult is approximately 80 to 100 mm Hg, with a range of 60 to 150 mm Hg. The CPP must be maintained near 80 mm Hg to provide adequate blood supply to the brain. If the CPP drops below this point, ischemia may develop. A sustained CPP of 30 mm Hg or less usually results in neuronal hypoxia and cell death. When the mean systemic arterial pressure equals the ICP, CBF may cease.[1-3]

Cerebral Oxygenation Monitoring

Cerebral Metabolism

The measurements of CBF and CPP do not address the brain's metabolic need for oxygen. Active neurons require greater amounts of oxygen than those that are inactive. The determination that CBF matches the brain's metabolic needs is expressed as *cerebral metabolic rate* ($CMRo_2$), the normal value of which is 3.4 ml per 100 g brain tissue per minute. Neuronal demand for oxygen is governed by their metabolic rate. This value is not easily attained for technical reasons, although it can be calculated. It is the product of the measured CBF and calculated arteriojugular oxygen difference ($AJDo_2$):[20]

$$CMRo_2 = CBF \times AJDo_2$$

CBF can be measured using a variety of complex techniques (e.g., positron emission tomography [PET] and single-proton emission computed tomography [SPECT] scans) Most recently, continuous bedside monitoring of regional cerebrocortical blood flow has become available.[8] Arteriojugular oxygen difference is the amount of oxygen extracted by the brain and is reflected in the difference between the arterial oxygen content and the jugular venous oxygen content. The normal value is 5.0 to 7.5 vol%.[20]

Jugular Venous Oxygen Saturation

One method of measuring CBF allows continuous measurement of oxygenation within the jugular venous system through the use of the jugular bulb monitor. Jugular venous oxygen saturation ($SjvO_2$) can be used to reflect cerebral oxygen supply and demand balance. Any disorder that increases $CMRo_2$ or decreases oxygen delivery may decrease $SjvO_2$, and conversely any disorder that that decreases $CMRo_2$ or increases oxygen delivery may increase $SjvO_2$.[20,21]

To measure $SjvO_2$ a fiberoptic catheter placed retrograde through the internal jugular vein into the jugular bulb and attached to a bedside monitor. The normal value is 60% to 80%. Patients with values less than 50% and 55% are either hypoxemic or oligemic (low cerebral blood flow as compared with metabolic rate). Oligemia occurs as a result of decreased blood flow due to hypotension, vasospasm, or intracranial hypertension or as a result of increased brain metabolic requirements due to fever or seizures.[20,21] $Sjvo_2$ values below 45% are indicative of severe cerebral hypoxia.[20] Patients with values above 75% to 80% are considered hyperemic (CBF high compared with metabolic need). $Sjvo_2$ will also rise if the brain is so severely injured the neurons are unable to extract oxygen.[20,21]

There are a number of limitations to $Sjvo_2$ monitoring. $Sjvo_2$ is a global measure of cerebral oxygenation and thus a normal $Sjvo_2$ does not mean that there are not localized areas of cerebral ischemia.[20,21] Readings are affected by the movement of the patient's head.[21] Up to 50% of the low $Sjvo_2$ readings are false and may be due to technical issues with the catheter, particularly due to catheter migration.[22] For accurate reading, the tip of the catheter must be within 1 cm of the jugular bulb.[21]

Brain Tissue Oxygen Pressure

Over the last few years a new device has become available to measure the partial pressure of oxygen within brain tissue ($Pbto_2$). The device consists of a monitoring probe, on the end of a catheter, which is inserted into the brain parenchyma and attached to a bedside monitor. The probe may be inserted into the damaged portion of the brain to measure regional oxygenation or inserted into the undamaged portion of the brain to measure global oxygenation. One risk associated with insertion of the catheter is bleeding with hematoma formation.[23] Although there is no consensus on normal values because they vary from device to device, normal values have been estimated to be between 20 and 40 mm Hg.[24] It has been concluded that the probability of death increases with prolonged periods of a $Pbto_2$ less than 15 mm Hg and any episode of a $Pbto_2$ less than 6 mm Hg.[23]

In the head-injured patient the goal of treatment is to maintain the $Pbto_2$ greater than 20 mm Hg. Factors that decrease $Pbto_2$ include tissue hypoxia, hypocapnia, hypovolemia, decreased blood pressure, low hemoglobin, intracranial hypertension, and hyperthermia.[25] Treatment is directed at the underlying cause.[24]

evolve To test your mastery of this chapter, try the Open-Book Quiz at http://evolve.elsevier.com/Urden/priorities/

REFERENCES

1. Barker E: *Neuroscience nursing: a spectrum of care*, ed 2, St Louis, 2002, Mosby.
2. Bader MK, Littlejohns LR: *AANN core curriculum for neuroscience nursing*, ed 4, St Louis, 2004, Elsevier.
3. Goetz CG: *Textbook of clinical neurology*, ed 2, St Louis, 2003, Elsevier.
4. Haymore J: A neuron in a haystack: advanced neurologic assessment, *AACN Clin Issues* 15:568, 2002.
5. Teasdale G, Jennett W: Assessment of coma and impaired consciousness—a practical scale, *Lancet* 2:81, 1974.
6. Juarez VJ, Lyons M: Interrater reliability of the Glasgow Coma Scale, *J Neurosci Nurs* 27:283, 1995.
7. Fischer J, Mathieson C: The history of the Glasgow Coma Scale: implications for practice, *Crit Care Nurs Q* 23(4):52, 2001.
8. Barnwell P: Assessing motor and sensory function: —a focused survey, *Aust Emerg Nurs J* 2(3):16, 1999.
9. O'Hanlon-Nichols T: Neurologic assessment, *Am J Nurs* 99(6):44, 1999.
10. Bishop BS: Pathologic pupillary signs: self-learning module, part I, *Crit Care Nurs* 11(6):58, 1991.
11. Bishop BS: Pathologic papillary signs: self-learning module, part II, *Crit Care Nurs* 11(7):58, 1991.
12. Marshall LF et al: The oval pupil: clinical significance and relationship to intracranial hypertension, *J Neurosurg* 58:566, 1983.
13. Chesnut RM: Management of brain and spine injuries, *Crit Care Clin* 20:25, 2005.
14. Keller C, Williams A: Cardiac dysrhythmias associated with central nervous system dysfunction, *J Neurosci Nurs* 25:349, 1993.
15. March K: Intracranial pressure monitoring: why monitor, *AACN Clin Issues* 16:456, 2005.
16. American Association of Neuroscience Nurses: *Guide to the care of the patient with intracranial pressure monitoring*, Glen View, Ill, 2005, The Association.
17. Arbour R: Intracranial hypertension: monitoring and nursing assessment, *Crit Care Nurse* 24(5):19, 2004.
18. March K: Intracranial pressure monitoring and assessing intracranial compliance in brain injury, *Crit Care Nurs Clin North Am* 12:429, 2000.
19. Kirkness CJ et al: Intracranial pressure waveform analysis: clinical and research implications, *J Neurosci Nurs* 32:271, 2000.
20. Smythe PR, Samra SK: Monitors of cerebral oxygenation, *Anesthesiol Clin North Am* 20:293, 2002.
21. Kidd JC, Criddle L: Using jugular venous catheters in patients with traumatic brain injury, *Crit Care Nurse* 21(6):16, 2001.

22. Coplin WM et al: Accuracy of continuous jugular bulb oximetry in the intensive care unit, *Neurosurgery* 42:533, 1998.
23. Littlejohn LR, Bader MK, March K: Brain tissue oxygen monitoring in severe brain injury. I. Research and usefulness in critical care, *Crit Care Nurse* 23(4):17, 2003.
24. Bader MK: Recognizing and treating ischemic insults to the brain: the role of brain tissue oxygen monitoring, *Crit Care Nurs Clin North Am* 18:243, 2006.
25. Littlejohn LR, Bader MK, March K: Brain tissue oxygen monitoring in severe brain injury. II. Implications for critical care teams and case study, *Crit Care Nurse* 23(4):17, 2003.

CHAPTER

18 Neurologic Disorders and Therapeutic Management

KATHLEEN M. STACY

OBJECTIVES

- Describe the etiology and pathophysiology of selected neurologic disorders.
- Identify the clinical manifestations of selected neurologic disorders.
- Explain the treatment of selected neurologic disorders.
- Discuss the nursing priorities for managing a patient with selected neurologic disorders.
- Discuss the concept of cerebral autoregulation.
- Describe the therapies commonly used to treat intracranial hypertension.
- List the four supratentorial herniation syndromes.

An understanding of the pathology of a disease or condition, the areas of assessment on which to focus, and the usual medical management allows the critical care nurse to more accurately anticipate and plan nursing interventions. Although a wide array of neurologic disorders exists, only a few routinely require care in the critical care environment.

COMA

Normal consciousness requires both awareness and arousal. Awareness is the combination of cognition (mental and intellectual) and affect (mood) that can be construed based on the patient's interaction with the environment. Thus, alterations of consciousness may be the result of deficits in awareness, arousal, or both.[1] Box 18-1 lists the descending states of consciousness.

Coma is the deepest state of unconsciousness in which both arousal and awareness are lacking.[1,2] The patient cannot be aroused and does not demonstrate any purposeful response to the surrounding environment. Coma is actually a symptom, rather than a disease, and it occurs as a result of some underlying process.[1] The incidence of coma is difficult to ascertain because a wide variety of conditions can produce coma.[2] This state of unconsciousness is unfortunately very common in critical care and will be the focus of the following discussion.

ETIOLOGY

The causes of coma can be divided into two general categories: structural or surgical and metabolic or medical. Structural causes of coma include ischemic stroke, intracerebral hemorrhage, trauma, and brain tumors.[3] Metabolic causes of coma include drug overdose, infectious diseases, endocrine disorders, and poisonings.[3] Approximately 85% of coma is caused by metabolic disorders and 15% by structural disorders.[4] Table 18-1 provides a brief list of the possible causes of coma.

Box 18-1

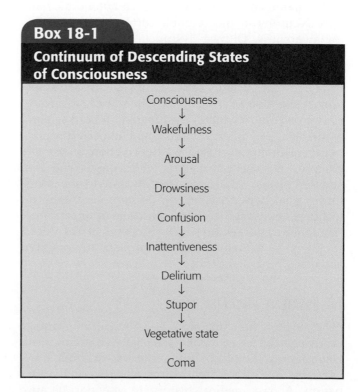

Continuum of Descending States of Consciousness

Consciousness
↓
Wakefulness
↓
Arousal
↓
Drowsiness
↓
Confusion
↓
Inattentiveness
↓
Delirium
↓
Stupor
↓
Vegetative state
↓
Coma

Table 18-1
Etiologies of Coma

STRUCTURAL/ SURGICAL COMA	METABOLIC/MEDICAL COMA
Trauma	Infection
Epidural hematoma	Meningitis
Subdural hematoma	Encephalitis
	Metabolic
Diffuse axonal injury	Metabolic conditions
	Hypoglycemia
Brain contusion	Hyperglycemia
Intracerebral hemorrhage	Hyperosmolar
	Uremia
Subarachnoid hemorrhage	Hepatic encephalopathy
	Hypertensive encephalopathy
Posterior fossa hemorrhage	Hypoxic encephalopathy
	Hyponatremia
Supratentorial hemorrhage	Hypercalcemia
	Myxedema
Hydrocephalus	Intoxication
Ischemic stroke	Narcotic overdose
Tumor	Alcohol
Other	Poisonings
	Psychogenic

Pathophysiology

Consciousness involves both arousal, or wakefulness, and awareness. Neither of these functions is present in the patient in coma. Ascending fibers of the reticular activating system (ARAS) in the pons, hypothalamus, and thalamus maintain arousal as an autonomic function. Neurons in the cerebral cortex are responsible for awareness. Diffuse dysfunction of both cerebral hemispheres and/or diffuse or focal dysfunction of the reticular activating system will produce coma.[5,6] Structural etiologies usually cause compression or dysfunction in the area of the ARAS, whereas most medical etiologies lead to general dysfunction of both cerebral hemispheres.[7] Diffuse brain dysfunction can be due to neuronal damage caused by deprivation of oxygen, glucose, or metabolic factors, endogenous and exogenous toxins, endocrine and electrolyte disorders, intracranial hypertension, central nervous system infections, neuronal disorders, disorders of temperature regulation, and seizures.[4] Dysfunction of the ARAS can be due to hemorrhage, infarction, tumors, and abscesses.[4]

Assessment and Diagnosis

Diagnosis of the coma state is a clinical one, readily established by assessment of the level of consciousness. Determining the full nature and cause of coma, however, requires a thorough history and physical examination. A past medical history is essential, because events immediately preceding the change in level of consciousness can often provide valuable clues as to the origin of the coma. When limited information is available and the coma is profound, the response of the patient to emergency treatment may provide clues to the underlying diagnosis, such as the patient who becomes responsive with the administration of naloxone can be presumed to have ingested some type of opiate.[6]

Detailed serial neurologic examinations are essential for all patients in coma. Assessment of pupillary size and reaction to light (normal, sluggish, or fixed), extraocular eye movements (normal, asymmetric, or absent), motor response to pain (normal, decorticate, decerebrate, or flaccid), and breathing pattern are important clues to determining whether the etiology of the coma is structural or metabolic.[3,5]

The areas of the brain stem that control consciousness and pupillary responses are anatomically adjacent. The sympathetic and parasympathetic nervous systems control pupillary dilatation and constriction, respectively. The anatomic directions of these pathways are known, and thus changes in pupillary responses can help identify where a lesion may be located. For example, if damage occurs in the midbrain region, pupils will be slightly enlarged and unresponsive to light. Lesions that compress the third nerve result in a fixed and dilated pupil on the same side as the insult. Pupillary responses are usually preserved when the etiology of the coma is metabolic in origin. Pupillary light responses are often the key to differentiating between structural and metabolic causes of coma.[3,5,8]

Areas of the brain stem adjacent to those responsible for consciousness also control the oculomotor eye movement. The ability to maintain conjugate gaze requires preservation of the internuclear connections of cranial nerves 3, 6, and 8 via the medial longitudinal fasciculus (MLF).[6,8] As with pupillary responses, structural lesions that impinge on these pathways will cause oculomotor dysfunction such as a disconjugate gaze. Thus deficits in extraocular eye movements usually accompany a structural etiology.[3,5,8]

Focal or asymmetrical motor deficits usually also indicate structural lesions.[3,5] Abnormal motor movements may also help pinpoint the location of a lesion. Decorticate posturing (abnormal flexion) can be seen with damage to the diencephalon. Decerebrate posturing (abnormal extension) can be seen with damage to the midbrain and pons. Flaccid posturing is an ominous sign and can be seen with damage to the medulla.[8]

Abnormal breathing patterns may also assist in differentiating structural from metabolic etiologies of coma. Cheyne-Stokes respirations are seen in patients with cerebral hemispheric dysfunction and metabolic conditions. Central neurogenic hyperventilation occurs with damage to the midbrain and upper pons.

Apneustic breathing may occur with damage to the pons, hypoglycemia, and anoxia. Ataxic breathing occurs with damage to the medulla. Agonal breathing occurs with failure of the respiratory centers in the medulla.[8]

In addition to physical assessment, laboratory studies and diagnostic procedures are done. Structural causes of coma are usually readily apparent with computerized tomography (CT) or magnetic resonance imaging (MRI). Laboratory studies are also used to identify metabolic or endocrine abnormalities.[6] Occasionally, the cause of coma is never clearly determined.

Medical Management

The goal of medical management of the patient in a coma is identification and treatment of the underlying cause of the condition. Initial medical management includes emergency measures to support vital functions and prevent further neurologic deterioration. Protection of the airway and ventilatory assistance are often needed. Administration of thiamine (at least 100 mg), glucose, and a narcotic antagonist is suggested whenever the cause of coma is not immediately known.[4-6] Thiamine is administered before glucose because the coma produced by thiamine deficiency, Wernicke's encephalopathy, can be precipitated by a glucose load.[5] The cervical neck is stabilized until traumatic injury is ruled out.[4]

The patient who remains in coma after emergency treatment requires supportive measures to maintain physiologic body functions and prevent complications. Continued airway protection and nutritional support are essential. Fluid and electrolyte management is often complex because of alterations in the neurohormonal system. Anticonvulsant therapy may be necessary to prevent further ischemic damage to the brain.[5,9]

The health care team and the patient's family jointly make decisions regarding the level of medical management to be provided. Family members require informational support in terms of probable cause of the coma and prognosis for recovery of both consciousness and function. Prognosis depends on the cause of the coma and the length of time unconsciousness persists. Sixty percent of patients in nontraumatic coma persisting for 6 or more hours die; 12% remain in a vegetative state.[10] The recovery rate for patients who are in coma for more than 1 week is only 3%.[10] As a general rule, metabolic coma has a better prognosis than coma caused by a structural lesion, and traumatic coma generally has a better outcome than nontraumatic.[6]

Much research has been directed toward identifying prognostic indicators for the patient in a coma after a cardiopulmonary arrest. As with all types of coma, the best prognosis is associated with early arousal. There is a 20% to 30% chance of survival with a good outcome in the comatose patient who responds to pain with reflex posturing (decorticate or decerebrate) within 1 to 3 hours after an arrest. In one study the presence of speech at 24 hours after arrest predicted complete neurologic recovery.[11] Survival is unlikely in the coma patient who has absent pupillary light reflexes for more than 6 hours after cardiopulmonary resuscitation.[11] These statistics are helpful in guiding decision making. However, it must always be remembered that regardless of the cause or duration of coma, outcome for an individual cannot be predicted with 100% accuracy.[5]

Box 18-2

NURSING DIAGNOSIS PRIORITIES

Coma

- Ineffective Airway Clearance related to excessive secretions or abnormal viscosity of mucus, p. A-33
- Ineffective Breathing Pattern related to decreased lung expansion, p. A-34
- Imbalanced Nutrition: Less Than Body Requirements related to lack of exogenous nutrients or increased metabolic demand, p. A-28
- Risk for Aspiration
- Compromised Family Coping related to critically ill family member, p. A-11

Nursing Management

Nursing management of the patient in a coma incorporates a variety of nursing diagnoses (Box 18-2) and is directed by the specific etiology of the coma, although some common interventions are used. One of the most important things to remember is that the patient in a coma is totally dependent on the health care team. **Nursing priorities are directed toward (1) monitoring for changes in neurologic status, (2) supporting all body functions, (3) maintaining surveillance for complications, (4) providing comforting and emotional support, and (5) initiating rehabilitation measures.**[5] Measures to support body functions include promoting pulmonary hygiene, maintaining skin integrity, initiating range of motion, managing bowel and bladder functions, and ensuring adequate nutritional support.[5]

Eye Care

The blink reflex is often diminished or absent in the comatose patient. The eyelids may be flaccid and dependent on body positioning to remain in a closed position, and edema may prevent complete closure. Loss of these protective mechanisms results in drying and ulceration of the cornea, which can lead to permanent scarring and blindness.[5]

Two interventions that are commonly used to protect the eyes are instilling saline or methylcellulose lubricating drops and taping the eyelids in the shut position. There is evidence suggesting that an alternative technique may be more effective in preventing corneal epithelial breakdown. In addition to instilling saline drops every 2 hours, a polyethylene film is taped over the eyes, extending beyond the orbits and eyebrows. The film creates a moisture chamber around the cornea and assists in keeping the eyes moist and in the closed position.[12] This technique also prevents damage to the eyes that results from tape or gauze placed directly on the delicate skin of the eyelids.[12]

Coma Stimulation Therapy

Coma stimulation has been used in rehabilitation settings for many years. This therapy is based on the belief that structured brain stimulation fosters brain recovery. The purpose of coma stimulation is to stimulate the reticular activating system and increase the patient's level of alertness. Based on the belief that maximal reorganization of the brain takes place in the early weeks after an insult, coma stimulation therapy must begin in the critical care unit to increase the possibility for maximal recovery.[13]

Coma stimulation therapy is the application of a stimulus, either auditory, visual, olfactory, gustatory, tactile, or kinesthetic, that is designed to elicit a meaningful, behavioral response from the patient.[13] The methods of stimuli used in coma stimulation therapy and the anticipated neurologic responses are listed in Boxes 18-3 and 18-4, respectively. Simple auditory and tactile stimulation are used most often in the critical care environment. However, a review of the research on sensory stimulation programs has concluded that there is no evidence to support the use of these programs.[14]

Collaborative management of the patient in a coma is outlined in Box 18-5.

STROKE

Stroke is a descriptive term for the onset of acute neurologic deficit persisting for more than 24 hours and caused by the interruption of blood flow to the brain. Stroke is the third leading cause of death in the United States, preceded by heart disease and cancer, and the leading cause of adult disability.[15] Approximately 700,000 people experience a stroke each year with 500,000 of these as first attacks and 200,000 as recurrent attacks.[15]

Strokes are generally classified as either ischemic or hemorrhagic. Although approximately 80% of all strokes are ischemic, hemorrhagic strokes have a higher mortality rate. Approximately 8% to 12% of ischemic strokes and 37% to 38% of hemorrhagic strokes result in death within 30 days.[15] Hemorrhage strokes can be further categorized as subarachnoid hemorrhages (SAHs) or intracerebral hemorrhages (ICHs). In 2007 the estimated annual cost for care and loss of productivity reached $62.7 billion.[15]

Ischemic Stroke

Ischemic stroke results from low cerebral blood flow, usually because of occlusion of a blood vessel. The

Box 18-3

Sensory Stimuli Used in Coma Stimulation Therapy

AUDITORY	VISUAL	OLFACTORY	GUSTATORY	TACTILE	KINESTHETIC
Verbal orientation	Photographs	Vinegar	Mouthwash swabs	Hand holding	Turning
Music	Penlight	Spices	Lemon juice	Rubbing lotion	Range of motion
Bells	Familiar objects	Perfume	Sweet or salty solutions	Heat/cold	Chair
Clapping	Faces	Potpourri		Cotton balls	Tilt table
Tuning fork	Flashcards	Orange/lemon peel		Rough surfaces	
				Familiar object	

From Sosnowski C, Ustik M: *J Neurosci Nurs* 26:336, 1994.

Box 18-4

Responses to Stimulation

AUDITORY	VISUAL	OLFACTORY	GUSTATORY	TACTILE	KINESTHETIC
Startle reaction	Eye blink	Grimacing	Grimacing	Localization	Spasticity of joints
Visual tracking toward sound	Visual tracking	Tearing	Spitting	Withdrawal	Assisted range of motion
Follows commands	Head turning	Swallowing	Posturing	Follows commands	

From Sosnowski C, Ustik M: *J Neurosci Nurs* 26:336, 1994.

occlusion can be either thrombotic or embolic in nature. Hypoperfusion resulting from hypotension also produces ischemic stroke. Eighty to eighty-five percent of all strokes are ischemic in nature.[16,17]

Strokes are preventable. Most thrombotic strokes are the result of the accumulation of atherosclerotic plaque in the vessel lumen, especially at bifurcations, or curves, of the vessel. The pathogenesis of cerebrovascular disease is identical to that of coronary vasculature. The greatest risk factor for ischemic stroke is hypertension.[6,16] Other risk factors are diabetes, elevated blood lipids, carotid artery disease, alcohol consumption, and smoking.[15,18] Common sites of atherosclerotic plaque are the bifurcation of the common carotid artery, the origins of the middle and anterior cerebral arteries, and the origins of the vertebral arteries.[6] Ischemic strokes secondary to vertebral artery dissection have been reported after chiropractic manipulation of the cervical spine.[19]

Etiology

An embolic stroke occurs when an embolus from the heart or lower circulation travels distally and lodges in a small vessel, resulting in loss of blood supply. At least 30% of ischemic strokes are attributed to a cardioembolic phenomenon.[6] The presence of valvular heart disease triples the risk for stroke.[20] Other risk factors include atrial fibrillation, myocardial infarction, ventricular aneurysm, and cardiomyopathy.[18] Embolic strokes also arise from atherosclerosis of the ascending aorta.[21] Recent research has linked chronic inflammation, evidenced by elevated serum C-reactive protein,[22] and chronic periodontitis with significantly increased risk for stroke.[23]

Box 18-5

Collaborative Management

Coma

- Identify and treat underlying cause
- Protect airway
- Provide ventilatory assistance as required
- Support circulation as required
- Initiate nutritional support
- Provide eye care
- Protect skin integrity
- Initiate range of motion
- Maintain surveillance for complications
  - Infections
  - Metabolic alterations
  - Cardiac dysrhythmias
  - Temperature alterations
- Provide comfort and emotional support
- Plan for rehabilitation program

Pathophysiology

Ischemic stroke is a cerebral hemodynamic insult. When cerebral blood flow is reduced to a level insufficient to maintain neuronal viability, ischemic injury occurs. In focal stroke, an area of marginally perfused tissue, the ischemic penumbra, surrounds a core of ischemic cells.[6] Sustained anoxic insult initiates a chain of events producing brain infarction. Irreversible neuronal injury soon follows. If infarction occurs, the affected brain tissue eventually softens and liquefies.[16]

The phenomenon of a focal ischemic stroke is identical to that associated with myocardial infarction, hence the term "brain attack" being used in public education strategies. Often a history of transient ischemic attacks (TIAs), brief episodes of neurologic symptoms, or reversible ischemic neurologic deficit (RIND), which lasts less than 24 hours, offers a warning that stroke is likely to occur. Sudden onset indicates embolism as the final insult to flow.[6,16,18] The size of the stroke depends on the size and location of the occluded vessel and the availability of collateral blood flow. Global ischemia results when severe hypotension or cardiopulmonary arrest produces a transient drop in blood flow to all areas of the brain.[24,25]

Cerebral edema sufficient to produce clinical deterioration develops in 10% to 20% of patients with ischemic stroke and can result in intracranial hypertension. The edema results from a loss of normal metabolic function of the cells and peaks at 3 to 5 days. This process is commonly the cause of death during the first week after a stroke.[25] Secondary hemorrhage at the site of the stroke lesion, known as *hemorrhagic conversion,* and seizures are the two other major acute neurologic complications of ischemic stroke.[6] Mortality rates in the first 20 days after ischemic stroke range from 8% to 30%.[13]

Assessment and Diagnosis

The characteristic sign of an ischemic stroke is the sudden onset of focal neurologic signs persisting for more than 24 hours. These signs usually occur in combination. Box 18-6 lists common patterns of neurologic symptoms associated with an ischemic stroke. Hemiparesis, aphasia, and hemianopia are common. Changes in level of consciousness usually occur only with brain stem or cerebellar involvement, seizure, hypoxia, hemorrhage, or elevated intracranial pressure (ICP). These changes may be exhibited as stupor, coma, confusion, and agitation.[5] The reported frequency of seizures in patients with ischemic stroke is variable, ranging from 5% to 20%. If seizures occur, they are usually seen within 24 hours of insult.[26]

The National Institutes of Health Stroke Scale (NIHSS) is often used as the basis of the focused neurologic examination (Table 18-2). The scale has six major categories: (1) overall level of consciousness,

Box 18-6

Neurologic Abnormalities in Acute Ischemic Strokes

Left (Dominant) Hemisphere
Aphasia; right hemiparesis, right-sided sensory loss, right visual field defect, poor right conjugate gaze; dysarthria; difficulty in reading, writing, or calculating

Right (Nondominant) Hemisphere
Neglect of left visual space, left visual field defect, left hemiparesis, left-sided sensory loss, poor left conjugate gaze, extinction of left-sided stimuli; dysarthria; spatial disorientation

Brain Stem/Cerebellum/Posterior Hemisphere
Motor or sensory loss in all four limbs, crossed signs, limb or gait ataxia, dysarthria, dysconjugate gaze, nystagmus, amnesia, bilateral visual field defects

Small Subcortical Hemisphere or Brain Stem

Pure Motor Stroke
Weakness of face and limbs on side of body without abnormalities of higher brain function, sensation, or vision

Pure Sensory Stroke
Decreased sensation of face and limbs on one side of body without abnormalities of higher brain function, motor function, or vision

From Adams HP et al: *Circulation* 90:1588, 1994.

(2) visual function, (3) motor skills, (4) sensation and neglect, (5) language, and 6) cerebellar integrity. The score ranges from 0 to 42 points with the higher the score, the more neurologically impaired the patient.[16,17]

Confirmation of the diagnosis of ischemic stroke is the first step in the emergent evaluation of these patients. Differentiation from intracranial hemorrhage is vital. Noncontrast CT scanning is the method of choice for this purpose and is considered the most important initial diagnostic study. In addition to excluding intracranial hemorrhage, CT can also assist in identifying early neurologic complications and the etiology of the insult.[17] An MRI will demonstrate actual infarction of cerebral tissue earlier than a CT but is less useful in the emergent differential diagnosis. Because of the strong correlation between acute ischemic stroke and heart disease, 12-lead electrocardiography, chest x-ray examination, and continuous cardiac monitoring are suggested to detect a cardiac etiology or coexisting condition. Echocardiography is valuable in identifying a cardioembolic phenomenon when a sufficient index of suspicion warrants.[27] Laboratory evaluation of hematologic function, electrolyte and glucose levels, and renal and hepatic function is also recommended. Arterial blood gas analysis is performed if hypoxia is suspected, and an electroencephalogram is obtained if seizures are suspected. Lumbar puncture is performed only if subarachnoid hemorrhage is suspected and the CT is negative.[28]

Box 18-7

Indications and Contraindications to Thrombolytic Therapy in Acute Ischemic Stroke

Indications
- Acute ischemic stroke within 3 hours from symptom onset
- Age greater than 18 years old (rt-PA has not been studied in pediatric stroke)

Contraindications
- Evidence of intracranial hemorrhage on pretreatment evaluation
- Suspicion of subarachnoid hemorrhage
- Recent stroke, intracranial or intraspinal surgery, or serious head trauma in the past 3 months
- Major surgery or serious trauma in the previous 14 days*
- Arterial puncture at a noncompressible site or lumbar puncture in the last 7 days
- Major symptoms that are rapidly improving or only minor stroke symptoms (NIHSS <4)*
- History of intracranial hemorrhage
- Uncontrolled hypertension at the time of treatment
- Seizure at the stroke onset
- Active internal bleeding
- Intracranial neoplasm, arteriovenous malformation, or aneurysm
- Known bleeding diathesis including but not limited to:
  - Current use of anticoagulants or an international normalized ratio (INR) >1.7 or a prothrombin time (PT) >15 seconds
  - Administration of heparin within 48 hours preceding the onset of stroke and an elevated activated partial thromboplastin time at presentation
  - Platelet count <100,000/mm^3

From Thurman RJ, Jauch EC: *Emerg Med Clin North Am* 20:609, 2002.
*In the NINDS trial, not present in current package insert.
rt-PA, Recombinant tissue plasminogen activator; *NIHSS,* National Institutes of Health Stroke Scale; *NINDS,* National Institute of Neurologic Disorders and Stroke.

MEDICAL MANAGEMENT

Major changes have taken place in the medical management of ischemic stroke since 1996. Based on results of the National Institute of Neurologic Disorders and Stroke (NINDS) rt-PA Stroke Study, thrombolytic therapy with intravenous recombinant tissue plasminogen activator (rt-PA) is now recommended within 3 hours of onset of ischemic stroke.[29,30] Indications and contraindication to thrombolysis are listed in Box 18-7. Confirmation of diagnosis with CT must be accomplished before rt-PA administration. The recommended dose of rt-PA is 0.9 mg/kg up to a maximum dose of 90 mg. Ten percent of the total dose is administered as an initial intravenous bolus over 1 minute, and the remaining 90% is administered by intravenous infusion over 60 minutes.[31]

The desired result of thrombolytic therapy is to dissolve the clot and reperfuse the ischemic brain. The goal is to reverse or minimize the effects of stroke. The major risk and complication of rt-PA therapy is

Table 18-2

National Institutes of Health Stroke Scale

1.a.	Level of consciousness:	0: Alert 1: Not alert, but arousable with minimal stimulation 2: Not alert, requires repeated stimulation to attend 3: Coma
1.b.	Ask patient the month and their age:	0: Answers both correctly 1: Answers one correctly 2: Both incorrect
1.c.	Ask patient to open and close eyes and to grip and release hand	0: Obeys both correctly 1: Obeys one correctly 2: Both incorrect
2.	Best gaze (only horizontal eye movement):	0: Normal 1: Partial gaze palsy 2: Forced deviation
3.	Visual field testing:	0: No visual field loss 1: Partial hemianopia 2: Complete hemianopia 3: Bilateral hemianopia (blind including cortical blindness)
4.	Facial paresis (ask patient to show teeth or raise eyebrows and close eyes tightly):	0: Normal symmetrical movement 1: Minor paralysis (flattened nasolabial fold, asymmetry on smiling) 2: Partial paralysis (total or near total paralysis of lower face) 3: Complete paralysis of one or both sides (absence of facial movement in the upper and lower face)
5.	Motor function—arm (right and left): Right arm ________ Left arm ________	0: Normal (extends arms 90 [or 45] degrees for 10 seconds without drift) 1: Drift 2: Some effort against gravity 3: No effort against gravity 4: No movement UN: Untestable (joint fused or limb amputated)
6.	Motor function—leg (right and left): Right leg ________ Left leg ________	0: Normal (hold leg 30 degrees position for 5 seconds) 1: Drift 2: Some effort against gravity 3: No effort against gravity 4: No movement UN: Untestable (joint fused or limb amputated)
7.	Limb ataxia:	0: No ataxia 1: Present in one limb 2: Present in two limbs
8.	Sensory (use pinprick to test arms, legs, trunk and face—compare side to side):	0: Normal 1: Mild to moderate decrease in sensation 2: Severe to total sensory loss
9.	Best language (describe picture, name items, read sentences)	0: No aphasia 1: Mild to moderate aphasia 2: Severe aphasia 3: Mute
10.	Dysarthria (read several words):	0: Normal articulation 1: Mild to moderate slurring of words 2: Near unintelligible or unable to speak UN: Intubated or other physical barrier
11.	Extinction and inattention:	0: Normal 1: Inattention or extinction to bilateral simultaneous stimulation in one of the sensory modalities 2: Severe hemi-inattention or hemi-inattention to more than one modality

From the National Institutes of Health, http://www.ninds.nih.gov/doctors/index.htm.
UN, Untestable.

bleeding, especially intracranial hemorrhage. Unlike thrombolytic protocols for acute myocardial infarction, subsequent therapy with anticoagulant or antiplatelet agents is *not* recommended after rt-PA administration in ischemic stroke. Persons receiving thrombolytic therapy for stroke should not receive aspirin, heparin, warfarin, ticlopidine, or any other antithrombotic or antiplatelet aggregating drugs for at least 24 hours after treatment.[32]

Other emergent care of the patient with ischemic stroke must include airway protection and ventilatory assistance to maintain adequate tissue oxygenation.[17] Hypertension often is present in the early period as a compensatory response and in most cases must not be lowered (Table 18-3). For the patient who has not received thrombolytic therapy, antihypertensive therapy is considered only if the diastolic blood pressure (BP) is greater than 120 mm Hg or the systolic BP is greater than 220 mm Hg.[33] Criteria differ for the patient who has received rt-PA. The BP for these patients is kept below 180/105 mm Hg to prevent intracranial hemorrhage. Intravenous labetalol or sodium nitroprusside is used to achieve BP control.[33] Body temperature and glucose levels also must be normalized.[23]

Medical management also must include the identification and treatment of acute complications, such as cerebral edema or seizure activity. Prophylaxis for these complications is not recommended. Surgical decompression is recommended if a large cerebellar infarction compresses the brain stem.[34]

Subarachnoid Hemorrhage

SAH is bleeding into the subarachnoid space, usually caused by rupture of a cerebral aneurysm or arteriovenous malformation (AVM). Subarachnoid hemorrhage accounts for 4.5% to 13% of all strokes[15]—with nontraumatic SAH affecting more than 30,000 Americans each year.[34] The incidence of SAH is greater in women and increases with age with a the peak incidence between 55 and 60 years.[35] The rate of significant morbidity approximates 50% to 60% of all survivors.[15] Unfortunately, no appreciable decrease in the incidence of SAH has occurred over time. Approximately 5% of the general population is believed to have an unruptured cerebral aneurysm,[36] the congenital anomaly responsible for most cases of SAH. The risk for rupture is 1% to 2% annually.[36] The known risk factors for

Table 18-3
Blood Pressure Management for Stroke (American Stroke Association Guidelines)

BLOOD PRESSURE*	TREATMENT
Nonthrombolytic Candidates	
DBP >140 mm Hg	Sodium nitroprusside (0.5 mcg/kg/min); aim for 10%-20% reduction in DBP
SBP >220 mm Hg, DBP 121-140 mm Hg, or MAP† >130 mm Hg	10-20 mg labetalol‡ IV push over 1-2 min; may repeat or double labetalol every 20 min to a maximum dose of 300 mg
SBP < 220 mm Hg, DBP = 120 mm Hg, or MAP† <130 mm Hg	Emergency antihypertensive therapy is deferred in the absence of aortic dissection, acute myocardial infarction, severe congestive heart failure, or hypertensive encephalopathy
Thrombolytic Candidates	
Pretreatment	
SBP >185 mm Hg or DBP >110 mm Hg	1-2 inches of nitroglycerine paste (Nitropaste) or 1-2 doses of 10-20 mg labetalol‡ IV push; if BP is not reduced and maintained to <185/110 mm Hg, the patient should not be treated with TPA
During and After Treatment	
Monitor BP	BP is monitored every 15 min for 2 hr, then every 30 min for 6 hr, and then hourly for 16 hr
DBP >140 mm Hg	Sodium nitroprusside (0.5 mcg/kg/min)
SBP >230 mm Hg or DBP 121-140 mm Hg	10 mg labetalol‡ IVP over 1-2 min; may repeat or double labetalol every 10 min to a maximum dose of 300 mg or give initial labetalol bolus and then start a labetalol drip at 2-8 mg/min If BP not controlled by labetalol, consider sodium nitroprusside
SBP 180-230 mm Hg or DBP 105-120 mm Hg	10 mg labetalol‡ IVP; may repeat or double labetalol every 10-20 min to a maximum dose of 300 mg or give initial labetalol bolus and then start a labetalol drip at 2-8 mg/min

From Bader MK, Littlejohns LR: *AANN core curriculum for neuroscience nursing,* ed 4, St Louis, 2004, Elsevier.

DBP, Diastolic blood pressure; *SBP,* systolic blood pressure; *MAP,* mean arterial pressure; *IV,* intravenous; *BP,* blood pressure; *TPA,* tissue plasminogen activator; *IVP,* intravenous push.

*All initial blood pressures should be verified before treatment by repeating reading in 5 minutes.

†As estimated by one third the sum of systolic and double diastolic pressure.

‡Labetalol should be avoided in patients with asthma, cardiac failure, or severe abnormalities in cardiac conduction. For refractory hypertension, alternative therapy may be considered with sodium nitroprusside or enalapril.

SAH include hypertension, smoking, alcohol use, and stimulant use. As in ischemic stroke, the single most important risk factor is hypertension.[15]

Etiology

Cerebral aneurysm rupture accounts for approximately 85% of all cases of spontaneous SAH.[6] An aneurysm is an outpouching of the wall of a blood vessel that results from weakening of the wall of the vessel (Table 18-4). Ninety percent of aneurysms are congenital—the cause of which is unknown. The other 10% can be the result of traumatic injury (that stretches and tears the muscular middle layer of the arterial vessel), infectious material (most often from infectious vegetation

Table 18-4

Aneurysm Classification According to Type, Shape, Location, and Common Characteristics

TYPES OF ANEURYSMS	CHARACTERISTICS
Berry or saccular 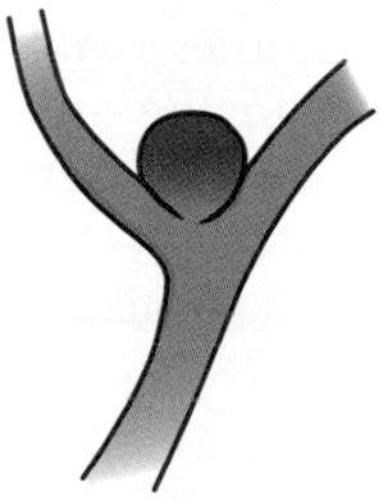	Most common type, usually congenital; appears at a bifurcation in the anterior circulation, primarily at the base of the brain or the circle of Willis and its branches; grows from the base of the arterial wall with a neck or stem; contains blood; thinned dome is usually the site of rupture
Giant or fusiform 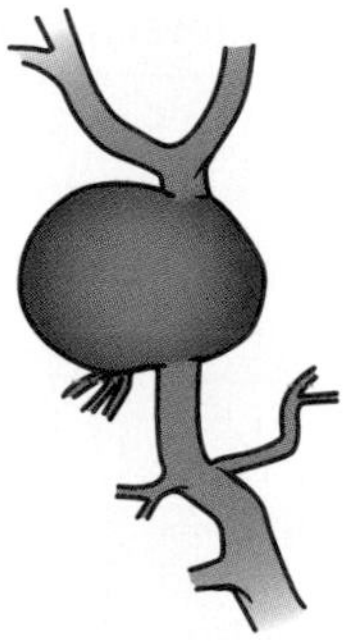	Can be irregular in shape and larger than 2.5 cm and atherosclerotic; involves mainly the internal carotid or vertebrobasilar artery; rarely ruptures; has no stem; can act like a space-occupying lesion in the brain; and is difficult to manage
Mycotic 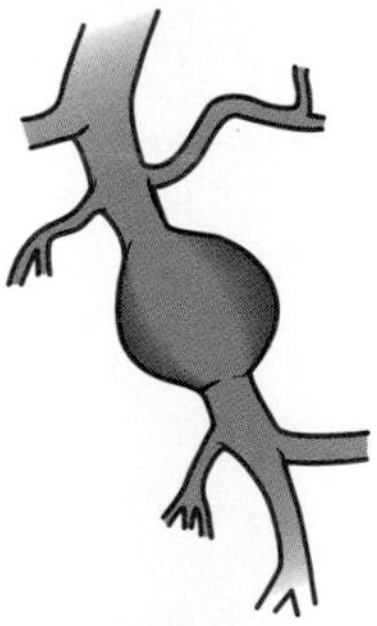	Rare form; usually occurs from septic emboli, usually secondary to bacterial infection, which weaken the vessel wall, causing dilation involving the distal branches of the middle cerebral arteries
Dissecting 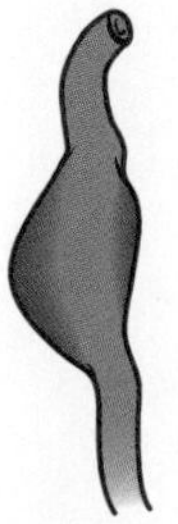	May occur during angiography, secondary to trauma, syphilis, or arteriosclerosis, or when blood is forced between layers of the arterial wall; the intima is pulled away from the medial layer, allowing blood to enter
Traumatic	Sometimes called a "pseudoaneurysm," which may resolve following trauma
Charcot-Bouchard	Small aneurysm that can be seen in the area of the basal ganglia and/or the brain stem in individuals with a history of hypertension; chronic hypertension causes fibrinoid necrosis in the penetrating and subcortical arteries, weakening the arterial walls and causing formation of small aneurismal outpouching[16]

on valves of the left side of the heart after bacterial endocarditis) that lodges against a vessel wall and erodes the muscular layer, or of undetermined cause.[5] Multiple aneurysms occur in 20% to 25% of the cases and often are bilateral, occurring in the same location on both sides of the cerebral vascular system.[6] It is possible for an individual to live a full life span with an unruptured cerebral aneurysm. Aneurysm rupture usually occurs during the fifth and sixth decades of life.[36]

Arteriovenous malformation rupture is responsible for less than 2% of all SAHs.[37] An AVM is a tangled mass of arterial and venous blood vessels that shunt blood directly from the arterial side into the venous side, bypassing the capillary system. AVMs may be small focal lesions or large diffuse lesions that occupy almost an entire hemisphere.[37] They are always congenital, though the exact embryonic cause for these malformations is unknown. They also occur in the spinal cord and renal, gastrointestinal, and integumentary systems. Small superficial AVMs are seen as port-wine stains of the skin. In contrast to the middle-age population with SAH from aneurysm, SAH from an AVM usually occurs in the second to fourth decades of life.[6]

Pathophysiology

The pathophysiology of the two most common causes of SAH is distinctly different.

Cerebral Aneurysm. As the individual with a congenital cerebral aneurysm matures, blood pressure rises and more stress is placed on the poorly developed and thin vessel wall. Ballooning out of the vessel occurs, giving the aneurysm a berrylike appearance. Most cerebral aneurysms are saccular or berrylike with a stem or neck. Aneurysms are usually small, 2 to 7 mm in diameter, and often occur at the base of the brain on the circle of Willis (Figure 18-1). Most cerebral aneurysms occur at the bifurcation of blood vessels.[5,6]

The aneurysm becomes clinically significant when the vessel wall becomes so thin that it ruptures, sending arterial blood at a high pressure into the subarachnoid space. For a brief moment after the aneurysm ruptures, intracranial pressure is believed to approach mean arterial pressure and cerebral perfusion falls. In other situations, the unruptured aneurysm expands and places pressure on surrounding structures. This is particularly true with posterior communicating artery aneurysms, because they put pressure on the oculomotor nerve (CN III), causing ipsilateral pupil dilation and ptosis.[5,6]

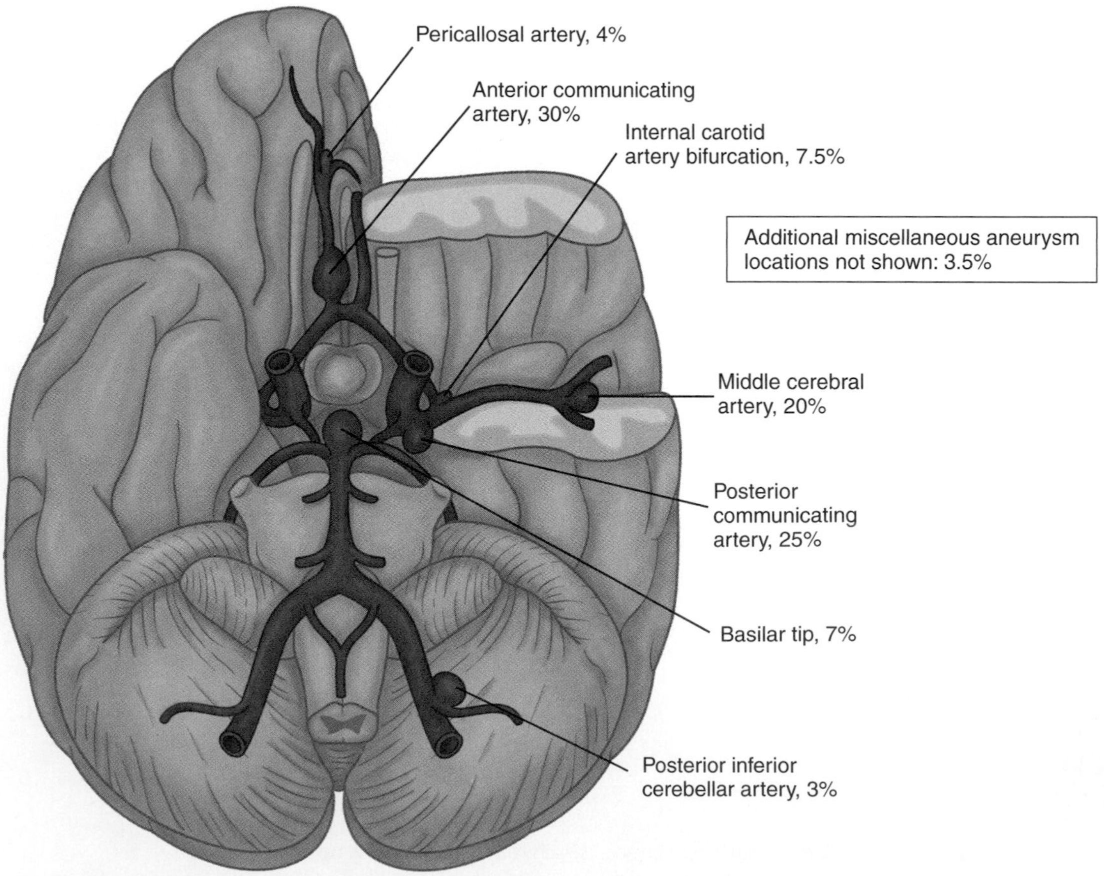

FIGURE 18-1. The most common locations of intracranial aneurysms. (From Brisman JL, Song JK, Newell DW: Medical progress: cerebral aneurysms, *N Engl J Med* 355:928, 2006.)

Arteriovenous Malformation. The pathophysiologic features of an AVM are related to the size and location of the malformation. One or more cerebral arteries, also known as *feeders*, feed an AVM. These feeder arteries tend to enlarge over time and increase the volume of blood shunted through the malformation, as well as increase the overall mass effect. Large, dilated, tortuous draining veins also develop as a result of increasing arterial blood flow being delivered at a higher than normal pressure. Normal vascular flow has a mean arterial pressure of 70 to 80 mm Hg, a mean arteriole pressure of 35 to 45 mm Hg, and a mean capillary pressure that drops from 35 to 10 mm Hg as it connects with the venous side. Lack of this capillary bridge allows blood with a mean pressure of 35 to 45 mm Hg to flow into the venous system. Because a vein has no muscular layer as does an artery, the veins become extremely engorged and rupture easily. Cerebral atrophy is also present sometimes in the patient with an AVM. It is the result of chronic ischemia because of the shunting of blood through the AVM and away from normal cerebral circulation.[5,6,37]

Assessment and Diagnosis

The patient with an SAH characteristically has an abrupt onset of pain, described as the "worst headache of my life." A brief loss of consciousness, nausea, vomiting, focal neurologic deficits, and a stiff neck may accompany the headache.[34,35] The SAH may result in coma or death.

Patient history may reveal one or more incidences of sudden onset of headache with vomiting in the weeks preceding a major SAH. These are "warning leaks" of an aneurysm in which small amounts of blood ooze from the aneurysm into the subarachnoid space. The presence of blood is an irritant to the meninges, particularly the arachnoid membrane. This irritation causes headache, stiff neck, and photophobia. These small "warning leaks" seldom are detected because the condition is not severe enough for the patient to seek medical attention. If a neurologic deficit, such as third cranial nerve palsy, develops before aneurysm rupture, medical intervention is sought and the aneurysm may be surgically secured before the devastation of a rupture can occur. Symptoms of unruptured AVM—headaches with dizziness or syncope or fleeting neurologic deficits—also may be found in the history.[6]

Diagnosis of SAH is based on clinical presentation, CT scan, and lumbar puncture. Noncontrast CT is the cornerstone of definitive SAH diagnosis.[38-40] In 92% of the cases, CT scan can demonstrate a clot in the subarachnoid space, if performed within 24 hours of the onset of the hemorrhage. On the basis of the appearance and the location of the SAH, diagnosis of cause—aneurysm or AVM—may be made from the CT scan. MRI is relatively insensitive for detecting blood in the subarachnoid space.

If the initial CT scan is negative, a lumbar puncture is performed to obtain cerebral spinal fluid (CSF) for analysis.[35] CSF after SAH is bloody in appearance with a red blood cell count greater than 1000/mm^3. If the lumbar puncture is performed more than 5 days after the SAH, CSF fluid is xanthochromic (dark amber), because the blood products have broken down.[38] Cloudy CSF usually indicates some type of infectious process, such as bacterial meningitis, not a subarachnoid hemorrhage.[6]

Once the SAH has been documented, cerebral angiography is necessary to identify the exact cause of the SAH. If a cerebral aneurysm rupture is the cause, angiography is also essential for identifying the exact location of the aneurysm in preparation for surgery.[38-40] Once the aneurysm has been located, it is graded using the Hunt and Hess classification scale. This scale categorizes the patient based on the severity of the neurologic deficits associated with the hemorrhage (Box 18-8).[11] If AVM rupture is the cause, angiography is necessary to identify the feeding arteries and draining veins of the malformation.

Medical Management

SAH is a medical emergency, and time is of the essence. Preservation of neurologic function is the goal. Initial treatment must always support vital functions. Airway management and ventilatory assistance may be necessary. Early diagnosis is also essential. A ventriculostomy is performed to control ICP if the patient's level of consciousness is depressed.[38]

Evidence suggests that only 19% of the deaths attributable to aneurysmal SAH are related to the direct effects of the initial hemorrhage.[42] Research has shown that rebleeding accounts for 22% of deaths from aneurysmal SAH, cerebral vasospasm for 23%, and nonneurologic medical complications for 23%.[42] Principal

Box 18-8

Classification of Subarachnoid Hemorrhage

Grade I	Asymptomatic or minimal headache Slight nuchal rigidity
Grade II	Moderate to severe headache Nuchal rigidity No neurologic deficit other than cranial nerve palsy
Grade III	Drowsiness Confusion Mild focal deficit
Grade IV	Stupor Moderate to severe hemiparesis Possible early decerebrate rigidity Vegetative disturbances
Grade V	Deep coma Decerebrate rigidity Moribund appearance

nonneurologic causes of death are systemic inflammatory response syndrome (SIRS) and secondary organ dysfunction.[43] Once initial intervention has provided necessary support for vital physiologic functions, medical management of acute SAH is aimed primarily toward the prevention and treatment of the complications of SAH that can produce further neurologic damage and death.

Rebleeding. Rebleeding is the occurrence of a second SAH in an unsecured aneurysm or, less commonly, an AVM.[6] The incidence of rebleeding during the first 24 hours following the first bleed is 4%, with a 1% to 2% chance per day for the following month. Mortality with aneurysmal rebleeding is approximately 70%.[35]

Historically, conservative measures to prevent rebleeding have included BP control and SAH precautions (see section on nursing management of stroke). An elevation in BP is a normal compensatory response to maintain adequate cerebral perfusion after a neurologic insult. In the belief that hypertension contributes to rebleeding, nitroprusside, metoprolol, or hydralazine has been commonly used to maintain a systolic BP no greater than 150 mm Hg.[44] Individualized guidelines must be determined based on clinical condition and preexisting values of the patient. Evidence suggests that rebleeding has more to do with variations in BP than it does with absolute values and that BP control does not lower the incidence of rebleeding.[39] Prophylactic anticonvulsant therapy is recommended to prevent seizures.[35,39]

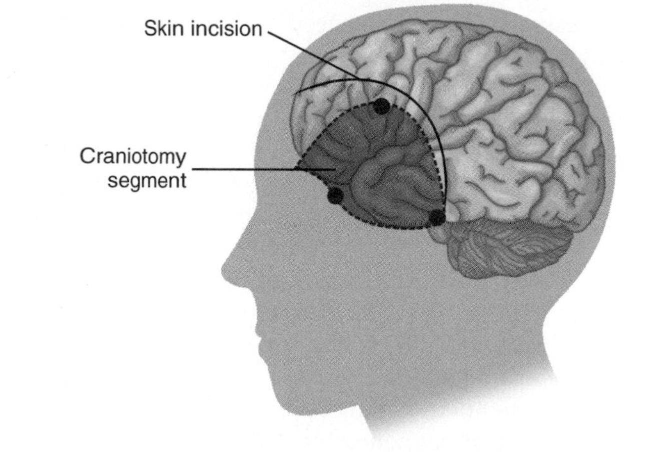

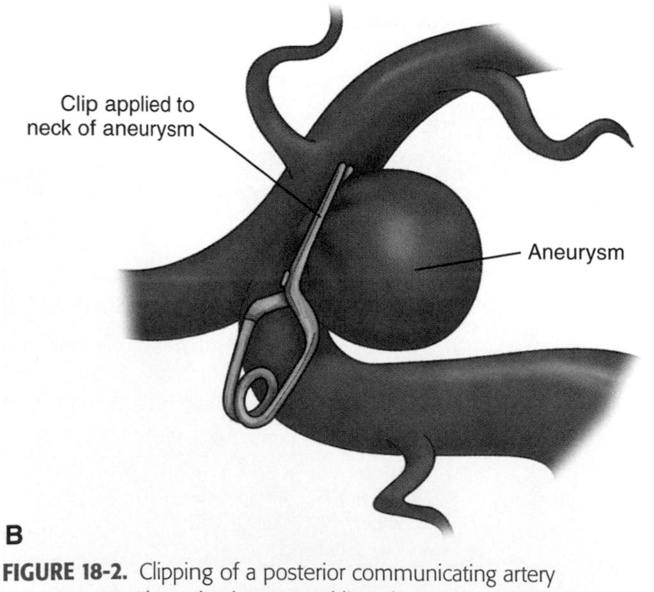

FIGURE 18-2. Clipping of a posterior communicating artery aneurysm. **A,** The unbroken curved line shows the typical skin incision, and the dashed lines show the craniotomy location. **B,** Application of the clip to the aneurysm.

Surgical Aneurysm Clipping. Definitive treatment for the prevention of rebleeding is surgical clipping with complete obliteration of the aneurysm. Timing of the surgery is a key medical management issue. Since the introduction of microsurgery and improved surgical techniques, patients commonly are taken to the operating room within the first 48 hours after rupture. This early surgical intervention to secure the aneurysm eliminates the risk of rebleeding and allows more aggressive therapy to be used in the postoperative period for the treatment of vasospasm.[38] Early surgery also allows the neurosurgeon to flush out the excess blood and clots from the basal cisterns (reservoir of CSF around the base of the brain and circle of Willis) to reduce the risk of vasospasm.[45] Early surgery is recommended for patients with a grade I or grade II SAH and some patients with grade III. In patients with a grade III SAH, the initial hemorrhage did not produce significant neurologic deficit, but the risk of rebleeding with a tragically high incidence of mortality is present until the aneurysm is secured. Because of the patient's clinical condition and the technical difficulty of the surgery, early surgical repair of the aneurysm is not always possible. Early surgery continues to be controversial for patients with grade IV or V SAH and those demonstrating vasospasm. However, recent studies have not supported the fear of worse ischemic sequelae with early surgery in these patients.[46] Careful consideration of the patient's clinical situation is necessary in determining the optimal time for surgery.

The surgical procedure involves a craniotomy to expose and isolate the area of aneurysm. A clip is placed over the neck of the aneurysm to eliminate the area of weakness (Figure 18-2). This is a technically difficult procedure that requires the skill of an experienced neurosurgeon. It is not uncommon, particularly in early surgery, for the clot to break away from the aneurysm as it is surgically exposed. Extensive hemorrhage into the craniotomy site results, and cessation of the hemorrhage often causes increased neurologic deficits. Deficits also may occur as a result of surgical manipulation to gain access to the site of the aneurysm.[5]

Surgical AVM Excision. Management of AVM traditionally has involved surgical excision or conservative management of such symptoms as seizures and headache. The decision for surgical excision depends on the location and size of the AVM. Some malformations are located so deep in the cerebral structures (the thalamus or midbrain) that attempts to remove the AVM would cause severe neurologic deficits. History of a previous hemorrhage and the patient's age and overall condition are also taken into account when making the decision regarding surgical intervention.[37]

Surgical excision of large AVMs includes the risk of reperfusion bleeding. As feeding arteries of the AVM are clamped off, the arterial blood that usually flowed into the AVM is now diverted into the surrounding circulation. In many cases the surrounding tissue has been in a state of chronic ischemia and the arterial vessels feeding these areas are maximally dilated. As arterial blood begins to flow at a higher volume and pressure into these dilated arteries, seeping of blood from the vessels may occur. Evidence of reperfusion bleeding in the operating room is an indication that no more arterial blood can be diverted from the AVM without risk of serious intracerebral hemorrhage. In the postoperative phase, a low blood pressure is maintained to prevent further reperfusion bleeding. In large AVMs, two to four stages of surgery may be required over 6 to 12 months.[6]

Embolization. Embolization is used to secure a cerebral aneurysm or AVM that is surgically inaccessible because of size, location, or medical instability of the patient. Embolization involves several new interventional neuroradiology techniques. All of the techniques use a percutaneous transfemoral approach in a manner similar to an angiogram. Under fluoroscopy, the catheter is threaded up to the internal carotid artery. Specially developed microcatheters are then manipulated into the area of the vascular anomaly, and embolic materials are placed endovascularly.[36,37] Two different embolization techniques are used, depending on the underlying pathologic derangement.

The first type of embolization is used to embolize an AVM. Glue, polyvinyl alcohol particles, detachable coils, or liquid polymers are slowly introduced into the vessels feeding the AVM. Blood flow then carries the material to the site, and embolization is achieved. This procedure may be used in combination with surgery. One to three sessions of embolization of the feeding vessels are performed to reduce the size of the lesion before a craniotomy is performed for total excision.[37] The primary risk of this procedure is lodging of the embolic substance in a vessel that feeds normal tissue. This occurrence creates an embolic stroke with the immediate onset of neurologic symptoms.[5,6]

The second type of embolization involves placement of one or more detachable coils into an aneurysm to produce an endovascular thrombus (Figure 18-3). The advantage of this technique is that an electrical current creates positive charging of the coil, which induces electrothrombosis. Complications include embolic stroke, coil migration, overproduction of the clot, subtotal occlusion and intraprocedural rupture of the vasculature, and death.[36]

Cerebral Vasospasm. The presence or absence of cerebral vasospasm significantly affects the outcome of aneurysmal SAH. This complication does not occur with SAH resulting from AVM rupture. Cerebral vasospasm is a narrowing of the lumen of the cerebral arteries, possibly in response to subarachnoid blood clots coating the outer surface of the blood vessels. Inasmuch as aneurysms occur at the circle of Willis, the major vessels responsible for feeding the cerebral circulation are affected by vasospasm. Depending on the arterial vessels involved in the vasospasm reaction, decreased arterial flow occurs in large areas of the cerebral hemispheres.[6]

It is estimated that 90% of all SAH patients develop vasospasm, which is demonstrable by angiography.[47] Thirty-two percent of these patients develop symptomatic vasospasm, resulting in ischemic stroke and/or death for 15% to 20% of them despite the use of maximal therapy. The onset of vasospasm is usually 4 to 12 days after the initial hemorrhage.[45]

Hypertensive, Hypervolemic, Hemodilution Therapy. Hypertensive, hypervolemic, hemodilution (HHH) therapy involves increasing the patient's blood pressure and cardiac output with vasoactive medications and diluting the patient's blood with fluid and volume expanders. Systolic BP is maintained between 150 and 160 mm Hg. The increase in volume and pressure forces blood through the vasospastic area at higher pressures. Hemodilution facilitates flow through the area by reducing blood viscosity. Many anecdotal reports exist of patients' neurologic deficits improving as systolic pressure increases from 130 mm Hg to between 150 and 160 mm Hg.[48] The Stroke Council of the American Heart Association (AHA) has recommended this therapy for prevention and treatment of vasospasm.[39] However, a review of the recent research on this therapy has indicated that there is not enough evidence to support the use of this therapy as a preventive measure and that further research is needed to support its use as treatment for symptomatic vasospasm.[47]

Nimodipine. Nimodipine is strongly recommended to reduce the poor outcomes associated with vasospasm. The exact nature of the effect of nimodipine is not clear, but use of the drug has demonstrated consistently positive effects on outcome without any demonstrable effect on the incidence or severity of vasospasm.[35,49] Sixty milligrams of nimodipine is given orally every 4 hours for 21 days.[35,38] Nimodipine may produce hypotension, especially when administered concurrently with other antihypertensive agents.

Cerebral Angioplasty. Cerebral angioplasty is used when pharmacologic management of cerebral vasospasm

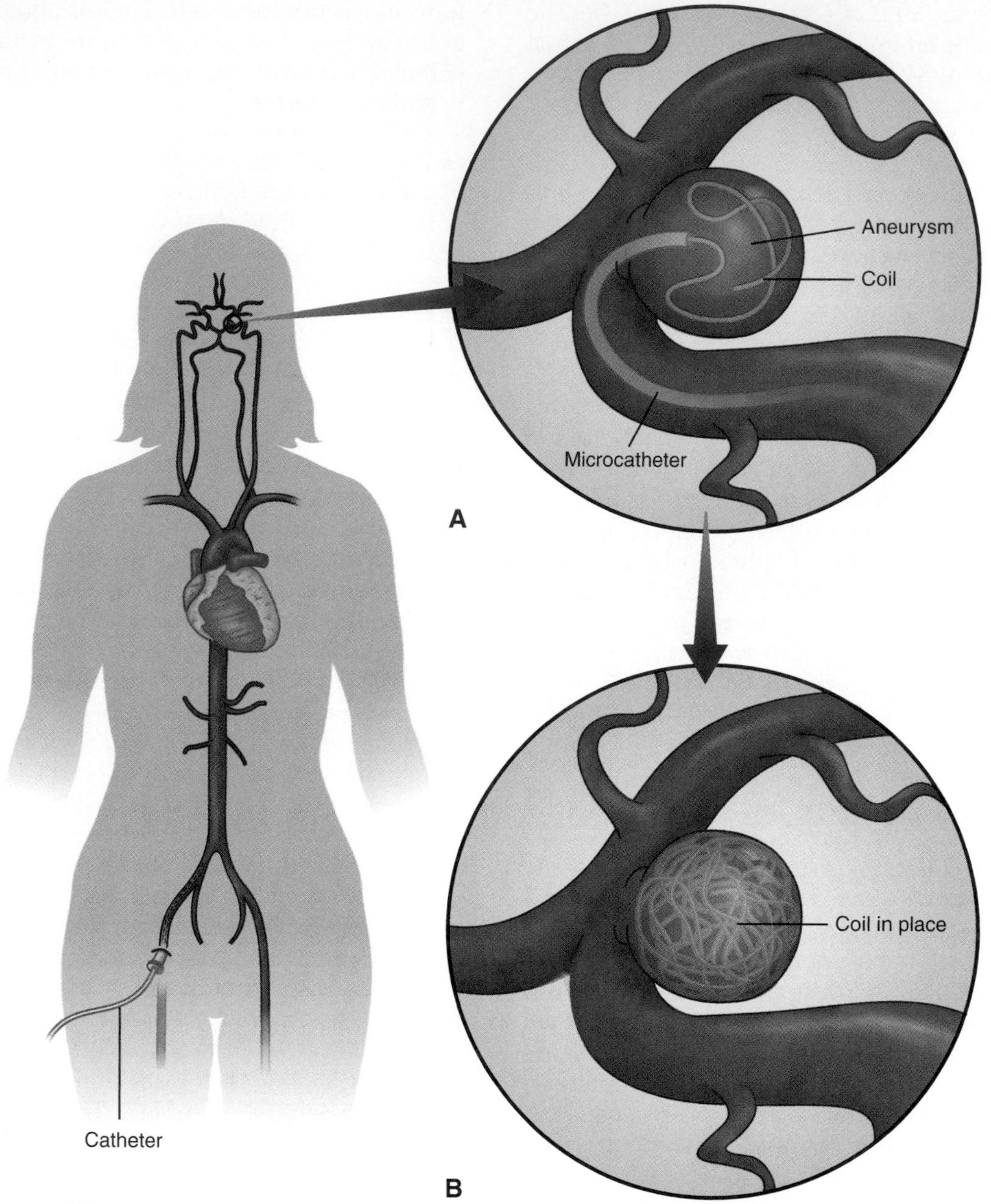

FIGURE 18-3. Endovascular occlusion of a posterior communicating artery aneurysm. **A,** Insertion of the microcatheter into the aneurysm via the right femoral artery, aorta, and left carotid artery. **B,** Occlusion of the aneurysm with coils.

has failed.[47] It is performed only when CT or MRI provides evidence that infarction has not yet occurred. An interventional neuroradiologist performs the procedure, and the patient is under local, general, or neuroleptic analgesia. The technique of cerebral angioplasty is very similar to that used in the coronary vasculature. Risks include intimal perforation or rupture, cerebral artery thrombosis or embolism, recurrence of stenosis, and severe diffuse vasospasm unresponsive to therapy. Hemorrhage at the femoral site also may occur. This procedure is recommended when conventional therapy is unsuccessful.[35,39,47]

Hyponatremia. Hyponatremia develops in 10% to 43% of patients with SAH as the result of a central salt-wasting syndrome. It usually occurs around the same time frame as vasospasm, several days after initial hemorrhage.[35] There is strong evidence that the use of fluid restriction to treat hyponatremia is associated with poor outcome in the SAH patient. The AHA Stroke Council has strongly recommended that fluid restriction not be used in this instance and instead recommends sodium replenishment with isotonic fluids.[39]

Hydrocephalus. Hydrocephalus is a late complication that occurs in approximately 15% to 20% of the patients after SAH.[35] Blood that has circulated in the subarachnoid space and has been absorbed by the arachnoid villi may obstruct the villi and reduce the rate of CSF absorption. Over time, increasing volumes of CSF in the intracranial space produce communicating hydrocephalus. Treatment consists of placing a drain to remove CSF. This can be accomplished temporarily by performing a ventriculostomy or permanently by placing a ventriculoperitoneal shunt.[39]

Intracerebral Hemorrhage

ICH is bleeding directly into cerebral tissue. ICH destroys cerebral tissue, causes cerebral edema, and increases ICP. The source of intracerebral bleeding is usually a small artery, but it can result also from rupture of an AVM or aneurysm. The most important cause of spontaneous ICH is hypertension, so this section concentrates on spontaneous hypertensive ICH.[50]

Spontaneous ICH is more than twice as common as SAH. The likeliness of death or disability is higher with ICH than with either ischemic stroke or SAH.[51] Approximately 15% of all hemorrhagic strokes are due to ICH. ICH has a 50% mortality rate at 6 months.[50]

Etiology

ICH can be categorized as either primary or secondary. Primary ICH is most often caused by hypertensive rupture of a cerebral vessel, resulting from a long-standing history of hypertension (HTN). Secondary ICH is caused by anticoagulation or thrombolytic therapy, coagulation disorders, drug abuse, brain tumors, rupture of a cerebral aneurysm or AVM, and cerebral infarct.[50] Many patients develop headache and neurologic symptoms after straining to have a bowel movement. Often on questioning, the patient with a hypertensive hemorrhage admits to having discontinued antihypertensive medication 2 to 3 weeks before the hemorrhage.

Pathophysiology

The pathophysiology of intracerebral hemorrhage is caused by continued elevated blood pressure exerting force against smaller arterial vessels that have become damaged from arteriosclerotic changes. Eventually these arteries break, and blood bursts from the vessels into the surrounding cerebral tissue, creating a hematoma. ICP rises precipitously in response to the increase in overall intracranial volume.[5,6,52]

Assessment and Diagnosis

Initial assessment usually reveals a critically ill patient who often is unconscious and requires ventilatory support. History from a relative or significant other describes a sudden onset of focal deficit often accompanied by severe headache, nausea, vomiting, and rapid neurologic deterioration. Approximately 50% of patients sustain early loss of consciousness, a key differential feature from ischemic stroke.[53] More than half of the patients with ICH present with a smooth progression of neurologic symptoms, an uncommon finding in either ischemic stroke or SAH.[53] One third of the patients have maximal symptoms at onset. Vital signs usually reveal a severely elevated blood pressure (200/100 to 250/150 mm Hg). Signs of increased ICP are often present by the time the patient arrives in the emergency department. Diagnosis is established easily with CT. Angiography is recommended only in patients considered surgical candidates without a clear cause of hemorrhage.[51,53]

Medical Management

ICH is a medical emergency. Initial management requires attention to airway, breathing, and circulation. Intubation is usually necessary. Blood pressure management must be based on individual factors. Reduction in BP is usually necessary to decrease ongoing bleeding, but lowering BP too much or too rapidly may compromise cerebral perfusion pressure, especially in the patient with elevated ICP. National guidelines recommend keeping the *mean* arterial BP below 130 mm Hg in patients with a history of HTN and below 110 mm Hg after surgical treatment for ICH.[53] Vasopressor therapy, following fluid replenishment, is recommended if systolic BP falls below 90 mm Hg.[50,51,53]

Increased ICP is common with ICH and is a major contributor to mortality. Recommended management includes mannitol when indicated, hyperventilation, and neuromuscular blockade with sedation. Steroids are avoided. Cerebral perfusion pressure (CPP) must be kept greater than 70 mm Hg.[53]

The goal for fluid management is euvolemia with a recommended pulmonary occlusion pressure of 10 to 14 mm Hg. Body temperature is kept at less than 38.5° C using acetaminophen or cooling blankets. Short-acting benzodiazepines or propofol is recommended to treat agitation or hyperactivity. Pneumatic compression devices are used to decrease risk of pulmonary embolism. Prophylactic antiepileptic therapy is sometimes used.[53]

The benefit of surgical treatment of spontaneous ICH is unclear. Recommendations for surgical removal of the clot depend on the size and location of the hematoma, the patient's ICP, and other neurologic symptoms. Medical treatment is recommended if the hemorrhage is small or neurologic deficit is minimal. Numerous techniques are being investigated to lessen the risk of brain damage associated with craniotomy for ICH.[50,53]

Nursing Management

Nursing management of the patient with stroke incorporates a variety of nursing diagnoses (Box 18-9).

Box 18-9

NURSING DIAGNOSIS PRIORITIES

Stroke

- Ineffective Cerebral Tissue Perfusion related to decreased cerebral blood flow, p. A-36
- Ineffective Cerebral Tissue Perfusion related to hemorrhage, p. A-36
- Unilateral Neglect related to perceptual disruption, p. A-48
- Impaired Verbal Communication related to cerebral speech center injury, p. A-32
- Impaired Swallowing related to neuromuscular impairment, fatigue, and limited awareness, p. A-31
- Disturbed Body Image related to actual change in body structure, function, or appearance, p. A-20
- Deficient Knowledge: Discharge Regimen related to lack of previous exposure to information (see Patient Education: Stroke), p. A-18

PATIENT EDUCATION

Stroke

- Pathophysiology of disease
- Specific etiology
- Risk factor modification
- Importance of taking medications
- Activities of daily living
- Measures to prevent injuries of impaired limbs
- Measures to compensate for residual deficits
- Basic rehabilitation techniques
- Importance of participating in neurologic rehabilitation program and/or support group

Nursing priorities are directed toward (1) monitoring the patient for changes in neurologic signs and symptoms, (2) maintaining surveillance for complications, and (3) providing comfort and emotional support, and (4) educating the patient and family.

Monitoring for Changes in Neurologic Signs and Symptoms

The goal of frequent monitoring of the patient's neurologic status is early recognition of deterioration or increased loss of function. Close monitoring of the patient's neurologic signs and vital signs is essential and requires almost continuous observation. Automatic noninvasive devices, such as a blood pressure cuff and a pulse oximeter, are helpful. Seizure activity must be identified and treated immediately. It is essential that all personnel working with the patient be aware of the desired hemodynamic and neurologic parameters set by the physician and that the physician be notified at the first sign of any changes.

Maintaining Surveillance for Complications

The patient with stroke should be monitored closely for signs of bleeding, vasospasm, and increased intracranial pressure. Other complications of stroke include aspiration, malnutrition, pneumonia, deep vein thrombosis, pulmonary embolism, decubitus ulcers, contractures, and joint abnormalities.[5] Nursing measures to prevent these complications are well known.

Additional complications that may be seen in the patient with stroke are related to the area of the brain that has been damaged. Damage to the temporoparietal area can create a variety of disturbances that affect the patient's ability to interpret sensory information. Damage to the dominant hemisphere (usually left) produces problems with speech and language and abstract and analytical skills. Damage to the nondominant hemisphere (usually right) produces problems with spatial relationships. The resulting deficits include agnosia, apraxia, and visual field defects. Perceptual deficits are not as readily noticeable as are motor deficits, but they may be more debilitating and can lead to the inability to perform skilled or purposeful tasks. In addition, the patient may develop impaired swallowing.[5]

Bleeding and Vasospasm. In the patient with a cerebral aneurysm, sudden onset of or an increase in headache, nausea and vomiting, increased BP, and changes in respiration herald the onset of rebleeding. The first indication of vasospasm is usually the appearance of new focal or global neurologic deficits. SAH precautions must be implemented to prevent any stress or straining that could potentially precipitate rebleeding. Precautions include BP control; bed rest; a dark, quiet environment; and stool softeners.[37] Short-acting analgesics and sedatives are used to relieve pain and anxiety. The patient must be kept calm. Limb restraints cause straining and must be avoided. If restraint is necessary, only a vest or jacket type of restraint is used. The head of the bed should be elevated to 35 to 45 degrees at all times. The patient is taught to avoid any activities that create the Valsalva maneuver, such as pushing with the legs to move up in bed, straining for a bowel movement, or holding his or her breath during procedures or discomfort. Deep vein thrombosis precautions are routinely implemented. Collaboration with the patient and family is used to establish a visitation plan to meet patient and family needs. Often, family members at the bedside can assist the patient with remaining calm.[5,16]

Increased Intracranial Pressure. Numerous signs and symptoms of increased ICP can be noted. A change in level of consciousness is the most sensitive indicator. Others include unequal pupil size; decreased pupillary response to light; headache; projectile vomiting; altered breathing patterns; Cushing's triad (bradycardia, systolic hypertension, and widening pulse pressure);

diminished brain stem reflexes; papilledema; and abnormal extension (decerebrate posturing) or flexion (decorticate posturing).[5,16]

Impaired Swallowing. Normal swallowing occurs in four phases that are controlled by the cranial nerves. Damage to the brain, brain stem, or cranial nerves can result in a variety of swallowing deficits that can place the patient at risk for aspiration. The stroke patient is observed for signs of dysphagia including drooling; difficulty handling oral secretions; absence of gag, cough, or swallowing reflexes; moist, gurgling voice quality; decreased mouth and tongue movements; and the presence of dysarthria. A speech therapy consult is initiated if any of these signs are present, and the patient must not be orally fed. In the absence of these warning signs, the patient may be fed, as ordered by the physician, though he or she must be continually monitored for signs of aspiration.[6,54]

Educating the Patient and Family

Rehabilitation starts in the critical care area, with a multidisciplinary team designing and implementing an individualized plan for maximizing the patient's potential for neurologic rehabilitation. Early in the patient's hospital stay, the patient and family must be taught about stroke, its etiologies, and its treatment. As the patient moves toward discharge, teaching focuses on the interventions necessary for preventing the reoccurrence of the event and on maximizing the patient's rehabilitation potential. The patient's family must be encouraged to participate in the patient's care; learn how to feed, dress, and bathe the patient; and learn some basic rehabilitation techniques. In addition, the importance of participating in a neurologic rehabilitation program and/or a support group must be stressed.

Collaborative management of the patient with a stroke is outlined in Box 18-10.

Box 18-10

Collaborative Management

Stroke

- Differentiate the cause of the stroke
  - Ischemic
  - Subarachnoid hemorrhage
  - Cerebral aneurysm
  - Arteriovenous malformation (AVM)
  - Intracerebral bleed
- Implement treatment according to cause of bleed
  - Ischemic
    - Thrombolytic therapy
    - Blood pressure control
  - Subarachnoid hemorrhage
    - Surgical aneurysm clipping or AVM excision
    - Embolization
  - Intracerebral bleed
    - Blood pressure control
- Protect patient's airway
- Provide ventilatory assistance as required
- Perform frequent neurologic assessments
- Maintain surveillance for complications
  - Cerebral edema
  - Cerebral ischemia/vasospasm
  - Rebleeding
  - Impaired swallowing
  - Neurologic deficits
- Provide comfort and emotional support
- Design and implement appropriate rehabilitation program
- Educate patient and family

GUILLAIN-BARRÉ SYNDROME

Description and Etiology

Guillain-Barré syndrome (GBS), once thought to be a single entity characterized by inflammatory peripheral neuropathy, is now understood to be a combination of clinical features with varying forms of presentation and multiple pathologic processes. A full discussion of the current understanding of this complex condition is beyond the scope of this text. Most cases of GBS do not require admission to a critical care unit. However, the prototype of GBS, known as *acute inflammatory demyelinating polyradiculoneuropathy (AIDP),* involves a rapidly progressive, ascending peripheral nerve dysfunction leading to paralysis that may produce respiratory failure. Because of the need for ventilatory support, AIDP is one of the few peripheral neurologic diseases that necessitates a critical care environment.[55] For the sake of this discussion, all references to GBS will pertain to the AIDP prototype.

The annual incidence of GBS is 1.8 per 100,000 persons.[55] It occurs more often in males and is the most commonly acquired demyelinating neuropathy.[56] Occasionally, clusters of cases are reported, such as occurred following the 1977 swine flu vaccinations.[57]

Etiology

The precise cause of GBS remains unknown, but the syndrome involves an immune-mediated response involving both cell-mediated immunity and development of IgG antibodies. Most patients report a viral infection 1 to 3 weeks before the onset of clinical manifestations, usually involving the upper respiratory tract.[55]

Numerous antecedent causes, or triggering events, have now been associated with GBS. These include viral infections (influenza; cytomegalovirus; hepatitis A, B, or C; Epstein-Barr virus; human immunodeficiency virus), bacterial infections (gastrointestinal *Campylobacter jejuni* and *Mycoplasma pneumoniae*), vaccines (rabies, tetanus, influenza), lymphoma, surgery, and trauma.[55,56]

Pathophysiology

This disease affects the motor and sensory pathways of the peripheral nervous system, as well as the autonomic nervous system functions of the cranial nerves. The major finding in GBS (AIDP type) is a segmental demyelination process of the peripheral nerves. GBS is believed to be an autoimmune response to antibodies formed in response to a recent physiologic event. T cells migrate to the peripheral nerves, resulting in edema and inflammation. Macrophages then invade the area and break down the myelin. Inflammation around this demyelinated area causes further dysfunction. Some axonal damage also occurs.[55,56]

The myelin sheath of the peripheral nerves is generated by Schwann's cells and acts as an insulator for the peripheral nerve. Myelin promotes rapid conduction of nerve impulses by allowing the impulses to jump along the nerve via nodes of Ranvier. Disruption of the myelin fiber slows and may eventually stop the conduction of impulses along the peripheral nerves. In GBS, the more thickly myelinated fibers of motor pathways and the cranial nerves are more severely affected than are the thinly myelinated sensory fibers of cutaneous pain, touch, and temperature.[6]

Once the temporary inflammatory reaction stops, myelin-producing cells begin the process of reinsulating the demyelinated portions of the peripheral nervous system. When remyelination occurs, normal neurologic function should return. In some instances the axon may be damaged during the inflammatory process. The degree of axonal damage is responsible for the degree of neurologic dysfunction that persists after recovery.[55]

Assessment and Diagnosis

Symptoms of GBS include motor weakness; paresthesias and other sensory changes; cranial nerve dysfunction (especially oculomotor, facial, glossopharyngeal, vagal, spinal accessory, and hypoglossal); and some autonomic dysfunction. The usual course of GBS begins with an abrupt onset of lower extremity weakness that progresses to flaccidity and ascends over a period of hours to days. Motor loss usually is symmetric, bilateral, and ascending. In the most severe cases, complete flaccidity of all peripheral nerves, including spinal and cranial nerves, occurs.[6]

The patient is admitted to the hospital when lower extremity weakness prevents mobility. Admission to the critical care unit is necessary when progression of the weakness threatens respiratory muscles. As the patient's weakness progresses, close observation is essential. Frequent assessment of the respiratory system, including ventilatory parameters such as inspiratory force and tidal volume, is necessary. The most common cause of death in patients with GBS is from respiratory arrest. As the disease progresses and respiratory effort weakens, intubation and mechanical ventilation are necessary. Continued, frequent assessment of neurologic deterioration is required until the patient reaches the peak of the disease and plateau occurs.[58]

The diagnosis of GBS is based on clinical findings plus CSF analysis and nerve conduction studies. The diagnostic finding is elevated CSF protein with normal cell count.[58] The increased protein count is usually present after the first week but does not occur in approximately 10% of all cases. Nerve conduction studies that test the velocity at which nerve impulses are conducted show significant reduction, as the demyelinating process of the disease suggests.

Medical Management

With no curative treatment available, the medical management of GBS is limited. The disease simply must run its course, which is characterized by ascending paralysis that advances over 1 to 3 weeks and then remains at a plateau for 2 to 4 weeks.[58] The plateau stage is followed by descending paralysis and return to normal or near-normal function. The main focus of medical management is the support of bodily functions and the prevention of complications.

Both plasmapheresis and intravenous immune globulin (IVIg) are used to treat GBS.[55,56,58] They have been shown to be equally effective.[59] Plasmapheresis involves the removal of venous blood via a catheter, separation of plasma from blood cells, and reinfusion of the cells plus autologous plasma or another replacement solution. Though the number of exchanges may vary, usually four to six exchanges are performed over 5 to 8 days.[55]

Nursing Management

The nursing management of the patient with GBS incorporates a variety of nursing diagnoses and interventions (Box 18-11). The goal of nursing management is to support all normal body functions until the patient can do so on his or her own. Although the condition is reversible, the patient with GBS requires extensive long-term care, because recovery can be a long process. **Nursing priorities are directed toward (1) maintaining surveillance for complications, (2) initiating rehabilitation, (3) facilitating nutritional support, (4) providing comfort and emotional support, and (5) educating the patient and family.**

Maintaining Surveillance for Complications

Continuous assessment of the progressive paralysis associated with GBS is essential to timely intervention and the prevention of respiratory arrest and further neurologic insult. Once the patient is intubated and placed on mechanical ventilation, close observation for pulmonary complications, such as atelectasis, pneumonia, and pneumothorax, is necessary. Autonomic dysfunction, dysautonomia, in the GBS patient can produce variations in heart rate and blood pressure that can reach extreme values.[60,61] Hypertension and tachycardia may require β-blocker therapy. All GBS patients must be observed for this phenomenon.

Initiating Rehabilitation

In patients with GBS, immobility may last for months. The usual course of GBS involves an average of 10 days of symptom progression and 10 days of maximal level of dysfunction, followed by 2 to 48 weeks of recovery. Although GBS is usually completely reversible, the patient will require physical and occupational rehabilitation because of the problems of long-term immobility. Rehabilitation starts in the critical care area, with a multidisciplinary team designing and implementing an individualized plan for maximizing the patient's potential for rehabilitation.

Facilitating Nutritional Support

Nutritional support is implemented early in the course of the disease. Because GBS recovery is a long process, adequate nutritional support will be a problem for an extended period. Nutritional support usually is accomplished through the use of enteral feeding.

Providing Comfort and Emotional Support

Pain control is another important component in the care of the patient with GBS. Although patients may have minimal to no motor function, most sensory functions remain, causing patients considerable muscle ache and pain. Because of the length of this illness, a safe, effective, long-term solution to pain management must be identified. These patients also require extensive psychologic support. Although the illness is almost 100% reversible, lack of control over the situation, constant pain or discomfort, and the long-term nature of the disorder create coping difficulties for the patient. GBS does not affect the level of consciousness or cerebral function. Patient interaction and communication are essential elements of the nursing management plan.

Educating the Patient and Family

Early in the patient's hospital stay, the patient and family must be taught about GBS and its different treatments. As the patient moves toward discharge, teaching focuses on the interventions to maximize the patient's rehabilitation potential. The patient's family must be encouraged to participate in the patient's care and to learn some basic rehabilitation techniques. In addition, the importance of participating in a neurologic rehabilitation program (if necessary) must be stressed.

Collaborative management of the patient with Guillain-Barre syndrome is outlined in Box 18-12.

Box 18-11

NURSING DIAGNOSIS PRIORITIES

Guillain-Barré Syndrome

- Ineffective Breathing Pattern related to musculoskeletal fatigue or neuromuscular impairment, p. A-34
- Acute Pain related to transmission and perception of cutaneous, visceral, muscular, or ischemic impulses, p. A-47
- Activity Intolerance related to prolonged immobility or deconditioning, p. A-2
- Imbalanced Nutrition: Less Than Body Requirements related to lack of exogenous nutrients or increased metabolic demand, p. A-28
- Powerlessness related to lack of control over current situation and/or disease progression, p. A-44
- Deficient Knowledge: Discharge Regimen related to lack of previous exposure to information (see Patient Education: Guillain-Barré Syndrome), p. A-18

PATIENT EDUCATION

Guillain-Barré Syndrome

- Pathophysiology of disease
- Importance of taking medications
- Measures to compensate for residual deficits
- Basic rehabilitation techniques
- Importance of participating in neurologic rehabilitation program (if necessary)

Box 18-12

Collaborative Management

Guillain-Barré Syndrome

- Support bodily functions
  - Protect airway
  - Provide ventilatory assistance as required
- Initiate treatments to limit duration of the syndrome
  - Plasmapheresis
  - Intravenous immunoglobulin
- Initiate nutritional support
- Maintain surveillance for complications
  - Infections
  - Cardiac dysrhythmias
  - Blood pressure alterations
  - Temperature alterations
- Provide comfort and emotional support
- Design and implement appropriate rehabilitation program
- Educate patient and family

CRANIOTOMY

TYPES OF SURGERY

A craniotomy is performed to gain access to portions of the CNS inside the cranium, usually to allow removal of a space-occupying lesion, such as a brain tumor (Table 18-5). Common procedures include tumor resection or removal, cerebral decompression, evacuation of hematoma or abscess, and clipping or removal of an aneurysm or arteriovenous malformation. Most patients who undergo craniotomy for tumor resection or removal do not require care in a critical care unit. Those patients who do usually need intensive monitoring or are at greater risk of complications because of underlying cardiopulmonary dysfunction or the surgical approach used. Box 18-13 provides definitions of common neurosurgical terms.[62] This section provides a generalized discussion of craniotomy care.

PREOPERATIVE CARE

Protection of the integrity of the CNS is a major priority of care for the patient awaiting a craniotomy. Optimal arterial oxygenation, hemodynamic stability, and cerebral perfusion are essential to maintaining adequate cerebral oxygenation. Management of seizure activity is essential to controlling metabolic needs.

Detailed assessment and documentation of the patient's preoperative neurologic status are imperative for accurate postoperative evaluation. Specific attention is placed on identifying and describing the nature and extent of any preoperative neurologic deficits. When pituitary surgery is planned, thorough evaluation of endocrine function is necessary to prevent major intraoperative and postoperative complications.[63]

Current trends in health care demand judicious use of routine preoperative studies. Depending on the type of surgery to be performed and the general health of the patient, preoperative screening may include a complete blood count (CBC), blood urea nitrogen (BUN), creatinine level, fasting blood sugar (FBS) level, chest x-ray examination, and electrocardiogram. A type and crossmatch for blood may also be ordered.[62]

Preoperative teaching is necessary to prepare both the patient and family for what to expect in the postoperative period. A description of the intravascular lines and intracranial catheters used during the postoperative period allows the family to focus on the patient, rather than be overwhelmed by masses of tubing. Some or all of the patient's hair is shaved off in the operating room, and a large, bulky, turbanlike craniotomy dressing is applied. Most patients experience some degree of postoperative eye or facial swelling and periorbital ecchymosis. An explanation of these temporary changes in appearance helps alleviate the shock and fear many patients and families experience in the immediate postoperative period.

All craniotomy patients require instruction to avoid activities known to produce sudden changes in intracranial pressure. These activities include bending, lifting, straining, and the Valsalva maneuver. Patients commonly elicit the Valsalva maneuver during repositioning in bed by holding their breath and straining with a closed epiglottis. Teaching the patient to continue to breathe deeply through the mouth during all position changes is an effective deterrent.

The patient undergoing transsphenoidal surgery requires preparation for the sensations associated with nasal packing. The patient often awakens with alarm because of the inability to breathe through the nose. Preoperative instruction in mouth breathing and avoidance of coughing, sneezing, or blowing of the nose facilitates postoperative cooperation.

The psychosocial issues associated with the prospect of neurosurgery cannot be overemphasized. Few procedures are as threatening as those involving the brain or spinal cord. For some patients the fear of permanent neurologic impairment may be as or more ominous than the fear of death. Steps to meet the needs of the patient, as well as the family, include collaboration with clergy and social services personnel, patient-controlled visitation, and provision of as much privacy as the patient's condition permits. Both the patient and the family must be provided with the opportunity to express their fears and concerns apart from each other as well as jointly.[62]

Box 18-13

Operative Terms

Burr hole: Hole made into the cranium using a special drill
Craniotomy: Surgical opening of the skull
Craniectomy: Removal of a portion of the skull without replacing it
Cranioplasty: Plastic repair of the skull
Supratentorial: Above the tentorium, separating the cerebrum from the cerebellum
Infratentorial: Below the tentorium; includes the brain stem and the cerebellum; an infratentorial surgical approach may be used for temporal or occipital lesions

SURGICAL CONSIDERATIONS

Whereas the emphasis in surgical approach for most other types of surgery is to gain adequate exposure of the surgical site, the neurosurgeon must select a route that also produces the least amount of disruption to the intracranial contents. Neural tissue is unforgiving. A significant portion of neurologic trauma and postoperative deficits is related to the surgical pathway through the brain tissue, rather than to the procedure performed at the site of the pathologic condition.

Table 18-5
Tumor Types and Characteristics

TUMOR	CLINICAL FEATURES	TREATMENT/PROGNOSIS
Glioblastoma multiforme (GM)	Often presents with nonspecific complaints and increased ICP As tumor grows, focal deficits develop	Rapidly progressive course, with poor prognosis Total surgical removal usually not possible; response to radiation poor
Astrocytoma	Presentation similar to GM, but course more protracted, often over several years; cerebellar astrocytoma, especially in children, may have more benign course	Variable prognosis By diagnosis, total excision usually impossible; tumor often not radiosensitive In cerebellar astrocytoma, total excision often possible
Medulloblastoma	Glioma most often seen in children Generally arises from roof of fourth ventricle and leads to increased ICP, with brain stem and cerebellar signs; may seed subarachnoid space	Treatment consists of surgery with radiation therapy and chemotherapy
Ependymoma	Glioma arising from ependyma of ventricle, especially fourth; leads early to signs of increased ICP; arises also from central canal of spinal cord	Tumor not radiosensitive and best treated surgically, if possible
Oligodendroglioma	Slow-growing glioma, usually arises in cerebral hemisphere in adults Calcification may be visible on radiograph	Treatment is surgical and usually successful
Brain stem glioma	Presents in childhood with cranial nerve palsies, then long-tract signs in limbs; signs of increased ICP occur late in course	Tumor is inoperable Treatment with irradiation and shunt for increased ICP
Cerebellar hemangioblastoma	Presents with disequilibrium, ataxia of trunk or limbs, and signs of increased ICP; at times familiar; may be associated with retinal and spinal lesions; polycythemia, and hypernephroma	Treatment is surgical
Pineal tumor	Presents with increased ICP, at times associated with impaired upward gaze (Parinaud's syndrome) and other deficits indicating midbrain lesion	Ventricular decompression by shunting, followed by surgical approach to tumor Irradiation if tumor malignant Prognosis depends on histopathologic findings and tumor extent
Craniopharyngioma	Originates from remnants of Rathke's pouch above sella turcica, depressing optic chiasm May present at any age but usually in childhood with endocrine dysfunction and bitemporal field deficits	Treatment is surgical, but total removal may not be possible
Acoustic neuroma	Most common initial symptom is ipsilateral hearing loss; subsequent symptoms may include tinnitus, headache, vertigo, facial weakness or numbness, and long-tract signs May be familial and bilateral when related to neurofibromatosis Most sensitive screening tests are MRI and brain-stem AEP	Treatment is by excision by translabyrinthine approach, craniectomy, or combination Prognosis usually good
Meningioma	Originates from dura mater or arachnoid; compresses rather than invades adjacent neural structures Increasingly common with advancing age Tumor size varies greatly; symptoms vary with tumor site* Tumor usually benign; readily detected by CT; may lead to calcification and bone erosion visible on plain skull radiographs	Treatment is surgical Tumor may recur if removal is incomplete; patient may receive radiation with incomplete excision to decrease risk of recurrence
Primary central lymphoma	Associated with AIDS and other immunodeficiency states Presentation may be with focal deficits or disturbances of cognition and consciousness; may be indistinguishable from cerebral toxoplasmosis	Treatment is by whole-brain irradiation Chemotherapy may have adjunctive role Prognosis depends on CD4 cell count at diagnosis

From Gawlinski A, Hamwi D, editors: *Acute care nurse practitioner: clinical curriculum and certification review,* Philadelphia, 1999, Saunders.

*For example, unilateral exophthalmos (sphenoidal ridge), anosmia and optic nerve compression (olfactory groove).

ICP, Intracranial pressure; *MRI,* magnetic resonance imaging; *AEP,* Auditory-evoked potential; *CT,* computed tomography; *AIDS,* acquired immunodeficiency syndrome.

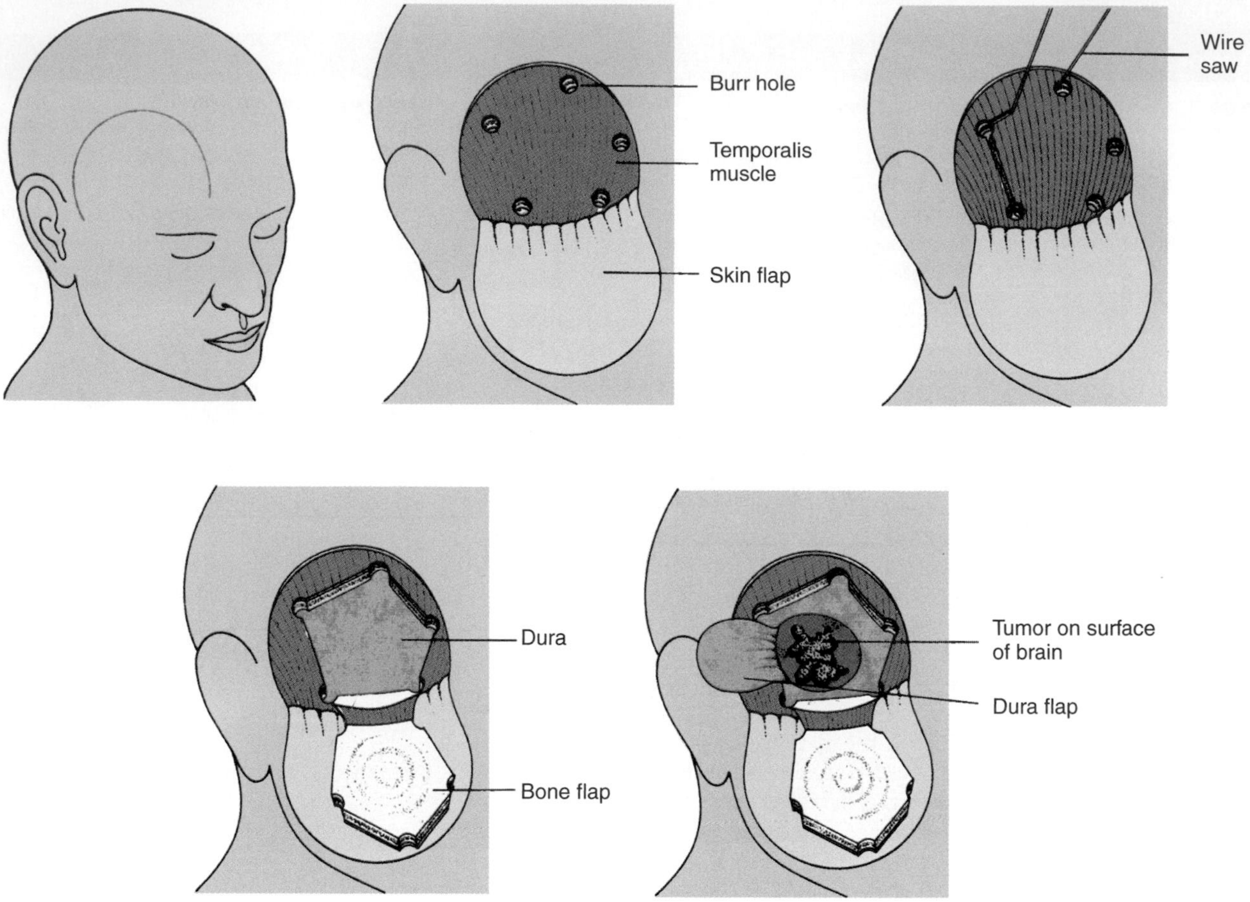

FIGURE 18-4. Craniotomy. (From Beare PG, Myers JL: *Principles and practice of adult health nursing,* ed 2, St Louis, 1994, Mosby.)

Depending on the location of the lesion and the surgical route decided on, either a transcranial or a transsphenoidal approach is used to open the skull.

Transcranial

In the transcranial approach, a scalp incision is made and a series of burr holes are drilled into the skull to form an outline of the area to be opened (Figure 18-4). A special saw is then used to cut between the holes. In most cases the bone flap is left attached to the muscle to create a hinge effect. In some cases the bone flap is removed completely and either placed in the abdomen for later retrieval and implantation or discarded and replaced with synthetic material. Next the dura is opened and retracted. After the intracranial procedure, the dura and the bone flap are closed, the muscles and scalp are sutured, and a turbanlike dressing is applied.[62]

Transsphenoidal

The transsphenoidal approach is the technique of choice for removal of a pituitary tumor without extension into the intracranial vault (Figure 18-5).[63] This approach involves making a microsurgical entrance into the cranial vault via the nasal cavity. The sphenoid sinus is entered to reach the anterior wall of the sella turcica. The sphenoid bone and the dura are then opened to gain intracranial access. After removal of the tumor, the surgical bed is packed with a small section of adipose tissue grafted from the patient's abdomen or thigh. After closure of the intranasal structures, nasal splints and soft packing or nasal tampons impregnated with antibiotic ointment are placed in the nasal cavities. Occasionally, epistaxis balloons are used instead. A nasal drip pad or mustache type of dressing is placed at the base of the nose to catch surgical drainage.[62]

The patient may be placed in a supine, prone, or even sitting position for a craniotomy procedure. A skull clamp connected to skull pins is used to position and secure the patient's head throughout the surgery. During a transsphenoidal approach or a transcranial approach into the infratentorial area, the patient's head is elevated during the surgery. This position places the patient at risk for an air embolism. Air can enter the vascular system either through the edges of the dura or a venous opening. Continuous monitoring of the patient's heart sounds by Doppler signal allows immediate recognition of this complication. If it occurs, an attempt may be made to withdraw the

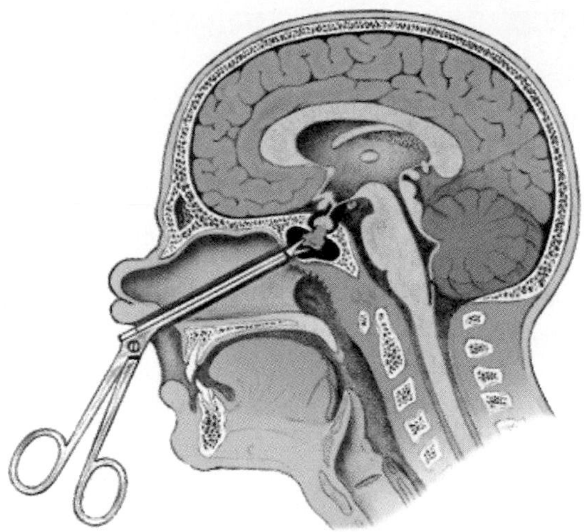

FIGURE 18-5. Transsphenoidal hypophysectomy.

embolus from the right atrium through a central line. Flooding the surgical field with irrigation fluid and placing a moistened sterile surgical sponge over the surgical site creates an immediate barrier to any further air entrance.[62]

Postoperative Medical Management

Definitive management of the postoperative neurosurgical patient will vary depending on the underlying reason for the craniotomy. During the initial postoperative period, management is usually directed toward the prevention of complications. Complications associated with a craniotomy include intracranial hypertension, surgical hemorrhage, fluid imbalance, CSF leak, and deep vein thrombosis.

Intracranial Hypertension

Postoperative cerebral edema is expected to peak 48 to 72 hours after surgery. If the bone flap is not replaced at the time of surgery, intracranial hypertension will produce bulging at the surgical site. Close monitoring of the surgical site is important so that integrity of the incision can be maintained. Postcraniotomy management of intracranial hypertension is usually accomplished through CSF drainage, patient positioning, and steroid administration.[5]

Surgical Hemorrhage

Surgical hemorrhage after a transcranial procedure can occur in the intracranial vault and is manifested by signs and symptoms of increasing ICP. Hemorrhage after a transsphenoidal craniotomy may be evident from external drainage, patient complaint of persistent postnasal drip, or excessive swallowing. Loss of vision after pituitary surgery is also indicative of evolving hemorrhage. Postoperative hemorrhage requires surgical reexploration.[63]

Fluid Imbalance

Fluid imbalance in the postcraniotomy patient usually results from a disturbance in production or secretion of antidiuretic hormone (ADH). ADH is secreted by the posterior pituitary (neurohypophysis) gland. It stimulates the renal tubules and collecting ducts to retain water in response to low circulating blood volume or increased serum osmolality. Intraoperative trauma or postoperative edema of the pituitary gland or hypothalamus can result in insufficient ADH secretion. The outcome is unabated renal water loss even when blood volume is low and serum osmolality is high. This condition is known as *diabetes insipidus (DI)*. The polyuria associated with DI is often greater than 200 ml/hr. Urine specific gravity of 1.005 or less and elevated serum osmolality provide evidence of insufficient ADH. The loss of volume may produce hypotension and inadequate cerebral perfusion. DI is usually self-limiting, with fluid replacement being the only necessary therapy. In some cases, however, it may be necessary to administer vasopressin intravenously to control the loss of fluid.[5]

The syndrome of inappropriate antidiuretic hormone (SIADH) commonly occurs with neurologic insult and results from excessive ADH secretion. SIADH is manifested by inappropriate water retention with hyponatremia in the presence of normal renal function. Urine specific gravity is elevated, and urine osmolality is greater than serum osmolality. The dangers associated with SIADH include circulating volume overload and electrolyte imbalance, both of which may impair neurologic functioning. SIADH is usually self-limiting, with the mainstay of treatment being fluid restriction.[5]

CSF Leak

Leakage of CSF fluid results from an opening in the subarachnoid space, as evidenced by clear fluid draining from the surgical site. When this complication occurs after transsphenoidal surgery, it is evidenced by excessive, clear drainage from the nose or persistent postnasal drip. To differentiate CSF drainage from postoperative serous drainage, a specimen is tested for glucose content. A CSF leak is confirmed by glucose values of 30 mg/dl or greater. Management of the patient with a CSF leak includes bed rest and head elevation. Lumbar puncture or placement of a lumbar subarachnoid catheter may be used to reduce CSF pressure until the dura heals. The risk of meningitis associated with CSF leak necessitates surgical repair to reseal the opening if necessary.[5,63]

Deep Vein Thrombosis

Deep vein thrombosis (DVT) has been reported to occur in 29% to 46% of all neurosurgical patients, as compared with a 25% incidence in general surgical patients. Early research demonstrated a greater risk after removal of a supratentorial tumor and a twofold

Box 18-14

NURSING DIAGNOSIS PRIORITIES

Craniotomy

- Decreased Intracranial Adaptive Capacity related to failure of normal intracranial compensatory mechanisms, p. 15
- Ineffective Cerebral Tissue Perfusion related to decreased blood flow, p. A-36
- Ineffective Cerebral Tissue Perfusion related to hemorrhage, p. A-38
- Acute Pain related to transmission and perception of cutaneous, visceral, muscular, or ischemic impulses, p. A-7
- Disturbed Body Image related to actual change in body structure, function, or appearance, p. A-20
- Deficient Knowledge: Discharge Regimen related to lack of previous exposure to information (see Patient Education: Craniotomy), p. A-18

risk in patients whose surgery lasted for more than 4 hours.[64] Recent research has demonstrated numerous additional risk factors significantly associated with DVT development: preoperative leg weakness, longer preoperative intensive care unit (ICU) stay, longer recovery room time, longer postoperative ICU stay, more days on bed rest, and delay of postoperative mobility and activity.[65] Clinical manifestations of DVT include leg or calf pain, edema, localized tenderness, and pain with dorsiflexion or plantar flexion (Homans' sign). Unfortunately the patient with a DVT is often asymptomatic, and the diagnosis is not made until the patient experiences a pulmonary embolus.

The primary treatment for DVT is prophylaxis. In the neurosurgery patient sequential (intermittent) pneumatic compression boots or stockings have been demonstrated to be effective in reducing the incidence of DVT. Effectiveness is enhanced when these devices are initiated in the preoperative period. Low-dose unfractionated heparin or low-molecular-weight heparin may also be used prophylactically in high-risk patients.[44]

POSTOPERATIVE NURSING MANAGEMENT

The nursing management of the neurosurgical patient incorporates a variety of nursing diagnoses (Box 18-14). As in preoperative care, the primary goal of postcraniotomy nursing management is protection of the integrity of the CNS. **Nursing priorities are directed toward (1) preserving adequate cerebral perfusion pressure, (2) promoting arterial oxygenation, (3) providing comfort and emotional support, (4) maintaining surveillance for complications, (5) initiating early rehabilitation, and (6) educating the patient and family.** Frequent neurologic assessment is necessary to evaluate accomplishment of these objectives and to identify and quickly intervene if complications do arise. Often a ventriculostomy is placed to facilitate ICP monitoring and/or CSF drainage.

PATIENT EDUCATION

Craniotomy

Before Surgery

- Pathophysiology and expected outcome of underlying disease
- Need for intensive care management after surgery
- Routine postoperative surgical care

After Surgery

- Routine postoperative surgical care
- Discharge medications—purpose, dose, and side effects
- Incisional care
- Signs and symptoms of infection
- Signs and symptoms of increased intracranial pressure
- Measures to compensate for residual deficits
- Basic rehabilitation techniques
- Importance of participating in neurologic rehabilitation program

Preserving Adequate Cerebral Perfusion

Nursing interventions to preserve cerebral perfusion include patient positioning, fluid management, and avoidance of postoperative vomiting and fever.

Positioning. Patient positioning is an important component of care for the craniotomy patient. The head of the bed should be elevated 30 to 45 degrees at all times to reduce the incidence of hemorrhage, facilitate venous drainage, and control ICP. Other positioning measures to control ICP include maintaining the patient's head in a neutral position at all times and avoiding neck or hip flexion. It is vital to adhere to these rules of positioning throughout all nursing activities, including linen changes and transporting the patient for diagnostic evaluation. Most craniotomy patients can still be turned from side to side within these restrictions, using pillows for support, except in some cases of extensive tumor removal, cranioplasty, and when the bone flap is not replaced. Specific orders from the surgeon must be obtained in these instances. The patient with an infratentorial incision may be restricted to only a very small pillow under the head to prevent strain on the incision. Avoidance of anterior or lateral neck flexion also protects the integrity of this type of incision.

Fluid Management. Fluid management is another important component of postcraniotomy care. Hourly monitoring of fluid intake and output facilitates early identification of fluid imbalance. Urine specific gravity must be measured if DI is suspected. Fluid restriction may be ordered as a routine measure to lessen the severity of cerebral edema or as treatment for the fluid and electrolyte imbalances associated with SIADH.

Vomiting and Fever. Postoperative vomiting must be avoided to prevent sharp spikes in ICP and possibly surgical hemorrhage. Antiemetics are administered as soon as nausea is apparent. Early nutrition in the neurosurgical patient is beneficial. If the patient is unable to eat, enteral hyperalimentation via feeding tube is the preferred method of nutritional support and can be initiated as early as 24 hours after surgery.[62] Postoperative fever may also adversely affect ICP and increase the metabolic needs of the brain. Acetaminophen is administered orally, rectally, or via a feeding tube. External cooling measures, such as a hypothermia blanket, may also be necessary.

Promoting Arterial Oxygenation

Routine pulmonary care is used to maintain airway clearance and prevent pulmonary complications. To prevent dangerous elevations in ICP, this care must be performed using proper technique and at time intervals that are adequately spaced from other patient care activities. If pulmonary complications do arise, consideration must be given to maintaining adequate oxygenation during repositioning. It may be necessary to restrict turning to only the side that places the good lung down.

Providing Comfort and Emotional Support

Pain management in the postcraniotomy patient primarily involves control of headache. Small doses of intravenous morphine are used in the intensive care setting. As soon as oral analgesics can be tolerated, acetaminophen with codeine is used. Both of these analgesics cause constipation. Administration of stool softeners and initiation of a bowel program are important components of postcraniotomy care. Constipation is hazardous, because straining to have a bowel movement can create significant elevations in blood pressure and ICP.

Maintaining Surveillance for Complications

The postoperative neurosurgical patient is at risk for infection, corneal abrasions, and injury from falls or seizures.

Infection. Care of the incision and surgical dressings is institution- and physician-specific. The rule of thumb for a craniotomy dressing is to reinforce it as needed and change it only with a physician's order. Often a drain is left in place to facilitate decompression of the surgical site. If a ventriculostomy is present, it is treated as a component of the surgical site. All drainage devices must be secured to the dressing to prevent unintentional displacement with patient movement. Sterile technique is required to prevent infection and resultant meningitis.

Corneal Abrasions. Routine eye care may be necessary to prevent corneal drying and ulceration. Periorbital edema interferes with normal blinking and eyelid closure, which are essential to adequate corneal lubrication. Saline drops are instilled every 2 hours. If the patient remains in a coma state, covering the eyes with a polyethylene film extending over the orbits and eyebrows may be beneficial.[12]

Injury. The postcraniotomy patient may also experience periods of altered mentation. Protection from injury may require use of restraint devices. The side rails of the bed must also be padded to protect the patient from injury. Having a family member stay at the bedside and/or use of music therapy is often helpful to keep the patient calm during periods of restlessness. In rare circumstances, neuromuscular blockade and sedation may be necessary to control patient activity and metabolic needs on a short-term basis.

Initiating Early Rehabilitation

Increased patient activity, including ambulation, is begun as soon as tolerated in the postoperative period. Rehabilitation measures and discharge planning may begin in the critical care unit but are beyond the scope of this text. Transfer to a general care or rehabilitation unit is usually accomplished as soon as the patient is considered to be stable and without complication.

Educating the Patient and Family

Preoperatively the patient and family should be taught about the precipitating event necessitating the need for the craniotomy and its expected outcome. The severity of the disease and the need for intensive care management postoperatively must be stressed. As the patient moves toward discharge, teaching focuses on medication instructions, incisional care, including the signs of infection, and the signs and symptoms of increased intracranial pressure. If the patient has neurologic deficits, teaching focuses on the interventions to maximize the patient's rehabilitation potential and the patient's family must be encouraged to participate in the patient's care and to learn some basic rehabilitation techniques. In addition, the importance of participating in a neurologic rehabilitation program must be stressed.

INTRACRANIAL HYPERTENSION

PATHOPHYSIOLOGY

The intracranial space comprises three components: brain substance (80%), CSF (10%), and blood (10%). Under normal physiologic conditions, the ICP is maintained below 15 mm Hg mean pressure.[8] Essential to understanding the pathophysiology of ICP, the Monro-Kellie hypothesis proposes that an increase in volume of one intracranial component must be compensated by a decrease in one or more of the other components so that total volume remains fixed. This compensation, although limited, includes displacing CSF from

Table 18-6
Mechanisms of Intracranial Pressure Elevation

PATHOPHYSIOLOGY	EXAMPLE	TREATMENT
Disorders of CSF Space		
Overproduction of CSF	Choroid plexus papilloma	Diuretics, surgical removal
Communicating hydrocephalus from obstructed arachnoid	Old subarachnoid hemorrhage	Surgical drainage from lumbar drain
Noncommunicative hydrocephalus	Posterior fossa tumor obstructing aqueduct	Surgical drainage by ventricular drain
Interstitial edema	Any of above	Surgical drainage of CSF
Disorders of Intracranial Blood		
Intracranial hemorrhage causing increased ICP	Epidural hematoma	Surgical drainage
Vasospasm	Subarachnoid hemorrhage	Hypervolemia and hypertensive therapy
Vasodilation	Elevated $Paco_2$	Hyperventilation
Increasing cerebral blood volume and ICP	Hypoxia	Adequate oxygenation
Disorders of Brain Substance		
Expanding mass lesion with local vasogenic edema causing increased ICP	Brain tumor	Steroids Surgical removal
Ischemic brain injury with cytotoxic edema increasing ICP	Anoxic brain injury from cardiac or respiratory arrest	Resistant to therapy
Increased cerebral metabolic rate increasing cerebral blood flow and ICP	Seizures, hyperthermia	Anticonvulsant medications to control fever

CSF, Cerebrospinal fluid; *ICP,* intracranial pressure.

the intracranial vault to the lumbar cistern, increasing CSF absorption, and compressing the low-pressure venous system.[66] Pathophysiologic alterations that can elevate ICP are outlined in Table 18-6.

Volume-Pressure Curve

When capable of compliance, the brain can tolerate significant increases in intracranial volume without much increase in ICP. The amount of intracranial compliance, however, does have a limit. Once this limit has been reached, a state of decompensation with increased ICP results. As the ICP rises, the relationship between volume and pressure changes, and small increases in volume may cause major elevations in ICP (Figure 18-6).[67] The exact configuration of the volume-pressure curve and the point at which the steep rise in pressure occurs vary among patients. The configuration of this curve also is influenced by the cause and the rate of volume increases within the intracranial vault; for example, neurologic deterioration occurs more rapidly in a patient with an acute epidural hematoma than in a patient with a meningioma of the same size.[5] Regardless of how fast the pressure increases, intracranial hypertension occurs when ICP is greater than 20 mm Hg.[67]

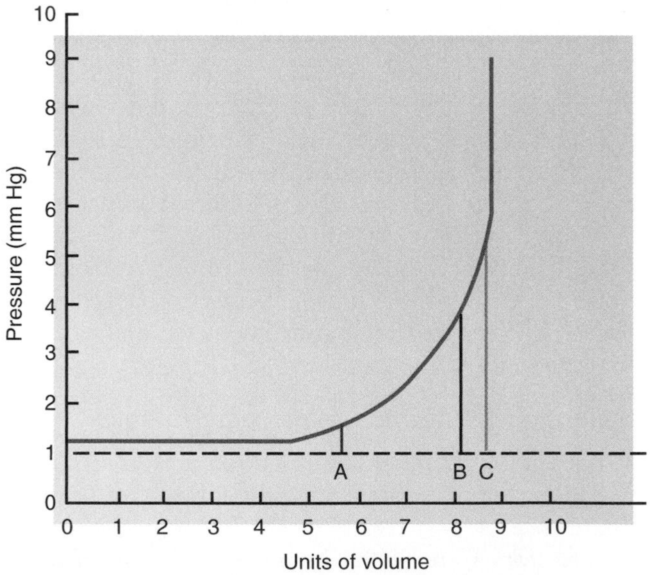

FIGURE 18-6. Intracranial volume-pressure curve. *A,* Pressure is normal, and increases in intracranial volume are tolerated without increases in intracranial pressure. *B,* Increases in volume may cause increases in pressure. *C,* Small increases in volume may cause larger increases in pressure.

Cerebral Blood Flow and Autoregulation

Cerebral blood flow (CBF) corresponds to the metabolic demands of the brain and is normally 50 ml per 100 g of brain tissue per minute. Although the brain makes up only 2% of body weight, it requires 15% to 20% of the resting cardiac output and 15% of the body's oxygen demands. The normal brain has a complex capacity to maintain constant CBF, despite wide ranges in systemic arterial pressure—an effect known as *autoregulation.* Mean arterial pressure (MAP) of 50 to 150 mm Hg does not alter CBF when autoregulation is present. Outside the limits of this autoregulation,

CBF becomes passively dependent on the perfusion pressure.[68]

Factors other than arterial blood pressure that affect CBF are conditions that result in acidosis, alkalosis, and changes in metabolic rate. Conditions that cause acidosis (e.g., hypoxia, hypercapnia, and ischemia) result in cerebrovascular dilation. Conditions causing alkalosis (e.g., hypocapnia) result in cerebrovascular constriction. Normally, a reduction in metabolic rate (e.g., from hypothermia or barbiturates) decreases CBF, and increases in metabolic rate (e.g., from hyperthermia) increase CBF.[68,69]

Arterial blood gases exert a profound effect on CBF. Carbon dioxide, which affects the pH of the blood, is a potent vasoactive substance. Carbon dioxide retention (hypercapnia) leads to cerebral vasodilation, with increased cerebral blood volume, whereas hypocapnia leads to cerebral vasoconstriction and a reduction in cerebral blood volume. Prolonged hypocapnia, however, especially at an arterial partial pressure of carbon dioxide ($Paco_2$) level less than 20 mm Hg, can produce cerebral ischemia. Low arterial partial pressure of oxygen (Pao_2) levels, especially below 40 mm Hg, lead to cerebral vasodilation, which increases the intracranial blood volume and can contribute to increased ICP. High Pao_2 levels have not been shown to affect CBF in either direction.[68,69]

Metabolic activity in the brain significantly influences CBF. Normally, when cerebral metabolic activity increases, CBF also increases to meet the demand. Any pathologic process that decreases CBF could lead to a mismatch between metabolic demand and blood supply, resulting in cerebral ischemia.[68]

ASSESSMENT AND DIAGNOSIS

The numerous signs and symptoms of increased ICP include decreased level of consciousness; Cushing's triad (bradycardia, systolic hypertension, and widening pulse pressure); diminished brain stem reflexes; papilledema; decerebrate posturing (abnormal extension); decorticate posturing (abnormal flexion); unequal pupil size; projectile vomiting; decreased pupillary reaction to light; altered breathing patterns; and headache.[70] Patients may exhibit one or all of these symptoms, depending on the underlying cause of the elevation in ICP. One of the earliest and most important signs of increased ICP is a decrease in level of consciousness. This change must be reported immediately to the physician.[67]

In the patient with suspected intracranial hypertension, a monitoring device may be placed within the cranium to quantify ICP. Under normal physiologic conditions, ICP is maintained below 15 mm Hg mean pressure. The device is used to monitor serial intracranial pressures and assist with the management of intracranial hypertension. An increase in intracranial pressure can cause a decrease in blood flow to the brain, causing brain damage. The monitor can also provide a sterile access for draining excess CSF. The four sites for monitoring ICP are the intraventricular space, the subarachnoid space, the epidural space, and the parenchyma. Each site has advantages and disadvantages for monitoring ICP. The type of monitor chosen depends on both the suspected pathologic condition and physician's preferences.[67,71] See Chapter 17 for further discussion of ICP monitoring.

MEDICAL AND NURSING MANAGEMENT

Once intracranial hypertension is documented, therapy must be prompt to prevent secondary insults. Although the exact pressure level denoting intracranial hypertension remains uncertain, most current evidence suggests that ICP generally must be treated when it exceeds 20 mm Hg.[68] All therapies are directed toward reducing the volume of one or more of the components (blood, brain, CSF) that lie within the intracranial vault. A major goal of therapy is to determine the cause of the elevated pressure and, if possible, to remove the cause.[68] In the absence of a surgically treatable mass lesion, intracranial hypertension is treated medically. Nurses play an important role in rapid assessment and implementation of appropriate therapies for reducing ICP.

Positioning and Other Nursing Activities

Positioning of the patient is a significant factor in the prevention and treatment of intracranial hypertension. Head elevation has long been advocated as a conventional nursing intervention to control ICP, presumably by increasing venous return. One recent study found that elevation of the bed at least 30 degrees did result in improvement in both ICP and CPP.[72] Other studies have suggested that while elevating the head of the bed does decrease ICP it can also decrease MAP and thus have an overall negative effect on CPP. Therefore the recent trend is to individualize the head position to maximize CPP and minimize ICP measurements.[73]

Positions that impede venous return from the brain cause elevations in ICP. Obstruction of jugular veins or an increase in intrathoracic or intraabdominal pressure is communicated as increased pressure throughout the open venous system, thereby impeding drainage from the brain and increasing ICP. Positions that decrease venous return from the head (e.g., Trendelenburg, prone, extreme flexion of the hips, angulation of the neck) must be avoided if possible. If changes to positions such as Trendelenburg are necessary to provide adequate pulmonary care, critical care nurses must closely monitor ICP and vital signs.[5,14]

Some routine nursing activities do affect ICP and can be harmful. Use of positive end-expiratory pressure

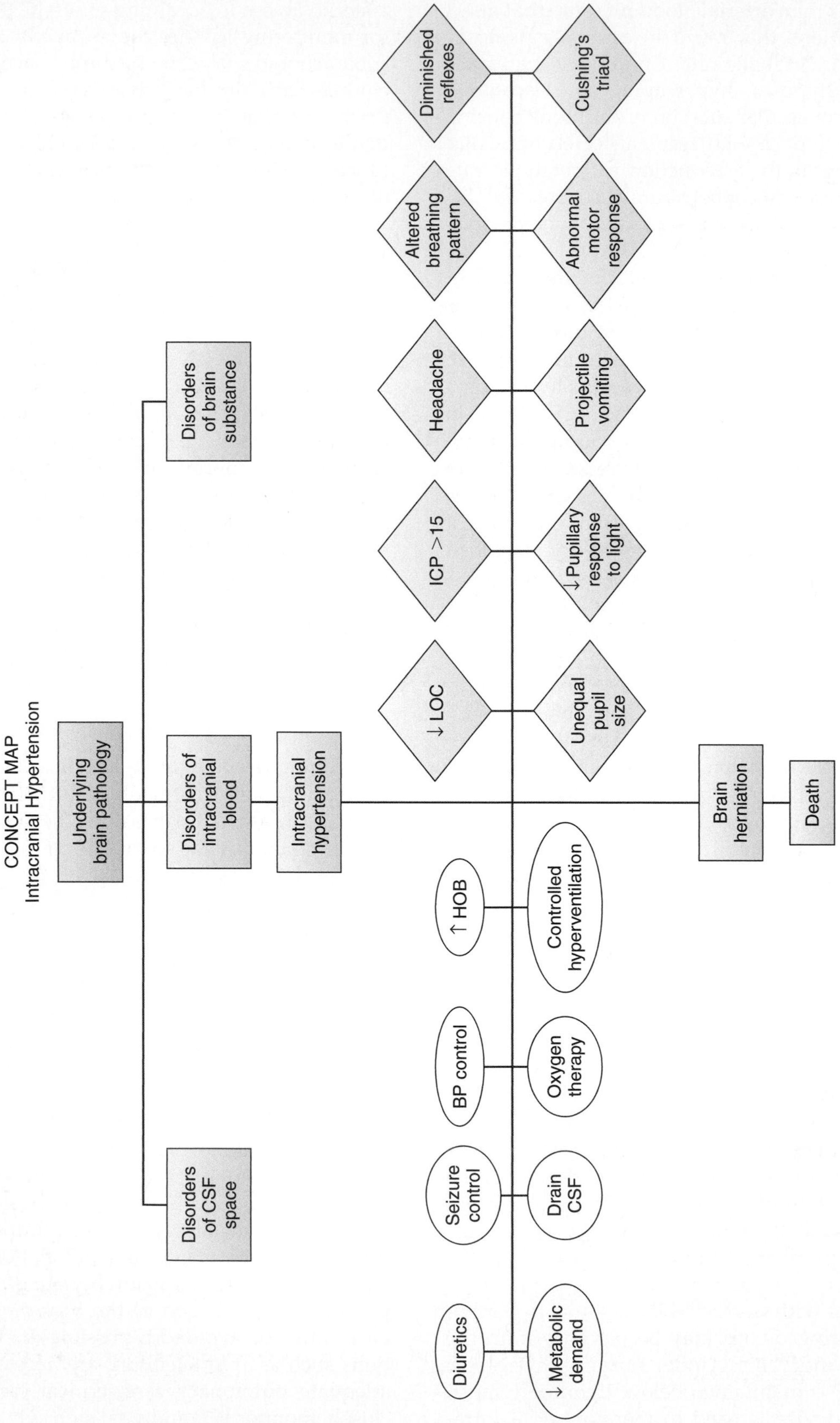
CONCEPT MAP
Intracranial Hypertension
Underlying brain pathology
Disorders of CSF space
Disorders of intracranial blood
Disorders of brain substance
Intracranial hypertension
↓ LOC
ICP >15
Headache
Altered breathing pattern
Diminished reflexes
Unequal pupil size
↓ Pupillary response to light
Projectile vomiting
Abnormal motor response
Cushing's triad
Diuretics
Seizure control
BP control
↑ HOB
↓ Metabolic demand
Drain CSF
Oxygen therapy
Controlled hyperventilation
Brain herniation
Death

(PEEP) greater than 20 cm H_2O pressure, coughing, suctioning, tight tracheostomy tube ties, and the Valsalva maneuver have been associated with ICP increases. Cumulative increases in ICP have been reported when care activities are performed one after another. Conversely, family contact and gentle touch have been associated with decreases in ICP.[5,73,74]

Hyperventilation

Controlled hyperventilation has been an important adjunct of therapy for the patient with increased ICP. The rationale employed in hyperventilation is that if the $Paco_2$ can be reduced from its normal level of 35 to 40 mm Hg to a range of 25 to 30 mm Hg in the patient with intracranial hypertension, vasoconstriction of cerebral arteries, reduction of cerebral blood flow, and increased venous return will result. This practice is currently being reexamined. More and more research has indicated that severe or prolonged hyperventilation can actually reduce cerebral perfusion and lead to cerebral ischemia and infarction. Rather, the trend now is to maintain $Paco_2$ levels on the lower side of normal (35 ± 2 mm Hg) by carefully monitoring arterial blood gas measurements and by adjusting ventilator settings.[66,75,76]

Although hypoxemia must obviously be avoided, excessively high levels of oxygen offer no benefits. In fact, increasing inspired oxygen concentrations above 60% may lead to toxic changes in lung tissue. The use of pulse oximetry has led to greater awareness of the circumstances, such as pain and anxiety, which can cause oxygen desaturation and therefore elevate ICP.[16,77]

Temperature Control

Directly proportional to body temperature, cerebral metabolic rate increases 7% per degree centigrade of increase in body temperature.[76] This fact is significant because as the cerebral metabolic rate increases, blood flow to the brain must increase to meet the tissue demands. To avoid the increase in blood volume associated with an increased cerebral metabolic rate, nurses must prevent hyperthermia in the patient with a brain injury. Antipyretics and cooling devices must be used when appropriate while the source of the fever is being determined.[14,76,77]

Conversely, hypothermia reduces cerebral metabolic rate. Research done in patients with severe head injury who were unresponsive to barbiturate therapy for control of intractable intracranial hypertension demonstrated a significant decrease in ICP when subjected to mild hypothermia between 32° C and 35° C.[76]

Blood Pressure Control

Maintenance of arterial blood pressure in the high normal range is essential in the brain-injured patient. Inadequate perfusion pressure decreases the supply of

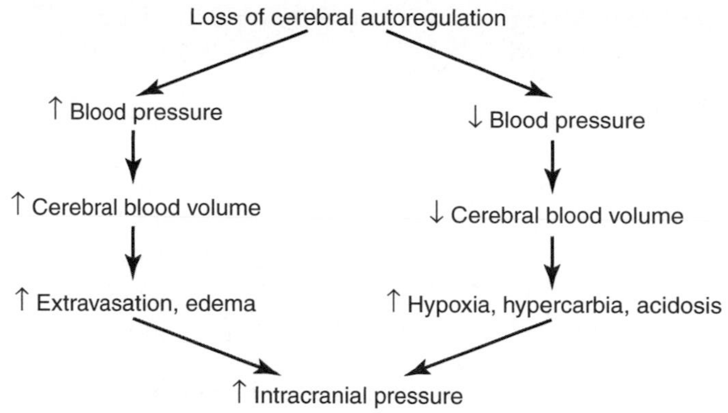

FIGURE 18-7. Loss of pressure autoregulation.

nutrients and oxygen requirements for cerebral metabolic needs. On the other hand, a blood pressure too high increases cerebral blood volume and may increase ICP (Figure 18-7).[14,76]

Control of systemic hypertension may require nothing more than the administration of a sedative agent. Small, frequent doses may be sufficient to blunt noxious stimuli and prevent them from triggering rises in blood pressure. When sedation proves inadequate in controlling systemic arterial hypertension, antihypertensive agents are used. Care must be taken in choosing these agents because many of the peripheral vasodilators (e.g., nitroprusside and nitroglycerin) also are cerebral vasodilators. However, all antihypertensives are believed to cause some degree of cerebral vasodilation. To reduce this vasodilating effect, cotreatment with β-blockers (e.g., metoprolol and labetalol) may be beneficial.[5]

Systemic hypotension should be treated aggressively with fluids to maintain a systolic blood pressure greater than 90 mm Hg.[5] Crystalloids, colloids, and blood products can be used depending on the patient's condition.[74] Recent studies have demonstrated a positive effect on ICP and CPP with hypertonic saline.[78] If fluids fail to adequately elevate the patient's blood pressure, than inotrope agents may be necessary.[76]

Seizure Control

The incidence of posttraumatic seizures in the head-injured population has been estimated at 5%. Because of the risk of a secondary ischemic insult associated with seizures, many physicians prescribe anticonvulsant medications prophylactically. Seizures cause metabolic requirements to increase, which results in elevation of cerebral blood flow, cerebral blood volume, and ICP, even in paralyzed patients. If blood flow cannot match demand, ischemia develops, cerebral energy stores are depleted, and irreversible neuronal destruction occurs. The usual anticonvulsant regimen for seizure control includes phenytoin or phenobarbital, or both, in therapeutic doses.[77] Fast-acting, short-duration agents such as lorazepam may be indicated for breakthrough seizures until therapeutic drug levels can be achieved.

Lidocaine

Various forms of sensory stimulation (e.g., tracheal intubation and endotracheal suctioning) may provoke marked increases in ICP and MAP. One therapy used to prevent cerebral ischemia and acute intracranial hypertension has been the administration of lidocaine through an endotracheal tube or through intravenous infusion before nasotracheal suctioning.[79] Lidocaine is believed to be effective in blunting ICP spikes secondary to tracheal stimulation. Studies have found that peak lidocaine concentrations are linearly related to the administered dose and that the rate of absorption depends on the vascularity of the site of administration.[79] It also has been documented that lidocaine is initially distributed to the lungs, then to the heart and kidneys, and then to muscle and adipose tissue.

Prophylactic administration of lidocaine before endotracheal suctioning is widely practiced. Lidocaine protects the patient from the associated increases in ICP that occur with suctioning. To prevent hypoxemia, suctioning should be limited to only if necessary. Suctioning should be preceded with hyperventilation using 100% oxygen, followed by a 10-second pass and limited to no more than two passes.[80]

Cerebrospinal Fluid Drainage

Cerebrospinal fluid drainage for intracranial hypertension may be used with other treatment modalities. CSF drainage is accomplished by the insertion of a pliable catheter into the anterior horn of the lateral ventricle (ventriculostomy), preferably on the nondominant side. Such drainage can help support the patient through periods of cerebral edema by controlling spikes in ICP. One of the major advantages of the ventriculostomy is its dual role as both a monitoring device and a treatment modality. Because CSF provides a favorable medium for the development of infection, flawless aseptic technique must be followed during insertion and maintenance of the system. The ventricular system is connected to a drainage bag and is then maintained as a closed system for the period the ventriculostomy remains in place—usually 3 to 5 days (Figures 18-8 and 18-9).[81]

Diuretics

Osmotic Agents. Clinicians have known for decades that osmotic agents effectively reduce ICP. The mechanism by which these diuretics reduce ICP continues to be a subject of investigational interest. One theory is that these agents act by remaining relatively impermeable to the blood-brain barrier, thereby drawing water from normal brain tissue to plasma. The direction of flow is from the hypoconcentrated tissue to the

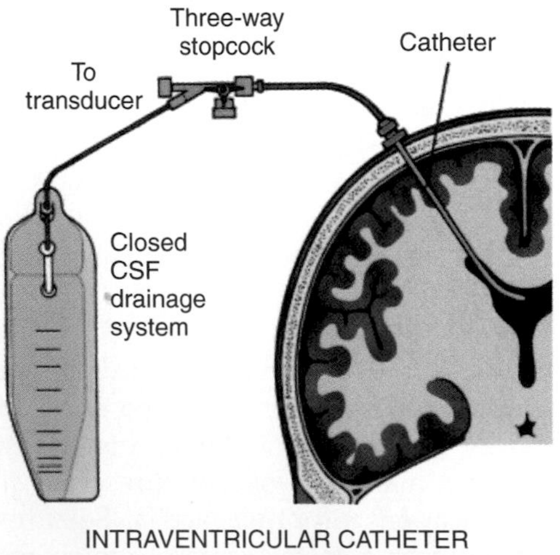

FIGURE 18-8. Intermittent drainage system. Intermittent drainage involves draining cerebrospinal fluid (CSF) via a ventriculostomy when intracranial pressure (ICP) exceeds the upper pressure parameter set by the physician. Intermittent drainage involves opening the three-way stopcock to allow CSF to flow into the drainage bag for brief periods (30 to 120 seconds) until the pressure is below the upper pressure parameter. (From Barker E: *Neuroscience nursing,* ed 2, St Louis, 2002, Mosby.)

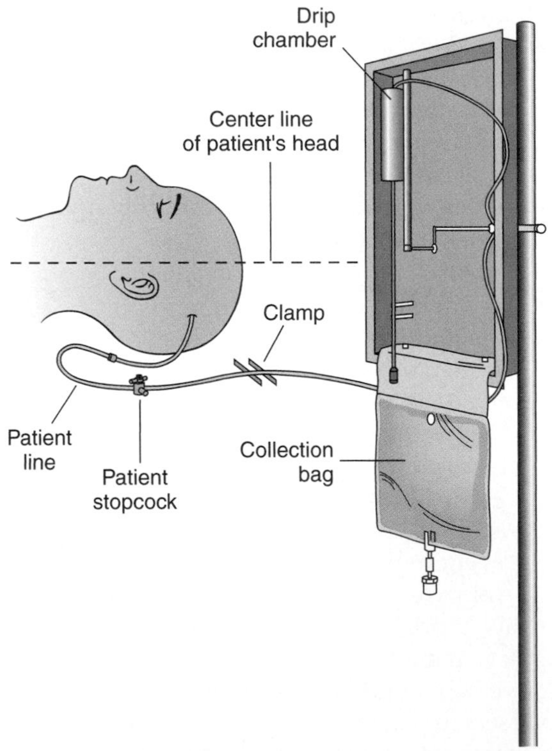

FIGURE 18-9. Continuous drainage system. Continuous drainage involves placing the drip chamber of the drainage system at a specified level above the foramen of Monro (usually 15 cm). The system is left open to allow continuous drainage of cerebrospinal fluid (CSF) into the chamber (which drains into a collection bag) against a pressure gradient that prevents excessive drainage and ventricular collapse. (Courtesy Codman/Johnson & Johnson Professional Inc, Raynham, Mass.)

hyperconcentrated cerebral vasculature. If the situation becomes reversed and the tissue becomes hyperconcentrated in relation to the cerebral vasculature, a rebound phenomenon could occur. These agents have little direct effect on edematous cerebral tissue situated in an area of defective blood-brain barrier; instead, they require an intact blood-brain barrier for osmosis to occur.[66,82]

The most widely used osmotic diuretic is mannitol, a large molecule that is retained almost entirely in the extracellular compartment and has little to no rebound effect noted with other osmotic diuretics. Mannitol may improve perfusion to ischemic areas of the brain, producing cerebral vasoconstriction and resulting in a reduction of ICP.[66,82]

Perhaps the most common difficulty associated with the use of osmotic agents is the production of electrolyte disturbances. Careful attention must be paid to body weight and fluid and electrolyte stability. Serum osmolality must be kept between 300 and 320 mOsm/L. Hypernatremia and hypokalemia often are associated with repeated administration of osmotic agents. Central venous pressure readings must be monitored to prevent hypovolemia. Smaller doses of mannitol simplify fluid and electrolyte management, and their use is encouraged whenever possible.[77,82]

Nonosmotic Agents. Loop diuretics have also been used to decrease ICP. Furosemide, one such nonosmotic diuretic, may act differently from osmotic agents by pulling sodium and water from edematous areas and, perhaps, by decreasing CSF production. One advantage of furosemide administration over the use of osmotic diuretics is that its effect is not generally associated with increases in serum osmolality. Therefore electrolyte imbalances may not be as severe with the use of nonosmotic diuretics.[14,77]

Volume Maintenance. Administration of osmotic and loop diuretics can contribute to dehydration, thus precipitating a decrease in cerebral perfusion pressure. Optimally the patient should be maintained in an euvolemic state to optimize cerebral perfusion. Volume replacement strategies include fluid boluses, fluid replacements, and albumin administration. Intravenous fluids administered are typically isotonic and low in glucose to prevent gradient shifts across the blood-brain barrier in the traumatically brain-injured patient.[74]

Control of Metabolic Demand

Any treatment modality that increases the incidence of noxious stimulation to the patient carries with it the potential for increasing ICP. Such noxious stimuli include pain, the presence of an endotracheal tube, coughing, suctioning, repositioning, bathing, and many other routine nursing interventions. Agents used to reduce metabolic demands include the use of benzodiazepines such as midazolam and lorazepam, intravenous sedative-hypnotics such as propofol, opioid narcotics such as fentanyl and morphine, and neuromuscular blocking agents such as vecuronium and atracurium. These agents may be administered separately or in combination, via continuous drip or as an intravenous bolus on an as-needed basis. The preferred treatment regimen begins with the administration of benzodiazepines for sedation and narcotics for analgesia. If these agents fail to blunt the patient's response to noxious stimuli, propofol and/or a neuromuscular blocking agent is added. The use of these medications is recommended only in patients who have an ICP monitor in place, because sedatives, narcotics, and neuromuscular blocking agents affect the reliability of neurologic assessment. The use of neuromuscular blocking agents without sedation is not recommended because these agents can cause skeletal muscle paralysis and thus have no analgesic effect and do not adequately protect the patient from pain and the physiologic responses that can occur from pain-producing procedures.[74,77] If these agents fail to control the patient's ICP, barbiturate therapy is considered.

Barbiturate Therapy. Barbiturate therapy is a treatment protocol developed for the management of uncontrolled intracranial hypertension that has not responded to the conventional treatments previously described.[83] The two most commonly used drugs in high-dose barbiturate therapy are pentobarbital and thiopental. The goal with either of these drugs is a reduction of ICP to 15 to 20 mm Hg while a MAP of 70 to 80 mm Hg is maintained. Patients are maintained on high-dose barbiturate therapy until ICP has been controlled within the normal range for 24 hours. Barbiturates must never be stopped abruptly but are tapered slowly over approximately 4 days.[5]

Complications of high-dose barbiturate therapy can be disastrous unless a specific and organized approach is used. The most common complications are hypotension, hypothermia, and myocardial depression. If any complications occur and are allowed to persist unchecked, they may cause secondary insults to an already damaged brain. Hypotension, the most common complication, results from peripheral vasodilation and can be compounded in an already dehydrated patient who has received large doses of an osmotic diuretic in an attempt to control ICP. Careful monitoring of fluid status by central venous pressure or a pulmonary artery catheter can help prevent this complication. Myocardial depression results from cardiac muscle suppression and can be avoided by frequent monitoring of fluid status, cardiac output, and serum drug levels. If an adequate cardiac output cannot be maintained in the presence of normothermia, barbiturates must be reduced, regardless of serum levels.[5,83]

Collaborative management of the patient intracranial hypertension is outlined in Box 18-15.

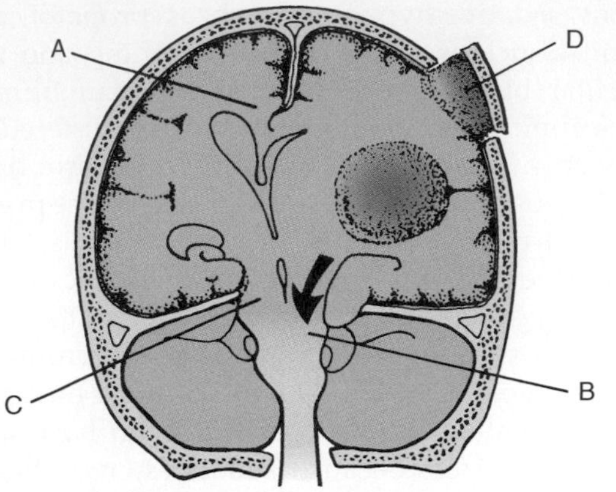

FIGURE 18-10. Supratentorial herniation. *A*, Cingulate. *B*, Uncal. *C*, Central. *D*, Transcalvarial.

Box 18-15

Collaborative Management

Intracranial Hypertension

- Position patient to achieve maximal ICP reduction
- Reduce environmental stimulation
- Maintain normothermia
- Control ventilation to ensure a normal $Paco_2$ level (35 ± 2 mm Hg)
- Administer diuretic agents, anticonvulsants, sedation, analgesia, paralytic agents, and vasoactive medications to ensure CPP >70 mm Hg
- Drain cerebrospinal fluid for ICP >20 mm Hg

ICP, Intracranial pressure; *$Paco_2$*, arterial partial pressure of carbon dioxide; *CPP*, cerebral perfusion pressure.

HERNIATION SYNDROMES

The goal of neurologic evaluation, ICP monitoring, and treatment of increased ICP is to prevent herniation. Herniation of intracerebral contents results in the shifting of tissue from one compartment of the brain to another and places pressure on cerebral vessels and vital function centers of the brain. If unchecked, herniation rapidly causes death as a result of the cessation of cerebral blood flow and respirations.

Supratentorial Herniation

The four types of supratentorial herniation syndrome are uncal; central, or transtentorial; cingulate; and transcalvarial (Figure 18-10).

Uncal Herniation. Uncal herniation is the most-often noted herniation syndrome. In uncal herniation, a unilateral, expanding mass lesion, usually of the temporal lobe, increases ICP, causing lateral displacement of the tip of the temporal lobe (uncus). Lateral displacement pushes the uncus over the edge of the tentorium, puts pressure on the oculomotor nerve (cranial nerve III) and posterior cerebral artery ipsilateral to the lesion, and flattens the midbrain against the opposite side. Clinical manifestations of uncal herniation include ipsilateral pupil dilation, decreased level of consciousness, respiratory pattern changes leading to respiratory arrest, and contralateral hemiplegia leading to decorticate or decerebrate posturing. If no intervention occurs, uncal herniation results in fixed and dilated pupils, flaccidity, and respiratory arrest.[5,84]

Central Herniation. In central, or transtentorial, herniation an expanding mass lesion of the midline, frontal, parietal, or occipital lobes results in downward displacement of the hemispheres, basal ganglia, and diencephalon through the tentorial notch. Central herniation often is preceded by uncal and cingulate herniation. Clinical manifestations of central herniation include loss of consciousness; small, reactive pupils progressing to fixed, dilated pupils; respiratory changes leading to respiratory arrest; and decorticate posturing progressing to flaccidity. In the late stages, uncal and central herniation syndromes affect the brain stem similarly.[5,84]

Cingulate Herniation. Cingulate herniation occurs when an expanding lesion of one hemisphere shifts laterally and forces the cingulate gyrus under the falx cerebri. Cingulate herniation occurs often. Whenever a lateral shift is noted on computed tomography (CT) scan, cingulate herniation has occurred. Little is known about the effects of cingulate herniation, and no clinical manifestations are present to assist in its diagnosis. Cingulate herniation is not in itself life-threatening, but if the expanding mass lesion that caused cingulate herniation is not controlled, uncal or central herniation will follow.[5,84]

Transcalvarial Herniation. Transcalvarial herniation is the extrusion of cerebral tissue through the cranium. In the presence of severe cerebral edema, transcalvarial herniation occurs through an opening from a skull fracture or craniotomy site.[5]

Infratentorial Herniation

The two infratentorial herniation syndromes are upward transtentorial herniation and downward cerebellar herniation.

Upward Transtentorial Herniation. Upward transtentorial herniation occurs when an expanding mass lesion of the cerebellum causes protrusion of the vermis (central area) of the cerebellum and the midbrain upward through the tentorial notch. Compression of the third cranial nerve and diencephalon occurs. Blockage of the central aqueduct and distortion of the third ventricle obstruct CSF flow. Deterioration progresses rapidly.[5,84]

Downward Cerebellar Herniation. Downward cerebellar herniation occurs when an expanding lesion of the cerebellum exerts pressure downward, sending the cerebellar tonsils through the foramen magnum. Compression and displacement of the medulla oblongata occur, rapidly resulting in respiratory and cardiac arrest.[5,84]

evolve To test your mastery of this chapter, try the Open-Book Quiz at http://evolve.elsevier.com/Urden/priorities/

REFERENCES

1. Olson DM, Graffagnino C: Consciousness, coma, and caring for the brain-injured patient, *AACN Clin Issues* 16:441, 2005.
2. Laureys S, Owen AM, Schiff ND: Brain function in coma, vegetative state, and related disorders, *Lancet Neurol* 3:537, 2004.
3. Malik K, Hess DC: Evaluating the comatose patient: rapid neurologic assessment is key to appropriate management, *Postgrad Med* 111(2):38, 2002.
4. Marx JA et al: *Rosen's emergency medicine: concepts and clinical practice*, ed 5, St Louis, 2002, Mosby.
5. Barker E: *Neuroscience nursing: a spectrum of care*, ed 2, St Louis, 2002, Mosby.
6. Goetz CG: *Textbook of clinical neurology*, ed 2, St Louis, 2003, Elsevier.
7. Berger JR: Clinical approach to stupor and coma. In Bradley WG et al, editors: *Neurology in clinical practice*, ed 3, Boston, 2000, Butterworth Heinemann.
8. McCance KL, Huether SE: *Pathophysiology: the biologic basis for disease in adults and children*, ed 5, St Louis, 2006, Mosby.
9. Wijdicks EFM: Coma in the critically ill. II. The transplant patient; management overview, *J Crit Illness* 15:646, 2000.
10. Stevens RD, Bhardwaj A: Approach to the comatose patient, *Crit Care Med* 34:31, 2006.
11. Jorgensen EO, Holm S: Prediction of neurological outcome after cardiopulmonary resuscitation, *Resuscitation* 41:145, 1999.
12. Cortese D, Capp L, McKinley S: Moisture chamber versus lubrication for the prevention of corneal epithelial breakdown, *Am J Crit Care* 4:425, 1995.
13. Gerber CS: Understanding and managing coma stimulation: are we doing everything we can? *Crit Care Nurs Q* 28:94, 2005.
14. Lombardi F et al.: Sensory stimulation of brain-injured individuals in coma or vegetative state: results of a Cochrane systematic review, *Clin Rehabil* 16:464, 2002.
15. American Heart Association. *Heart disease and stroke statistics—2007 update,* Dallas, 2005, The Association.
16. Bader MK, Littlejohns LR: *AANN core curriculum for neuroscience nursing*, ed 4, St Louis, 2004, Elsevier.
17. Singh V: Critical care assessment and management of acute ischemic stroke, *J Vasc Interv Radiol* 15:S21, 2004.
18. Frizzell JP: Acute stroke: pathophysiology, diagnosis, and treatment, *AACN Clin Issues* 16:421, 2005.
19. Chen WL et al: Vertebral artery dissection and cerebellar infarction following chiropractic manipulation *Emerg Med J* 23(1):e1, 2006.
20. Petty GW et al: Rates and predictors of cerebrovascular events among patients with valvular heart disease: a population-based study, *Stroke* 31:279A, 2000.
21. van der Linden J, van der Linden W: Role of calcium in the aortic atherosclerosis/stroke relation *Am J Cardiol* 96:1753, 2005.
22. Kushner I, Rzewnicki D, Samols D: What does minor elevation of C-reactive protein signify? *Am J Med* 119:166, 2006.
23. Offenbacher S, Beck JD: A perspective on the potential cardioprotective benefits of periodontal therapy, *Am Heart J* 149:950, 2005.
24. American Association of Neuroscience Nursing: *Guide to the care of the patient with ischemic stroke*, Glenview, IL, 2005, The Association.
25. Samples SD, Krieger DW: Acute ischemic stroke, *Curr Opin Crit Care* 6:77, 2000.
26. Silverman IE, Restrepo L, Mathews G: Poststroke seizures, *Arch Neurol* 59:195, 2002.
27. Muir KW et al: Imaging of acute stroke, *Lancet Neurol* 5:755, 2006.
28. Becker K: Intensive care unit management of the stroke patient, *Neurol Clin* 18:439, 2000.
29. Adams JP et al: Guidelines for thrombolytic therapy for acute stroke: a supplement to the guidelines for the management of patients with acute ischemic stroke, *Circulation* 94:1167, 1996.
30. Mullen MT, McGarvey ML, Kasner SE: Safety and efficacy of thrombolytic therapy in postoperative cerebral infarctions, *Neurol Clin* 24:783, 2006.
31. Albers GW et al: Antithrombotic and thrombolytic therapy for ischemic stroke: the Seventh ACCP Conference on Antithrombotic and Thrombolytic Therapy, *Chest* 126:483S, 2004.
32. Adams HP: Emergent use of anticoagulation for treatment of patients with ischemic stroke, *Stroke* 33:856, 2002.
33. Adams HP et al: Guidelines for the early management of patients with acute ischemic stroke: a statement from the Stroke Council of the American Stroke Association, *Stroke* 34:1056, 2003.
34. Swadron SP et al: The acute cerebrovascular event: surgical and other interventional therapies, *Emerg Med Clin N Am* 21:847, 2003.
35. Brisman JL, Song JK, Newell DW: Medical progress: cerebral aneurysms, *N Engl J Med* 355:928, 2006.
36. Brettler S: Endovascular coiling for cerebral aneurysms, *AACN Clin Issues* 16:515, 2005.
37. Choi JH, Mohr JP: Brain arteriovenous malformations in adult, *Lancet Neurol* 4:299, 2005.
38. Manno EM: Subarachnoid hemorrhage, *Neurol Clin* 22:347, 2004.
39. Mayberg MR et al: Guidelines for the management of aneurysmal subarachnoid hemorrhage: a statement for healthcare professionals from a special writing group of the Stroke Council, American Heart Association, *Circulation* 25:2315, 1994.
40. Shpritz DW: Neurodiagnostic studies, *Nurs Clin North Am* 34:593, 1999.
41. Hunt WE, Hess RM: Surgical risks as related to time of intervention in the repair of intracranial aneurysms, *J Neurosurg* 28:14, 1968.
42. Solenski NJ et al: Medical complications of aneurysmal subarachnoid hemorrhage: a report of the multicenter, cooperative aneurysm study, *Crit Care Med* 23:1007, 1995.
43. Classen J et al: Effect of acute physiologic derangements on outcome after subarachnoid hemorrhage, *Crit Care Med* 32:832, 2004.

44. Lefevre F, Woolger JM: Surgery in the patient with neurologic disease, *Med Clin North Am* 87:257, 2003.
45. Oyama K, Criddle L: Vasospasm after aneurysmal subarachnoid hemorrhage, *Crit Care Nurse* 24(5):58, 2004.
46. Bendo AA: Intracranial vascular surgery, *Anesthesiol Clin North America* 20:377, 2002.
47. Naval NS et al: Controversies in the management of aneurysmal subarachnoid hemorrhage, *Crit Care Med* 34:511, 2006.
48. Sen J et al: Triple-H therapy in the management of aneurysmal subarachnoid haemorrhage, *Lancet Neurol* 2:614, 2003.
49. Suarez JI: Outcome in neurocritical care: advances in monitoring and treatment and effect of a specialized neurocritical care team, *Crit Care Med* 34(9 suppl):S232, 2006.
50. Hsieh PC et al: Current updates in perioperative management of intracerebral hemorrhage, *Neurol Clin* 24:745, 2006.
51. Panagos PD, Jauch EC, Broderick JP: Intracerebral hemorrhage, *Emerg Med Clin North Am* 20:631, 2002.
52. Xi G, Keep RF, Hoff JT: Mechanisms of brain injury after intracerebral haemorrhage, *Lancet Neurol* 5:53, 2006.
53. Mayer SA, Rincon F: Treatment of intracerebral haemorrhage, *Lancet Neurol* 4:662, 2005.
54. Ashley J, Duggan M, Sutcliffe N: Speech, language, and swallowing disorders in the older adult, *Clin Geriatr Med* 22:291, 2006.
55. Chitnis T, Khoury SJ: Immunologic neuromuscular disorders, *J Allergy Clin Immunol* 111:S659, 2003.
56. Newswanger DL, Warren CR: Guillain-Barré syndrome, *Am Fam Physician* 69:2405, 2004.
57. Keenlyside R, Brezman D: Fatal Guillain-Barré syndrome after the national influenza immunization program, *Neurology* 30:929, 1980.
58. Marinelli WA, Leatherman JW: Neuromuscular disorders in the intensive care unit, *Crit Care Clin* 18:915, 2002.
59. Hughes RA et al: Intravenous immunoglobulin for Guillain-Barré syndrome, *Cochrane Database Syst Rev* CD002063, 2004.
60. Kihara M et al: A dysautonomia case of Guillain-Barré syndrome with recovery: monitored by composite autonomic scoring scale, *J Auton Nerv Syst* 73:186, 1998.
61. Pfeiffer G et al: Indicators of dysautonomia in severe Guillain-Barré syndrome, *J Neurol* 246:1015, 1999.
62. Rothrock JC: *Alexander's care of the patient in surgery*, ed 12, St Louis, 2003, Mosby.
63. Vance ML: Perioperative management of patients undergoing pituitary surgery, *Endocrinol Metab Clin North Am* 32:355, 2003.
64. Valladeres JB, Hankinson J: Incidence of lower extremity deep vein thrombosis in neurosurgical patients, *Neurosurgery* 6:138, 1980.
65. Warbel A, Lewicki L, Lupica K: Venous thromboembolism: risk factors in the craniotomy patient population, *J Neurosci Nurs* 31:180, 1999.
66. Eigsti J, Henke K: Anatomy and physiology of neurological compensatory mechanisms, *Dimens Crit Care Nurs* 25:197, 2006.
67. Arbour, R: Intracranial hypertension: monitoring and nursing assessment, *Crit Care Nurse* 24(5):19, 2004.
68. Littlejohns L, Bader MK: Prevention of secondary brain injury: targeting technology, *AACN Clin Issues* 16:501, 2005.
69. Vavilala MS, Lee LA, Lam AM: Cerebral blood flow and vascular physiology, *Anesthesiol Clin North Am* 20:247, 2002.
70. Wall BM, Philips JP, Howard JC: Validation of increased intracranial pressure and high risk for increased intracranial pressure, *Nurs Diag* 5:74, 1994.
71. American Association of Neuroscience Nurses: *Guide to the care of the patient with intracranial pressure monitoring*, Glenview, IL, 2005, The Association.
72. Winkleman C: Effect of backrest position on intracranial and cerebral perfusion pressures in traumatically brain-injured adults, *Am J Crit Care* 9:373, 2000.
73. Simmons BJ: Management of intracranial hemodynamics in the adult: a research analysis of head positioning and recommendations for clinical practice and future research, *J Neurosci Nurs* 29:44, 1997.
74. Bader MK, Palmer S: Keeping the brain in the zone: applying the severe head injury guidelines to practice, *Crit Care Nurs Clin North Am* 12:413, 2000.
75. Coles JP et al: Effect of hyperventilation on cerebral blood flow in traumatic head injury: clinical relevance and monitoring correlates, *Crit Care Med* 30:1950, 2002.
76. Wong FWH: Prevention of secondary brain injury. *Crit Care Nurse* 20(5):18, 2000.
77. Arbour R: Aggressive management of intracranial dynamics, *Crit Care Nurse* 18(3):30, 1998.
78. Qureshi AI, Suarez JI: Use of hypertonic saline solutions in treatment of cerebral edema and intracranial hypertension, *Crit Care Med* 28:3301, 2000.
79. Brucia JJ, Owen DC, Rudy EB: The effects of lidocaine on intracranial hypertension, *J Neurosci Nurs* 24:205, 1992.
80. Kerr M et al: Head-injured adults: recommendations for endotracheal suctioning, *J Neurosci Nurs* 25:86, 1993.
81. Cummings R: Understanding ventricular drainage, *J Neurosci Nurs* 24:84, 1992.
82. Paczynski RP: Osmotherapy: basic concepts and controversies, *Crit Care Clin* 13:105, 1997.
83. Bader MK, Arbour R: Refractory increased intracranial pressure in severe traumatic brain injury, *AACN Clin Issues* 16:526, 2005.
84. Morrison CAM: Brain herniation syndromes, *Crit Care Nurs* 7(5):34, 1987.

CHAPTER 19

Renal Clinical Assessment and Diagnostic Procedures

MARY SCHIRA

OBJECTIVES

- Describe the priorities of the renal nursing assessment.
- Identify ways in which alterations of hemoglobin and hematocrit levels can signal fluid volume deficit or excess.
- Explain why elevation of blood urea nitrogen and serum creatinine signal kidney dysfunction.

A renal history begins with a description of the chief complaint, stated in the patient's own words. A description of the chief complaint includes the onset, location, duration, and factors or strategies that lessen and/or aggravate the problem.[1] The individual should be encouraged to describe the effects of any treatment for the problem thus far, medications taken to alleviate symptoms (both prescription and nonprescription), efforts taken to determine the cause of the problem, and/or procedures performed to improve the problem. A careful history that explores symptoms fully is an essential component of the clinical assessment.

Predisposing factors for acute kidney dysfunction are also elicited during the history, including the use of over-the-counter medicines, recent infections requiring antibiotic therapy, antihypertensive medicines, and any diagnostic procedures performed using radiopaque contrast media.[2] Nonsteroidal antiinflammatory drugs (such as ibuprofen), antibiotics (especially aminoglycosides), antihypertensives (especially medicines that block angiotensin), and iodine-based dyes may cause an acute or chronic decline in kidney function. A history of recent onset of nausea and vomiting or appetite loss caused by taste changes (uremia often causes a metallic taste) may also provide clues to the rapid onset of kidney problems.[2] And finally, symptoms that indicate rapid fluid volume gains are explored. For example, weight gains of more than 2 pounds per day, sleeping on additional pillows, and sitting in a chair to sleep are signals of volume overload and potential kidney dysfunction. The patient and/or family or significant other must be asked to provide as much detail about previous kidney function and problems as possible.

PHYSICAL EXAMINATION

In the critical care area, nursing assessment does not routinely include a full physical examination of the kidneys and associated renal system. However, many of the assessment parameters for the renal system provide information related to the volume status of the individual and are helpful in a large number of patients regardless of kidney function or status. Although assessment is not often performed in the depth described in the following sections, the critical care nurse must be aware of how to perform a thorough renal assessment in stable patients and as needed in patients with kidney dysfunction.

INSPECTION

Nursing priorities for inspection of the patient with kidney dysfunction focus on (1) bleeding, (2) volume depletion or overload, and (3) edema.

Bleeding

Visual inspection related to the kidneys generally focuses on the flank and abdomen. Kidney trauma is suspected if a purplish discoloration is present on the flank (Grey-Turner's sign) or near the posterior eleventh or twelfth ribs.[1] Bruising, abdominal distention, and abdominal guarding may also signal renal trauma or a hematoma around a kidney. Blood in the urine is not a common sign of kidney trauma and is more likely to indicate a urologic (e.g., bladder injury) rather than kidney etiology.

Volume Depletion/Overload

Inspection is especially helpful in looking for signs of volume depletion or overload that might signal kidney problems. Fluid volume assessment begins with an inspection of the patient's neck veins. The supine position facilitates normal venous distention. An absence of distention (or flat neck veins) indicates hypovolemia. Assessment continues with the head of the bed elevated 45 to 90 degrees.[1] If the neck veins remain distended more than 2 cm above the sternal notch when the bed is at 45 degrees, fluid overload may be present.[3]

Hand vein inspection may be helpful in assessing volume status and is performed by observing for venous distention when the hand is held in the dependent position. Venous filling that takes longer than 5 seconds suggests hypovolemia. When the hand is elevated, the distention should disappear within 5 seconds. If distention does not disappear within 5 seconds after the hand is elevated, fluid overload is suspected.

Assessment of skin turgor provides additional data for identifying fluid-related problems. To assess turgor, the skin over the forearm is picked up and released. Normal elasticity and fluid status allow an almost immediate return to shape once the skin is released. In fluid volume deficit, however, the skin remains raised ("tented") and does not return to its normal position for several seconds. Because of the loss of skin elasticity in elderly persons, skin turgor assessment is not an accurate fluid assessment for this age-group.

Finally, inspection of the oral cavity provides clues to fluid volume status. When a fluid volume deficit exists, the mucous membranes of the mouth become dry. However, mouth breathing and some medicines (such as antihistamines) can also dry the mucous membranes temporarily. Therefore a more accurate way to assess the oral cavity is to inspect the mouth using a tongue blade. Dryness of the oral cavity is more indicative of fluid volume deficit than are complaints of a dry mouth.[3]

Edema

Edema is the presence of excess fluid in the interstitial space and can be a sign of volume overload. In the presence of volume excess, edema may be present in dependent areas of the body, such as the feet and legs of an ambulatory person or the sacrum of an individual confined to bed. The presence of edema, however, does not always indicate fluid volume overload. A loss of albumin from the vascular space can cause peripheral edema in the presence of hypovolemia or normal fluid states. A critically ill patient may have a low serum albumin level (hypoalbuminemia) because of inadequate nutrition after surgery, a burn, or a head injury and may exhibit edema as a result of the loss of plasma oncotic pressure and not as a result of volume overload. In addition, edema may signal circulatory difficulties. An individual who is fluid balanced but who has poor venous return may experience pedal edema after prolonged sitting in a chair with the feet dependent. Similarly, an individual with heart failure may experience edema because the left ventricle is unable to pump blood effectively through the vessels. A key feature that distinguishes edema due to excess volume or hypoalbuminemia from circulatory compromise is that the edema does not reverse with elevation of the extremity.

Edema can be assessed by applying fingertip pressure on the skin over a bony prominence, such as the ankles, pretibial areas (shins), and sacrum. If the indentation made by the fingertip does not disappear within 15 seconds, "pitting" edema is present. Pitting edema indicates increased interstitial volume and is generally not evident until a weight gain of approximately 10% has occurred.[4] Edema also may appear in the hands and feet, around the eyes, and in the cheeks. Dependent areas, such as the feet and sacrum, are the areas most likely to demonstrate edema in patients confined to a wheelchair or bed. One way of measuring the extent of edema is by using a subjective scale of 1 to 4, with 1 indicating only minimal pitting and 4 indicating severe pitting (Table 19-1).[1]

Table 19-1
Pitting Edema Scale

RATING	APPROXIMATE EQUIVALENT
+1	2-mm depth
+2	4-mm depth (lasting up to 15 sec)
+3	6-mm depth (lasting up to 60 sec)
+4	8-mm depth (lasting longer than 60 sec)

AUSCULTATION

Nursing priorities in auscultation of the patient with kidney dysfunction focus on (1) the heart, (2) blood pressure, and (3) the lungs.

Heart

Auscultation of the heart requires not only assessing rate and rhythm but also listening for extra sounds. Fluid overload is often accompanied by a third or fourth heart sound, which may be heard with the bell of the stethoscope.[1] Increased heart rate alone provides little information about fluid volume, but combined with a low blood pressure it may indicate hypovolemia. The heart also is auscultated for the presence of a pericardial friction rub. A rub can best be heard at the third intercostal space to the left of the sternal border, with the individual leaning slightly forward.[1] The presence of a pericardial friction rub indicates pericarditis and may result from uremia in a patient with kidney failure.

Box 19-1

Orthostatic Hypotension Assessment

1. Take BP and HR with patient lying down.
2. Assist patient to sitting position.
   Monitor patient for complaints of dizziness, imbalance.
   Take BP and HR immediately and record.
   Take BP and HR after 3 minutes and record.
3. Assist patient to standing position (if patient not dizzy, imbalanced).
   Assess as above.

BP, Blood pressure; *HR,* heart rate.

Blood Pressure

Blood pressure and heart rate changes are very useful in assessing fluid volume deficit. In stable critically ill patients or in patients on a telemetry unit, orthostatic vital sign measurements provide clues to blood loss, dehydration, unexplained syncope, and the effects of some antihypertensive medications.[5,6] A drop in systolic blood pressure of 20 mm Hg or more, a drop in diastolic blood pressure of 10 mm Hg or more, or a rise in pulse rate of more than 15 beats/min from lying to sitting or from sitting to standing represents orthostatic hypotension. Box 19-1 describes how to assess for orthostatic hypotension. The drop in blood pressure occurs because a sufficient preload is not immediately available after the position change. The heart rate increases in an attempt to maintain cardiac output and circulation. Orthostatic hypotension produces subjective feelings of weakness, dizziness, or faintness. Although orthostatic hypotension is often a sign of hypovolemia, peripheral vascular disease may also be responsible.

Lungs

Lung assessment also is extremely important in gauging fluid status. Crackles indicate fluid overload. Dyspnea with mild exertion, dyspnea at night that prevents sleeping in a supine position (orthopnea), or dyspnea that awakens the individual from sleep (paroxysmal nocturnal dyspnea) may indicate pooling of fluid in the lungs. Shallow, gasping breaths with periods of apnea reflect severe acid-base imbalances.

PALPATION

Nursing priorities in percussion of the patient with kidney dysfunction focus on determining the shape and the size of the kidneys.

Determining Kidney Size/Shape

Although rarely performed in critically ill patients, palpation of the kidneys in stable patients provides information about the kidneys' size and shape. Palpation of the kidneys is achieved through the bimanual capturing approach. Capturing is accomplished by placing one hand posteriorly under the flank of the supine patient with fingers pointing to the midline, while placing the opposite hand just below the rib cage anteriorly.[1,4] The patient is asked to inhale deeply while pressure is exerted to bring the hands together. As the patient exhales, the examiner may feel the kidney between the hands (Figure 19-1). After each kidney is palpated in this manner, the two should be compared for size and shape. Each kidney should be firm, smooth, and of equal size. The examiner is usually unable to palpate a normal left kidney. The right kidney is more easily palpated because of its lower position, being displaced downward by the liver. Problems should be suspected if a mass (cancer) or an irregular surface (polycystic kidneys) is palpated, a size difference is detected, the kidney extends significantly lower than the rib cage on either side, or there is evidence of recent blunt trauma.[1,7]

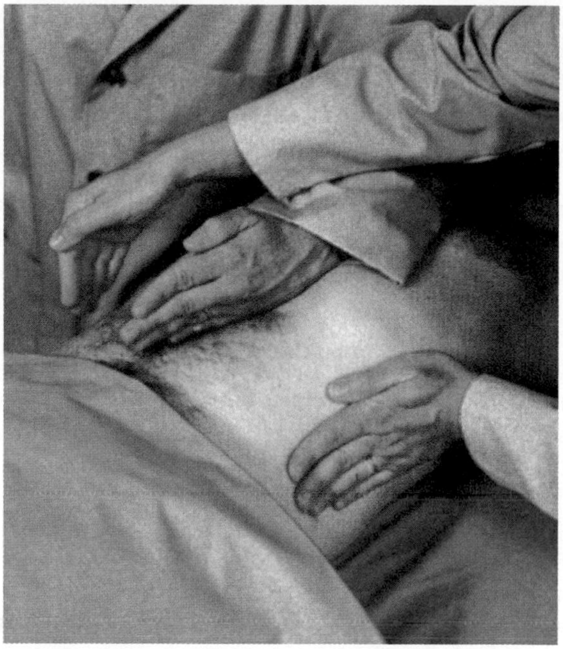

FIGURE 19-1. Palpation of the kidney. (From Barkauskas V, Baumann V, Darling-Fisher C: *Health & physical assessment,* ed 3, St Louis, 2002, Mosby.)

PERCUSSION

Nursing priorities in percussion of the patient with kidney dysfunction focus on (1) the kidneys and (2) the abdomen.

Kidneys

Percussion of a kidney is performed with the patient in a side-lying or sitting position, with the examiner's hand placed over the costovertebral angle (lower border of the rib cage on the flank).[1] Striking the back of the hand with the opposite fist produces a dull thud, which is normal. Pain may indicate infection (such as a urinary tract infection that has extended into the kidneys) or injury resulting from trauma. Traumatic injury to the kidneys should be assessed in the presence of a penetrating abdominal wound, with blunt abdominal trauma, or with a fractured pelvis or ribs.[7,8]

Abdomen

Observation and percussion of the abdomen are of value in assessing fluid status. Percussing the abdomen with the patient in the supine position generally yields a dull sound (solid bowel contents or fluid) or a hollow sound (gaseous bowel).[1]

Ascites, or severe fluid distention of the abdominal cavity, is an important observation in determining fluid overload. Differentiating ascites from distortion caused by solid bowel contents is accomplished by producing a fluid wave. A fluid wave is elicited by exerting pressure to the abdominal midline while one hand is placed on the right or left flank.[1,4] Tapping the opposite flank produces a wave in the accumulated fluid that can be felt under the hands (Figure 19-2). Other signs of ascites include a protuberant, rounded abdomen and abdominal striae.[1]

Individuals with kidney failure may have ascites caused by volume overload, which forces fluid into the abdomen because of increased capillary hydrostatic pressures. However, ascites may or may not represent fluid volume excess. Severe ascites in persons with liver dysfunction results from decreased plasma proteins and elevated portal vein pressure.

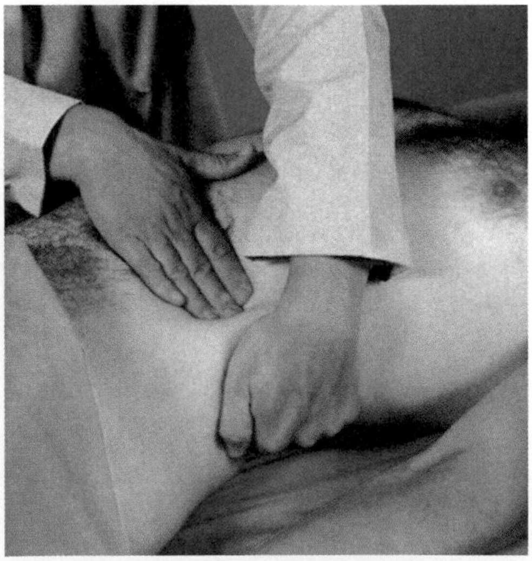

FIGURE 19-2. Test for the presence of a fluid wave. (From Barkauskas V, Baumann V, Darling-Fisher C: *Health & physical assessment,* ed 3, St Louis, 2002, Mosby.)

ADDITIONAL ASSESSMENT PARAMETERS

Nursing priorities for the patient undergoing fluid balance assessment focus on (1) weight, (2) intake and output, and (3) hemodynamic monitoring.

Weight

One of the most important assessments of kidney and fluid status is the patient's weight as it relates to fluid volume status. Significant fluctuations in body weight over a 1- to 2-day period indicate fluid gains and losses. Rapid weight gains or losses of greater than 2 pounds per day are generally caused by fluid rather than nutritional factors. One liter of fluid equals 1 kg, or approximately 2.2 pounds.

Whenever possible, the patient is weighed during admission to the critical care unit. It is important to note whether the current weight differs significantly from the weight 1 to 2 weeks before admission. The patient is weighed daily for comparison with the previous day's weight. The weight is obtained at the same time each day, with the patient wearing the same amount of clothing. The individual's weight is of critical importance to the dialysis nurse caring for a patient with acute or chronic kidney failure. The differences in weight from day to day are used to calculate the amount of fluid to remove during a dialysis treatment.[9]

Intake and Output

Like patient weight, intake and output are monitored on all patients in the critical care unit. Intake and output can be compared with the patient's weight to more accurately evaluate fluid gains or losses. Urinary output plus insensible fluid losses (perspiration, stool, and water vapor from the lungs) can vary from 750 to 2400 ml/day. When intake exceeds output (excessive intravenous fluid, decreased urine output), a positive fluid balance exists. In impaired kidney function, the positive fluid balance results in fluid volume overload. Conversely, if output exceeds intake (fever, increased respiration, profuse sweating, vomiting, diarrhea, gastric suction, diuretic therapy), a negative fluid balance exists and volume deficit results. During a 24-hour period, fever can increase skin and respiratory losses by as much as 75 ml per degree of Fahrenheit temperature rise.

Individuals with acute renal failure (ARF) often exhibit a decrease in urine output, or oliguria (less than 30 ml/hr or 400 ml/day in adults; less than 1 ml/kg/hr in infants and young children). However, there may be a fairly normal or only slightly decreased urine output that reflects water removal without solute removal in the early phases of ARF. Therefore kidney function cannot be accurately determined by urine output alone.

Hemodynamic Monitoring

Body fluid status is most accurately reflected in measurements of cardiovascular hemodynamics. Measurements such as central venous pressure (CVP), pulmonary artery occlusion pressure (PAOP), cardiac index (CI), and mean arterial pressure (MAP) provide a clear picture of the increases or decreases in vascular volume returning to and being ejected from the heart.[10] Indeed, both volume depletion and overload are easily detected by use of central venous or arterial catheters from which pressure measurements can be obtained. The most frequent cause of acute renal failure that requires hemodynamic monitoring in critical care is severe sepsis and septic shock.[10]

LABORATORY ASSESSMENT

Serum Tests

Blood Urea Nitrogen

In addition to history and physical examination, laboratory data are extremely helpful in the diagnosis, management, and ongoing evaluation of kidney system dysfunction. Blood urea nitrogen (BUN) is a by-product of protein and amino acid metabolism.[11] The normal value for BUN is 5 to 25 mg/dl and is increased when kidney function deteriorates.[12] With kidney dysfunction, the BUN is elevated because of a decrease in the glomerular filtration rate (GFR) and a fall in urea excretion. Severe elevations in the BUN can be correlated with the clinical manifestations of uremia; as the BUN rises, symptoms of uremia become more pronounced.[2] However, a drop in the GFR and therefore an increase in the BUN also may be caused by hypovolemia and dehydration,[13] nephrotoxic drugs, or a prolonged hypotensive episode. An unexpected decrease in BUN may represent poor nutrition status and is therefore not representative of kidney function. Thus, the BUN is never evaluated in isolation and is always considered with a known serum creatinine level.

Creatinine

Creatinine is a by-product of muscle and normal cell metabolism and appears in serum in amounts proportional to the body muscle mass. Although slightly higher in males than females, the normal serum creatinine level is about 0.5 to 1.5 mg/dl.[12] Creatinine is easily excreted by the renal tubules and is not significantly resorbed or secreted in the tubules.[2] Measuring the creatinine clearance—the amount of creatinine in the excreted urine and the amount of creatinine in the blood over 24 hours—provides a reliable and accurate estimate of glomerular filtration and therefore of kidney function.[2] The normal value for creatinine clearance is 110 to 120 ml/min; values less than 50 ml/min indicate significant kidney dysfunction. The creatinine clearance in the urine is measured using a 12- or 24-hour urine collection and blood sample. The creatinine clearance can also be estimated from the serum creatinine level and is expressed as eGFR (estimated glomerular filtration rate) (Box 19-2).[14,15] As kidney function declines, creatinine clearance decreases and is a useful marker to monitor the severity, progression, and recovery of kidney function. Although there are some limitations to using the formulas, the estimated/calculated creatinine clearance is widely used to determine changes in drug dosing with kidney dysfunction because many drugs are excreted by the kidneys.[15] Creatinine levels are fairly constant and are affected by fewer factors than BUN. A typical ratio of BUN to creatinine is approximately 10:1. A change in this ratio generally indicates kidney dysfunction and is very useful in identifying the etiology of the acute kidney dysfunction.[12,15]

Osmolarlity

The serum osmolarlity reflects the concentration or dilution of vascular fluid and measures the dissolved

Box 19-2

Creatinine Clearance Calculations

Measured: 12- or 24-Hour Urine

(Urine creatinine × Volume of urine) ÷ Serum creatinine

Estimated: Adults-Cockcroft-Gault Formula

[(140 − Age) × Body weight (kg)] ÷ [72 × Plasma creatinine (mg/dl)]

For women, multiply above by 0.85.

Estimated: Children

BODY WEIGHT (kg)	FORMULA
<10	0.45 × Height (cm) ÷ Serum creatinine (mg/dl)
>10, <70	0.55 × Height (cm) ÷ Serum creatinine (mg/dl)
>70	[1.55 × Age (yr)] + 0.5 × Height (cm) ÷ Serum creatinine (mg/dl)

Estimated: Abbreviated or Modified Modification of Diet in Renal Disease (MDRD) Formula

186 × (plasma creatinine) − 1.154 × (age in years) − 0.203

For females, the above result is multiplied by 0.742.

For African Americans, the above result is multiplied by 1.210.

The MDRD formula is complex (due to the negative log algebra functions); as a result, a calculator is needed to compute the creatinine clearance. However, the MDRD formula is generally considered a more accurate estimate of creatinine clearance than the Cockcroft-Gault formula because of the inclusion of additional variables. Many clinicians and reference books use the Cockcroft-Gault equation because of ease of calculation.

Data from National Kidney Foundation: *Am J Kid Dis* 39(suppl 2):S1, 2002, http://www.kidney.org/professionals/KDOQI/guidlelines.

particles in the vascular fluid. The normal serum osmolarlity is 275 to 295 mOsm/L.[3] An elevated osmolarlity indicates hemoconcentration or dehydration, whereas a decreased osmolarlity indicates hemodilution or volume overload. When the serum osmolarlity level increases, antidiuretic hormone (ADH) is released from the posterior pituitary gland and stimulates increased water resorption in the kidney tubules. This expands the vascular space, brings the serum osmolarlity back to normal, and results in more concentrated urine (and thus an elevated urine osmolarlity). The opposite occurs with a decreased serum osmolarlity level, which inhibits the production of ADH. The decreased ADH results in increased excretion of water in the tubules, producing dilute urine with a low osmolarlity, and brings the serum osmolarlity back to normal. Sodium accounts for 85% to 95% of the serum osmolarlity; therefore doubling the serum sodium gives an estimate of the serum osmolarlity.[12] A bedside value of the serum osmolarlity can be calculated from the following formula:

$$(2 \times \text{Na}) + (\text{BUN}/3) + (\text{Glucose}/18)$$

Anion Gap

The anion gap is a calculation of the difference between the measurable extracellular cations (primarily sodium) and the measurable extracellular anions (chloride and bicarbonate).[3] The value represents the remaining unmeasurable ions present in the extracellular fluid (phosphates, sulfates, ketones, lactate). The formula generally used in the calculation of the anion gap is as follows:

$$Na^+ - (Cl^- + HCO_3^-)$$

A normal anion gap is 1 to 12 mEq/L and generally does not exceed 14 mEq/L. An increased anion gap level reflects overproduction or decreased excretion of acid products and indicates metabolic acidosis; a decreased anion gap indicates metabolic alkalosis.

Hemoglobin and Hematocrit

The hemoglobin (Hgb) and hematocrit (Hct) levels can indicate increases or decreases in intravascular fluid volume.[11] Both Hgb and Hct vary between genders, with the Hgb in males normally 13.5 to 17.5 g/dl and in females 12 to 16 g/dl. The Hct ranges from 40% to 54% in males and 37% to 47% in females. Hct values are higher in newborns (up to 65%) and decrease to adult ranges between the ages of 4 and 10 years.[12] Hgb transports oxygen and carbon dioxide and is important in maintaining cellular metabolism and acid-base balance.[3]

The Hct is the proportion or concentration of red blood cells (RBCs) in a volume of whole blood and is expressed as a percentage.[12] Hematocrit is approximately three times the Hgb if the individual is in a normal fluid balance. An increase in the Hct often indicates a fluid volume deficit, which results in hemoconcentration. Conversely, a decreased Hct can indicate fluid volume excess because of the dilutional effect of the extra fluid load. Decreases, however, also can result from anemias, blood loss, liver damage, or hemolytic reactions.[12] Hgb and Hct are always evaluated together in the critically ill patient.

Albumin

Slightly more than 50% of the total plasma protein is serum albumin. It is manufactured in the liver, with a normal blood level of 3.5 to 5 g/dl.[12] Albumin is primarily responsible for the maintenance of colloid osmotic pressure, which functions to hold fluid in the vascular space. The blood vessel walls, because of their impermeability to plasma proteins, prevent albumin from leaving the vascular space. However, in some disease states such as severe burns (cell membrane destruction), sepsis, or ARF resulting from the nephrotic syndrome (increased glomerular capillary permeability to protein), albumin is lost from the vascular space. Decreased albumin levels in the vascular space result in a plasma-to-interstitium fluid shift, creating peripheral edema. A decreased albumin level can occur as a result of protein-calorie malnutrition, which occurs in many critically ill patients in whom available stores of albumin are depleted. A decrease in the plasma oncotic pressure results, and fluid shifts from the vascular space to the interstitial space. Liver disease or severe injury to the liver also causes a fall in albumin levels as the diseased liver fails to synthesize sufficient albumin. Furthermore, severe portal hypertension can force albumin and other plasma proteins into the abdominal cavity, resulting in ascites.

Increased albumin levels are rare. The body uses a fixed amount of protein for energy and body cell replacement and converts excess protein into stored fat. If all plasma protein levels are elevated, fluid volume deficit (hemoconcentration) is suspected.

Urine Analysis

Analysis of the urine provides excellent information about the patient's kidney function and condition relative to fluids and electrolytes. Specific tests and abnormal indications are presented in Table 19-2.[16-19] In some cases, urinalysis in the critically ill patient aids in locating the site of kidney damage or disease and therefore guides therapeutic management of the patient's care.

RADIOLOGIC ASSESSMENT

Although laboratory assessment is used most often in diagnosing kidney problems in the critically ill patient,

Table 19-2
Urinalysis Results

TEST	NORMAL	POSSIBLE CAUSES FOR INCREASED VALUES	POSSIBLE CAUSES FOR DECREASED VALUES
pH	4.5-8.0	Alkalosis	Acidosis Intrarenal ARF
Specific gravity	1.003-1.030	Volume deficit Glycosuria Proteinuria Prerenal ARF (>1.020)	Volume overload Intrarenal ARF
Osmolarlity	300-1200 mOsm/L	Volume deficit Prerenal ARF (urine > serum osmolarlity)	Volume excess Intrarenal ARF (urine < serum osmolarlity)
Protein	30-150 mg/24 hr	Trauma Infection Intrarenal ARF Transient with exercise Glomerulonephritis	
Sodium	40-220 mEq/24 hr	High-sodium diet Intrarenal ARF	Prerenal ARF
Creatinine	1-2 g/24 hr		Intrarenal ARF Chronic kidney failure
Urea	6-17 g/24 hr		Intrarenal ARF Chronic kidney failure
Myoglobin	Absent	Crush injury Rhabdomyolysis	
RBCs	0-5	Trauma Intrarenal ARF Infection Strenuous exercise Renal artery thrombus	
WBCs	0-5	Infection	
Bacteria	None-few	Infection	
Casts	None-few	RBC: glomerular disease WBC: pyelonephritis Glomerular disease Nephrotic syndrome Epithelial: glomerular disease	

ARF, Acute renal failure; *RBCs,* red blood cells; *WBCs,* white blood cells.

radiologic assessment can confirm or clarify causes of particular disorders. Radiologic assessment ranges from basic to more complex (Table 19-3) and provides information about abnormal masses, abnormal fluid collection, obstructions, vascular supply alterations, and other disorders of the kidneys and urinary tract.[2,20,21]

Some of the radiologic studies require the use of contrast medium or injection of a radiopaque dye. Many of the dyes used in radiology are potentially nephrotoxic. Therefore dyes must be used carefully in patients with ARF or chronic kidney disease. For example, an individual with ARF undergoing a test using contrast medium may experience a further worsening of kidney function caused by the dye. In general, to prevent nephrotoxicity, adequate hydration before and after the test and careful monitoring of renal status are indicated any time a contrast medium is used.

KIDNEY BIOPSY

Kidney biopsy is the definitive tool for diagnosing disease processes of the kidney. Two methods are used: closed biopsy and open biopsy. Percutaneous needle biopsy (closed method) involves inserting a needle via the flank to obtain a specimen of cortical and medullary kidney tissue. An open biopsy is a surgical procedure and is rarely done in critically ill patients. In either case, biopsy is often the last choice for diagnostic assessment in the critically ill patient because of the postprocedural risks of bleeding, hematoma formation, and infection.

evolve To test your mastery of this chapter, try the Open-Book Quiz at http://evolve.elsevier.com/Urden/priorities/

Table 19-3

Renal Imaging Tests

TEST	COMMENTS
Kidney-ureter-bladder (KUB)	Flat plate x-ray film of abdomen; determines position, size, and structure of kidneys and urinary tract and pelvis; useful to evaluate presence of calculi and masses Usually followed by additional tests
Intravenous pyelogram (IVP)	Intravenous (IV) injection of contrast medium with x-ray film; allows visualization of internal kidney tissues
Renal angiography	Injection of contrast medium into arterial blood perfusing the kidneys; allows visualization of renal blood flow May also visualize stenosis, cysts, clots, trauma, and infarctions
Renal computed tomography (CT)	Radioisotope administered by IV route and absorbed by kidneys; scintillation photography is then performed in several planes; spiral or helical CT allows rapid imaging. Spiral CT is especially useful in determining the presence/location of calculi. Density of the image helps evaluate kidney vessels, perfusion, tumors, cysts, hemorrhage, necrosis, and trauma
Renal ultrasound	High-frequency sound waves are transmitted to the kidneys and urinary tract, and image is viewed on an oscilloscope; noninvasive Identifies fluid accumulation or obstruction, cysts, and masses Useful to evaluate kidney size and shape before biopsy
Magnetic resonance imaging (MRI)	A scanner produces three-dimensional images in response to the application of high-energy radiofrequency waves to the tissues Produces clear images; the density of the image may indicate trauma, cysts, masses, malformation of the vessels or tubules, and necrosis

REFERENCES

1. Seidel HM et al: *Mosby's guide to physical examination,* ed 5, St Louis, 2003, Mosby.
2. Richard C: Assessment of renal structure and function. In Lancaster L, editor: *Core curriculum for nephrology nursing,* ed 4, Pitman, NJ, 2001, American Nephrology Nurses Association.
3. Metheny NM: *Fluid and electrolyte balance-nursing considerations,* ed 4, Philadelphia, 2000, Lippincott.
4. Malasanos L, Barkauskas V, Stoltenberg-Allen K: *Health assessment,* ed 4, St Louis, 1990, Mosby.
5. Ejaz AA et al: Characteristics of 100 consecutive patients presenting with orthostatic hypotension, *Mayo Clin Proc* 79(7):890, 2004.
6. Irvin D: The importance of accurately assessing orthostatic hypotension, *Geriatr Nurs* 25(2):99, 2004.
7. Bozeman C et al: Selective operative management of major blunt renal trauma, *J Trauma* 57(2):305, 2004.
8. Knudson MM et al: Outcome after major renovascular injuries: a Western trauma association multicenter report, *J Trauma* 49(6):1116, 2000.
9. Purcell W et al: Accurate dry weight assessment: reducing the incidence of hypertension and cardiac disease in patients on hemodialysis, *Nephrol Nurs J* 31(6):631, 2004.
10. Subramanian S, Ziedalski TM: Oliguria, volume overload, Na^+ balance, and diuretics, *Crit Care Clin* 21(20):291, 2005.
11. Robinson BE, Weber H: Dehydration despite drinking: beyond the BUN/creatinine ratio, *J Am Med Dir Assoc* 5(2 suppl):S67, 2004.
12. Kee J: *Handbook of laboratory & diagnostic tests with nursing implications,* ed 5, Upper Saddle River, NJ, 2005, Pearson Prentice-Hall.
13. Thomas DR et al: Physician misdiagnosis of dehydration in older adults, *J Am Med Dir Assoc* 5(2 suppl):S30, 2004.
14. Miller D et al: Challenges for nephrology nurses in the management of children with chronic kidney disease, *Nephrol Nurs J* 31(3):287, 2004.
15. Simonson M: Measurement of glomerular filtration rate. In Hricik DE et al, editors: *Nephrology secrets,* ed 2, Philadelphia, 2003, Hanley & Belfus.
16. Ganz M: Urinalysis. In Hricik DE et al, editors: *Nephrology secrets,* ed 2, Philadelphia, 2003, Hanley & Belfus.
17. Hanson K: Laboratory studies in the evaluation of urologic disease, part I, *Urol Nurs* 23(6):400, 2004.
18. Simonson M: Measurement of urinary protein. In Hricik DE et al, editors: *Nephrology secrets,* ed 2, Philadelphia, 2003, Hanley & Belfus.
19. Russell T: Acute renal failure related to rhabdomyolysis: pathophysiology, diagnosis, and collaborative management, *Nephrol Nurs J* 27(5):567, 2000.
20. Hanson K: Diagnostic tests and tools in the evaluation of urologic disease, part II, *Urol Nurs* 23(6):405, 2004.
21. Elashi E et al: Renal imaging techniques. In Hricik DE et al, editors: *Nephrology secrets,* ed 2, Philadelphia, 2003, Hanley & Belfus.

CHAPTER

20 Renal Disorders and Therapeutic Management

MARY E. LOUGH

OBJECTIVES

- List the etiologies of acute renal failure.
- Describe the stages of acute tubular necrosis.
- Identify the priorities of nursing management in acute renal failure.
- Discuss the differences among hemodialysis, peritoneal dialysis, and continuous renal replacement therapy.
- Explain the differences between a living and cadaver kidney donor.
- Describe the priorities of postoperative management following kidney transplantation.

ACUTE RENAL FAILURE

Acute renal failure (ARF) is characterized by a sudden decline in glomerular filtration rate (GFR), with subsequent retention of products in the blood that are normally excreted by the kidneys; this disrupts electrolyte balance, acid-base homeostasis, and fluid volume equilibrium.

CRITICAL ILLNESS AND ARF

Once ARF has occurred in the critically ill patient, the risk of death rises dramatically.[1] Mortality ranges from 38% to 80%.[2] One of the reasons for the high mortality is that critical care patients often have coexisting nonrenal health problems that increase their susceptibility to the development of ARF. High-risk conditions include heart failure, shock, respiratory failure, and sepsis.[1,2] The increasing number of comorbid conditions found in critically ill patients is changing the spectrum of acute renal failure. A recent observational study that examined the incidence and course of ARF in six academic medical centers in the United States found that acute renal failure was accompanied by extrarenal organ failure in most patients, even those who did not require dialysis.[1] In this study of 618 patients with ARF, 64% of patients required dialysis, the in-hospital mortality was 37%, and the rate of nonrecovery of the kidney and/or death was 50%.[1] The clinicians' conclusion is that mortality in the critically ill patient with ARF is related to the severity of the extrarenal disease.[1] Mortality rates exceeded 50% when four or more systems had failed.[1]

The high mortality related to ARF has not changed for over four decades in spite of increasingly complex technologies to treat acute renal failure.[1] One could argue that today patients with acute renal failure often have associated multiple organ dysfunction syndrome (MODS) and have more complex illnesses and comorbidities compared with patients 40 years ago. More critical care patients are receiving dialysis therapies in the critical care unit.[1]

Typically a patient is not admitted to the critical care unit with a diagnosis of acute renal failure alone; there is always coexisting hemodynamic, cardiac, pulmonary, or neurologic compromise. Many individuals come into the hospital with preexisting renal insufficiency (elevated serum creatinine level), although they may be nonsymptomatic and unaware of their renal compromise.[3] This lack of renal reserve places them at increased risk of acute renal failure should complications occur in any of the other major organ systems. As a result, the picture of acute renal failure in the modern critical care unit has changed to encompass patients with renal failure who also have multisystem nonrenal diseases that complicate their clinical course.[1]

DEFINITION OF ARF

At this time there is no standardized definition of acute renal failure that may be applied to the critically ill.[4] Some researchers suggest that ARF be described according to whether it was community- or hospital-acquired, or by the speed of the rise of the serum creatinine level.[2] Others focus on the etiology of the

Box 20-1

Etiologies of Acute Renal Failure

Prerenal
Prolonged hypotension (sepsis, vasodilation)
Prolonged low cardiac output (heart failure, cardiogenic shock)
Prolonged volume depletion (dehydration, hemorrhage)
Renovascular thrombosis (thromboemboli)

Intrarenal
Renal ischemia (advanced stage of prerenal failure)
Endogenous toxins (rhabdomyolysis, tumor lysis syndrome)
Exogenous toxins: (radiocontrast dye, nephrotoxic drugs)
Infection (acute glomerulonephritis, interstitial nephritis)

Postrenal
Obstruction (urethra/prostate/bladder)
Rare to be cause of ARF in critical care

acute renal failure.[1] For the purposes of understanding the etiology of acute renal dysfunction in this chapter, ARF is classified into three categories according to location of the insult relative to the kidney: prerenal, intrarenal, and postrenal (Box 20-1).

Prerenal ARF

Any condition that decreases blood flow, blood pressure (BP), or renal perfusion before arterial blood reaches the kidney can cause prerenal failure. When renal hypoperfusion due to low cardiac output, hemorrhage, vasodilation, thrombosis, or other cause reduces the blood flow to the kidney, glomerular filtration decreases and consequently urine output decreases (see Box 20-1). This is a major reason that the critical care nurse monitors the urine output on an hourly basis. Initially, in prerenal states the integrity of the kidney's nephron structure and function is preserved. If normal perfusion and cardiac output are restored quickly, the kidney will not suffer any permanent injury. However, if the prerenal insult is not corrected, the GFR will decline, the blood urea nitrogen (BUN) will rise, and the patient will develop oliguria and risk significant kidney damage. *Oliguria*, or a urine output less than 400 ml/day, is a classic finding in ARF.[2] Prerenal ARF is seen frequently in the critically ill. In a study of hospitalized elderly patients with renal failure, prerenal ARF occurred in 58% of the patients.[2] This compares with 34% intrarenal and 8% postrenal causes in the same study.[2]

Intrarenal ARF

Any condition that produces an ischemic or toxic insult directly at the site of the nephron places the patient at risk for development of intrarenal failure (see Box 20-1). Ischemic damage may be caused by prolonged hypotension or low cardiac output. Toxic injury reaction may occur in response to substances that damage the renal tubular endothelium such as some antimicrobial drugs and the contrast dye used in radiology diagnostic studies. The insult may involve both the glomeruli and the tubular epithelium. When the internal filtering structures are affected, this is known as *acute tubular necrosis (ATN)*.[5]

Postrenal ARF

Any obstruction that hinders the flow of urine from beyond the kidney through the remainder of the urinary tract may lead to postrenal failure. This is not a frequent cause of kidney failure in the critically ill. When monitoring of the urine output reveals a sudden decrease in the patient's urine output from the urinary catheter, a blockage may be responsible. Sudden development of *anuria* (urine output below 100 ml/24 hr) should prompt verification that the urinary catheter is not occluded.

Azotemia

The term *azotemia* is used to describe an acute rise in BUN. *Uremia* is another term used to describe an elevated BUN.

ACUTE TUBULAR NECROSIS

ATN results from either nephrotoxic or ischemic injury that damages the renal tubular epithelium and, in severe cases, extends to the basement membrane. Injury that is limited to the epithelial layer recovers sooner than injury that also involves the basement membrane. Over 90% of episodes of acute renal failure are due to ATN as result of toxic and or ischemia exposure.[5]

Epidemiology and Etiology

Damage to the cells in the glomerular and tubular structures prevents normal concentration of urine, filtration of wastes, and regulation of acid-base, electrolyte, and water balance. The renal tubular cells are constantly at risk for damage because of their normally high blood flows, high oxygen requirements, and the constant resorption and secretion of metabolites. A number of disorders can result in ATN, and several contributing factors often work together to bring about tubular damage. Common causes of ATN are divided into two categories: ischemic injury and nephrotoxic injury (Box 20-2).

Ischemic Acute Tubular Necrosis

Ischemic damage secondary to inadequate perfusion impairs tubular endothelial function, causing nonuni-

Box 20-2

Ischemic Versus Nephrotoxic Acute Tubular Necrosis

Ischemic Injury
Advanced stage of prerenal injury
Massive hemorrhage
Severe volume loss
Severe dehydration
Severe, prolonged hypotension
Shock: cardiogenic, hypovolemic, septic
Sepsis
Anaphylaxis

Nephrotoxic Injury
Endogenous Toxins*
Rhabdomyolysis
Tumor lysis syndrome

Exogenous Toxins*
Radiocontrast dye

Nephrotoxic Antimicrobials
Aminoglycosides: gentamicin, tobramycin
Cephalosporins: cefazolin
Antifungals: amphotericin B
Antivirals: acyclovir

Nephrotoxic Immunosuppressants
Cyclosporin
Tacrolimus (FK506)

Nephrotoxic Chemotherapeutics
5-Azacitidine
Cisplatin
Methotrexate

Nephrotoxic Street Drugs
Heroin
Amphetamines
Phencyclidine (PCP)

Nephrotoxic Analgesics
Nonsteroidal antiinflammatory drugs (NSAIDs)

*Only represents a partial list of potential nephrotoxic medications.

form patchy areas of tubular cell damage and cast formation. Ischemic necrosis occurs as a result of vasodilation associated with sepsis and when hypotension or a low-cardiac-output episode is prolonged; it is worsened by renal hypoperfusion or dehydration. In other words, prerenal low perfusion can develop into intrarenal ischemic ATN (see Box 20-2). In the multicenter study of critical care patients with ARF by Mehta et al,[1] 50% of the patients had ischemic ATN, which was largely precipitated by hypotension (20%) and sepsis (19%).

Toxic Acute Tubular Necrosis

Nephrotoxic damage results from damage by drugs and chemical agents. A common cause of toxic ATN is the radiopaque (contrast) dye administered during an interventional or diagnostic radiologic study. Complications from the contrast will cause ARF in 9% to 14% of patients.[1,6] In affected patients, the serum creatinine levels typically begin to rise 48 to 72 hours after the study, peak at 3 to 5 days, and return to baseline within another 3 to 5 days.[6] The renal dysfunction can persist up to 3 weeks after the procedure. Although patients with normal renal function are not considered to be at risk, those with elevated serum creatinine levels, diabetes, or microvascular disease are highly vulnerable.[6]

Toxic damage causes uniform, widespread injury to the renal endothelium. Because the basement membrane is not injured as severely as with ischemic ATN, the healing is more rapid, the layer of the membrane can regenerate, and full recovery from ATN and resumption of renal function is more likely (see Box 20-2).

Pathophysiology

The mechanisms responsible for tubular dysfunction in ischemic ATN are multifactorial. When "cellular debris" accumulates in the nephron tubular lumen, an obstruction will occur if there is not adequate flow of filtrate through the nephron. The obstruction is made up of casts and sloughing tissue and is exacerbated by interstitial edema. Filtration ceases when tubular hydrostatic pressure rises to match GFR. This decreases the formation of urine because of the lack of filtrate to process. The result is more tubular cell swelling, obstruction, decreased capillary blood flow, and finally, further ischemia and cell injury. The clinical course of ATN progresses through four phases.

Phases of Acute Tubular Necrosis

Onset Phase

The onset (initiating) phase is the period from when an insult occurs until cell injury. Ischemic injury is evolving during this time. The GFR is decreased because of impaired renal blood flow and decreased glomerular ultrafiltration pressure. This disrupts the integrity of the tubular epithelium, which back-leaks the glomerular filtrate. This phase lasts from hours to days, depending on the cause, with toxic factors causing the phase to last longer. If treatment is initiated during this time, irreversible damage can be alleviated. A longer course of recovery reflects the presence of more extensive tubular injury.

Oliguric/Anuric Phase

The oliguric/anuric phase, the second phase of ATN, lasts 5 to 8 days in the nonoliguric patient and 10 to 16 days in the oliguric patient.[7] The accumulation of necrotic cellular debris in the tubular space blocks the flow of urine and causes damage to the tubular wall

Table 20-1

Initial Urine Laboratory Analysis Findings in Acute Renal Failure*

	PRERENAL†	INTRARENAL‡	POSTRENAL§
Urine volume	Normal	Oliguria or nonoliguria	Oliguria to anuria
Urine specific gravity	>1.020	1.010	1.000-1.010
Urine osmolality (mOsm/kg)	>350	<300	300-400
Urine sodium (mEq/L)	<20	>30	20-40
FENa (%)	<1	>2-3	1-3
BUN/Cr ratio	20:1	Ischemic: 20:1 Toxic: 10:1	10:1
Urine microscopy (sediment)	Normal	ATN: dark granular casts, hyaline casts, renal epithelial cells	Normal

*Results of urine laboratory tests are only valid in the absence of diuretics.
†Urine in prerenal failure is concentrated, with low sodium.
‡Urine in intrarenal failure shows kidney damage because the nephron cannot concentrate urine or conserve sodium, and evidence of renal damage (casts) is seen.
§Urine test results in postrenal failure are variable, because initially the findings depend on the hydration status of the patient rather than the status of the kidney.
Oliguria, Urine volume 100 to 400 ml/24 hr; *anuria,* urine volume less than 100 ml/24 hr; *FENa,* fractional excretion of sodium; *BUN,* blood urea nitrogen; *Cr,* creatinine; *ATN,* acute tubular necrosis.

and basement membranes. Also, a back-leak phenomenon occurs because damage in the tubular wall causes the glomerular filtrate to flow passively into the renal tissue rather than be passed out as urine through the ureters and bladder. Oliguria is encountered more often in ischemic damage and is a sign that the damage is more extensive and severe. During the oliguric/anuric phase, GFR is greatly reduced, which leads to increased levels of BUN (azotemia), elevated serum creatinine levels, electrolyte abnormalities (hyperkalemia, hyperphosphatemia, hypocalcemia), and metabolic acidosis.

Diuretic Phase

The third phase, the diuretic phase, lasts 7 to 14 days and is characterized by an increase in GFR and sometimes polyuria with a urine output as high as 2 to 4 L/day. If the patient is receiving hemodialysis during this phase, the polyuria will not be evident because excess volume will be removed by dialysis. During the diuretic phase the tubular obstruction has passed, but edema and scarring are present. In this situation, the GFR returns before the ability of the tubules to function normally and the kidney can remove volume but not solutes.

Recovery Phase

The last phase of ATN is the recovery, or convalescent, phase. Both oliguric and nonoliguric patients will demonstrate increased urine output if they enter the recovery stage. During this stage, renal function slowly returns to normal or near normal, with a GFR that is 70% to 80% of normal within 1 to 2 years.[8] However, if significant renal parenchymal damage has occurred, BUN and creatinine levels may never return to normal. For patients surviving ATN, approximately 62% will recover normal renal function, 33% will be left with residual renal insufficiency, and at least 5% will require long-term hemodialysis.[8]

Table 20-2

Normal Serum Electrolyte Values

ELECTROLYTE	NORMAL VALUE
Sodium	135-145 mEq/L
Potassium	3.5-4.5 mEq/L
Chloride	98-108 mEq/L
Calcium	8.5-10.5 mg/dl *or* 4.5-5.8 mEq/L
Phosphorus	2.7-4.5 mg/dl
Magnesium	1.5-2.5 mEq/L
Bicarbonate	24-28 mEq/L

ASSESSMENT AND DIAGNOSIS

Laboratory Assessment

Once acute renal disease is suspected, the presence or degree or renal dysfunction is assessed by blood serum analysis and less frequently by urinalysis. Table 20-1 lists the range of initial urinalysis findings in ARF; note if the patient has received diuretics, the urine values are affected by the forced diuresis and are not considered reliable for diagnostic purposes. Table 20-2 lists the normal serum electrolyte values. Serum electrolyte derangements occur as ARF develops, particularly elevated levels of potassium and phosphate. Electrolyte changes also occur consequent to other disease states, and clinical signs associated with specific electrolyte abnormalities are listed in Table 20-3.

Acidosis

Acidosis (pH below 7.5) is one of the trademarks of acute renal failure.[9] Metabolic acidosis occurs as a result of the accumulation of unexcreted waste products.

Table 20-3
Serum Electrolytes in Acute Renal Failure

ELECTROLYTE DISTURBANCE	SERUM VALUE	CLINICAL FINDINGS
Potassium		
Hypokalemia	<3.5 mEq/L	Muscular weakness Cardiac irregularities on ECG Abdominal distention and flatulence Paresthesia Decreased reflexes Anorexia Dizziness, confusion Increased sensitivity to digitalis
Hyperkalemia	>4.5 mEq/L	Irritability and restlessness Anxiety Nausea and vomiting Abdominal cramps Weakness Numbness and tingling (fingertips and circumoral) Cardiac irregularities on ECG
Sodium		
Hyponatremia	<135 mEq/L	Disorientation Muscle twitching Nausea/vomiting, abdominal cramps Headaches, dizziness Seizures, postural hypotension Cold, clammy skin Decreased skin turgor Tachycardia Oliguria
Hypernatremia	>145 mEq/L	Extreme thirst Dry, sticky mucous membranes Altered mentation Seizures (later stages)
Calcium		
Hypocalcemia	<8.5 mg/dl *or* <4.5 mEq/L	Irritability Muscular tetany, muscle cramps Decreased cardiac output (decreased contractions) Bleeding (decreased ability to coagulate) ECG changes Positive Chvostek's/Trousseau's signs
Hypercalcemia	>10.5 mg/dl *or* >5.8 mEq/L	Deep bone pain Excessive thirst Anorexia Lethargy, weakened muscles
Magnesium		
Hypomagnesemia	<1.5 mEq/L	Choroid/athetoid muscle activity Facial tics, spasticity Cardiac dysrhythmias
Hypermagnesemia	>2.5 mEq/L	CNS depression Respiratory depression Lethargy Coma Bradycardia ECG changes
Phosphate		
Hypophosphatemia	<2.7 mg/dl	Hemolytic anemias Depressed white cell function Bleeding (decreased platelet aggregation) Nausea/vomiting Anorexia
Hyperphosphatemia	>4.5 mg/dl	Tachycardia Nausea, diarrhea, abdominal cramps Muscle weakness, flaccid paralysis Increased reflexes
Chloride		
Hypochloremia	<98 mEq/L	Hyperirritability Tetany or muscular excitability Slow respirations
Hyperchloremia	>108 mEq/L	Weakness, lethargy Deep, rapid breathing Possible unconsciousness (later stages)

ECG, Electrocardiogram; *CNS,* central nervous system.

The acid waste products consist of strong negative ions (anions), elevated serum phosphorus (hyperphosphatemia), and other normally "unmeasured ions" (sulfate, urate, lactate, and others) that decrease the serum pH.[9] A low serum albumin level, often present in ARF, has a slight alkalinizing effect, but not enough to offset the metabolic acidosis.[9] Even though respiratory compensation may be present, or the patient may receive mechanical ventilatory support, this is rarely sufficient to reverse the metabolic acidosis.

Blood Urea Nitrogen

BUN is not a reliable indicator of kidney damage.[10] Although it reflects cellular damage, BUN is easily changed by protein intake, blood in the gastrointestinal (GI) tract, and cell catabolism and is diluted by fluid administration. A BUN/creatinine ratio may be calculated to determine the cause of the acute renal dysfunction (see Table 20-1). The BUN/creatinine ratio is most useful in diagnosing prerenal failure (often described as prerenal azotemia) where the BUN level is greatly elevated relative to the serum creatinine value.

Serum Creatinine

Creatinine is a by-product of muscle metabolism that is formed from nonenzymatic dehydration of creatine in the liver[10]; 98% of creatine is in the muscles,[10] and it is almost totally excreted by the renal tubules. Thus, if the kidneys are not working, the creatinine level will rise in the serum. When the serum creatinine level doubles (for example from 0.75 to 1.5 mg/dl), this reflects a decrease of approximately 50% in the GFR.[10] Serum creatinine level is assessed daily to follow the trend of renal function and answer the question, is kidney function stable, getting better, or getting worse?[10]

Creatinine Clearance

If the patient is making sufficient urine, the urinary creatinine clearance can be measured. A normal urine creatinine clearance is 120 ml/min, but this value decreases with renal failure. Critical care patients in ARF are oliguric, and the urine creatinine clearance is infrequently measured.

Fractional Excretion of Sodium

The fractional excretion of sodium (FENa) in the urine is measured early in the ARF course to differentiate between a prerenal condition and ATN (intrarenal). A FENa value below 1% (in the absence of diuretics) suggests prerenal compromise, because resorption of almost all the filtered sodium is an appropriate response to decreased renal perfusion. If diuretics are administered, the test is meaningless. A FENa value above 2% implies the kidney cannot concentrate the sodium and that the damage is intrarenal (ATN).

Urinary Sodium

Urinary sodium is measured in milliequivalents per liter (mEq/L). The interpretation of results is similar to the FENa. For example, urinary sodium less than 10 mEq/L (low) indicates a prerenal condition. Urinary sodium greater than 40 mEq/L (high) suggests an intrarenal cause (see Table 20-1). As with other urinalysis tests, the use of diuretics invalidates any results. This is because the diuretics alter resorption of water and produce dilute urine and the test result will not reflect actual kidney function.

Radiologic Findings

A computed tomography (CT) scan of the abdomen is useful to evaluate the anatomic status of the kidney in the critically ill. Angiography is used more cautiously because of the association between use of contrast media and nephrotoxic renal failure.[6]

"AT RISK" DISEASE STATES AND ACUTE RENAL FAILURE

Many patients come into the critical care unit with disease states that predispose them to the development of acute renal failure. There are also many individuals who already have kidney damage but are unaware of this condition.[3]

Underlying Chronic Kidney Disease

The incidence of chronic kidney disease (CKD) in United States is estimated to be 11% (19.2 million adults).[11] Recent clinical practice guidelines for management of end-stage kidney disease (ESKD) have classified renal dysfunction into five stages.[12] Because of the large numbers of adults with renal dysfunction (diagnosed or not), kidney function must be assessed on all critically ill patients at risk for fluid and electrolyte imbalance. The glomerular filtration rate associated with each stage and the numeric population estimates in each stage of kidney dysfunction are shown in Table 20-4.

Most people in the early stages of renal disease are unaware of their condition.[3] A national health survey queried individuals whether they had ever been told by their physician that they had "weak or failing kidneys." The answer to this question was then correlated with the individual's GFR and the presence of albuminuria by urine test to stratify them according to the five stages of kidney failure (see Table 20-4). The results showed that over half the respondents were unaware that they had kidney dysfunction until they reached stage 5 or end-stage kidney disease when they would become dialysis dependent.[3] The results categorized by stage of kidney failure are listed in Table 20-4.

Risk of Acute Renal Failure

A classification to determine risk of developing acute renal failure in critically ill patients has been proposed by a multinational group of nephrologists.[13] The classification uses the acronym *RIFLE: r*isk, *i*njury, *f*ailure, *l*oss, and *E*SKD (end-stage kidney disease).[13] The RIFLE system classifies patients into categories of risk, based on GFR criteria, urine output, or previous

Table 20-4

Decreased Kidney Function by Stage in Adult U.S. Population

STAGE*	POPULATION AFFECTED*	GFR† AND DIAGNOSIS*	PERCENT WHO KNOW THEY HAVE KIDNEY DYSFUNCTION (%)‡
1	9 million (3.3%)	Normal; persistent albuminuria	40.5
2	5.3 million (3.0%)	60 to 89; persistent albuminuria	29.3
3	7.6 million (4.3%)	30 to 59	22.0
4	400,000 (0.2%)	15 to 29	44.5
5	300,000 (0.2%)	Below 15; end-stage kidney disease	100

*Data from Coresh J et al: *Am J Kidney Dis* 41(1):1, 2003.
†Glomerular filtration rate (GFR) in ml/min /1.73 m^2 body surface area.
‡Data from Nickolas TL et al: *Am J Kidney Dis* 44(2):185, 2004.

Table 20-5

RIFLE Criteria for Acute Renal Dysfunction

RIFLE	SERUM CR/GFR CRITERIA	URINE OUTPUT CRITERIA
*R*isk	Serum Cr increased 1.5 times above normal ***or*** GFR decreased more than 25%	<0.5 ml/kg/hr for 6 hours
*I*njury	Serum Cr increased 2 times above normal ***or*** GFR decreased more than 50%	<0.5 ml/kg/hr for 12 hours
*F*ailure	Serum Cr increased 3 times above normal ***or*** GFR decreased more than 75% ***or*** Serum Cr ≥ 4 mg/dl ***or*** Serum Cr acute rise ≥ 0.5 mg/dl	<0.3 ml/kg/hr for 24 hours ***or*** anuria for 12 hours
*L*oss	Persistent acute renal failure (ARF); complete loss of kidney function for more than 4 weeks	
*E*SKD	End-stage kidney disease for >3 months	

Data from Bellomo R et al: *Crit Care* 8(4):R204, 2004.
Cr, Creatinine; *GFR,* glomerular filtration rate; *anuria,* urine volume less than 100 ml/24 hr.

loss of renal function[13] (Table 20-5). If acute renal failure is superimposed on a kidney that is already compromised, the researchers recommend adding the term chronic to the RIFLE criteria to denote an "acute-on-chronic" renal failure etiology.[13]

Older Age and ARF

Older age appears to be a risk factor for development of chronic kidney disease, because 11% of individuals older than 65 years *without* hypertension or diabetes have stage 3 or worse CKD.[11] In the presence of diabetes or hypertension, the risk of developing chronic kidney disease increases substantially.

Heart Failure And ARF

There is a strong association between kidney failure and cardiovascular disease. In studies of critically ill patients with acute renal failure, 54%[1] to 63%[2] have both acute renal failure and heart failure. Hypertension, a major contributor to the development of heart failure, is also a major risk factor for the development of CKD.[14] Unfortunately, the presence of hypertension and diabetes predisposes an individual to development of chronic kidney disease and exposes him or her to a higher risk of death.[11,15-17] As the patient's GFR declines, the risks of cardiovascular disease, myocardial infarction, and death increase, especially for patients with stage 3 or worse CKD.[18,19]

Respiratory Failure and ARF

There is a significant association between respiratory failure and kidney failure. In studies of critically ill patients with renal failure, 54% to 88% have respiratory failure.[1-2] The range in values is due to how the renal failure was classified. For example, in one study 57% have respiratory and renal failure but were not treated with dialysis,[1] and 88% have respiratory and renal failure and were given dialysis treatment with continuous renal replacement therapy (CRRT).[2] (See later section for a description of CRRT.) Prolonged mechanical ventilation in critically ill patients is associated with an increased incidence of acute renal failure.[20,21]

Sepsis and ARF

Sepsis and septic shock create hemodynamic instability and decrease renal perfusion.[21,22] The mechanism is presumed to be prerenal. Sepsis caused 19% of ARF in one study[1] and 55% of ARF in a population of elderly hospitalized patients.[2] Clinical guidelines for hemodynamic support in sepsis emphasize the need for adequate fluid resuscitation, because in 40% to 50% of cases reversal of hypotension and restoration of hemodynamic stability can be achieved with fluids alone.[22] Unfortunately, in severely septic patients, inflammation increases vascular permeability and much of this fluid may move into the third space (interstitial space).[22] If the BP remains low, the use of vasopressors is recommended to raise refractory low BP. Vasopressors raise BP, increase systemic vascular resistance (SVR), and presumably also increase intrarenal vascular re-sistance. Other practices aimed at reversing the deleterious effects of sepsis include maintaining the patient's hemoglobin level over 8 mg/dl and achieving a pulmonary artery occlusion pressure (PAOP), or wedge pressure, between 12 and 15 mm Hg.[22]

Trauma and ARF

Trauma patients with major crush injuries have an elevated risk of kidney failure because of the release of creatine and myoglobin from damaged muscle cells.[23] Myoglobin in large quantities is toxic to the kidney. Overall survival from rhabdomyolysis is 77%.[23]

Creatine kinase (CK), a marker of systemic muscle damage, will rise with rhabdomyolysis. One trauma service reported that out of 2,083 critical care trauma admissions, 85% had elevated CK levels and 10% developed acute renal failure secondary to rhabdomyolysis.[24] A CK level of 5000 units/L was the lowest abnormal value present in patients who developed ARF associated with rhabdomyolysis.[24]

Volume resuscitation is the primary treatment to preserve adequate kidney function and prevent development of acute renal failure. In many hospitals the intravenous (IV) fluids are alkalinized by the addition of sodium bicarbonate, and the urine output is increased by IV administration of the diuretic mannitol.[23] A bicarbonate/mannitol regimen is utilized to try to prevent acidosis and hyperkalemia, both frequent complications of rhabdomyolysis. Close attention is paid to urine output, CK, any rise in serum creatinine level, and any signs of compartment syndrome in all patients admitted with this diagnosis.

Contrast-Induced Nephrotoxic Injury and ARF

Over 1 million diagnostic studies or interventional procedures that involve use of IV radiocontrast are performed every year.[6] Approximately 1% of those patients will require dialysis as a result of contrast-induced nephrotoxicity, with prolongation of the hospital stay to an average of 17 days.[6] Patients at risk are those with a baseline serum creatinine level over 1.5 mg/dl, known diabetes, heart failure, or volume depletion.[25] A clinical definition of contrast-induced nephrotoxicity is a rise in serum creatinine level of 0.5 mg/dl or more, or a 25% rise from the patient's baseline, within 48 to 72 hours of contrast medium exposure.[6,25] High- molecular-weight contrast medium is a potential cause of nephrotoxicity.[6,26] One strategy to prevent contrast-induced nephrotoxicity involves use of a lower quantity of contrast per study and use of nonionic, low-osmolar or isoosmolar (iohexol) contrast media that are less nephrotoxic.[26] Research studies are still needed to determine how to avoid this complication. The best method of prevention is aggressive hydration with IV normal saline both during and after the procedure.[5] Research results are mixed on the use of the oral drug N-acetylcysteine (NAC),[27-29] and IV infusions of dopamine and fenoldopam are described as neutral—neither beneficial nor harmful.[5,6,27] Patients undergoing radiologic studies with contrast represent a major at-risk population, and more research on the optimal treatment strategy is required to prevent contrast-induced nephrotoxicity.[5]

Hemodynamic Monitoring and Fluid Balance

Hemodynamic monitoring is important for the analysis of fluid volume status in the critically ill patient with ARF.

Hemodynamic Monitoring

Hemodynamic monitoring includes surveillance of central venous pressure (CVP), PAOP, cardiac output (CO), and cardiac index (CI).

Daily Weight

Less "high-tech" but also important is a daily weight and focused physical assessment.[30] The "daily weight," combined with accurate "intake and output" monitoring, is a powerful indicator of fluid gains or losses over 24 hours. A 1-kg weight gain over 24 hours represents 1000 ml of additional fluid retention.

Physical Assessment

Physical assessment signs and symptoms are used to assess fluid balance. Signs that suggest extracellular fluid (ECF) depletion include thirst, decreased skin turgor, and lethargy. Signs that imply intravascular fluid volume overload include pulmonary congestion, increasing heart failure, and rising blood pressure. The patient with untreated ARF is edematous. Several factors contribute to this state:

1. Fluid is retained because of the inadequate urine output.
2. Low serum albumin creates a lower oncotic pressure in the vasculature, and more fluid seeps

out into the interstitial spaces as peripheral edema.

3. Inflammation associated with ARF or a coexisting nonrenal disease increases vascular permeability to the movement of water into the tissues.

In critical illness, even though there is peripheral edema, and the patient may have gained 8 L over his or her "dry-weight" baseline, the patient may remain "intravascularly dry" and hemodynamically unstable. This is because the retained fluid is not inside a vascular compartment and thus cannot contribute to maintenance of hemodynamic stability. The patient in ARF is assessed frequently for pitting edema over bony prominences and in dependent body areas.

Electrolyte Balance

Potassium

Electrolyte levels require frequent observation, especially in the critical phases of renal failure (see Table 20-3). Potassium may quickly reach levels of 6.0 mEq/L and above. Specific electrocardiogram (ECG) changes are associated with hyperkalemia, specifically peaked T waves, a widening of the QRS interval, and ultimately, ventricular tachycardia or fibrillation. If hyperkalemia is present, all potassium supplements are stopped.[31] If the patient is producing urine, IV diuretics can be administered. Acute hyperkalemia can be treated temporarily by IV administration of insulin and glucose. An infusion of 50 ml of 50% dextrose accompanied by 10 units of regular insulin forces potassium out of the serum and into the cells.

Finally, sodium polystyrene sulfonate (Kayexalate), a cation-exchange resin, is mixed in water and sorbitol and given orally, rectally, or through a nasogastric (NG) tube. The resin binds potassium in the bowel, which eliminates it in the feces. Kayexalate and dialysis are the only permanent methods of potassium removal.[31]

Sodium

Dilutional hyponatremia, associated with renal failure, is an expected finding (see Table 20-3). It can be corrected over a few days with fluid restriction. More rapidly, sodium levels may be raised during dialysis by changing the amount of sodium in the dialysate bath.

Calcium and Phosphorus

Serum calcium levels are reduced *(hypocalcemia)* in renal failure (see Table 20-3). This reduction results from multiple factors, including *hyperphosphatemia*. Chronically elevated serum phosphorus levels (greater than 5.5 to 6.5 mEq/L) are associated with higher mortality in renal failure.[12,32] At the renal level, calcium and phosphorus are regulated in part by parathyroid hormone (PTH). Normally, PTH helps calcium be resorbed back into the bloodstream at the proximal tubule and distal nephron and promotes excretion of phosphorus by the kidney to maintain homeostasis. In renal failure this mechanism is nonfunctional; thus the serum phosphorus level rises in the bloodstream, and the serum calcium level falls.

Calcium Replacement

Most calcium in the bloodstream is bound to protein. This can be measured as a total serum calcium level. The metabolically active, non–protein-bound portion is known as the *ionized calcium*. Without adequate levels of serum calcium, a compensatory mechanism "steals" calcium from the bones, making the patient with kidney failure more vulnerable to fractures.[33] Maintaining adequate calcium stores in the body is important and is achieved by administration of calcium supplements, vitamin D preparations, and synthetic calcitriol.

Dietary-Phosphorus–Binding Drugs

A second method used in tandem with calcium supplements to achieve normal calcium levels is to lower the level of phosphorus in the bloodstream. Phosphorus occurs in many foods, and to eliminate all phosphorus-containing foods from the diet would make it unpalatable.[34] Foods that contain particularly high levels of phosphorus include dairy products, processed meats, some carbonated drinks, and nuts.[34] Unfortunately, once eaten, free phosphorus passes from the GI tract into the bloodstream and raises the serum level. Medications that bind dietary phosphorus in the GI tract are administered orally or via NG tube. The binding agent must be taken at the same time as a meal.[34] Once the dietary phosphorus is bound to the binding substance in the bowel, it is eliminated from the intestine with stool. This lowers the serum phosphorus level.

The types of dietary-phosphorus binders used have changed over the years. The original binders were aluminum salts (aluminum hydroxide) that bound dietary phosphorus effectively in the GI tract but conferred aluminum toxicity because some of the aluminum metal was also absorbed.[34] For this reason, aluminum binders have largely been abandoned.[34]

The second generation of dietary-phosphorus–binding agents that are most widely prescribed use calcium salts (calcium carbonate; calcium acetate [PhosLo]) to bind dietary phosphorus in the GI tract. Calcium-based drugs are safer, but elevated serum calcium levels and calcium deposits in other areas of the body (extraosseous calcification) are a problem.[34]

A third generation of dietary-phosphorus–binding medications has recently become available. These medications are not aluminum or calcium based.

They include sevelamer hydrochloride (Renagel) and lanthanum carbonate (Fosrenol).[34]

Medical Management

Treatment goals for patients experiencing ARF focus on prevention, compensation for the deterioration of renal function, and regeneration of the remaining kidney functional capacity. Over the past four decades, mortality from acute renal failure has remained at more than 50%.[1,2] Key areas that are evaluated include prevention strategies, fluid balance, anemia, medications, and electrolyte imbalance.

Prevention

The only truly effective remedy for ARF is prevention.[5] For effective prevention the patient's risk for development of ARF must be assessed. Knowledge of the most frequent causes of ARF in the critically ill is essential if prevention strategies are to be enacted. The critical care team collaborates closely with the clinical pharmacist to avoid drugs with nephrotoxic side effects in patients with renal insufficiency or chronic kidney disease.[11,12] Nonsteroidal antiinflammatory drugs (NSAIDs) for pain relief are avoided in patients with elevated creatinine level, those taking antibiotics, or those recovering from major surgery.[35] The use of intravascular contrast dye is delayed until the patient is fully rehydrated.[5,6]

Fluid Resuscitation

Prerenal failure is caused by decreased perfusion and flow to the kidney. It is often associated with trauma, hemorrhage, hypotension, and major fluid losses. If contrast dye is used, aggressive fluid resuscitation with 0.9% normal saline (NaCl) is recommended.[5,6] Fluid replacement is the only treatment shown to prevent renal tubular injury.[36] The objectives of volume replacement are to replace fluid and electrolyte losses and to prevent ongoing loss. Maintenance IV fluid therapy is initiated when oral (PO) fluid intake is inadvisable. Maintenance fluids are calculated with consideration for individual body surface area. Adults require approximately 1500 $ml/m^2/24$ hr; fever, burns, and trauma significantly increase fluid requirements. Other important criteria when calculating fluid volume replacement include baseline metabolism, environmental temperature, and humidity. The rate of replacement depends on cardiopulmonary reserve, adequacy of renal function, urine output, fluid balance, ongoing loss, and type of fluid replaced.

Crystalloids and Colloids

Crystalloids and colloids refer to two different types of IV fluids used for volume management in critically ill patients. These IV solutions are used on all types of patients, not just those with acute renal failure. Which IV fluid to select to most successfully resuscitate hemodynamically unstable patients has been a controversial topic in critical care. The major debate centers on the differences between crystalloid versus colloid solutions.

Crystalloids. Crystalloid solutions, which are balanced salt solutions, are in widespread use for both maintenance infusion and replacement therapy. Crystalloid fluids include normal saline solution (0.9% NaCl), half-strength saline solution (0.45% NaCl), and lactated Ringer's (LR) solution (Table 20-6). LR solution is generally avoided in patients with renal failure because it contains potassium. A noncrystalloid solution that may be infused is dextrose (5% or 10%) in water (D_5W, $D_{10}W$).

Colloids. Colloids are solutions containing oncotically active particles that are used to expand intravascular volume to achieve and maintain hemodynamic stability. Albumin (5% and 25%) and hetastarch are colloid solutions (see Table 20-6). Colloids expand intravascular volume, and the effect can last as long as 24 hours. The goal is to optimize PAOP or "wedge" pressure, raise mean arterial pressure (MAP), and increase CO and the CI to a therapeutic level.

The controversy over resuscitation fluids is not resolved, and some recent research study results have reopened the debate. The SAFE study was a randomized, prospective, double-blind trial that examined whether the selection of resuscitation fluid in the critical care unit affected survival at 28 days. SAFE stands for *s*aline versus *a*lbumin *f*luid *e*valuation.[37] This was a huge study, with almost 7000 critical care patients randomized into two similar groups. One group received 4% albumin, and the other group received 0.9% normal saline (NaCl) for fluid resuscitation.[37] The patients in both groups were very similar in terms of organ dysfunction, mechanical ventilator support (64% of patients), and renal replacement therapy (1% of patients). The SAFE results showed that there was that there was no difference in mortality (death rate), time in the critical care unit, ventilator days, or renal replacement therapy days.[37] The researchers conclude that albumin and saline should be considered clinically equivalent treatments for intravascular volume expansion in critically ill patients.[37]

The findings of the SAFE study investigators have been validated by a meta-analysis of 71 studies that compared albumin with other IV solutions for fluid volume resuscitation.[38] These authors went further and declared that albumin reduces morbidity (complications) in acutely ill hospitalized patients.[38] The authors state that many of the previous studies were flawed because albumin was administered to both the investigational and the control group, thus invalidating many studies.[38] The authors are careful to point out that every patient is an individual, that clinical situations are often unique, and that their findings

Table 20-6
Frequently Used Intravenous Solutions

SOLUTION	ELECTROLYTES	INDICATIONS
Dextrose Solutions		
Dextrose in water (D_5W)—isotonic	None	Maintain volume Replace mild volume loss Provide minimal calories
Crystalloids*		
Normal saline solution (0.9% NaCl)	Sodium 154 mEq/L Chloride 154 mEq/L Osmolality 308 mEq/L	Maintain volume Replace mild loss Correct mild hyponatremia
Half-strength saline solution (0.45% NaCl)	Sodium 77 mEq/L Chloride 77 mEq/L	Free water replacement Correct mild hyponatremia Free water/electrolyte replacement (fluid/electrolyte-restricted conditions)
Lactated Ringer's solution	Sodium 130 mEq/L Potassium 4 mEq/L Calcium 2.7 mEq/L Chloride 107 mEq/L Lactate 27 mEq/L pH 6.5	Fluid and electrolyte replacement (contraindicated for patients with renal or liver disease or in lactic acidosis)
Colloids		
5% Albumin (Albumisol)	Albumin 50 g/L Sodium 130-160 mEq/L Potassium 1 mEq/L Osmolality 300 mOsm/L Osmotic pressure 20 mm Hg pH 6.4 to 7.4	Volume expansion Moderate protein replacement Achievement of hemodynamic stability in shock states
25% Albumin (salt-poor)	Albumin 240 g/L Globulins 10 g/L Sodium 130-160 mEq/L Osmolality 1500 mOsm/L pH 6.4 to 7.4	Concentrated form of albumin sometimes used with diuretics to move fluid from tissues into the vascular space for diuresis
Hetastarch	Sodium 154 mEq/L Chloride 154 mEq/L Osmolality 310 mOsm/L Colloid osmotic pressure 30-35 mm Hg	Synthetic polymer (6% solution) used for volume expansion Hemodynamic volume replacement after cardiac surgery, burns, sepsis
Low-molecular-weight dextran (LMWD)	Glucose polysaccharide molecules with average molecular weight of 40,000; no electrolytes	Volume expansion and support (contraindicated for patients with bleeding disorders)
High-molecular-weight dextran (HMWD)	Glucose polysaccharide molecules with average molecular weight of 70,000; no electrolytes	Used prophylactically in some cases to prevent platelet aggregation; available in either saline or glucose solutions

*For the crystalloid solutions that contain electrolytes, specific concentrations of electrolytes and pH will vary according to the manufacturer.

would not necessarily apply to every clinical situation.[38] Nonetheless, these studies are certain to make clinicians reevaluate the use of both albumin and normal saline as resuscitation fluids for the critically ill patient.

Fluid Restriction. Fluid restriction constitutes a large part of the medical treatment for acute renal failure. Fluid restriction is used to prevent circulatory overload and the development of interstitial edema when the kidneys cannot remove excess volume. The fluid requirements are calculated on the basis of daily urine volumes and insensible losses. Obtaining daily weight measurements and keeping accurate intake and output records are essential. Renal failure patients are usually restricted to 1 L of fluid per 24 hours if urine output is 500 ml or less. Insensible losses range from 500 to 750 ml/day.

Fluid Removal. Acute renal failure promotes increased amounts of water, solutes, and potential toxins into the circulation; thus prompt measures are needed to decrease their levels. Diuretics are used to stimulate the urine output. However, renal replacement therapies (RRTs), either hemodialysis or hemofiltration, are the treatment of choice, particularly if volume overload exacerbates pulmonary and heart failure.

Pharmacologic Management

The first step is to eliminate any nephrotoxic medications. Second, if drugs are eliminated through the kidneys, it is important to decrease the frequency of administration (e.g., from every 6 hours to every 12 hours) or to decrease the dose and to monitor the serum concentration by measuring serum drug levels.[35]

Diuretics

Diuretics are used to stimulate urinary output in the fluid-overloaded patient with functioning kidneys. Care must be taken in their use to avoid the creation of secondary electrolyte abnormalities (Table 20-7). Diuretics are used in many patient populations, not only those with incipient renal failure.

Loop Diuretics. The loop diuretic *furosemide* (Lasix) is the most frequently used diuretic in critical care patients. It may be prescribed as a bolus dose or as a continuous infusion. Electrolytic abnormalities are frequently encountered. Close monitoring of serum potassium, magnesium, and sodium is essential. Although many patients in the ICU receive loop diuretics to reduce volume overload, there is no evidence that they reduce the risk of developing acute renal failure.[5]

Thiazide Diuretics. Diuretics may be prescribed in combination. A thiazide diuretic such as chlorothiazide (Diuril) or metolazone (Zaroxolyn) may be administered followed by a loop diuretic, to take advantage of the fact that these drugs work on different parts of the nephron.

Osmotic Diuretics. Osmotic diuretics (mannitol) are also prescribed to decrease fluid overload and improve urine output. It is important to use an in-line 5-μ filter when administering this drug. Mannitol is frequently prescribed for patients with brain injury and increased intracranial pressure (ICP). There is no firm research evidence that mannitol prevents the development of ARF in the critically ill.[5]

Heart Failure. In patients with heart failure the natriuretic peptides (atrial natriuretic peptide [ANP] and brain natriuretic peptide [BNP]) may be prescribed to increase urine output. These drugs work by stimulating natriuretic receptors in the atrium (ANP) and ventricular myocardium (BNP). In a randomized controlled trial low-dose recombinant ANP has been shown to reduce the development of acute renal failure in cardiac surgical patients.[5] However, ANP has not

Table 20-7
Pharmacologic Management: Renal Drugs

DRUG	DOSAGE	ACTIONS	SPECIAL CONSIDERATIONS
Diuretics			
Loop Diuretics			
Furosemide (Lasix)	20-80 mg/day (Lasix) 0.5-2 mg/day (Bumex)	Acts on loop of Henle to inhibit sodium and chloride	Ototoxicity if administered too rapidly or with other ototoxic drugs Monitor intake/output, hydration, watch for hypotension
Thiazide Diuretics			
Chlorothiazide (Diuril)	500 mg-2 g/day	Inhibit sodium, chloride resorption in distal tubule	Enhanced with low-sodium diet Synergistic effect with loop diuretics
Potassium-Sparing Diuretics			
Aldactone	100 mg/day for 5 days	Exert effects on collecting tubule; reduce potassium, hydrogen and increase sodium	Weak diuretic effect, so given with other diuretics Potassium supplements not required; monitor for hyperkalemia Used as an "aldosterone blocker" to treat heart failure
Osmotic Diuretics			
Mannitol	0.25-2.0 g/kg IV infusion as a 15%-20% solution over 30-90 min	Increases urine output because of increased plasma osmolality, increasing flow of water from tissues Increases sodium, potassium	Often used in head injury to decrease cerebral edema Can be used to promote urinary secretion of toxic substances Use in-line 5-μ IV filter with >20% solutions

IV, Intravenous.

proved to be effective at preventing ARF in other populations.[5]

The potassium-sparing diuretic Aldactone is also used in heart failure as an "aldosterone agonist," not as a diuretic. Most heart failure patients also require significant dosages of loop diuretics. One method of diuresis is to administer 50 ml of IV 25% albumin followed by a loop diuretic. The rationale is that the albumin will pull fluid from the tissues into the bloodstream and the diuretic will increase the water excretion.

Controversies. The use of diuretics continues to be controversial in the critically ill. This is a topic that is under active investigation. Mehta et al[39] published an observational study that showed that once ARF with oliguria was present, loop diuretics increased mortality and delayed kidney recovery in critically ill patients with established ARF. A subsequent study found that furosemide helped maintain urine output but had no more impact on survival and renal recovery than a placebo.[40] Finally, a third research trial found that furosemide (Lasix) neither helped nor worsened ARF in the critically ill.[41] Undoubtedly, the debate and the research studies will continue, but for now it appears that loop diuretics increase the urine output, which makes clinicians feel better, but have no impact on the outcome of oliguric ARF.[5]

Dopamine

Low-dose dopamine (2 to 3 mcg/kg/min), also known as "renal-dose dopamine," is frequently infused to stimulate renal blood flow. Dopamine is effective in increasing urine output in the short term, but dopamine-renal-receptor tolerance to the drug is theorized to develop in the critically ill patients who are most at risk for development of ARF.[42] A meta-analysis of related research studies determined that renal-dose dopamine did not prevent onset of ARF and did not decrease the need for dialysis or reduce mortality.[43] At this point the support for routine use of low-dose dopamine for the prevention of renal failure remains anecdotal only.[44]

Acetylcysteine

N-acetylcysteine (Mucomyst, Mucosil) is an N-acetyl derivative of the amino acid L-cysteine.[5] It has been used for many years as a mucolytic agent to assist with expectoration of thick pulmonary secretions. It is now frequently prescribed for patients with mildly elevated serum creatinine level before a radiology study or procedure involving contrast dye.[5] Acetylcysteine is believed to work directly in the kidney to both vasodilate the tubule and "scavenge" oxygen free radicals. The recommended dosage is 600 mg orally twice a day (morning and evening), on the day before and the day of any procedure that involves administration of IV radiopaque contrast. Research studies of patients undergoing angioplasty have shown a decreased incidence of contrast-induced nephrotoxicity when acetylcysteine plus hydration was used.[5]

Fenoldopam

Fenoldopam mesylate (Corlopam) is a dopamine-1 (D_1) receptor agonist similar in structure to dopamine and dobutamine. It is used to lower blood pressure but has not been shown helpful to prevent contrast-induced nephrotoxicity.[5]

Other pharmacologic interventions that are recommended to reduce the impact of contrast dye on the kidney include stopping all diuretics on the day of the procedure to prevent volume depletion[6]; stopping administration of the hypoglycemic drug metformin (Glucophage) because of its association with nephrotoxicity and lactic acidosis on rare occasions; limiting the quantity of contrast dye administered[45]; and providing adequate rehydration after the procedure.[5,6]

Dietary-Phosphorus Binders

Many patients with renal failure will be prescribed a dietary-phosphorus binding medication (see earlier section on calcium/phosphorus).[34] There are many dietary-phosphorus binding drugs available; some important issues concern all of them. The dietary-phosphorus binder must be taken at the time of the meal. If it is taken 2 hours later, it will only increase the level of the binding substance (such as calcium) in the bloodstream, and will not lower the serum phosphorus level. Other related issues such as the quantity of phosphorus in the diet should be discussed with a clinical nutritionist (dietitian).

NUTRITION

The diet for the patient with renal problems restricts the electrolytes potassium, sodium, and phosphorus. It also limits protein intake to control azotemia (increased BUN level). Fluids are limited. By contrast, carbohydrates are encouraged, to provide energy for metabolism and healing.[46]

NURSING MANAGEMENT

Nursing management of ARF patients involves a variety of nursing diagnoses (Box 20-3). **Nursing priorities for the patient with acute renal disease are directed toward (1) recognizing risk factors for development of acute renal failure, (2) preventing infectious complications, (3) optimizing fluid balance, (4) avoiding electrolyte imbalance, (5) preventing anemia, and (6) providing patient education.**

Recognizing Risk Factors for Acute Renal Failure

Some individuals have an increased risk of developing ARF as a complication during their hospitalization, and the alert critical care nurse recognizes potential

Box 20-3

NURSING DIAGNOSIS PRIORITIES

Acute Renal Failure

- Excess Fluid Volume related to renal dysfunction, p. A-24
- Ineffective Renal Tissue Perfusion related to decreased renal blood flow, p. A-42
- Anxiety related to threat to biologic, psychologic, and/or social integrity, p. A-9
- Decreased Cardiac Output related to decrease in preload, p. A-12
- Risk for Infection risk factors: protein-calorie malnourishment, invasive monitoring devices, p. A-46
- Disturbed Body Image related to functional dependence on life-sustaining technology, p. A-20
- Ineffective Coping related to situational crisis and personal vulnerability, p. A-38
- Insomnia related to fragmented sleep, p. A-43
- Deficient Knowledge: Fluid Restriction, Reportable Symptoms, and Medications related to lack of previous exposure to information, p. A-18

risk factors and acts as a patient advocate.[11,12] Patients at risk include elderly persons because their GFR may be decreased,[2] dehydrated patients because hypoperfusion of the kidneys may lead to ischemic ATN, patients with increased creatinine levels before their hospitalization,[13] and patients undergoing a radiology procedure involving contrast dye.[5,6]

Preventing Infectious Complications

The critical care patient with ARF is at risk for infectious complications. Signs of infection such as increased white blood cell (WBC) count, redness at a wound or IV site, or increased temperature are always a cause for concern. A urinary catheter is inserted to facilitate accurate urine measurement and patient comfort. However, any indwelling catheter is a potential source for infection. Therefore, when the patient no longer makes large quantities of urine, the catheter is removed and a scheduled "straight catheterization" is performed to minimize the risk of infection from an indwelling catheter and drainage system. This method allows the patient's bladder to be emptied, but the catheter does not remain in place. Pulmonary hygiene is maintained by asking the patient to cough and deep-breathe frequently if he or she is awake and alert. If the patient is intubated and ventilated, frequent turning, endotracheal suctioning, and frequent mouth care become mandatory. If the patient is immobile, changes of position and observation of potential sites for skin breakdown help avoid creating sites for infection.

Optimizing Fluid Balance

Intravascular fluid balance is often assessed on an hourly basis for the critically ill patient who has hemodynamic lines inserted. Hemodynamic values (heart rate [HR], BP, CVP, PAOP, CO, and CI) and daily weight measurements are correlated with the intake and output. Urine output is measured hourly, via a urinary catheter and drainage bag, throughout all phases of ARF, particularly in response to diuretics. Any fluid removed with dialysis is recorded in the fluid balance section of the nursing flow sheet. Recognition of the clinical signs and symptoms of fluid overload is important. Excess fluid will move from the vascular system into the peripheral tissues (dependent edema), abdomen (ascites), the lungs (crackles, pulmonary edema, and pulmonary effusions), around the heart (pericardial effusions), and into the brain (increased intracranial swelling).

Avoiding Electrolyte Imbalance

Hyperkalemia, hypocalcemia, hyponatremia, hyperphosphatemia, and acid-base imbalances all occur during ARF (see Table 20-3). Clinical manifestations of these electrolyte imbalances must be prevented and their associated side effects controlled. The potential imbalances that are the most likely are hyperkalemia and hypocalcemia, which can result in life-threatening cardiac dysrhythmias. Dilutional hyponatremia may develop as fluid overload worsens in the patient with oliguria. Monitoring the serum sodium level is important to prevent this complication. Hyperphosphatemia results in severe pruritus. Nursing care is directed at soothing the itching by performing frequent skin care with emollients, discouraging scratching, and administering phosphate-binding medications.[34] The acid-base imbalances that occur with renal failure are monitored by arterial blood gas (ABG) analysis. The goal of treatment is to maintain the pH within the normal range.

Preventing Anemia

Anemia is an expected side effect of renal failure that occurs because the kidney no longer produces the hormone *erythropoietin*.[33] Thus the bone marrow is not stimulated to produce red blood cells (RBCs). Care is taken to prevent blood loss in the patient with ARF, and blood withdrawal is minimized as much as possible. Irritation of the GI tract from metabolic waste accumulation is expected, and GI bleeding is a possibility. Stool, NG drainage, and emesis are routinely tested for occult blood. Anemia is treated pharmacologically by the administration of recombinant human erythropoietin (r-HuEPO), epoetin alfa (Procrit, Epogen), to stimulate erythrocyte production by the bone marrow, and if required by RBC transfusion.[33,47] Treatment of anemia early in the course of ARF (predialysis) appears to slow the progression of the renal failure and delays the initiation of renal replacement therapies.[33,48] Even in anemic critically ill patients without renal failure, administration of r-HuEPO weekly significantly decreases the number of blood transfusions.[49]

Box 20-4

Collaborative Management

Acute Renal Failure (ARF)

- Assess risk of renal failure.
  - Assess baseline renal function on all patients at risk for development of ARF.
- Protect the kidneys.
  - If patient has preexisting renal dysfunction, avoid nephrotoxic drugs, limit exposure to radiologic contrast dye, and prevent both hypotension and hypovolemia.
- Monitor urine output.
  - Intervene for low urine output before patient is oliguric or anuric for several hours (see Table 20-1).
- Supply nutrition.
  - Oral, enteral, or parenteral nutrition is needed to combat catabolism in critically ill patient with renal dysfunction.
- Provide renal replacement.
  - If patient has lost renal function during acute illness, replace kidney function with intermittent hemodialysis or CRRT as indicated.

Box 20-5

Indications and Contraindications for Hemodialysis

Indications

Blood urea nitrogen (BUN) level exceeds 90 mg/dl
Serum creatinine level 9 mg/dl
Hyperkalemia
Drug toxicity
Intravascular and extravascular fluid overload
Metabolic acidosis
Symptoms of uremia
- Pericarditis
- Gastrointestinal bleeding

Changes in mentation
Contraindications to other forms of dialysis

Contraindications

Hemodynamic instability
Inability to anticoagulate
Lack of access to circulation

Providing Patient Education

It is vital to provide accurate and uncomplicated information to the patient and family about ARF, including its prognosis, treatment, and possible complications.[3] Education of the patient can be challenging because elevations of BUN and creatinine can negatively affect level of consciousness. Also, sleep-rest disorders and emotional upset often occur as complications of ARF and can disrupt short-term memory. Encouraging the patient and family to voice concerns, frustrations, or fears and allowing the patient to control personal aspects of the acute care environment also are essential.

Collaborative Management

Management of the patient with acute renal dysfunction is complex and requires the expertise of many different health care clinicians (Box 20-4). Recently developed clinical guidelines[12,13] can be used to guide the health care team in determining priority interventions for this high-risk group of patients.

RENAL REPLACEMENT THERAPY—DIALYSIS

A range of RRTs is available for the treatment of ARF. These include intermittent hemodialysis (IHD) therapy, continuous renal replacement therapy (CRRT), and peritoneal dialysis (PD).

Hemodialysis

Hemodialysis roughly translates as "separating from the blood." Indications and contraindications for hemodialysis are listed in Box 20-5. As a treatment, hemodialysis literally separates and removes from the blood the excess electrolytes, fluids, and toxins by use of a hemodialyzer (Figure 20-1). Although hemodialysis is efficient in removing solutes, it does not remove all metabolites. Furthermore, electrolytes, toxins, and fluids increase between treatments, necessitating hemodialysis on a regular basis. Hemodialysis therapy is always intermittent; each dialysis treatment takes 3 to 4 hours. In the acute phases of renal failure, dialysis is performed daily.[50] The dialysis frequency gradually decreases to three times per week as the patient moves into a more chronic phase of kidney failure.

Hemodialyzer

Hemodialysis works by circulating blood outside the body through synthetic tubing to a dialyzer, which consists of hollow-fiber tubes. The dialyzer is sometimes described as an "artificial kidney" (Figure 20-2). While the blood flows through the membranes, which are semipermeable, a fluid "dialysate bath" bathes the membranes and, through osmosis and diffusion, performs exchanges of fluid, electrolytes, and toxins from the blood to the bath, where toxins and dialysate then pass out of the artificial kidney. The blood and the dialysate bath are shunted in opposite directions (countercurrent flow) through the dialyzer to match the osmotic and chemical gradients at the most efficient level for effective dialysis.

Ultrafiltration

To remove fluid, a positive hydrostatic pressure is applied to the blood and a negative hydrostatic pressure is applied to the dialysate bath. The two forces together create *transmembrane pressure,* to simultaneously push

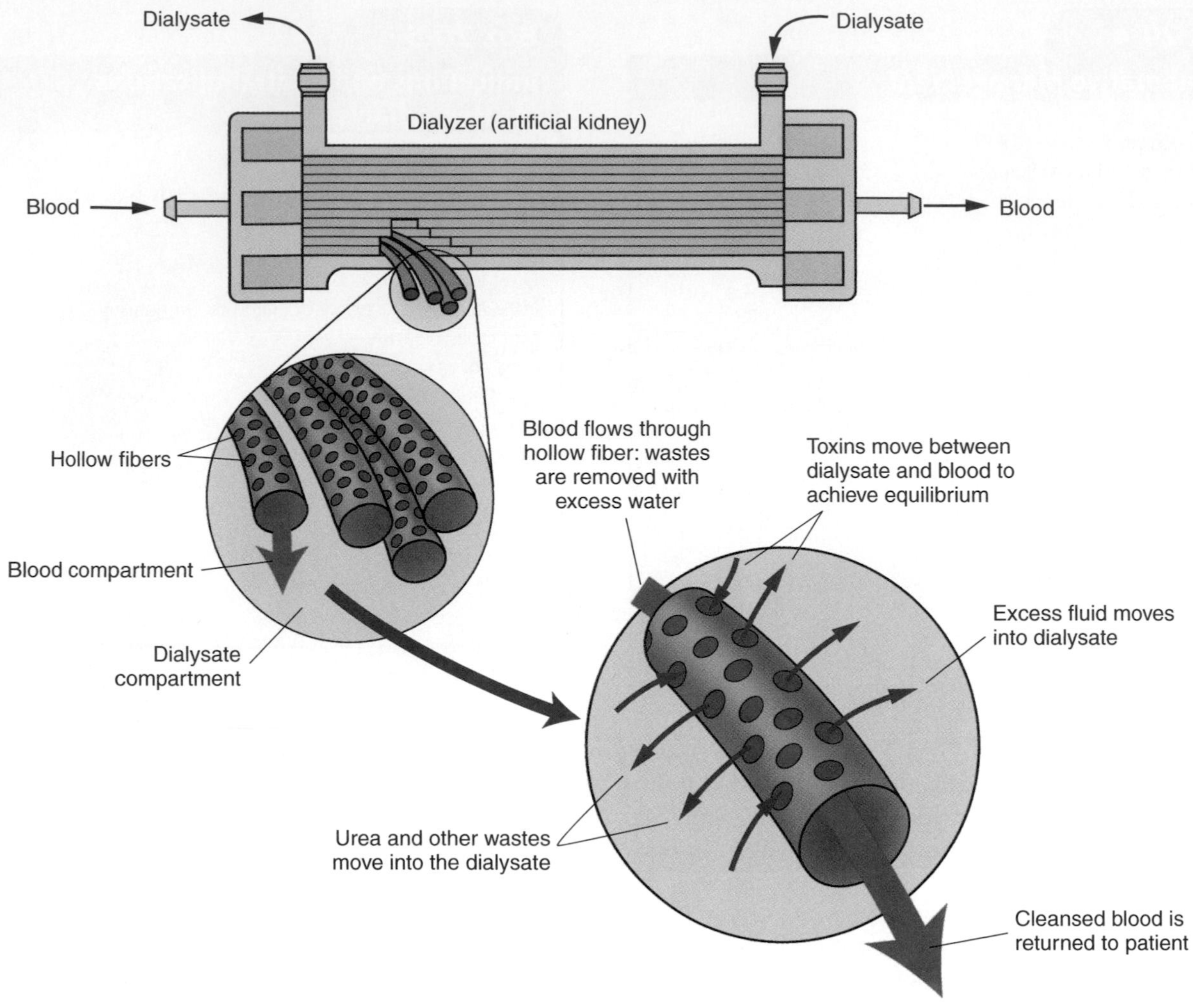

FIGURE 20-1. Hemodialyzer.

and pull the excess fluid from the blood. The difference between the two values (expressed in millimeters of mercury [mm Hg]) represents the transmembrane pressure and results in fluid extraction, known as *ultrafiltration,* from the vascular space.

Anticoagulation

Either heparin or sodium citrate is added to the system just before the blood enters the dialyzer to anticoagulate the blood within the dialysis tubing. Without an anticoagulant the blood will clot because its passage through the foreign tubular substances of the dialysis machine activates the clotting mechanism. Heparin can be administered either by bolus injection or intermittent infusion. It has a short half-life, and its effects subside within 2 to 4 hours. If necessary, the effects of heparin are reversed with the antidote protamine sulfate. When there is concern about the development of heparin-induced thrombocytopenia (HIT),[51] alternative anticoagulants can be used. Citrate (trisodium citrate) can also be infused as an anticoagulant via intermittent bolus or continuous infusion.[52]

Vascular Access

Hemodialysis requires access to the bloodstream. Various types of temporary and permanent devices are in clinical use. It is important for patient safety to be able to recognize these different vascular access devices and to properly care for them. The following section discusses temporary vascular access catheters used in the acute care hospital environment and permanent methods used for long-term hemodialysis.

Temporary Acute Access. *Subclavian* and *femoral* veins are catheterized when short-term access is required or when vascular access is nonfunctional in a patient requiring immediate hemodialysis. Both subclavian and femoral catheters are routinely inserted at the bedside. Most temporary catheters are venous only. Blood flows out toward the dialyzer and flows back to the patient via the same vein. A dual-lumen venous catheter is the most commonly seen. It has a central partition running the length of the catheter. The outflow catheter section pulls the blood flow through openings that are proximal to the inflow openings on the opposite side (Figure 20-3). This design helps

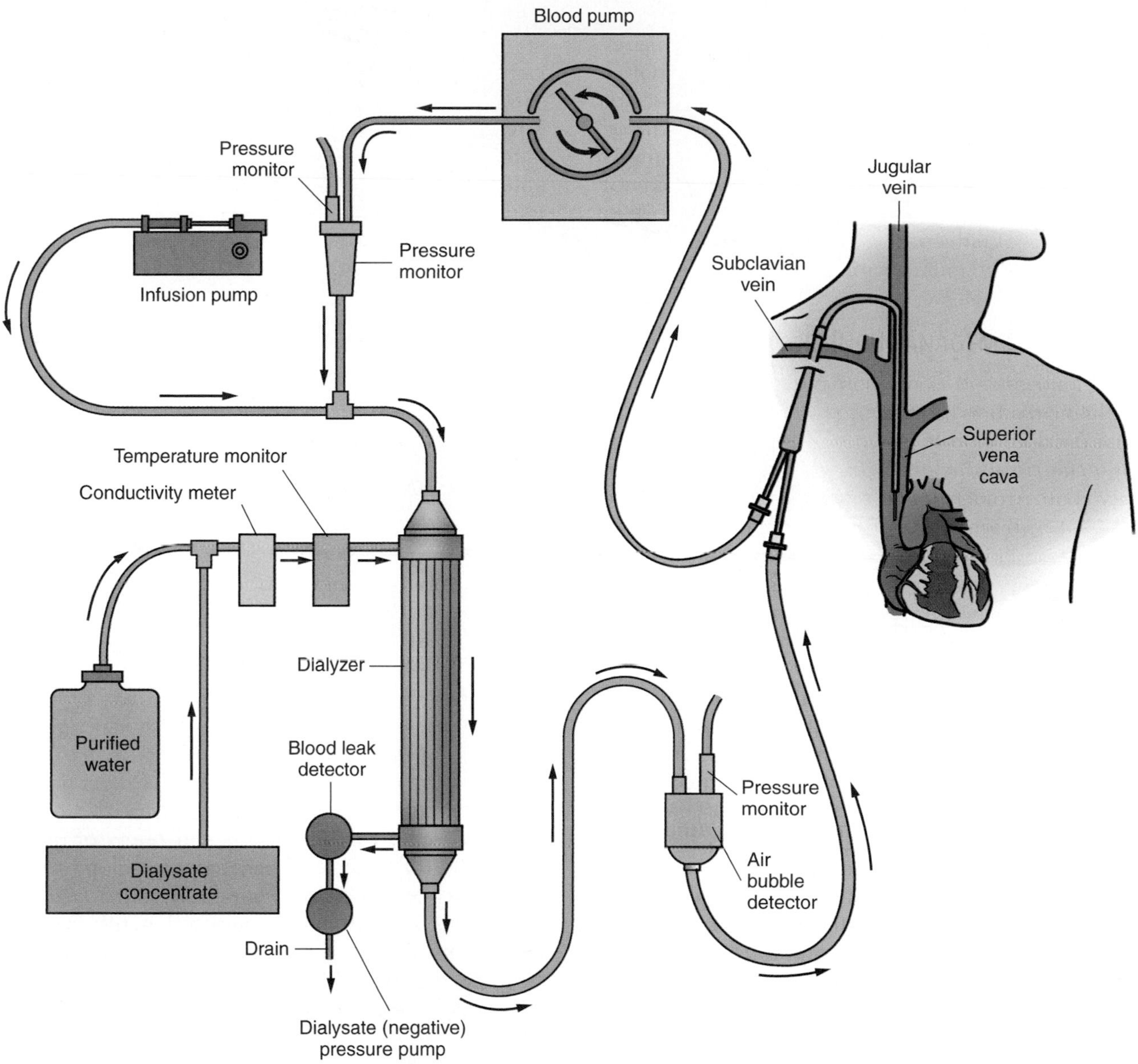

FIGURE 20-2. Components of a hemodialysis system.

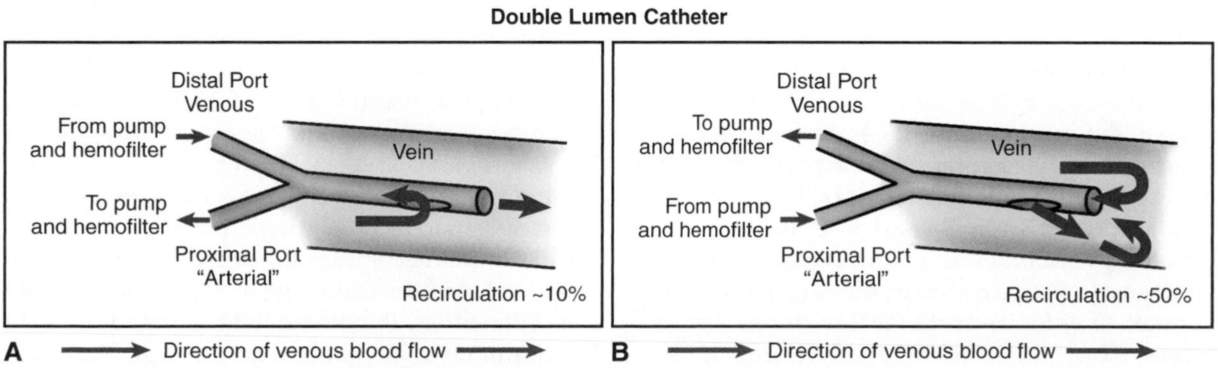

FIGURE 20-3. Temporary dialysis venous access catheter.

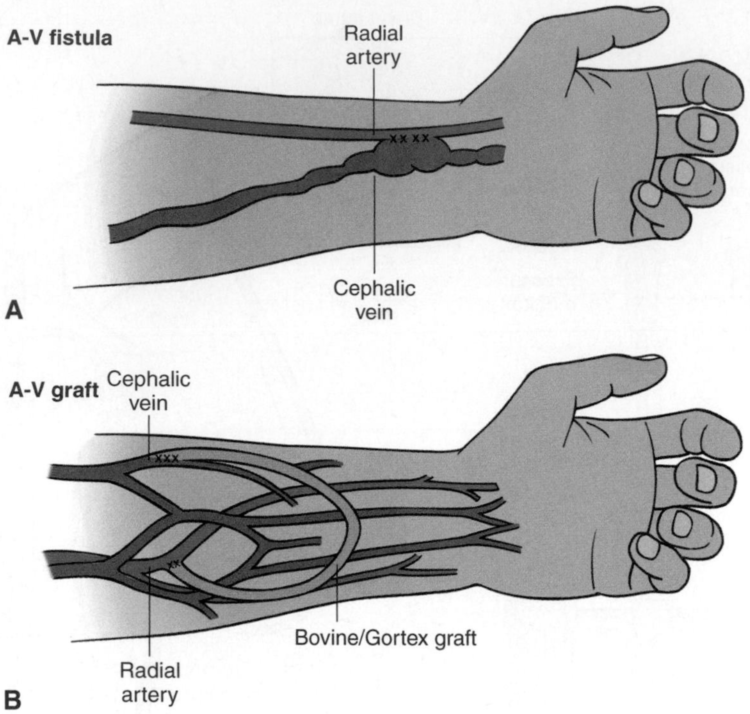

FIGURE 20-4. Methods of vascular access for hemodialysis. **A,** Arteriovenous fistula between vein and artery. **B,** Internal synthetic graft connects artery and vein.

prevent dialyzing the same blood just returned to the area (recirculation), which would severely reduce the procedure's efficiency. A silicone rubber, dual-lumen catheter with a polyester cuff designed to decrease catheter-related infections is also available.

Permanent Vascular Access. The common denominator in permanent vascular access devices is a connection to the arterial circulation and a return conduit to the venous circulation.

Arteriovenous Fistula. The arteriovenous (AV) fistula is created by surgically exposing a peripheral artery and vein, creating a side-by-side opening in the artery and the vein, and joining the two vessels together. The high arterial flow creates a swelling of the vein, or a pseudoaneurysm, at which point (when healed) a large-bore needle can be inserted to obtain arterial outflow to the dialyzer. Inflow is accomplished through a second large-bore needle inserted into a peripheral vein distal to the fistula (Figure 20-4, *A*). If the patient's vessels are adequate, fistulas are the preferred mode of access because of the durability of blood vessels, relatively few complications, and less need for revision compared with other access methods.[12] An initial disadvantage of a fistula concerns the time required for development of sufficient arterial flow to enlarge the new access. The minimum reported length of time before a fistula can be cannulated is 14 days,[53] but the time lag for many patients is longer, as much as weeks to possibly months.[54]

In caring for a patient with a fistula, there are some important nursing priorities to ensure the ongoing viability of the vascular access and safety of the limb (Table 20-8). The critical care nurse frequently assesses the quality of blood flow through the fistula. A patent fistula has a thrill when palpated gently with the fingers and a bruit if auscultated with a stethoscope. The extremity should be pink and warm to the touch. No blood pressure measurements, IV infusions, or laboratory phlebotomy are performed on the arm with the fistula.

The AV fistula is the preferred long-term access for hemodialysis.[12] However, in the United States only 27% of hemodialysis patients have an AV fistula; 47% have a synthetic graft; and 23% have a tunneled hemodialysis catheter.[55] An AV fistula provides the most favorable long-term patency for hemodialysis access and is recommended if patients require long-term hemodialysis.[12]

Arteriovenous Grafts. AV grafts are vascular access devices for treating chronic kidney failure. The graft is a tube made of synthetic material, which is surgically implanted inside the limb. The area is surgically opened, and an artery and a vein are located. A tunnel is created in the tissue where the graft is placed. Anastomoses are made with the graft ends connected to the artery and vein. The blood is allowed to flow through the graft, and the surgical area is closed. The graft creates a raised area that looks like a large periph-

Table 20-8

Complications and Nursing Management of Arteriovenous Fistula/Graft

TYPE	COMPLICATIONS	NURSING MANAGEMENT
Fistula	Thrombosis	Teach patients to avoid wearing constrictive clothing on limbs containing access.
	Infection	Teach patients to avoid sleeping on or bending accessed limb for prolonged periods.
	Pseudoaneurysm	Use aseptic technique when cannulating access.
	Vascular steal syndrome	Avoid repetitious cannulation of one segment of access.
	Venous hypertension	Offer comfort measures, such as warm compresses and ordered analgesics, to lessen pain of vascular steal.
	Carpal tunnel syndrome	Teach patients to develop blood flow in the fistulas through exercises (squeezing a rubber ball) while applying mild impedance to flow just distal to the access (at least once per day for 10-15 minutes).
	Inadequate blood flow	Avoid too-early cannulation of new access.
Graft	Bleeding	Teach patients to avoid wearing constrictive clothing on accessed limbs.
	Thrombosis	Avoid repeated cannulation of one segment of access.
	False aneurysm formation	Use aseptic technique when cannulating access.
	Infection	Monitor for changes in arterial or venous pressure while patients are on dialysis.
	Arterial or venous stenosis	Provide comfort measures to reduce pain of vascular steal (e.g., warm compresses, analgesics as ordered).
	Vascular steal syndrome	

eral vein just under the skin and peripheral tissue layers (Figure 20-4, *B*). Two large-bore needles are used for outflow and inflow to the graft. For both grafts and fistulas, after needle removal at the end of the hemodialysis treatment, firm pressure must be applied to stop any bleeding (see Table 20-8).

Tunneled Catheters. While waiting for the fistula or graft to mature to be ready for access, some patients may have a long-term Silastic catheter tunneled under the skin and inserted into the jugular or subclavian vein. These catheters are not common in critical care.

Medical Management

Medical management involves the decision to place a vascular access device and then to choose the most appropriate type and location for each patient. Patients in the critical care setting who require vascular access for hemodialysis usually use a temporary hemodialysis catheter. The exact quantity of fluid and/or solute removal to be achieved via hemodialysis is determined individually for each patient by clinical examination and review of all relevant laboratory results.

Nursing Management

A non–critical care nurse who is specially trained in dialysis manages the intermittent hemodialysis. The dialysis nurse typically comes to the patient's bedside with the hemodialysis machine. During the acute phase of treatment, hemodialysis occurs daily. The frequency is reduced to 3 days a week as the patient becomes hemodynamically stable. The essential role of the critical care nurse during dialysis is to monitor the patient's hemodynamic stability. The ARF patient on hemodialysis is dependent on a viable venous access catheter. When not in use the catheter is "heparin-locked" to preserve patency. The critical care nurse provides education about the disease process and treatment plan to patient and family.

Continuous Renal Replacement Therapy

Continuous renal replacement therapy (CRRT) is a newer mode of dialysis that has many similarities to traditional hemodialysis. CRRT has the advantage of being a continuous therapy, lasting 12 hours to several days, where the venous blood is circulated through a highly porous hemofilter.[56,57] As with traditional hemodialysis, it is rare to use an artery-to-vein setup; both access and return of blood are through a large venous catheter (venovenous) as shown in Figure 20-3. The advantage of the CRRT system is the continuous removal of fluid from the plasma. The fluid removal rate ranges from 5 to 45 ml/min, depending on the particular CRRT system used, plus removal of solutes (urea, creatinine, and electrolytes) as listed in Table 20-9. The removed fluid is described as *ultrafiltrate.* In an ideal situation the hydrostatic pressure exerted by a MAP greater than 70 mm Hg would propel a continuous flow of blood through the hemofilter to remove fluid and solute. However, because many critically ill patients are hypotensive and cannot provide adequate flow through the hemofilter, an electric roller pump "milks" the tubing to augment flow. If large amounts

Table 20-9
Comparison of Continuous Renal Replacement Therapy Methods

TYPE	ULTRAFILTRATION RATE	FLUID REPLACEMENT	METHOD OF SOLUTE REMOVAL	INDICATION
SCUF	100-300 ml/hr	None	None	Fluid removal
CVVH	500-800 ml/hr	Predilution or postdilution, calculating hourly net loss	Convection	Fluid removal, moderate solute removal
CVVHD	500-800 ml/hr	Predilution or postdilution, subtracting dialysate, then calculating hourly net loss	Diffusion	Fluid removal, maximum solute removal
CVVHDF		Predilution or postdilution, subtracting dialysate, then calculating hourly net loss	Convection and diffusion	Maximal fluid removal, maximum solute removal

SCUF, Slow continuous ultrafiltration; *CVVH,* continuous venovenous hemofiltration; *CVVHD,* continuous venovenous hemodialysis; *CVVHDF,* continuous venovenous hemodiafiltration.

Box 20-6
Indications and Contraindications for CRRT

Indications

Need for large fluid volume removal in hemodynamically unstable patient
Hypervolemic or edematous patients unresponsive to diuretic therapy
Patients with multiple organ dysfunction syndrome
Ease of fluid management in patients requiring large daily fluid volume
- Replacement for oliguria
- TPN administration

Contraindication to hemodialysis and peritoneal dialysis
Inability to be anticoagulated

Contraindications

Hematocrit >45%
Terminal illness

CRRT, Continuous renal replacement therapy; *TPN,* total parenteral nutrition.

of fluid are to be removed, IV replacement solutions are infused. Indications and contraindications for CRRT are described in Box 20-6.

Because controlled removal and replacement of fluid is possible over many hours or days with CRRT, hemodynamic stability is maintained. This makes CRRT highly advantageous for use in the patient with multisystem problems. There are several CRRT methods used in critical care units:

1. Slow continuous ultrafiltration (SCUF)
2. Continuous venovenous hemofiltration (CVVH)
3. Continuous venovenous hemodialysis (CVVHD)
4. Continuous venovenous hemodiafiltration (CVVHDF)

The decision as to which type of therapy to initiate is based on myriad factors, including clinical assessment, metabolic status, severity of uremia, and whether a particular treatment modality is available at that institution.

CRRT Terminology

In CRRT, solutes are removed from the blood by *diffusion* or *convection.* Both processes remove fluid, and they remove molecules of different sizes depending on the method chosen.

Diffusion. Diffusion describes the movement of solutes along a *concentration gradient* from "high" concentration to a "low" concentration across a semipermeable membrane. This is the main mechanism used in hemodialysis. Solutes such as creatinine and urea cross the dialysis membrane from the blood to the dialysis fluid compartment.

Convection. Convection occurs when a pressure gradient is set up so that the water is pushed or pumped across the dialysis filter and carries the solutes from the bloodstream with it. This method of solute removal is known as *"solvent drag"* and is commonly employed in CRRT.

Absorption. The filter attracts solute, and molecules attach (absorb) to the dialysis filter.

The size of solute molecules is measured in *daltons.* The different sizes of molecules that can be removed by convection or diffusion methods are shown in Table 20-10. Very tiny molecules such as urea and creatinine are removed by both diffusion and convection (all methods). As the molecular size increases (above 500 daltons), convection is the more efficient method.

Ultrafiltrate Volume. The fluid that is removed each hour is not called *urine;* it is known as *ultrafiltrate.*

Replacement Fluid. Typically some of the ultrafiltrate is replaced via the CRRT circuit by a sterile "replacement fluid." This replacement fluid can be added before the filter (prefilter dilution) or after the filter (postfilter dilution). The purpose is to increase the volume of fluid passing through the hemofilter and improve convection of solute.

Anticoagulation. Because the blood outside the body is in contact with artificial tubing and filters, the coagulation cascade and complement cascades are activated. To prevent the hemofilter from becoming

Table 20-10

Size of Molecules Cleared by CRRT

TYPE OF MOLECULE	SIZE OF MOLECULE	SOLUTES	SOLUTE REMOVAL METHOD
Small	Below 500 daltons	Urea, creatinine	Convection, diffusion
Middle	500-5000 daltons	Vancomycin	Convection better than diffusion
Low-molecular-weight (small) proteins	5000-50,000 daltons	Cytokines, complement	Convection or absorption onto hemofilter
Large proteins	Over 50,000 daltons	Albumin	Minimal removal

CRRT, Continuous renal replacement therapy.

obstructed by clotting, or clotting off, low-dose anticoagulation must be used. The dose should be low enough to have no effect on patient anticoagulation parameters. Systemic anticoagulation is not the goal. Typical anticoagulant choices include unfractionated heparin (UFH) and sodium citrate.

Because of the design of the CRRT machine it is not possible to look at the outside and follow the flow of blood and, if used, dialysate. The following section describes each of the CRRT methods and uses diagrams to clearly show the mechanism of CRRT that is used.

Slow Continuous Ultrafiltration

SCUF, as the name implies, slowly removes fluid, 100 to 300 ml/hr, through a process of ultrafiltration (Figure 20-5, *A*). This consists of a movement of fluid across a semipermeable membrane. SCUF has minimal impact on solute removal. Because small amounts of fluid are removed via this process, it was initially hoped it would be a suitable choice for edematous patients with acute heart failure and diminished renal perfusion who were unresponsive to diuretics. In reality, SCUF is an infrequent clinical choice because it requires both arterial and venous access for effective functioning. In addition, the SCUF system is more likely to thrombose (clot off) than other CRRT methods that use higher flows.

Continuous Venovenous Hemofiltration

CVVH is indicated when the patient's clinical condition warrants removal of significant volumes of fluid and solutes. Fluid is removed by ultrafiltration in volumes of 5 to 20 ml/min or up to 7 to 30 L/24 hr. Removal of solutes such as urea, creatinine, and other small non–protein-bound toxins is accomplished by convection. The replacement fluid rate of flow through the CRRT circuit can be altered to achieve desired fluid and solute removal without causing hemodynamic instability. Replacement fluid can be added via the addition of a prehemofilter replacement fluid (Figure 20-5, *B*) or posthemofilter replacement fluid.

As with other CRRT systems, the blood outside the body is anticoagulated and the ultrafiltrate is drained off either by gravity or by the addition of negative-pressure suction into a large drainage bag. Because large volumes of fluid may be removed in CVVH, some of the removed ultrafiltrate volume must be replaced hourly with a continuous infusion (replacement fluid) to avoid intravascular dehydration. Replacement fluids may consist of standard solutions of bicarbonate, potassium-free LR solution, acetate, or dextrose. Electrolytes such as potassium, sodium, calcium chloride, magnesium sulfate, and sodium bicarbonate also may be added. The formula used to calculate the volume removed from the patient follows with an example:

Ultrafiltrate in bag + other output – (CVVH replacement fluid + IV/oral/NG intake) = Output

Example: 1000 ml – 800 ml = 200 ml/hr output

Continuous Venovenous Hemodialysis

CVVHD is technically more like traditional hemodialysis and removes solute via diffusion because of a slow (15 to 30 ml/min) countercurrent drainage flow on the membrane side of the hemofilter (Figure 20-5, *C*). Countercurrent flow is through the hemofilter. *Countercurrent* means the blood flows in one direction and the dialysate flows in the opposite direction. As with other types of CRRT and hemodialysis, although arterial access is always possible, venovenous vascular access is the most common choice today.

CVVHD is indicated for patients who require large-volume removal for severe uremia or critical acid-base imbalances or for those who are diuretic resistant. A MAP of at least 70 mm Hg is desirable for effective volume removal and dialysis, and it is most effective when used over days, not hours. The use of replacement fluid is optional and depends on the patient's clinical condition and plan of care. The critical care nurse is responsible for calculating the hourly intake and output, noting fluid trends, and replacing excessive losses. This therapy is ideal for hemodynamically unstable patients in the critical care setting because they do not experience the abrupt fluid and solute changes that can accompany standard hemodialysis treatments.

Continuous Venovenous Hemodiafiltration

CVVHDF is another CRRT option CVVHDF combines two of the previously described methods (CVVH + CVVHD) to achieve maximal fluid and solute removal.

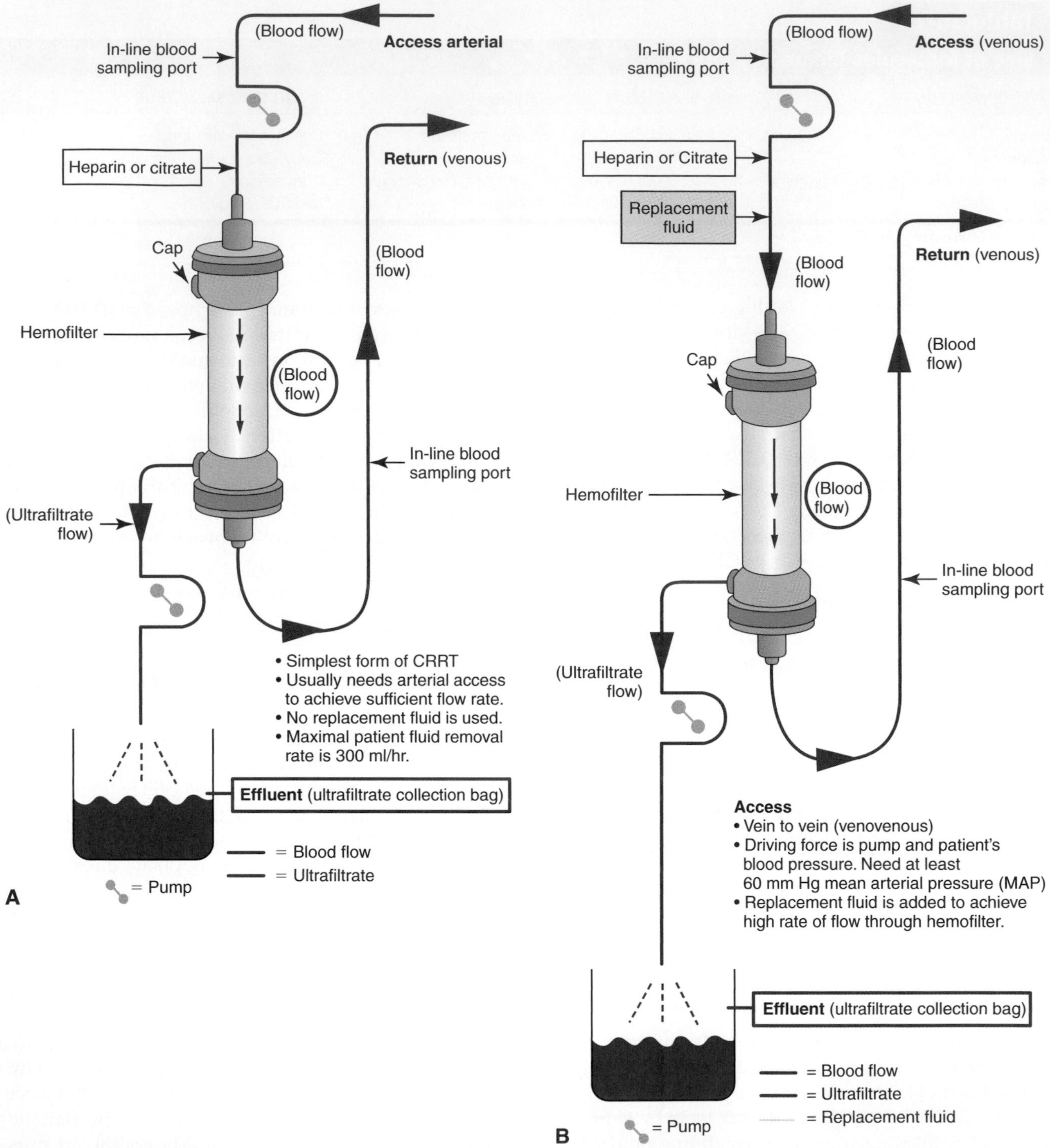

FIGURE 20-5. Continuous renal replacement therapy (CRRT) systems. **A,** Slow continuous ultrafiltration (SCUF). **B,** Continuous venovenous hemofiltration (CVVH).

Continued

A strong transmembrane pressure is applied to the hemofilter to push water across the filter, and a negative pressure is applied at the other side to pull fluid across the membrane and produce large volumes of ultrafiltrate, and also create a "solvent drag." In addition, the blood and the dialysate are circulated in a countercurrent flow pattern to remove fluid and solutes by diffusion. Thus CVVHDF can remove large volumes of fluid and solute because it employs both diffusion gradients and convection.

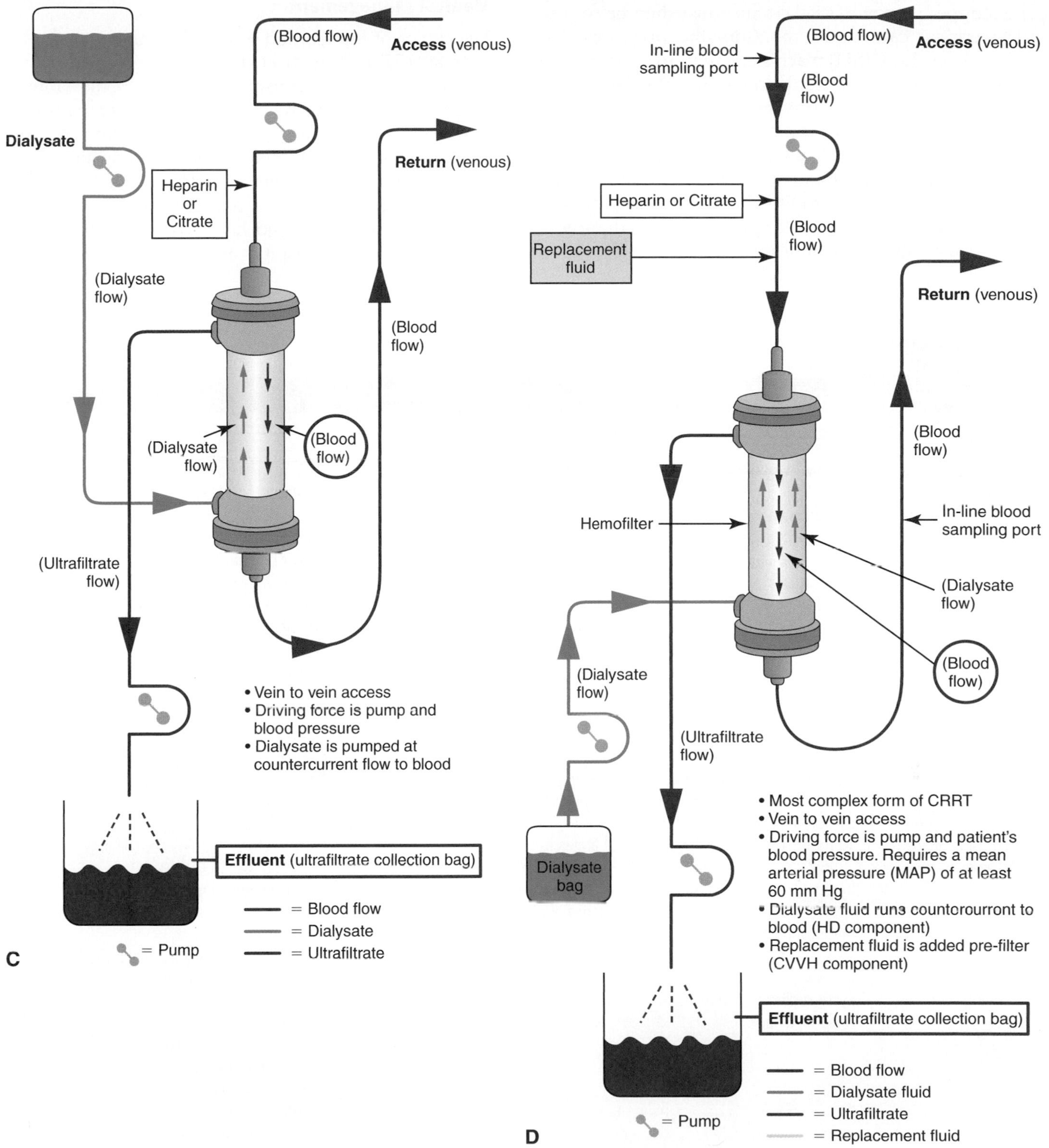

FIGURE 20-5, *cont'd.* **C,** Continuous venovenous hemofiltration dialysis (CVVHD). **D,** Continuous venovenous hemodiafiltration (CVVHDF).

Complications

Potential problems associated with CRRT and appropriate nursing interventions are listed in Table 20-11. Complications are often related to the rate of flow through the system. If the patient becomes hypotensive, or the access lines remain kinked, the ultrafiltration rate will decrease. This in turn can lead to increased clot formation within the hemofilter. As the surface of the hemofilter becomes more clotted, it will not provide effective fluid or solute clearance and CRRT will be stopped; a new CRRT circuit must then be set up. The critical care nurse monitors the pressures displayed on the CRRT machine screen to monitor the positive pressure of fluid going into the hemofilter (inflow) and the pressures coming out of the hemofilter to ensure that resistance to the negative pressure "pull" of the fluid across the hemofilter membrane has not developed. Other patient-related complications include fluid and electrolyte alterations, bleeding secondary to anticoagulation, or problems with the access site such as dislodgment or infection.

Medical Management

The choice of the method of blood purification to use to treat ARF is a medical decision. There is no clear clinical or research consensus as to whether intermittent or continuous renal replacement therapy is the most beneficial.[56] Age, gender, and preexisting chronic conditions are of little help in determining the need for hemofiltration or hemodialysis. Often the acute clinical diagnosis, physician preference, availability of the CRRT machine, and knowledgeable physicians and nurses at the hospital are the deciding factors.

Table 20-11

Complications Associated With CRRT

PROBLEM	ETIOLOGY	CLINICAL MANIFESTATIONS	NURSING MANAGEMENT
Decreased ultrafiltration rate	Hypotension Dehydration Kinked lines Bending of catheters Clotting of filter	Ultrafiltration rate decreased Minimal flow through blood lines	Observe filter and arteriovenous system Control blood flow Control coagulation time Position patient on back Lower height of collection container
Filter clotting	Obstruction Insufficient heparinization	Ultrafiltration rate decreased, despite height of collection container being lower	Control anticoagulation (heparin/citrate) Maintain continuous system anticoagulation Call physician Remove system Prime catheters with anticoagulated solution Prime new system; connect it Start predilution with 1000 ml saline 0.9% solution per hour Do not use three-way stopcocks
Hypotension	Increased ultrafiltration rate Blood leak Disconnection of one of lines	Bleeding Call physician	Control amount of ultrafiltration Control access sites Clamp lines
Fluid and electrolyte changes	To much/too little removal of fluid Inappropriate replacement of electrolytes Inappropriate dialysate	Changes in mentation, ↑ or ↓ CVP, ↑ or ↓ PAOP, ECG change, ↑ or ↓ BP and heart rate Abnormal electrolyte levels	Observe for: • Changes in CVP/PAOP • Changes in vital signs • ECG changes resulting from electrolyte abnormalities Monitor output values every hour Control ultrafiltration
Bleeding	System disconnection Anticoagulation	Oozing from catheter insertion site or connection	Monitor ACT no less than once every hour (heparin) Adjust heparin dose within specifications to maintain ACT Monitor serum calcium if using citrate as an anticoagulant Observe dressing on vascular access for blood loss Observe for blood in filtrate (filter leak)
Access dislodgment or infection	Catheter or connections not secured Break in sterile technique Excessive patient movement	Bleeding from catheter site or connections Inappropriate flow/infusion Fever Drainage at catheter site	Observe access site at least once every 2 hours Ensure that clamps are available within easy reach at all times Observe strict sterile technique when dressing vascular access

CRRT, Continuous renal replacement therapy; *CVP,* central venous pressure; *PAOP,* pulmonary artery occlusion pressure or "wedge" pressure; *ECG,* electrocardiogram; *BP,* blood pressure; *ACT,* activated coagulation time.

Infectious complications are associated with a grave prognosis. Dialysis is prescribed for almost anyone who develops severe ARF, unless the patient is clearly dying.

Intermittent hemodialysis or CCRT is usually begun before the BUN level exceeds 90 mg/dl or the creatinine level exceeds 9 mg/dl. In many hospitals the threshold to begin is considerably lower. Whether daily treatment is more effective than treatment every other day is controversial. The patient's serum creatinine, BUN, and fluid volume status are the deciding factors. CCRT is often prescribed when the BUN level is approximately 60 mg/dl. CRRT is more effective in the early stages of ARF. If severe electrolyte imbalance or fluid overload is present, even earlier intervention may be required.

Nursing Management

Critical care nurses play a vital role in monitoring the patient receiving CRRT. In many critical care units, the CRRT system is set up by the dialysis staff but is run on a 24-hour basis by critical care nurses with additional training. Complications can occur related to the CRRT circuit, the CRRT pump, the catheter, or the patient, as listed in Box 20-7. The critical care nurse monitors fluid intake and output, prevents and detects potential complications (e.g., bleeding, hypotension), trends electrolyte laboratory values, supervises safe operation of the CRRT equipment, and provides patient and family education about the patient's condition inclusive of CRRT.

Peritoneal Dialysis

PD is a modality used in patients with chronic kidney disease.[58] Only 8.4% of patients with ESKD are treated with PD.[59] When a PD-dependent patient is admitted to the critical care unit with a nonrenal acute illness, peritoneal dialysis may be continued. Peritoneal dialysis involves the introduction of sterile dialyzing fluid through an implanted catheter into the abdominal cavity. The dialysate bathes the peritoneal membrane, which covers the abdominal organs and overlies the capillary beds that support the organs.[58] By the processes of osmosis, diffusion, and active transport, excess fluid and solutes travel from the peritoneal capillary fluid through the capillary walls, through the peritoneal membrane, and into the dialyzing fluid. After a selected period the fluid is drained out of the abdomen by gravity (Figure 20-6). The process is then repeated at regular prescribed intervals.[60]

Indications for peritoneal dialysis include renal failure, volume overload, electrolyte imbalances, hemodynamic instability, lack of access to circulation, and removal of high-molecular-weight toxins. (Box 20-8).

The peritoneal membrane's structure and capillary blood flow to the peritoneum account for the relatively slow nature of PD. The small capillary pores, the

Box 20-7

Complications of CRRT

Catheter
Dislodgment
Hemorrhage
Infection

Circuit
Air embolism
Clotted hemofilter
Blood leaks

Pump
Circuit pressure alarms
Access (inflow) pressure alarm
Filter pressure alarm
Effluent pressure alarm
Return (outflow) pressure
Air bubble detector alarm
Excess fluid removal
Incorrect weight change alarm

Patient
Dehydration
Hypotension
Electrolyte imbalances
Acid-base imbalances

CRRT, Continuous renal replacement therapy.

Box 20-8

Indications and Contraindications for Peritoneal Dialysis

Indications
Uremia
Volume overload
Electrolyte imbalances
Hemodynamic instability
Lack of access to circulation
Removal of high-molecular-weight toxins
Patients with nonrenal critical illness receiving peritoneal dialysis for chronic kidney failure
Severe cardiovascular disease
Inability to anticoagulate
Contraindication to hemodialysis

Contraindications
Recent abdominal surgery
History of abdominal surgeries with adhesions and scarring
Significant pulmonary disease
Need for rapid fluid removal
Peritonitis

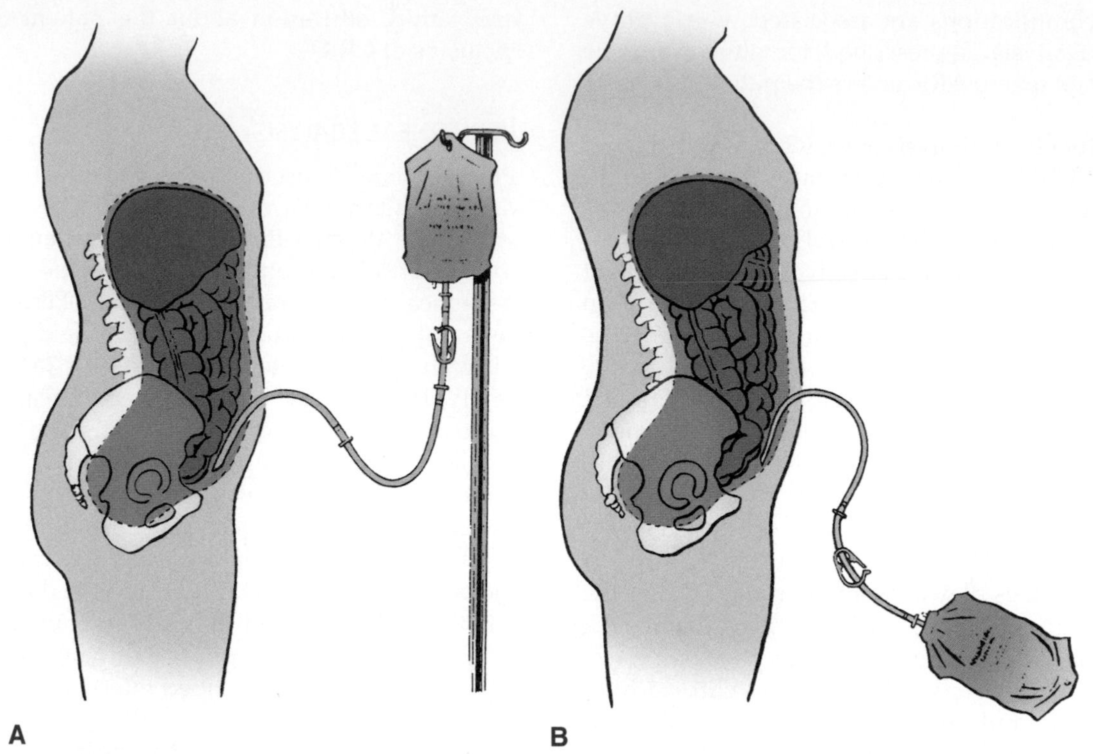

FIGURE 20-6. Peritoneal dialysis. **A,** Inflow. **B,** Outflow (drains by gravity). (From Thompson JM et al: *Mosby's clinical nursing,* ed 5, St Louis, 2002, Mosby.)

capillary membrane, the interstitium, the mesothelium of the peritoneum, and the fluid film layers in the capillary and the peritoneal cavity provide formidable barriers to fluid and solute passage. If needed, a "peritoneal equilibration test" can be performed to determine the level of solute clearance for a specific patient.[58]

The volume of dialysate instilled into the abdomen affects the clearance. Normally the PD-dependent patients are well versed in the amount, type, and frequency of dialysate to be infused into their abdomen, with subsequent drainage by gravity into a "waste" bag. The primary nursing consideration is to avoid contamination of the access point and monitor the patient's vital signs during this process. The dialysate should be instilled at body temperature to be comfortable, provide some vasodilation, and provide increased solute transport in the peritoneum. The length of time the solution remains in the peritoneal cavity *(dwell time)* and the solution composition affect the outcome. The dwell time affects the amount of fluid removed from the peritoneal capillaries, although a longer dwell time will not remove proportionately more fluid because of osmotic equilibration across the membranes. The various glucose concentrations of the dialysate provide for different rates of fluid removal.[58,61]

Catheter Placement

Most catheters have four segments: an external segment outside the abdomen, a tunnel segment that passes through subcutaneous tissue and muscle, a cuff for stabilization at the peritoneal membrane, and an internal segment with numerous holes for fast delivery and drainage of dialysate (Figure 20-7). The infusion and removal of the dialysate fluid are sterile procedures.

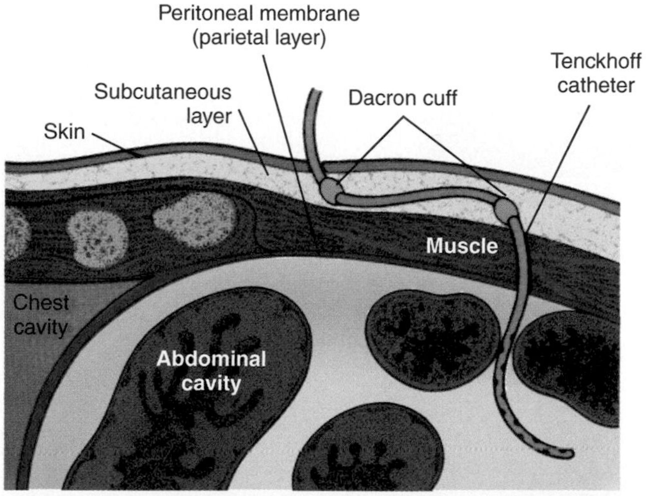

FIGURE 20-7. Tenckhoff catheter used in peritoneal dialysis. (From Lewis SM, Heitkemper MM, Dirksen SR: *Medical-surgical nursing assessment and management of clinical problems,* ed 6, St Louis, 2004, Mosby.)

Infection

The most significant risk to the patient with peritoneal dialysis is development of peritonitis secondary to catheter contamination and infection. Infection accounts for about two thirds of all PD catheter losses.[58] PD catheter infection results in peritonitis in 25% to 50% of cases.[58] Serious infection is also a reason a patient who uses PD would be admitted to the hospital.[58] The critical care nurse must be acutely aware of the signs and symptoms of systemic infection, such as a sudden rise in the WBC count, increased temperature, and malaise. At the same time, clinicians remain vigilant for signs of localized catheter or abdominal infection manifested by catheter site redness, site swelling, cloudy dialysis effluent following the dwell time, and abdominal tenderness or pain, which is present 75% of the time when infection is present.[58]

Medical Management

PD is used for long-term end-stage kidney failure. It is never used as a first-line acute care intervention. If a patient uses PD at home, PD will continue during the acute care hospitalization, provided the condition precipitating the admission is unrelated to the kidneys or abdomen.

Nursing Management

Nursing management of the patient receiving peritoneal dialysis is complex. Nurses are vigilant about prevention and detection of complications related to PD (Table 20-12). The critical care nurse observes for signs and symptoms of infection, monitors fluid volume status, infuses the dialysate fluid, observes drainage of the ultrafiltrate fluid, prevents complications associated with the PD catheter, and provides patient and family education. Patients who use PD are partners in the maintenance of their health because of the huge commitment they make in self-management of their peritoneal dialysis care.[59-62]

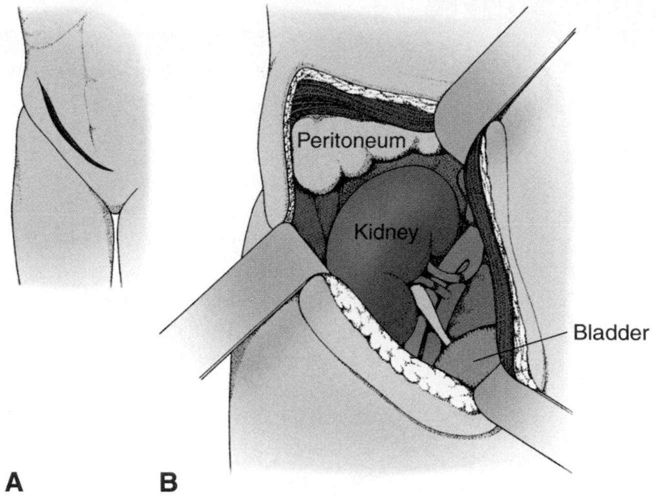

FIGURE 20-8. Placement of the kidney graft into the iliac fossa. **A,** The incision depicted is for the right side of the abdomen, representing kidney graft implantation in the right iliac fossa. **B,** The iliac vessels are exposed. (Modified from Smith SL: *AACN tissue and organ transplantation: implications for professional nursing practice*, St Louis, 1990, Mosby.)

KIDNEY TRANSPLANT

Kidney Transplant Surgical Procedure

When the kidney to be transplanted is removed from the donor—whether living or cadaveric—the ureter, renal vein, and renal artery are dissected, leaving as much length as possible.

Living Donor Surgery

A kidney from a living donor is the most frequent donor source today.[63] Most living donors are related to the recipient, although about 30% of donors are genetically unrelated, either as a spouse, friend, or part of a donor-pair exhange.[63] The kidney procurement can take place either as a laparoscopic procedure or as an open procedure. Once the kidney is secured, it is flushed with a cold electrolyte preservative solution until the venous return is clear. This usually requires approximately 500 ml of solution. The kidney is then transported into the recipient's operating room to be transplanted.

Cadaver Donor Surgery

If the donor is a cadaver donor, the kidney is flushed with a cold, electrolyte preservative solution and simultaneously cooled externally as quickly as possible. It can be transported either on a kidney perfusion machine or packed in an iced preservation solution. After it is procured and placed in the hypothermic solution, it can be maintained for 48 to 72 hours before it must be transplanted. However, most transplant centers attempt to transplant the organ as soon after procurement as possible to avoid both cold ischemic injury and ATN. At the time of procurement, the kidney is visualized in situ to note color, shape, and form. It is palpated to determine firmness, and a biopsy is often taken to rule out undiagnosed renal dysfunction or other disease.

Recipient Surgery

The patient is anesthetized in the usual manner, and a urinary catheter is placed. A curvilinear incision is made 3 to 4 cm above the symphysis pubis that extends to the iliac crest (Figure 20-8, *A*). The kidney is to be placed in the extraperitoneal space of either the right or left iliac fossa.[64] The muscles and fascia are divided and retracted medially to expose the iliac vessels. The renal artery is anastomosed end-to-side or end-to-end to the external iliac artery, and the vein is sutured end-to-side or end-to-end to the common iliac vein (Figure 20-8, *B*). During the surgery, a CVP ranging

Table 20-12
Complications Associated With Peritoneal Dialysis

COMPLICATION	NURSING MANAGEMENT
Peritonitis	Assess for signs and symptoms: cloudy effluent, abdominal pain, rebound tenderness, nausea and vomiting, fever. Obtain effluent sample for culture. Administer antibiotics as ordered. Teach patient/family signs and symptoms and prevention.
Exit site infection	Monitor site daily for signs and symptoms of infection: induration, erythema, purulence, hyperthermia. Increase daily cleaning of site. Apply topical antibiotics as ordered (controversial). Teach patient/family to avoid agents such as creams and lotions around exit site.
Catheter-tunnel infection	Assess for signs and symptoms of infection: pain along tunnel, induration for several centimeters away from catheter, erythema leading away from exit site, drainage at exit site or as tunnel is "milked" toward exit site. Teach patient/family signs and symptoms of infection. Teach patient/family to avoid pulls or tugs on catheter or trauma to exit site. Emphasize need to maintain cleansing regimen at exit site.
Fluid obstruction	Change position of patient (standing, lying, side-lying, knee-chest). Relieve patient's constipation. Irrigate the catheter. Ensure that sufficient fluid is in abdomen (sometimes requires a residual reservoir of approximately 50 ml).
Rectal pain	Ensure a sufficient reservoir of fluid. Use slow infusion rate.
Shoulder pain	Ensure that all air is primed from infusion tubing. Attempt draining the effluent with patients in knee-chest position. Administer mild analgesics as ordered.
Hernia	Monitor for increase in size of or pain in area of hernia. Decrease volume of exchanges as ordered. Dialyze with patients in the supine position. Use abdominal binder or support for patients (as long as not binding on catheter exit site). Avoid initiation of peritoneal dialysis until exit site healing has taken place (approximately 1 to 2 weeks) if possible.
Fluid overload	Increase use of hypertonic solutions. Decrease oral (PO) fluid intake. Shorten dwell times. Weigh patients frequently. Monitor lung sounds and peripheral edema.
Dehydration	Assess patients for decreased skin turgor, muscle cramps, hypotension, tachycardia, and dizziness. Discontinue hypertonic solutions. Increase oral fluid intake. Lengthen dwell times.
Blood-tinged effluent	Monitor for change in effluent color (clear yellow to pink or rusty). Administer heparin, as ordered, to prevent fibrin formation. Obtain patient history about catheter trauma and patient activity before appearance of complication.

from 8 to 16 mm Hg must be maintained and a systolic blood pressure at or above the patient's baseline should be maintained to ensure adequate perfusion of the transplanted kidney. After the revascularization procedures are completed, the ureteral anastomosis is done.

Posttransplant Medical Management and Nursing Care

After the transplant is completed and the patient is stable and ready for discharge from the recovery room, most transplant centers admit the patient directly to the organ transplant unit or to the critical care unit. Serious complications can occur in the immediate postoperative period, and a sound knowledge base of postoperative nursing care, renal function, anatomy, and immunosuppressive medications is imperative for the nurse.[64]

Fluid Status

If the transplanted organ is working well, fluid status in the patient, monitored by CVP, patient weight, and vital signs observation, must be regulated very closely. Adequate hydration is an absolute necessity for continued graft function in the immediate postoperative period. Hypovolemia can lead to compromised blood flow to the kidney, ATN, and possible graft failure. The new kidney will be producing large amounts of urine, and replacement fluids, usually maintained at a "1 ml:1 ml" (one-to-one) ratio, must be sustained.

If the kidney is not functioning in the immediate postoperative period, the patient's fluid status must be monitored very closely. Hypervolemia may be so great that respiratory compromise occurs. Output monitoring and bladder decompression are maintained. If significant fluid overload or respiratory compromise occurs, oxygen therapy and dialysis treatments may be necessary for several days.

Electrolyte Balance

Electrolyte balance is also of grave concern. Because of the large volumes of urine produced, the potential exists for hypokalemia, hypomagnesemia, and hypocalcemia, leading to possible cardiac compromise. These electrolytes must be monitored at least every 4 to 6 hours and replaced as necessary. Assessment of the BUN and creatinine levels is also necessary every 4 to 6 hours to monitor graft function and determine the need for dialysis.

Bleeding Risk

The complete blood count and platelet count should be monitored every 4 to 6 hours. Blood loss during the operation is minimal, generally 500 ml or less. Abrupt decreases or continuously falling counts may indicate hemorrhage at an anastomosis site, requiring a return to the operating room for repair. Despite minimal blood loss during surgery, transfusion of blood products after the surgery is often necessary. Frequent observation and assessment of the surgical incision is needed to evaluate for drainage and swelling.

Urine Output

Urine output volume and color should be monitored at least every 30 minutes. The bladder anastomosis is fragile, and clots occluding the catheter are not uncommon. The bladder must remain decompressed for several days to promote proper healing. If clots occlude the end of the catheter, gentle irrigation/aspiration may be necessary. If the clot cannot be dislodged or aspirated out, it may be necessary to change the catheter. Painful bladder spasms also can occur and require the use of pain medications and opiates to relax the bladder, usually in the form of a belladonna and opium suppository.

Immunosuppressive Therapy

Initiation of induction immunosuppressant therapy begins at the time of transplant, usually in the form of a polyclonal antithymocyte/antilymphocyte IV compound or IV monoclonal antibody compound. These compounds remove the lymphocytes from the patient's system, preventing rejection and suppressing the immune system until oral agents can be safely administered and blood levels are sufficient to allow the IV agent to be discontinued. Immunosuppression protocols often include drugs from three drug groups: *calcineurin inhibitors* (e.g., cyclosporin, tacrolimus), *antiproliferative agents* (e.g., azathioprine, mycophenolate mofetil) and *steroids* (prednisolone). Because the kidney transplant recipient is immunocompromised, strict aseptic technique is required to prevent infection. Thorough hand washing, aseptic dressing changes, discontinuation of any unnecessary invasive lines, and limiting the number of visitors are necessary protective mechanisms.

Infection Risk

Because of the patient's immunocompromised status, subtle changes in the patient's temperature, white blood cell counts, and wound drainage can signal an active infection. Patients also are susceptible to opportunistic native organisms such as *Candida,* pneumocystis pneumonia, cytomegalovirus (CMV), Epstein-Barr virus (EBV), and *herpes simplex* infections.

The average length of stay in the hospital for an uncomplicated kidney transplant is 5 to 7 days. In the first few days after transplant, the patient is guided in self-care management of the new kidney. Medication regimens are complex, and most centers initiate a self-medication program at the patient's bedside as a training tool. Patients are taught the signs and symptoms of infection and graft rejection, transplant clinic protocols, and new dietary limitations. It is important the recipient understand the importance of strict adherence to the immunosuppressive drug regimen.[65] Frequent transplant clinic visits to check the functioning of the organ and to adjust down the doses of immunosuppressant medications are necessary for the first few months after transplantation.

Rejection

Rejection of the organ is of ongoing concern for all transplant patients. Graft function is monitored closely, and if rejection is suspected, a biopsy is performed. If the biopsy reveals acute rejection, rescue therapy is initiated. This therapy can be in the form of high-dose IV steroids in the case of mild rejection or IV monoclonal antibody for moderate to severe rejection. Long-term, if the biopsy reveals chronic rejection, the oral immunosuppressant medications are increased to the higher doses used immediately after transplant. No two patients' immune systems are exactly alike. The immunosuppressant medication regimen required to prevent rejection must be tailored to each patient individually. The goal is to create a balance among medications that allows the patient to fight off most infections and yet avoid rejection of the transplanted kidney.

evolve To test your mastery of this chapter, try the Open-Book Quiz at http://evolve.elsevier.com/Urden/priorities/

REFERENCES

1. Mehta RL et al: Spectrum of acute renal failure in the intensive care unit: the PICARD experience, *Kidney Int* 66(4):1613, 2004.
2. Sesso R et al: Prognosis of ARF in hospitalized elderly patients, *Am J Kidney Dis* 44(3):410, 2004.
3. Nickolas TL et al: Awareness of kidney disease in the U.S. population: findings from the National Health and Nutrition Examination Survey (NHANES) 1999 to 2000, *Am J Kidney Dis* 44(2):185, 2004.
4. Kellum JA et al: Developing a consensus classification system for acute renal failure, *Curr Opin Crit Care* 8(6):509, 2002.
5. Venkataraman R, Kellum J: Prevention of acute renal failure, *Chest* 131(1):300, 2007.
6. Asif A, Epstein M: Prevention of radiocontrast-induced nephropathy, *Am J Kidney Dis* 44(1):12, 2004.
7. Sheridan AM, Bonventre JV: Cell biology and molecular mechanisms of injury in ischemic acute renal failure, *Curr Opin Nephrol Hypertens* 9(4):427, 2000.
8. Liano F et al: The spectrum of acute renal failure in the intensive care unit compared with that seen in other settings: The Madrid Acute Renal Failure Study Group, *Kidney Int Suppl* 66:S16, 1998.
9. Rocktaeschel J et al: Acid-base status of critically ill patients with acute renal failure: analysis based on Stewart-Figge methodology, *Crit Care* 7(4):R60, 2003.
10. Bellomo R, Kellum JA, Ronco C: Defining acute renal failure: physiological principles, *Intensive Care Med* 30(1):33, 2004.
11. Coresh J et al: Prevalence of chronic kidney disease and decreased kidney function in the adult U.S. population: Third National Health and Nutrition Examination Survey, *Am J Kidney Dis* 41(1):1, 2003.
12. K/DOQI clinical practice guidelines for chronic kidney disease: evaluation, classification, and stratification, *Am J Kidney Dis* 39(2 suppl 1):S1, 2002.
13. Bellomo R et al: Acute renal failure—definition, outcome measures, animal models, fluid therapy and information technology needs: the Second International Consensus Conference of the Acute Dialysis Quality Initiative (ADQI) Group, *Crit Care* 8(4):R204, 2004.
14. Warnock DG, Textor SC: Hypertension, *Am J Kidney Dis* 44(2):369, 2004.
15. K/DOQI clinical practice guidelines on hypertension and antihypertensive agents in chronic kidney disease, *Am J Kidney Dis* 43(5 suppl 1):S1, 2004.
16. Mitch WE et al: Detecting and managing patients with type 2 diabetic kidney disease: proteinuria and cardiovascular disease, *Kidney Int Suppl* 92:S97, 2004.
17. Keith DS et al: Longitudinal follow-up and outcomes among a population with chronic kidney disease in a large managed care organization, *Arch Intern Med* 164(6):659, 2004.
18. Go AS et al: Chronic kidney disease and the risks of death, cardiovascular events, and hospitalization, *N Engl J Med* 351(13):1296, 2004.
19. Anavekar NS et al: Relation between renal dysfunction and cardiovascular outcomes after myocardial infarction, *N Engl J Med* 351(13):1285, 2004.
20. Vieria J et al: Effect of acute kidney injury on weaning from mechanical ventilation in critically ill patients, *Critical Care Medicine* 35(1):184, 2007.
21. Dellinger RP et al: Surviving Sepsis Campaign guidelines for management of severe sepsis and septic shock, *Crit Care Med* 32(3):858, 2004.
22. Hollenberg SM et al: Practice parameters for hemodynamic support of sepsis in adult patients: 2004 update, *Crit Care Med* 32(9):1928, 2004.
23. Criddle LM: Rhabdomyolysis: pathophysiology, recognition, and management, *Crit Care Nurse* 23(6):14, 2003.
24. Brown CV et al: Preventing renal failure in patients with rhabdomyolysis: do bicarbonate and mannitol make a difference? *J Trauma* 56(6):1191, 2004.
25. Kandzari DE et al: Contrast nephropathy: an evidence-based approach to prevention, *Am J Cardiovasc Drugs* 3(6):395, 2003.
26. Aspelin P et al: Nephrotoxic effects in high-risk patients undergoing angiography, *N Engl J Med* 348(6):491, 2003.
27. Durham JD et al: A randomized controlled trial of N-acetylcysteine to prevent contrast nephropathy in cardiac angiography, *Kidney Int* 62(6):2202, 2002.
28. Guru V, Fremes SE: The role of N-acetylcysteine in preventing radiographic contrast-induced nephropathy, *Clin Nephrol* 62(2):77, 2004.
29. Kshirsagar AV et al: N-acetylcysteine for the prevention of radiocontrast induced nephropathy: a meta-analysis of prospective controlled trials, *J Am Soc Nephrol* 15(3):761, 2004.
30. El-Shahawy MA, Agbing LU, Badillo E: Severity of illness scores and the outcome of acute tubular necrosis, *Int Urol Nephrol* 32(2):185, 2000.
31. Ahee P, Crowe AV: The management of hyperkalemia in the emergency department, *J Accid Emerg Med* 17(3):188, 2000.
32. Levey AS et al: National Kidney Foundation practice guidelines for chronic kidney disease: evaluation, classification, and stratification, *Ann Intern Med* 139(2):137, 2003.
33. Leavey SF, Weitzel WF: Endocrine abnormalities in chronic renal failure, *Endocrinol Metab Clin North Am* 31(1):107, 2002.
34. Emmett M: A comparison of clinically useful phosphorus binders for patients with chronic kidney failure, *Kidney Int Suppl* 90:S25, 2004.
35. Haney SL: Drug use in renal failure, *Crit Care Nurs Clin North Am* 14(1):77, 2002.
36. Mehta RL, Clark WC, Schetz M: Techniques for assessing and achieving fluid balance in acute renal failure, *Curr Opin Crit Care* 8(6):535, 2002.
37. Finfer S et al: A comparison of albumin and saline for fluid resuscitation in the intensive care unit, *N Engl J Med* 350(22):2247, 2004.
38. Vincent JL, Navickis RJ, Wilkes MM: Morbidity in hospitalized patients receiving human albumin: a meta-analysis of randomized, controlled trials, *Crit Care Med* 32(10):2029, 2004.
39. Mehta RL et al: Diuretics, mortality, and nonrecovery of renal function in acute renal failure, *JAMA* 288(20):2547, 2002.

40. Cantarovich F et al: High-dose furosemide for established ARF: a prospective, randomized, double-blind, placebo-controlled, multicenter trial, *Am J Kidney Dis* 44(3):402, 2004.
41. Uchino S et al: Diuretics and mortality in acute renal failure, *Crit Care Med* 32(8):1669, 2004.
42. Ichai C et al: Prolonged low-dose dopamine infusion induces a transient improvement in renal function in hemodynamically stable, critically ill patients: a single-blind, prospective, controlled study, *Crit Care Med* 28(5):1329, 2000.
43. Kellum JA: Use of dopamine in acute renal failure: a meta-analysis, *Crit Care Med* 29(8):1526, 2001.
44. Bellomo R et al: Low-dose dopamine in patients with early renal dysfunction: a placebo-controlled randomised trial. Australian and New Zealand Intensive Care Society (ANZICS) Clinical Trials Group, *Lancet* 356(9248):2139, 2000.
45. Freeman RV et al: Nephropathy requiring dialysis after percutaneous coronary intervention and the critical role of an adjusted contrast dose, *Am J Cardiol* 90(10):1068, 2002.
46. Druml W: Nutritional management of acute renal failure, *Am J Kidney Dis* 37(1 suppl 2):S89, 2001.
47. Pearl RG, Pohlman A: Understanding and managing anemia in critically ill patients, *Crit Care Nurse* suppl:1, 2002.
48. Gouva C et al: Treating anemia early in renal failure patients slows the decline of renal function: a randomized controlled trial, *Kidney Int* 66(2):753, 2004.
49. Corwin HL et al: Efficacy of recombinant human erythropoietin in critically ill patients: a randomized controlled trial, *JAMA* 288(22):2827, 2002.
50. Schiffl H, Lang SM, Fischer R: Daily hemodialysis and the outcome of acute renal failure, *N Engl J Med* 346(5):305, 2002.
51. Warkentin TE, Greinacher A: Heparin-induced thrombocytopenia: recognition, treatment, and prevention: the Seventh ACCP Conference on Antithrombotic and Thrombolytic Therapy, *Chest* 126(3 suppl):311S, 2004.
52. Monchi M et al: Citrate vs. heparin for anticoagulation in continuous venovenous hemofiltration: a prospective randomized study, *Intensive Care Med* 30(2):260, 2004.
53. Rayner HC et al: Creation, cannulation and survival of arteriovenous fistulae: data from the Dialysis Outcomes and Practice Patterns Study, *Kidney Int* 63(1):323, 2003.
54. Beathard GA et al: Aggressive treatment of early fistula failure, *Kidney Int* 64(4):1487, 2003.
55. Asif A et al: Arteriovenous fistula creation: should US nephrologists get involved? *Am J Kidney Dis* 42(6):1293, 2003.
56. Kellum JA et al: Continuous versus intermittent renal replacement therapy: a meta-analysis, *Intensive Care Med* 28(1):29, 2002.
57. Rempher KJ: Continuous renal replacement therapy for management of overhydration in heart failure, *AACN Clin Issues* 14(4):512, 2003.
58. Teitelbaum I, Burkart J: Peritoneal dialysis, *Am J Kidney Dis* 42(5):1082, 2003.
59. Curtin RB, Johnson HK, Schatell D: The peritoneal dialysis experience: insights from long-term patients, *Nephrol Nurs J* 31(6):615, 2004.
60. Kelley KT: How peritoneal dialysis works, *Nephrol Nurs J* 31(5):481, 2004.
61. Crawford-Bonadio TL, Diaz-Buxo JA: Comparison of peritoneal dialysis solutions, *Nephrol Nurs J* 31(5):499, 2004.
62. Maaz DE: Troubleshooting non-infectious peritoneal dialysis issues, *Nephrol Nurs J* 31(5):521, 2004.
63. Davis CL, Delmonica FL: Living-donor kidney transplantation: a review of the current practices for the live donor, *J Am Soc Nephrol* 16:2098, 2005.
64. Barone C, Lightfoot ML, Barone G: The postanesthesia care of an adult renal transplant recipient, *J Perianesthesia Nurs* 18(1):32, 2003.
65. Russell CL et al: Medication adherence patterns in adult renal transplant recipients, *Res Nurs Health* 29:521, 2006.

CHAPTER 21

Gastrointestinal Assessment and Diagnostic Procedures

KATHLEEN M. STACY

OBJECTIVES

- Identify the components of a gastrointestinal history.
- Describe inspection, palpation, percussion, and auscultation of the patient with gastrointestinal dysfunction.
- Delineate the clinical significance of selected laboratory tests used in the assessment of gastrointestinal disorders.
- Identify key diagnostic procedures used in assessment of the patient with gastrointestinal dysfunction.
- Discuss the nursing management of a patient undergoing a gastrointestinal diagnostic procedure.

Assessment of the critically ill patient with gastrointestinal (GI) dysfunction includes a review of the patient's health history, a thorough physical examination, and an analysis of the patient's laboratory data. Numerous invasive and noninvasive diagnostic procedures may also be performed to assist in the identification of the patient's disorder. This chapter focuses on priority clinical assessments, laboratory studies, and diagnostic tests for the critically ill patient with gastrointestinal dysfunction.

CLINICAL ASSESSMENT

A thorough clinical assessment of the patient with GI dysfunction is imperative for the early identification and treatment of GI disorders. Once completed, the assessment serves as the foundation for developing the management plan for the patient. The assessment process can be brief or can involve a detailed history and examination, depending on the nature and immediacy of the patient's situation.[1]

HISTORY

Taking a thorough and accurate history is extremely important to the assessment process. The patient's history provides the foundation and direction for the rest of the assessment. The overall goal of the patient interview is to expose key clinical manifestations that will facilitate the identification of the underlying cause of the illness. This information will then assist in the development of an appropriate management plan.[2]

The initial presentation of the patient determines the rapidity and direction of the interview. For a patient in acute distress, the history should be curtailed to just a few questions about the patient's chief complaint and precipitating events. For a patient in no obvious distress, the history focuses on four different areas: (1) review of the patient's present illness, (2) overview of the patient's general gastrointestinal status including previous GI diagnostic studies or interventional procedures, (3) examination of the patient's personal and social history including dietary habits, nutritional status, bowel characteristics (stool descriptions), alcohol intake, and dependence on laxatives or enemas, and (4) survey of the patient's family history including metabolic disorders, malabsorption syndromes, and cancer of the GI tract.[3,4]

PHYSICAL EXAMINATION

The physical assessment helps establish baseline data about the physical dimensions of the patient's situation. The physical examination helps establish baseline data about the physical dimensions of the patient's situation.[3] The abdomen is divided into four quadrants (left upper, right upper, left lower, and right lower), with the umbilicus as the middle point, to facilitate the identification of the location of examination findings (Figure 21-1 and Box 21-1). The assessment proceeds when the patient is as comfortable as possible and in the supine position; however, the position may need readjustment if it elicits pain. To prevent stimulation of GI activity, the order for the assessment should be

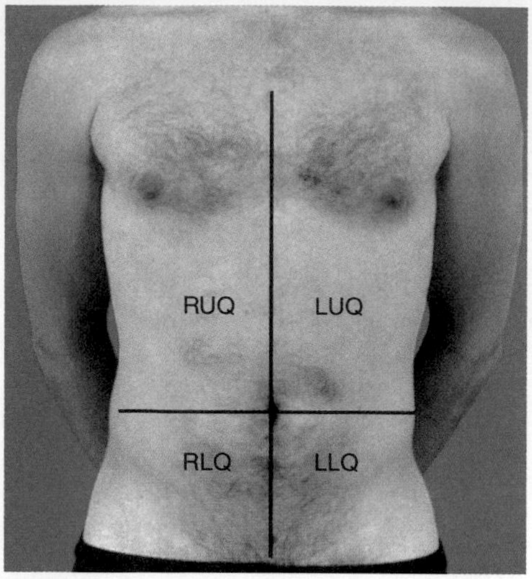

FIGURE 21-1. Anatomic mapping of the four quadrants of the abdomen. *RUQ,* Right upper quadrant; *LUQ,* left upper quadrant; *RLQ,* right lower quadrant; *LLQ,* left lower quadrant. (From Barkauskas V et al: *Health and physical assessment,* ed 3, St Louis, 2002, Mosby.)

changed to inspection, auscultation, percussion, and palpation.[4]

Inspection

Nursing priorities in inspection of the patient with gastrointestinal dysfunction focus on (1) oral cavity, (2) skin over the abdomen, and (3) shape of the abdomen. Inspection should be performed in a warm, well-lighted environment with the patient in a comfortable position with the abdomen exposed. Although assessment of the GI system classically begins with inspection of the abdomen, the patient's oral cavity also must be inspected to determine any unusual findings. Abnormal findings of the mouth include joint tenderness, inflammation of the gums, missing teeth, dental caries, ill-fitting dentures, and mouth odor.[5]

The skin is observed for pigmentation, lesions, striae, scars, petechiae, signs of dehydration, and venous pattern. Pigmentation may vary considerably within normal range because of race and ethnic background, although the abdomen is generally lighter in color than other, exposed areas of the skin. Abnormal findings include jaundice, skin lesions, and a tense and glistening appearance of the skin. Old striae (stretch marks) are generally silver in color, whereas pink-purple striae may be indicative of Cushing's syndrome.[4] A bluish discoloration of the umbilicus (Cullen's sign) or of the flank (Turner's sign) is indicative of intraperitoneal bleeding.[1]

The abdomen is observed for contour (noting if it is flat, slightly concave, or slightly round), for symmetry, and for movement. Marked distention is an abnormal finding. In particular, ascites may cause generalized distention and bulging flanks. Asymmetric distention may be indicative of organ enlargement or a mass. Peristaltic waves should not be visible except in very thin patients. In the case of intestinal obstruction, hyperactive peristaltic waves may be noted. Pulsation in the epigastric area is frequently a normal finding, but increased pulsation may be indicative of an aortic aneurysm. Symmetric movement of the abdomen with respirations is usually seen in men.[4,5]

Box 21-1

Anatomic Correlates of Four Abdominal Quadrants

Right Upper Quadrant
Liver and gallbladder
Pylorus
Duodenum
Head of pancreas
Right adrenal gland
Portion of right kidney
Hepatic flexure of colon
Portions of ascending and transverse colon

Right Lower Quadrant
Lower pole of right kidney
Cecum and appendix
Portion of ascending colon
Bladder (if distended)
Ovary and salpinx
Uterus (if enlarged)
Right spermatic cord
Right ureter

Left Upper Quadrant
Left lobe of liver
Spleen
Stomach
Body of pancreas
Left adrenal gland
Portion of left kidney
Splenic flexure of colon
Portions of transverse and descending colon

Left Lower Quadrant
Lower pole of left kidney
Sigmoid colon
Portion of descending colon
Bladder (if distended)
Ovary and salpinx
Uterus (if distended)
Left spermatic cord
Left ureter

From Barkauskas V et al: *Health and physical assessment,* ed 3, St Louis, 2002, Mosby.

Auscultation

Nursing priorities in auscultation of the patient with gastrointestinal dysfunction focus on (1) bowel

Table 21-1
Abnormal Abdominal Sounds

SOUND	DESCRIPTION	CAUSES
Borborygmi	Hyperactive bowel sounds; loud and prolonged	Hunger Gastroenteritis Early intestinal obstruction
Bowel sounds	High-pitched, tinkling sounds	Intestinal air/fluid under pressure; characteristic of early intestinal obstruction
Decreased bowel sounds	Hypoactive bowel sounds; infrequent, abnormally faint	Possible peritonitis or ileus
Absence of bowel sounds	Confirmed only after auscultation of all four quadrants and continuous auscultation for 5 minutes	Temporary loss of intestinal motility, as with complete ileus
Friction rubs	High-pitched sounds over liver/spleen (RUQ/LUQ), synchronous with respiration	Pathologic conditions (e.g., tumors, infection) that cause inflammation of organ's peritoneal covering
Bruits	Audible swishing sounds over aorta, iliac, renal, and femoral arteries	Abnormality of blood flow (requires additional evaluation to determine specific disorder)
Venous hum	Low-pitched, continuous sound	Increased collateral circulation between portal and systemic venous systems

From Doughty DB, Jackson DB: *Gastrointestinal disorders,* St Louis, 1993, Mosby.
RUQ, Right upper quadrant; *LUQ,* left upper quadrant.

sounds and (2) presence of bruits. Auscultation of the abdomen provides clinical data regarding the status of the motility of the bowel. Initially, the examiner must listen with the diaphragm of the stethoscope below and to the right of the umbilicus. Proceeding methodically through all four quadrants, the examiner lifts and places the diaphragm of the stethoscope lightly against the abdomen. Normal bowel sounds include high-pitched, gurgling sounds that occur approximately every 5 to 15 seconds or at a rate of 5 to 34 times each minute. Colonic sounds are low pitched and have a rumbling quality. A venous hum may also be audible at times.[6] See Table 21-1 for list of abnormal abdominal sounds.

Abnormal findings include the absence of bowel sounds throughout a 5-minute period,[7] extremely soft and widely separated sounds, and increased sounds with a high-pitched, loud rushing sound (peristaltic rush). Absent bowel sounds may occur as a result of inflammation, ileus, electrolyte disturbances, and ischemia. Bowel sounds may be increased with diarrhea and early intestinal obstruction.[6] The abdomen should also be auscultated for the presence of bruits using the bell of the stethoscope. Bruits are created by turbulent flow over a partially obstructed artery and are always considered an abnormal finding. The aorta, right and left renal arteries, and iliac arteries should be auscultated.[5,6]

PERCUSSION

Nursing priorities in percussion of the patient with gastrointestinal dysfunction focus on assessment of the deep organs. Percussion is used to elicit information about deep organs, such as the liver, spleen, and pancreas. Because the abdomen is a sensitive area, muscle tension may interfere with this part of the assessment. Because percussion often helps relax tense muscles, it is performed before palpation. Percussion, in the absence of disease, is most helpful in delineating the position and size of the liver and spleen, and it also assists in the detection of fluid, gaseous distention, and masses in the abdomen.[5]

Percussion should proceed systemically and lightly in all four quadrants. Normal findings include tympany over the stomach when empty, tympany or hyperresonance over the intestine, and dullness over the liver and spleen. Abnormal areas of dullness may indicate an underlying mass. Solid masses, enlarged organs, and a distended bladder also produce areas of dullness. Dullness over both flanks may be indicative of ascites and requires further assessment.[6]

PALPATION

Nursing priorities in palpation of the patient with gastrointestinal dysfunction focus on (1) light palpation and (2) deep palpation of the abdominal area. Palpation is the assessment technique most useful in detecting abdominal pathologic conditions. Both light and deep palpation of each organ and quadrant should be completed. Light palpation assesses the depth of skin and fascia and has a depth of palpation of approximately 1 cm. Deep palpation assesses the rectus abdominis muscle and is performed bimanually to a depth of 4 to 5 cm. Deep palpation is most helpful in detecting abdominal masses. Areas in which the patient complains of tenderness should be palpated last.[6]

Table 21-2
Selected Laboratory Studies of Gastrointestinal Function

TEST	NORMAL FINDINGS	CLINICAL SIGNIFICANCE OF ABNORMAL FINDINGS
Stool studies	Resident microorganisms: clostridia, enterococci, *Pseudomonas,* a few yeasts	Detection of *Salmonella typhi* (typhoid fever), *Shigella* (dysentery), *Vibrio cholerae* (cholera), *Yersinia* (enterocolitis), *Escherichia coli* (gastroenteritis), *Staphylococcus aureus* (food poisoning), *Clostridium botulinum* (food poisoning), *Clostridium perfringens* (food poisoning), *Aeromonas* (gastroenteritis)
	Fat: 2-6 g/24 hr	Steatorrhea (increased values) from intestinal malabsorption or pancreatic insufficiency
	Pus: none	Large amounts of pus associated with chronic ulcerative colitis, abscesses, anal-rectal fistula
	Occult blood: none (orthotolidine, guaiac test)	Positive tests associated with bleeding
	Ova and parasites: none	Detection of *Entamoeba histolytica* (amebiasis), *Giardia lamblia* (giardiasis), worms
D-Xylose absorption	5-hr urinary excretion: 4.5 g/L	Differentiation of pancreatic steatorrhea (normal D-xylose absorption) from intestinal steatorrhea (impaired D-xylose absorption)
	Peak blood level: >30 mg/dl	
Gastric acid stimulation	11-20 mEq/hr after stimulation	Detection of duodenal ulcers, Zollinger-Ellison syndrome (increased values); gastric atrophy, gastric carcinoma (decreased values)
Culture and sensitivity of duodenal contents	No pathogens	Detection of *Salmonella typhi* (typhoid fever)

Modified from McCance KL, Huether SE: *Pathophysiology: the biologic basis for disease in adults and children,* ed 4, St Louis, 2002, Mosby.

Table 21-3
Common Laboratory Studies of Liver Function

TEST	NORMAL VALUE	INTERPRETATION
Serum Enzymes		
Alkaline phosphatase	13-39 units/ml	Increases with biliary obstruction and cholestatic hepatitis
Aspartate transferase (AST)*	5-40 units/ml	Increases with hepatocellular injury
Alanine transferase (ALT)†	5-35 units/ml	Increases with hepatocellular injury
Lactate dehydrogenase (LDH)	200-500 units/ml	Isoenzyme LD_5 elevated with hypoxic and primary liver injury
5′-Nucleotidase	2-11 units/ml	Increases with increased alkaline phosphatase, cholestatic disorders
Bilirubin Metabolism		
Serum bilirubin		
• Indirect (unconjugated)	<0.8 mg/dl	Increases with hemolysis (lysis of red blood cells)
• Direct (conjugated)	0.2-0.4 mg/dl	Increases with hepatocellular injury or obstruction
Total	<1.0 mg/dl	Increases with biliary obstruction
Urine bilirubin	0	Decreases with biliary obstruction
Urine urobilinogen	0-4 mg/24 hr	Increases with hemolysis or shunting of portal blood flow
Serum Proteins		
Albumin	3.3-5.5 g/dl	Reduced with hepatocellular injury
Globulin	2.5-3.5 g/dl	Increases with hepatitis
Total	6-7 g/dl	
Albumin/globulin (A/G) ratio	1.5:1-2.5:1	Ratio reverses with chronic hepatitis or other chronic liver disease
Transferrin	250-300 mcg/dl	Liver damage with decreased values; iron deficiency with increased values
Alpha-fetoprotein (AFP)	6-20 ng/ml	Elevated values in primary hepatocellular carcinoma
Blood-Clotting Functions		
Prothrombin time (PT)	11.5-14 seconds or 90%-100% of control	Increases with chronic liver disease (cirrhosis) or vitamin K deficiency
Partial thromboplastin time (PTT)	25-40 seconds	Increases with severe liver disease or heparin therapy
Bromsulphalein (BSP) excretion	<6% retention in 45 minutes	Increased retention with hepatocellular injury

From McCance KL, Huether SE: *Pathophysiology: the biologic basis for disease in adults and children,* ed 4, St Louis, 2002, Mosby.

*Also aspartate aminotransferase; previously serum glutamic-oxaloacetic transaminase (SGOT).

†Also alanine aminotransferase; previously serum glutamic-pyruvic transaminase (SGPT).

Normal findings include no areas of tenderness or pain, no masses, and no hardened areas. Persistent involuntary guarding may indicate peritoneal inflammation, particularly if it continues even after relaxation techniques are used. Rebound tenderness, in which pain increases with quick release of palpated area, is indicative of an inflamed peritoneum.[4]

LABORATORY STUDIES

The value of various laboratory studies used to diagnose and treat diseases of the GI system has been emphasized often. No single study, however, provides an overall picture of the various organs' functional state. Also, no single value is predictive by itself. Laboratory studies used in the assessment of GI function, liver function, and pancreatic function are found in Tables 21-2, 21-3, and 21-4, respectively.

DIAGNOSTIC PROCEDURES

Table 21-5 presents an overview of the various diagnostic procedures used to evaluate the patient with GI dysfunction.

Table 21-4
Common Laboratory Studies of Pancreatic Function

TEST		NORMAL VALUE / CLINICAL SIGNIFICANCE
Serum amylase	60-180 Somogyi units/ml	Elevated levels with pancreatic inflammation
Serum lipase	1.5 Somogyi units/ml	Elevated levels with pancreatic inflammation May be elevated with other conditions; differentiates with amylase, isoenzyme study
Urine amylase	35-260 Somogyi units/hr	Elevated levels with pancreatic inflammation
Secretin test	Volume 1.8 ml/kg/hr HCO_3^- concentration: >80 mEq/L HCO_3^- output: >10 mEq/L/30 sec	Decreased volume with pancreatic disease (secretin stimulates pancreatic secretion)
Stool fat	2-5 g/25 hr	Measures fatty acids; decreased pancreatic lipase increases stool fat

From McCance KL, Huether SE: Pathophysiology: the biologic basis for disease in adults and children, ed 4, St Louis, 2002, Mosby.
HCO_3^-, Bicarbonate.

Table 21-5
Abdominal Diagnostic Procedures

PROCEDURE	EVALUATES	COMMENTS
Barium enema (also called lower GI series)*	Visualizes movement, position, and filling of various segments of colon after installation of barium by enema Diagnoses colorectal lesions, diverticulitis, inflammatory bowel disease, strictures, fistulas Evaluates colon size, length, patency	Low-fiber diet for 1-3 days before study. Bowel preparation with bowel irrigation (e.g., GoLytely) and cathartics. NPO for 8-12 hours before study. Cathartics must be given after study. Contraindicated if bowel perforation or obstruction exists.
Barium swallow, upper GI series, and small bowel follow-through*†	Visualizes position, shape, and activity of esophagus, stomach, duodenum, and jejunum Diagnoses esophageal lesions/varices or motility disorders, hiatal hernia, gastric ulcers/tumors, small bowel obstruction small bowel lesions, Crohn's disease Evaluates gastric and small bowel motility	Bowel preparation with bowel irrigation (e.g., GoLYTELY) and cathartics. NPO for 8-12 hours before study. Cathartics must be given after study. Contraindicated if bowel perforation or obstruction exists.
Angiography (celiac or mesenteric)	Evaluates portal vasculature Diagnoses source of GI bleeding Evaluates cirrhosis, portal hypertension, vascular damage resulting from trauma, intestinal ischemia, tumors	Bowel preparation (e.g., cathartics) as prescribed. NPO for 8 hours before study. Sedative usually prescribed before procedure.

Continued

Table 21-5

Abdominal Diagnostic Procedures—*cont'd*

PROCEDURE	EVALUATES	COMMENTS
	May be used to treat GI bleeding using vasopressin	If contrast media used: • Check for allergy to iodine before study. • Monitor for allergic reaction after procedure. • Ensure hydration after procedure. After procedure, keep affected extremity (catheter placed) immobilized in straight position for 6-12 hours. Monitor arterial puncture point for hemorrhage or hematoma. Monitor neurovascular status of affected limb. Monitor for indications of systemic emboli.
Cholecystography (oral, intravenous, common bile duct)	Assesses gallbladder function, patency of biliary system, and presence of gallstones	PTC contraindicated in patients with bleeding disorders.
Percutaneous transhepatic cholangiography (PTC)	Diagnoses extrahepatic/intrahepatic jaundice, biliary calculi, biliary obstruction, common bile duct injury	Fatty meal day before study, but fat-free evening meal. Enema may be given evening before study. NPO 8-12 hours before study. Check for allergy to iodine before study. Contrast medium administered orally evening before study; intravenously immediately before study; injected percutaneously into bile duct or directly into common bile duct during surgery. Monitor for allergic reaction after procedure. Ensure hydration after procedure. After PTC, monitor for clinical indications of bile leakage, hemorrhage, or peritonitis.
Computed tomography (CT) of abdomen	Diagnoses tumors, pancreatic cancer or cysts, pancreatitis, biliary tract disorders, obstructive versus nonobstructive jaundice, cirrhosis, liver metastases, ascites, lymph node metastases, aneurysm	No special preparation required.
	Evaluates vasculature and focal points found on nuclear scans	Contrast medium may be used; if used:
	Used to direct biopsy of tumors or aspiration of abscess	• Check for allergy to iodine before study. • Monitor for allergic reaction after procedure. • Ensure hydration after procedure.
Endoscopic retrograde cholangio-pancreatography (ERCP)	Diagnoses biliary stones, ductal stricture, ductal compression, neoplasms of pancreas and biliary system	Same as for esophagogastroduodenoscopy.
	Evaluates patency of biliary and pancreatic ducts, jaundice, pancreatitis, cholecystitis, hepatitis	Contraindicated if patient uncooperative or if bilirubin >3.5 mg/dl. Monitor for clinical indications of pancreatitis (most common complication) after study. Monitor for clinical indications of sepsis.
Endoscopy • Esophagogastro-duodenoscopy (EGD) • Colonoscopy	Directly visualizes mucosa of areas in GI tract EGD can be extended to visualize pancreas and gallbladder EGD diagnoses esophagitis, esophageal ulcers/strictures/varices, hiatal hernia, gastritis, gastric ulcers, pyloric obstruction, pernicious anemia, foreign bodies, duodenal inflammation/ulcers; evaluates esophageal/gastric motility, bleeding, lesions, anastomoses	Sedation may be prescribed, especially for colonoscopy. Bowel preparation with gastric irrigation (e.g., GoLYTELY) and cathartics required before lower GI endoscopy. NPO 4-8 hours before study.
• Proctosigmoidoscopy	Esophagoscopy or gastroscopy used therapeutically: sclerosis of varices	Keep NPO until gag reflex returns if sedated.

Table 21-5
Abdominal Diagnostic Procedures—*cont'd*

PROCEDURE	EVALUATES	COMMENTS
	Proctosigmoidoscopy diagnoses rectosigmoid cancer, strictures, polyps, inflammatory processes, hemorrhoids; evaluates bleeding from rectosigmoid area and surgical anastomoses Colonoscopy diagnoses diverticular disease, obstruction, strictures, radiation injury, polyps, neoplasms, bleeding, ischemia Colonoscopy or sigmoidoscopy used therapeutically: polyp removal Biopsies may be taken during any endoscopic procedure	Monitor closely after procedure for clinical indications of perforation and hemorrhage.
Flat plate of abdomen	Diagnoses perforated viscus, paralytic ileus, mechanical obstruction, intraabdominal mass Evaluates distribution of visceral gas (and identifies free air in peritoneum indicative of bowel perforation) Evaluates organ size	No preparation required.
Liver biopsy	Obtains tissue specimen for microscopic evaluation Diagnoses liver disease or malignancy	May be performed open or closed. • Open biopsy done in surgery. • Closed biopsy may be done at bedside; contraindicated if platelets <100,000/mm^3. Clotting profile evaluated before procedure. Patient must be cooperative because must take deep breath and hold for closed biopsy. Type/crossmatch 2 units blood before procedure. NPO for 4-8 hours before study. After procedure, position patient on right side for 2 hours; apply pressure dressing, and patient on bed rest for 24 hours. Observe for: • Hemorrhage: hypotension, dyspnea (subphrenic hematoma) • Pneumothorax: dyspnea, chest pain, diminished breath sounds on right, hypoxemia • Sepsis: fever, leukocytosis, rebound tenderness
Liver scan	Diagnoses cirrhosis, hepatitis, tumors, abscesses, cysts, tuberculosis	No preparation required.
Magnetic resonance imaging (MRI)	Evaluates liver, biliary tree, pancreas, spleen Differentiates cyst from solid mass Diagnoses hepatic metastasis Cannot be done if patient mechanically ventilated. Evaluates abscesses, fistulas, source of GI bleeding Used for staging of colorectal cancer	Cannot be used in patients with implanted metallic device, including pacemakers. No special preparation required.
Paracentesis	Analysis of fluid removed during peritoneal tap Diagnoses intraperitoneal bleeding with diagnostic peritoneal lavage	After tap, monitor for: • Peritoneal leakage • Clinical indications of infection, peritonitis
Percutaneous transhepatic portography	Diagnoses esophageal varices and visualizes portal venous circulation	As for angiography.
Radionuclide imaging (hepatobiliary scintigraphy) • HIDA scan • PIPIDA scan	Diagnoses hepatocellular disease, hepatic metastasis, biliary disease, lower GI bleeding, gastric reflux	NPO 2 hours before study.
Schilling test	Evaluates ileal absorption of vitamin B_{12}	Intramuscular (IM) vitamin B_{12} and oral radioactive B_{12} are given, and 24-hour urine specimen is collected.

Continued

Table 21-5
Abdominal Diagnostic Procedures—*cont'd*

PROCEDURE	EVALUATES	COMMENTS
	Diagnoses pernicious anemia caused by intrinsic factor deficiency and inadequate ileal absorption of intrinsic factor–vitamin B_{12} complex	
Ultrasound of abdomen	Evaluates pancreas, biliary ducts, gallbladder, liver Identifies tumor, abdominal abscesses, hepatocellular disease, splenomegaly, pancreatic or splenic cysts Differentiates obstructive from nonobstructive jaundice	All barium must have been cleared from GI tract before ultrasonography. NPO for 8 hours before study. If for evaluation of gallbladder: fat-free meal evening before study.

From Dennison RD: *Pass CCRN!,* ed 2, St Louis, 2000, Mosby.

GI, Gastrointestinal; *NPO,* nothing by mouth, *HIDA,* hepatobiliary iminodiacetic acid; *PIPIDA,* paraisopropyl iminodiacetic acid.

*Meglumine diatrizoate (Gastrografin) may be used, especially if bowel perforation is suspected.

†Ordered according to which area or areas need to be evaluated (e.g., "upper GI with small bowel follow-through" means stomach, pylorus, duodenum; "barium swallow with upper GI" means esophagus, stomach, pylorus).

Nursing Management

The nursing management of a patient undergoing a diagnostic procedure involves a variety of interventions. **Priorities are directed toward preparing the patient psychologically and physically for the procedure, monitoring the patient's responses to the procedure, and assessing the patient after the procedure.** Preparing the patient includes teaching the patient about the procedure, answering any questions, and transporting and/or positioning the patient for the procedure. Monitoring the patient's responses to the procedure includes observing the patient for signs of pain, anxiety, or hemorrhage and monitoring vital signs. Assessing the patient after the procedure includes observing for complications of the procedure and medicating the patient for any postprocedure discomfort. Any evidence of gastrointestinal bleeding should be immediately reported to the physician, and emergency measures to maintain circulation must be initiated.

evolve To test your mastery of this chapter, try the Open-Book Quiz at http://evolve.elsevier.com/Urden/priorities/

REFERENCES

1. O'Toole MT: Advanced assessment of the abdomen and gastrointestinal problems, *Nurs Clin North Am* 24:771, 1990.
2. Gehring PE: Physical assessment begins with a history, *RN* 54(11):26, 1991.
3. Seidel HM et al: *Mosby's guide to physical examination,* ed 6, St Louis, 2006, Mosby.
4. Barkauskas V et al: *Health and physical assessment,* ed 3, St Louis, 2002, Mosby.
5. Thompson JM et al: *Mosby's clinical nursing,* ed 5, St Louis, 2002, Mosby.
6. O'Hanlon-Nicholas T: Basic assessment series: gastrointestinal system, *Am J Nurs* 98(4):48, 1998.
7. Solomon KH, Wilson CM: (2002) A case study approach for abdominal assessment, *Clin Excellence Nurse Pract* 6(1):3, 2002.

CHAPTER

22 Gastrointestinal Disorders and Therapeutic Management

DEBORAH BARNES

OBJECTIVES

- Describe the etiology and pathophysiology of the major gastrointestinal (GI) disorders seen in the critical care unit.
- Identify the clinical manifestations of GI disorders.
- Explain the treatment of GI disorders.
- Discuss the nursing priorities for managing a patient with GI dysfunction.
- Outline the use and care of GI tubes.
- Depict the postoperative nursing management of a patient undergoing GI surgery or liver transplantation.

Understanding the pathology of a disease, the areas of assessment on which to focus, and the usual medical management allows the critical care nurse to anticipate and plan nursing interventions more accurately. This chapter focuses on gastrointestinal disorders commonly seen in the critical care environment.

ACUTE GASTROINTESTINAL HEMORRHAGE

DESCRIPTION

Gastrointestinal (GI) hemorrhage is a medical emergency that remains a very common complication of critical illness[1] and results in almost 300,000 hospital admissions yearly.[2] Despite advances in medical knowledge and nursing care, the mortality rate for patients with acute GI bleeding has not changed in more than 50 years; it remains between 5% and 35%.[2,3]

ETIOLOGY

GI hemorrhage occurs from bleeding in the upper or lower GI tract. The ligament of Treitz is the anatomic division used to differentiate between the two sites. Thus bleeding proximal to the ligament is considered to be upper GI in origin, and bleeding distal to the ligament is considered to be lower GI in origin.[4] The various causes of acute GI hemorrhage are listed in Box 22-1.[1,3,5] Only the three main causes of GI hemorrhage commonly seen in the intensive care unit (ICU) are discussed further.

Peptic Ulcer Disease

Peptic ulcer disease (gastric and duodenal ulcers), resulting from the breakdown of the gastromuscosal lining, is the leading cause of upper GI hemorrhage, accounting for approximately 50% of the cases.[3,6]

Box 22-1

Etiology of Acute Gastrointestinal (GI) Hemorrhage

Upper GI
- Peptic ulcer disease
- Stress ulcers
- Esophagogastric varices
- Mallory-Weiss tear
- Esophagitis
- Neoplasm
- Aortoenteric fistula
- Angiodysplasia

Lower GI
- Diverticulosis
- Angiodysplasia
- Neoplasm
- Inflammatory bowel disease
- Trauma
- Infectious colitis
- Radiation colitis
- Ischemia
- Aortoenteric fistula
- Hemorrhoids

Normally, protection of the gastric mucosa from the digestive effects of gastric secretions is accomplished in several ways. First, the gastroduodenal mucosa is coated by a glycoprotein mucus barrier that that protects the surface of the epithelium from hydrogen ions and other noxious substances present in the gut lumen.[7] Adequate gastric mucosal blood flow is necessary to maintain this mucosal barrier function. Second, gastroduodenal epithelial cells are protected structurally against damage from acid and pepsin because they are connected by tight junctions that help prevent acid penetration. Lastly, prostaglandins and nitric oxide protect the mucosal barrier by stimulating mucus and bicarbonate secretion and inhibiting the secretion of acid.[7,8]

Peptic ulceration occurs when these protective mechanisms cease to function, thus allowing gastroduodenal mucosal breakdown. Once the mucosal lining is penetrated, gastric secretions autodigest the layers of the stomach or duodenum, leading to injury of the mucosal and submucosal layers. This results in damaged blood vessels and subsequent hemorrhage.[7] The two main causes of disruption of gastroduodenal mucosal resistance are nonsteroidal antiinflammatory drugs[9] and the bacterial action of *Helicobacter pylori*.[10]

Stress Ulcers

Stress ulcers is a term used to describe the gastric mucosal abnormalities often found in the critically ill patient that develop in response to severe stress in other organ systems. These abnormalities develop rapidly within hours of admission. They range from superficial mucosal erosions to deep ulcers and are usually limited to the stomach. Stress ulcers occur via the same pathophysiologic mechanisms as peptic ulcer disease, but the main cause of disruption of gastric mucosal resistance is increased acid production and decreased mucosal blood flow resulting in ischemia and degeneration of the mucosal lining.[11] Patients at risk include those in high physiologic stress situations, such as occur with mechanical ventilation, extensive burns, severe trauma, major surgery, shock, or acute neurologic disease.[12] GI hemorrhage is estimated to occur in 1% to 4% of patients who develop stress ulcers.[11]

Esophagogastric Varices

Esophagogastric varices are engorged and distended blood vessels of the esophagus and proximal stomach that develop as a result of portal hypertension secondary to hepatic cirrhosis, a chronic disease of the liver that results in damage to the liver sinusoids (Figure 22-1). Without adequate sinusoid function, resistance to portal blood flow is increased and pressures within the liver are elevated. This leads to a rise in portal venous pressure (portal hypertension), causing collateral circulation to divert portal blood from areas of high pressure within the liver to adjacent areas of low pressure outside the liver, such as into the veins of the esophagus, spleen, intestines, and stomach. The tiny, thin-walled vessels of the esophagus and proximal stomach that receive this diverted blood

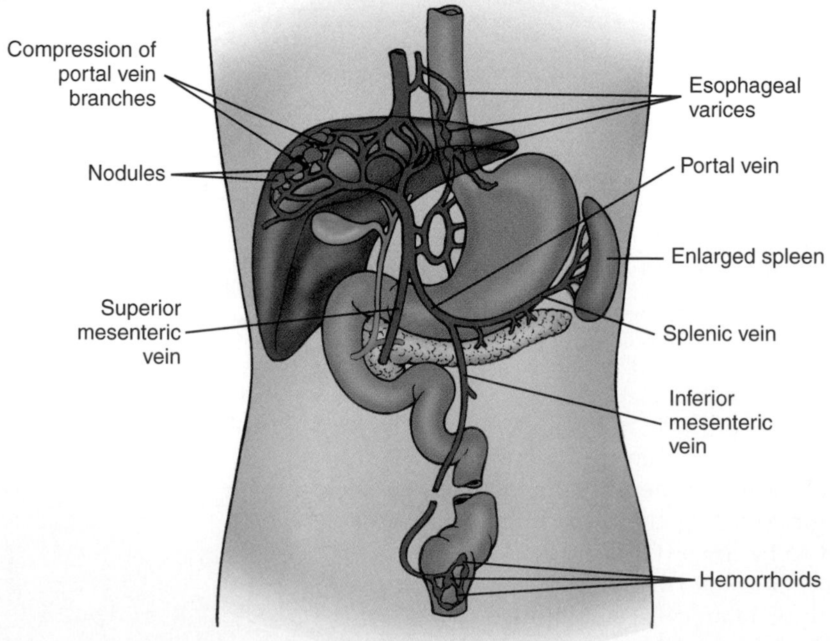

FIGURE 22-1. Esophageal varices caused by cirrhosis. (Modified from Powell LW, Piper DW: *Fundamentals of gastroenterology*, Sydney, 1991, McGraw-Hill.)

lack sturdy mucosal protection. The vessels become engorged and dilated, forming esophagogastric varices that are vulnerable to damage from gastric secretions and may result in subsequent rupture and massive hemorrhage.[13] The risk of variceal bleeding increases with disease severity and variceal size, but overall, bleeding occurs in 16% to 44% of the patients.[13]

Pathophysiology

GI hemorrhage is a life-threatening disorder that is characterized by acute, massive GI bleeding. Regardless of the cause, acute GI hemorrhage results in hypovolemic shock, initiation of the shock response, and the development of multiple organ dysfunction syndrome if left untreated (Figure 22-2 and the Concept Map).[2,14] However, the most common cause of death in GI hemorrhage is exacerbation of the underlying disease, not intractable hypovolemic shock.

Assessment and Diagnosis

The initial clinical presentation of the patient with acute GI hemorrhage is that of a patient in hypovolemic shock; the clinical presentation will vary depending on the amount of blood lost (Table 22-1).[8] Hematemesis (bright-red or brown/coffee-ground emesis), hematochezia (bright-red stools), and melena (black, tarry, or dark-red stools) are the hallmarks of GI hemorrhage.[2]

Table 22-1

Clinical Classification of Hemorrhage

CLASS	BLOOD LOSS (%)	CLINICAL SIGNS/SYMPTOMS
1	≤15	Pulse rate: normal or <100 beats/min (supine) Capillary refill: <3 sec Urine output: adequate (30-35 ml/hr) Orthostatic hypotension Apprehensive
2	15-30	Pulse rate: increased (>100 beats/min) Capillary refill: sluggish Pulse pressure: decreased Blood pressure: normal (supine) Tachypnea Urine output: low (25-30 ml/hr)
3	30-40	Pulse rate: 120+ beats/min (supine) Hypotension Skin: cool, pale Confused Hyperventilating Urine output: low (5-15 ml/hr)
4	≥40	Profoundly hypotensive Pulse rate: 140+ beats/min Confused, lethargic Urine output minimal

From Klein DG: *AACN Clin Issues Crit Care Nurs* 1:508, 1990.

Hematemesis

The patient who is vomiting blood is usually bleeding from a source above the duodenojejunal junction because reverse peristalsis is seldom sufficient to cause hematemesis if the bleeding point is below this area. The hematemesis may be bright red or coffee-ground in appearance, depending on the amount of gastric contents at the time of bleeding and the length of time the blood has been in contact with gastric secretions. Gastric acid converts bright-red hemoglobin to brown hematin, accounting for the coffee-ground appearance of the emesis. Bright-red emesis results from profuse bleeding with little contact with gastric secretions.[2]

Hematochezia and Melena

The presence of blood in the GI tract results in increased peristalsis and diarrhea. Hematochezia (bright red stool) occurs from massive lower GI hemorrhage and, if rapid enough, upper GI hemorrhage. Melena (black, tarry, or dark red stool) occurs from digestion of blood from an upper GI hemorrhage and may take several days to clear after the bleeding has stopped.[2]

Laboratory Studies

Laboratory tests can help determine the extent of bleeding, although it is important to realize that the patient's hemoglobin and hematocrit are poor indicators of the severity of blood loss if the bleeding is acute. As whole blood is lost, plasma and red blood cells are lost in the same proportion; thus if the patient's hematocrit is 45% before a bleeding episode, it will still be 45% several hours later.[8] It may take as long as 72 hours for the redistribution of plasma from the extravascular space to the intravascular space to occur and cause the patient's hemoglobin and hematocrit to drop.[2,15] A platelet count and prothrombin time should also be obtained.[2]

Diagnostic Procedures

To isolate and treat the source of bleeding, an urgent fiberoptic endoscopy is usually undertaken. Endoscopy is able to identify the source of hemorrhage in more than 90% of lesions.[16] Before the endoscopy, the patient must be hemodynamically stabilized and the area that is to be visualized must be cleared of blood.[2,16] A tagged red blood cell and/or an angiogram may be done to assist with localizing and treating a bleeding lesion in the GI tract when it is impossible to clearly view the GI tract because of continued active bleeding.[3]

Medical Management

To reduce mortality related to GI hemorrhage, patients at risk should be identified early and interventions should be implemented to reduce gastric acidity and support the gastric mucosal defense mechanisms.

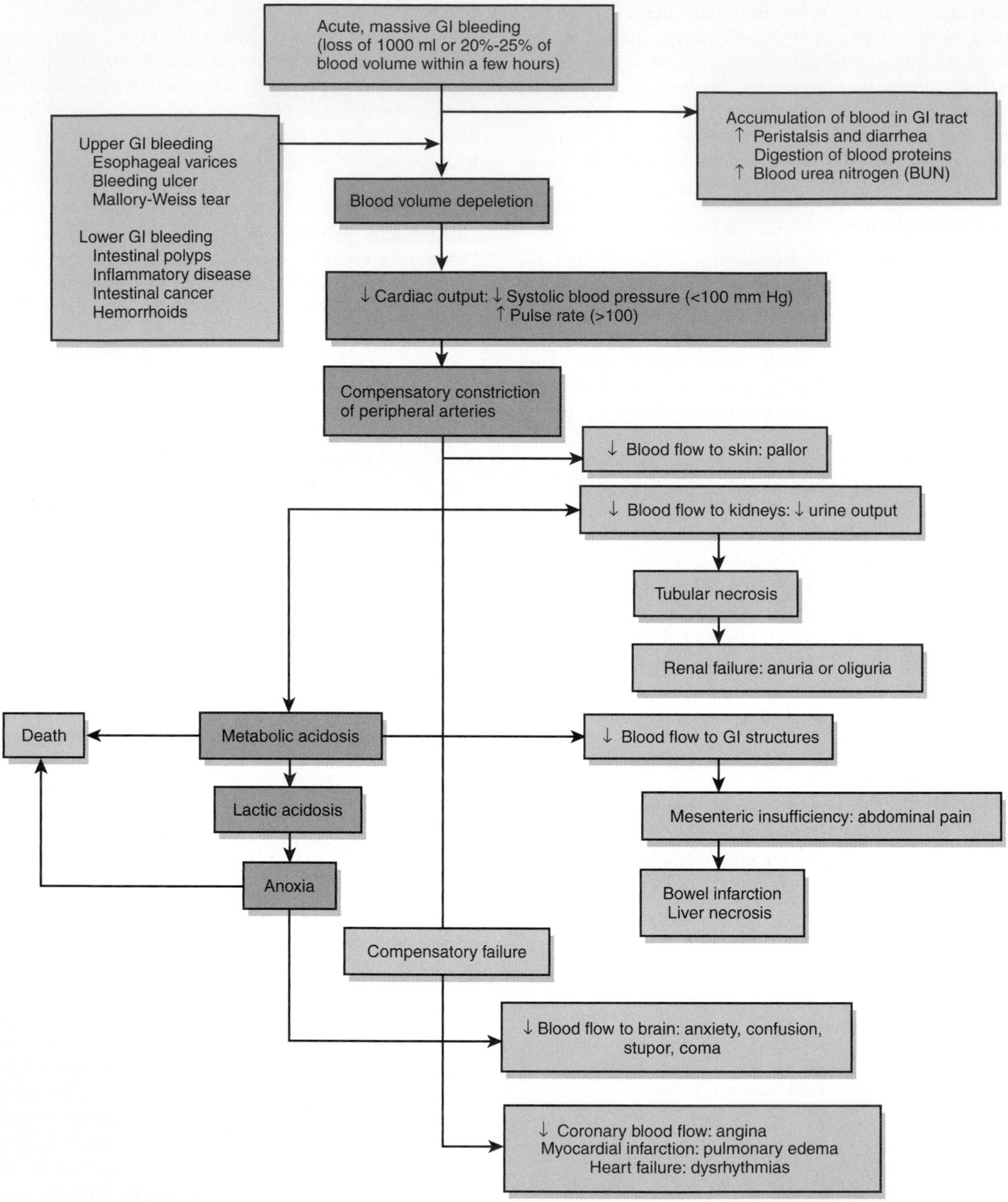

FIGURE 22-2. Pathophysiology of acute gastrointestinal hemorrhage. (From Huether SE, McCance KL, Tarmina MS: Alterations of digestive function. In McCance KL, Huether SE, editors: *Pathophysiology: the biologic basis for disease in adults and children,* ed 4, St Louis, 2002, Mosby.)

Management of the patient at risk for GI hemorrhage should include prophylactic administration of pharmacologic agents for gastric acid neutralization. These agents include antacids, histamine$_2$ (H_2) antagonists, cytoprotective agents, and proton pump inhibitors.[7]

Priorities in the medical management of the patient with GI hemorrhage include airway protection, fluid resuscitation to achieve hemodynamic stability, correction of comorbid conditions (coagulopathy), therapeutic procedures to control and/or stop bleeding, and

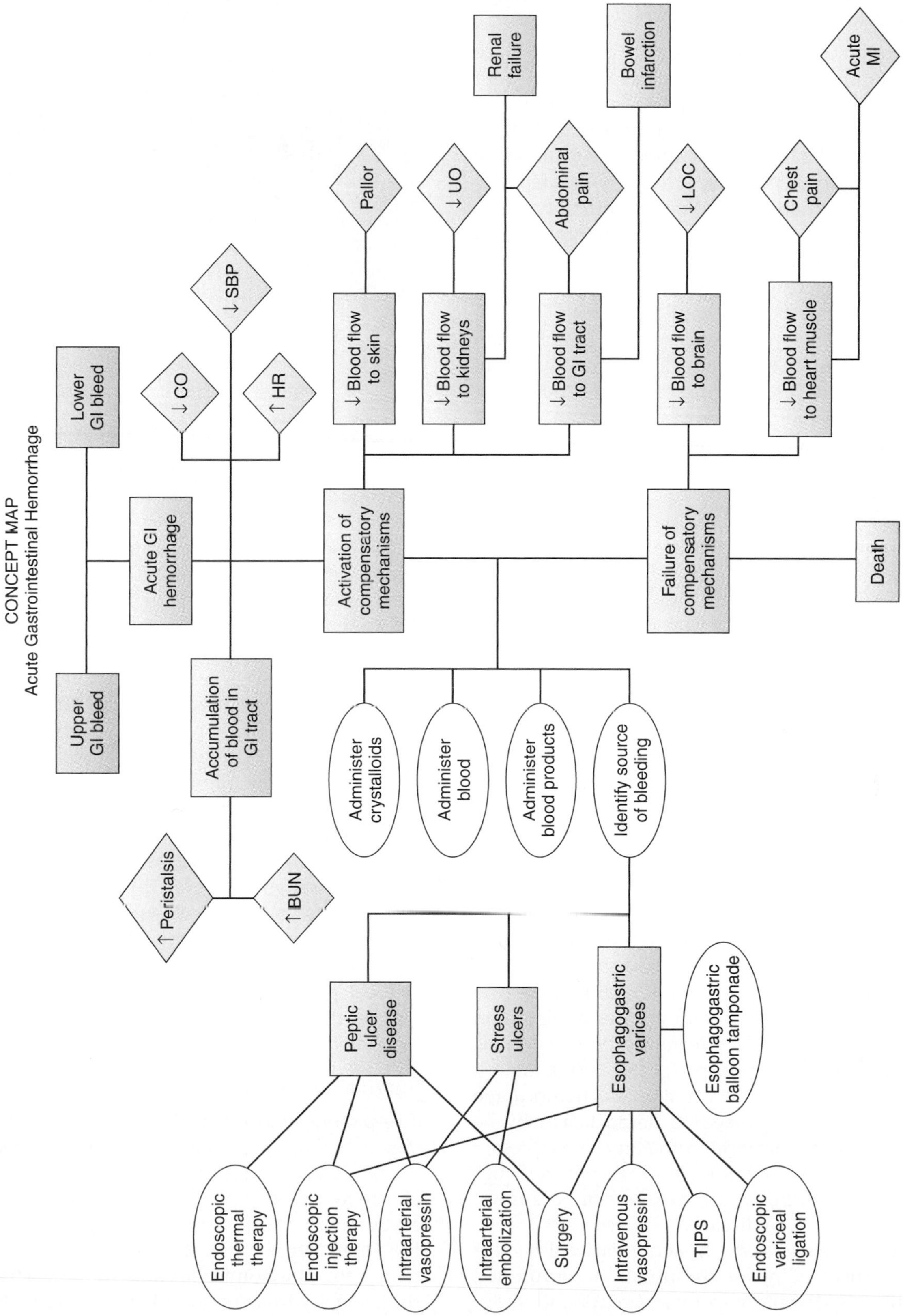
CONCEPT MAP
Acute Gastrointestinal Hemorrhage
Upper GI bleed
Lower GI bleed
Acute GI hemorrhage
Accumulation of blood in GI tract
↑ Peristalsis
↑ BUN
↓ CO
↓ SBP
↑ HR
Activation of compensatory mechanisms
↓ Blood flow to skin
↓ Blood flow to kidneys
↓ Blood flow to GI tract
↓ Blood flow to brain
↓ Blood flow to heart muscle
Pallor
↓ UO
Abdominal pain
↓ LOC
Chest pain
Renal failure
Bowel infarction
Acute MI
Failure of compensatory mechanisms
Death
Administer crystalloids
Administer blood
Administer blood products
Identify source of bleeding
Peptic ulcer disease
Stress ulcers
Esophagogastric varices
Esophagogastric balloon tamponade
Endoscopic thermal therapy
Endoscopic injection therapy
Intraarterial vasopressin
Intraarterial embolization
Surgery
Intravenous vasopressin
TIPS
Endoscopic variceal ligation

diagnostic procedures to determine the exact etiology of the bleeding.[2]

Stabilization

The initial treatment priority is the restoration of adequate circulating blood volume to treat or prevent shock. This is accomplished with the administration of intravenous infusions of crystalloids, blood, and blood products.[2,17] A central venous catheter or pulmonary artery catheter may be necessary to guide fluid replacement therapy, particularly in those patients at risk for developing cardiac failure.[17] Supplemental oxygen therapy is initiated to increase oxygen delivery and improve tissue perfusion.[17] Intubation may be necessary in the patient at risk for aspiration or to facilitate gastric lavage.[2,17] A large nasogastric (NG) tube may be inserted to confirm the diagnosis of active bleeding and to prepare the esophagus, stomach, and proximal duodenum for endoscopic evaluation.[18] A urinary drainage catheter should be inserted to monitor urine output.[2,17]

Control Bleeding

Interventions to control bleeding are the second priority for the patient with GI hemorrhage.

Peptic Ulcer Disease. In the patient with GI hemorrhage related to peptic ulcer disease, bleeding hemostasis may be accomplished endoscopically. Endoscopic therapies include thermal, injection, and mechanical.[2,16] Endoscopic thermal therapy uses heat to cauterize the bleeding vessel, whereas injection therapy uses a variety of agents, such as hypertonic saline, epinephrine, ethanol, and sclerosants, to induce localized vasoconstriction of the bleeding vessel. Mechanical therapy uses endoscopic clips to compress the bleeding vessel at the base of the ulcer.[2,16] Intraarterial infusion of vasopressin into the gastric artery or intraarterial injection of an embolizing agent (Gelfoam pledgets, stainless steel coils, platinum microcoils, and polyvinyl alcohol particles) can also be performed during arteriography to control bleeding once the site has been identified.[2,6] Intraarterial administration of vasopressin is less effective for duodenal lesions because of the dual blood supply of the duodenum.[2]

Stress Ulcers. In the patient with GI hemorrhage caused by stress ulcers, bleeding hemostasis may be accomplished via intraarterial infusion of vasopressin and intraarterial embolization. Endoscopic therapies have been shown to be of minimal benefit because of the diffuse nature of the disease.[2]

Esophagogastric Varices. In acute variceal hemorrhage, control of bleeding may be initially accomplished through the use of pharmacologic agents and endoscopic therapies. Intravenous vasopressin, somatostatin, and octreotide have been shown to reduce portal venous pressure and slow variceal hemorrhaging by constricting the splanchnic arteriolar bed.[19] Two commonly used endoscopic therapies are injection therapy and variceal ligation. Endoscopic injection therapy (also referred to as sclerotherapy) controls bleeding via the injection of a sclerosing agent in or around the varices. This creates an inflammatory reaction that induces vasoconstriction and results in the formation of a venous thrombosis. During endoscopic variceal band ligation, bands are placed around the varices to create an obstruction to stop the bleeding.[2,19]

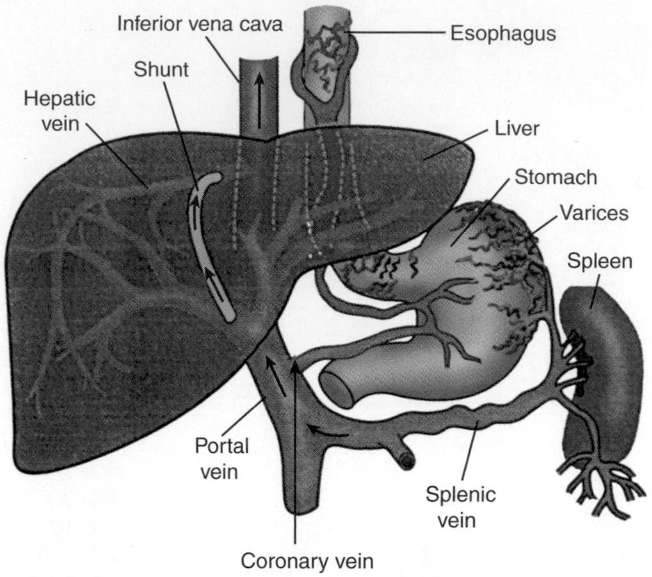

FIGURE 22-3. Anatomic location of the transjugular intrahepatic portosystemic shunt (TIPS). (From Vargas HE, Gerber D, Abu-Elmagd K: *Surg Clin North Am* 79:1, 1999.)

If these initial therapies fail, esophagogastric balloon tamponade or transjugular intrahepatic portosystemic shunting (TIPS) may be necessary. Balloon tamponade tubes (Sengstaken-Blakemore, Linton, and Minnesota tubes) stop hemorrhaging by applying direct pressure against bleeding vessels while decompressing the stomach.[20] In a TIPS procedure, a channel between the systemic and portal venous systems is created to redirect portal blood, thereby reducing portal hypertension and decompressing the varices to control bleeding (Figure 22-3).[2,19,20]

Surgical Intervention

The patient who remains hemodynamically unstable despite volume replacement may need urgent surgery.

Peptic Ulcer Disease. The operative procedure of choice to control bleeding from peptic ulcer disease is a vagotomy and pyloroplasty. During this procedure the vagus nerve to the stomach is severed, thus eliminating the autonomic stimulus to the gastric cells and reducing hydrochloric acid production. Because the vagus nerve also stimulates motility, a pyloroplasty is performed to provide for gastric emptying.[14]

Stress Ulcers. There are several operative procedures to control bleeding from stress ulcers. A total

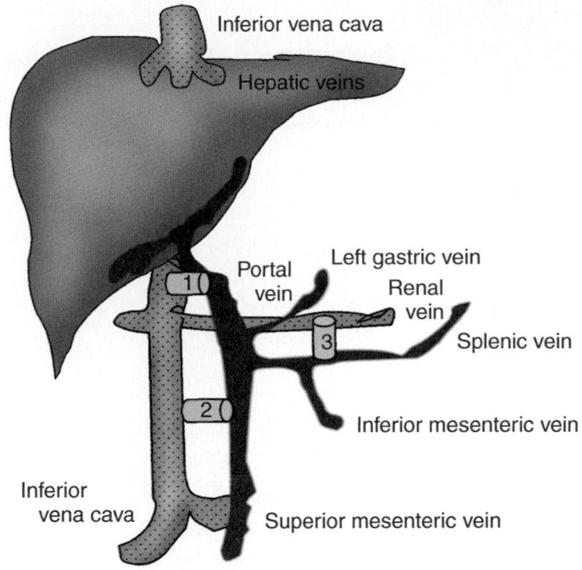

FIGURE 22-4. The anatomy of the portal venous system and the sites in which surgical anastomoses are made to shunt blood from the portal *(dark)* to the systemic *(light)* venous circulation. Sites used for surgical portal decompression: (1) portacaval shunt; (2) mesocaval shunt; (3) splenorenal shunt. (From Luketic VA, Sanyal AJ: *Gastroenterol Clin North Am* 29:387, 2000.)

gastrectomy is performed when bleeding is generalized. An oversew of the ulcers is performed when bleeding is localized. A total gastrectomy involves the complete removal of the stomach with anastomosis of the esophagus to the jejunum. During an oversew of the ulcers, the bleeding vessel is ligated and the ulcer crater is closed.[14]

Esophagogastric Varices. The Operative procedures to control bleeding gastroesophageal varices include portacaval shunt, mesocaval shunt, and splenorenal shunt (Figure 22-4).[2,20,21] These shunt procedures are also referred to as decompression procedures because they result in the diversion of portal blood flow away from the liver and decompression of the portal system. The portacaval shunt procedure has two variations. An end-to-side portacaval shunt procedure involves the ligation of the hepatic end of the portal vein with subsequent anastomosis to the vena cava. During a side-to-side portacaval shunt procedure, the side of the portal vein is anastomosed to the side of the vena cava. A mesocaval shunt procedure involves the insertion of a graft between the superior mesenteric artery and the vena cava. During a distal splenorenal shunt procedure, the splenic vein is detached from the portal vein and anastomosed to the left renal vein.[21]

Nursing Management

All critically ill patients should be considered at risk for stress ulcers and therefore GI hemorrhage. It is imperative that the nurse ensure the patient is receiving appropriate stress ulcer prophylaxis. Nursing actions also include the correct and timely administration of the selected pharmacologic agent.[22] Patients at risk should be assessed for the presence of bright-red or coffee-ground emesis, bloody NG aspirate, and bright-red, black, or dark-red stools.[2,22] Any signs of bleeding should be promptly reported to the physician.[22]

Nursing management of a patient experiencing acute GI hemorrhage incorporates a variety of nursing diagnoses (Box 22-2). **Nursing priorities are directed toward (1) administering volume replacement, (2) providing comfort and emotional support, (3) maintaining surveillance for complications, and (4) educating the patient and family.**

Box 22-2

NURSING DIAGNOSIS PRIORITIES

Acute Gastrointestinal Hemorrhage

- Deficient Fluid Volume related to absolute loss, p. A-16
- Decreased Cardiac Output related to alterations in preload, p. A-12
- Powerlessness related to health care environment or illness-related regimen, p. A-44
- Deficient Knowledge: Discharge Regimen related to lack of previous exposure to information (see Patient Education: Acute Gastrointestinal Hemorrhage), p. A-18

PATIENT EDUCATION

Acute Gastrointestinal Hemorrhage

- GI hemorrhage
- Specific etiology
- Precipitating factor modification
- Interventions to reduce further bleeding episodes
- Importance of taking medications
- Lifestyle changes
- Stress management
- Diet modifications
- Alcohol cessation
- Smoking cessation

Administering Volume Replacement

Measures to facilitate volume replacement include obtaining intravenous access and administering prescribed fluids and blood products. Two large-diameter peripheral IV catheters should be inserted to facilitate the rapid administration of prescribed fluids.[2]

Maintaining Surveillance for Complications

The patient should also be continuously observed for signs of gastric perforation. Although a rare complication, gastric perforation constitutes a surgical emergency. Signs and symptoms include sudden, severe,

Box 22-3

Collaborative Management

Acute Gastrointestinal Hemorrhage
- Initiate fluid resuscitation to achieve hemodynamic stability
  - Crystalloids
  - Colloids
  - Blood and blood products
- Determine the etiology of the bleeding
  - Gastric lavage
- Control bleeding
  - Endoscopic interventions
  - Vasopressin, somatostatin, octreotide
  - Esophagogastric balloon tube
  - Transjugular intrahepatic portosystemic shunting
  - Surgery
- Provide comfort and emotional support
- Maintain surveillance for complications
  - Hypovolemic shock
  - Gastric perforation

generalized abdominal pain with significant rebound tenderness and rigidity. Perforation should be suspected when fever, leukocytosis, and tachycardia persist despite adequate volume replacement.[2]

Patient Education

Early in the hospital stay, the patient and family should be taught about acute GI hemorrhage and its causes and treatments. As the patient moves toward discharge, teaching should focus on the interventions necessary for preventing the recurrence of the precipitating disorder. If an alcohol abuser, the patient should be encouraged to stop drinking and be referred to an alcohol cessation program.

Collaborative management of the patient with acute GI hemorrhage is outlined in Box 22-3.

ACUTE PANCREATITIS

DESCRIPTION

Acute pancreatitis is an inflammation of the pancreas that produces exocrine and endocrine dysfunction that may also involve surrounding tissues and/or remote organ systems. The clinical course can range from a mild, self-limiting disease to a systemic process characterized by organ failure, sepsis, and death. In approximately 75% to 85% of patients it takes the milder form of *edematous interstitial pancreatitis*, whereas the other 15% develop severe *acute necrotizing pancreatitis*. Reported mortality rates for acute pancreatitis vary from less than 1% for patients with mild pancreatitis to 10% to 24% in patients with severe disease.[23] Several prognostic scoring systems have been developed to predict the severity of acute pancreatitis. One of the most commonly used is Ranson's criteria (Box 22-4). If the patient has up to two factors present, predicted mortality is 1%; with three or four factors, 15% to 20% mortality; with five or six factors, 40% mortality; and with seven or eight factors, 100% predicted mortality.[24]

Box 22-4

Ranson's Criteria for Estimating the Severity of Acute Pancreatitis

At Admission

Age >55 years
Hypotension
Abnormal pulmonary findings
Abdominal mass
Hemorrhagic or discolored peritoneal fluid
Increased serum LDH levels (>350 units/L)
AST >250 units/L
Leukocytosis (>16,000/mm^3)
Hyperglycemia (>200 mg/dl; no diabetic history)
Neurologic deficit (confusion, localizing signs)

During Initial 48 Hours of Hospitalization

Fall in hematocrit >10% with hydration or hematocrit <30%
Necessity for massive fluid and colloid replacement
Hypocalcemia (<8 mg/dl)
Arterial Po_2 <60 mm Hg with or without acute respiratory distress syndrome
Hypoalbuminemia (<3.2 mg/dl)
Base deficit >4 mEq/L
Azotemia

From Latifi R, McIntosh JK, Dudrick SJ: *Surg Clin North Am* 71:583, 1991.
LDH, Lactate dehydrogenase; *AST*, aspartate aminotransferase; *Po_2*, partial pressure of oxygen.

ETIOLOGY

The two most common causes of acute pancreatitis are gallstones and alcoholism. Together they account for approximately 80% of cases. Other less common causes are quite diverse and include surgical trauma, hypercalcemia, various toxins, ischemia, infections, and the use of certain drugs (Box 22-5). In 10% to 20% of patients with acute pancreatitis, no etiologic factor can be determined.[24]

PATHOPHYSIOLOGY

In acute pancreatitis the normally inactive digestive enzymes become prematurely activated within the pancreas itself leading to autodigestion of pancreatic tissue. The enzymes become activated through various mechanisms, including obstruction or damage to the pancreatic duct system, alterations in the secretory processes of the acinar cells, infection, ischemia, and/or other unknown factors.[24,25]

Trypsin is the enzyme that becomes activated first and initiates the autodigestion process by triggering

Box 22-5

Etiology of Acute Pancreatitis

- Toxins—ethyl alcohol, methyl alcohol, scorpion, venom, parathion
- Biliary disease—stones, sludge, common bile duct obstruction
- Drugs—sulfonamides, thiazide diuretics, furosemide, estrogens, tetracycline, pentamidine, procainamide, salicylates, steroids, cyclosporine, amphetamines, nonsteroidal antiinflammatory agents, valproic acid, azathioprine, allopurinol
- Hypercalcemia—hyperparathyroidism
- Hyperlipidemia
- Tumors
- Infections—bacterial, viral, parasitic
- Trauma—abdominal, surgical, endoscopic
- Ischemia
- Transplant
- Vasculitis
- Pregnancy
- Hypothermia
- Sphincter of Oddi dysfunction
- Systemic lupus erythematosus
- Ampullary stenosis
- Idiopathic

Data from Steer ML: Acute pancreatitis. In Taylor MB, editor: *Gastrointestinal emergencies,* Baltimore, 1992, Williams & Wilkins.

Box 22-6

Presenting Clinical Manifestations of Acute Pancreatitis

- Pain
- Vomiting
- Nausea
- Fever
- Abdominal distention
- Abdominal guarding
- Abdominal tympany
- Hypoactive/absent bowel sounds
- Severe disease
  Peritoneal signs
  Ascites
  Jaundice
  Palpable abdominal mass
  Grey Turner's sign
  Cullen's sign
  Signs of hypovolemic shock

From Krumberger JM: *Crit Care Nurs Clin North Am* 5:185, 1993.

the secretion of proteolytic enzymes kallikrein, chymotrypsin, elastase, phospholipase A, and lipase. Release of kallikrein and chymotrypsin results in increased capillary membrane permeability, leading to leakage of fluid into the interstitium and the development of edema and relative hypovolemia. Elastase activation is the most harmful enzyme in terms of direct cell damage. It causes dissolution of the elastic fibers of blood vessels and ducts, leading to hemorrhage. Phospholipase A, in the presence of bile, destroys the phospholipids of cell membranes, causing severe pancreatic and adipose tissue necrosis. Lipase flows into the damaged tissue and is absorbed into the systemic circulation, resulting in fat necrosis of the pancreas and surrounding tissues.[24,25]

The extent of injury to the pancreatic cells determines which form of acute pancreatitis will develop. If injury to the pancreatic cells is mild and without necrosis, edematous pancreatitis develops. The acinar cells appear structurally intact, and blood flow is maintained through small capillaries and venules. This form of acute pancreatitis is self-limiting. If injury to the pancreatic cells is severe, acute necrotizing pancreatitis develops. Cellular destruction in pancreatic injury results in the release of toxic enzymes and inflammatory mediators into the systemic circulation and causes injury to vessels and other organs distant from the pancreas; this may result in systemic inflammatory response syndrome (SIRS), multiorgan failure, and/or death. Local tissue injury results in infection, abscess and pseudocyst formation, disruption of the pancreatic duct, and severe hemorrhage with shock.[24,25]

Assessment and Diagnosis

The clinical manifestations of acute pancreatitis range from mild to severe and often mimic other disorders (Box 22-6). Epigastric to midabdominal pain may vary from mild and tolerable to severe and incapacitating. Many patients report a twisting or knifelike sensation that radiates to the low dorsal region of the back. Nausea and vomiting is present in more than 80% of patients. The patient may obtain some comfort by leaning forward or assuming a semifetal position. Other clinical findings include fever, diaphoresis, weakness, tachypnea, hypotension, and tachycardia. Depending on the extent of fluid loss and hemorrhage, the patient may exhibit signs of hypovolemic shock.[24,26]

Physical Examination

The results of physical assessment usually reveal hypoactive bowel sounds and abdominal tenderness, guarding, distention, and tympany. Findings that could indicate pancreatic hemorrhage include Grey Turner's sign (gray-blue discoloration of the flank) and Cullen's sign (discoloration of the umbilical region); however, they are rare and would generally be seen several days into the illness.[24,27,28] A palpable abdominal mass is indicative of the presence of a pseudocyst or abscess.[28]

Laboratory Studies

Assessment of laboratory data usually demonstrates elevated levels of serum amylase and lipase. Serum lipase is more pancreas-specific than amylase and a more accurate marker for acute pancreatitis. Amylase is present in other body tissues, and other disorders (intraabdominal emergencies, renal insufficiency, salivary gland trauma, liver disease) may contribute to an elevated level. Unlike other serum enzymes, however, amylase is excreted in urine, and this clearance increases with acute pancreatitis. Measurement of urinary versus serum amylase should be considered in light of the patient's creatinine clearance. In addition, serum amylase may be elevated for only 3 to 5 days; if the patient delays seeking treatment, a normal level (false-negative) may be noted. Leukocytosis, hypocalcemia, hyperglycemia, hyperbilirubinemia, and hypoalbuminemia may also be present (Table 22-2).[8,24,28]

Diagnostic Procedures

An abdominal ultrasound is obtained as part of the diagnostic evaluation to determine the presence of biliary stones. A contrast-enhanced computed tomography (CT) scan is considered the gold standard for diagnosing pancreatitis as well as for ascertaining the overall degree of pancreatic inflammation and necrosis.[29]

Table 22-2

Laboratory Tests and Diagnostic Procedures in Acute Pancreatitis

STUDY	FINDING IN PANCREATITIS
Laboratory	
Serum amylase	Elevated
Serum isoamylase	Elevated
Urine amylase	Elevated
Serum lipase (if available)	Elevated
Serum triglycerides	Elevated
Glucose	Elevated
Calcium	Decreased
Magnesium	Decreased
Potassium	Decreased
Albumin	Decreased or increased
White blood cell count	Elevated
Bilirubin	May be elevated
Liver enzymes	May be elevated
Prothrombin time	Prolonged
Arterial blood gases	Hypoxemia, metabolic acidosis
Radiographic	
Abdominal	
Ultrasonography	
Magnetic resonance imaging	
ERCP	
Abdominal films (flat plate and upright or decubitus)	
Chest films (posteroanterior and lateral)	

From Krumberger JM: *Crit Care Nurs Clin North Am* 5:185, 1993.
ERCP, Endoscopic retrograde cholangiopancreatograph.

Medical Management

Initial management of the patient with severe acute pancreatitis includes ensuring adequate fluid and electrolyte replacement, providing nutritional support, and correcting metabolic alterations. In addition, careful monitoring for systemic and local complications is critical.[24,29]

Fluid Management

Because pancreatitis is often associated with massive fluid shifts, intravenous crystalloids and colloids are administered immediately to prevent hypovolemic shock and maintain hemodynamic stability. In severe forms of acute pancreatitis, the use of a pulmonary artery catheter may be used to guide ongoing fluid management.[24,27,29] Electrolytes are monitored closely, and abnormalities such as hypocalcemia, hypokalemia, and hypomagnesemia are corrected.[22,29] If hyperglycemia develops, exogenous insulin may be required.[29]

Nutritional Support

Until recently, conventional nutritional management was to place the patient on a nothing by mouth (NPO) regimen and institute intravenous hydration. The rationale was to rest the inflamed pancreas and prevent enzyme release. Oral feeding was only initiated when the attack had subsided and enzymes had normalized. Total parenteral nutrition (TPN) was started on patients anticipated to have oral feedings held for greater than 5 days. Although this practice is still followed in many hospitals, recent randomized clinical trials have demonstrated that enteral feeding (gastric or jejunal) is safe, cost-effective, associated with fewer septic and metabolic complications, and should be considered. TPN, however, still has a role in the critically ill patient with acute pancreatitis, especially in the presence of paralytic ileus or duodenal obstruction.[23,29] In the past, nasogastric suction was also recommended, but this intervention has not been shown to be of benefit and should only be instituted if the patient has persistent vomiting, obstruction, or gastric distention.[23]

Systemic Complications

Acute pancreatitis can affect every organ system, and recognition and treatment of systemic complications are crucial to management of the patient (Box 22-7). The most serious complications are hypovolemic shock, acute lung injury (ALI), acute renal failure (ARF), and GI hemorrhage. Hypovolemic shock is the result of relative hypovolemia resulting from third spacing of intravascular volume and vasodilation caused by the release of inflammatory immune mediators. These mediators also contribute to the development of ALI and ARF. Other possible pulmonary complications include pleural effusions, atelectasis, and pneumonia.

Stress ulcers and bleeding gastroesophageal varices (in the alcoholic patient) can precipitate the development of GI hemorrhage.[24,30]

Local Complications

Local complications include the development of infected pancreatic necrosis and pancreatic pseudocyst.[30] The necrotic areas of the pancreas can lead to the development of a widespread pancreatic infection (infected pancreatic necrosis), which significantly increases the risk of death. Prophylactic antibiotics have been shown to reduce sepsis and mortality and are initiated in patients suspected of having necrotizing pancreatitis. Once the patient develops infected necrosis, however, surgical debridement is necessary. The procedure of choice is a necrosectomy, which entails careful debridement of the necrotic tissue in and around the pancreas. It often requires postoperative lavage and multiple reexplorations with further debridement to remove all the necrotic tissue.[31] A pancreatic pseudocyst is a collection of pancreatic fluid enclosed by a nonepithelialized wall. Cyst formation may result from liquefaction of a pancreatic fluid collection or from direct obstruction in the main pancreatic duct. A pancreatic pseudocyst may (1) resolve spontaneously; (2) rupture, resulting in peritonitis; (3) erode a major blood vessel, resulting in hemorrhage; (4) become infected, resulting in abscess; or (5) invade surrounding structures, resulting in obstruction. Treatment involves drainage of the pseudocyst either surgically, endoscopically, or percutaneously.[30]

Nursing Management

Nursing management of the patient with pancreatitis incorporates a variety of nursing diagnoses (Box 22-8). **Nursing priorities are directed toward (1) providing pain relief and emotional support, (2) maintaining surveillance for complications, and (3) educating the patient and family.**

Box 22-8
NURSING DIAGNOSIS PRIORITIES
Acute Pancreatitis

- Acute Pain related to transmission and perception of cutaneous, visceral, muscular, ischemia impulses, p. A-7
- Deficient Fluid Volume related to relative fluid loss, p. A-16
- Decreased Cardiac Output related to alterations in preload, p. A-12
- Anxiety related to threat to biologic, psychologic, and/or social integrity, p. A-9
- Deficient Knowledge: Discharge Regimen related to lack of previous exposure to information (see Patient Education: Acute Pancreatitis), p. A-18

Box 22-7
Complications of Acute Pancreatitis

Respiratory
Early hypoxemia
Pleural effusion
Atelectasis
Pulmonary infiltration
ALI
Mediastinal abscess

Cardiovascular
Hypotension
Pericardial effusion
ST-T changes

Renal
Acute tubular necrosis
Oliguria
Renal artery or vein thrombosis

Hematologic
DIC
Thrombocytosis
Hyperfibrinogenemia

Endocrine
Hypocalcemia
Hypertriglyceridemia
Hyperglycemia

Neurologic
Fat emboli
Psychosis
Encephalopathy

Ophthalmic
Purtscher's retinopathy—sudden blindness

Dermatologic
Subcutaneous fat necrosis

GI/Hepatic
Hepatic dysfunction
Obstructive jaundice
Erosive gastritis
Paralytic ileus
Duodenal obstruction
Pancreatic
- Pseudocyst
- Phlegmon
- Abscess
- Ascites

Bowel infarction
Massive intraperitoneal bleed
Perforation
- Stomach
- Duodenum
- Small bowel
- Colon

From Ranson JHC: Complications of pancreatitis. In Taylor MB, editor: *Gastrointestinal emergencies,* Baltimore, 1992, Williams & Wilkins.
ALI, Acute lung injury; *DIC,* disseminated intravascular coagulation; *GI,* gastrointestinal.

PATIENT EDUCATION

Acute Pancreatitis

- Pancreatitis
- Specific etiology
- Precipitating factor modification
- Interventions to reduce further episodes
- Importance of taking medications
- Lifestyle changes
- Diet modification
- Stress management
- Alcohol cessation
- Diabetes management (if present)

Box 22-9

Signs and Symptoms of Pancreatic Infection

Symptoms
Persistent abdominal pain
Abdominal tenderness

Signs
Prolonged fever
Abdominal distention
Palpable abdominal mass
Vomiting

Diagnostics
Laboratory
- Increased white blood cell count
- Persistent elevation of serum amylase
- Hyperbilirubinemia
- Elevated alkaline phosphatase
- Positive culture and Gram's stain

Radiography/CT
- Pancreatic inflammation or enlargement
- Necrosis
- Cystic or mass lesions
- Fluid accumulations
- Pseudocyst abscess

From Krumberger JM: *Crit Care Nurs Clin North Am* 5:185, 1993.
CT, Computed tomography.

Providing Comfort and Emotional Support

Pain management is a major priority in acute pancreatitis. Administration of analgesics to achieve pain relief is essential. For years, meperidine (Demerol) was considered to be the preferred agent in the patient with acute pancreatitis because morphine produced spasms at the sphincter of Oddi. Recent studies, however, have demonstrated that all opioids have a spasmogenic effect on the sphincter of Oddi. Therefore, there is no evidence to indicate that morphine is contraindicated for use in acute pancreatitis, and it may provide more effective analgesia with less side effects than meperidine.[23] Relaxation techniques and positioning the patient in the knee-chest position can also assist in pain control.[24]

Maintaining Surveillance for Complications

The patient must be routinely monitored for signs of local or systemic complications (see Box 22-7). Intensive monitoring of each of the organ systems is imperative because organ failure is a major indicator of the severity of the disease.[24] In addition, the patient must be closely monitored for signs and symptoms of pancreatic infection, which include increased abdominal pain and tenderness, fever, and increased white blood cell count (Box 22-9).[26]

Patient Education

Early in the patient's hospital stay, the patient and family should be taught about acute pancreatitis and its causes and treatment. As the patient moves toward discharge, teaching should focus on the interventions necessary for preventing the recurrence of the precipitating disorder. If the patient has sustained permanent damage to the pancreas, the patient will require teaching specific to diet modification and supplemental pancreatic enzymes. Diabetes education may also be necessary. If an alcohol abuser, the patient should be encouraged to stop drinking and be referred to an alcohol cessation program.[26]

Box 22-10

Collaborative Management

Acute Pancreatitis
- Ensure adequate circulating volume
- Provide nutritional support
- Correct metabolic alterations
- Minimize pancreatic stimulation
- Provide comfort and emotional support
- Maintain surveillance for complications
- Multiple organ dysfunction syndrome

Collaborative management of the patient with pancreatitis is outlined in Box 22-10.

FULMINANT HEPATIC FAILURE

Description

Fulminant hepatic failure (FHF) is a life-threatening condition characterized by severe and sudden liver cell dysfunction, coagulopathy, and hepatic encephalopathy.[32,33] Although uncommon, FHF is associated with a mortality rate as high as 80% and generally occurs in patients without preexisting liver disease.[32] Because liver transplantation is one of the few definitive treatments for FHF, the patient with FHF should

Box 22-11

Causes of Fulminant Hepatic Failure

Infections
Hepatitis A, B, C, D, E, non-A, non-B, non-C
Herpes simplex virus (types 1 and 2)
Epstein-Barr virus
Varicella-zoster virus
Dengue fever virus
Rift Valley fever virus

Drugs/Toxins
Industrial substances (chlorinated hydrocarbons, phosphorus)
Amanita phalloides (mushrooms)
Aflatoxin (herb)
Medications (isoniazid, rifampin, halothane, methyldopa, tetracycline, valproic acid, monoamine oxidase inhibitors, phenytoin, nicotinic acid, tricyclic antidepressants, isoflurane, ketoconazole, trimethoprim-sulfamethoxazole, sulfasalazine, pyrimethamine, octreotide)
Acetaminophen toxicity
Cocaine

Hypoperfusion
Venous obstructions
Budd-Chiari syndrome
Veno-occlusive disease
Ischemia

Metabolic Disorders
Wilson's disease
Tyrosinemia
Heat stroke
Galactosemia

Surgery
Jejunoileal bypass
Partial hepatectomy
Liver transplant failure

Other
Reye's syndrome
Acute fatty liver of pregnancy
Massive malignant infiltration
Autoimmune hepatitis

be transferred to a critical care unit and strongly considered for referral to a major medical center where transplant services are available.[32,33]

Etiology

The causes of FHF include infections, drugs, toxins, hypoperfusion, metabolic disorders, and surgery (Box 22-11); however, acetaminophen toxicity is the predominant cause in the United States.[33,34] Patients are usually healthy before the onset of symptoms because FHF tends to occur in patients with no known liver history. Therefore, a thorough medication and health history is imperative to determine a possible etiology. The patient should be questioned about exposure to environmental toxins, hepatitis, intravenous drug use, and sexual history. Viral hepatitis, drug toxicity, poisoning, and metabolic disorders, such as Reye's syndrome and Wilson's disease, should be considered.[33]

Pathophysiology

FHF is a syndrome characterized by the development of acute liver failure over 1 to 3 weeks, followed by the development of hepatic encephalopathy within 8 weeks, in a patient with a previously healthy liver. Generally the interval between the actual failure of the liver and the onset of hepatic encephalopathy is less than 2 weeks.[34] The underlying cause is massive necrosis of the hepatocytes.[32-34]

Acute liver failure results in a number of derangements, including impaired bilirubin conjugation, decreased production of clotting factors, depressed glucose synthesis, and decreased lactate clearance. This results in jaundice, coagulopathies, hypoglycemia, and metabolic acidosis.[33] Other effects of acute liver failure include increased risk of infection and altered carbohydrate, protein, and glucose metabolism.[32] Hypoalbuminemia, fluid and electrolyte imbalances, and acute portal hypertension contribute to the development of ascites.[32] Hepatic encephalopathy is thought to result from failure of the liver to detoxify various substances in the bloodstream and may be worsened by metabolic and electrolyte imbalances.[32,35]

The patient may also experience a variety of other complications, including cerebral edema, cardiac dysrhythmias, acute respiratory failure, sepsis, and acute renal failure. Cerebral edema and increased intracranial pressure (ICP) develops as a result of breakdown of the blood-brain barrier and astrocyte swelling. Circulatory failure that mimics sepsis is common in FHF and may exacerbate low cerebral perfusion pressure (CPP). Hypoxemia, acidosis, electrolyte imbalances, and/or cerebral edema can precipitate the development of cardiac dysrhythmias. Acute respiratory failure, progressing to ALI, can result from pulmonary edema, aspiration pneumonia, and atelectasis. Acute renal failure may be caused by acute tubular necrosis, hypotension, or hemorrhage.[32,35]

Assessment and Diagnosis

Early recognition of FHF is extremely important. The diagnosis should include potentially reversible conditions (e.g., autoimmune hepatitis) and should differentiate FHF from decompensating chronic liver disease. Prognostic indicators, such as coma grade, serum bilirubin, prothrombin time (PT), coagulation factors, and pH, should be noted and potential etiologies investigated.[33]

Signs and symptoms of FHF include headache, hyperventilation, jaundice, mental status changes,

Box 22-12

Staging of Hepatic Encephalopathy

I	Euphoria or depression, mild confusion, slurred speech, disordered sleep rhythm; slight asterixis and normal EEG
II	Lethargy, moderate confusion; marked asterixis and abnormal EEG
III	Marked confusion, incoherent speech, sleeping but arousable; asterixis present and abnormal EEG
IV	Coma; initially responsive to noxious stimuli, later unresponsive; asterixis absent and abnormal EEG

EEG, Electroencephalogram.

palmar erythema, spider nevi, bruises, and edema. The patient should be evaluated for the presence of asterixis or "liver flaps," best described as the inability to voluntarily sustain a fixed position of the extremities. Asterixis is best demonstrated by having the patient extend the arms and dorsiflex the wrists, resulting in downward flapping of the hands. Hepatic encephalopathy is assessed using a grading system that stages the encephalopathy according to the patient's clinical manifestations (Box 22-12).[35,36] Diagnostic findings include elevated serum bilirubin, aspartate aminotransferase (AST), alkaline phosphatase, and serum ammonia levels, and decreased serum albumin level. Arterial blood gas (ABG) values reveal respiratory alkalosis and/or metabolic acidosis. Hypoglycemia, hypokalemia, and hyponatremia also may be present.[33,35]

Factors I (fibrinogen), II (prothrombin), V, VII, IX, and X are produced exclusively by the liver. Of these, prothrombin time may be the most useful test in the evaluation of acute FHF because levels may be 40 to 80 seconds above control values. Decreased levels of plasmin and plasminogen and increased levels of fibrin and fibrin-split products also are noted. Platelet counts may be decreased to 80,000/mm^3 or less.[33,35]

Medical Management

Medical interventions are directed toward management of the multiple system impact of FHF.

Ammonia Levels

Neomycin or lactulose is administered to remove or decrease production of nitrogenous wastes in the large intestine. Neomycin, given orally or rectally, reduces bacterial flora of the colon. This aids in decreasing ammonia formation by decreasing bacterial action on protein in the feces. Side effects include renal toxicity and hearing impairment. Lactulose, a synthetic ketoanalog of lactose split into lactic acid and acetic acid in the intestine, is given orally, via NG tube, or as a retention enema. The result is the creation of an acidic environment that decreases bacterial growth. Lactulose also traps ammonia and has a laxative effect that promotes expulsion.[35] Various experimental therapies such as exchange transfusion, charcoal hemoperfusion, and plasmapheresis have been used to lower ammonia levels, but have not improved survival.[35]

Complications

Bleeding is best controlled through prevention. Because these patients are at risk for acute GI hemorrhage, stress ulcer prophylaxis is essential.[35] If an invasive procedure (central line placement, ICP monitor) will be performed or the patient develops active bleeding, vitamin K, fresh frozen plasma (to maintain reasonable prothrombin time), and platelet transfusions are necessary.[35] Metabolic disturbances such as hypoglycemia, metabolic acidosis, hypokalemia, and hyponatremia should be monitored and treated appropriately. Prophylactic antibiotic administration may be initiated because the patient is at high risk for an infection.[35]

The development of cerebral edema necessitates the need for ICP monitoring. Mannitol is the only treatment shown to be of benefit in managing increased ICP in the patient with FHF but must be used with caution in patients with renal failure.[32,35] Other interventions to control intracranial hypertension include elevating the head of the bed to 20 to 30 degrees, treating fever and hypertension, minimizing noxious stimulation, and correcting hypercapnia and hypoxemia.[35] If renal failure develops, continuous renal replacement therapy (CRRT) should be initiated. Intubation and mechanical ventilation may be necessary as hypoxemia develops.[34,35] Hemodynamic instability is a common complication requiring fluid administration and vasoactive medications to avoid prolonged episodes of hypotension. A pulmonary artery catheter may be used to guide clinical management.[35]

If FHF continues and the patient shows no immediate signs of improvement or reversal, the patient should be considered for a liver transplant. Prompt referral to a transplant center should be a high priority for patients experiencing fulminant hepatic failure.[35]

Nursing Management

Nursing management of the patient with FHF incorporates a variety of nursing diagnoses (Box 22-13). **Nursing priorities are directed toward (1) protecting the patient from injury, (2) providing comfort and emotional support, (3) maintaining surveillance for complications, and (4) educating the patient and family.**

Protecting the Patient From Injury

Use of benzodiazepines and other sedatives is discouraged in the FHF patient because of the "masking" of pertinent neurologic changes and further potentiation of hepatic encephalopathy.[32] These patients are

Box 22-13

NURSING DIAGNOSIS PRIORITIES

Fulminant Hepatic Failure

- Ineffective Breathing Pattern related to decreased lung expansion, p. A-34
- Impaired Gas Exchange related to ventilation/perfusion mismatching or intrapulmonary shunting, p. A-29
- Decreased Cardiac Output related to alterations in preload, p. A-12
- Decreased Intracranial Adaptive Capacity related to failure of normal compensatory mechanisms, p. A-15
- Ineffective Renal Tissue Perfusion related to decreased renal blood flow, p. A-42
- Disturbed Body Image related to actual change in body structure, function, or appearance, p. A-20
- Deficient Knowledge: Discharge Regimen related to lack of previous exposure to information (see Patient Education: Fulminant Hepatic Failure), p. A-18

PATIENT EDUCATION

Fulminant Hepatic Failure

- Specific etiology
- Precipitating factor modification
- Interventions to reduce further episodes
- Importance of taking medications
- Lifestyle changes
- Diet modification
- Alcohol cessation

often very difficult to manage because they may be extremely agitated and combative. Physical restraint is generally required to prevent patient injury.

Maintaining Surveillance for Complications

As the neurologic condition worsens, respiratory depression and arrest can occur quickly. Continuous pulse oximetry monitoring and ABG analysis are helpful in assessing adequacy of respiratory efforts. A thorough neurologic assessment should be performed at least every hour.[32]

Educating Patient and Family

Early in the patient's hospital stay, the patient and family should be taught about fulminant hepatic failure and its causes and treatment. As the patient moves toward discharge, teaching should focus on the interventions necessary for preventing the recurrence of the precipitating etiology. If the patient is considered a liver transplant candidate, the patient and family will need specific information regarding the procedure and care. Liver transplant evaluation may include screening for medical contraindications, human immunodeficiency virus (HIV) serology, anticipated compliance, and assessment of the social support system. Psychiatric and other specialty team consults are necessary for a thorough evaluation of the patient's suitability for a transplant.[35]

Collaborative management of the patient with fulminant hepatic failure is outlined in Box 22-14.

Box 22-14

Collaborative Management

Fulminant Hepatic Failure

- Decrease ammonia levels
- Control bleeding
- Correct metabolic alterations
- Prevent infection
- Prepare patient for liver transplantation if necessary
- Protect patient from injury
- Provide comfort and emotional support
- Maintain surveillance for complications
  - Cerebral edema
  - Renal failure

THERAPEUTIC MANAGEMENT

GASTROINTESTINAL INTUBATION

Because GI intubation is used so often in critical care units, it is important for nurses to know the clinical indications and responsibilities inherent in tube use. The four categories of GI tubes are based on function: NG suction tubes, long intestinal tubes, feeding tubes, and esophagogastric balloon tamponade tubes (see Patient Safety: Tubing Misconnections—A Persistent and Potentially Deadly Occurrence).

Nasogastric Suction Tubes

NG tubes remove fluid regurgitated into the stomach, prevent accumulation of swallowed air, may partially decompress the bowel, and reduce the patient's risk for aspiration. NG tubes also can be used for collecting specimens, assessing for the presence of blood, and administering tube feedings. The most common NG tubes are the single lumen Levin tube and the double-lumen Salem sump. The Salem sump has one lumen that is used for suction and drainage and another that allows air to enter the patient's stomach and prevents the tube from adhering to the gastric wall and damaging the mucosa. The tube is passed through the nose into the nasopharynx and then down through the pharynx into the esophagus and stomach. The length of time the NG tube remains in place depends on its use. The tube is then placed to gravity, low intermittent suction, or low continuous suction, or in rare instances is clamped.[36]

PATIENT SAFETY PRIORITIES

Tubing Misconnections—A Persistent and Potentially Deadly Occurrence

Tubing and catheter misconnection errors are an important and under-reported problem in health care organizations. In addition, these errors are often caught and corrected before any injury to the patient occurs. Given the reality of and potential for life threatening consequences, increased awareness and analysis of these errors—including averted errors—can lead to dramatic improvement in patient safety.

To date, nine cases involving tubing misconnections have been reported to the Joint Commission's Sentinel Event Database. These resulted in eight deaths and one instance of permanent loss of function, and affected seven adults and two infants. Reports in the media and to organizations such as ECRI, the Food and Drug Administration (FDA), the Institute for Safe Medication Practices (ISMP), and United States Pharmacopela (USP) indicate that misconnection errors occur with significant frequency and, in a number of instances, lead to deadly consequences.

Types of Misconnections

The types of tubes and catheters involved in the cases reported to the Joint Commission included central intravenous catheters, peripheral intravenous catheters, nasogastric feeding tubes, percutaneous enteric feeding tubes, peritoneal dialysis catheters, tracheostomy cuff inflation tubes, and automatic blood pressure cuff insufflation tubes. The specific misconnections involved an enteric tube feeding into an intravenous catheter (4 cases); injection of barium sulfate (GI contrast medium) into a central venous catheter (1 case); an enteric tube feeding into a peritoneal dialysis catheter (1 case); a blood pressure insufflator tube connected to an intravenous catheter (2 cases); and injection of intravenous fluid into a tracheostomy cuff inflation tube (1 case).

A review by USP of more than 300 cases reported to its databases found misconnection errors involving the following:

- Intravenous infusions connected to epidural lines, and epidural solutions (intended for epidural administration) connected to peripheral or central IV catheters.
- Bladder irrigation solutions using primary intravenous tubing connected as secondary infusions to peripheral or central IV catheters.
- Infusions intended for IV administration connected to an indwelling bladder (foley) catheter.
- Infusions intended for IV administration connected to nasogastric (NG) tubes.
- Intravenous solutions administered with blood administration sets, and blood products transfused with primary intravenous tubing.
- Primary intravenous solutions administered through various other functionally dissimilar catheters, such as external dialysis catheters, a ventriculostomy drain, an amnio-infusion catheter, and the distal port of a pulmonary artery catheter.

Many of the misconnection cases involved luer connectors—small devices used in the connection of many medical components and accessories. There are two types of luer connectors—slips and locks. A luer slip connector consist of a tapered "male" fitting that slips into a wider "female" fitting to create a secure connection. The luer lock connector has a threaded collar on the "male" fitting and a flange on the "female" fitting that screw together to create a more secure connection. Examples of misconnections involving luer connectors include the following:

- Capnography sampling tube to an intravenous cannula.
- Enteral feeding set to a central venous catheter.
- Enteral feeding set to a hemodialysis line.
- Noninvasive blood pressure (NIBP) insufflation tube to a needleless IV port.
- Oxygen tubing to a needleless IV port.
- Sequential compression device (SCD) hose to needleless "piggy-back" port of an IV administration set.

Root Causes Identified

The basic lesson from these cases is that if it can happen, it *will* happen. Luer connectors are implicated in or contribute to many of these errors because they enable functionally dissimilar tubes or catheters to be connected. Other identified causes include the routine use of tubes or catheters for unintended purposes, such as using IV extension tubing for epidurals, irrigation, drains, and central lines, or to extend enteric feeding tubes; and the positioning of functionally dissimilar tubes used in patient care in close proximity to one another. In the cases reported to the Sentinel Event Database, contributing factors included movement of the patient from one setting or service to another, and staff fatigue associated with working consecutive shifts.

Risk Reduction Strategies

There are currently no published standards that specifically restrict the use of luer connectors to certain medical devices. Consequently, a broad range of medical devices, which have different functions and access the body through different routes, are often outfitted with luer fittings that can be easily misconnected. Organizations in Europe and the U.S. are now developing standards to restrict the types of devices that use luer fittings in an attempt to mitigate misconnection hazards. According to Jim Keller, vice president, Health Technology Evaluation and Safety for ECRI, and Stephanie Joseph, project engineer for ECRI, the solution to reducing—even eliminating—misconnection errors lies in both engineering controls respecting how products and devices are designed ("incompatibility by design"), and in re-engineering work practices.

"A well-designed device should prevent misconnections and should prompt the user to take the correct action," explains Joseph, author of a guidance article published in the March 2006 issue of ECRI's *Health Devices* journal. As a first step in prevention, Joseph urges hospitals to avoid buying non-intravenous equipment (such as nebulizers, NIBP devices, and enteral feeding sets) that can mate with the luer connectors on patient IV lines. In addition, Joseph emphasizes that the single most important work practice solution for clinicians is to trace all lines back to their origin before connecting or disconnecting any devices or infusions.

GI, Gastrointestinal; *IV,* intravenous.

PATIENT SAFETY PRIORITIES

Tubing Misconnections—A Persistent and Potentially Deadly Occurrence—*cont'd*

Other solutions include specific education and training regarding this problem for all clinicians and having practitioners take simple precautions such as turning on the light in a darkened room before connecting or reconnecting tubes or devices. The risk of waking a sleeping patient is minimal by comparison. Errors have also occurred when patients or family members attempt to disconnect and reconnect equipment themselves. Staff should emphasize to all patients the importance of contacting a clinical staff member for assistance when there is an identified need to disconnect or reconnect devices.

Other approaches to reducing the risk of misconnections that have been identified also have significant potential for unintended consequences. These include:

- Labeling all tubes and catheters—This may not always be practical and may therefore lead to inconsistent implementation. However, the labeling of certain high-risk catheters (epidural, intrathecal, arterial) should always be done.
- Color-coding tubes and catheters—This can lead users to rely on the color coding rather than assuring a clear understanding of which tubes and catheters are connected correctly to which body inlets. In addition, the training and educating of all staff (including temporary agency and travel staff) about the institution's color-coding system requires continuing attention. Finally, color-coding schemes often vary across institutions in the same community, creating increased risk when agency and travel staff are used.

Joint Commission Recommendations

The Joint Commission offers the following recommendations and strategies to health care organizations to reduce tubing misconnection errors:

1. Do not purchase non-intravenous equipment that is equipped with connectors that can physically mate with a female luer IV line connector.
2. Conduct acceptance testing (for performance, safety and usability) and, as appropriate, risk assessment (e.g., failure mode and effect analysis) on new tubing and catheter purchases to identify the potential for misconnections and take appropriate preventive measures.
3. Always trace a tube or catheter from the patient to the point of origin before connecting any new device or infusion.
4. Recheck connections and trace all patient tubes and catheters to their sources upon the patient's arrival to a new setting or service as part of the hand-off process. Standardize this "line reconciliation" process.
5. Route tubes and catheters having different purposes in different, standardized directions (e.g., IV lines routed toward the head; enteric lines toward the feet). This is especially important in the care of neonates.
6. Inform non-clinical staff, patients and their families that they must get help from clinical staff whenever there is a real or perceived need to connect or disconnect devices or infusions.
7. For certain high-risk catheters (e.g., epidural, intrathecal, arterial), label the catheter and do not use catheters that have injection ports.
8. Never use a standard luer syringe for oral medications or enteric feedings.
9. Emphasize the risk of tubing misconnections in orientation and training curricula.
10. Identify and manage conditions and practices that may contribute to health care worker fatigue, and take appropriate action.

In addition, the Joint Commission urges product manufacturers to implement "designed incompatibility," as appropriate, to prevent dangerous misconnections of tubes and catheters.

Resources

FDA Patient Safety News, Show #31, September 2004; Show #20, October 2003; Show #46, December 2005

"Fatal Air Embolism Caused by the Misconnection of a Medical Device Hoses to Needleless Luer Ports on IV Administration Sets" [hazard report], ECRI, *Health Devices,* June 2004; 33(6): 223-5

"Misconnected Flowmeter Leads to Two Deaths" [special report], ECRI, *Health Devices Alerts,* January 25, 2003

"Preventing Misconnections of Lines and Cables," ECRI, *Health Devices,* March 2006; 35(3): 81-95

"Safe Systems, Safe Patients: Common Connectors Pose a Threat to Safe Practice." *Texas Board of Nursing Bulletin,* 37(2):6-7, April 2006

From the Joint Commission: Sentinel Event Alert, Issue 36–April 3,2006, http://www.jointcommision.org/SentinelEvents/SentinelEventAlert/sea–36.htm.

Nursing management is focused on preventing complications common to this therapy, such as ulceration and necrosis of the nares, esophageal reflux, esophagitis, esophageal erosion and stricture, gastric erosion, and dry mouth and parotitis from mouth breathing. In addition, interference with ventilation and coughing, aspiration, and loss of fluid and electrolytes can be critical problems. Interventions include irrigating the tube every 4 hours with normal saline, ensuring the blue air vent of the Salem sump is patent and maintained above the level of the patient's stomach, and providing frequent mouth and nares care.[37]

Long Intestinal Tubes

Miller-Abbott, Cantor, and Anderson tubes are examples of long, weighted-tip, intestinal tubes that are placed either preoperatively or intraoperatively. The long length allows removal of contents from the intestine to treat an obstruction that cannot be accomplished by an NG tube. These tubes can decompress the small bowel and can splint the small bowel intraoperatively or postoperatively. Because progression of the tubes depends on bowel peristalsis, their use is contraindicated in patients with paralytic ileus and severe mechanical bowel obstructions. Older tubes like the Cantor and Miller-Abbott are rarely used today because the balloon and the distal end is filled with mercury; the newer Anderson tube has a preweighted tungsten tip and is a safer option.[36]

Interventions used in the care of the patient with a long intestinal tube are similar to those with an NG tube. The patient should be observed for (1) gaseous distention of the balloon section, which makes removal difficult; (2) rupture of the balloon or spillage of mercury into the intestine; (3) overinflation of the balloon, which can lead to intestinal rupture; and (4) reverse intussusception if the tube is removed rapidly. Intestinal tubes should be removed slowly; usually 6 inches of the tube is withdrawn every hour.

Feeding Tubes

Small-diameter (8 Fr to 12 Fr) flexible feeding tubes, such as Dobhoff tubes, are commonly placed at the bedside for patients who cannot take nourishment by mouth. The feeding tube may be inserted orally or nasally so that the tip ends up in either the stomach or duodenum. To facilitate passage into the gastrointestinal tract, these tubes generally have a weighted tungsten tip and need a guidewire to prevent them from curling up in the back of the patient's throat. An x-ray film must be obtained to verify correct placement of the tube before initiating feeding. The tube should also be marked with indelible ink where it exits the mouth/nares so that the nurse can later verify that the tube has not been dislodged.[36]

Nursing management of the patient with a feeding tube includes prevention of complications and monitoring the tolerance of feeding. Before administering medications or feedings, it is important to make sure that the tube is in the patient's stomach or duodenum. Assessing the exit point marked on the tube helps to determine if the tube has maintained the same position. Looking for coiling in the mouth or throat can help detect upward displacement that may have occurred as a result of vomiting. The traditional practice of confirming placement by auscultating air inserted through the tube over the epigastrium is not reliable and is not recommended. If there is any doubt as to the position of the tube, a repeat x-ray film should be obtained. During feedings, the head of the bed should be elevated 30 to 45 degrees to minimize the risk of aspiration, and gastric residuals should be checked at least every 8 hours. Increased residuals (greater than 150 ml), cramping, and abdominal distention may indicate intolerance of feeding and the physician should be notified. Other interventions include nares/oral care and flushing the tube with normal saline or water to maintain patency.[37]

Esophagogastric Balloon Tamponade Tubes

Tamponade tubes may be used stop bleeding in patients when endoscopic therapy fails or while waiting for surgical intervention. Although effective in 80% to 90% of patients, they are only a temporizing measure until definitive treatment can occur and over 50% will rebleed when the balloon is deflated.[38] Currently three different types of balloon tamponade tubes are available. The *Sengstaken-Blakemore* tube has three lumens: one for the gastric balloon, one for the esophageal balloon, and one for the gastric suction (Figure 22-5, *A*). The Linton-Nachlas tube also has three lumens: for the gastric balloon, gastric suction, and esophageal suction (Figure 22-5, *B*). The Minnesota tube has four lumens: for the gastric balloon, esophageal balloon, gastric suction, and esophageal suction (Figure 22-5, *C*). The Sengstaken-Blakemore and Minnesota tubes are considered the standard for tamponade therapy; however, the Minnesota tube is preferable because it offers both a gastric and an esophageal balloon and allows suction to be applied both above and below the balloons (in the stomach and in the esophagus).[39]

Balloon tamponade tubes are inserted by the physician. Once the tube is passed into the stomach and placement is confirmed by gastric aspirate, the gastric balloon is slowly inflated to a total of 500 ml of air (or as specified by the tube manufacturer). After x-ray confirmation of placement, the tube is then secured and placed under tension so that the gastric balloon places pressure on the gastroesophageal junction. One to three pounds of tension are usually applied using a helmet with a constant-traction spring device. If bleeding continues, the esophageal balloon is inflated to a pressure of 25 to 45 mm Hg. Low intermittent suction is applied to both the gastric and esophageal ports. Typically balloons are deflated after 24 hours to prevent tissue necrosis; however, the gastric balloon may be inflated for up to 72 hours if needed. When discontinuing tamponade therapy, the esophageal balloon pressure should be gradually decreased and the patient observed for evidence of bleeding. If no bleeding is noted, the gastric balloon may be deflated. If no further bleeding occurs, the tube is removed 4 hours later.[39]

Nursing management of the patient with a balloon tamponade tube includes monitoring for rebleeding and observing for complications of the tube. The most common complication is pulmonary aspiration, which can be limited by emptying the stomach and placing an endotracheal tube before passing the balloon tamponade tube. Additional complications include esopha-

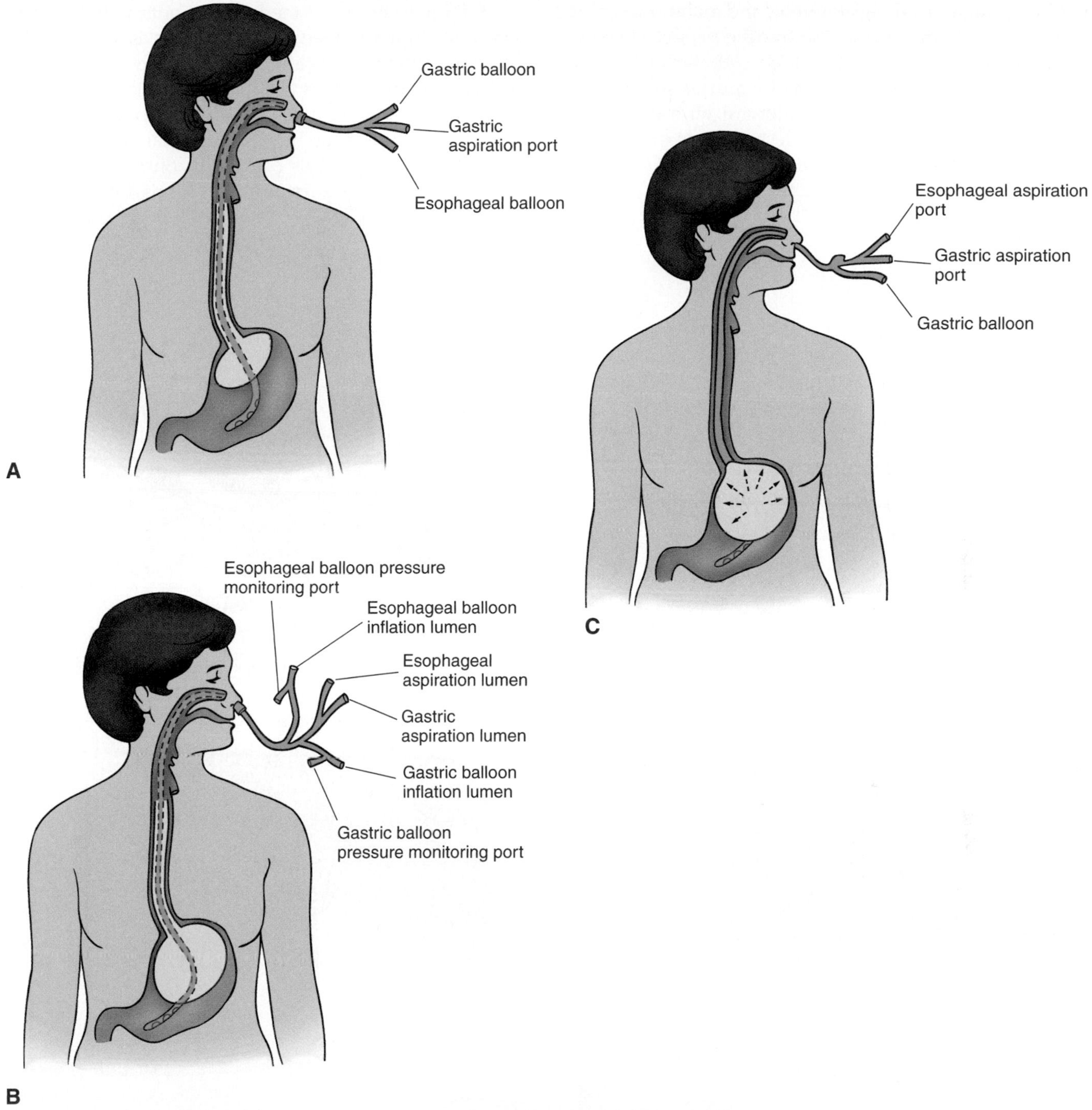

FIGURE 22-5. Esophageal tamponade tubes. **A,** Sengstaken-Blakemore tube. **B,** Linton-Nachlas tube. **C,** Minnesota tube.

geal erosion and rupture, balloon migration, and nasal necrosis.[39]

Transjugular Intrahepatic Portosystemic Shunt

A transjugular intrahepatic portosystemic shunt (TIPS) is an angiographic interventional procedure for decreasing portal hypertension. Recent data suggest that TIPS is advocated in (1) patients with portal hypertension who are also experiencing active bleeding or have poor liver reserve, (2) transplant patients, or (3) patients with other operative risks. The TIPS procedure is usually performed by a gastroenterologist, vascular surgeon, or interventional radiologist.[40]

Portal hypertension is first confirmed via direct measurement of the pressure in the portal vein (gradient greater than 10 mm Hg). Cannulation is achieved through the internal jugular vein, and an angiographic catheter is advanced into the middle or right hepatic vein. The midhepatic vein is then catheterized, and a new route is created connecting the portal and hepatic veins, using a needle and guidewire with a dilating balloon. An expandable stainless steel stent is then placed in the liver parenchyma to maintain that connection (Figure 22-6). The increased resistance in the liver is therefore bypassed.[21,40]

TIPS may be performed on patients with bleeding varices, refractory bleeding varices, or as a "bridge" to liver transplant if the candidate becomes hemodynamically unstable. Postprocedure care should include observation for overt (cannulation site) or covert (intrahepatic site) bleeding, hepatic or portal vein laceration (resulting in rapid loss of blood volume), and inadvertent puncture of surrounding organs. Other complications include bile duct trauma, stent migration, and

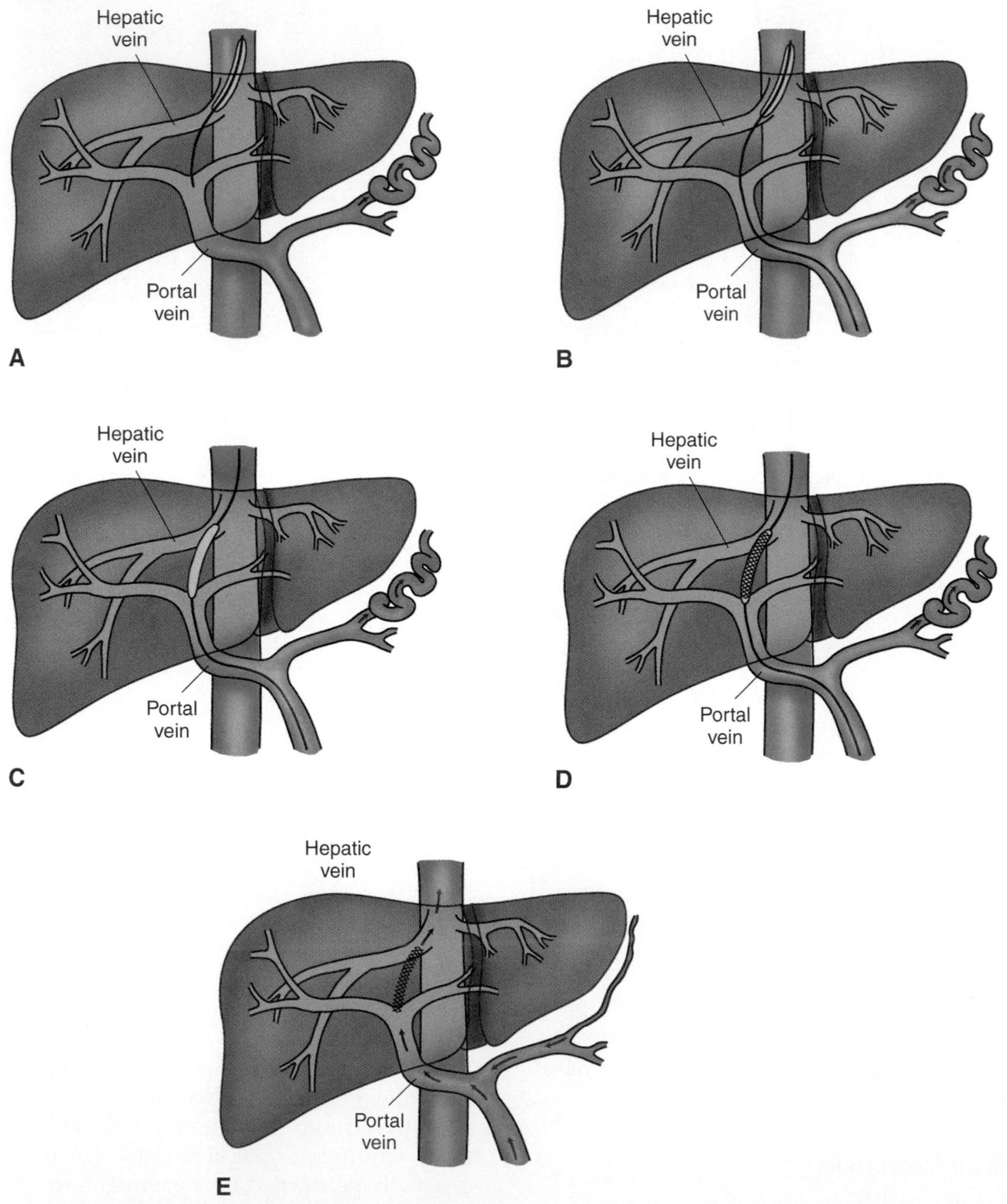

FIGURE 22-6. Transjugular intrahepatic portosystemic shunt (TIPS). **A,** Needle directed though liver parenchyma to portal vein. **B,** Needle and guidewire passed down to midportal vein. **C,** Balloon dilation. **D,** Deployment of stent. **E,** Intrahepatic shunt from portal to hepatic vein. (From Zemel G et al: *JAMA* 266:391, 1991. ©1991 American Medical Association.)

stent thrombosis.[21] Portal hypertension recurs almost universally after TIPS, whereas stent stenosis occurs in 3% to 10% of patients.[21,40]

Gastrointestinal Surgery

Gastrointestinal surgery refers to a wide variety of surgical procedures that involve the esophagus, stomach, intestine, liver, pancreas, or biliary tract. Indications for gastrointestinal surgery are numerous and include bleeding or perforation from peptic ulcer disease, obstruction, trauma, inflammatory bowel disease, and malignancy. Patients may be admitted to the ICU for monitoring after GI surgery as a result of their underlying medical condition; however, this portion of the chapter will focus only on several surgical procedures that commonly require postoperative critical care.

Types of Surgery

Esophagectomy is usually performed for cancer of the distal esophagus and gastroesophageal junction. The procedure involves the removal of part or the entire esophagus, part of the stomach, and lymph nodes in the surrounding area. The stomach is then pulled up into the chest and connected to the remaining part of the esophagus. If the entire esophagus and stomach must be removed, part of the bowel may be used to form the esophageal replacement.[41,42]

The standard operation for pancreatic cancer is a pancreaticoduodenectomy, or Whipple procedure. In the Whipple procedure the pancreatic head, duodenum, part of the jejunum, common bile duct, gallbladder, and part of the stomach are removed. The continuity of the GI tract is restored by anastomosing the remaining portion of the pancreas, bile duct, and stomach to the jejunum (Figure 22-7).[41]

Preoperative Care

A thorough preoperative evaluation should be conducted to evaluate the patient's physical status and identify risk factors that may affect the postoperative course. Before esophagectomy or pancreaticoduodenectomy, the patient may undergo multiple diagnostic tests, such as CT, positron emission tomography (PET), and endoscopic ultrasound (EUS), to determine the invasiveness of the tumor.[41]

Surgical Considerations

Two approaches may be used for esophageal resection, transhiatal or transthoracic (Figure 22-8). In both approaches, the stomach is mobilized through an abdominal incision then transposed into the chest. The anastomosis of the stomach to the esophagus is then performed either in the chest (transthoracic) or in the neck (transhiatal). The approach selected depends upon the location of the tumor, the patient's overall health and pulmonary function, and the experience

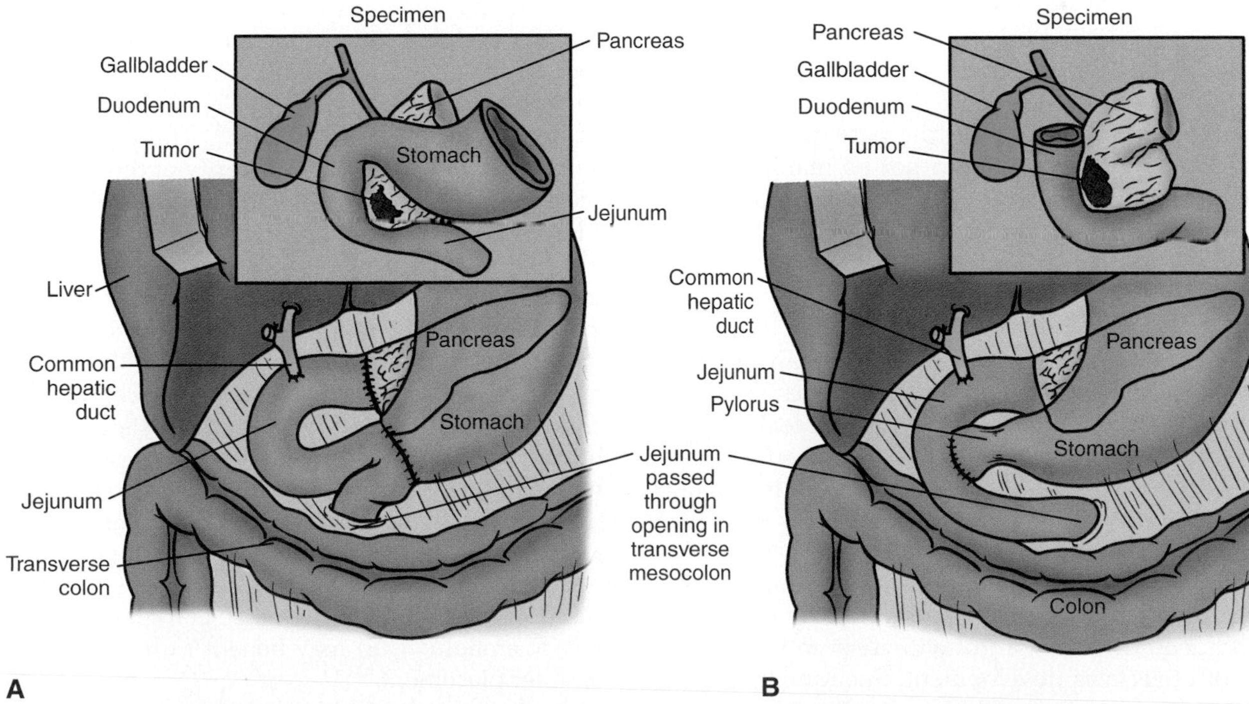

FIGURE 22-7. Standard and pylorus-preserving Whipple procedures. **A,** The "standard Whipple" involves resection of the gastric antrum, head of pancreas, distal bile duct, and entire duodenum with reconstruction as shown. **B,** The "pylorus-preserving Whipple" does not include resection of the distal stomach, pylorus, or proximal duodenum. (From Cameron JL: Current status of the Whipple operation for periampullary carcinoma, *Surg Rounds* 77, 1998.)

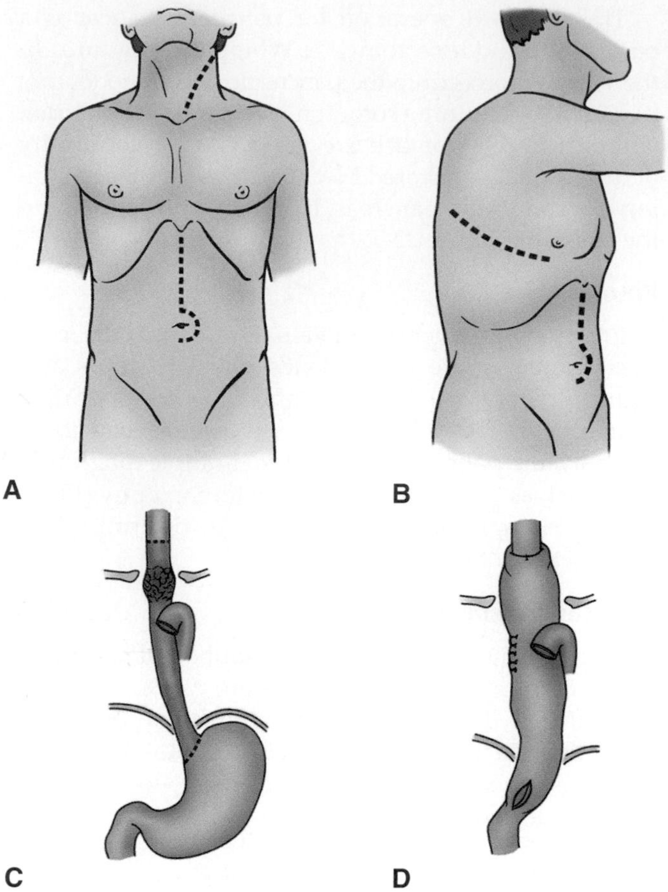

FIGURE 22-8. Overview of transhiatal esophagectomy **A,** and right thoracotomy **B,** with gastric mobilization **C,** and gastric pull-up **D,** for cervical-esophagogastric anastomosis. (Modified from Ellis F: *Surg Clin North Am* 60:275, 1980.)

of the surgeon. Postoperatively the patient will have an NG tube in place that should not be manipulated because of the potential to cause damage to the anastomosis. Those who undergo transthoracic esophagectomy will have one or more chest tubes.[41,42]

Complications and Medical Management

A number of complications are associated with GI surgery. They include, but are not limited to, respiratory failure, atelectasis, pneumonia, anastomotic leak, deep vein thrombosis, pulmonary embolus, and bleeding.[41,42]

Pulmonary Complications. The risk for pulmonary complications and adverse respiratory events such as atelectasis and pneumonia is substantial after GI surgery. Aggressive pulmonary toilet should be initiated in the immediate postoperative period. Early ambulation and adequate pain control will assist in reducing the risk of atelectasis development. Suctioning, chest physiotherapy, or bronchodilators may be needed to optimize pulmonary function. Patients should be closely monitored for developing problems with oxygenation. Treatment should be aimed at supporting adequate ventilation and gas exchange. Mechanical ventilation may be required in the event of respiratory failure.

Anastomotic Leak. An anastomotic leak is a severe complication of GI surgery. It occurs when there is a breakdown of the suture line in a surgical anastomosis and results in leakage of gastric or intestinal contents into the abdomen or mediastinum (transthoracic esophagectomy).[41,43] The clinical signs and symptoms of a leak can be very subtle and often go unrecognized. They include tachycardia, tachypnea, fever, abdominal pain, anxiety, and restlessness. In the patient with an esophagectomy, a leak of the esophageal anastomosis may manifest itself as subcutaneous emphysema in the chest and neck.[41] If undetected, a leak can result in sepsis, multiorgan failure, and death. Patients with progressive tachycardia and tachypnea should have a radiologic study (upper GI or CT scan) with contrast to rule out an anastomotic leak.[43] The type of treatment is dependent upon the severity of the leak. If the leak is small and well contained, it may be managed conservatively by making the patient NPO, administering antibiotics, and draining the fluid percutaneously. If the patient is deteriorating rapidly, an urgent laparotomy is indicated in order to repair the defect.[43]

Deep Vein Thrombosis/Pulmonary Embolus. Pulmonary embolism is a very serious complication of any surgical procedure. Deep vein thrombosis (DVT) prophylaxis should be initiated before surgery and continue until the patient is fully ambulatory to reduce the risk of clot development. Typically a combination of sequential compression devices and subcutaneous unfractionated heparin or low-molecular-weight heparin is used. Patients determined to be at high risk for pulmonary embolus (PE) may benefit from prophylactic IVC filter placement.[41]

Bleeding. Upper GI bleeding is an uncommon but life-threatening complication of GI surgery. Early bleeding generally occurs at the site of the anastomosis and can usually be treated through endoscopic intervention. Surgical revision may be needed for persistent,

Box 22-15

NURSING DIAGNOSIS PRIORITIES

Gastrointestinal Surgery

- Ineffective Breathing Pattern related to decreased lung expansion, p. A-34
- Acute Pain related to transmission and perception of cutaneous, visceral, muscular, or ischemic impulses, p. A-7
- Anxiety related to threat to biologic, psychologic, and/or social integrity, p. A-9
- Disturbed Body Image related to actual change in body structure, function, or appearance, p. A-20
- Deficient Knowledge related to cognitive/perceptual learning limitations, p. A-18

uncontrolled bleeding. Late bleeding is usually a result of ulcer development. Medical therapy is aimed at the prevention of this complication through administration of H_2 antagonists or proton pump inhibitors.[41]

Postoperative Nursing Management

Nursing care of the patient who has had GI surgery incorporates a number of nursing diagnoses (Box 22-15). **Nursing priorities are directed toward (1) optimizing oxygenation and ventilation, (2) providing comfort and emotional support, and (3) maintaining surveillance for complications.**

Optimizing Oxygenation and Ventilation. Nursing interventions in the postoperative period are focused on promoting ventilation, adequate oxygenation, and preventing complications such as atelectasis and pneumonia. After the patient is extubated, deep-breathing exercises and incentive spirometry should be initiated and then performed regularly. Early ambulation is encouraged to promote maximal lung inflation and thereby reduce the risk of pulmonary complications, as well as reduce the potential for pulmonary embolus.

Providing Comfort and Emotional Support. It is imperative to appropriately manage the patient's pain after GI surgery. Adequate analgesia is necessary to promote mobility of the patient and decrease pulmonary complications. Initial pain management may be accomplished by IV opioid (e.g., morphine or hydromorphone) administration via a patient-controlled analgesia (PCA) pump or through continuous epidural infusion of an opioid and local anesthetic (e.g., bupivacaine).[42] Oral pain medications can be started after an anastomosis leak is ruled out. Nonpharmacologic interventions such as positioning, application of heat/cold, and distraction may also be used. If the patient's pain is not being sufficiently relieved, the pain management service should be consulted.

Liver Transplantation

Indications and Selection

Liver transplantation must be considered for any patient who suffers from irreversible acute or chronic liver disease that is progressive and has no therapy of established efficacy. Box 22-16 lists the most common diseases seen in patients who undergo liver transplantation. In the United States, most common indications for liver transplantation in adults are alcohol-induced liver disease and chronic viral hepatitis C.[44] Current patient survival rates for liver transplantation are approximately 85% at 1 year and greater than 70% at 5 years.[45]

Candidate selection is an important aspect of transplantation. The patient must not be so ill as to be unable to survive the surgery but yet is experiencing deterioration in the quality of life. In general, liver transplantation is not to be offered to patients who would

Box 22-16

End-Stage Liver Diseases Commonly Treated With Liver Transplantation

Cholestatic Liver Diseases
Biliary atresia
Primary sclerosing cholangitis
Primary biliary cirrhosis

Chronic Hepatocellular Diseases
Viral hepatitis (types A, B, C, D, E)
Alcoholic liver disease (Laënnec's disease)
Autoimmune hepatitis
Cryptogenic cirrhosis
Drug-induced liver disease

Vascular Diseases
Budd-Chiari syndrome
Veno-occlusive disease

Fulminant and Subfulminant Hepatic Failure
Viral hepatitis (types A, B, C, D, E)
Drug-induced (acetaminophen, isoniazid overdoses)
Fulminant Wilson's disease

Inborn Metabolic Disorders
Wilson's disease
α_1-Antitrypsin deficiency
Hemochromatosis
Tyrosinemia
Glycogen storage disease, types I and II

Primary Hepatic Malignancies
Hepatocellular carcinoma
Hemangioendothelioma
Hepatoblastoma

Box 22-17

Liver Transplantation Contraindications

Absolute Contraindications
Brain death
Metastatic malignancies
Extrahepatic malignancy
Active drug or alcohol abuse
Advanced cardiopulmonary disease
Acquired immunodeficiency syndrome (AIDS)
Extrahepatic sepsis

Relative Contraindications
Physiologic age
Advanced renal disease
Multiple hepatic malignancies
Moderate cardiopulmonary disease
Peripheral vascular disease
Psychosocial behaviors indicating noncompliance to medical regimens
HIV-positive

HIV, Human immunodeficiency virus.

not likely survive major surgery or the effects of long-term immunosuppression, who have a disease that is likely to recur quickly, and those who are not willing to comply with long-term and sometimes difficult and demanding medical regimens. The absolute and relative contraindications for liver transplantation are listed in Box 22-17.[46]

Recipient Evaluation. The candidate for liver transplant undergoes a thorough evaluation to determine the etiology and severity of the liver disease, to establish the need for transplantation rather than other interventions, and to identify objective indications and contraindications. Evaluation begins with a carefully elicited patient history. A comprehensive approach includes laboratory, radiographic, and diagnostic testing and multidisciplinary consultations (Box 22-18). Placement on the waiting list is determined by blood type, weight, and patient urgency. Patients with acute fulminant hepatic failure are considered in most urgent need.[46]

Pretransplant Phase. The patient with end-stage liver disease awaiting a transplant may be one of the most challenging to care for in the critical care unit. Hepatic encephalopathy, coagulopathies, portal hypertension, severe fluid and electrolyte imbalances, cardiac compromise, and renal deterioration are not uncommon. Frequent mental status assessments of the patient are important in determining continued candidacy for transplant. Hepatic encephalopathy may improve with administration of antibiotics and laxatives or may proceed to stage IV coma. Protection of the airway is especially important in an encephalopathic patient who is not intubated. In these circumstances, if hematemesis or vomiting occurs, intubation and use of paralytic agents may be necessary to protect the patient's airway. Diagnostic studies may be needed to evaluate the possibility of intracranial bleed. Maintain the elevation of the head of the patient's bed at 30 to 45 degrees to avoid even slight increases in intracranial pressure. Patients who have chronic liver disease also have nutritional deficits. They require supplements of the fat-soluble vitamins (A, D, E, and K), may be on protein restrictions to reduce serum ammonia levels, and may experience severe muscle wasting.[46]

Determining Donor Suitability. The two criteria necessary for matching a donor liver to a recipient are blood type and body size. Human lymphocyte antigen (HLA) tissue typing is not used in the matching of donor livers because this has not been shown to significantly affect patient outcomes. Donors are carefully screened for infectious diseases and metastatic carcinomas because these can be transmitted to the recipient. The transplant center is notified by an organ procurement organization that a liver is available.[47] If the organ is accepted, the transplant team contacts the patient. In very urgent situations the donor blood type may not be compatible with the recipient's; for example, an A-type donor and an O-type recipient. Despite this incompatibility, liver transplantation can be successful. There may be some early postoperative complications, such as mild hemolysis, but long-term

Box 22-18
Sample of a Pretransplant Evaluation for Liver Transplantation

Laboratory Tests

Liver function profiles: Transaminases (AST, ALT, GGT); alkaline phosphatase; bilirubin; albumin; prothrombin time; partial thromboplastin time; clotting factors; cholesterol; triglycerides

Renal function profile with electrolytes: Blood urea nitrogen, creatinine, sodium, potassium, carbon dioxide, chloride

Hematology: CBC, reticulocytes, erythrocyte sedimentation rate

Thyroid function: T_3RIA; T_4RIA; thyroid-stimulating hormone; T_4, T_3 uptake

Serologic studies for hepatic viruses and other infectious diseases: Viral hepatitis (A, B, C, D, E), cytomegalovirus, Epstein-Barr virus, herpes I and II, parvovirus, RPR, HIV

Blood type and antibody screen

Immunologic profiles: Antinuclear antibody; antimitochondrial antibody; anti–smooth muscle antibody; immunoglobulins (A, G, M)

Nutritional profiles: Vitamin levels (A, D, E, B_{12}, folate), iron studies with ferritin

Tumor markers: α-Fetoprotein, CEA, PSA, CA 19-9

Miscellaneous: Ceruloplasmin, α_1-antitrypsin level and phenotype

Urine

24-Hour protein and electrolytes, cultures, creatinine clearance, urinalysis, copper

Stool

Ova, cysts, parasites, occult blood, 48-hour fecal fats, cultures

Gastrointestinal Work-Up

Endoscopy, colonoscopy, endoscopic retrograde cholangiopancreatography, liver biopsy

Pulmonary Profile

Arterial blood gases, pulmonary function studies

Radiographic and Diagnostic Tests

Chest x-ray, ultrasound of liver including vascular studies

Other, Optional Tests

Doppler studies; sinus x-ray examination; computed tomography (abdomen, chest, head); electrocardiogram; echocardiogram; cardiac stress test; cardiac catheterization; mammogram; peripheral vascular studies; carotid ultrasound; abdominal angiography; percutaneous cholangiogram; bone mineral density

AST, Aspartate transaminase; *ALT,* alanine aminotransferase; *GGT,* γ-glutamyltransferase; *CBC,* complete blood count; *T_3RIA,* serum triiodothyronine (T_3); *T_4RIA,* serum triiodothyronine (T_4); *RPR,* rapid plasma reagin; *HIV,* human immunodeficiency virus; *CEA,* carcinoembryonic antigen; *PSA,* prostate specific antigen; *CA 19-9,* investigational cancer antigen.

follow-up of patients with recipient-donor ABO incompatibility has been favorable.[48] Once a donor liver becomes available, it is necessary to expedite the preoperative preparation of the recipient.[47]

Surgical Procedure

Liver transplant surgery is lengthy and technically difficult, often lasting 4 to 12 hours. The procedure involves the combined efforts of surgeons, anesthesiologists, nurse anesthetists, operating room nurses and technicians, perfusionists, and personnel from the blood bank and laboratory and radiology departments, to name a few. The patient is taken to the operating room for anesthesia induction, insertion of large-bore intravenous catheters that allow high-volume fluid infusion, and insertion of a pulmonary artery catheter for hemodynamic monitoring. Other devices such as an arterial line, a nasogastric tube, and a urinary drainage catheter are also inserted. The patient is positioned on the operating room table in such a way as to minimize pressure that may cause ischemia and chronic injury to tissue and peripheral nerves. The surgery can be divided into three stages: (1) recipient hepatectomy, (2) vascular anastomoses with donor liver, and (3) biliary anastomosis.[49]

Stage 1 is the longest and most difficult part of the surgery because it involves removal of the native liver. It is complicated even more by coagulopathies, adhesions, portal hypertension, and venous collaterals. Before completion of this stage, the patient may be put on venovenous bypass (Figure 22-9). A centrifugal pump cycles the blood out via iliac and portal vein cannulas and returns it to the central circulation via the axillary or subclavian vein. Advances in surgical techniques, anesthesia, and fluid management have shortened the length of surgery enough to warrant not using venovenous bypass on all liver transplants.[49]

Stage 2 comprises the four vascular anastomoses: suprahepatic inferior vena cava, infrahepatic vena cava, hepatic artery, and portal vein. Many variations and adaptations, such as vascular patches, are used depending on both donor and recipient anatomy. If venovenous bypass is used, it is removed after the infrahepatic vena cava anastomosis and before the hepatic artery anastomosis.[49]

Stage 3, biliary anastomosis, can be achieved in two ways: choledochojejunostomy (bile duct to jejunum) and choledochocholedochostomy (bile duct to bile

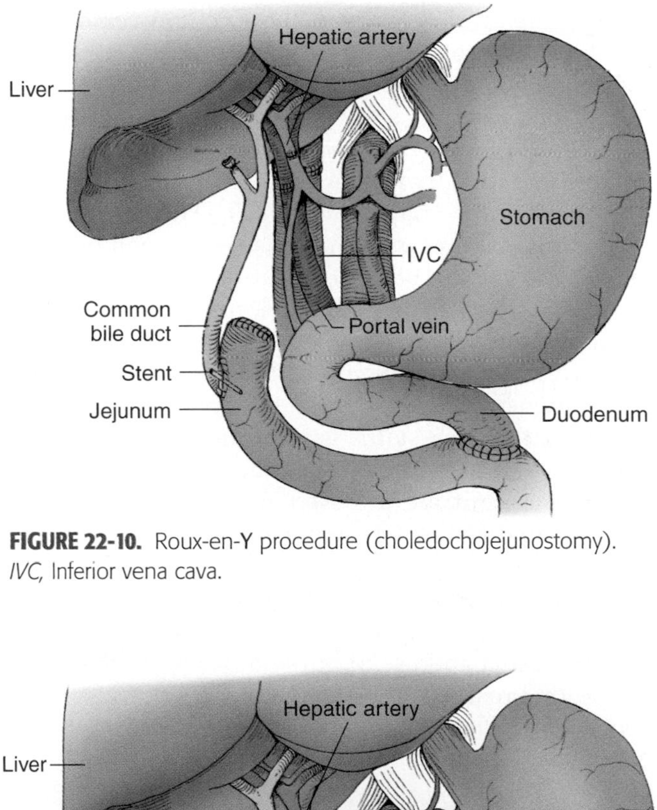

FIGURE 22-10. Roux-en-Y procedure (choledochojejunostomy). *IVC*, Inferior vena cava.

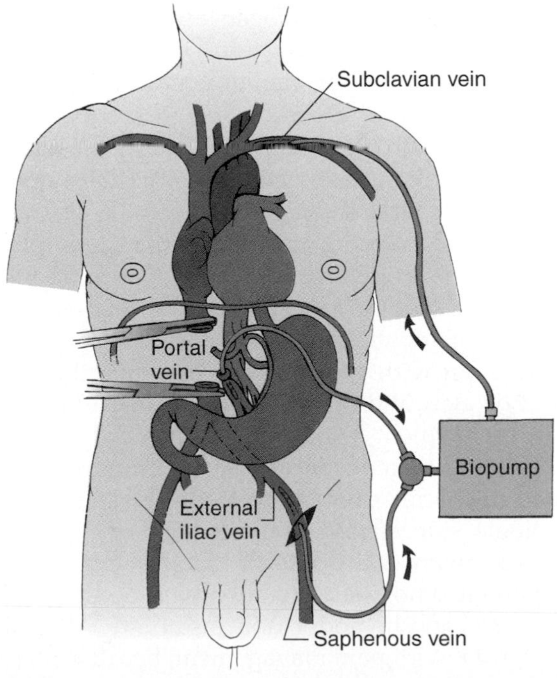

FIGURE 22-9. Venovenous bypass during removal of the native liver. The portal and iliac veins are cannulated, and blood is circulated via a centrifugal pump to the subclavian vein.

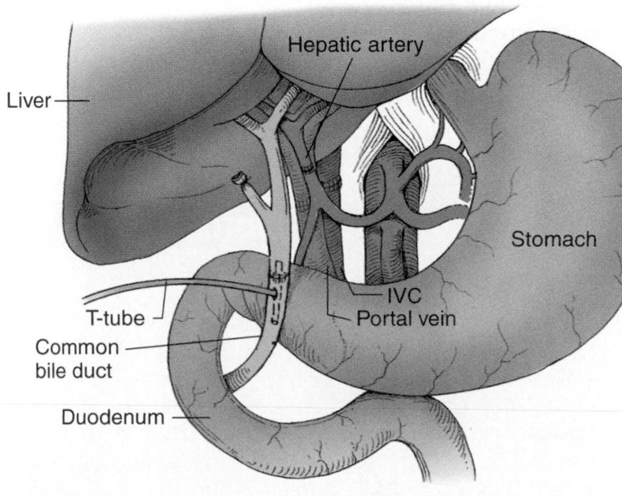

FIGURE 22-11. Choledochocholedochostomy procedure. *IVC*, Inferior vena cava.

duct). Choledochojejunostomy is done in patients with diseased bile ducts such as those with biliary atresia or sclerosing cholangitis. It is also known as a *Roux-en-γ* procedure and is shown in Figure 22-10. The choledochocholedochostomy is performed when the patient has a healthy and intact common bile duct and is shown in Figure 22-11. The patient returns from surgery with or without an external stent or T-tube. If an external stent or T-tube is present, it is connected to a bag into which bile drains. Patients who do not have external biliary tubes present may have an internal stent inserted in the bile duct across the biliary anastomosis. Eventually the internal stent moves and is passed with the stool.[49]

Postoperative Collaborative Management

The common nursing diagnoses associated with liver transplantation are listed in Box 22-19. After surgery, some patients may be extubated before arriving in the critical care unit. But most will arrive unreversed from anesthesia. **Immediate priorities include (1) reestablishment of normal body temperature, (2) hemodynamic stabilization, and (3) maintenance of adequate oxygenation and ventilation.**

Postoperative hypothermia is common after an orthotopic liver transplant (OLT). The critical care nurse must achieve rewarming safely by methods such as using warming blankets, heating lamps, and head covers. Hemodynamic stabilization is a particular challenge, because the patient may arrive hypervolemic, euvolemic, or hypovolemic and also be hypertensive or hypotensive. Assessment of total body fluids versus intravascular fluid status is important. Accurate measurements of hemodynamic function, urinary output, and bile output are assessed frequently to evaluate true volume status. Choice of replacement fluid and pharmacologic agent for correcting volume and blood pressure abnormalities is transplant center–specific. These protocols vary as to use of albumin or fresh-frozen plasma and use of intravenous renal-dose dopamine or prostaglandin, as well as other agents and solutions. Still, the goals are all the same: optimize tissue perfusion and deliver oxygen to all tissues, especially the newly transplanted graft.

Electrolyte abnormalities can occur after OLT. Disturbances in potassium and magnesium levels are common. High serum levels are usually associated with renal impairment; low levels can be the result of drug side effects, such as diuretic therapy. The patient also may be hypernatremic or hyponatremic, which will complicate correction of volume status and replacement fluids.

Ventilatory support of the patient is maintained until anesthesia has been metabolized and cleared by the new liver and the patient awakens. Frequent measurement of arterial blood gas levels, continuous pulse oximetry, and assessment of breath sounds are needed. The patient may require changes in ventilatory settings, suctioning to remove secretions, or administration of pharmacologic agents to correct acid-base imbalances. Pulmonary complications are common. After extubation, patients must be encouraged to perform incentive spirometry exercises and to turn and deep breathe frequently to help prevent atelectasis and pneumonia.[46]

Management of coagulopathies is important in the early postoperative phase. Careful measurement of drain output and drainage from incisions is needed along with other nursing assessments of blood loss, such as signs of hypovolemia, tachypnea, tachycardia, or poor peripheral oxygenation. A sudden increase in sanguineous nasogastric output or black, tarry stools are hallmarks of bleeding problems and must be reported immediately. Laboratory monitoring to assess blood loss and coagulopathies includes hematocrit, hemoglobin, platelet count, prothrombin time, partial thromboplastin time, fibrinogen, and fibrin split products. Reversal of coagulopathies is done judiciously with consideration for the potential to thrombose newly anastomosed blood vessels in the liver. Blood products such as platelets, fresh-frozen plasma, and specific factors can be given along with pharmacologic agents such as vitamin K.

Neurologic assessment of the patient is important in the early postoperative phase to determine mental status and graft function. Patients who preoperatively were encephalopathic will generally be slower to clear mentally. But with good hepatic function, the patient should be alert and oriented within 1 to 2 days. Neurologic assessment also can be influenced by certain pharmacologic agents, including the immunosuppressants, which can cause both peripheral and central neurologic side effects. The critical care nurse must always be aware of the potential for intracranial bleeds in a patient who has coagulopathies, serum sodium imbalances, and hemodynamic instability. All of these can interfere with pain management, because pharmacologic agents used for pain can mask deterioration in mental status. Medications to relieve pain are administered, but other nonpharmacologic nursing interventions also must be used.[46]

Box 22-19

NURSING DIAGNOSIS PRIORITIES

Liver Transplantation

- Risk for Infection, p. A-46
- Imbalanced Nutrition: Less Than Body Requirements related to lack of exogenous nutrients or increased metabolic demand, p. A-28
- Deficient Fluid Volume related to absolute loss, p. A-16
- Disturbed Body Image related to actual change in body, structure, function, or appearance, p. A-20
- Deficient Knowledge related to lack of previous exposure to information, p. A-18

Renal function can be altered after a liver transplant because of acute tubular necrosis, intrinsic kidney disease, or poor liver function. Some studies estimate 21% to 73% of OLT patients develop renal failure.[50] Patients are managed with attention to fluid and electrolyte imbalances; avoidance of nephrotoxic drugs; and occasionally continuous renal replacement therapy or intermittent hemodialysis. With good liver function, kidney function usually improves. But certain immunosuppressive agents and antibiotics can deleteriously affect renal function. Adjustments in doses or avoidance of use must be balanced with assessment of kidney and liver function.[46]

Immunosuppressive therapy places the transplant patient at an increased risk of infection. Infectious complications continue to be the leading cause of death in the OLT patient,[51] and the potential for infection is greatest when patients receive high doses of immunosuppressants.[46] Good hand-washing techniques and standard precautions must be practiced by all persons who come into contact with the transplant patient throughout the hospitalization. Infections are treated with appropriate antibiotics specific to the invading organism. Prophylactic therapies are commonly used as well.[51]

Careful attention to any external biliary drain line is important. If the patient has an external biliary drain, the critical care nurse documents color, character, and amount of drainage and reports any changes. Biliary complications can occur after OLT.[46] Posttransplant complications, including biliary ones, are listed in Box 22-20.

Box 22-20

Common Complications After Liver Transplant

Pulmonary Complications
- Pleural effusion
- Pulmonary edema
- Pneumonia
- Pneumothorax or hemothorax
- Atelectasis
- Paralysis of right diaphragm

Biliary Complications
- Leaks
- Strictures
- Obstruction
- Infection (cholangitis)
- Breakdown of anastomosis

Gastrointestinal Complications
- Bleeding/ulceration
- GI infections (cytomegalovirus, *Candida, Clostridium difficile*)
- Bowel perforations

Vascular Complications
- Hepatic artery thrombosis
- Portal vein thrombosis
- Vena caval thrombosis
- Peripheral and/or central line sepsis
- Hepatic vein thrombosis

GI, Gastrointestinal.

Posttransplant Assessment of Liver Function. The standard laboratory measures used to follow graft function are serum aspartate aminotransferase (AST/SGOT), alanine aminotransferase (ALT/SGPT), alkaline phosphatase, and γ-glutamyltransferase (GGT), serum bilirubin, and prothrombin times. In the first few postoperative days, the serum levels may continue to rise before peaking and subsequently falling. These liver function tests (LFTs) are measured frequently in the first few days after surgery. As liver function improves, the frequency of laboratory testing decreases.

The patient with suspected primary nonfunction of the graft will demonstrate (1) hemodynamic instability, (2) progressive renal deterioration, (3) coagulopathies and abnormal serum liver function laboratory test results, (4) hypoglycemia, (5) continued ventilatory dependence, and (6) an inability to awaken from anesthesia. Continued nonfunction of the graft will necessitate relisting the patient for another donor liver. Early signs of optimal graft function include improving kidney function, mental alertness, a high to normal serum glucose, and early extubation. The serum ALT, AST, GGT, and alkaline phosphatase levels may peak on the third or fourth day but subsequently will decrease. The serum bilirubin may take 1 week before beginning to fall and may have a mild elevation when the external biliary drainage tube is clamped or following a blood transfusion. Early mobilization and physical therapy are encouraged.[52]

The nasogastric tube is removed when its output is minimal, bowel sounds return, and the patient is extubated. If the patient is expected to be intubated longer than several days, TPN may be started. Otherwise, nutrition may begin orally or by feeding tube as soon as bowel function returns. The diet is slowly advanced as tolerated. Central venous catheters and arterial lines are removed. The urinary catheter is removed as soon as the patient is awake enough to be continent. Drain lines are removed as drainage outputs become minimal. As the patient begins to participate in self-care, plans are made to transfer the patient out of the critical care unit to the transplant nursing unit.

On the transplant unit, laboratory data and vital signs continue to be monitored on a routine basis. Self-care protocols are promoted.[53] Increasing levels of physical therapy are encouraged and diet is advanced, and much of the nurse's effort is spent teaching the patient and family.

Rejection Surveillance. Acute rejection in OLT is a cellular-mediated event and is suspected any time the serum LFTs become elevated over the previous levels. An elevation of the LFTs usually precedes any other sign of acute rejection of the liver allograft. Sometimes the patient also exhibits fever, a drop in bile output (if a T-tube is still connected to a drainage bag), and a change in the color and viscosity of the bile. At first the patient may not have any other physical symptoms, but eventually malaise may occur and the urine may darken and stools become clay-colored. An acute elevation in LFTs can signal rejection of the liver graft. However, certain infections, such as cytomegalovirus, may also cause LFTs to increase. A liver biopsy may be indicated to determine cause of liver dysfunction. Acute rejection can occur anytime after transplant, but most commonly it occurs in the first few months and even as early as in the first week. The majority of liver transplant patients experience at least one acute rejection episode. Treatment of acute rejection requires increasing immunosuppression (i.e., an increase in tacrolimus or steroid dose, possibly an addition of monoclonal or polyclonal antilymphocyte antibodies, or other newer pharmacologic agents). Immunosuppressant protocols vary from center to center and are usually very successful at reversing acute rejection.[52]

Chronic rejection is a humoral event and is progressive and nonreversible. Chronic rejection in a liver transplant patient usually requires retransplantation if the patient is still considered a candidate.[52]

Patient Education. Considerable attention is focused on patient education and discharge planning. Discharge booklets are helpful in the education process. It is important for the patient to learn how to self-administer medications, monitor vital signs, care for incision and T-tube (if present), prevent infections, and identify problems that must promptly receive medical attention. Because it is not uncommon for patients to be discharged within 2 weeks after an OLT, it is important for discharge instructions to begin as soon as the patient is mentally alert. Patients discharged early may require home health care nurse referrals to assist with follow-up of incision care, intravenous therapies, and more. In addition, education must be provided about rejection surveillance, signs and symptoms of infection, lifestyle changes if needed, long-term transplant medication considerations, and the follow-up visit schedule.

evolve To test your mastery of this chapter, try the Open-Book Quiz at http://evolve.elsevier.com/Urden/priorities/

REFERENCES

1. Conrad SA: Acute upper gastrointestinal bleeding in critically ill patients: causes and treatment modalities, *Crit Care Med* 30:S365, 2002.
2. Hamoui N, Docherty SD, Crookes PF: Gastrointestinal hemorrhage: is the surgeon obsolete? *Emerg Med Clin North Am* 21:1017, 2003.
3. Esrailian E, Gralnek IM: Nonvariceal upper gastrointestinal bleeding: epidemiology and diagnosis, *Gastroenterol Clin North Am* 34:589, 2005.
4. Wong RC: Acute GI bleeding: upper and lower, but is there a "middle kingdom"? *Gastrointest Endosc* 58:409, 2003.
5. Bounds BC, Friedman LS: Lower gastrointestinal bleeding, *Gastroenterol Clin North Am* 32:1107, 2003.
6. Huang CS, Lichtenstein DR: Nonvariceal upper gastrointestinal bleeding, *Gastroenterol Clin North Am* 32:1053, 2003.
7. Eswaran S, Roy MA: Medical management of acid-peptic disorders of the stomach, *Surg Clin North Am* 85:895, 2005.
8. McCance KL, Huether SE: *Pathophysiology: the biologic basis for disease in adults and children,* ed 5, St Louis, 2006, Mosby.
9. Peura DA: Prevention of nonsteroidal anti-inflammatory drug–associated gastrointestinal symptoms and ulcer complications, *Am J Med* 117(suppl 5A):63S, 2004.
10. Gerrits MM et al: *Helicobacter pylori* and antimicrobial resistance: molecular mechanisms and clinical implications, *Lancet Infect Dis* 6:699, 2006.
11. Fennerty MB: Pathophysiology of the upper gastrointestinal tract in the critically ill patient: rationale for the therapeutic benefits of acid suppression, *Crit Care Med* 30(6 suppl):S351, 2002.
12. Sung JJ: The role of acid suppression in the management and prevention of gastrointestinal hemorrhage associated with gastroduodenal ulcers, *Gastroenterol Clin North Am* 32(3 suppl):S11, 2003.
13. Zaman A: Portal hypertension-related bleeding: management of difficult cases, *Clin Liver Dis* 10:353, 2006.
14. Martin RF: Surgical management of ulcer disease, *Surg Clin North Am* 85:907, 2005.
15. Velayos F: Upper and lower gastrointestinal bleeding in the critically ill patient. In Parsons PE, Wiener-Kronish JP, editors: *Critical care secrets: questions and answers reveal the secrets to effective critical care,* ed 3, Philadelphia, 2003, Hanley & Belfus.
16. Ferguson CB, Mitchell RM: Nonvariceal upper gastrointestinal bleeding: standard and new treatment, *Gastroenterol Clin North Am* 34:607, 2005.
17. Holmes CL, Walley KR: The evaluation and management of shock, *Clin Chest Med* 24:775, 2003.
18. Leung FW: The venerable nasogastric tube, *Gastrointest Endosc* 59:255, 2004.
19. Zaman A, Chalasani N: Bleeding caused by portal hypertension, *Gastroenterol Clin North Am* 34:623, 2005.
20. Dib N, Oberti F, Calès P: Current management of the complications of portal hypertension: variceal bleeding and ascites, *CMAJ* 174:1433, 2006.
21. Comar KM, Sanyal AJ: Portal hypertensive bleeding, *Gastroenterol Clin North Am* 32:1079, 2003.
22. Flannery J, Tucker DA: Pharmacologic prophylaxis and treatment of stress ulcers in critically ill patients, *Crit Care Nurs Clin North Am* 14:39, 2002.
23. Mayerle J, Simon P, Lerch MM: Medical treatment of acute pancreatitis, *Gastroenterol Clin North Am* 33:855, 2004.
24. Gavaghan M: The pancreas: hermit of the abdomen, *AORN J* 75:1110, 2002.
25. Papachristou GI, Whitcomb DC: Inflammatory markers of disease severity in acute pancreatitis, *Clin Lab Med* 25:17, 2005.

26. Hughes E: Understanding the care of patients with acute pancreatitis, *Nurs Stand* 18:45, 2003.
27. Bowyer MW: Acute pancreatitis. In Parsons PE, Wiener-Kronish JP, editors: *Critical care secrets: questions and answers reveal the secrets to effective critical care,* ed 3, Philadelphia, 2003, Hanley & Belfus.
28. Flasar MH, Goldberg E: Acute abdominal pain, *Med Clin North Am* 90:481, 2006.
29. Nathens AB et al: Management of the critically ill patient with severe pancreatitis, *Crit Care Med* 32:2524, 2004.
30. Law NM, Freeman ML: Emergency complications of acute and chronic pancreatitis, *Gastroenterol Clin North Am* 32:1169, 2003.
31. Cothren C, Burch JM: Acute pancreatitis. In Harken AH, Moore EE, editors: *Abernathy's surgical secrets: questions and answers reveal the secrets to successful surgery,* ed 5, Philadelphia, 2004, Hanley & Belfus.
32. Han MK, Hyzy R: Advances in critical care management of hepatic failure and insufficiency, *Crit Care Med* 34(9 suppl):S225, 2006.
33. Khan SA et al: Acute liver failure: a review, *Clin Liver Dis* 10:239, 2006.
34. Sass DA, Shakil AO: Fulminant hepatic failure, *Gastroenterol Clin North Am* 32:1195, 2003.
35. Krasko A, Deshpande K, Bonvino S: Liver failure, transplantation, and critical care, *Crit Care Clin* 19:155, 2003.
36. Cottrell DB, Asturi E: Gastric intubation: assessment and intervention, *Crit Care Nurs Clin North Am* 16:489, 2004.
37. Kowalak JP, Hughes AS, Mills JE: *Best practices: a guide to excellence in nursing care,* Philadelphia, 2003, Lippincott Williams & Wilkins.
38. Stotland BR, Ginsberg GG: Upper gastrointestinal bleeding. In Lanken PN, Hanson CW, Manaker SM, editors: *The intensive care unit manual,* Philadelphia, 2001, Saunders.
39. Day MW: Esophagogastric tamponade tube. In Lynn-McHale DJ, Carlson KK, editors, *The AACN procedure manual for critical care,* ed 5, Philadelphia, 2005, Saunders
40. Shah VH, Kamath PS: Portal hypertension and gastrointestinal bleeding. In Feldman M, Friedman LS, Brandt LJ, editors: *Sleisenger & Fordtran's gastrointestinal and liver disease,* ed 8, Philadelphia, 2006, Saunders.
41. Mackenzie DJ, Popplewell PK, Billingsley KG: Care of patients after esophagectomy, *Crit Care Nurse* 24:16, 2004.
42. Jaffe RA, Samuels SI: *Anesthesiologist's manual of surgical procedures,* ed 3, Philadelphia, 2004, Lippincott Williams & Wilkins.
43. Rubesin SE, Levine MS: Radiologic diagnosis of gastrointestinal perforation, *Radiol Clin North Am* 41:1095, 2003.
44. Bloom RD et al: An overview of solid organ transplantation, *Clin Chest Med* 26:529, 2005.
45. Cupples SA, Ohler L: *Transplantation nursing secrets,* Philadelphia, 2003, Hanley & Belfus
46. Krasko A, Deshpande K, Bonvino S: Liver failure, transplantation, and critical care, *Crit Care Clin* 19:155, 2003.
47. Keeffe EB: Liver transplantation at the millennium: past, present, and future, *Clin Liver Dis* 4:241, 2000.
48. Farges O et al: Long-term results of ABO-incompatible liver transplantation, *Transplant Proc* 27:1701, 1995.
49. Saggi BH et al: Surgical advances in liver and bowel transplantation, *Anesthesiology Clin N Am* 22:713, 2004.
50. Ojo A et al: Chronic renal failure after transplantation of a non-renal organ. *N Engl J Med* 349(10):931, 2003.
51. Preksaitis J, Green M, Avery R: Guidelines for the prevention and management of infectious complications of solid organ transplant, *Am J Transplant* 4 (suppl 10):66, 2004.
52. Burton JR, Rose HR: Diagnosis and management of allograft failure, *Clin Liver Dis* 10:407, 2006.
53. Randolf S, Sholtz K: Self care guidelines: finding a common ground. *J Transplant Coordination* 9(3):156, 1999.

CHAPTER 23

Endocrine Assessment and Diagnostic Procedures

MARY E. LOUGH

OBJECTIVES

- Identify the components of an endocrine history.
- Describe clinical findings in patients with pancreatic and posterior pituitary dysfunction.
- Explain the clinical significance of laboratory and diagnostic tests of pancreatic dysfunction.
- Explain the clinical significance of laboratory and diagnostic tests of posterior pituitary dysfunction.

ENDOCRINE ASSESSMENT AND DIAGNOSTIC PROCEDURES

Assessment of the patient with endocrine dysfunction is a systematic process that incorporates both the history and the physical examination. Most of the endocrine glands are deeply encased in the human body. Although the placement of the glands provides security for the glandular functions, their resulting inaccessibility limits clinical examination. Nevertheless, the endocrine glands can be assessed indirectly. The critical care nurse who understands the metabolic actions of the hormones produced by endocrine glands assesses the physiology of the gland by monitoring that gland's target tissue as listed in Figure 23-1. This chapter describes clinical and diagnostic evaluation of the pancreas and the posterior pituitary.

HISTORY

The initial presentation of the patient determines the rapidity and direction of the interview. For a patient in acute distress the history is curtailed to only a few questions about the chief complaint and precipitating events. For the patient without obvious distress the endocrine history focuses on four areas: (1) current health status, (2) history of present illness, (3) past history and general endocrine status, and (4) family history.

PANCREAS

PHYSICAL ASSESSMENT

Insulin, which is produced by the pancreas, is responsible for glucose metabolism. The clinical assessment provides information about pancreatic functioning. Clinical manifestations of abnormal glucose metabolism often manifest as hyperglycemia, which is the initial assessment priority for the patient with pancreatic dysfunction.[1-4] Patients with hyperglycemia may ultimately be diagnosed with either type 1 or type 2 diabetes[4] or be hyperglycemic in association with a severe critical illness.[1,5] Data collection in the endocrine history for diabetes complications is outlined in Box 23-1.

Hyperglycemia

Because severe hyperglycemia affects a variety of body systems, all systems are assessed. The patient may complain of blurred vision, headache, weakness, fatigue, drowsiness, anorexia, nausea, and abdominal pain. On *inspection* the patient has flushed skin, polyuria, polydipsia, vomiting, and evidence of dehydration. Progressive deterioration in the level of consciousness, from alert to lethargic or comatose, is observed as the hyperglycemia exacerbates. If ketoacidosis occurs, the patient's breathing becomes deep and rapid (Kussmaul respirations), and the breath may have a fruity odor. *Auscultation* of the abdomen reveals hypoactive bowel sounds. *Palpation* elicits abdominal tenderness. *Percussion* reveals diminished deep tendon reflexes. Because hyperglycemia results in osmotic diuresis, the patient's fluid volume status is assessed. Signs of dehydration include tachycardia, orthostatic hypotension, and poor skin turgor.

LABORATORY STUDIES

Pertinent laboratory tests for pancreatic function measure the short-term (plasma glucose) and long-term (glycolated hemoglobin) blood glucose levels, which can identify and diagnose diabetes.

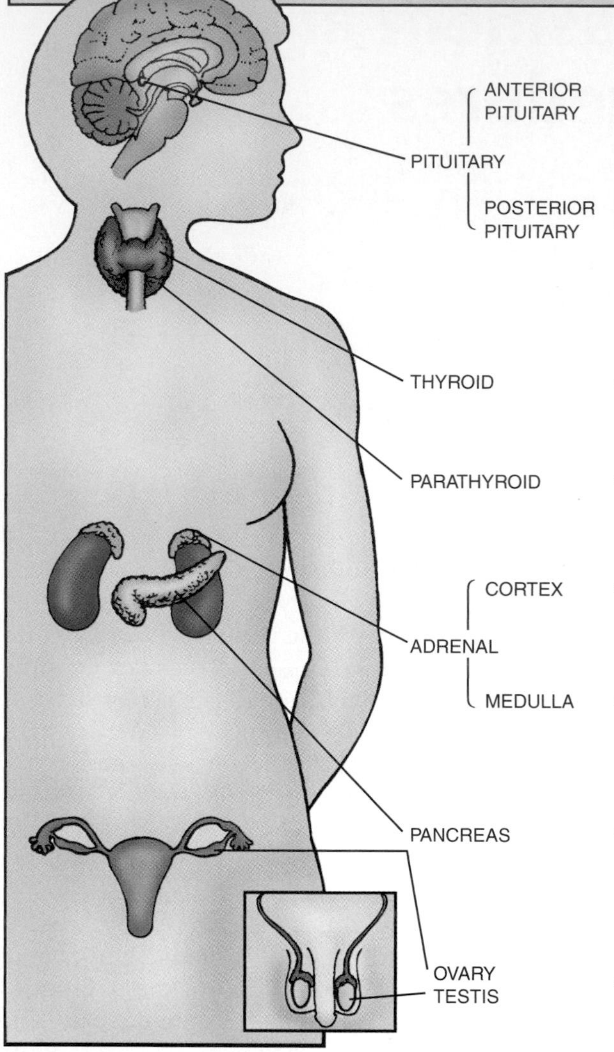

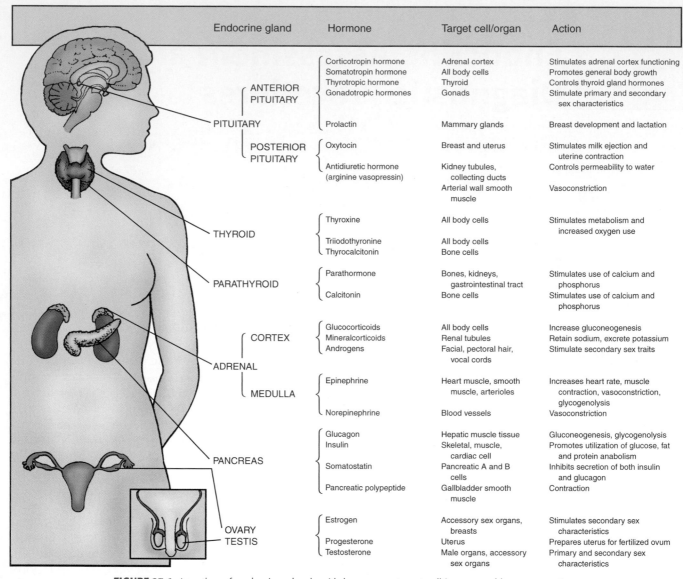

Endocrine gland	Hormone	Target cell/organ	Action
Pituitary – Anterior pituitary	Corticotropin hormone	Adrenal cortex	Stimulates adrenal cortex functioning
	Somatotropin hormone	All body cells	Promotes general body growth
	Thyrotropic hormone	Thyroid	Controls thyroid gland hormones
	Gonadotropic hormones	Gonads	Stimulate primary and secondary sex characteristics
	Prolactin	Mammary glands	Breast development and lactation
Pituitary – Posterior pituitary	Oxytocin	Breast and uterus	Stimulates milk ejection and uterine contraction
	Antidiuretic hormone (arginine vasopressin)	Kidney tubules, collecting ducts	Controls permeability to water
		Arterial wall smooth muscle	Vasoconstriction
Thyroid	Thyroxine	All body cells	Stimulates metabolism and increased oxygen use
	Triiodothyronine	All body cells	
	Thyrocalcitonin	Bone cells	
Parathyroid	Parathormone	Bones, kidneys, gastrointestinal tract	Stimulates use of calcium and phosphorus
	Calcitonin	Bone cells	Stimulates use of calcium and phosphorus
Adrenal – Cortex	Glucocorticoids	All body cells	Increase gluconeogenesis
	Mineralcorticoids	Renal tubules	Retain sodium, excrete potassium
	Androgens	Facial, pectoral hair, vocal cords	Stimulate secondary sex traits
Adrenal – Medulla	Epinephrine	Heart muscle, smooth muscle, arterioles	Increases heart rate, muscle contraction, vasoconstriction, glycogenolysis
	Norepinephrine	Blood vessels	Vasoconstriction
Pancreas	Glucagon	Hepatic muscle tissue	Gluconeogenesis, glycogenolysis
	Insulin	Skeletal, muscle, cardiac cell	Promotes utilization of glucose, fat and protein anabolism
	Somatostatin	Pancreatic A and B cells	Inhibits secretion of both insulin and glucagon
	Pancreatic polypeptide	Gallbladder smooth muscle	Contraction
Ovary / Testis	Estrogen	Accessory sex organs, breasts	Stimulates secondary sex characteristics
	Progesterone	Uterus	Prepares uterus for fertilized ovum
	Testosterone	Male organs, accessory sex organs	Primary and secondary sex characteristics

FIGURE 23-1. Location of endocrine glands with hormones, target cell/organ, and hormone action.

Blood Glucose

Fasting plasma glucose (FPG) is assessed by a simple blood test when the person has not eaten for 8 hours. A normal FPG is between 70 and 110 mg/dl. A fasting glucose level between 110 and 126 mg/dl identifies a person with *impaired glucose tolerance,* that is, one who is *prediabetic.* Even prediabetic individuals are at increased risk for developing complications of diabetes such as coronary heart disease and stroke. An FPG level of greater than 126 mg/dl (7 mmol/L) is diagnostic of diabetes (Table 23-1). Following a meal the glucose level rises in the bloodstream. It is recommended that postprandial glucose levels not exceed 180 mg/dl (10 mmol/L).[6] A plasma blood glucose below 70 mg/dl is indicative of hypoglycemia.[1]

All hospitalized patients must have their blood glucose level monitored frequently while in the hospital.[1] Clinical practice recommendations emphasize maintaining blood glucose as close to normal as possible for all critically ill patients, whether or not they have a diagnosis of diabetes. If a continuous insulin drip is infused to normalize blood glucose levels, point-of-care blood glucose testing is performed hourly by the critical care nurse until the blood glucose is within the target range.[1,5]

Before discharge home, diabetic patients should be taught to self-monitor their blood glucose levels.[1,6] Maintaining blood glucose within the normal range is associated with fewer diabetes-related complications and a lower rate of complications of diabetes.[4] Laboratory tests or point-of-care or self-monitoring of blood glucose levels represent the standard of care for management of diabetes.[4] Unfortunately, home monitoring of blood glucose levels is not the norm, in spite of research evidence that maintaining blood glucose levels as close to normal as possible prolongs life and

Box 23-1

Taking a Health History for Diabetic Complications

Current Health Status

The body may not be able to adjust to increased insulin needs resulting from sudden physiologic changes such as infection, injury, or surgery, among others. The nurse would assess whether the patient had a severe infection, surgical wound, or traumatic injury.

Recent/current signs and symptoms
- Unexplained changes in weight, thirst, hunger
- Headache, blurred vision
- Long-standing, unhealed infection
- Vaginitis, pruritus
- Leg pain, numbness

Unexplained change in urinary patterns (i.e., daytime and nighttime, frequency, and volume)
- Energy/stamina changes
- Endurance level
- Weakness
- Unexplained, excessive fatigue

Behavior/mental changes (also ask family member or significant other for input)
- Memory loss
- Orientation

History of Present Illness—Onset, Characteristics, Course

Chronic illness—physiologic or psychologic stress could increase endogenous glucose

Recent treatments that could be a source of exogenous glucose
- Hyperalimentation
- Peritoneal dialysis
- Hemodialysis

Medications—prescription and over-the-counter preparations (Pharmacologic agents can alter pancreatic function by either increasing or decreasing release of the endocrine hormones. Drugs also may interfere with hormonal action at the receptor site on the target cell.)

Past History

Previous pancreatic surgery?

Ever been told any of the following applied to you:
- Too much sugar in the urine?
- Too much sugar in the blood?
- Would probably develop too much sugar later in life?

If "yes" answer to any of the above, what treatment, if any, was prescribed?

Are you currently following such a treatment?

Family History

Has a family member ever been diagnosed with diabetes/sugar in the blood?

If so, how did he or she treat the condition?

Table 23-1

Plasma Blood Glucose Levels

PATIENT STATUS	mg/dl	mmol/L
Hypoglycemia	Below 70	Below 3.9
Normal FPG	70-110	3.9-6.1
Impaired FPG	110-126	6.1-7.0
FPG diagnostic of diabetes	Above 126	Above 7.0
Non-FPG diagnostic of diabetes	Above 200	Above 11.1

Data from American Diabetes Association: *Diabetes Care* 30(suppl 1):S4, 2007.
FPG, Fasting plasma glucose.

reduces complications. Only 40% of patients with type 1 diabetes and 26% of patients with type 2 diabetes monitor their blood glucose level at least once a day.[6]

Urine Glucose

Testing the urine for glucose is not recommended for diabetic patients because there is too much variation in the renal threshold for glucose when kidney damage secondary to diabetes has occurred.[6] Urine glucose measurements are affected by variation in fluid intake, reflect an average glucose level and not a specific point in time, and are altered by some drugs.[6] The other limitation of urine glucose testing is that it does not offer any help in the identification of hypoglycemia.[6] For all of these reasons urine testing is not recommended.

Glycated Hemoglobin

Blood testing of glucose is useful for daily management of diabetes. However, a different blood test is used to achieve an objective measure of blood glucose over an extended period of time. The glycated hemoglobin test (also known as the glycosylated hemoglobin, or HbA_{1c} or A_{1c}), provides information about the average amount of glucose that has been present in the patient's bloodstream over the previous 3 to 4 months.[6] During the 120-day life span of red blood cells (erythrocytes), the hemoglobin within each cell binds to the available blood glucose through a process known as *glycosylation.* Typically 4% to 6% of hemoglobin contains the glucose group hemoglobin A_{1c}. A normal hemoglobin A_{1c} level is 4% to 6%, with an acceptable target level for diabetic patients below 7%.[4] The hemoglobin A_{1c} value correlates with specific blood glucose levels as shown in Table 23-2. Not all clinical laboratories use the same analytical techniques to measure the glycated hemoglobin A_{1c}, and methods to standardize the reporting of results worldwide are underway.[6,7]

Table 23-2

Correlation Between Hemoglobin (HbA_{1c}) and Blood (Plasma) Glucose

HbA_{1c} (%)	MEAN PLASMA GLUCOSE (mg/dl)	(mmol/L)
6	135	7.5
7	170	9.5
8	205	11.5
9	240	13.5
10	275	15.5
11	310	17.5
12	345	19.5

Data from American Diabetes Association: *Diabetes Care* 30(suppl 1):S4, 2007.

Blood Ketones

In a serum blood test, normal ketone level is 2 to 4 mg/dl of blood and normal acetone 0.3 to 2.0 mg/dl of blood. Ketones are by-products of fat metabolism. In most cases when the body uses carbohydrate as its main source of energy, the liver completes fat metabolism and minimal or no ketones are found in the blood. Elevated blood ketone levels (ketonemia) are also detected by a fruity, sweet-smelling odor on the exhaled breath. This odor is the result of the body's attempt to keep the pH within the normal range. A sweet-smelling breath occurs when the patient exhales in an attempt to decrease the accumulated acids.

Urine Ketones

Urine ketone monitoring is important, particularly in patients with type 1 diabetes.[6] The presence of ketones may signify impending or established ketoacidosis. In diabetic ketoacidosis (DKA), fat breakdown (lipolysis) occurs so rapidly that fat metabolism is incomplete, and ketone bodies (acetone, β-hydroxybutyric acid, and acetoacetic acid) accumulate in the blood *(ketonemia)* and are excreted in the urine *(ketonuria)*. It is recommended that all diabetic patients self-test or have their urine tested for the presence of ketones during any acute illness or stress; with a blood glucose level greater than 300 mg/dl (16.7 mmol/L); with symptoms of nausea, vomiting, or abdominal pain; and for women during pregnancy.[6]

Normally, in healthy nonfasting individuals only minute quantities of ketones are present in the urine, and the levels are so low they are below the threshold of detectability with routine testing methods.[6] In fasting and starvation states, ketones may be present in the urine.[6]

PITUITARY GLAND

The pituitary gland, recessed in the base of the cranium, is not accessible to physical assessment. The critical care nurse must therefore be aware of the systemic effects of a normally functioning pituitary to be able to identify dysfunction. One essential hormone formed in the hypothalamus but secreted through the posterior pituitary gland is *antidiuretic hormone* (ADH), also known as *vasopressin*.

PHYSICAL ASSESSMENT

ADH controls the amount of fluid lost and retained within the body. Acute dysfunction of the posterior pituitary or the hypothalamus can result in insufficient or excessive ADH production. Thus the clinical signs of posterior pituitary dysfunction often manifest as fluid volume deficit (insufficient ADH production) or fluid volume excess (excessive ADH production).

Hydration Status

The nurse determines the effectiveness of ADH production by conducting a hydration assessment. A hydration assessment includes observations of skin integrity, skin turgor, and buccal membrane moisture. Moist, shiny buccal membranes indicate satisfactory fluid balance. Skin turgor that is resilient and returns to its original position in less than 3 seconds after being pinched or lifted indicates adequate skin elasticity. Skin over the forehead, clavicle, and sternum is the most reliable for testing tissue turgor because it is less affected by aging and thus more easily assessed for changes related to fluid balance. A well-hydrated patient has skin in the groin and axilla that is slightly moist to touch. In elderly patients these "typical" assessment findings may be absent. Elderly persons, especially women, experience a as much as a 50% decreases in total body water content by age 75.[8]

Other indicators that the patient's hydration status is adequate for metabolic demands include a balanced intake and output and absence of thirst. Absence of thirst, however, is not a reliable indicator of dehydration in those with decreased thirst mechanisms, such as the elderly or critically ill patients. Absence of abrupt changes in mental status may also indicate normal hydration. Other indicators of normal hydration include absence of edema, stable weight, and urine specific gravity that falls within the normal range (1.005 to 1.030).

Vital Signs

Changes in heart rate, blood pressure (BP), and central venous pressure (when available) are useful to determine fluid volume status. BP and pulse are monitored frequently. Decreased BP with increased pulse is characteristic of hypovolemia, whereas elevated blood pressure and a rapid, bounding pulse may indicate hypervolemia. In contrast, orthostatic hypotension, which occurs when intravascular fluid volume decreases, is identified by a drop in systolic BP of 20 millimeters of mercury (mm Hg) or a drop in diastolic BP of 10 mm Hg when the patient changes position from lying to standing.

Weight and Intake/Output

Daily weight changes coincide with fluid retention and fluid loss. Sudden changes in weight could result from a change in fluid balance; 1 L of fluid lost or retained is equal to approximately 2.2 pounds, or 1 kg, of weight gained or lost. To use weight as a true determinant of the fluid balance, all extraneous variables are eliminated, and the same scale is used at the same time each day. Precise measurement and notation of intake and output are used as criteria for fluid replacement therapy.

LABORATORY ASSESSMENT

No single diagnostic test identifies dysfunction of the posterior pituitary gland. Diagnosis usually is made through laboratory tests combined with the clinical profile of the patient.

Serum Antidiuretic Hormone

The result of a blood test for normal levels of serum ADH is 1 to 5 picogram per milliliter (pg/ml).[8] Testing for ADH levels is not typical in critical care. If a blood test to measure ADH levels is going to be drawn, all drugs that may alter the release of ADH must be withheld for a minimum of 8 hours. Common medications that affect ADH levels include morphine sulfate, lithium carbonate, chlorothiazide, carbamazepine, oxytocin, nicotine, alcohol, and selective serotonin reuptake inhibitors (SSRIs).[9] Mechanical ventilation (positive-pressure and negative-pressure) and emotional stress also influence ADH levels and must be considered in the interpretation of values.

The test, read by comparing serum ADH levels with the blood and urine osmolarity, is helpful in differentiating the *syndrome of inappropriate antidiuretic hormone* (SIADH) from central *diabetes insipidus* (DI). The presence of increased ADH in the bloodstream compared with a low serum osmolarity and elevated urine osmolarity confirms the diagnosis of SIADH. Reduced levels of serum ADH in a patient with high serum osmolarity, hypernatremia, and reduced urine concentration signal central DI.

Urine and Serum Osmolarity

Values for serum osmolarity in the bloodstream range from 275 to 295 milliosmoles per liter of solution. *Osmolarity* measurements determine the concentration of dissolved particles in a solution. In a healthy person a change in the concentration of solutes triggers a chain of events to maintain adequate serum dilution. Urine osmolarity in the person with normal kidneys is highly dependent on fluid intake. With high fluid intake, particle dilution is low but will increase if fluids are restricted, and therefore the expected range for urine osmolarity is wide, ranging from 50 to 1400 mOsm/kg.

Increased serum osmolarity stimulates the release of ADH, which in turn reduces the amount of water lost through the kidney. Body fluid thereby is retained to dilute the particle concentration in the bloodstream. Decreased serum osmolarity inhibits the release of ADH, the kidney tubules increase their permeability, and fluid is eliminated from the body in an attempt to regain normal concentration of particles in the bloodstream. The most accurate measures of the body's fluid balance are obtained when urine and blood samples are collected simultaneously.

Antidiuretic Hormone Test

The ADH test is used to differentiate between *neurogenic* DI (central) and *nephrogenic* (kidney) DI. The patient is challenged with 0.05 to 1 ml intranasally administered ADH in the form of desmopressin (DDAVP).[10] An intravenous (IV) line is inserted before the ADH; urine volume and osmolarity are measured every 30 minutes for 2 hours before and after the ADH challenge. The patient with normal posterior pituitary functioning responds to the exogenous ADH by resorbing water at the renal tubule and raising the urine osmolarity slightly. In severe central DI, where the pituitary is affected, the urine osmolarity shows a significant rise (becomes more concentrated), which indicates that the cell receptor sites on the renal tubules are responsive to vasopressin. Test results in which urine osmolarity remains unchanged indicate nephrogenic DI, suggesting renal dysfunction because the kidneys are no longer responsive to ADH. This test is rarely performed in the critical care unit because of the unstable hemodynamic and volume status of most patients.[10]

DIAGNOSTIC PROCEDURES

In addition to laboratory tests, radiographic examination, computed tomography (CT), and magnetic resonance imaging (MRI) are used to diagnose structural lesions such as cranial bone fractures, tumors, or blood clots in the region of the pituitary. Although these procedures do not diagnose DI or SIADH, they are useful in uncovering the likely underlying cause.[8]

Radiographic Examination

A basic x-ray examination of the inferior skull views the sella turcica and surrounding bone formation. Bone fractures or tissue swelling at the base of the brain, which are apparent on a radiograph, suggest interference with the vascular supply and nerve impulses to the hypothalamic-pituitary system. Dysfunction can occur if the hypothalamus, infundibular stalk, or pituitary is impaired.

Computed Tomography

CT scan of the base of the skull identifies pituitary tumors, blood clots, cysts, nodules, or other soft tissue masses. This rapid procedure causes no discomfort except that it requires the patient to lie perfectly still. CT studies can be performed with radiopaque contrast (sodium iodine solution) or "without contrast." The contrast dye is given intravenously to highlight the hypothalamus, infundibular stalk, and pituitary gland. This dye may cause allergic reactions in iodine-sensitive persons, and the patient must be carefully questioned about iodine allergy before the test. Size and shape of sella turcica and position of hypothalamus, infundibular stalk, and pituitary are identified.

Magnetic Resonance Imaging

MRI enables the radiologist to visualize internal organs and cellular characteristics of specific tissue. MRI uses a magnetic field rather than radiation to produce high-resolution cross-sectional images. The soft brain tissue and surrounding cerebrospinal fluid (CSF) make the brain especially suited to MRI scanning. Although not a definitive diagnostic test for posterior pituitary hormonal imbalance, MRI may identify anatomic disruption of the gland and the surrounding area to uncover a primary cause of DI or SIADH.

evolve To test your mastery of this chapter, try the Open-Book Quiz at http://evolve.elsevier.com/Urden/priorities/

REFERENCES

1. American Diabetes Association: Standards of medical care in diabetes—2007, *Diabetes Care* 30(suppl 1):S4, 2007.
2. Clement S et al: Diagnosis and classification of diabetes mellitus, *Diabetes Care* 27(suppl 1):S5, 2004.
3. Clement S et al: Screening for type 2 diabetes, *Diabetes Care* 27(suppl 1):S11, 2004.
4. Dungan K et al: Glucose measurement: Confounding issues in setting targets for inpatient management, *Diabetes Care* 30(2):403, 2007.
5. ACE/ADA Taskforce on inpatient diabetes, American College of Endocrinology and American Diabetes Association consensus statement on inpatient diabetes and glycemic control, *Diabetes Care* 29(8):1955, 2006.
6. Goldstein DE et al: Tests of glycemia in diabetes, *Diabetes Care* 27(7):1761, 2004.
7. Jeffcoate SL: Diabetes control and complications: the role of glycated haemoglobin, 25 years on, *Diabet Med* 21(7):657, 2004.
8. Janicic N, Verbalis JG: Evaluation and management of hypo-osmolality in hospitalized patients, *Endocrinol Metab Clin North Am* 32(2):459, 2003.
9. Rottmann CN: SSRI and the syndrome of inappropriate antidiuretic hormone secretion, *Am J Nurs* 107(1):51, 2007.
10. Holcomb S: Diabetes insipidus, *Dimens Crit Care Nurs* 21(3):94, 2002.

CHAPTER

24 Endocrine Disorders and Therapeutic Management

MARY E. LOUGH

OBJECTIVES

- Summarize the role of the hypothalamic-pituitary-adrenal axis, liver, pancreas, and thyroid in responses to the stress of critical illness.
- Discuss the assessment and management of adrenal dysfunction in critical illness.
- Describe the management of hyperglycemia associated with critical illness.
- Compare and contrast the etiology and management of type 1 and type 2 diabetes.
- Describe the use of intensive insulin therapy in the critical care unit.
- Compare and contrast the management of diabetic ketoacidosis and hyperglycemic hyperosmolar syndrome.
- Discuss the nursing priorities for managing a patient with diabetes insipidus.
- List three causes of the syndrome of inappropriate secretion of antidiuretic hormone.

The endocrine system is almost invisible when it functions well and causes widespread upset whenever an organ is suppressed, hyperstimulated, or under physiologic stress. This results in a wide spectrum of possible disorders; some are rare, whereas others are frequently encountered in the critical care unit. This chapter focuses on the neuroendocrine stress associated with critical illness and disorders of two major endocrine glands: the pancreas and the posterior pituitary.

NEUROENDOCRINOLOGY OF STRESS AND CRITICAL ILLNESS

Major neurologic and endocrine changes occur when an individual is confronted with physiologic stress caused by critical illness,[1-3] sepsis,[4] burns,[5] major surgery,[6] stroke,[7] cardiovascular disease,[8] or cardiac arrest.[9] The normal "fight or flight" response that is initiated in times of physiologic stress is exacerbated in critical illness through activation of the neuroendocrine system, specifically the hypothalamic-pituitary-adrenal axis (HPA),[4,9] thyroid,[10] and pancreas.[1] HPA influence on the course of critical illness is just beginning to be understood. Hormonal neuroendocrine output is very active at the beginning of a critical insult but greatly diminishes if the critical illness is prolonged.[11-12] All endocrine organs are affected by acute critical illness, as shown in Table 24-1. How much influence hormonal fluctuations have on morbidity and mortality remains the focus of ongoing research.

ACUTE NEUROENDOCRINE RESPONSE TO CRITICAL ILLNESS

The initial "fight or flight" acute response to physiologic threat is a rapid discharge of the catecholamines *norepinephrine* and *epinephrine* into the bloodstream.[9] Norepinephrine is released from the nerve endings of the sympathetic nervous system (SNS).[9]

Hypothalamic-Pituitary-Adrenal Axis in Acute Stress

Epinephrine, also known as *adrenaline*, is released from the medulla of the adrenal glands. Epinephrine increases cerebral blood flow and cerebral oxygen consumption and may be the trigger for recruitment of the hypothalamic-pituitary axis.[9]

The pituitary gland has two parts (anterior and posterior) that function under control of the hypothalamus. As a response to stress the *posterior pituitary gland* releases antidiuretic hormone (ADH), also known as *arginine vasopressin*. This hormone is an antidiuretic with a powerful vasoconstrictive effect on blood vessels.[9] The combination of epinephrine and vasopressin raises blood pressure quickly and also decreases gastric motility.[9] Epinephrine increases heart rate, causes ventricular dysrhythmias in susceptible patients, and

Table 24-1
Endocrine Responses to Stress

GLAND/ORGAN	HORMONE	RESPONSE/PHYSICAL EXAMINATION
Adrenal cortex	Cortisol	↑ Insulin resistance → ↑ glycogenolysis → ↑ glucose circulation
		↑ Hepatic gluconeogenesis → ↑ glucose available
		↑ Lipolysis
		↑ Protein catabolism
		↑ Sodium → ↑ water retention to maintain plasma osmolarity by movement of extravascular fluid to intravascular space
		↓ Connective tissue fibroblasts → poor wound healing
	Glucocorticoid	↓ Histamine release → suppresses immune system
		↓ Lymphocytes, monocytes, eosinophils, basophils
		↑ Polymorphonuclear leukocytes → ↑ infection risk
		↑ Glucose
		↓ Gastric acid secretion
	Mineralocorticoids	↑ Aldosterone → ↓ sodium excretion → ↓ water excretion → ↑ intravascular volume
		↑ Potassium excretion → hypokalemia →
		↑ Hydrogen ion excretion → metabolic acidosis
Adrenal medulla	Epinephrine	↑ Endorphins → ↓ pain
	Norepinephrine, epinephrine	↑ Metabolic rate to accommodate stress response
		↑ Live glycogenolysis → ↑ glucose
		↑ Insulin (cells are insulin resistant)
		↑ Cardiac contractility
		↑ Cardiac output
		↑ Dilation of coronary arteries
		↑ Blood pressure
		↑ Heart rate
		↑ Bronchodilation → ↑ respirations
		↑ Perfusion to heart, brain, lungs, liver, and muscle
		↓ Perfusion to periphery of body
		↓ Peristalsis
	Norepinephrine	↑ Peripheral vasoconstriction
		↑ Blood pressure
		↑ Sodium retention
		↑ Potassium excretion
Pituitary	All hormones	↑ Endogenous opioids → ↓ pain
Anterior pituitary	Adrenocorticotropic hormone	↑ Aldosterone → ↓ sodium excretion → ↑ water excretion → ↑ intravascular volume
		↑ Cortisol to ↑ blood volume
	Growth hormones	↑ Protein anabolism of amino acids to protein
		↑ Lipolysis → ↑ gluconeogenesis
Posterior pituitary	Antidiuretic hormone	↑ Vasoconstriction
		↑ Water retention → restoration of circulating blood volume
		↓ Urine output
		↑ Hypoosmolality
Pancreas	Insulin	Insulin resistance → hyperglycemia
	Glucagon	Directly opposes action of insulin → ↑ glycolysis
		↑ Glucose for fuel
		↑ Glycogenolysis
		↑ Gluconeogenesis
		↑ Lipolysis
Thyroid	Thyroxine	↓ Routine metabolic demands during stress
Gonads	Sex hormones	Energy and oxygen supply diverted to brain, heart, muscles, and liver

↑, Increased; →, causes; ↓, decreased.

provides some analgesia or lack of pain awareness during acute physical stress.[9]

The *anterior pituitary gland* is also under the control of the hypothalamus. In acute physiologic stress, "pulses" of growth hormone (GH) are released from the anterior pituitary gland to boost serum GH levels.[12] In critical illness the anterior pituitary actively secretes hormone, but the quantity may be insufficient for extreme physiologic needs. A different problem is that peripheral tissues may be "resistant" and unable to use the anabolic (tissue building) growth hormone.[13] The anterior pituitary gland also produces *corticotrophin,* which stimulates release of *cortisol* from the adrenal cortex.[14]

Cortisol release is an important protective response to stress, and serum levels will increase six-fold with normal adrenal function.[14] High cortisol levels alter carbohydrate, fat, and protein metabolism so that energy is immediately and selectively available to vital organs such as the brain.[12]

Liver and Pancreas in Acute Stress

The liver releases the hormone *glucagon* to stimulate the liver to pour additional glucose into the bloodstream. This greatly raises blood glucose levels.[4] Paradoxically the pancreas does not produce more insulin. Serum insulin levels remain normal, even with the increased metabolic demand associated with critical illness or sepsis. Cells become *insulin resistant.*[4] In other words, the tissues are unable to use the available insulin to transport glucose inside the cells for normal metabolism. This raises blood glucose levels, causing persistent hyperglycemia. Continuous infusion of insulin to return and maintain blood glucose levels within the normal range significantly reduces morbidity and mortality.[1] Management of hyperglycemia for the nondiabetic critically ill patient is discussed in detail in a later section.

Thyroid Gland in Acute Stress

Within 2 hours of trauma or surgery serum levels of triiodothyronine (T_3) decrease.[12] The greater the decrease of T_3 in the first 24 hours, the more severe the critical illness. Thyroid-stimulating hormone (TSH) and thyroxine (T_4) briefly increase and then return to normal levels. In the acute phase of critical illness a high serum cortisol level or a low serum T_3 level is associated with a poor prognosis.[12]

A systemic illness that does not directly involve the thyroid gland, but alters thyroid gland metabolism, is referred to as a *nonthyroidal illness syndrome,* or *sick euthyroid syndrome.*[10] The significance of altered thyroid function in critical illness is unknown at this time.[10]

Prolonged Neuroendocrine Response to Critical Illness

If critical illness is prolonged, the neuroendocrine response changes dramatically. The initially high hormonal levels are greatly reduced, and output is decreased from all the major endocrine glands.

Hypothalamic-Pituitary-Adrenal Axis in Prolonged Critical Illness Stress

When critical illness is prolonged over 7 to 10 days, the production of hormones from the pituitary gland is significantly lessened.

Normally the posterior pituitary gland produces ADH, or vasopressin. The impact of prolonged critical illness on vasopressin production has not been reported.

GH from the anterior pituitary is greatly decreased and lacks the "pulses" or bolus doses delivered during the initial acute phase.[12] Growth hormone levels are low when compared with the high levels seen as part of the initial stress response (see preceding paragraphs).[12] Unexpectedly, when critically ill patients were given high-dose GH as part of a large multicenter study, the morbidity increased and the mortality doubled.[12] Because of this finding, exogenous administration of growth hormone is not recommended.

Adrenal dysfunction is common in prolonged critical illness that lasts more than 7 to 10 days.[12] Serum adrenocorticotropic hormone (ACTH) level decreases, whereas the cortisol level remains high.[12] The reason for this paradoxical effect is unknown. Some researchers believe that an alternative metabolic pathway, as yet unidentified, may be stimulating the adrenal cortex to produce cortisol outside of the normal channels.[12] With time, all pathways fail as indicated by a twentyfold increase in adrenal failure seen in critically ill patients over 50 years of age who spend more than 14 days in a critical care unit.[12] If the critical illness is prolonged and the patient remains hypotensive, vasopressor dependent, and mechanically ventilated, adequacy of adrenal function must be evaluated. Even if a corticotropin test was performed earlier in the hospitalization, it is important to repeat the test because the adrenal gland may have been initially normal but has since failed as a result of the stress of the critical illness.[14] Older patients are particularly susceptible to adrenal failure.[12,14,15]

Liver-Pancreas in Prolonged Critical Illness Stress

Hyperglycemia is often persistent. Gluconeogenesis (the metabolism of glucose from fat or protein) and proteolysis (protein breakdown) continue throughout the catabolic phase of critical illness.[13] Critically ill patients can lose up to 10% of their lean body mass per week.[13] The addition of adequate supplemental nutrition is recommended, in addition to an intravenous (IV) insulin infusion, to reduce hyperglycemia and provide additional substrate other than the patient's own body tissues.[1] Insulin is an anabolic hormone and can improve protein synthesis and reduce protein breakdown.[13] While the critical illness is ongoing, nutrition and insulin seem to limit rather than stop the loss of lean body mass.

Thyroid Gland in Prolonged Critical Illness Stress

The thyroid gland appears to follow a similar pattern to the pituitary gland when critical illness is prolonged. The serum levels of T_3, T_4, and TSH are greatly reduced.[12] Also, the normal pulses of TSH are flattened.[12] The significance of this is unknown, and investigation of the impact of thyroid hormone infusions is underway.[12]

Adrenal Dysfunction in Critical Illness

Diminished adrenal gland function may result from one or more causes during critical illness:

- *Primary hypoadrenalism* describes an intrinsic failure of the adrenal gland to produce normal endogenous glucocorticosteroid hormones such as cortisol. Absolute adrenal failure is rare and occurs in 0.01% to 3% of critically ill patients.[16,17]
- *Secondary hypoadrenalism* occurs as a result of the administration of therapeutic steroids. In response to exogenous glucocorticosteroids the adrenal glands stop production of intrinsic hormones. Patients who have taken steroids before their admission to the hospital will need their dosage increased. One recommendation is to double the dose for a febrile illness.[14]
- *Relative adrenal insufficiency* describes a situation where the adrenal gland produces glucocorticosteroids but the quantity is insufficient for the disease process. Estimates of the frequency of adrenal insufficiency in critical illness range from 0% to 77% but are as high as 50% to 75% in septic shock.[16]
- *Peripheral adrenal resistance* is thought to occur in severe sepsis and septic shock.[16] In septic patients, inflammatory cytokines induce cellular resistance to cortisol; low-dose, short-term replacement corticosteroids may be required.[14,16]

Assessment of Adrenal Function

Clinical assessment of adrenal dysfunction is difficult in the critically ill, and a specialized laboratory assay is necessary for an accurate diagnosis. First, a baseline serum cortisol level is obtained. Adrenal failure is likely if the cortisol level is below 15 mcg/dl and suspected if the level is above 15 but below 34 mcg/dl.[14]

Further confirmation may be obtained by performance of a corticotropin stimulation test *(cosyntropin test)*.[14,16] Cosyntropin is a medication made from the first 24 amino acids of corticotropin.[14] In the test, 250 mcg cosyntropin is administered by IV route, and serum blood levels are measured 30 and 60 minutes later. If the serum cortisol level rise from baseline is less than 9 mcg/dl after 30 to 60 minutes, this denotes inability of the adrenal gland to respond to a stress stimulus (nonresponder).[14,16] When the cortisol level rise is greater than 18 mcg/dl in response to corticotropin stimulation, this indicates normally functioning adrenal glands (responder).[17] Corticosteroids are only given to nonresponders.[17]

The combination of a low baseline cortisol value (below 15 mcg/dl) with minimal or no rise in cortisol level (below 9 mcg/dl) after the cosyntropin test is firm evidence of adrenal failure.[14] The cosyntropin test is particularly helpful to determine level of adrenal dysfunction in patients whose serum cortisol level falls between 15 and 34 mcg/dl. One study demonstrated that after surgery, older patients with cortisol levels below 30 mcg/dl and who were vasopressor dependent were successfully weaned off the vasopressor drips following cortisol replacement (hydrocortisone).[15] Further clinical trials will be required to fully explore the role of short-term corticosteroids in critical illness.

Corticosteroid Replacement

Clinical guideline recommendations promote short-term provision of low-dose hydrocortisone for patients with depleted cortisol levels who do not demonstrate a rise in cortisol level following corticotropin stimulation and have a diagnosis of septic shock.[12,14,16] Hydrocortisone is the recommended replacement because it is the pharmacologic steroid that most resembles endogenous cortisol.[16] One suggested replacement regimen is 50 mg of hydrocortisone (glucocorticoid) every 6 hours (200 mg/day total), plus an optional 50 mg of fludrocortisone (mineralocorticoid) via a nasogastric (NG) tube once per day.[14,16] Fludrocortisone can only be taken by mouth or via a feeding tube.[16] Steroid replenishment is recommended as early as possible once septic shock with depleted cortisol levels is identified, but only if the septic patient is vasopressor dependent.[16] High-dose steroid replacement is never recommended in management of sepsis.[16]

The role of corticosteroid replacement with other diagnoses is less well defined, but the current trend is to supplement low cortisol levels in critically ill patients. Corticosteroids are never discontinued abruptly and must be tapered gradually over several days.

Hyperglycemia in Critical Illness

When hyperglycemia is actively managed with an insulin drip and blood glucose is maintained within the normal range, clinical outcomes are better for both diabetic and nondiabetic patients. Plasma blood glucose in the normal range (70-110 mg/dl) is associated with a lower morbidity and mortality.[1,18] The landmark study of "tight glucose control" by van den Berghe et al found that for every 20 mg/dl serum glucose level was elevated above normal, mortality rose 30%.[1,18]

Hospitalized Patients Who Are Diabetic

Not all patients who are hyperglycemic in the critical care unit have a previous diagnosis of diabetes. Estimates of the number of in-hospital patients who are diabetic ranges from 12% to 25%.[18] This wide range is due to the different methodologies used to define diabetes in hospitalized patients—sometimes by the serum glucose level and sometimes by discharge diagnosis.[18] The range is also an indication that no one is really tracking how many hospitalized patients have diabetes as a primary or secondary diagnosis.

Hyperglycemia and the Cardiovascular System

Many patients who are admitted to the hospital with acute complications of cardiovascular disease are also diabetic. The connection between acute cardiovascular events and diabetes is perhaps due to inflammatory changes in the vessel wall that are driven by hyperglycemia.[18] Phagocytic white blood cells (WBCs) that are exposed to high serum glucose levels produce inflammatory mediators—tumor necrosis factor (TNF) and interleukin-6 (IL-6)—that are known to be damaging to endothelial tissue.[18] It has been suggested that elevated blood glucose level contributes to acute cardiovascular events because hyperglycemia inhibits vasodilation by blocking the action of nitric oxide (NO), a vasodilator normally released by the vascular endothelium.[18]

Hyperglycemia and the Neurologic System

Acute hyperglycemia is associated with increased neuron damage following brain ischemia or ischemic stroke.[7,18] Most at risk is the *penumbra*—the potentially viable area of brain tissue around the ischemic core. More than one third of patients admitted with acute stroke are hyperglycemic when they arrive at the hospital.[19] Hyperglycemia decreases cerebral blood flow and increases brain lactate production.[20] If the hyperglycemia is not controlled after the stroke, the potentially viable penumbra (ischemic brain tissue) is more likely to progress to infarction.[21] Thus, the area of brain tissue affected is larger in patients with acute hyperglycemia at the time of an ischemic stroke.[19,21]

Hyperglycemia and Infection

Elevated serum blood glucose level is associated with an increased incidence of infection and sepsis.[1,18] In cardiac surgery patients, many of whom are diabetic, hyperglycemia increases the incidence of deep sternal wound infections[22] and increases mortality.[18]

Insulin Management in the Critically Ill

A profound shift in the management of the hyperglycemic critically ill ventilated patient has recently taken place.[18] As a result of the research that has highlighted the deleterious effects of hyperglycemia in critical illness, most hospitals have developed an institution-specific "tight glucose control" algorithm to lower blood glucose level into the normal range. Many of these protocols are now published to enable others to use and adapt the developed algorithims.[22,23] The vigilance of the critical care nurse is pivotal to the success of any intervention to lower blood glucose level using a continuous insulin infusion.

Some clinical interventions increase the likelihood that the patient will receive exogenous insulin. Infusion of total parental nutrition (TPN) typically requires a continuous insulin infusion to normalize blood glucose levels. In a study of critically ill surgical patients with preexisting type 2 diabetes who did not previously require insulin, 77% of patients needed insulin to control the blood glucose level while receiving TPN.[18] Some enteral nutrition formulas are high in carbohydrates and will increase blood glucose levels in the same way. In this situation, either the composition of the enteral feeding is altered or the insulin dosage is increased to achieve normal blood glucose levels. It is important to provide nutrition, and insulin can be a powerful adjunct to nutritional support.

Frequent Blood Glucose Level Checks

Monitoring the blood glucose level using a point-of-care glucometer is the basis of targeted glucose control. As part of the comprehensive initial assessment the blood glucose level is measured either by a standard laboratory sample or by a "finger-stick" capillary blood sample. In many institutions if the blood glucose level is greater than 130 mg/dl (although the initial value will vary between hospitals), the patient is started on a continuous IV insulin infusion. In critically ill catabolic patients the initial blood glucose level can be well above 200 mg/dl. While the glucose is elevated, blood sample measurements are generally tested hourly to allow titration of the insulin drip to lower blood glucose levels. Once the patient is stable, blood glucose measurements can be spaced every 2 hours, although the actual time intervals will vary based on individual hospital protocols.

Several different blood-sampling methods are available. A capillary finger stick is one option, although the fingers can become noticeably marked if there are numerous sticks over several days. Trauma to the fingers is also exacerbated if there is diminished peripheral perfusion. If a central venous catheter (CVC) or an arterial line with a blood conservation system attached is in place, this can be a highly efficient system because there is no blood wastage. If there is not a blood conservation setup attached, the venous/arterial catheter access method is unacceptable because of the amount of waste blood that would be discarded.

Continuous Insulin Infusion

Many hospitals use insulin infusion protocols for management of stress-induced hyperglycemia that are implemented by the critical care nurse.[1,8,23] Effective glucose protocols gauge the insulin infusion rate based on two parameters:

1. The immediate blood glucose result
2. The rate of change in the blood glucose level since the last hourly measurement

The following three examples illustrate this concept:

- Patient A receives 3 units of continuous IV regular insulin per hour and has a blood glucose measurement of 110 mg/dl, but 1 hour ago it was 190 mg/dl; the insulin rate must be decreased to avoid sudden hypoglycemia.
- Patient B receives 3 units of continuous IV regular insulin per hour and has a blood glucose measurement of 110 mg/dl, but an hour before it was 112 mg/dl; in this situation, no change is made in the insulin infusion rate.
- Patient C receives 3 units of continuous IV regular insulin per hour and has a blood glucose measurement of 190 mg/dl, and 1 hour ago it was 197 mg/dl; in this situation, the insulin rate must be increased to more rapidly move the patient's blood glucose level toward normoglycemia.

The important point to emphasize is that the *rate of change* of the blood glucose is as important as the *most recent* blood glucose measurement. Each of the patients described may have the same insulin infusion rate, depending on their catabolic state, but individualization between different patients with different diagnoses can be safely achieved as long as the rate of change is also considered. A person's insulin requirement often fluctuates over the course of his or her illness. This occurs in response to changes in the clinical condition such as development of an infection, caloric alterations caused by stopping or starting enteral nutrition or TPN, administration of therapeutic steroids, or because the person is less catabolic.[18] A method to allow for corrective incremental changes (up or down) to adapt to the reality of clinical developments and maintain the glucose level within the target range is essential.[18] Some protocols alter only the infusion rates, and others incorporate bolus insulin doses when the glucose is above a preestablished threshold such as 180 mg/dl. Typically, when the blood glucose level has remained within target range for a number of hours (varies with hospital protocol from 4 to 12 hours), the time interval between blood glucose monitoring is extended to every 2 hours.

Transition From Continuous to Intermittent Insulin Coverage

The transition from a continuous insulin infusion to intermittent insulin coverage must be handled with care to avoid large fluctuations in blood glucose levels. Before the conversion the regular insulin infusion should be at a stable and preferably low rate and the patient's blood glucose level maintained consistently within the target range. Even after the IV infusion has been turned off the insulin effect in the tissues extends for at least 30 minutes beyond circulating plasma insulin levels.[24] Recommended methods to facilitate the transition from IV to subcutaneous (Sub-Q) insulin administration include the following[18,24]:

- Administer short-acting insulin Sub-Q 1 to 2 hours before discontinuation of the continuous IV infusion. *Example:* Regular insulin.
- Administer intermediate-acting insulin Sub-Q 2 to 4 hours before stopping the continuous IV infusion. *Example:* NPH and Lente insulin.
- Administer long-acting insulin Sub-Q 4 to 6 hours before stopping the continuous IV infusion. *Example:* Lantus (glargine) insulin.

Clinicians use various methods to calculate the quantity of insulin to prescribe during the transition to maintain stable blood glucose levels. Figure 24-1 depicts hypothetical examples of how a combination of basal and bolus insulin regimens (prandial insulin) can work in clinical practice. Acute hyperglycemic crisis is generally managed by an infusion of regular insulin. However, the types of insulin available for Sub-Q administration are more extensive, as shown in Table 24-2. An ongoing area of controversy is the transition from IV to Sub-Q insulin. One transition method is described below for Alice Smith, a 67-year-old patient recovering from critical illness and recently extubated.

1. Mrs. Smith is in stable condition on a regular insulin drip at 1 unit/hr. She is ready to be transitioned to Sub-Q insulin. Mrs. Smith is now going to be taking food and liquids by mouth. Her total insulin requirement over the previous 24 hours was 24 units. Mrs. Smith will require both *basal* coverage (provided by Sub-Q intermediate or long-acting insulin) and *nutritional* coverage for mealtimes (provided by short-acting Sub-Q insulin).
2. The 24 units of insulin infused during the previous 24 hours is her required insulin dose. Half of this (12 units) will be administered Sub-Q as intermediate or long-acting insulin; the other half will be administered as short-acting insulin to coincide with meals (4 units insulin Sub-Q with each meal—12 units total).
3. Insulin administration options (Sub-Q):
   - *Basal insulin:* 12 units once a day (***or*** 6 units twice a day) of Neutral Protamine Hagedorn (NPH) Sub-Q; ***or*** glargine 12 units once a day.[22]
   - *Prandial/nutritional insulin:* 4 units regular insulin Sub-Q before each meal (short-acting), ***or*** 4 units lispro or aspart Sub-Q with meals (ultra–short-acting insulin).[22]
   - *Supplemental correction dosages:* A sliding insulin scale can be used to cover any hyperglycemia above target, combined with scheduled blood glucose measurement.[22-24]

Subsequently the Sub-Q insulin dosage is adjusted to the individual patient's needs. In a stable *insulin-*

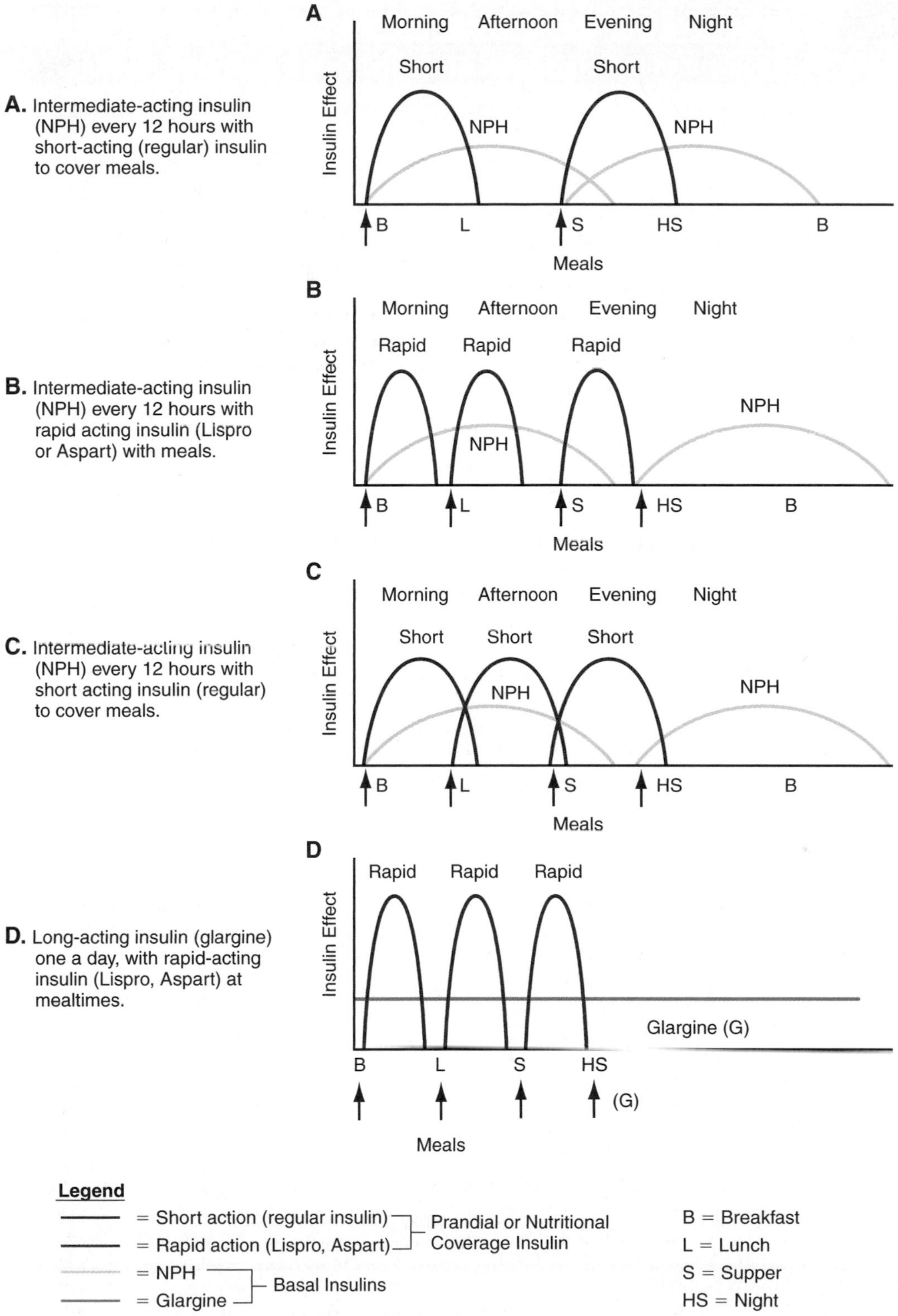

FIGURE 24-1. Basal–nutritional bolus insulin combinations.

sensitive patient 1 unit of short-acting insulin will lower the blood glucose level by 50 to 100 mg/dl.[18] In critical care patients greater quantities of insulin are typically required to reduce blood glucose levels because of the stress of the critical illness.[22]

Intermittent Insulin Coverage

As the critical illness resolves and the glucose levels become more predictable and stable, the patient can be transitioned to intermittent insulin using a "sliding scale." These scales can be either IV or Sub-Q. The

Table 24-2

Pharmacologic Management of Hyperglycemic Crisis and Type 1 Diabetes: Insulins

INSULIN*	ROUTE	ACTION	ONSET/PEAK/DURATION	SPECIAL CONSIDERATIONS
Ultra–Short-Acting Insulins				
Lispro (Humalog)	Sub-Q†	Insulin replacement, rapid onset	10-15 min/0.5-2.5 hr/3-6.5 hr	First available synthetic insulin (human insulin analog), almost *immediately* absorbed **Must be taken with food** Shorter duration of action than regular insulin; should be used with basal longer-acting insulin See Figure 24-1, *B* and *D*.
Aspart (NovoLog)	Sub-Q†	Insulin replacement, rapid onset	10-20 min/1-3 hr/3-5 hr	Insulin analog almost *immediately* absorbed **Must be taken with food** Insulin appearance should be clear Must be used in combination with intermediate-acting or long-acting basal insulin regimen See Figure 24-1, *B* and *D*.
Short-Acting Insulin				
Regular (Humulin R or Novolin R)	IV or Sub-Q	Insulin replacement therapy	IV: Under 15 minutes Sub-Q: In under 1 hr/2-4 hr/5-8 hr	Only type of insulin suitable for IV continuous infusion or IV bolus administration
Intermediate-Acting Insulins				
Neutral Protamine Hagedorn (NPH)	Sub-Q†	Insulin replacement Intermediate action	3-4 hr/6-12 hr/18-28 hr	
Zinc suspension (Ultralente)	Sub-Q†	Insulin replacement Extended action	4-6 hr/18-24 hr/36 hr	Also available as extended insulin zinc, human See Figure 24-1, *A* and *C*.
Long-Acting Insulins				
Glargine (Lantus)	Sub-Q†	Long-acting basal insulin analog Longer-acting than NPH or Ultralente	Does not produce peak concentrations; relatively constant concentrations over 24 hr	Synthetic insulin (human insulin analog), differs from human insulin by three amino acids, slowing release over 24 hours No peak Decrease dose by 20% if switching from NPH to glargine Must not be diluted or mixed with other insulins See Figure 24-1, *D*.
Combination (Premixed) Insulins				
Various	Sub-Q†	Rapid plus intermediate or long-acting insulin combination	Varies according to combination used, and many other combinations exist **Long-acting component/short-acting component** –70% NPH with 30% regular (70/30 regular) –70% aspart-protamine suspension with 30% aspart (NovoLog mix 70/30) –75% lispro-protamine suspension with 25% lispro (Humalog mix 75/25)	

Dosages are individualized according to patient's age and size.
IV, Intravenous; *Sub-Q,* subcutaneous.
*Trade names are in parentheses.
†Not for IV use.

intermittent scales are generally not as proactive as the continuous IV infusion method and should be reserved for the stable patient. A frequent criticism of "sliding scale" therapy is that the dosages are rarely reevaluated or adjusted once established.[18] A second criticism is that the scales treat hyperglycemia only after it has occurred. They are not proactive in the manner of continuous insulin infusions.[18]

Box 24-1

NURSING DIAGNOSIS PRIORITIES

Managing Hyperglycemia Associated With Stress of Critical Illness

- Risk for Imbalanced Fluid Volume related to critical illness
- Risk for Injury related to metabolic stress related to critical illness
- Imbalanced Nutrition: Less Than Body Requirements related to increased metabolic demands, p. A-28
- Risk for Infection, p. A-46
- Ineffective Tissue Perfusion: endocrine alterations in critical illness
- Compromised Family Coping related to critically ill family member, p. A-11

Hypoglycemia Management

It is important to have a protocol for the management of hypoglycemia, defined as a plasma blood glucose level below 70 mg/dl.[25] The major drawback to use of intensive insulin protocols, as described above, is the potential for hypoglycemia. Whenever hypoglycemia is detected, it is important to *stop* any continuous infusion of insulin. An example of one protocol to reverse hypoglycemia is described below:

- *Blood glucose level below 40 mg/dl:* Administer an IV bolus of 50 ml dextrose 50% in water ($D_{50}W$).
- *Blood glucose level 40 to 60 mg/dl:* Administer an IV bolus of 25 ml $D_{50}W$.
- *Blood glucose level 60 to 80 mg/dl:* Supplementary bolus glucose is not generally required; continue to monitor blood glucose level.

In all cases of hypoglycemia the blood glucose level is monitored every 15 to 20 minutes until the blood glucose level has risen into a safe range. Some protocols use the patient's level of consciousness as a guide to glucose replacement with hypoglycemia. A different protocol suggests the following for a plasma glucose level below 60 mg/dl[22]:

- *Blood glucose level below 60 mg/dl and patient is awake and responsive:* Administer IV push 25 ml $D_{50}W$.
- *Blood glucose level below 60 mg/dl and patient is unresponsive:* Administer IV push 50 ml $D_{50}W$.

Nursing Management

Nursing management of the patient with hyperglycemia associated with critical illness incorporates a variety of nursing diagnoses (Box 24-1). **Nursing priorities are directed toward (1) monitoring the glycemic side effects of vasopressor, corticosteroid, and nutritional therapy; (2) monitoring effectiveness of insulin therapy; (3) maintaining surveillance for complications; and (4) providing education to the patient's family and supportive others.**

Monitoring Glycemic Side Effects of Vasopressor, Corticosteroid, and Nutritional Therapy

Two vasopressors frequently used as continuous infusions to counteract hypotension in the critically ill also raise blood glucose levels. Epinephrine and, to a lesser extent, norepinephrine stimulate an increase in gluconeogenesis (creation of new glucose), an increase of skeletal muscle and hepatic glycogenolysis (increased glucose production), an increase in lipolysis (increased fat breakdown), direct suppression of insulin secretion, and an increase in peripheral insulin resistance.[25] All of these actions serve to raise the serum glucose level in the bloodstream. If hyperglycemia develops while a patient is receiving vasopressor therapy, IV insulin and a dextrose infusion should be instituted.[1,18]

Critically ill patients with below-normal cortisol levels are prescribed low-dose hydrocortisone IV. Therapeutic steroids raise blood glucose levels, making glycemic control more difficult. Frequent monitoring of the blood glucose level is necessary to guide treatment of hyperglycemia in the patient receiving IV corticosteroids. Ongoing monitoring for presence of new infection is mandatory, although short-term use of therapeutic steroids does confer greater benefit than harm in the septic patient population.[14]

When an insulin infusion is started to lower blood glucose level, some protocols add a 10% dextrose infusion if the patient is not receiving other nutritional support (enteral or TPN).[24] Although the 10% dextrose will further increase the blood glucose level and the need for insulin, it offers the advantage of carbohydrate calories for metabolism, limits fluctuations in the blood glucose level, and reduces the risk of hypoglycemia. Once the patient's metabolic condition is stable, introduction of nonglucose nutrition (protein and fat) is preferable.

Monitoring Effectiveness of Insulin Therapy

Hyperglycemia is associated with an increase in both morbidity and mortality in the critically ill patient.[1,8,18] The critical care nurse is responsible for the hourly monitoring of blood glucose levels and titration of the insulin infusion according to the hospital's established protocol while the patient is hyperglycemic. The use of standardized protocols makes possible a systematic approach to the control of blood glucose. This results in improved glycemic control and lower rates of hypoglycemia.[8] It is essential and recommended that nurses receive effective and ongoing education about the anabolic impact of insulin therapy in critical illness.[8]

Providing Patient Education

When the patient is acutely ill, the majority of the educational interventions are directed to the family and supportive friends at the bedside. Numerous explications are required to describe the IV medications, the nutritional needs, the purpose of insulin, the role of steroids (if applicable), the ongoing nursing care, prevention of complications, risk of multiple organ dysfunction syndrome (MODS), and management of the underlying disease process.

Collaborative Management

It is well established that standardized protocols designed to manage the complications of critical illness result in a lower morbidity and mortality for the patients.[8] Optimally, all disciplines concerned with the endocrine status of the patient have participated in design of these guidelines in each critical care area. The guideline that will apply to most patients is the use of tight glucose control. Many professional organizations endorse the importance of normalizing blood glucose levels in the hospitalized patient as described in Evidence-Based Collaborative Practice: Managing Hyperglycemia Associated With Stress of Critical Illness.

EVIDENCE-BASED COLLABORATIVE PRACTICE

Managing Hyperglycemia Associated With Stress of Critical Illness

Summary of evidence and evidence-based recommendations for controlling symptoms related to physiologic stress of critical illness

Strong Evidence to Support the Following:

- Maintenance of normal blood glucose levels
  - Maintaining blood glucose levels between 80 and 110 mg/dl reduces patient morbidity and mortality.
  - For patients who are eating, maintain preprandial blood glucose level below 110 mg/dl; maintain peak postprandial blood glucose level below 180 mg/dl.
  - Use of continuous intravenous (IV) insulin to control hyperglycemia is safe for critical care patients who have tight monitoring of their blood glucose.
- Use of a multidisciplinary team approach
  - Use of a multidisciplinary team that implements institutional guidelines, protocols, and standardized order-sets for the hospital results in fewer hypoglycemic and hyperglycemic events.

Moderate Evidence to Support the Following:

- Maintenance of normal cortisol levels.
- In septic patients with depleted cortisol levels, hydrocortisone IV is administered short-term.

Data from Garber AJ et al: *Endocr Pract* 10(suppl 2):4, 2004; Clement S et al: *Diabetes Care* 27(2): 553, 2004; and Keh D, Sprung CL: *Crit Care Med* 32(11):S527, 2004.

DIABETES MELLITUS

Diabetes mellitus is a progressive endocrinopathy associated with carbohydrate intolerance and insulin dysregulation.[6] It is a chronic illness that requires intensive patient self-management and interventions and education from a multidisciplinary health care team to prevent complications.[25]

Morbidity and Mortality Associated with Diabetes Mellitus

Diabetes is the sixth most common cause of death in U.S. adults as reported by the U.S. Centers for Disease Control and Prevention (CDC).[26] Heart disease and stroke are the first and third leading causes of death among U.S. adults.[26] This data must be interpreted in light of the knowledge that adults with diabetes have a risk for dying from cardiovascular diseases that is two to four times greater than adults without diabetes.[27] Although the annual incidence of deaths attributed to cardiovascular diseases has decreased substantially, the decline is less among those with diabetes.[27] Age-adjusted prevalence of heart disease and stroke is approximately two to three times greater among adults with diabetes than among those without.[27] Diabetes is associated with an increased risk of cancer.[26] The CDC reports that diabetes is an independent predictor of mortality from cancer of the colon, the pancreas, the female breast, and, in men, of the liver and the bladder.[28] Annual cost for hospital care per capita for persons with diabetes is $6,309, compared with $2,971 for persons without diabetes.[18] This represents a cost ratio of 2:1.[18]

Diagnosis of Diabetes

Diabetes mellitus is diagnosed by measurement of the fasting plasma glucose (FPG), also known as a fasting blood glucose (FBG) or fasting blood sugar (FBS).[29] The benchmarks for "normal" FPG levels have been progressively lowered in recent years as more knowledge has been gained about the benefits of maintaining the plasma glucose level as close to normal as possible.

The FPG values endorsed by the American Diabetes Association (ADA)[29] are listed below:

- FPG below 100 mg/dl (5.6 mmol/L) signifies normal fasting glucose.
- FPG between 100 and 125 mg/dl (5.6 and 6.9 mmol/L) implies impaired fasting glucose (IFG).
- FPG above 126 mg/dl (7 mmol/L) provides a diagnosis of diabetes (result is verified by testing more than once).

Two fasting blood glucose values of 126 mg/dl or higher confirm the diagnosis of diabetes.[29] For the acutely ill patient, hyperglycemia is actively treated with insulin to lower the blood glucose level to within

Understanding Diabetes Mellitus and Its Treatment

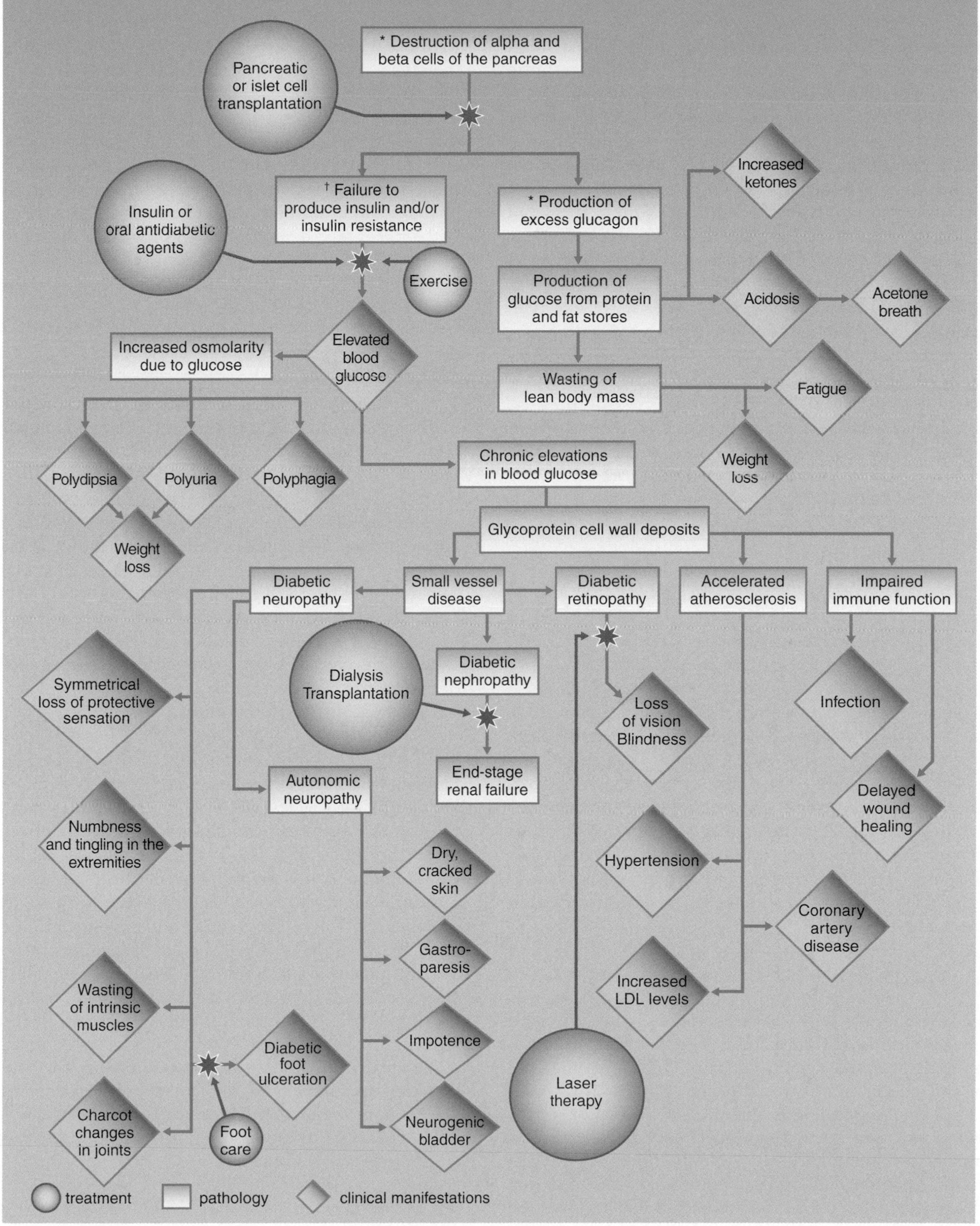

*Type 1 diabetes.
†Type 2 diabetes.

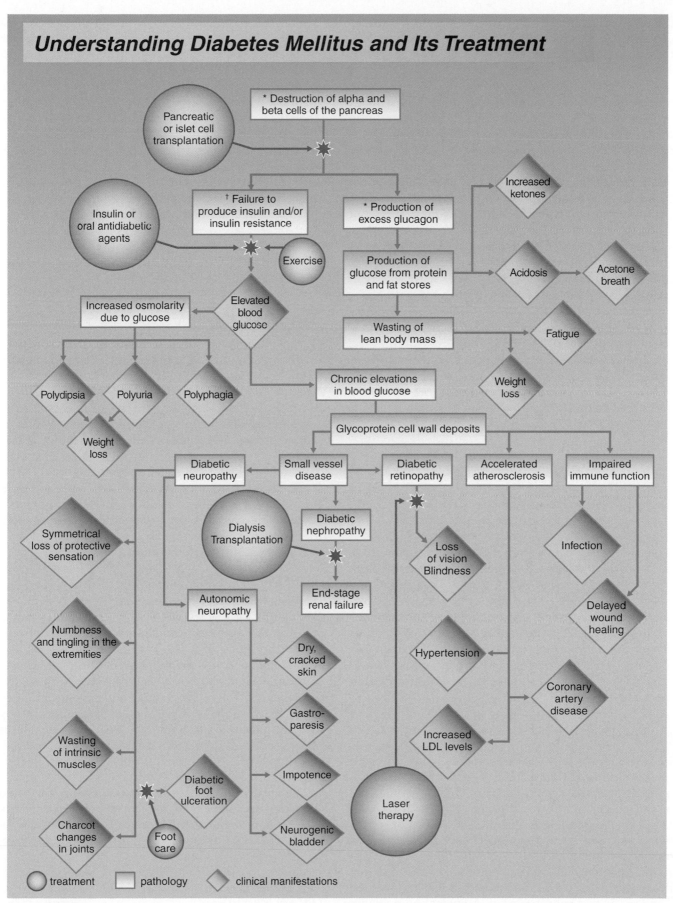

the normal range.[1] There are differences in the values of plasma versus whole blood glucose measurements. Plasma glucose values are 10% to 15% higher than whole blood glucose values, and it is essential that health care clinicians and people with diabetes know whether their monitor and strips provide whole blood or plasma results, especially when results from more than one setting (laboratory or monitor) are being compared.[30] Most laboratories measure plasma glucose levels (red cells are separated out). In contrast, most home-monitoring units measure glucose using whole blood from a finger stick.[31] In the critical care unit, point-of-care units measure glucose from a sample of blood from an indwelling arterial or venous catheter.[32]

The benefit and importance of maintaining blood glucose at levels as close to normal as possible was conclusively demonstrated in patients with both type 1 and type 2 diabetes.[31] The Diabetes Control and Complications Trial (DCCT) of 1995 on type 1 diabetes and the United Kingdom Prospective Diabetes Study (UKPDS), published in 1998 on type 2 diabetes, demonstrated that lifestyle changes and use of medications that lead to consistently normal glucose levels reduce microvascular diabetes-related complications and decrease mortality.[31]

Types of Diabetes

There are two distinct types of diabetes that will be discussed in this chapter[25]:

- Type 1 diabetes results from β-cell destruction, usually leading to absolute insulin deficiency.
- Type 2 diabetes results from a progressive insulin secretory defect in addition to insulin resistance.

The two diseases are different in nature, etiology, treatment, and prognosis.[29] A further category of *prediabetes* has recently been added to describe patients with impaired fasting glucose (FPG value between 100 and 125 mg/dl) who are likely to develop diabetes at some time in the future and are also at increased risk for coronary artery disease and stroke.[29] Other conditions such as gestational diabetes are not discussed in this chapter.

Glycated Hemoglobin

For individuals with diabetes, maintenance of blood glucose levels within a tight normal range is fundamental to avoid development of microvascular and neuropathic secondary conditions. Although the fasting plasma glucose level produces a "snapshot" of the blood glucose level at a single point in time, the *glycated hemoglobin* (hemoglobin A_{1c}), also known as a *glycosylated hemoglobin,* identifies a percentage of glucose that the red cells have absorbed from the plasma over the previous 3- to 4-month period. A normal hemoglobin A_{1c} value falls between 4% and 6%.[29] The target for diabetic patients is an A_{1c} value below 7%.[29] Long-term studies have shown that for every 1% increase in the hemoglobin A_{1c} there is an approximate 30% increase in microvascular complications.[33] A clinical study is underway to determine if a more stringent A_{1c} target of 6% or less will reduce complications even further for those with diabetes.[29] Additional information about the glycosylated hemoglobin and the correlation with the plasma glucose level is shown in Table 23-2. Currently the hemoglobin A_{1c} is not recommended as a diagnostic tool for new diabetics; it is recommended only for those with known diabetes as a means to track their degree of glycemic control.[29] However, it is obvious that in the newly admitted critical care patient with an elevated hemoglobin A_{1c} value that the hyperglycemia has been present before admission.[29] This situation offers an opportunity to reevaluate and manage the ongoing hyperglycemia.

Type 1 Diabetes

Type 1 diabetes mellitus accounts for only about 5% to 10% of the diabetic population.[29] Older names for this condition include insulin-dependent diabetes mellitus (IDDM) and juvenile diabetes. Type 1 diabetes is a cellular-mediated autoimmune disease that causes progressive destruction of the β-cells of the islets of Langerhans in the pancreas. Autoantibodies that falsely identify "self" as a foreign invader to be destroyed can now be detected by laboratory analysis.[29] Over time the autoantibodies render the pancreatic β-cells incapable of secreting insulin and regulating intracellular glucose. In type 1 diabetes, the rate of β-cell destruction is highly variable. It occurs rapidly in some individuals and slowly in others.

Management of Type 1 Diabetes

Patients with type 1 diabetes must receive IV or Sub-Q insulin therapy. Treatment with exogenous insulin replacement restores normal entry of glucose into the cells. The range of insulin replacements available is expanding, and it is essential that critical care nurses are knowledgeable about this class of medications. All therapeutic insulins used today are analogs of human insulin. An analog insulin is manufactured using recombinant DNA technology.[34] Regular IV insulin is also produced by rDNA (trade names Humulin R or Novolin R). Examples of Sub-Q insulins include lispro (Humalog), aspart (NovoLog), glargine (Lantus), as described in Table 24-2. Without insulin, the rapid breakdown of noncarbohydrate substrate, particularly fat, leads to ketonemia, ketonuria, and diabetic ketoacidosis (DKA), a life-threatening complication associated with type 1 diabetes.

Type 2 Diabetes

The estimated prevalence of type 2 diabetes among adults in the United States was 8.7% in 2002.[35] Almost

90% to 95% of those with diabetes have type 2 diabetes.[29] Most patients with this type of diabetes are older and obese, and many also have a condition known as *metabolic syndrome*.[29] Up to one third of people who have diabetes are undiagnosed. Patients at high risk of developing type 2 diabetes include those who meet the following criteria[35]:

- A family history of type 2 diabetes in first- and second-degree relatives[35]
- Member of racial or ethnic groups known to be at greater risk of developing type 2 diabetes: Native Americans, African Americans, Hispanic Americans, Asians/South Pacific Islanders[35]
- Have signs of *insulin resistance syndrome* or conditions associated with insulin resistance such as hypertension, dyslipidemia, polycystic ovary syndrome, or metabolic syndrome[35,36]

In type 2 diabetes, pancreatic β-cells are present and functioning, but the amount of insulin they produce is highly variable in different patients:

- In some patients the pancreatic β-cells do not produce sufficient insulin to meet the metabolic need. In these patients there is evidence that the β-cells may be in decline for years before the appearance of clinical symptoms. This is termed an *inadequate insulin response*.
- In other individuals the pancreas may produce sufficient insulin or even more than is needed (hyperinsulinemia), but the tissues are resistant to the effects of the insulin. This is known as *insulin resistance syndrome*.[36]
- Some patients may have a combination of the above, a lower than normal level of insulin production and a heightened insulin resistance at the cellular level.

Insulin resistance describes a complex metabolic situation where organ and tissue cells deny entry to insulin and glucose. This creates the clinical paradox in which elevated serum insulin levels and hyperglycemia are present at the same time. Abdominal obesity increases insulin resistance.[29] Insulin resistance has a strong association with type 2 diabetes. Until researchers clarify the exact nature of insulin resistance, many labels are used to describe similar clusters of symptoms, including insulin resistance syndrome and metabolic syndrome.[36-38]

Metabolic Syndrome

The major known stimuli for development of metabolic syndrome are obesity and disorders of insulin resistance.[38] Any three of the following factors are diagnostic of metabolic syndrome:

- Waist measurement greater than 40 inches in men and over 35 inches in women
- Triglyceride levels higher than 150 mg/dl
- High-density lipoprotein (HDL) cholesterol levels below 40 mg/dl in men and below 35 mg/dl in women
- Blood pressure higher than 130/85 mg Hg
- Fasting plasma glucose level higher than 100 mg/dl

Screening for Type 2 Diabetes

The ADA uses the fasting plasma glucose cut-off point of 100 mg/dl in order to identify individuals who are prediabetic, not only those who are diabetic.[38] The ADA recommends screening individuals at risk for type 2 diabetes at 3-year intervals beginning at age 45, particularly those who are overweight or obese (body mass index [BMI] of 25 kg/m^2 or greater).[35] With the rise of obesity in the United States the incidence of type 2 diabetes in children and adolescents has also increased dramatically in the last decade.[29]

Lifestyle Management With Type 2 Diabetes

The majority of adults with type 2 diabetes are overweight or obese as demonstrated by a BMI that exceeds 25 kg/m^2 (overweight) or 30 kg/m^2 (obese). Most patients with type 2 diabetes are recommended a program of weight reduction, increased physical exercise, and a change in diet pattern. Diets that contain large quantities of carbohydrate are discouraged.[38] The diet should contain less than 30% of calories from fat, reduced sugar intake, low levels of saturated and trans fats, and an increased quantity of whole grains, vegetables, and fruits. "Crash diets" are not recommended, and a gradual program of weight loss, if needed, is preferred.[38] The exercise program is tailored to the individual but might start with 30 minutes of brisk walking each day if the person was previously sedentary.

Pharmacologic Management of Type 2 Diabetes

If lifestyle changes are unsuccessful in reversing the pattern of type 2 diabetes, oral antihyperglycemic medications are prescribed. Table 24-3 contains a description of specific oral medications used in the treatment of Type 2 diabetes.[33] These drugs are not oral forms of insulin, because insulin would be destroyed by gastric juices. There are six major classes of oral agents: sulfonylureas, meglitinides, phenylalanine derivatives, biguanides, thiazolidinediones, and α-glucosidase inhibitors. These medications can also be classified by their mechanism of action to lower plasma glucose levels (Box 24-2).[33]

Insulin Secretagogues. The *insulin secretagogues* stimulate pancreatic secretion of insulin and decrease hyperglycemia. Three classes of drugs have this action: the sulfonylureas (glyburide, glipizide, and glimepiride), the meglitinides (repaglinide), and phenylalanine derivatives (nateglinide).[33] The sulfonylurea drugs are taken once or twice a day, lower hyperglycemia, and have a long duration of action but little effect on postprandial hyperglycemia. Both of the other drugs are taken with meals, lower hyperglycemia, and also lower postprandial blood glucose levels.[33]

Table 24-3
Pharmacologic Management of Type 2 Diabetes: Oral Medications

DRUG	DOSAGE	ACTION	ONSET/PEAK/DURATION	SPECIAL CONSIDERATIONS
Insulin Secretagogues				
First-Generation Antihyperglycemics				
Tolbutamide (Orinase)	0.5-2 g bid-tid	Stimulates release of insulin	Rapid absorption 30 min-1 hr/ 3-5 hr/6-12 hr	Metabolized in liver; excreted in kidneys Renal insufficiency: start with lower dose; observe for signs of hypoglycemia Contraindicated in pregnancy Numerous drug interactions
Tolazamide (Tolinase)	0.1-1 g single dose or bid	Stimulates release of insulin	4 hr/4 hr/10 hr	
Chlorpropamide (Diabinese)	0.1-0.5 g single dose	Stimulates release of insulin Antidiuretic	1 hr/2-4 hr/48 hr	Frequent monitoring for patients with fluid retention or cardiac dysfunction
Second-Generation Antihyperglycemics				
Glipizide (Glucotrol, Glucotrol XL)	5-10 mg bid 5-20 mg bid	Stimulates release of insulin	1 hr/1-3 hr/12-24 hr	
Glyburide (Micronase, DiaBeta, Glynase)	5 mg single dose or bid	Stimulates release of insulin	1 hr/4 hr/18-24 hr Prestab	3-6 mg daily
Glimepiride (Amaryl)	1-4 mg daily	Stimulates release of insulin	Duration 24 hr	
Phenylalanine Derivatives				
Nateglinide (Starlix)	120 mg tid (1-30 min before meals)	Stimulates release of insulin	Peak < 1 hr	*Contraindications:* • Pregnancy, breast-feeding • Children • Hepatic disorders Dose may need to be adjusted with increased glucose during times of stress (infection, surgery, trauma)
Meglitinides				
Repaglinide (Prandin)	0.5-4 mg before meals	Binds to potassium on pancreatic β-cells; increases insulin secretion	Useful in patients with sulfa allergies	
Insulin Sensitizers				
Biguanide				
Metformin (Glucophage)	Max: 500-2550 mg divided dose	Sensitizer Antihyperglycemic Suppresses hepatic glucose production	1-3 hr/24 hr/24-48 hr	Lowers serum glucose by reducing hepatic glucose output Decreases peripheral insulin resistance Temporarily withhold if patient having contrast radiography Adverse effects: lactic acidosis, GI upset Promotes weight loss Contraindications: • Pregnancy • Renal insufficiency • Acute/chronic acidosis • Diabetic ketoacidosis • Hepatic dysfunction • Excessive alcohol intake

Table 24-3

Pharmacologic Management of Type 2 Diabetes: Oral Medications—*cont'd*

DRUG	DOSAGE	ACTION	ONSET/PEAK/DURATION	SPECIAL CONSIDERATIONS
Thiazolidinediones				
Pioglitazone (Actos)	15-45 mg	Enhances insulin action by increasing cell receptors to exogenous and endogenous insulin	Peak 2-3 hr	Decreases insulin resistance and decreases hepatic glucose production Take with meals to increase absorption
Rosiglitazone (Avandia)	4-8 mg			Reduces BP and triglycerides Administration with oral contraceptives reduces efficacy of both drugs by 30%
Carbohydrate Inhibitors				
α-Glucosidase Inhibitors				
Acarbose (Precose)	100 mg tid with meals	Inhibits activity of intestinal enzymes that metabolize carbohydrate Reduces postprandial glucose mobilization	Peak 2-3 hr	Take with "first bite" each meal First drug to reduce effectively postprandial glucose Delays carbohydrate digestion by blocking absorption of complete carbohydrates in small intestine Does not promote weight loss; carbohydrate absorbed in distal small intestine and perhaps colon No apparent effect on lactose absorption, so lactose (not sucrose) substances should be used to treat hypoglycemia Side effects: flatulence, abdominal pain, diarrhea; minimized with slow titration Not recommended in severe renal impairment; safety in pregnancy not established
Miglitol (Glyset)	50-100 mg tid Initial 25 mg daily, adjust biweekly per GI tolerance		Peak 2-3 hr	Same as for acarbose Administration with digoxin reduces average plasma concentration of digoxin Administration with propranolol or ranitidine greatly reduces bioavailability of these two drugs Do not take concomitantly with digestive enzymes (e.g., amylase, pancreatin)
Combination				
Glyburide and metformin (Glucovance)	1.25 mg/250 mg 2.5 mg/500 mg 5 mg/500 mg	Initial or second-line therapy Glyburide stimulates insulin secretion Metformin decreases glucose production and absorption		See Glyburide and Metformin Common side effects: diarrhea, nausea, upset stomach

Second-generation hypoglycemics in this table are considered second-generation *oral* hypoglycemics and are more potent. Dosage is lower than for the first-generation drugs, but fewer side effects are associated with the second-generation agents.
bid, Twice daily; *tid,* three times daily; *GI,* gastrointestinal; *BP,* blood pressure.

Box 24-2

Oral Antihyperglycemic Drug Classes

Drugs That Stimulate the Pancreas to Make More Insulin (Insulin Secretagogues)
Sulfonylureas
Meglitinides
Phenylalanine derivatives

Drugs That Sensitize the Body to Insulin (Insulin Sensitizers)
Biguanides
Thiazolidinediones

Drugs That Delay Carbohydrate Absorption
α-Glucosidase inhibitors

Insulin Sensitizers. The *insulin sensitizers* work at two locations in the body. The drugs increase insulin sensitivity in the liver, increasing the ability of insulin to suppress endogenous glucose production, and also increase insulin sensitivity at the peripheral cellular level, allowing an increased uptake of glucose.[39] This class of drugs is considered first-line therapy for patients with type 2 diabetes. Two separate drug classes work in different ways to increase insulin sensitivity. The biguanide drugs (metformin) increase insulin sensitivity in the liver and have only a minor effect on skeletal muscle. In contrast, the thiazolidinedione drugs (pioglitazone and rosiglitazone) are about 70% more effective at increasing peripheral insulin sensitivity compared with metformin.[33] Both of these drug classes have rare but significant side effects that must be recognized if they occur. Metformin is associated with a risk of metabolic acidosis, especially for patients with elevated creatinine clearance.[40,41] The thiazolidinediones cause fluid gain and pedal edema in 3% to 5% of patients and heart failure in under 1%.[42] Of greater concern is when the thiazolidinedione drugs are combined with insulin therapy, the incidence of heart failure rises to between 2% and 3%.[42] The reasons for this occurrence are not yet known.

Carbohydrate Inhibitors. The third group of drugs slows digestion of ingested carbohydrates, delays glucose absorption, and reduces postprandial (after meals) hyperglycemia.[33] These are the *α-glucosidase inhibitors*. The drugs in this class are acarbose and miglitol.[33] A review of the physiology of carbohydrate digestion is helpful to understand how these drugs work. Carbohydrates are broken down to absorbable components in the duodenum and upper jejunum. The carbohydrates are digested to *oligosaccharides* in the small intestine by pancreatic lipase; then, the oligosaccharides are cleaved to *monosaccharides* by the *α-glucosidase* group of enzymes. The *monosaccharides* are then available to be absorbed from the intestine into the bloodstream. The α-glucosidase inhibitor drugs work by decreasing the conversion of carbohydrates from oligosaccharides to monosaccharides, thus limiting the blood glucose rise that occurs after eating. The most frequently prescribed drug in this class is acarbose, which is nonabsorbable.[33]

Combination therapy, either by prescription of drugs from more than one class or use of a drug that combines two different methods of action, is the treatment of choice in most patients with type 2 diabetes.[33] The number of oral antihyperglycemic agents is increasing rapidly, and the critical care nurse must be familiar with these categories of drugs. See Table 24-3 for more specific details related to oral antihyperglycemic drugs. Pancreatic β-cell decline occurs as type 2 diabetes progresses, and eventually, for many patients, oral agents alone will fail to control hyperglycemia. Insulin may be added to the drug regimen to maintain normal blood glucose levels.[33,43] At this stage, many patients with type 2 diabetes take oral medications and receive Sub-Q insulin.[33] Some patients convert entirely to type 1 diabetes.[43] When a patient with type 2 diabetes is admitted to the critical care unit, he or she is often switched to either Sub-Q or IV insulin and the oral medications are temporarily stopped.[44]

Other Complications

Patients who have type 2 diabetes are prone to a wide range of other complications that increase morbidity and mortality. Thus, in addition to antihyperglycemic drugs, patients with type 2 diabetes often require medications to lower their blood pressure,[45] lower their cholesterol and triglyceride levels,[46] and treat ischemic heart disease.[47]

A serious complication of type 2 diabetes that, if present, mandates admission to a critical care unit is hyperglycemic hyperosmolar syndrome (HHS). This severe, sustained elevation of glucose levels leads to a serum hyperosmolarity and, if left untreated, progresses toward cellular dehydration, coma, and death. HHS is discussed in a later section.

DIABETIC KETOACIDOSIS

Epidemiology and Etiology

DKA is a life-threatening complication of diabetes mellitus[48-52] Type 1 diabetics who are dependent on insulin are typically affected. Some elderly patients with type 2 diabetes can develop DKA, but this is not as frequently encountered.[50,51] The diagnostic criteria for DKA are as follows[49]:

- Blood glucose level greater than 250 mg/dl
- Arterial pH below 7.3
- Serum bicarbonate level below18 mEq/L
- Moderate ketonemia or ketonuria

The annual incidence of DKA ranges from 4.6 to 8 episodes per 1,000 patients with diabetes.[49] This represents about 68,000 emergency department visits for DKA in the United States.[48] Annual hospital costs for patients with DKA exceed $1 billion per year.[49]

Infection is the major reason that diabetic patients develop and progress to DKA. Symptoms of fatigue and polyuria may precede the development of full-blown DKA, which can develop in under 24 hours, in a person with type 1 diabetes.[49] In an undiagnosed diabetic patient, it is unknown how long it may take to develop as the pancreatic β-cells gradually fail. About 20% of hospital admissions for DKA are related to diagnosis of new-onset type 1 diabetes.[51] Mortality in DKA is below 5% in patients with type 1 diabetes when patients are managed by clinicians experienced in treatment of this disorder.[49]

Changes in the type of insulin, change in dosage, or increased metabolic demand can precipitate DKA in individuals with type 1 diabetes.[49] Life cycle changes, such as growth spurts in the adolescent, require an increase in insulin intake, as do surgery, infection, and trauma. In young persons with diabetes, psychologic problems combined with eating disorders may be a contributing factor in up to 20% of recurrent ketoacidosis.[49]

Ketoacidosis also occurs with acute pancreatitis. In addition to elevated glucose level and acidosis, the serum amylase and lipase levels are abnormally high, which helps to establish the diagnosis as separate from type 1 diabetes.[51] Other nondiabetes causes of ketoacidosis are *starvation ketoacidosis* and *alcoholic ketoacidosis.* Both of these are distinguished from classical DKA by clinical history and, usually, by a plasma glucose level below 200 mg/dl.[49]

PATHOPHYSIOLOGY

Insulin Deficiency

Insulin is the metabolic key to the transfer of glucose from the bloodstream into the cell, where it can be used immediately for energy or stored for use at a later time. Without insulin, glucose remains in the bloodstream, and cells are deprived of their energy source. A complex pathophysiologic chain of events follows (Figure 24-2). The release of glucagon from the liver is stimulated when insulin is ineffective in providing the cells with glucose for energy. Glucagon increases the amount of glucose in the bloodstream by breaking down stored glucose (glycogenolysis). In addition, noncarbohydrates (fat and protein) are converted into glucose (gluconeogenesis). Blood glucose levels for the patient in DKA typically range from 300 to 800 mg/dl of blood. The reason the plasma glucose is not higher is because of the short time period in which DKA develops. Elevated serum glucose level, ketonemia, and metabolic acidosis with an increased anion gap define DKA.[49]

Hyperglycemia

Hyperglycemia increases the plasma osmolarity, and blood volume becomes hyperosmolar. Cellular dehydration occurs as the hyperosmolar extracellular fluid draws the more dilute intracellular and interstitial fluid into the vascular space in an attempt to return the plasma osmolality to normal. Dehydration stimulates catecholamine production in an effort to provide emergency support. Catecholamine output stimulates further glycogenolysis, lipolysis, and gluconeogenesis, pouring glucose into the bloodstream.

Fluid Volume Deficit

Excessive urination *(polyuria)* and *glycosuria* (glucose in the urine) occur as a result of the osmotic particle load that occurs with DKA. The excess glucose, filtered at the glomeruli, cannot be resorbed at the renal tubule and is then detectable in the urine. The unresorbed solute exerts its own osmotic pull in the renal tubules, and less water is returned to circulation through the collecting ducts. As a result, large volumes of water, along with sodium, potassium, and phosphorus, are excreted in the urine, causing a fluid volume deficit. Serum sodium may be decreased because of the movement of water from the intracellular to the extracellular (vascular) space.[49]

Ketoacidosis

In the healthy individual, the presence of insulin in the bloodstream suppresses the manufacture of ketones. In insulin deficiency states, fat is rapidly converted into glucose (gluconeogenesis). Ketoacidosis occurs when free fatty acids are metabolized into ketones: acetoacetate, β-hydroxybutyrate, and acetone make up the three ketone bodies that are produced.[50] During normal metabolism the ratio of β-hydroxybutyrate to acetoacetate is 1:1, with acetone present in only small amounts. In insulin deficiency the quantity of all three ketone bodies increases substantially, and the ratio of β-hydroxybutyrate to acetoacetate increases by as much as 10:1.[50] β-Hydroxybutyrate and acetoacetate are the ketones responsible for acidosis in DKA. Acetone does not cause acidosis and is safely excreted in the lungs, causing the characteristic "fruity" odor.[50] Ketones are measurable in the bloodstream (ketonemia). Blood tests that measure the quantity of β-hydroxybutyric acid, the predominant ketone body, are the most useful.[30] Because ketones are excreted via the kidney, they are also measurable in the urine *(ketonuria).* Ketone blood tests are preferred over urine tests for diagnosis and monitoring of DKA.[30] When the blood and urine are clear of ketones, the DKA is resolved.

Acid-Base Balance

The acid-base balance will vary depending on the severity of the DKA. The patient with DKA typically has a pH below 7.30.[49] Acid ketones dissociate and yield hydrogen ions (H^+) that accumulate and precipitate a fall in serum pH. The level of serum bicarbonate also decreases consistent with a diagnosis of metabolic acidosis. Breathing becomes deep and rapid (Kussmaul respirations) to release carbonic acid in the form of carbon dioxide.

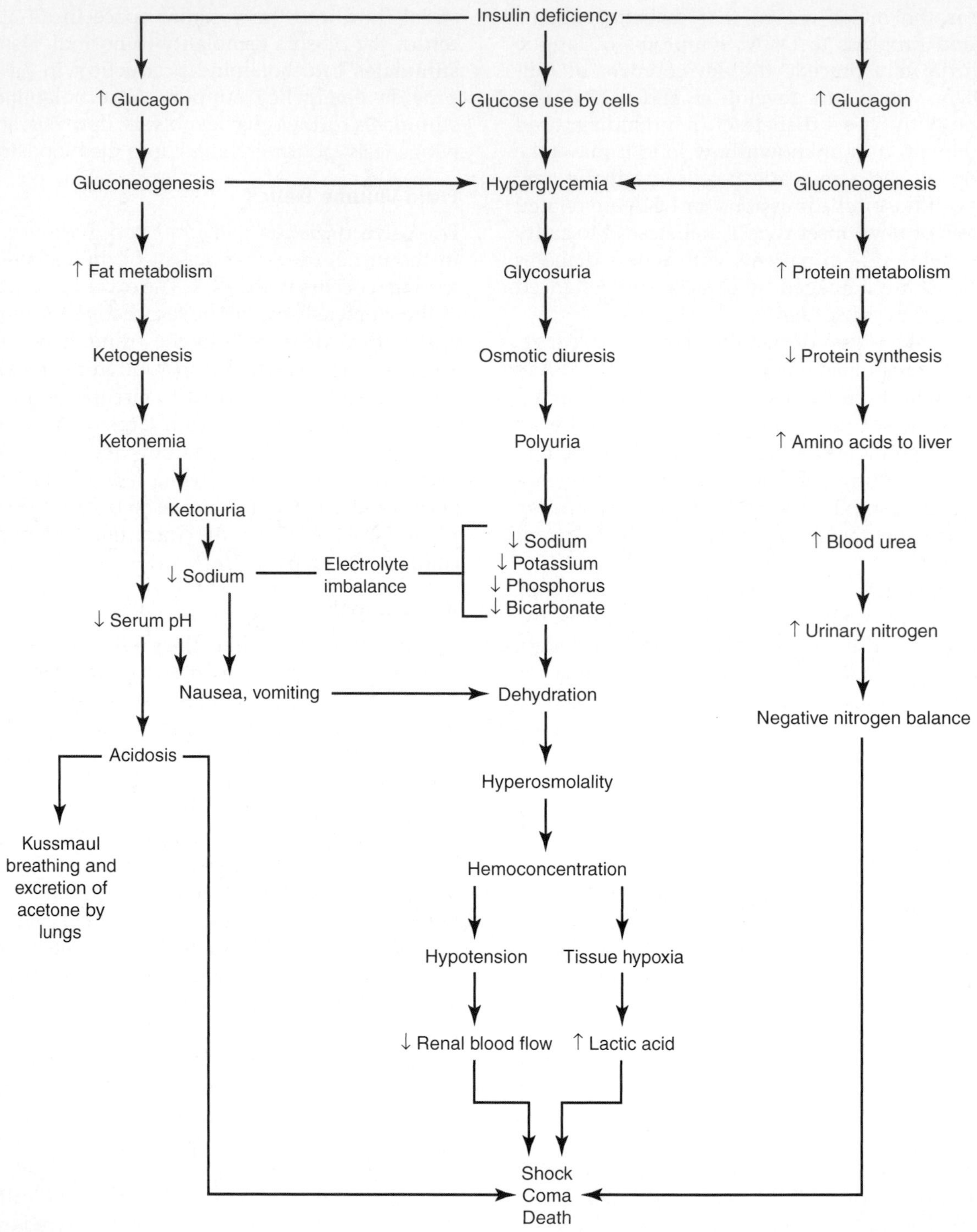

FIGURE 24-2. Pathophysiology of diabetic ketoacidosis (DKA).

Gluconeogenesis

Gluconeogenesis is the process of breaking down fat or protein to make new glucose. Fat is metabolized to ketones as described above. Protein used for gluconeogenesis leaves no reserve protein available for synthesis and repair of vital body tissues. Nitrogen accumulates as protein is metabolized to urea. Urea, added to the bloodstream, increases the osmotic diuresis and accentuates the dehydration.

ASSESSMENT AND DIAGNOSIS

Clinical Manifestations

DKA has a predictable clinical presentation. It is usually preceded by patient complaints of malaise, headache, polyuria (excessive urination), polydipsia (excessive thirst), and polyphagia (excessive hunger). Nausea, vomiting, extreme fatigue, dehydration, and weight loss follow. Central nervous system depression, with changes in the level of consciousness, can lead quickly to coma.[49,50,52]

The patient with DKA may be stuporous or unresponsive, depending on the degree of fluid-balance disturbance. The physical examination reveals evidence of dehydration, including flushed dry skin, dry buccal membranes, and skin turgor that takes longer than 3 seconds to return to its original position after the skin has been lifted. Often, "sunken eyeballs," resulting from the lack of fluid in the interstitium of the eyeball, are observed. Tachycardia and hypotension may signal profound fluid losses. *Kussmaul respirations* are present, and the fruity odor of acetone may be detected.

Laboratory Studies

Considering the complexity and potential seriousness of DKA, the laboratory diagnosis is straightforward. With a known diabetic patient, the presence of urine ketones and hyperglycemia on bedside finger stick provide rapid diagnostic confirmation of DKA. If a blood gas sample is obtained, this can confirm the acid-base imbalance. Other clues may be gleaned from the blood chemistry panel. If the laboratory panel measures CO_2, this value will be low in the presence of uncompensated metabolic acidosis, and the anion gap will be elevated. Serum sodium level may be low as a result of the movement of water from the intracellular space into the extracellular (vascular) space.[49] The serum potassium level is often normal. However, if the serum potassium level is low, this indicates a severe total-body potassium deficiency.[49]

Medical Management

Diagnosis of DKA is based on the combination of presenting symptoms, patient history, medical history (type 1 diabetes), precipitating factors if known, and results of serum glucose and urine ketone testing. Once diagnosed, DKA requires aggressive clinical management to prevent progressive decompensation. The goals of treatment are the following:

- Reverse dehydration
- Replace insulin
- Reverse ketoacidosis
- Replenish electrolytes

Reverse Hydration

The patient with DKA is dehydrated and may have lost 5% to 10% of body weight in fluids. A fluid deficit up to 6 L can exist in severe dehydration. Aggressive fluid replacement is provided to rehydrate both the intracellular and the extracellular compartments and prevent circulatory collapse as detailed in Figure 24-3.[49] An assessment of hydration is an important first step. Isotonic saline (0.9% NaCl) IV is infused to replenish the vascular deficit and to reverse hypotension. For the severely dehydrated patient, 1 L of normal saline is infused immediately.[49] Laboratory assessment of the serum osmolarity and of serum sodium level can help guide the subsequent interventions. If the serum sodium level is low, 0.9% NaCl is infused. If the serum osmolarity is elevated and serum sodium is high (hypernatremia), infusions of hypotonic sodium chloride (0.45% NaCl) will follow the initial saline replacement (see Figure 24-3). The replacement infusion typically includes 20 to 30 mEq potassium per liter to restore the intracellular potassium debt, provided kidney function is normal.[49] Fluid replacement should correct intravascular volume deficits within 24 hours.[49] In patients without normally functioning kidneys or with cardiopulmonary disease, very careful attention must be paid to the volume of fluid replacement to avoid fluid overload.

Once the serum glucose level decreases to 200 mg/dl, the infusing solution is changed to a 50/50 mix of 5% dextrose (D_5W) and hypotonic saline (0.45% NaCl).[49] Dextrose is added to replenish depleted cellular glucose as the circulating serum glucose level falls. Dextrose infusion will also prevent unexpected hypoglycemia when the insulin drip is continued, but before the patient can take in sufficient carbohydrate from an oral diet.

Replace Insulin

In moderate to severe DKA, an initial IV bolus of regular insulin at 0.1 units for each kg (units/kg) of body weight is administered.[49] Subsequently, a continuous infusion of regular insulin at 0.1 units/kg/hr is infused simultaneously with IV fluids.[49] For example, in a 70-kg adult this would represent 7 units of regular insulin per hour. If the plasma glucose level does not fall by 50 to 70 mg/dl in the first hour of treatment, recheck the glucose measurement and reevaluate the hydration status of the patient. The insulin infusion should be adjusted until a steady glucose decline between 50 and 70 mg/dl is achieved.[49] See Figure 24-3 for a diagrammatic representation of both IV and Sub-Q insulin administration options in DKA. Frequent assessment of the patient's blood glucose level is mandatory in moderate to severe DKA. Initially blood glucose tests are performed hourly; frequency decreases to every 2 to 4 hours as the patient's blood glucose levels stabilize and approach normal. Once the blood glucose level has decreased to 200 mg/dl, acidosis is corrected, and dehydration is achieved, it will be possible to decrease the insulin infusion rate to 0.05 to 0.1 unit per kg body weight, hourly.[49] This usually represents 3 to 6 units/hr in an adult receiving a continuous IV insulin infusion. It is important

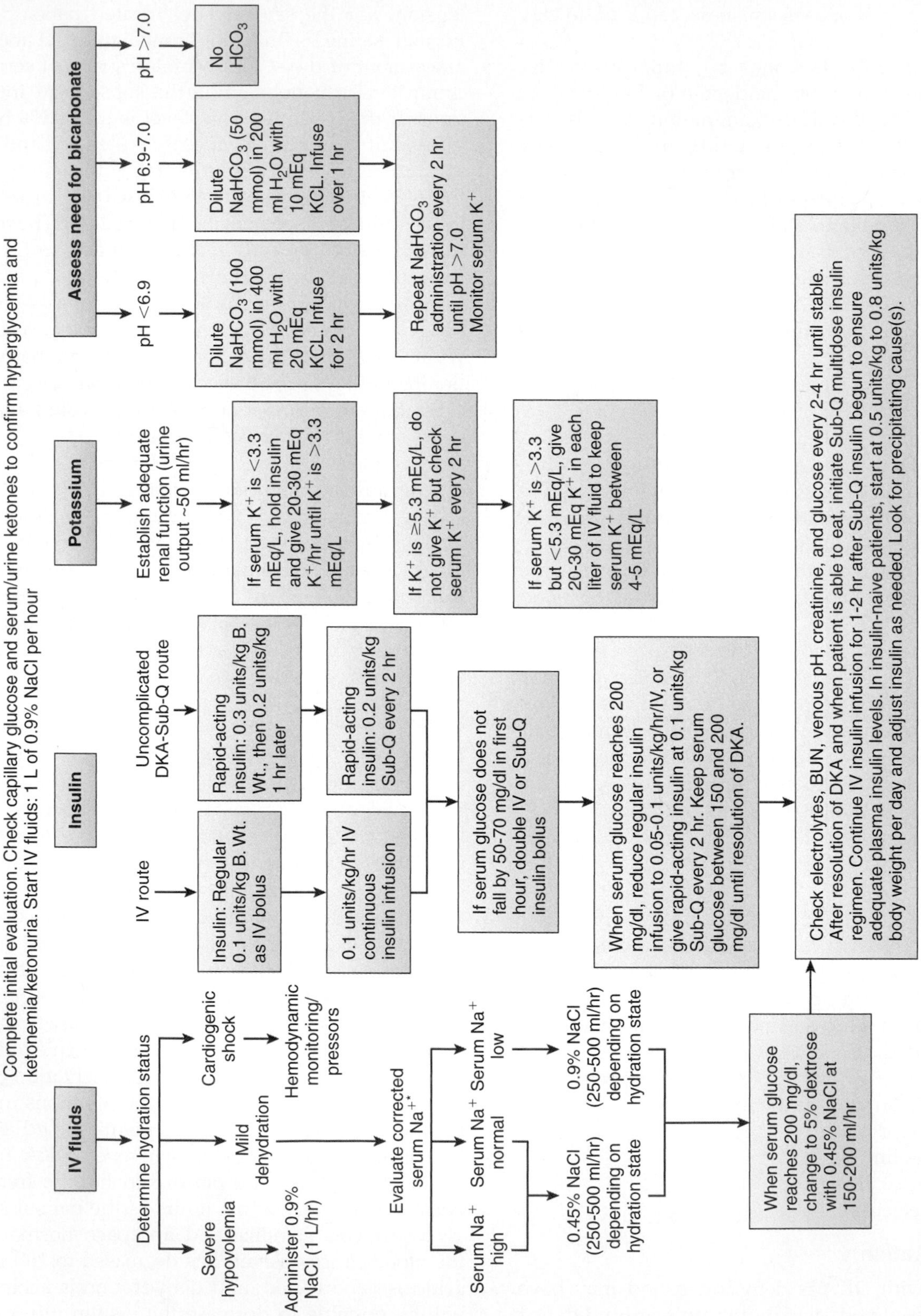
Complete initial evaluation. Check capillary glucose and serum/urine ketones to confirm hyperglycemia and ketonemia/ketonuria. Start IV fluids: 1 L of 0.9% NaCl per hour
IV fluids
Insulin
Potassium
Assess need for bicarbonate
Determine hydration status
Severe hypovolemia
Mild dehydration
Cardiogenic shock
Administer 0.9% NaCl (1 L/hr)
Hemodynamic monitoring/ pressors
Evaluate corrected serum Na+*
Serum Na+ high
Serum Na+ normal
Serum Na+ low
0.45% NaCl (250-500 ml/hr) depending on hydration state
0.9% NaCl (250-500 ml/hr) depending on hydration state
When serum glucose reaches 200 mg/dl, change to 5% dextrose with 0.45% NaCl at 150-200 ml/hr
IV route
Uncomplicated DKA-Sub-Q route
Insulin: Regular 0.1 units/kg B. Wt. as IV bolus
Rapid-acting insulin: 0.3 units/kg B. Wt., then 0.2 units/kg 1 hr later
0.1 units/kg/hr IV continuous insulin infusion
Rapid-acting insulin: 0.2 units/kg Sub-Q every 2 hr
If serum glucose does not fall by 50-70 mg/dl in first hour, double IV or Sub-Q insulin bolus
When serum glucose reaches 200 mg/dl, reduce regular insulin infusion to 0.05-0.1 units/kg/hr/IV, or give rapid-acting insulin at 0.1 units/kg Sub-Q every 2 hr. Keep serum glucose between 150 and 200 mg/dl until resolution of DKA.
Establish adequate renal function (urine output ~50 ml/hr)
If serum K+ is <3.3 mEq/L, hold insulin and give 20-30 mEq K+/hr until K+ is >3.3 mEq/L
If K+ is ≥5.3 mEq/L, do not give K+ but check serum K+ every 2 hr
If serum K+ is >3.3 but <5.3 mEq/L, give 20-30 mEq K+ in each liter of IV fluid to keep serum K+ between 4-5 mEq/L
pH <6.9
pH 6.9-7.0
pH >7.0
Dilute NaHCO3 (100 mmol) in 400 ml H2O with 20 mEq KCL. Infuse for 2 hr
Dilute NaHCO3 (50 mmol) in 200 ml H2O with 10 mEq KCL. Infuse over 1 hr
No HCO3
Repeat NaHCO3 administration every 2 hr until pH >7.0 Monitor serum K+
Check electrolytes, BUN, venous pH, creatinine, and glucose every 2-4 hr until stable. After resolution of DKA and when patient is able to eat, initiate Sub-Q multidose insulin regimen. Continue IV insulin infusion for 1-2 hr after Sub-Q insulin begun to ensure adequate plasma insulin levels. In insulin-naive patients, start at 0.5 units/kg to 0.8 units/kg body weight per day and adjust insulin as needed. Look for precipitating cause(s).

FIGURE 24-3. Protocol for the management of adult patients with diabetic ketoacidosis (DKA). (From Kitabchi AE et al: *Diabetes Care* 29[12]:2739, 2006).

to verify that the serum potassium is not below 3.3 mEq/L and to replace the serum potassium if necessary before administering the initial insulin bolus.[49]

Reverse Ketoacidosis

Replacement of fluid volume and insulin will interrupt the ketotic cycle and reverse the metabolic acidosis. In the presence of insulin, glucose will enter the cells, and the body will cease to convert fats into glucose. The ketoacidotic cycle is broken by the provision of fluid volume and insulin replacement.

Adequate hydration and insulin replacement will usually correct the acidosis and is sufficient treatment for many patients with DKA. As shown in Figure 24-3, replacement of bicarbonate is no longer routine except for the severely acidotic patient with a serum pH at or below 7.0.[49] An indwelling arterial catheter provides access for hourly sampling of arterial blood gases (ABGs) to evaluate pH, bicarbonate, and other laboratory values in the patient with severe DKA. If an arterial line is not available, the pH can be assessed using the venous pH.[49]

Hyperglycemia generally resolves before ketoacidemia. In one clinical report, patients with previously diagnosed type 1 diabetes in DKA took an average of 21 hours after being started on an IV insulin protocol to clear ketones from the urine; the IV insulin infusion was continued for 36 hours until the patients could tolerate an oral diet, and the patients received a total of 9.5 L of normal saline for rehydration.[51] It is important to be aware that patients who are newly diagnosed type 1 diabetics take longer to clear their urine ketones and require more insulin to achieve normal glycemic control.[51]

Replenish Electrolytes

Low serum potassium level (hypokalemia) will occur as insulin promotes the return of potassium into the cell and metabolic acidosis is reversed. Replacement of potassium using potassium chloride (KCl) begins as soon as the serum potassium falls below normal. Frequent verification of the serum potassium level is required for the DKA patient receiving fluid resuscitation and insulin therapy. The serum phosphate level is sometimes low (hypophosphatemia) in DKA. Insulin treatment may make this more obvious as phosphate is returned to the interior of the cell. If the serum phosphate level is below 1 mg/dl, phosphate replacement is recommended.[49] See Figure 24-3 for further information about potassium replacement options.

Nursing Management

Nursing management of the patient with diabetic ketoacidosis incorporates a variety of nursing diagnoses (Box 24-3). **Nursing priorities are directed toward (1) administering prescribed fluids, insulin, and electrolytes; (2) monitoring response to therapy; (3) maintaining surveillance for complications; and (4) providing patient education.**

Box 24-3

NURSING DIAGNOSIS PRIORITIES

Diabetic Ketoacidosis

- Decreased Cardiac Output related to alterations in preload, p. A-12
- Deficient Fluid Volume related to absolute loss, p. A-16
- Anxiety related to threat to biologic, psychologic, and/or social integrity, p. A-9
- Disturbed Body Image related to functional dependence on life-sustaining technology, p. A-20
- Ineffective Coping related to situational crisis and personal vulnerability, p. A-38
- Powerlessness related to lack of control over current situation and/or disease progression, p. A-44
- Deficient Knowledge: Discharge Regimen related to lack of previous exposure to information, p. A-18

Administering Fluids, Insulin, and Electrolytes

Rapid IV fluid replacement requires the use of a volumetric pump. Insulin is administered IV to patients who are severely dehydrated or have poor peripheral perfusion to ensure effective absorption. Patients with DKA are maintained on NPO status (nothing by mouth) until the blood glucose level is below 200 mg/dl. Throughout the insulin therapy, both patient response and laboratory data are assessed for changes relating to blood glucose levels. The critical care nurse is responsible for monitoring the rate of plasma glucose decline in response to insulin. The goal is to achieve a fall in glucose levels of approximately 50 to 70 mg/dl each hour.[49] The coordination involved in monitoring blood glucose, potassium, and often blood gas values on an hourly basis is considerable. When the blood glucose level falls to 200 mg/dl, a 5% dextrose solution is infused to prevent hypoglycemia.[49] At this time, it is likely the insulin dose per hour will also be decreased. The regular insulin drip is not discontinued until the ketoacidosis subsides, as identified by a normal pH on an arterial or venous blood gas.[49] Insulin is given subcutaneously when glucose levels, dehydration, hypotension, and acid-base balance are normalized and the patient is in stable condition and taking an oral diet.

Monitoring Response to Therapy

Accurate intake and output (I&O) measurements must be maintained to monitor reversal of dehydration. Measuring hourly urine output is an indicator of renal function and provides information to prevent overhydration or underhydration. Vital signs, especially heart rate (HR), hemodynamic values, and blood pressure (BP), are continuously monitored to assess

Box 24-4

Hydration Assessment

- Hourly intake
- Blood pressure changes
  - Orthostatic hypotension
  - Pulse pressure
  - Pulse rate, character, rhythm
- Neck vein filling
- Skin turgor
- Skin moisture
- Body weight
- Central venous pressure
- Pulmonary arterial occlusion pressure
- Hourly output
- Complaints of thirst

response to the fluid replacement. Evidence that fluid replacement is effective includes normal central venous pressure (CVP), decreased HR, and normal BP. Box 24-4 lists the standard features to be included in an assessment of hydration status. More invasive hemodynamic monitoring, such as a pulmonary artery catheter, is rarely needed. Further evidence of hydration improvement includes a change from a previously weak, thready pulse to a pulse that is strong and full and a change from hypotension to a gradual elevation of systolic BP. Respirations are assessed frequently for changes in rate, depth, and presence of the fruity acetone odor.

Blood glucose level is measured each hour in the initial period. Sometimes potassium level is measured just as frequently. Serum osmolarity and serum sodium level are evaluated, and blood urea nitrogen (BUN) and creatinine levels are assessed for possible renal impairment related to decreased kidney perfusion. The purpose of these frequent assessments is to determine that the patient's clinical status is improving. Once the patient has stable laboratory indicators and is awake and alert, the transition to Sub-Q insulin and an oral diet can be made. Hypoglycemia is a risk during the transition period. For example, in anticipation of discontinuing the insulin and IV dextrose infusion, a patient would receive a Sub-Q dose of insulin and would be expected to eat a meal. However, if the patient is then unable to eat an adequate amount, hypoglycemia results secondary to the Sub-Q insulin without adequate glucose.[51]

The markers for resolution of DKA include a blood glucose level below 200 mg/dl, serum bicarbonate level above 18 mEq/L, and a venous pH greater than 7.3.[49]

Maintaining Surveillance for Complications

The patient in DKA can experience a variety of complications, including risk for fluid volume overload, hypoglycemia, hypokalemia or hyperkalemia, hyponatremia, cerebral edema, and infection.

Fluid Volume Overload. Fluid overload from rapid volume infusion is a serious complication that can occur in the patient with a compromised cardiopulmonary system, renal system, or both. Neck vein engorgement, dyspnea without exertion, and pulmonary crackles on auscultation signal circulatory overload. Reduction in the rate and volume of infusion, elevation of the head of the bed, and provision of oxygen may be required to manage the increased intravascular volume. Hourly urine measurement is mandatory to assess renal output and adequacy of fluid replacement.

Hypoglycemia. Hypoglycemia is defined as plasma glucose level below 70 mg/dl.[25] Most acute care hospitals have specific procedures for management of the hypoglycemic patient. For example, if hypoglycemia is detected by finger-stick point-of-care testing at the bedside, a blood sample is sent to the laboratory for a verification, the physician is notified immediately, and replacement glucose is given either IV or by mouth. The route of administration is based on the patient's clinical condition, diagnosis, and level of consciousness.

Unexpected behavior change or decreased level of consciousness, diaphoresis, and tremors are physical warning signs that the patient has become hypoglycemic. These symptoms are especially important to recognize if the frequency of glucose testing has lengthened to 2- to 4-hour intervals. A comparison between the physical symptoms expected with hypoglycemia versus hyperglycemia is provided in Box 24-5.

Hypokalemia. Hypokalemia can occur within the first 4 hours of rehydration and insulin treatment. Continuous cardiac monitoring is required because low serum potassium level (hypokalemia) can cause ventricular dysrhythmias.

Hyperkalemia. Hyperkalemia occurs with acidosis or with overaggressive administration of potassium replacement in patients with renal insufficiency. Severe hyperkalemia is noted on the cardiac monitor by a large, peaked T wave, flattened P wave, and widened QRS complex. Ventricular fibrillation can follow.

Hyponatremia. Sodium is eliminated from the body as a result of the osmotic diuresis and compounded by the vomiting and diarrhea that occur during DKA. Clinical manifestations of hyponatremia include abdominal cramping, apprehension, postural hypotension, and unexpected behavioral changes. Sodium chloride is infused as the initial IV solution. Maintenance of the saline infusion depends on clinical manifestations of sodium imbalance plus serum laboratory values.

Risk for Cerebral Edema. Changes in the patient's neurologic status may be insidious. Alterations in level of consciousness, pupil reaction, and motor function may be the result of fluctuating glucose levels and

Box 24-5

Clinical Manifestations of Hypoglycemia and Hyperglycemia

HYPOGLYCEMIA	HYPERGLYCEMIA
• Restlessness	• Excessive thirst
• Apprehension	• Excessive urination
• Irritability	• Hunger
• Trembling	• Weakness
• Weakness	• Listlessness
• Diaphoresis	• Mental fatigue
• Pallor	• Flushed, dry skin
• Paresthesia	• Itching
• Headache	• Headache
• Hunger	• Nausea
• Difficulty thinking	• Vomiting
• Loss of coordination	• Abdominal cramps
• Difficulty walking	• Dehydration
• Difficulty talking	• Weak, rapid pulse
• Visual disturbances	• Postural hypotension
• Blurred vision	• Hypotension
• Double vision	• Acetone breath odor
• Tachycardia	• Kussmaul respirations
• Shallow respirations	• Rapid breathing
• Hypertension	• Changes in level of consciousness
• Changes in level of consciousness	• Stupor
• Seizures	• Coma
• Coma	

cerebral fluid shifts. Confusion and sudden complaints of headache are ominous signs that may signal cerebral edema. These observations require immediate action to prevent neurologic damage. Neurologic assessments are performed every hour or as needed during the acute phase of hyperglycemia and rehydration. Assessment of level of consciousness serves as the cerebral index of the patient's response to the rehydration therapy.

Risk for Infection. Skin care takes on new dimensions for the patient with DKA. Dehydration, hypovolemia, and hypophosphatemia interfere with oxygen delivery at the cell site and contribute to inadequate perfusion and tissue breakdown. Patients must be repositioned frequently to relieve capillary pressure and promote adequate perfusion to body tissues. The typical patient with type 1 diabetes is either of normal weight or underweight. Bony prominences must be assessed for tissue breakdown and the patient's body weight repositioned every 1 to 2 hours. Irritation of skin from adhesive tape, shearing force, and detergents should be avoided. Maintenance of skin integrity will prevent unwanted portals of entry for microorganisms.

Oral care, including toothbrushing and lip balm, helps keep lips supple and prevents cracking. Prepared sponge sticks or moist gauze pads can be used to moisten oral membranes of the unconscious patient. Swabbing the mouth moistens the tissue and displaces the bacteria that collect when saliva, which has a bacteriostatic action, is curtailed by dehydration. The conscious patient removes bacteria and provides oral comfort with frequent toothbrushing and oral rinsing.

Strict sterile technique is used to maintain all IV systems. All venipuncture sites are checked every 4 hours for signs of inflammation, phlebitis, or infiltration. Strict surgical asepsis is used for all invasive procedures. Sterile technique is used if urinary catheterization is necessary to obtain urine samples for testing. Urinary catheter care is provided every 8 hours.

Providing Patient Education

It is important to be aware of the knowledge level and adherence history of patients with previously diagnosed diabetes to formulate an appropriate teaching plan. Learning objectives include a discussion of target glucose levels, definition of hyperglycemia and its causes, harmful effects, and symptoms and how to manage insulin and diet when one is unwell and unable to eat.[51] Additional objectives include a definition of DKA and its causes, symptoms, and harmful consequences. The patient and family are also expected to learn the principles of diabetes management. Universal precautions must be emphasized for all family caregivers.[18] The patient and family must also learn the warning signs to report to the attention of a health care practitioner. Education of the patient, family, or other support persons to achieve knowledge-based, independent self-management of blood glucose level and avoidance of diabetes-related complications are the goals of the teaching process.

Collaborative Management

In all aspects of patient care management, health care professionals work as a team, with the major collaborative goal of providing the best possible outcome for each patient. Current guidelines related to collaborative management of patients with hyperglycemia crisis are listed in Evidence-Based Collaborative Practice: Diabetic Ketoacidosis.

HYPERGLYCEMIC HYPEROSMOLAR SYNDROME

Epidemiology and Etiology

HHS is a potentially lethal complication of type 2 diabetes. The hallmarks of HHS are extremely high levels of plasma glucose with resultant elevation in hyperosmolarity causing osmotic diuresis. Ketosis is absent or mild.[49] Inability to replace fluids lost through diuresis leads to profound dehydration and changes in level of consciousness. Overall mortality from HHS

EVIDENCE-BASED COLLABORATIVE PRACTICE

Diabetic Ketoacidosis

Summary of evidence and evidence-based recommendations for controlling symptoms related to diabetic ketoacidosis (DKA)

Strong Evidence to Support the Following:
- Rehydration.
- Regular insulin by continuous infusion, unless DKA is mild.
- Replace serum potassium if level is below 3.3 mEq/L.
- Replace serum phosphate if level is below 1.0 mg/dl.

Very Little Evidence to Support the Following:
- No support for use of routine bicarbonate to correct low serum pH. May be considered if pH is below 7.0.

Data from Kitabchi AE et al: *Diabetes Care* 29(12):2739, 2006.

is 11%,[49] although older patients with associated illnesses have increased risk of death.[50,51] When the mortality for diabetic patients is stratified by age, there is no difference in death rates based on the underlying hyperglycemic crisis (HHS or DKA).[50] For HHS patients less than 75 years of age, mortality is 10%; for patients ages 75 to 84, mortality is 19%; and for those older than 85 years, mortality is 35%.[50] The diagnostic criteria for HHS are as follows[30,49]:

- Blood glucose level above 600 mg/dl
- Arterial pH above 7.3
- Bicarbonate level greater than 15 mEq/L
- Minimal ketonemia and ketonuria (ketones in blood and urine)

Most patients with this level of metabolic disruption also experience visual changes, mental status changes, and potentially hypovolemic shock.

HHS occurs when the pancreas produces a relatively insufficient amount of insulin for the high levels of glucose that flood the bloodstream. HHS primarily affects older obese persons with underlying cardiovascular conditions. Infection is the primary reason that type 2 diabetics develop HHS. The patient may have type 2 diabetes treated with diet and oral hypoglycemic agents that is destabilized by an infection. The most common infections are pneumonia and urinary tract infections. Other precipitating causes of HHS include stroke, myocardial infarction, trauma, burns, or the stress of a major illness. Many classes of medications have been associated with the development of HHS, including corticosteroids, phenytoin, thiazide diuretics, β-blockers, dobutamine, and antipsychotics.[49,50]

Differences Between HHS and DKA

Clinically HHS is distinguished from DKA by the presence of extremely elevated serum glucose level, more profound dehydration, and minimal or absent ketosis (Table 24-4). There is another major difference between HHS and DKA. In HHS, protein and fats are not used to create new supplies of glucose as in DKA, and the ketotic cycle is either never started or does not occur until the glucose level is extremely elevated. In one third of adults with hyperglycemic crisis there is overlap between symptoms of DKA and HHS.[49] Generally, patients with type 1 diabetes do not develop HHS, but some patients with type 2 diabetes do develop DKA.[50, 51]

PATHOPHYSIOLOGY

HHS represents a deficit of insulin and an excess of glucagons (Figure 24-4). Reduced insulin levels prevent the movement of glucose into the cells, thus allowing glucose to accumulate in the plasma. The decreased insulin level triggers glucagon release from the liver, and hepatic glucose is poured into the circulation. As the number of glucose particles increases in the blood, serum hyperosmolarity increases. In an effort to decrease the serum osmolarity, fluid is drawn from the intracellular compartment (inside the cells) into the vascular bed. Profound intracellular volume depletion occurs if the patient's thirst sensation is absent or decreased. HHS may evolve over days or even weeks.[49]

Hyperglycemia persists despite removal of large amounts of glucose in the urine (glycosuria). The glomerular filtration and elimination of glucose by the kidney tubules is ineffective in reducing the serum glucose level sufficiently to maintain normal glucose levels. The hyperosmolarity and reduced blood volume stimulate release of antidiuretic hormone (ADH) to increase the tubular resorption of water. ADH, however, is unable to overcome the osmotic pull exerted by the glucose load. Excessive fluid volume is lost at the kidney tubule with simultaneous loss of potassium, sodium, and phosphate in the urine. This chain of events results in progressively worsening hypovolemia.

Hypovolemia reduces circulation to the kidneys, and oliguria develops. Although this process conserves water and preserves the blood volume, it prevents further glucose loss, and hyperosmolarity increases. Ketosis is absent or mild in HHS. However, the patient with HHS with an extremely elevated serum glucose level can develop a metabolic acidosis secondary to dehydration, poor tissue perfusion, and lactic acid accumulation.

The sympathetic nervous system reacts to the body's stress response to try to restore homeostasis. Epinephrine, a potent stimulus for gluconeogenesis,

Table 24-4

Comparison of Diabetic Ketoacidosis (DKA) and Hyperglycemic Hyperosmolar Syndrome (HHS)

	DKA	HHS
Cause	Insufficient exogenous glucose for glucose needs	Insufficient exogenous/endogenous insulin for glucose needs
Onset	Sudden (hours)	Slow, insidious (days, weeks)
Precipitating factors	Newly diagnosed type 1 diabetes Lack of adherence to insulin regimen in type 1 diabetes Type 1 diabetes with infection, illness, surgery	Elderly patients with recent acute illness; therapeutic procedures
Mortality	5%	11%
Population affected	Type 1 diabetes	Type 2 diabetes
Clinical manifestations	Dry mouth, polydipsia, polyuria, polyphagia, dehydration, dry skin, hypotension, weakness, mental confusion, tachycardia, changes in level of consciousness	
	Ketoacidosis; air hunger, acetone breath odor, respirations deep and rapid, nausea, vomiting	No ketosis, no breath odor, respirations rapid and shallow, usually mild nausea/vomiting
Laboratory Tests		
Glucose	>250 mg/dl	>600 mg/dl
Ketones	Strongly positive	Normal or mildly elevated
pH	<7.3	Normal*
Osmolarity	<350 mOsm/L	>350 mOsm/L
Sodium	Normal or low	Normal or elevated
Potassium (K^+)	Normal, low (total body K^+ depleted), or elevated	Low, normal, or elevated
Bicarbonate	<18 mEq/L	>15 mEq/L
Phosphorus	Low, normal, or elevated (may decrease after insulin therapy)	Low, normal, or elevated (may decrease after insulin therapy)
Urine acetone	Strong	None, or mild

*Except if lactic acidosis develops. With severe HHS, lactic acidosis may result from dehydration and severe tissue hypoperfusion and ischemia.

is released, and additional glucose is added to the bloodstream. Unless the glycemic diuresis cycle is broken by aggressive fluid replacement and insulin, intracellular dehydration negatively affects fluid and oxygen transport to the brain cells. Central nervous system dysfunction may result and lead to coma. Hemoconcentration increases the blood viscosity, which may result in clot formation, thromboemboli, and cerebral, cardiac, and pleural infarcts.

Assessment and Diagnosis

Clinical Manifestations

HHS has a slow, subtle onset and develops over several days. Initially the symptoms may be nonspecific and may be ignored or attributed to the patient's concurrent disease processes. History reveals malaise, blurred vision, polyuria, polydipsia (depending on patient's thirst sensation), weight loss, and advancing weakness.[50] Medical attention may not be obtained for these nonspecific, nonacute symptoms until the patient is unable to take sufficient fluids to offset the fluid losses. Progressive dehydration follows and leads to mental confusion, convulsions, and eventually coma, especially in the elderly.

The physical examination may reveal a profound fluid deficit. Signs of severe dehydration include longitudinal wrinkles in the tongue, decreased salivation, and decreased CVP, with increases in HR and rapid respirations (Kussmaul air hunger is not present). In elderly patients, assessment of clinical signs of dehydration is challenging. Neurologic status is affected as the serum glucose level climbs, especially above 1500 mg/dl. Without intervention, obtundation, coma, and death will occur.

Laboratory Studies

Laboratory findings are used to establish the definitive diagnosis of HHS. Plasma glucose levels are strikingly elevated with blood glucose above 600 mg/dl. Serum osmolarity is generally above 320 mOsm/L. Acidosis is absent with an arterial pH above 7.3, a serum bicarbonate greater than 15 mEq/L, and absent or mild ketonuria.[49-51] Elevated hematocrit and depleted serum potassium and phosphorus levels may also be noted.

Point-of-care finger stick or arterial catheter with a blood conservation system attached is used to facilitate frequent testing of blood glucose level at the bedside. Insulin replacement is then prescribed according to the blood glucose result. Some electrolytes also can be tested at the bedside (potassium, sodium, ionized calcium) and generally require an arterial line for frequent blood access. If point-of-care testing is not available, traditional serial laboratory tests keep the

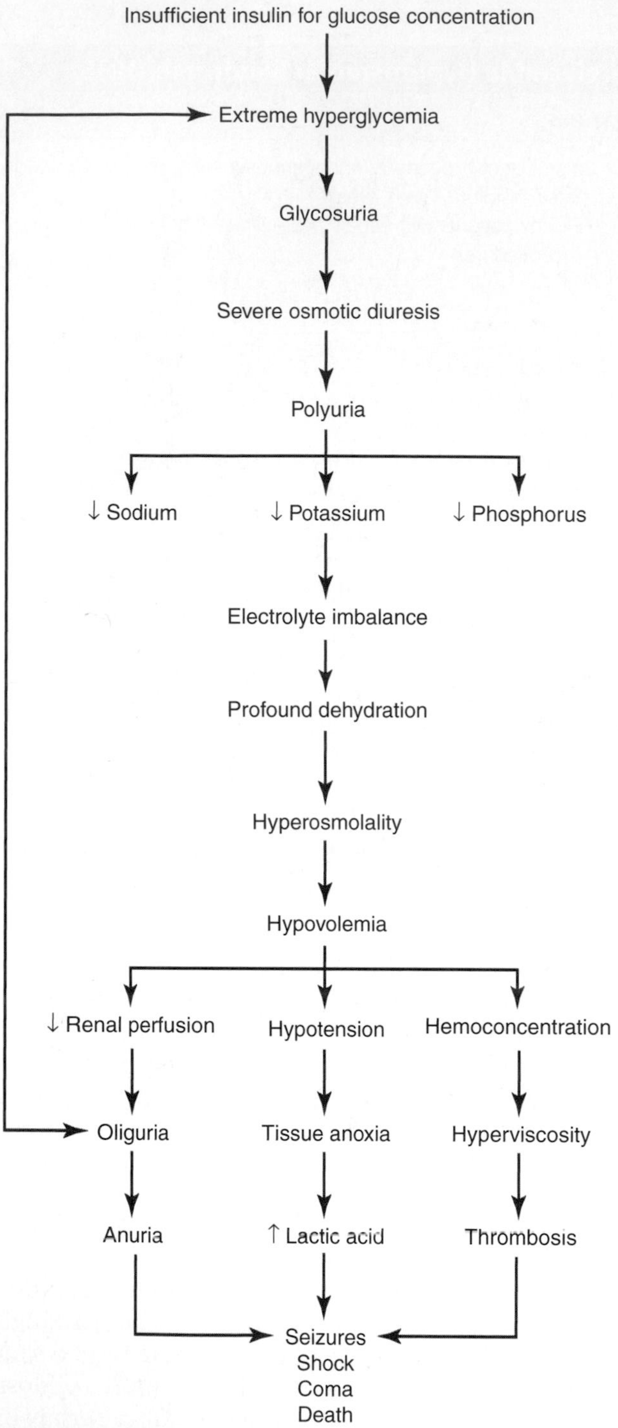

FIGURE 24-4. Pathophysiology of hyperglycemic hyperosmolar syndrome (HHS).

clinician apprised of the fluctuating serum electrolyte levels and provide the basis for electrolyte replacement. Intracellular potassium and phosphate levels usually are depleted as a result of dehydration.[49]

Elevated BUN and creatinine levels suggest kidney impairment as a result of the severe reduction in renal circulation. Metabolic acidosis usually is absent at lower glucose levels. Acidosis may result from starvation ketosis or an increase in lactic acid production secondary to poor tissue perfusion.

Medical Management

The goals of medical management are rapid rehydration, insulin replacement, and correction of electrolyte abnormalities, specifically potassium replacement. The underlying stimulus of HHS must be discovered and treated. The same basic principles used to treat DKA are used for the patient with HHS.

Rapid Rehydration

The primary intervention for HHS is rapid rehydration to restore intravascular volume. The average 150-pound adult can lose more than 7 L of fluid. The total body deficit of sodium and potassium may be as high as 500 to 700 mEq.[49] Physiologic saline solution (0.9%) is infused at 1 L/hr, especially for the patient in hypovolemic shock.[49] The patient may need replacement of 6 to 10 L of fluid in the first 10 hours to achieve a BP and CVP within normal range.

Serum sodium is the parameter that is monitored to determine when to change from isotonic (0.9%) to hypotonic (0.45%) saline. For example, patients with sodium levels below 140 mEq/L receive 0.9% normal saline solution. Patients with levels equal to or greater than 140 mEq/L receive 0.45% saline solution as shown in Figure 24-5. In reality it is difficult to assess serum sodium in the presence of hemoconcentration. Another recommendation is to calculate a *corrected sodium value.* To correct serum sodium in hyperglycemia, for each 100 mg/dl glucose greater than 100 mg/dl, add 1.6 mEq to the sodium value for the corrected serum sodium value.[49,50] Sodium input should not exceed the amount required to replace the losses. Careful monitoring of serum sodium is recommended to avoid a sodium-water imbalance and hemolysis as the hemoconcentration is gradually reduced.[53]

To prevent hypoglycemia, when the serum glucose level falls to the 200 to 250 mg/dl range, the hydrating solution is changed to 5% dextrose in water—0.45% saline solution (D_5W—0.45% NaCl) at 150 to 250 ml/hr.[49]

Insulin Administration

Volume resuscitation will lower serum glucose levels and improve symptoms even without insulin.[50] However, insulin replacement is recommended to treat HHS because of clinical reports that acidosis can develop when insulin is withheld.[50] Insulin is given to facilitate the cellular use of glucose.

Methods to lower the glucose level vary. One method is initially to administer an IV bolus of regular insulin (0.1 unit per kg body weight), followed by a continuous insulin drip. Regular insulin infusing at an initial rate calculated as 0.1 unit/kg/hour (7 units/hr for

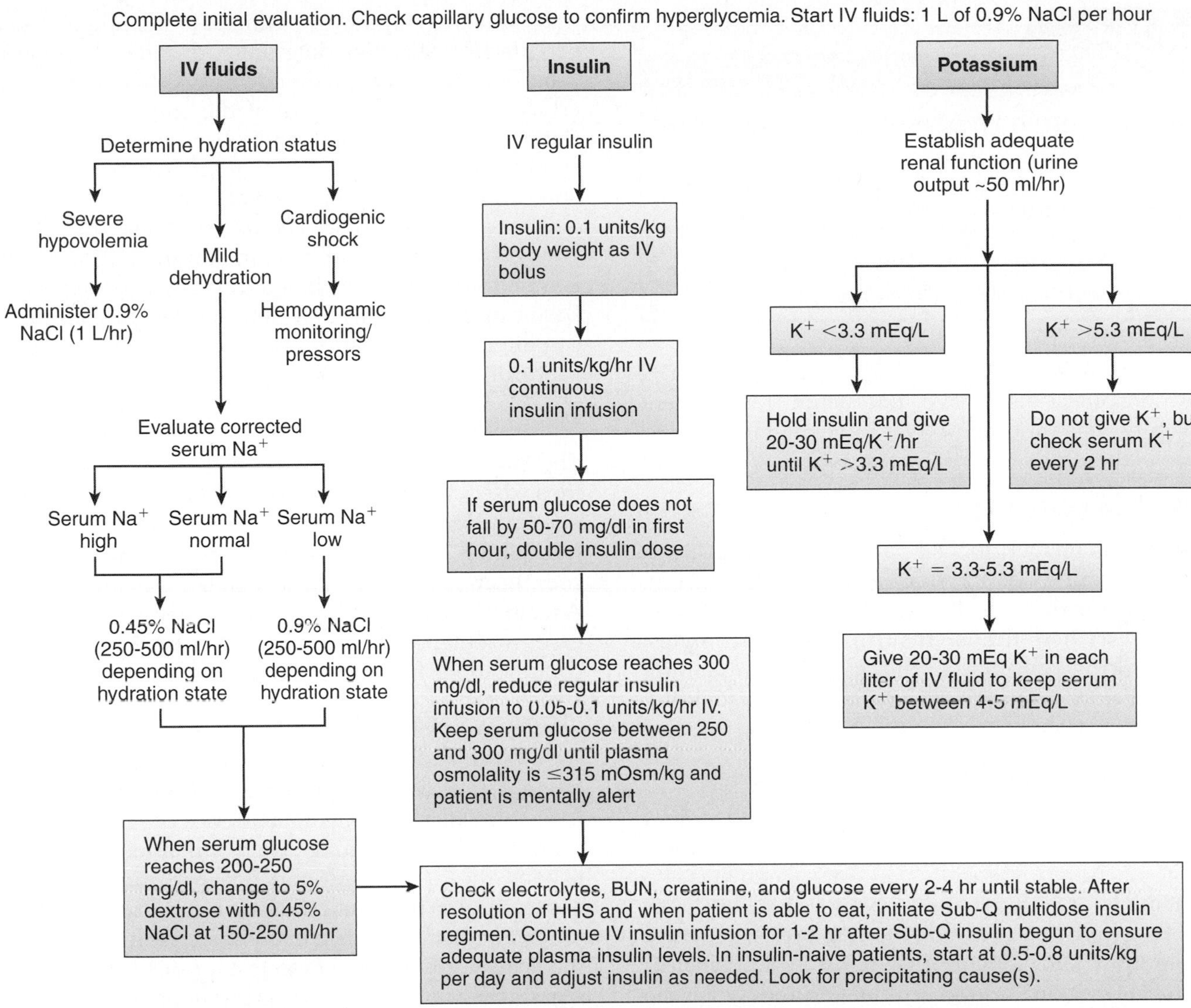
Complete initial evaluation. Check capillary glucose to confirm hyperglycemia. Start IV fluids: 1 L of 0.9% NaCl per hour
IV fluids
Insulin
Potassium
Determine hydration status
Severe hypovolemia
Mild dehydration
Cardiogenic shock
Administer 0.9% NaCl (1 L/hr)
Hemodynamic monitoring/ pressors
Evaluate corrected serum Na+
Serum Na+ high
Serum Na+ normal
Serum Na+ low
0.45% NaCl (250-500 ml/hr) depending on hydration state
0.9% NaCl (250-500 ml/hr) depending on hydration state
When serum glucose reaches 200-250 mg/dl, change to 5% dextrose with 0.45% NaCl at 150-250 ml/hr
IV regular insulin
Insulin: 0.1 units/kg body weight as IV bolus
0.1 units/kg/hr IV continuous insulin infusion
If serum glucose does not fall by 50-70 mg/dl in first hour, double insulin dose
When serum glucose reaches 300 mg/dl, reduce regular insulin infusion to 0.05-0.1 units/kg/hr IV. Keep serum glucose between 250 and 300 mg/dl until plasma osmolality is ≤315 mOsm/kg and patient is mentally alert
Establish adequate renal function (urine output ~50 ml/hr)
K+ <3.3 mEq/L
K+ >5.3 mEq/L
Hold insulin and give 20-30 mEq/K+/hr until K+ >3.3 mEq/L
Do not give K+, but check serum K+ every 2 hr
K+ = 3.3-5.3 mEq/L
Give 20-30 mEq K+ in each liter of IV fluid to keep serum K+ between 4-5 mEq/L
Check electrolytes, BUN, creatinine, and glucose every 2-4 hr until stable. After resolution of HHS and when patient is able to eat, initiate Sub-Q multidose insulin regimen. Continue IV insulin infusion for 1-2 hr after Sub-Q insulin begun to ensure adequate plasma insulin levels. In insulin-naive patients, start at 0.5-0.8 units/kg per day and adjust insulin as needed. Look for precipitating cause(s).

FIGURE 24-5. Protocol for the management of adult patients with hyperglycemic hyperosmolar syndrome (HHS). (From Kitabchi AE et al: *Diabetes Care* 29[12]:2739, 2006).

a person weighing 70 kg) should lower the plasma glucose by 50 to 70 mg/dl in the first hour of treatment.[49] If the measured glucose does not decrease by this amount, the insulin infusion rate may be doubled until the blood glucose is declining at a rate of 50 to 70 mg/dl per hour.[49]

When the serum glucose reaches 300 mg/dl, the regular insulin infusion is reduced to 0.5 to 1 unit/kg/hr to maintain the serum glucose level between 250 and 300 mg/dl until the serum osmolarity is below 315 mOsm/L and the person is mentally alert.[49]

Insulin Resistance. Patients with HHS have underlying type 2 diabetes; many will have metabolic syndrome and exhibit signs of *insulin resistance.*[38] In critical illness the presence of *counterregulatory hormones,* also known as *stress hormones* (cortisol, glucagon, growth hormone, epinephrine), will both increase glucose production and induce insulin resistance.[50] Patients with HHS may require very high doses of insulin to overcome the hyperglycemia and insulin resistance.[50] Hourly serial monitoring of the blood glucose will permit safe glycemic management and avoid the most common complication, which is hypoglycemia.[49] Once the patient is over the hyperglycemic crisis and the insulin is discontinued, oral agents designed to decrease insulin resistance in type 2 diabetics will be prescribed (see Table 24-3).

Electrolyte Replacement

Increasing the circulating levels of insulin with therapeutic doses of IV insulin will promote the rapid return of potassium and phosphorus into the cell. Serial laboratory tests keep the clinician apprised of the serum electrolyte levels and provide the basis for electrolyte replacement. Potassium is typically added to the IV infusion as shown in Figure 24-5. If the serum potassium level is below 3.3 mEq/L, it is essential to replenish the serum potassium before giving insulin.[49]

Box 24-6

NURSING DIAGNOSIS PRIORITIES

Hyperglycemic Hyperosmolar Syndrome

- Decreased Cardiac Output related to alterations in preload, p. A-12
- Deficient Fluid Volume related to absolute loss, p. A-16
- Anxiety related to threat to biologic, psychologic, and/or social integrity, p. A-9
- Deficient Knowledge: Discharge Regimen related to previous lack of exposure to information, p. A-18

Many hospitals also have potassium replacement algorithms that are used to treat hypokalemia.

Nursing Management

Nursing management of the patient with HHS incorporates a variety of nursing diagnoses (Box 24-6). **Nursing priorities are directed toward (1) administering prescribed fluids, insulin, and electrolytes; (2) monitoring response to therapy; (3) maintaining surveillance for complications; and (4) providing patient education.**

Administering Fluids, Insulin, and Electrolytes

Rigorous fluid replacement and continuous IV insulin replacement must be controlled with an electronic volumetric pump. Accurate I&O measurements are maintained to monitor fluid balance. I&O includes the total of all IV fluids and hourly losses, typically urine output and sometimes emesis. Hemodynamic monitoring may include an arterial line and CVP if the patient manifests signs of hypovolemic shock. Arterial line access is very helpful to monitor serial blood glucose and electrolyte values. The use of a blood conservation system on the arterial line is essential to avoid iatrogenic exsanguination of the patient. Most critical care units have developed protocols or guidelines to ensure that patients in hyperglycemic crisis are managed safely (see Figure 24-3). The major responsibility for delivery of insulin, hourly monitoring of blood glucose, and infusion of appropriate crystalloid solutions is with the critical care nurse. Many hospitals mandate a "double check" for medications such as insulin and potassium that have the potential to cause harm if wrongly administered.

Monitoring Response to Therapy

The BP, HR, and CVP are monitored to evaluate the degree of dehydration, the effectiveness of hydration therapy, and the patient's fluid tolerance. Because patients with HHS have underlying type 2 diabetes, many have preexisting illnesses such as heart failure and renal failure. Thus, it is important to monitor for symptoms of circulatory overload in susceptible individuals. Symptoms to anticipate include elevated CVP, tachycardia, bounding pulse, dyspnea, tachypnea, lung crackles, and engorged neck veins. The astute critical care nurse is aware of the clinical manifestations of fluid overload and observes for potential complications when rehydrating the patient with HHS and cardiac, pulmonary, or renal disease.

The serum glucose should decrease by 50 to 70 mg/dl per hour with insulin administration.[49] This is monitored by hourly blood glucose determinations. Based upon the glucose value the critical care nurse can alter the infusion of insulin based upon hospital protocol (see Figure 24-5).

Maintaining Surveillance for Complications

The potential complications in HHS are similar to those described in the previous section on DKA: hypoglycemia, hypokalemia or hyperkalemia, and infection. In addition, the patient with HHS is at risk for other complications specific to associated disease entities. A history of cardiovascular, pulmonary, or kidney disease, whether known or latent, creates a high risk of complications for HHS patients.

Providing Patient Education

As the patient's condition improves and the patient demonstrates readiness to learn, education about type 2 diabetes and avoiding a recurrence of HHS becomes a priority. Most teaching will occur after the patient has left the critical care unit. Teaching topics include a description of type 2 diabetes and how it relates to HHS, dietary restrictions, exercise requirements, medication protocols, home testing of blood glucose, signs and symptoms of hyperglycemia and hypoglycemia, foot care, and lifestyle modifications if cardiovascular disease is present.[53]

Collaborative Management

Because HHS is an acute condition superimposed upon the chronic health problem of type 2 diabetes, many health professionals provide care and work collaboratively to restore homeostasis for each patient as described in Evidence-Based Collaborative Practice: Hyperglycemic Hyperosmolar Syndrome.

DIABETES INSIPIDUS

Diabetes insipidus (DI) is recognized by the vast quantities of very dilute urine that are produced in susceptible patients. In the critically ill patient the extreme diuresis is most likely to be due to a lack of ADH. Any patient with head trauma or after neurosurgery incurs an increased risk of developing DI. Physiologically ADH is primarily released in response to even small elevations in serum osmolarity and secondarily in reaction to hypovolemia or hypotension.[54] ADH is also

EVIDENCE-BASED COLLABORATIVE PRACTICE

Hyperglycemic Hyperosmolar Syndrome

Summary of evidence and evidence-based recommendations for controlling symptoms related to hyperglycemic hyperosmolar syndrome (HHS)

Strong Evidence to Support the Following:

- Regular insulin by continuous infusion is recommended to normalize blood glucose level to 80 to 110 mg/dl (euglycemic levels).
- Replace serum phosphate if level is below 1 mg/dl.
- A multidisciplinary team approach to care reduces length of stay and improves clinical outcomes.
- Close follow-up after discharge is recommended to maintain hemoglobin A_{1c} below 7% and prevent diabetes-related complications.

Weak Evidence to Support the Following:

- Use of a "sliding insulin scale" alone is discouraged because it is associated with both hyperglycemia and hypoglycemia in hospitalized patients.

Data from Kitabchi AE et al: *Diabetes Care* 29(12):2739, 2006; Garber AJ et al: *Endocr Pract* 10(suppl 2):4, 2004; and Clement S et al: *Diabetes Care* 27(2):553, 2004.

Box 24-7

Etiology of Diabetes Insipidus

Central Diabetes Insipidus
Primary (Rare in Critical Care)
ADH deficiency from hypothalamic-hypophyseal malformation
- Congenital defect
- Idiopathic

Secondary (Most Common in Critical Care)
ADH deficiency from damage to the hypothalamic-hypophyseal system
- Trauma
- Infection
- Surgery
- Primary neoplasms
- Metastatic malignancies

Nephrogenic Diabetes Insipidus
Inability of kidney tubules to respond to circulating ADH
- Decrease or absence of ADH receptors
- Cellular damage to nephron, especially loop of Henle
- Kidney damage (e.g., hydronephrosis, pyelonephritis, polycystic kidney)
- Untoward response to drug therapy (e.g., lithium carbonate, demeclocycline)

Psychogenic Diabetes Insipidus
Rare form of water intoxication
- Compulsive water drinking

ADH, Antidiuretic hormone.

known by the name *vasopressin*.[55] DI can occur at any one of the physiologic steps listed below[55]:

- The hypothalamus produces insufficient ADH.
- The posterior pituitary fails to release ADH.
- The kidney nephron is resistant (unresponsive) to ADH.

Etiology

DI is categorized into three types according to cause: central, nephrogenic, and psychogenic (Box 24-7). Only central DI, also known as neurogenic DI because of the association with the brain, is encountered with any frequency in the critical care unit.

Central Diabetes Insipidus

In central diabetes insipidus, there is an inability to secrete an adequate amount of vasopressin in response to osmotic or nonosmotic stimuli, resulting in inappropriately dilute urine.[56] Either the synthesis of ADH is incomplete in the hypothalamus or the release of ADH from the pituitary is interrupted. Central DI can be congenital or idiopathic, but this is not typically seen in critical care. The most likely acute cause of central DI is secondary to neurosurgery, traumatic head injury,[57] tumors,[58] increased intracranial pressure (ICP), brain death, and infections such as encephalitis or meningitis.[56] In patients undergoing surgery on the pituitary gland, DI occurs in approximately 12% of patients and is permanent in 3%.[59] The degree of hormone replacement required following surgery is dependent on the quantity of pituitary tissue that is removed.[59] One clinical study reported the incidence of central DI to be almost 3% in patients with traumatic brain injury (TBI).[57]

Nephrogenic Diabetes Insipidus

Nephrogenic DI results from the inability of the kidney nephrons to respond to circulating ADH.[60] Nephrogenic DI is a rare disorder that occurs in the setting of kidney disease when V_2-receptors on the kidney tubule become nonresponsive to the action of ADH. Some drugs cause nephrogenic DI by decreasing the responsiveness of the kidney tubules to ADH. Long-term use of lithium carbonate, prescribed for bipolar disorder, is a frequent culprit.[60,61]

Psychogenic Diabetes Insipidus

Psychogenic DI is a rare form of the disease that occurs with compulsive drinking of more than 5 L of water a day. Long-standing psychogenic DI closely mimics nephrogenic DI because the kidney tubules become less responsive to ADH as a result of prolonged conditioning to hypotonic urine. It is uncommon to see this in the critical care unit.

PATHOPHYSIOLOGY

The purpose of ADH is to maintain normal serum osmolarity and circulating blood volume. Normally ADH binds to the V_2-receptors on the kidney collecting tubules, causing insertion of water channels known as *aquaporins*, along the luminal surface.[54] Even small (1% to 2%) increases in plasma osmolarlity are sufficient to stimulate ADH release.[54] Although there are several types of DI, this discussion focuses on neurogenic central DI, the condition encountered in the critical care unit following neurosurgery or head injury[57] (Figure 24-6).

In DI as free water is eliminated, the urine, osmolarity, and specific gravity decrease (dilute urine). By contrast, in the bloodstream, serum sodium level and serum osmolarity rise.[55] Normally, when the serum osmolarlity rises above 290 mOsm/L (290 mmol/L), this triggers the synthesis and release of ADH.[54] At 295 mOsm/L the thirst sensors are activated in the hypothalamus.[54] In central DI, however, no ADH is released, or the ADH released is insufficient. Without ADH, the kidney collecting tubules are incapable of concentrating urine and retaining water.

As the extracellular dehydration ensues, hypotension and hypovolemic shock occur. If the person is alert, extreme thirst will permit the individual to replace lost fluids by drinking lots of water. This excessive intake of water reduces the serum osmolarity to a more normal level and prevents dehydration. In the person with decreased level of consciousness, the polyuria leads to severe hypernatremia, dehydration, decreased cerebral perfusion, seizures, loss of consciousness, and death.

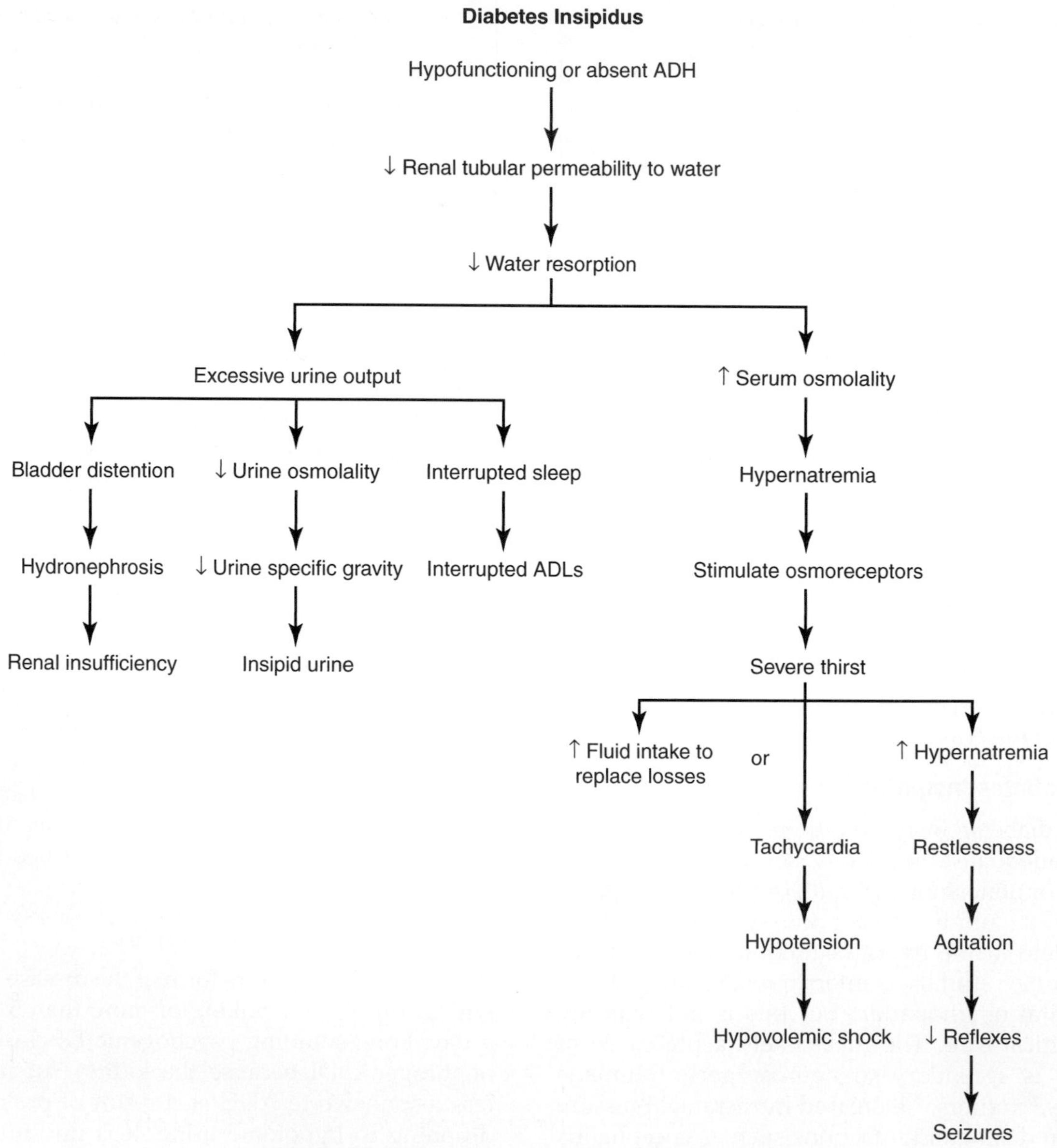

FIGURE 24-6. Pathophysiology of diabetes insipidus (DI).

Assessment and Diagnosis

Clinical Manifestations

The clinical diagnosis is made by the dramatic increase in dilute urine output in the absence of diuretics, a fluid challenge, or hyperglycemia. Central DI is anticipated in conditions where the underlying disease process is likely to disrupt pituitary function. If central DI occurs because of increasing ICP, this is life-threatening. It is imperative that the underlying condition be recognized and treated appropriately. In this situation medications that treat DI are not sufficient.

Laboratory Studies

The core diagnostic tests used to establish the presence of DI that evaluate the body's ability to balance fluid and electrolytes are not specific to the endocrine system. The most common tests are serum sodium level, serum osmolarity, and urine osmolarity (Table 24-5). In combination with an obvious clinical picture the presence of these three laboratory criteria is sufficient to diagnose central DI:

- Serum sodium level above 145 mEq/L
- Serum osmolarity above 295 mOsm/L (mmol/L)
- Urine osmolarity below 300 mOsm/L (mmol/L)

Serum Sodium. The normal serum sodium level is 140 mEq/L (range 135 to 145 mEq/L). In central DI the serum sodium level can rise precipitously due to the loss of free water. Hypernatremia is always associated with serum hyperosmolarity.[62]

Serum Osmolarity Test. Bedside calculation of osmotic activity, using the patient's laboratory data, is typically expressed in solution (osmolarity) as milliosmoles per liter (mOsm/L). The bedside calculation is described in Chapter 19. Serum osmolarity has a narrow normal range, 275 to 295 mOsm/L. Severe DI can raise serum osmolarity to greater than 320 mOsm/L.[54]

Urine Osmolarity. Urine osmolarity is low, below 300 mOsm/L (mmol/L) in patients with central DI. For greatest accuracy the urine sample should be collected and tested simultaneously with the blood sample. Normal urine ADH ranges from 500 to 1400 mOsm/L, although this will vary with fluid intake and hydration status.

Measurement of ADH. Measurement of the baseline serum ADH level is an additional diagnostic step. This is not always performed in critical care when the clinical circumstances (e.g., head injury with raised ICP) make further testing unnecessary. Normal ADH levels range from 1 to 5 pg/ml. Most hydrated people have a morning fasting serum level below 4 pg/ml.[63] ADH tests are rarely performed in the ICU because of the risk of causing hemodynamic instability.

In a stable patient exogenous ADH (vasopressin) may be administered to test for the underlying cause of the DI. An ADH plasma concentration of approximately 1 pg/ml will increase urinary concentration and decrease urine flow. Maximum antidiuresis occurs at an ADH (vasopressin) concentration of approximately 5 pg/ml.[56] ADH administration is used to distinguish between central DI and nephrogenic DI. If 1 mcg Sub-Q of desmopressin is administered, the following responses are diagnostic[62]:

- Urine output greatly decreased in response to ADH administration is diagnostic for central DI.
- Urine output unchanged in response to ADH administration suggests nephrogenic DI.

MEDICAL MANAGEMENT

Immediate management of the patient in DI requires an aggressive approach. Treatment goals include restoration of circulating fluid volume, pharmacologic ADH replacement, plus treatment of the underlying condition.

Volume Restoration

Fluid replacement is provided in the initial phase of the treatment to prevent circulatory collapse. Patients who are able to drink are given voluminous amounts of fluid orally to balance output. For those unable to take sufficient fluids orally, hypotonic IV solutions are rapidly infused and carefully monitored to restore the hemodynamic balance. The amount of fluid lost can be estimated, based on normal fluid stores and body weight, using the following formula:

$$0.6\ (\text{kg wt}) \times (\text{Serum sodium} - 140) \div 140 = \text{Total body water deficit in liters}$$

Table 24-5

Laboratory Values for Patients With DI and SIADH

Serum ADH	1-5 pg/ml	*Central DI:* decreased serum ADH level.	Elevated ADH level
Serum osmolarity	275-295 mOsm/L*	>295 mOsm/L*	<270 mOsm/L
Serum sodium	135-145 mEq/L	>145 mEq/L	<120 mEq/L
Urine osmolarity	300-1400 mOsm/L	<300 mOsm/L	Increased
Urine specific gravity	1.005-1.030	<1.005	>1.030
Urine output	1.0-1.5 L/day	1.0-1.5 L/hr	Below normal

*Some hospitals use 280-300 mOsm/L as their normal reference value.

DI, Diabetes insipidus; *SIADH,* syndrome of inappropriate antidiuretic hormone; *ADH,* antidiuretic hormone.

For example, the total body water deficit for a patient in DI with a serum sodium level of 160 mEq/L who weighs 135 kg is calculated as follows:

$$(0.6 \times 135 \text{ kg}) \times (160 - 140) \div 140 = \text{Total body water deficit in liters}$$

$$81 \times 20 \div 140 = 11.57 \text{ L water deficit}$$

The formula assumes that 60% of an individual's weight is fluid, although this is not always exact. The calculated liters of body water deficit can be used for planning replacement fluids to restore hemodynamic stability.

Medications

Central DI requires immediate pharmacologic management.[55] The most frequently prescribed medications used to treat the various forms of DI are shown in Table 24-6.

Medications Used for Central Diabetes Insipidus. Patients with central DI who are unable to synthesize ADH require replacement ADH *(vasopressin)* or an ADH analog. The most commonly prescribed drug is the synthetic analog of ADH, *desmopressin* (DDAVP). It is preferred over vasopressin (Pitressin) because it has a stronger antidiuretic action with little effect on

Table 24-6

Pharmacologic Management of Diabetes Insipidus

DRUG	DOSAGE	ACTIONS	SPECIAL CONSIDERATIONS
Central Diabetes Insipidus			
Desmopressin acetate (DDAVP available IV, as nasal spray, rhinal tube, rhinyle drops; Stimate)	Nasal: 10-40 mcg at bedtime or in divided doses Parenteral*: 2-4 mcg twice daily	*Central diabetes insipidus (DI)* Antidiuretic Increases water resorption in nephron Prevents and controls polydipsia, polyuria	Few side effects Observe for nasal congestion, upper respiratory infection, allergic rhinitis Monitor intake/output, urine osmolarity, serum sodium
Vasopressin (Pitressin Synthetic, Pressyn)	Intramuscular, intravenous, subcutaneous, intraarterial Topical: nasal mucosa	*Central DI* Antidiuretic Promotes resorption of water at kidney tubule Decreases urine output Increases urine osmolarity Diagnostic aid Increases gastrointestinal peristalsis	Monitor fluid volume often, especially in elderly patients Assess cardiac status May precipitate angina, hypertension, or myocardial infarction if increased dose given to patient with cardiac history Parenteral extravasation may cause skin necrosis
Lypressin (Diapid)	Intranasal: 1-2 sprays (7-14 mcg) each nostril 4 times daily	*Central DI* Synthetic antidiuretic hormone Increases resorption of sodium and water in nephron	Proper instillation important for absorption and action Patient sits upright while holding bottle upright for administration Repeat sprays (>2-3) ineffective, wasteful; if dose increased to 2-3 sprays, shorten time between dosing Cough, chest tightness, shortness of breath
Nephrogenic Diabetes Insipidus			
Thiazide diuretics	Varies according to diuretic chosen, patient's size and age	*Nephrogenic DI* Leads to mild fluid depletion Increased water/sodium resorbed in proximal nephron; less fluid travels to distal nephron, excreting less water	Varies according to diuretic chosen
Psychogenic Diabetes Insipidus			
Anti–compulsive disorder drugs, anxiolytics, psychopharmacologic agents; dosage varies	*Psychogenic DI*	Varies according to medication chosen	

*Parenteral indicates intravenous or subcutaneous.
IV, Intravenous.

blood pressure. DDAVP can be given IV, Sub-Q, or as a nasal spray. A typical DDAVP dose is 1 to 2 mcg IV or Sub-Q every 12 hours.[64] Sometimes only 0.5 mcg IV is used. The dosage is subsequently titrated according to the patient's antidiuretic response to the drug. In order to avoid a medication error it is important to be aware that DDAVP is also used to control hemorrhage caused by platelet disorders and that the dose ranges for all of these conditions are different.[64]

Vasopressin (Pitressin) 5 to 10 units intramuscularly (IM) every 3 to 4 hours will produce a reduction in urine output.[64] Vasopressin acts on the V_1-receptors in vascular smooth muscle and can elevate systemic blood pressure. Water intoxication also can occur if the dosage is higher than the therapeutic level. Because of the risk of hypertension this is not typically the first drug of choice for treating central DI.

Clinicians must be aware that vasopressin is also prescribed in septic shock states as an IV infusion, and in cardiac arrest, IV push.[65,66] Dosages for these conditions are very different from the dosage used to treat central DI. Extreme care must be taken to ensure that all drug dosages are accurate for each specific diagnosis.

Medications Used for Nephrogenic Diabetes Insipidus. The mainstay of therapy is to stop any medications that are inducing the ADH resistance. Nephrogenic DI is treated with hydrochlorothiazide 12.5 to 25 mg administered 1 or 2 times per day. The dosage is titrated according to the patient's antidiuretic response.

Nursing Management

Nursing management of the patient with diabetes insipidus incorporates a variety of nursing diagnoses (Box 24-8). Nursing priorities are directed toward **(1) administering fluids and medications, (2) evaluating response to therapy, (3) maintaining surveillance for complications, and (5) providing patient education.**

Administrating Fluids and Medications

Rapid IV fluid replacement requires the use of a volumetric pump. Initially a hypotonic IV solution is used to replace fluids lost and lower the serum hyperosmolality. ADH replacement is accomplished with extreme caution in the patient with a history of cardiac disease because ADH may cause hypertension and overhydration. At the first signs of cardiovascular impairment, the drug is discontinued and fluid intake restricted until urine specific gravity is less than 1.015 and polyuria resumes.

Evaluating Response to Therapy

Critical assessment and management of the fluid status are the most important initial concerns for the patient with DI. Monitoring of HR, BP, CVP, and pulmonary artery (PA) pressures (if PA catheter in place) provide early indications of response to fluid volume replacement. I&O measurement, condition of buccal membranes, skin turgor, daily weight measurements, presence of thirst, and temperature provide a basic assessment list that is vital for the patient unable to regulate fluid needs and losses. Placement of a urinary catheter is essential to accurate monitoring of the urinary output. Simultaneous urine and blood specimens for osmolarity, sodium, and potassium levels are collected and results relayed to the physician as necessary. The patient who is unable to satisfy sensations of thirst or to complete any task or self-care activity without the need to urinate may be confused and frightened. For patients who are able to verbalize their fears, having a caring nurse who is interested and nonjudgmental will help reduce the emotional turmoil associated with their condition.

Maintaining Surveillance for Complications

The most dangerous potential complication is hypertension and vasospasm of cardiac cerebral or mesenteric arterial vessels secondary to vasopressin (Pitressin) replacement. In most cases, DDAVP will be the ADH replacement selected to avoid this complication. A less serious complication from DI is constipation from fluid loss, treated with dietary fiber, stool softeners, or both. Conversely, diarrhea, abdominal cramping, and intestinal hyperactivity may accompany vasopressin therapy. Untoward effects can be mitigated by modification of the vasopressin dose.

Providing Patient Education

Educating the patient and the family about the disease process and how it affects thirst, urination, and fluid balance will encourage patients to participate in their care. For most critical care patients central DI is a temporary condition that resolves as the underlying medical condition, such as cerebral edema, improves. Patients who are discharged with DI are taught, along with their families, the signs and symptoms of dehydration and overhydration and procedures for accurate daily weight and urine specific gravity measurement. Printed information pertaining to drug actions, side

Box 24-8

NURSING DIAGNOSIS PRIORITIES

Diabetes Insipidus

- Deficient Fluid Volume related to compromised regulatory mechanism, p. A-16
- Decreased Cardiac Output related to alterations in preload, p. A-12
- Anxiety related to threat to biologic, psychologic, and/or social integrity, p. A-9
- Deficient Knowledge: Discharge Regimen related to lack of previous exposure to information, p. A-18

effects, dosages, and timetable is provided, as well as an outline of factors that must be reported to the physician.

Collaborative Management

Central DI is a life-threatening condition. The collaborative assessment and clinical skills of all health care professionals with a clear plan of care is essential to achieving optimal outcomes for each patient.

SYNDROME OF INAPPROPRIATE ANTIDIURETIC HORMONE

The opposing syndrome to DI is the syndrome of inappropriate antidiuretic hormone (SIADH). The patient with SIADH has an excess of ADH secreted into the bloodstream, more than the amount needed to maintain normal blood volume and serum osmolarity. Excessive water is resorbed at the kidney tubule, leading to dilutional hyponatremia.

Etiology

Numerous causes of SIADH are observed in patients who are critically ill (Box 24-9). Central nervous system injury, tumors, or diseases interfering with the normal functioning of the hypothalamic-pituitary system can cause SIADH. A common cause is malignant bronchogenic small cell carcinoma. This type of malignant cell is capable of synthesizing and releasing ADH regardless of the body's needs.[67] With much less frequency, other cancers that involve the brain, head and neck, gastrointestinal, gynecologic, and hematologic systems are capable of autonomous production of ADH.[54]

Some commonly used drugs may also cause SIADH. The thiazide diuretics are one such group.[68] Another group is the selective serotonin reuptake inhibitors (SSRIs), such as citalopram (Celexa), fluoxetine (Prozac), paroxetine (Paxil), and sertraline (Zoloft), which are used to treat depression and other conditions.[68,69] These drugs cause SIADH with hyponatremia in about 1% of patients.[69] Levels of ADH also rise with use of positive-pressure ventilators that decrease venous return to the thorax, simultaneously stimulating pulmonary baroreceptors to release more ADH.

Pathophysiology

ADH (arginine vasopressin) is a powerful, complex polypeptide. When released into the circulation by the posterior pituitary gland, ADH regulates water and electrolyte balance in the body. In SIADH, profound fluid and electrolyte disturbances result from the unsolicited, continuous release of the hormone into the bloodstream (Figure 24-7). Excessive ADH stimulates the kidney tubules to retain fluid regardless of need. This results in severe overhydration and dilutional hyponatremia.

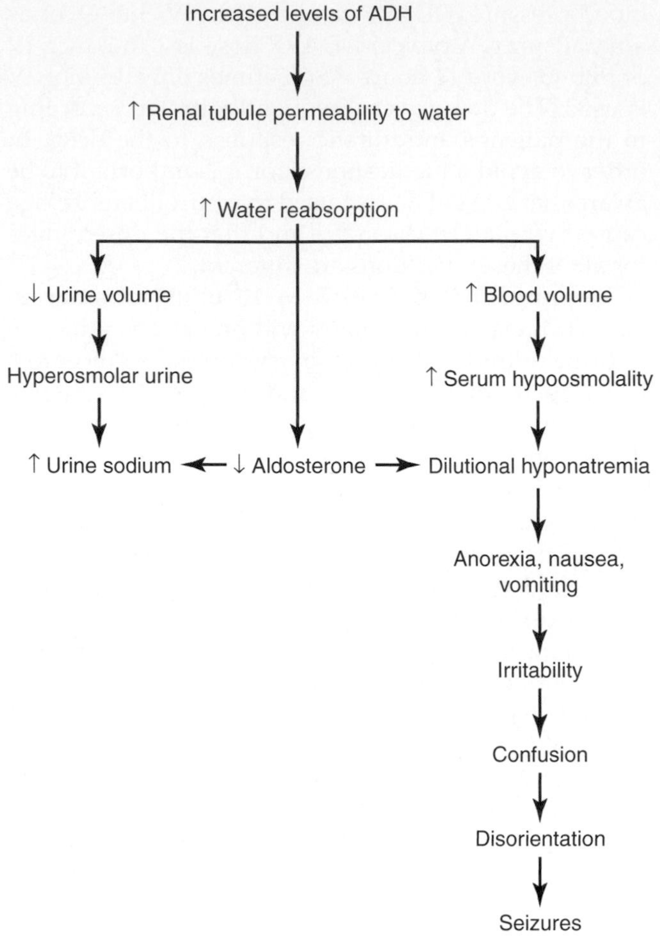

FIGURE 24-7. Pathophysiology of syndrome of inappropriate antidiuretic hormone (SIADH).

Excessive ADH dramatically alters the sodium balance in the extracellular vascular compartment. The increased circulating volume causes a dilutional hyponatremia and reduces the sodium concentration to critically low levels.[68] In the healthy adult, hyponatremia inhibits the release of ADH; however, in SIADH the increased levels of circulating ADH are unrelated to the serum sodium. Aldosterone production from the adrenal glands is also suppressed. Serum hypoosmolarity leads to a shift of fluid from the extracellular fluid space into the intracellular fluid compartment (inside the cells) in an attempt to equalize osmotic pressure. Because minimal sodium is present in this fluid, edema usually does not result. The urine has an increased osmolarity from the decreased water excretion. It is believed that despite the serum hyponatremia, the increased release of ADH promotes sodium loss through the kidneys into the urine.

Box 24-9

Etiology of Syndrome of Inappropriate Antidiuretic Hormone (SIADH)

- *Malignant disease* associated with autonomous production of ADH
  - Bronchogenic small cell carcinoma
  - Pancreatic adenocarcinoma
  - Duodenal, bladder, ureter, prostatic carcinomas
  - Lymphosarcoma, Ewing's sarcoma
  - Acute leukemia, Hodgkin's disease
  - Cerebral neoplasm, thymoma
- *Central nervous system diseases* that interfere with the hypothalamic-hypophyseal system and increase the production and/or release of ADH
  - Head injury
  - Brain abscess
  - Hydrocephalus
  - Pituitary adenoma
  - Subdural hematoma
  - Subarachnoid hemorrhage
  - Cerebral atrophy
  - Guillain-Barré syndrome
- *Neurogenic stimuli* capable of increasing ADH
  - Decreased glomerular filtration rate
  - Physical and/or emotional stress
  - Pain
  - Fear
  - Trauma
  - Surgery
  - Myocardial infarction
  - Acute infection
  - Hypotension
  - Hemorrhage
  - Hypovolemia
- *Pulmonary diseases* believed to stimulate the baroreceptors and increase ADH
  - Pulmonary tuberculosis
  - Viral and bacterial pneumonia
  - Empyema
  - Lung abscess
  - Chronic obstructive lung disease
  - Status asthmaticus
  - Cystic fibrosis
- *Endocrine disturbances* that hormonally influence ADH
  - Myxedema
  - Hypothyroidism
  - Hypopituitarism
  - Adrenal insufficiency—Addison's disease
- *Medications* that mimic, increase the release of, or potentiate ADH
  - Hypoglycemics
    - Insulin
    - Tolbutamide
    - Chlorpropamide
  - Thiazide diuretics
  - Tricyclic antidepressants
    - Imipramine
    - Amitriptyline
  - Phenothiazine
    - Fluphenazine
    - Thioridazine
  - Selective serotonin reuptake inhibitors
    - Citalopram (Celexa)
    - Escitalopram (Lexapro)
    - Fluvoxamine (Luvox)
    - Paroxetine (Paxil)
    - Sertraline (Zoloft)
  - Thioxanthenes
    - Thiothixene
    - Chlorprothixene
  - Chemotherapeutic agents
    - Vincristine
    - Cyclophosphamide
  - Opiates
  - Carbamazepine
  - Clofibrate
  - Acetaminophen
  - Nicotine
  - Oxytocin
  - Vasopressin
  - Anesthetics

ADH, Antidiuretic hormone.

Assessment and Diagnosis

Clinical Manifestations

The clinical manifestations of SIADH relate to the excess fluids in the extracellular compartment and the proportionate dilution of the circulating sodium. Edema usually is not present[70]; slight weight gain may occur from the expanded extracellular fluid volume. Early clinical manifestations of dilutional hyponatremia include lethargy, anorexia, nausea, and vomiting. Severe neurologic symptoms generally do not develop until the serum sodium level drops below 120 mEq/L.[62,70] Progressively deteriorating neurologic signs of hyponatremia then predominate, and the patient is admitted to the critical care unit. Symptoms of severe hyponatremia include inability to concentrate, mental confusion, apprehension, seizures, decreased level of consciousness, coma, and death.

Laboratory Values

SIADH presents with very dilute serum and very concentrated urine output. Laboratory values confirm this clinical picture. In SIADH the serum is hypoosmolar (less than 275 mOsm/L) with low serum sodium level and a urine osmolality greater than would be expected of such hypotonic blood.[62] A serum sodium level below 120 mEq/L is associated with severe neurologic symptoms.[62,68,70] An elevated urine sodium level, greater than 30 mEq/L, is congruent with the concentrated urine output of SIADH.[62,68] Use of diuretics negates the reliability of the urine sodium and urine osmolarity levels.[70] A comparison of the typical laboratory values associated with SIADH versus those in DI is presented in Table 24-5.

MEDICAL MANAGEMENT

In the critical care unit, SIADH often occurs as a secondary disease. Ideally, recognition and treatment of the primary disease will reduce the production of ADH. If the patient is receiving any of the medications suspected of causing the disease, discontinuing the drug may return ADH levels to normal. Several drugs that alter ADH levels are listed in Box 24-9.

Fluid Restriction

The medical therapy that is the most successful (along with treatment of the primary disease) is simple reduction of fluid intake.[62] This is achieved most successfully for the patient with a moderate increase in body fluid volume with hyponatremia. Although fluid restrictions are calculated on the basis of individual needs and losses, a general criterion is to restrict fluids to 500 ml less than average daily output.[54]

Sodium Replacement

Patients with severe hyponatremia (less than 120 mEq/L serum sodium) experience severe neurologic symptoms, even seizures. How rapidly the sodium level should be corrected and which sodium concentration to use remains controversial.[71] One recommended regimen is an IV rate that provides sufficient sodium to raise serum sodium levels by no more than 8 to 12 mEq/day for the first 24 hours,[68] with a total rise of 18 mEq/L in the initial 48 hours.[62] There are other regimens that are more aggressive,[62] and some that are less so.[72] Another option is to add furosemide (Lasix) to increase the diuresis of free water.[68]

An infusion of 3% hypertonic saline solution may be used to replenish the serum sodium without adding extra volume when hyponatremia is severe (below 120 mEq/L). It is imperative that clinicians be aware that hypertonic saline solution is dangerous if administered too quickly in hyponatremic patients and that calculation of the quantity of sodium that will be administered is advised. An example of one sodium replacement regimen is an infusion of 3% saline infusion at 35 ml/hr in a 70-kg patient, which will increase the serum sodium by approximately 0.5 mEq/L per hour (12 mEq per day).[62] Suggested end points at which to stop the acute sodium repletion include the following[62]:

- The patient's symptoms are abolished.
- A safe serum sodium level is achieved, generally greater than 120 mEq/L.
- A total correction of 20 mEq/L is achieved.

Too-rapid serum sodium correction must be avoided to reduce the risk of *osmotic demyelination,* previously known as *central pontine myelinolysis.*[72] The demyelination occurs in the pons and in other areas of the white matter of the brain.[54] The lesions may be detected on imaging studies (computed tomography [CT] and magnetic resonance imaging [MRI]), and severe neurologic damage or even death can result.[54] Patients with a baseline serum sodium level below 120 mEq/L are most at risk.[54] Serum sodium levels must be evaluated at least every 4 hours during the acute phase of sodium replacement.[62]

Medications

Medications are prescribed only if water restriction is ineffective in correcting the SIADH. Certain drugs decrease the output of ADH from the pituitary gland, and other medications increase the action of ADH on the V_2 tubule (aquaporin-2 receptors) in the kidney so that more water is excreted.

Medications That Increase Renal Water Excretion. The drug traditionally used to treat SIADH is demeclocycline, a derivative of tetracycline.[62] The required dosage range is from 600 to 1200 mg/day, and several days of therapy are necessary to achieve maximal effects.[62] Thus, it is advisable to wait several days before changing the initial dose regimen.[62] A new oral agent (tolvaptan) that binds directly to the V_2 tubule receptors to increase aquaresis (loss of free water) was recently approved by the U.S. Food and Drug Administration (FDA).[73]

NURSING MANAGEMENT

Nursing management of the patient with SIADH incorporates a variety of nursing diagnoses (Box 24-10). **Nursing priorities are directed toward (1) restricting fluids, (2) maintaining surveillance for complications, and (3) providing patient education.**

Box 24-10

NURSING DIAGNOSIS PRIORITIES

Syndrome of Inappropriate Antidiuretic Hormone

- Excess Fluid Volume related to comprised regulation mechanism, p. A-24
- Anxiety related to lack of control over current situation or disease progression, p. A-9
- Deficient Knowledge: Discharge Regimen related to lack of previous exposure to information, p. A-18

Restricting Fluids

Frequent assessment of the patient's hydration status is accomplished with serial measurements of urine output, serum sodium levels, and serum osmolarity. Accurate measurement of I&O is required to calculate fluid replacement for the patient with SIADH. All fluids are restricted. Intake that equals urine output may be given until serum sodium level returns to normal. Frequent mouth care through moistening the buccal membrane may provide comfort during the period of fluid restriction. The patient is weighed daily to gauge fluid retention or loss. Weight gain signifies continual fluid retention, whereas weight loss indicates loss of body fluid.

Constipation is a frequent complication of decreased fluid intake. Cathartics or low-volume hypertonic enemas may be given to stimulate peristalsis. Tap water or hypotonic enemas should never be given because the water in the enema solution may be absorbed through the bowel and potentiate water intoxication.

Maintaining Surveillance for Complications

The patient's neurologic status, especially level of consciousness, should be evaluated on an hourly basis if the serum sodium level is critically low, below 120 mEq/L. Seizure precautions for the patient with SIADH are provided regardless of the degree of hyponatremia. Serum sodium levels may fluctuate rapidly, and neurologic impairment may occur with no apparent warning. The patient's altered neurologic response also may be influenced by the acuity of the primary disease (central nervous system disease) and not solely by the result of low sodium levels. Seizure precautions include nursing actions to protect the patient from injury (padded side rails, bed in low position when patient is unattended) and to provide an open airway (oral airway, head turned to side without forcibly restraining the patient, suction apparatus). Oxygen may be required to maintain a saturation level greater than 92% if there is pulmonary congestion or edema that interferes with alveolar gas exchange.

Providing Patient Education

Rapidly occurring changes in the patient's neurologic status may frighten visiting family members. Sensitivity to the family's unspoken fears can be shown by words that express empathy and by providing time for the patient and family to communicate their feelings. The nurse may discuss the course of SIADH, its effect on water balance, and the reasons for fluid restrictions.

Collaborative Management

At this time there are no published guidelines that discuss acute collaborative care management of the patient with SIADH. This is a complex condition, and effective clinical management requires the skills of many health care professionals working as a team with goals that are clearly communicated to all team members.

SUMMARY

The endocrine system is complex, and assessment relies heavily on laboratory tests for confirmation of disease processes. As clinicians gain a more comprehensive understanding of the role of the endocrine system in critical illness, the tests of endocrine organ function will be more frequently requested as part of a complete critical care evaluation. Hormone deficiencies will be replenished if this practice is supported by adequate research. To fully participate in the care of these complex patients, it is imperative that critical care nurses be familiar with the intricacies of the endocrine system.

evolve To test your mastery of this chapter, try the Open-Book Quiz at http://evolve.elsevier.com/Urden/priorities/

REFERENCES

1. Van den Berghe G et al: Intensive insulin therapy in the critically ill patients, *N Engl J Med* 345(19):1359, 2001.
2. Van den Berghe G et al: Intensive insulin therapy in the medical ICU, *N Engl J Med* 354(5):449, 2006.
3. Laird AM et al: Relationship of early hyperglycemia to mortality in trauma patients, *J Trauma* 56(5):1058, 2004.
4. Marik PE, Raghavan M: Stress-hyperglycemia, insulin and immunomodulation in sepsis, *Intensive Care Med* 30(5):748, 2004.
5. Holm C et al: Acute hyperglycaemia following thermal injury: friend or foe? *Resuscitation* 60(1):71, 2004.
6. Coursin DB, Connery LE, Ketzler JT: Perioperative diabetic and hyperglycemic management issues, *Crit Care Med* 32(4 suppl):S116, 2004.
7. Capes SE et al: Stress hyperglycemia and prognosis of stroke in nondiabetic and diabetic patients: a systematic overview, *Stroke* 32(10):2426, 2001.
8. Garber AJ et al: American College of Endocrinology position statement on inpatient diabetes and metabolic control, *Endocr Pract* 10(suppl 2):4, 2004.
9. Wortsman J: Role of epinephrine in acute stress, *Endocrinol Metab Clin North Am* 31(1):79, 2002.
10. Langton JE, Brent GA: Nonthyroidal illness syndrome: evaluation of thyroid function in sick patients, *Endocrinol Metab Clin North Am* 31(1):159, 2002.
11. Van Den Berghe G: Neuroendocrine pathobiology of chronic critical illness, *Crit Care Clin* 18(3):509, 2002.
12. Van Den Berghe G: Endocrine evaluation of patients with critical illness, *Endocrinol Metab Clin North Am* 32(2):385, 2003.
13. Weekers F, Van Den Berghe G: Endocrine modifications and interventions during critical illness, *Proc Nutr Soc* 63(3):443, 2004.
14. Cooper MS, Stewart PM: Corticosteroid insufficiency in acutely ill patients, *N Engl J Med* 348(8):727, 2003.
15. Rivers EP et al: Adrenal insufficiency in high-risk surgical ICU patients, *Chest* 119(3):889, 2001.

16. Keh D, Sprung CL: Use of corticosteroid therapy in patients with sepsis and septic shock: an evidence-based review, *Crit Care Med* 32(11):S527, 2004.
17. Axelrod L: Perioperative management of patients treated with glucocorticoids, *Endocrinol Metab Clin North Am* 32(2):367, 2003.
18. Clement S et al: Management of diabetes and hyperglycemia in hospitals, *Diabetes Care* 27(2):553, 2004.
19. Baird TA et al: The influence of diabetes mellitus and hyperglycaemia on stroke incidence and outcome, *J Clin Neurosci* 9(6):618, 2002.
20. Parsons MW et al: Acute hyperglycemia adversely affects stroke outcome: a magnetic resonance imaging and spectroscopy study, *Ann Neurol* 52(1):20, 2002.
21. Baird TA et al: Persistent poststroke hyperglycemia is independently associated with infarct expansion and worse clinical outcome, *Stroke* 34(9):2208, 2003.
22. Moghissi E: Hospital management of diabetes: beyond the sliding scale, *Cleve Clin J Med* 71(10):801, 2004.
23. Clement S: Better glycemic control in the hospital: beneficial and feasible, *Cleve Clin J Med* 74(2):111, 2007.
24. Dinardo MM, Korytkowski MT, Siminerio LS: The importance of normoglycemia in critically ill patients, *Crit Care Nurs Q* 27(2):126, 2004.
25. American Diabetes Association: Standards of medical care in diabetes—2007, *Diabetes Care* 30(suppl 1):S4, 2007.
26. Anderson RN, Smith BL: Deaths: leading causes for 2001, *Natl Vital Stat Rep* 52(9):1, 2003.
27. Self-reported heart disease and stroke among adults with and without diabetes—United States, 1999-2001, *MMWR Morb Mortal Wkly Rep* 52(44):1065, 2003.
28. Coughlin SS et al: Diabetes mellitus as a predictor of cancer mortality in a large cohort of U.S. adults, *Am J Epidemiol* 159(12):1160, 2004.
29. American Diabetes Association: Diagnosis and classification of diabetes mellitus, *Diabetes Care* 30(suppl 1):S42, 2007.
30. Goldstein DE et al: Tests of glycemia in diabetes, *Diabetes Care* 27(suppl 1):S91, 2004.
31. Blake DR, Nathan DM: Point-of-care testing for diabetes, *Crit Care Nurs Q* 27(2):150, 2004.
32. Dungan K et al: Glucose measurement: confounding issues in setting targets for inpatient management, *Diabetes Care* 30(2):403, 2007.
33. Lebovitz HE: Oral antidiabetic agents: 2004, *Med Clin North Am* 88(4):847, 2004.
34. Richter B, Neises G, Bergerhoff K: Human versus animal insulin in people with diabetes mellitus: a systematic review, *Endocrinol Metab Clin North Am* 31(3):723, 2002.
35. Screening for type 2 diabetes, *Diabetes Care* 27(suppl 1): S11, 2004.
36. American Association of Clinical Endocrinologists: Position statement on the insulin resistance syndrome, *Endocr Pract* 9(S2):5, 2003.
37. Fletcher B, Lamendola C: Insulin resistance syndrome, *J Cardiovasc Nurs* 19(5):339, 2004.
38. Grundy SM et al: Clinical management of metabolic syndrome: report of the American Heart Association/National Heart, Lung, and Blood Institute/American Diabetes Association conference on scientific issues related to management, *Circulation* 109(4):551, 2004.
39. Yki-Jarvinen H: Thiazolidinediones, *N Engl J Med* 351(11):1106, 2004.
40. Kruse JA: Metformin-associated lactic acidosis, *J Emerg Med* 20(3):267, 2001.
41. Khan JK et al: Lactic acidemia associated with metformin, *Ann Pharmacother* 37(1):66, 2003.
42. Nesto RW et al: Thiazolidinedione use, fluid retention, and congestive heart failure: a consensus statement from the American Heart Association and American Diabetes Association, *Circulation* 108(23):2941, 2003.
43. Davis T, Edelman SV: Insulin therapy in type 2 diabetes, *Med Clin North Am* 88(4):865, 2004.
44. Lien LF, Angelyn Bethel M, Feinglos MN: In-hospital management of type 2 diabetes mellitus, *Med Clin North Am* 88(4):1085, 2004.
45. Toto RD: Lessons learned from recent clinical trials in hypertensive diabetics: what's good for the kidney is good for the heart and brain, *Am J Hypertens* 17(11 suppl): S7, 2004.
46. Krauss RM: Lipids and lipoproteins in patients with type 2 diabetes, *Diabetes Care* 27(6):1496, 2004.
47. Wilson Tang WH, Maroo A, Young JB: Ischemic heart disease and congestive heart failure in diabetic patients, *Med Clin North Am* 88(4):1037, 2004.
48. Ginde AA et al: National survey of U.S. emergency department visits with diabetic ketoacidosis, 1993-2003, *Diabetes Care* 29(9):2117, 2006.
49. Kitabchi AE et al: Hyperglycemic crises in adult patients with diabetes, *Diabetes Care* 29(12):2739, 2006.
50. Gaglia JL, Wyckoff J, Abrahamson MJ: Acute hyperglycemic crisis in the elderly, *Med Clin North Am* 88(4): 1063, 2004.
51. Newton CA, Raskin P: Diabetic ketoacidosis in type 1 and type 2 diabetes mellitus: clinical and biochemical differences, *Arch Intern Med* 164(17):1925, 2004.
52. Magee MF, Bhatt BA: Management of decompensated diabetes: diabetic ketoacidosis and hyperglycemic hyperosmolar syndrome, *Crit Care Clin* 17(1):75, 2001.
53. Buse JB et al: Primary prevention of cardiovascular disease in people with diabetes mellitus, *Diabetes Care* 30(1):162, 2007.
54. Janicic N, Verbalis JG: Evaluation and management of hypo-osmolality in hospitalized patients, *Endocrinol Metab Clin North Am* 32(2):459, 2003.
55. Holcomb S: Diabetes insipidus, *DCCN* 21(3):94, 2002.
56. Wong LL, Verbalis JG: Systemic diseases associated with disorders of water homeostasis, *Endocrinol Metab Clin North Am* 31(1):121, 2002.
57. Boughey JC, Yost MJ, Bynoe RP: Diabetes insipidus in the head-injured patient, *Am Surg* 70(6):500, 2004.
58. Verbalis JG: Management of disorders of water metabolism in patients with pituitary tumors, *Pituitary* 5(2):119, 2002.
59. Vance ML: Perioperative management of patients undergoing pituitary surgery, *Endocrinol Metab Clin North Am* 32(2):355, 2003.
60. Innis J: Treating nephrogenic diabetes insipidus: a case study, *DCCN* 21(3):98, 2002.
61. Olson DM, Meek LG, Lynch JR: Accurate patient history contributes to differentiating diabetes insipidus: a case study, *J Neurosci Nurs* 36(4):228, 2004.

62. Verbalis JG: Disorders of body water homeostasis, *Best Pract Res Clin Endocrinol Metab* 17(4):471, 2003.
63. Holmes CL et al: Physiology of vasopressin relevant to management of septic shock, *Chest* 120(3):989, 2001.
64. *Mosby's Drug Consult*, St Louis, 2004, Mosby.
65. Holmes CL, Landry DW, Granton JT: Science review: vasopressin and the cardiovascular system. I. Receptor physiology, *Crit Care* 7(6):427, 2003.
66. Holmes CL, Landry DW, Granton JT: Science review: vasopressin and the cardiovascular system. II. Clinical physiology, *Crit Care* 8(1):15, 2004.
67. Seute T et al: Neurologic disorders in 432 consecutive patients with small cell lung carcinoma, *Cancer* 100(4):801, 2004.
68. Bissram M. et al: Risk factors for symptomatic hyponatraemia: the role of pre-existing asymptomatic hyponatraemia, *Intern Med J* 37(3):149, 2007.
69. Rottmann CN: SRRIs and the syndrome of inappropriate antidiuretic secretion, *Am J Nurs* 107(1):51, 2007.
70. Freda BJ, Davidson MB, Hall PM: Evaluation of hyponatremia: a little physiology goes a long way, *Cleve Clin J Med* 71(8):639, 2004.
71. Johnson AL, Criddle LM: Pass the salt: indications for and implications of using hypertonic saline, *Crit Care Nurse* 24(5):36, 2004.
72. Rabinstein AA, Wijdicks EF: Hyponatremia in critically ill neurological patients, *Neurologist* 9(6):290, 2003.
73. Schrier RW et al: Tolvaptan, a selective oral vasopressin V2-receptor antagonist, for hyponatremia, *N Engl J Med* 355(20):2099, 2006.

CHAPTER 25

Trauma

KAREN L. JOHNSON ■ KARA L. ADAMS

OBJECTIVES

- Compare and contrast injuries associated with blunt and penetrating trauma.
- Discuss mechanism of injury, pathophysiology, assessment findings, medical management, and nursing management of traumatic injuries to the head, spinal cord, heart, lungs, and abdomen.
- Use assessment findings to identify potential complications and sequelae of traumatic injuries.

Trauma is the leading cause of death for all age-groups under the age of 44. Injury costs the United States hundreds of billions of dollars annually. It is one of the most pressing health problems in the United States today. However, the problem continues to go largely unrecognized.

Injury as a result of trauma is no longer considered to be an "accident." The term *motor vehicle accident (MVA)* has been replaced with *motor vehicle crash (MVC)*, and the term *accident* has been replaced with *unintentional injury*. Unintentional injury is no accident. Accident traditionally has implied an act of God or an unpredictable accident. Domestic violence and alcohol-related issues are priority prevention areas with which health care providers must be actively involved.

Domestic violence constitutes a major public health issue in the United States. It is unrecognized and underreported.[1] Domestic violence is the leading cause of injury to women in the United States, and it has been estimated that one million women every year are severely beaten or assaulted with weapons by male partners.[2] Domestic violence and alcohol abuse have a high prevalence among female trauma patients admitted to trauma centers.[1,3] Health care providers should consider routinely inquiring about domestic violence as part of the history, at a minimum for all female adolescents and adult patients.[4] Key points in prevention, recognition, and treatment of domestic violence summarized by Sisley, Jacobs, and People[5] are listed in Box 25-1.

An alcohol-related motor vehicle crash kills someone every 30 minutes and nonfatally injures someone every 2 minutes.[6] Each year, alcohol-related crashed in the United States cost about $51 billion.[7] To decrease the incidence of alcohol-related crashes, communities need to implement and enforce strategies that are known to be effective such as sobriety checkpoints, regulations limiting driving to those whose blood alcohol levels are below 0.08%, minimum legal drinking age laws, and "zero tolerance" for young drivers.[8,9] Alcohol screening and intervention have been recommended as routine components of trauma care.[10] CAGE, a screening questionnaire, has been recommended (Box 25-2).[11]

Over the past few decades, major advances have been made in the management of patients with traumatic injuries, and significant improvements have been made in their care in both prehospital and emergency department settings. The American College of Surgeons developed guidelines (Advanced Trauma Life Support [ATLS]) to guide rapid assessment, resuscitation, and definitive care for trauma patients in the emergency department.[12] This chapter reviews nursing management of patients with traumatic injuries, particularly in the critical care setting.

Box 25-1

Prevention, Recognition, and Treatment of Domestic Violence

- Development of a curriculum on domestic violence for health care providers and students
- Support for a policy of universal screening of all female patients for domestic violence
- Promotion of hospital-based domestic violence programs
- Advocacy for an increase in the number of beds available in battered women's shelters
- Development of intervention programs for children who witness domestic violence
- Treatment programs for batterers
- Development of a research agenda
- Support for the establishment of a national database for compiling incidence and other epidemiologic data on domestic violence

Box 25-2

CAGE Alcohol Screening Questionnaire

- Have you ever thought you should ***C***ut down on your drinking?
- Have you ever been ***A***nnoyed by other people's criticism of your drinking?
- Have you ever felt ***G***uilty about your drinking?
- Have you ever had an early morning drink (***E***ye opener) to steady your nerves?

MECHANISMS OF INJURY

Trauma occurs when an external force of energy impacts the body and causes structural or physiologic alterations, or "injuries." External forces can be radiation, electrical, thermal, chemical, or mechanical forms of energy. This chapter focuses on trauma from mechanical energy. Mechanical energy can produce either blunt or penetrating traumatic injuries. Knowledge of the mechanism of injury helps health care providers anticipate and predict potential internal injuries.

BLUNT TRAUMA

Blunt trauma is seen most often with MVCs, contact sports, blunt force injuries (e.g., trauma caused by a baseball bat), or falls. Injuries occur because of the forces sustained during a rapid change in velocity (deceleration). To estimate the amount of force a person would sustain in an MVC, multiply the person's weight by miles per hour of speed the vehicle was traveling. A 130-pound woman in a vehicle traveling at 60 miles per hour that hits a brick wall, for example, would sustain 7800 pounds of force within milliseconds. As the body stops suddenly, tissues and organs continue to move forward. This sudden change in velocity causes injuries that result in lacerations or crush injuries of internal body structures.

PENETRATING TRAUMA

Penetrating injuries occur with stabbings, firearms, or accidents resulting in impalement injuries that penetrate the skin and result in damage to internal structures. Damage occurs along the path of penetration. Penetrating injuries can be misleading inasmuch as the condition of the outside of the wound does not determine the extent of internal injury. Bullets can create internal cavities 5 to 30 times larger than the diameter of the bullet.[12] Once inside the body, the bullet can ricochet off bone and create further damage along its pathway. With penetrating stab wounds, factors that determine the extent of injury include the type and length of object used, as well as the angle of insertion.

PHASES OF TRAUMA CARE

PREHOSPITAL RESUSCITATION

The goal of prehospital care is immediate stabilization and transportation. This is achieved through airway maintenance, control of external bleeding and shock, immobilization of the patient, and immediate transport (ground or air) to the closest appropriate medical facility.[12] Personnel providing prehospital care should also communicate information needed for triage at the hospital. Nursing management of the patient with traumatic injuries begins the moment a call for help is received and continues throughout the trajectory of critical illness, rehabilitation, and return to work or school and is also supportive of the patient in the event of long-term disability or death.[13] Advance planning for care of the injured patient is essential.

EMERGENCY DEPARTMENT RESUSCITATION

Primary Survey

On arrival of the trauma patient in the emergency department, the primary survey is initiated. During this assessment, life-threatening injuries are discovered and treated. The five steps in the primary survey compose the ABCDEs (Table 25-1):

- **A**irway maintenance with cervical spine protection
- **B**reathing and ventilation
- **C**irculation with hemorrhage control
- **D**isability and neurologic status
- **E**xposure/environmental control

Resuscitation Phase

After the primary survey the resuscitation phase begins. Events that occur during the resuscitation phase can have a significant impact on later complications (Table 25-2). Hypovolemic shock is the most common type of shock that occurs in trauma patients.[12] Hemorrhage must be identified and treated rapidly. Two large-bore peripheral intravenous (IV) catheters (14- to 16-gauge) or a central venous catheter is inserted. During the initiation of IV lines, blood samples are drawn (Box 25-3). Intravenous therapy with Ringer's lactate solution should be administered rapidly. High-flow fluid warmers may be used to deliver warmed IV solutions at rates greater than 1000 ml/min. If the patient remains unresponsive to bolus intravenous therapy, O-negative blood or type-specific blood may be administered.[12] Transfusion of autologous salvaged blood (autotransfusion) also may be used to replace intravascular volume and to provide oxygen-carrying capacity.

Placement of urinary and gastric catheters is part of the resuscitation phase. An indwelling urinary catheter can help evaluate urine output as an indicator of volume status and renal perfusion. A gastric tube is inserted to reduce gastric distention and assist in reducing the risk of aspiration.[12]

Table 25-1
Primary Survey of the Trauma Patient

SURVEY COMPONENT	NURSING DIAGNOSIS	NURSING ASSESSMENT/ CARE
Airway	Ineffective Airway Clearance related to obstruction or actual injury	Immobilize cervical spine. *Look:* • Is there obvious airway trauma, tachypnea, accessory muscle use, tracheal shift? *Listen:* • Stridor, hyperresonance, dullness to percussion? *Feel:* • For air exchange over the mouth; insert finger sweep to clear foreign bodies. Secure airway. • Oropharyngeal • Nasopharyngeal • Endotracheal tube • Cricothyrotomy
Breathing	Ineffective Breathing Pattern related to actual injury Impaired Gas Exchange related to actual injury or disrupted tissue perfusion	Assess for: • Spontaneous breathing • Respiratory rate, depth, symmetry • Chest wall integrity *Absent breathing:* • Intubate, mechanical ventilation. *Breathing but ineffective:* • Assess life-threatening conditions (e.g., tension pneumothorax, flail chest). Administer supplemental oxygen. Initiate pulse oximetry.
Circulation	Decreased Cardiac Output related to actual injury Ineffective Tissue Perfusion related to actual injury or shock Deficient Fluid Volume related to actual loss of circulating volume	Assess pulse quality/rate. Maintain ECG monitoring. *No pulse:* • Initiate ACLS. *Pulse but ineffective:* • Assess and treat life-threatening conditions (uncontrolled bleeding, shock). Initiate two large-bore IVs or central catheter; obtain serum samples for laboratory tests. Initiate fluid replacement.
Disability	Ineffective Cerebral Tissue Perfusion Risk for Injury related to actual injury of brain or spinal cord	Assess Glasgow Coma Scale. Assess pupil size and reactivity.
Exposure/environmental control	Risk for Imbalanced Body Temperature	Remove all clothing to inspect all body regions. Prevent hypothermia.

ECG, Electrocardiogram; *ACLS,* advanced cardiac life support; *IV,* intravenous line.

Table 25-2
Impact of Trauma Resuscitation on Later Complications

ASPECT OF INJURY/RESUSCITATION	EFFECT ON ICU COURSE
Prolonged extrication time	Gives an indication of length of time patient may have been hypotensive and/or hypothermic before medical care
Period of respiratory or cardiac arrest	Effects of loss of perfusion to brain (anoxic injury), kidneys, and other vital organs may predispose patient to later organ dysfunction
Time on backboard	Potentiates risk of sacral or occipital breakdown
Number of units of blood; whether any were not fully cross-matched; packed cells versus whole blood used	Potentiates risk of infection, ARDS, MODS

ICU, Intensive care unit; *ARDS,* acute respiratory distress syndrome; *MODS,* multiple organ dysfunction syndrome.

Box 25-3

Serum Samples to Obtain With Intravenous Placement

- Complete blood cell (CBC) count
- Electrolyte profile (Na^+, K^+, Cl^-, CO_2, glucose, blood urea nitrogen [BUN], creatinine [Cr])
- Coagulation parameters: prothrombin time (PT); partial thromboplastin time (PTT)
- Type and screen (ABO compatibility)
- Amylase
- Toxicology screens
- Liver function studies
- Pregnancy test (for females of childbearing age)
- Lactate

The resuscitation phase begins in the emergency department and may continue well into the critical care phase. Resuscitation is aimed at ensuring adequate perfusion of tissues with oxygen and nutrients to support cellular function. Assessment of the patient's response to resuscitation is a priority nursing assessment because the patient's response to these efforts is key to determining subsequent therapy. Resuscitation end points (i.e., variables or parameters) must be viewed across the continuum of resuscitation from shock. During resuscitation from traumatic hemorrhagic shock, normalization of standard clinical parameters such as blood pressure, heart rate, and urine output are not adequate.[14] The optimal resuscitation end point is a major focus of research in trauma care. Current guidelines recommend that during resuscitation, attempts should be made to improve oxygen delivery to normalize base deficit, lactate or gastric pH_i during the first 24 hours after injury.[14]

Secondary Survey

The secondary survey begins when the primary survey is completed, resuscitation is well established, and the patient is demonstrating normalization of vital signs. During the secondary survey, a head-to-toe approach is used to thoroughly examine each body region. The history is one of the most important aspects of the secondary survey. Often head injury, shock, or the use of drugs or alcohol may preclude taking a good history, so the history must be pieced together from other sources. The prehospital care providers (paramedics, emergency medical technicians) usually can provide most of the vital information pertaining to the accident. Specific information that must be elicited pertaining to the mechanism of injury is summarized in Box 25-4. This information can help predict internal injuries and facilitate rapid intervention. The patient's pertinent past history can be assessed by use of the mnemonic AMPLE: ***A***llergies, ***M***edications currently used, ***P***ast medical illnesses/pregnancy, ***L***ast meal, and ***E***vents/environment related to the injury.

Box 25-4

History of Mechanism of Injury

Penetrating Trauma

Weapon used (handgun, shotgun, rifle, knife)
Caliber of weapon
Number of shots fired
Gender of assailant
Position of victim and assailant when injury occurred

Blunt Trauma

Height of fall
Motor vehicle crash (MVC) extrication time
Ejection
Steering wheel deformation
Location in automobile (passenger, driver, front seat, back seat)
Restraint status (lap belt, shoulder harness, or combination; unrestrained)
Speed of automobile(s)/direction of impact
Occupants (number and morbidity status)

During the secondary survey the nurse ensures the completion of special procedures, such as an electrocardiogram (ECG); radiographic studies (chest, cervical spine, thorax, and pelvis); diagnostic peritoneal lavage; and ultrasonography. Throughout this survey the nurse continuously monitors the patient's vital signs and response to medical therapies. Emotional support to the patient and family also is imperative.

Definitive Care/Operative Phase

Once the secondary survey has been completed, specific injuries usually have been diagnosed. Definitive care related to specific injuries is described throughout this chapter. Trauma is often referred to as a "surgical disease" because the nature and extent of injuries usually requires operative management. After surgery, depending on the patient's status, a transfer to the intensive care unit may be indicated.

Critical Care Phase

Critically ill trauma patients are admitted into the intensive care unit (ICU) as direct transfers from the emergency department (ED) or operating room (OR). Information the ICU nurse must obtain from the ED or OR nurse, or both, is summarized in Box 25-5. This information must be obtained before patient admission to the ICU to ensure availability of needed personnel, equipment, and supplies. This information also helps the ICU nurse to assess the impact of trauma resuscitation on the patient's ICU presentation and course.

Box 25-5

Nursing Report From Referring Area

- Mechanism of injury/injuries sustained
- Diagnostic tests completed and results
- Medications administered (particularly narcotics, sedatives, neuromuscular blocking agents)
- Diagnostic/therapeutic procedures performed (diagnostic peritoneal lavage [DPL], chest tube insertion, intravenous [IV] access)
- Vital signs
- Established airway/mechanical ventilation settings/O_2 flow devices
- Any loss of consciousness and its duration
- Current Glasgow Coma Scale score
- Fluid replacement (colloid and crystalloid)
- Fluid loss (urine output, chest tube drainage, estimated intraoperative blood loss)
- Laboratory tests (including blood alcohol and toxicology screen)
- Past medical/surgical history (including medications taken at home, allergies)
- Family members present (assessment of coping and current knowledge of nature and extent of injuries and treatment plan)

Modified from Johnson KL: Critical care of the trauma patient. In Neff JA, Kidd PS, editors: *Trauma nursing: the art and science,* St Louis, 1993, Mosby.

Table 25-3

Factors Predisposing the Trauma Patient to Impaired Oxygenation

FACTOR	IMPAIRMENT
Impaired ventilation	Injury to airway structures, loss of CNS regulation of breathing, impaired level of consciousness
Impaired pulmonary gas diffusion	Pneumothorax, hemothorax, aspiration of gastric contents Shifts to the left of the oxyhemoglobin dissociation curve (can be secondary to infusion of large volumes of banked blood, hypocarbia or alkalosis, or hypothermia)
Decreased oxygen supply	Reduced hemoglobin (secondary to hemorrhage) Reduced cardiac output (cardiovascular injury, decreased preload)
Increased oxygen supply	Increased metabolic demands (associated with the stress response to injury)

CNS, Central nervous system.

On the patient's arrival to the ICU, the nurse, using the primary and secondary surveys and resuscitative measures in accordance with ATLS guidelines, assesses the trauma patient's status. Priority nursing care during the critical care phase includes ongoing physical assessments and monitoring the patient's response to medical therapies. One of the most important nursing roles is assessment of the balance between oxygen delivery and oxygen demand (Table 25-3). Oxygen delivery must be optimized to prevent further system damage.[15]

Frequent and thorough nursing assessment of all body systems is important because these assessments are the cornerstone to the medical and nursing management of the critically ill trauma patient. The nurse can detect subtle changes and facilitate the implementation of timely therapeutic interventions to prevent complications often associated with trauma. The nurse must be knowledgeable about specific organ injuries, as well as their associated sequelae.

SPECIFIC TRAUMA INJURIES

TRAUMATIC BRAIN INJURIES

Over 1.5 million traumatic brain injuries (TBIs) occur annually in the United States,[16] with approximately 15% of those patients hospitalized as a result of their injury. Approximately 50,000 Americans die each year from TBI, which accounts for about one third of all trauma-related deaths.[16] Approximately 50% of all trauma deaths are associated with some type of head injury.[12] Of the patients with head trauma who are hospitalized, approximately 35% of the survivors will suffer long-term disability, posing a tremendous economic impact on society due to both health care costs and life years lost.[17]

Mechanism of Injury

TBIs occur when mechanical forces are transmitted to brain tissue. Mechanisms of injury include penetrating or blunt trauma to the head. Before 1990 the incidence of transportation-related TBI exceeded that of TBI related to firearm use. Since 1994 this has switched, with firearm-related TBIs exceeding injuries due to transportation, such as MVC.[16] Penetrating trauma can result from the penetration of a foreign object (e.g., a bullet) that causes direct damage to cerebral tissue. Blunt trauma can be the result of deceleration, acceleration, or rotational forces. Deceleration causes the brain to crash against the skull after it has hit something (e.g., the dashboard of a car). Acceleration injuries occur when the brain has been hit by something (e.g., a baseball bat). In many instances, TBIs can be caused by both acceleration and deceleration. Acceleration injuries occur when the skull is hit by a force that causes the brain to move forward to the point of impact;and then as the brain reverses direction and hits the other side of the skull, deceleration injuries occur.

Pathophysiology

The review of the pathophysiology of a TBI can be divided into two categories: primary injury and secondary injury. It is important that the critical care nurse understands this pathophysiology, because goals of ICU care include efforts to reduce morbidity and mortality from primary and secondary injuries.

Primary Injury. The primary injury occurs at the moment of impact as a result of mechanical forces to the head. The extent of and recovery from injury are related to whether the primary injury was localized to an area or was diffuse or widespread throughout the brain. Primary injuries may occur as direct damage to the parenchyma or as injury to the vessels that causes hemorrhage, compressing nearby structures. Examples of primary injuries include contusion, laceration, shearing injuries, and hemorrhage. Primary injury may be mild, with little or no neurologic damage, or severe, with major tissue damage. Immediately after injury, a cascade of neural and vascular processes is activated.

Secondary Injury. Secondary injury is the biochemical and cellular response to the initial trauma that can exacerbate the primary injury and cause loss of brain tissue not originally damaged.[18] Secondary injury can be caused by ischemia, hypercapnia, hypotension, cerebral edema, sustained hypertension, calcium toxicity, or metabolic derangements. Hypoxia or hypotension, the best-known culprits for secondary injury, typically are the result of extracranial trauma.[18] A self-perpetuating cycle develops that may result in the expansion of a relatively focal primary injury into uncontrolled, refractory secondary injury.[12,18] Tissue ischemia occurs in areas of poor cerebral perfusion as a result of hypotension and/or hypoxia. The cells in ischemic areas become edematous. Extreme vasodilation of the cerebral vasculature occurs in an attempt to supply oxygen to the cerebral tissue. This increase in blood volume increases intracranial volume and intracranial pressure (ICP).

Classification

Injuries of the brain are described by the functional changes or losses that occur. Some of the major functional abnormalities seen in head injury are described here.

Skull Fracture. Skull fractures are common, but they do not by themselves cause neurologic deficits. Skull fractures can be classified as open (dura is torn) or closed (dura is not torn), or they can be classified as those of the vault or those of the base. Common vault fractures occur in the parietal and temporal regions. Basilar skull fractures usually are not visible on conventional skull films, and a computerized tomography (CT) scan is typically required. Assessment findings may include cerebrospinal fluid otorrhea or rhinorrhea, Battle's sign (ecchymosis overlying the mastoid process), "raccoon eyes" (subconjunctival and periorbital ecchymosis), or palsy of the seventh cranial nerve.

The significance of a skull fracture is that it identifies the patient with a higher probability of having or developing an intracranial hematoma. Open skull fractures require surgical intervention to remove bony fragments and to close the dura. The major complications of basilar skull fractures are cranial nerve injury and leakage of cerebrospinal fluid (CSF). CSF leakage may result in a fistula, which increases the possibility of bacterial contamination and resultant meningitis. Because fistula formation may be delayed, patients with a basilar skull fracture are admitted to the hospital for observation and possible surgical intervention.

Concussion. A concussion is a brain injury accompanied by a brief loss of neurologic function, especially loss of consciousness.[17] If loss of consciousness occurs, it may last for seconds to an hour. The neurologic dysfunctions include confusion, disorientation, and sometimes a period of antegrade or retrograde amnesia. Other clinical manifestations that occur after concussion are headache, dizziness, nausea, irritability, inability to concentrate, impaired memory, and fatigue. The diagnosis of concussion is based on the loss of consciousness inasmuch as the brain remains structurally intact despite functional impairment.

Contusion. Contusion, or bruising of the brain, usually is related to acceleration-deceleration injuries, which result in hemorrhage into the superficial parenchyma, often the frontal and temporal lobes. Frontal or temporal contusions are most common and can be seen in a coup-contrecoup mechanism of injury (Figure 25-1). Coup injury affects the cerebral tissue directly under the point of impact. Contrecoup injury occurs in a line directly opposite the point of impact.

The clinical manifestations of contusion are related to the location of the contusion, the degree of contusion, and the presence of associated lesions. Contusions can be small, in which localized areas of dysfunction result in a focal neurologic deficit. Larger contusions can evolve over several days after injury as a result of edema and further hemorrhaging. A large contusion can produce a mass effect that can cause a significant increase in ICP. Contusions are almost always associated with subdural hematoma.[12]

Contusions of the tips of the temporal lobe are a common occurrence and are of particular concern. Because the inner aspects of the temporal lobe surround the opening in the tentorium where the midbrain enters the cerebrum, edema in this area can cause rapid deterioration of the patient's condition and can lead to herniation. Because of the location, this deterioration can occur with little or no warning at a deceptively low ICP. Diagnosis of contusion is made by CT scan. If the CT scan indicates contusion, especially in the temporal area, the nurse must pay particular atten-

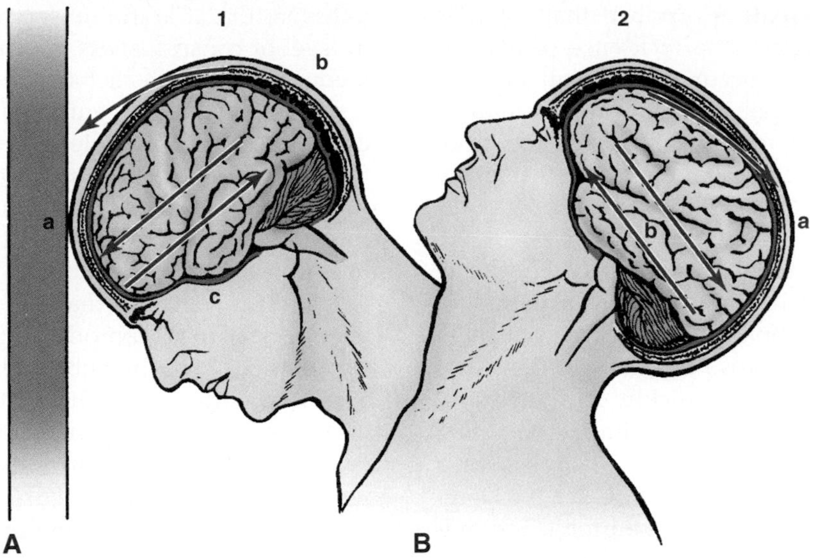

FIGURE 25-1. Coup and contrecoup head injury after blunt trauma. **A,** Coup injury: impact against object. ***a,*** Site of impact and direct trauma to brain; ***b,*** shearing of subdural veins; ***c,*** trauma to base of brain. **B,** Contrecoup injury: impact within skull. ***a,*** Site of impact from brain hitting opposite side of skull; ***b,*** shearing forces throughout brain. These injuries occur in one continuous motion—the head strikes the wall (coup), then rebounds (contrecoup).

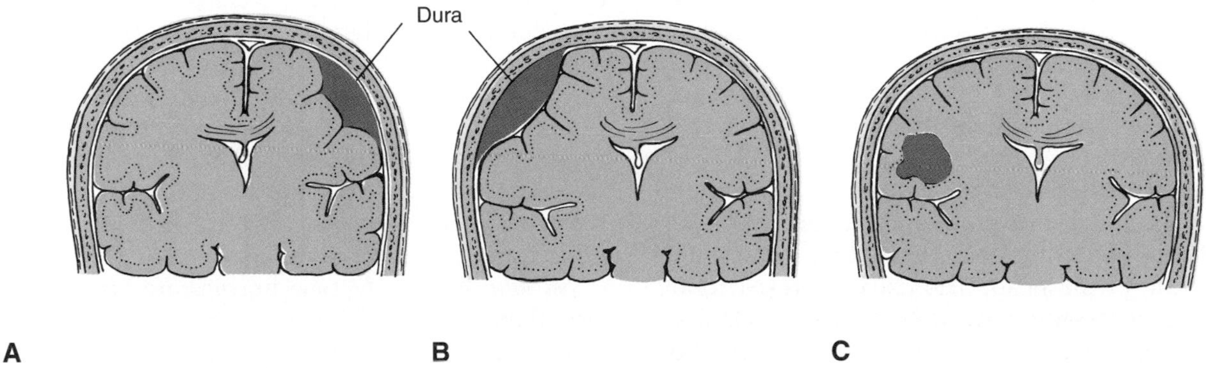

FIGURE 25-2. Types of hematomas. **A,** Subdural hematoma. **B,** Epidural hematoma. **C,** Intracerebral hematoma.

tion to neurologic assessments and look for subtle changes in pupillary signs or vital signs, irrespective of a stable ICP.

Medical management of cerebral contusions may consist of medical or surgical therapies. Because a contusion can progress over several days after injury, secondary injury may occur. If contusions are small, focal, or multiple, they are treated medically with serial neurologic assessments and possibly ICP monitoring. Larger contusions that produce considerable mass effect require surgical intervention to prevent the increased edema and intracranial pressure as the contusion matures. Outcome of cerebral contusion varies, depending on the location and the degree of contusion.

Cerebral Hematomas. Extravasation of blood produces a space-occupying lesion on the brain and leads to increased ICP. Three types of hematomas are discussed here (Figure 25-2). The first two hematomas, epidural and subdural, are extraparenchymal (outside of brain tissue) and produce injury by pressure effect and displacement of intracranial contents. The third type of hematoma, intracerebral, directly damages neural tissue and can produce further injury as a result of pressure and displacement of intracranial contents.

Epidural Hematoma. Epidural hematoma (EDH) is a collection of blood between the inner table of the skull and the outermost layer of the dura. EDHs are most often associated with patients with skull fractures and middle meningeal artery lacerations (two thirds of patients) or skull fractures with venous bleeding.[12] A blow to the head that causes a linear skull fracture on the lateral surface of the head may tear the middle meningeal artery. As the artery bleeds, it pulls the dura away from the skull, creating a pouch that expands into the intracranial space. The incidence of EDH is relatively low. EDH can occur as a result of low-impact injuries (such as falls) or high-impact injuries (such as motor vehicle crashes). EDH occurs from trauma to the skull and meninges rather than from the acceleration-deceleration forces seen in other types of head trauma.

The classic clinical manifestations of EDH include brief loss of consciousness followed by a period of lucidity. Rapid deterioration in level of consciousness should be anticipated because arterial bleeding into the epidural space can occur quickly. A dilated and fixed pupil on the same side as the impact area is a hallmark of EDH.[12] The patient may complain of a severe, localized headache and may be sleepy. Diagnosis of EDH is based on clinical symptoms and evidence of a collection of epidural blood identified on CT scan. Treatment of EDH involves surgical intervention to remove the blood and to cauterize the bleeding vessels.

Subdural Hematoma. Subdural hematoma (SDH), which is the accumulation of blood between the dura and the underlying arachnoid membrane, most often is related to a rupture in the bridging veins between the cerebral cortex and the dura.[19] Acceleration-deceleration and rotational forces are the major causes of SDH, which often is associated with cerebral contusions and intracerebral hemorrhage. SDH is common, representing about 30% of severe head injuries.

The three types of SDH are based on the time frame from injury to clinical symptoms: acute, subacute, and chronic. Acute SDHs are hematomas that occur after a severe blow to the head. The clinical presentation of acute SDH is determined by the severity of injury to the underlying brain at the time of impact and the rate of blood accumulation in the subdural space. In other situations the patient has a lucid period before deterioration. Careful observation for deterioration in level of consciousness or lateralizing signs, such as inequality of pupils or motor movements, is essential. Rapid surgical intervention, including craniectomy, craniotomy, or burr hole evacuation, and aggressive medical management can reduce mortality.

Subacute SDHs are hematomas that develop symptomatically 2 days to 2 weeks after trauma. In subacute hematomas the expansion of the hematoma occurs at a rate slower than that in acute SDH; therefore it takes longer for symptoms to become obvious. Clinical deterioration with subacute SDH usually is slower than that with acute SDH, but treatment by surgical intervention, when appropriate, is the same.

Intracerebral Hematoma. Intracerebral hematoma (ICH) results when bleeding occurs within cerebral tissue. Traumatic causes of ICH include depressed skull fractures, penetrating injuries (bullet, knife), or sudden acceleration-deceleration motion. The ICH can act as a rapidly expanding lesion; however, late ICH into the necrotic center of a contused area is also possible. Sudden clinical deterioration of a patient 6 to 10 days after trauma may be the result of ICH.

Medical management of ICH may include surgical or nonsurgical management. Generally it is believed that hemorrhages that do not cause significant ICP problems should be treated nonsurgically. Over time, the hemorrhage may be reabsorbed. If significant problems with ICP occur as a result of a mass effect produced by the ICH, surgical removal is necessary. Outcome from ICH depends greatly on the location of the hemorrhage. Size, mass effect, and displacement of other intracranial structures also affect the outcome.

Missile Injuries. Missile injuries are caused by objects that penetrate the skull to produce a significant focal damage but little acceleration-deceleration or rotational injury. The injury may be depressed, penetrating, or perforating (Figure 25-3). Depressed injuries

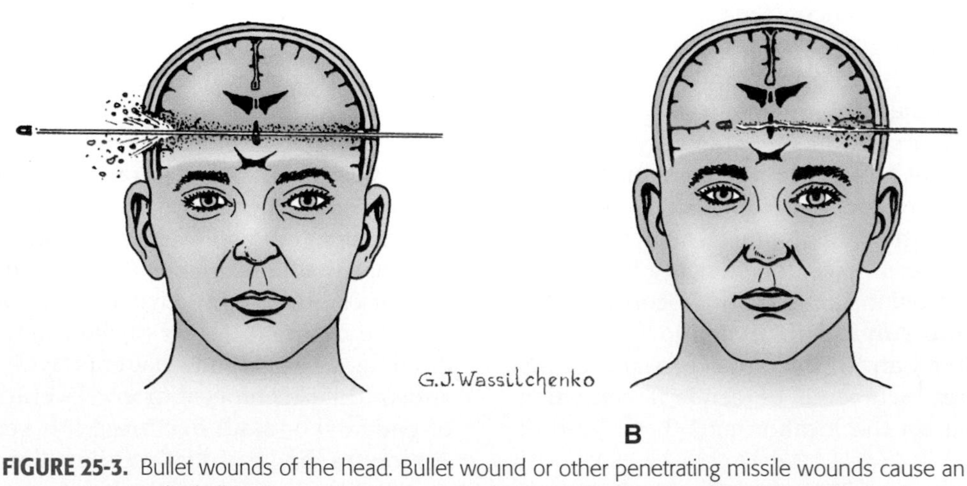

A B

FIGURE 25-3. Bullet wounds of the head. Bullet wound or other penetrating missile wounds cause an open (compound) skull fracture and damage to brain tissue. Shock wave effects are transmitted throughout the brain. **A,** Perforating injury. **B,** Penetrating injury.

are caused by fractures of the skull, with penetration of bone into cerebral tissue. Penetrating injury is caused by a missile that enters the cranial cavity but does not exit. A low-velocity penetrating injury (knife) may involve only focal damage and no loss of consciousness. A high-velocity missile (bullet) can produce shock waves that are transmitted throughout the brain, in addition to injury caused by the bullet. Perforating injuries are missile injuries that enter and then exit the brain. Perforating injuries have much less ricochet effect but are still responsible for significant injury.

Risk of infection and cerebral abscess is a concern in missile injuries. If fragments of the missile are embedded within the brain, careful consideration of the location and risk of increasing neurologic deficit is weighed against the risk of abscess or infection. The outcome after missile injury is based on the degree of penetration and the location of the injury, as well as the velocity of the missile.

Diffuse Axonal Injury. Diffuse axonal injury (DAI) is a term used to describe prolonged posttraumatic coma that is not due to a mass lesion, although DAI with mass lesions has also been reported.[19] DAI covers a wide range of brain dysfunction typically caused by acceleration/deceleration and rotational forces. DAI occurs as a result of damage to the axons or disruption of axonal transmission of the neural impulses.

The pathophysiology of DAI is related to the stretching and tearing of axons as a result of movement of the brain inside the cranium at the time of impact. The stretching and tearing of axons result in microscopic lesions throughout the brain, but especially deep within cerebral tissue and the base of the cerebrum. Disruption of axonal transmission of impulses results in loss of consciousness. Unless surrounding tissue areas are significantly injured, causing small hemorrhages, DAI may not be visible on CT scan or magnetic resonance imaging (MRI). DAI can be classified into three grades based on the extent of lesions: mild, moderate, or severe. The patient with mild DAI may be in a coma for 24 hours and may exhibit periods of decorticate and decerebrate posturing. Patients with moderate DAI may be in a coma for longer than 24 hours and may exhibit periods of decorticate and decerebrate posturing. Severe DAI is usually manifested as a prolonged deep coma with periods of hypertension, hyperthermia, and excessive sweating. Treatment of DAI includes support of vital functions and maintenance of ICP within normal limits. The outcome after severe DAI is poor because of the extensive dysfunction of cerebral pathways.

Assessment

The priorities in neurologic assessment after traumatic brain injury focus on (1) level of consciousness and (2) motor and sensory function. The neurologic assessment is the most important tool for evaluating the patient with a severe TBI, because it can indicate severity of injury, provide prognostic information, and dictate the speed with which further evaluation and treatment must proceed.[17] The cornerstone of the neurologic assessment is the Glasgow Coma Scale (GCS).[18] The GCS does not provide a complete neurologic examination, however. Pupillary and motor strength assessment must also be incorporated into the early and ongoing assessments. Once injuries are specifically identified, a more thorough, focused neurologic examination, extending for instance to the cranial nerves, is warranted. To assist with the initial assessment, TBIs are divided into three descriptive categories on the basis of the patient's GCS score and duration of the unconscious state.

Degree of Injury

Mild Injury. Mild TBI is described as a GCS score of 13 to 15, with a loss of consciousness that lasts up to 15 minutes. Patients with mild injury often are seen in the ED and discharged home with a family member who is instructed to evaluate the patient routinely and to bring the patient back to the hospital if any further neurologic symptoms appear.

Moderate Injury. Moderate TBI is described as a GCS score of 9 to 12, with a loss of consciousness for up to 6 hours. Patients with this type of TBI usually are hospitalized. They are at high risk for deterioration from increasing cerebral edema and ICP, and therefore serial clinical assessments are an important function of the nurse. Hemodynamic and ICP monitoring and ventilatory support often are not required in this group unless other systemic injuries make them necessary. A CT scan usually is performed on admission. Repeat CT scans are indicated if the patient's neurologic status deteriorates.

Severe Injury. Patients with a GCS score of 8 or less after resuscitation or those who deteriorate to that level within 48 hours of admission have a severe TBI. Patients with severe TBI often receive ventilatory support along with ICP and hemodynamic monitoring. A CT scan is performed to rule out any mass lesions that can be surgically removed. Patients are placed in a critical care setting for continual assessment, monitoring, and management.

Diagnostic Procedures. The cornerstone of diagnostic procedures for evaluation of TBI is the CT scan.[18] The CT scan is a rapid, noninvasive procedure that can provide invaluable information about the presence of mass lesions and cerebral edema. Serial CT scans may be used over a period of several days to assess areas of contusion and ischemia and to detect delayed hematomas. A nurse must always remain with a TBI patient during the CT scan to provide continued observation and monitoring during transport and scanning. Transporting the patient, moving the patient from the bed to the CT table, and positioning the head flat during the CT scan are all stressful events and could cause severe increases in ICP. Continuous monitoring allows for rapid intervention.

Electrophysiology studies can aid in ongoing assessments of neurologic function. Somatosensory evoked potentials may be used to evaluate injuries deep in the brain structures to gain prognostic information.[18] MRI is useful in detecting hematomas and cerebral edema.

Medical Management

Surgical Management. If a lesion, identified by CT scan, is causing a shift of intracranial contents or an increase in ICP, surgical intervention is necessary. A craniotomy is performed to remove the hematoma whether EDH, SDH, or large ICH. Occasionally, if an area of contusion is large, hemorrhagic, and associated with an elevated ICP, a craniotomy with removal of part of the skull may be performed to relieve pressure and prevent herniation. Patients who have had surgery for penetrating head trauma have an increased incidence of posttraumatic seizures and are prescribed anticonvulsants.

Nonsurgical Management. No longer is surgery the only mainstay of treatment of TBI because approximately 95% of management occurs in the intensive care unit.[18] Nonsurgical management includes management of ICP, maintenance of adequate cerebral perfusion pressure and oxygenation, and treatment of any complications (e.g., pneumonia or infection). The decision of when to initiate intracranial pressure monitoring is critical. ICP monitoring may be required for patients with a GCS less than 8 and abnormal findings on a head CT scan.[20,21]

Nursing Management

Nursing priorities in management of traumatic brain injury focus on (1) stabilizing vital signs, (2) preventing further injury, and (3) reducing increased ICP and maintaining adequate CPP (Box 25-6). Ongoing nursing assessments are the cornerstone to the care of patients with TBI. Such assessments are the primary mechanism for determining secondary brain injury from cerebral edema and increased ICP. In addition to astute neurologic assessments, it is crucial to monitor ventilatory and oxygenation requirements, to be knowledgeable about the impact of nursing procedures such as endotracheal suctioning on ICP (Box 25-7), to monitor fluid and electrolyte balance, hemodynamic stability, and nutrition, and to work with a multidisciplinary team to provide family support and education.

SPINAL CORD INJURIES

Approximately 10,000 new spinal cord injuries (SCIs) occur annually, with an overwhelming majority of injuries occurring in males between the ages of 16 and 30.[22] Of the new cases of SCI each year, about 4000 patients will die before arrival to the hospital and 1000 patients will die of complications of their SCI during the hospitalization.[22] The diagnosis of SCI begins with a detailed history of events surrounding the incident, precise evaluation of sensory and motor function, and radiographic studies of the spine.

Mechanism of Injury

The type of primary injury sustained depends on the mechanism of injury. Mechanisms of injury can include hyperflexion, hyperextension, rotation, axial loading (vertical compression), and missile or penetrating injuries.

Box 25-6

NURSING DIAGNOSIS PRIORITIES

Traumatic Brain Injury

- Ineffective Breathing Pattern related to neuromuscular impairment, perceptual/cognitive impairment, p. A-34
- Risk for Aspiration risk factors: impaired laryngeal sensation or reflex; impaired pharyngeal peristalsis or tongue function; impaired laryngeal closure or elevation; increased gastric volume; decreased lower esophageal sphincter pressure, p. A-45
- Impaired Gas Exchange related to ventilation/perfusion mismatching, p. A-29
- Imbalanced Nutrition: Less Than Body Requirements related to lack of exogenous nutrients and increased metabolic demand, p. A-28
- Disturbed Sensory Perception related to altered sensory reception or transmission (neurologic trauma)
- Powerlessness related to lack of control over current situation, p. A-44
- Decreased Intracranial Adaptive Capacity related to failure of normal compensatory mechanisms, p. A-15
- Impaired Physical Mobility related to perceptual/cognitive impairment
- Ineffective Cerebral Tissue Perfusion related to hemorrhage, cerebral edema, p. A-36

Box 25-7

Recommendations for Suctioning Patients With Traumatic Brain Injury

Pass the suction catheter for no longer than 10 seconds.
Limit the number of suction catheter passes, preferably to no more than 2 passes per suctioning episode.
Hyperoxygenate the patient before and after each passage of the suction catheter (e.g., deliver 4 ventilator breaths at 135% of the patient's tidal volume on 100% FIO_2, at a rate of 4 breaths in 20 seconds).
Minimize airway stimulation (i.e., stabilize endotracheal tube, avoid passing the suction catheter all the way to the carina).

From McQuillan KA, Mitchell PH: Traumatic brain injuries. In McQuillan KA et al, editors: *Trauma nursing: from resuscitation through rehabilitation,* ed 3, Philadelphia, 2002, WB Saunders.

Hyperflexion. Hyperflexion injury most often is seen in the cervical area, especially at the level of C5 to C6, because this is the most mobile portion of the cervical spine. This type of injury most often is caused by sudden deceleration motion, as in head-on collisions. Injury occurs from compression of the cord by fracture fragments or as a result of dislocation of the vertebral bodies. Instability of the spinal column occurs because of the rupture or tearing of the posterior muscles and ligaments.

Hyperextension. Hyperextension injuries involve backward and downward motion of the head. With this injury, often seen in rear-end collisions or diving accidents, the spinal cord itself is stretched and distorted. Neurologic deficits associated with this injury are often caused by contusion and ischemia of the cord without significant bony involvement. A mild form of hyperextension is the *whiplash* injury.

Rotation. Rotation injuries often occur in conjunction with a flexion or extension injury. Severe rotation of the neck or body results in tearing of the posterior ligaments and displacement (rotation) of the spinal column.

Axial Loading. Axial loading, or vertical compression, injuries occur from vertical force along the spinal cord. This is most commonly seen in a fall from a height in which the person lands on the feet or buttocks. Compression injuries cause burst fractures of the vertebral body that often send bony fragments into the spinal canal or directly into the spinal cord (Figure 25-4).

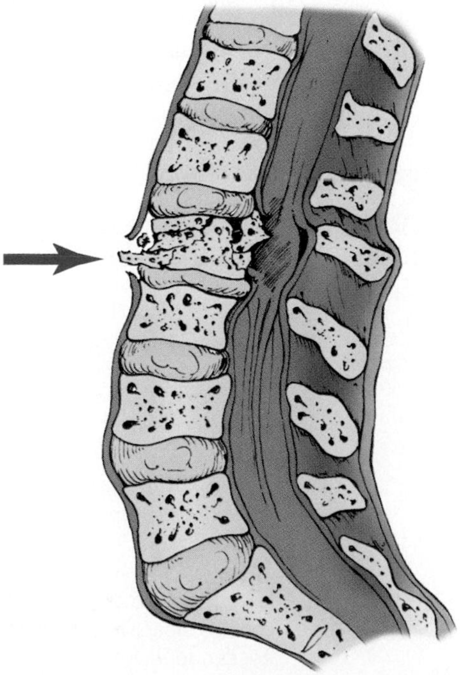

FIGURE 25-4. Spinal cord compression burst fractures. Compression injuries cause burst fractures of the vertebral body that often send bony fragments into the spinal canal or directly into the spinal cord.

Penetrating Injuries. Penetrating injury to the spinal cord can be caused by a bullet, knife, or any other object that penetrates the cord. These types of injury cause permanent damage by anatomically transecting the spinal cord.

Pathophysiology

Spinal cord injuries are the result of a mechanical force that disrupts neurologic tissue or its vascular supply, or both. Much like the pathophysiology of TBI, the injury process includes both primary and secondary injury mechanisms. Primary injury is the neurologic damage that occurs at the moment of impact. Secondary injury refers to the complex biochemical processes affecting cellular function. Secondary injury can occur within minutes of injury and can last for days to weeks.[22]

Several events after a spinal cord injury can lead to spinal cord ischemia and loss of neurologic function. A cascade of events is initiated that includes systemic and local vascular changes, electrolyte and biochemical changes, neurotransmitter accumulation, and local edema (Box 25-8). Collectively, these pathophysiologic events result in worsening of the injury, potentially extending the level of functional deficit, and worsening long-term outcome.[22] Knowledge of the pathophysiology of secondary processes has led to the development of new drugs, which target the cellular changes contributing to injury.[22] Despite ongoing research efforts at repairing the primary injury, minimizing damage through reducing secondary injury has shown the most promise.

Functional Injury of the Spinal Cord

Functional injury of the spinal cord refers to the degree of disruption of normal spinal cord function. This depends on what specific sensory and motor structures within the cord are damaged. SCIs are classified as complete or incomplete, but SCI cannot be accurately classified until spinal shock has resolved.

Complete Injury. Complete SCI results in a total loss of sensory and motor function below the level of injury. Regardless of the mechanism of injury, the result is a complete dissection of the spinal cord and its neurochemical pathways, resulting in one of two conditions: quadriplegia or paraplegia.

Quadriplegia. With quadriplegia the injury occurs from the C1 to T1 level. Residual muscle function depends on the specific cervical segments involved. The potential functional status resulting from different neurologic levels of injury is described in Table 25-4.

Paraplegia. With paraplegia the injury occurs in the thoracolumbar region (T2 to L1). Patients with injuries in this area may have full use of the arms and may need a wheelchair, although some may have limited ability to ambulate short distances with crutches and orthoses. Thoracic L1 and L2 injuries produce paraplegia with variable innervation to intercostal and abdominal muscles.

Incomplete Injury. Incomplete SCI results in a mixed loss of voluntary motor activity and sensation below the level of the lesion. Incomplete SCI exists if any function remains below the level of injury. Incomplete injuries can result in one of a variety of syndromes, which are classified according to the degree of motor and sensory loss below the level of injury. Incomplete injury offers the best prognosis for recovery.[23]

Spinal Shock. Spinal shock is a condition that can occur shortly after traumatic injury to the spinal cord. Spinal shock is the complete loss of all muscle tone and normal reflex activity below the level of injury.[12] Patients with spinal shock may appear to be completely without function below the area of the injury, although all of the area may not necessarily be destroyed.

Neurogenic Shock. Neurogenic shock results from injury to the descending sympathetic pathways in the spinal cord. This results from loss of vasomotor tone and sympathetic innervation to the heart. A relative hypovolemia and hypovolemic shock ensues, causing hypotension and a decreased systemic vascular resistance. Patients with SCI at T6 or above may have profound neurogenic shock as a result of interruption of the sympathetic nervous system and loss of vasoconstrictor response below the level of the injury. Blood vessels cannot constrict and the heart rate is slow, which results in hypotension, venous pooling, and decreased cardiac output. Cellular oxygenation is threatened as cardiac output falls secondary to both a decrease in stroke volume (hypovolemia) and heart rate (bradycardia). This shock state can persist for up to 1 month after injury. Blood pressure support may be required with the use of sympathomimetic drugs. Because hypotension is a problem, be cautious when adjusting backrest position or when repositioning a patient in bed, because orthostatic blood pressure changes can occur.

Box 25-8

Primary and Secondary Mechanisms of Acute Spinal Cord Injury

Primary Injury Mechanisms

Acute Compression
- Impact
- Missile
- Distraction
- Laceration
- Shear

Secondary Injury Mechanisms

Systemic Effects
- Heart rate: brief increase, then prolonged bradycardia
- Blood pressure: brief hypertension, then prolonged hypotension
- Decreased peripheral resistance
- Decreased cardiac output
- Increased catecholamines, then decreased
- Hypoxia
- Hyperthermia
- Injudicious movement of the unstable spine leading to worsening compression

Local vascular changes
- Loss of autoregulation
- Systemic hypotension (neurogenic shock)
- Hemorrhage (especially gray matter)
- Loss of microcirculation
- Reduction in blood flow
- Vasospasm
- Thrombosis

Electrolyte changes
- Increased intracellular calcium
- Increased intracellular sodium
- Increased sodium permeability
- Increased intracellular potassium

Biochemical Changes
- Neurotransmitter accumulation
- Catecholamines (e.g., norepinephrine, dopamine)
- Excitotoxic amino acids (e.g., glutamate)
- Arachidonic acid release
- Free radicals production
- Eicosanoid production
- Prostaglandins
- Lipid peroxidation
- Endogenous opioids
- Cytokines
- Edema
- Loss of energy metabolism
- Decreased adenosine triphosphate production
- Apoptosis

Modified from Sekhon LHS, Fehlings MG: Epidemiology, demographics, and pathophysiology of acute spinal cord injury, *Spine* 26(24S):S2, 2001.

Table 25-4

Quadriplegia Functional Status

NEUROLOGIC LEVEL OF COMPLETE INJURY (VERTEBRAE)	FUNCTIONAL ABILITY
C1-C4	Requires electric wheelchair with breath, head, or shoulder controls
C5	Needs electric wheelchair with hand control and/or manual wheelchair with rim projections; may require adaptive devices to assist with ADLs
C6	Independent in manual wheelchair on level surface; may need hand controls; adaptive devices may be needed for ADLs
C7	Requires manual wheelchair on most surfaces
C8-T1	May need adaptive devices

ADLs, Activities of daily living.

Autonomic Dysreflexia. Autonomic dysreflexia is a life-threatening complication that may occur with SCI. This condition is caused by a massive sympathetic response to a noxious stimulus (full bladder, line insertions, fecal impaction), which results in bradycardia, hypertension, facial flushing, and headache. Immediate intervention is needed to prevent cerebral hemorrhage, seizures, and acute pulmonary edema. Treatment is aimed at alleviating the noxious stimulus. A clinical algorithm for treatment of autonomic dysreflexia is provided in Box 25-9.[24] If symptoms persist, antihypertensive agents can be administered to reduce blood pressure. Prevention of autonomic dysreflexia is imperative and can be accomplished through the use of a good bowel and bladder program.

Box 25-9

Autonomic Dysreflexia

- If patient is supine, immediately sit the patient up.
- Begin frequent vital sign monitoring: perform every 5 minutes.
- Survey for instigating causes: begin with urinary system.
- Loosen clothing, constrictive devices.
- If indwelling catheter is not present, catheterize the patient:
  - Lidocaine jelly may be instilled 5 minutes before catheter insertion.
- If indwelling catheter is present:
  - Check system for kinks, obstructions to flow.
  - Irrigate bladder with small amount of fluid.
  - If not draining, remove catheter and replace.
- If systolic blood pressure is greater than 150 mm Hg, consider rapid-onset, short-duration antihypertensive agent.
- If acute symptoms persist, suspect fecal impaction:
  - Instill lidocaine jelly into rectum; wait at least 5 minutes.
  - Perform digital examination to check for presence of stool; if present, gently remove. If signs of autonomic dysreflexia persist, stop examination; instill additional lidocaine jelly, and wait 20 minutes to reexamine.
  - If no stool found and abdominal distention noted, consider administration of laxative.

Assessment

On admission to the ICU, attention to the ABCs is imperative in the patient with known or suspected SCI. **Nursing priorities in assessment after spinal cord injury focus on evaluation of the ABCs: (1) airway, (2) breathing pattern, (3) circulation, and (4) neurologic status.**

Stabilization of the spinal cord is mandatory to prevent further injury, and spinal precautions are maintained until the spine is cleared of injury. Stabilization in the ICU may include the use of bed rest with log-rolling maneuvers and a hard cervical collar until definitive stabilization is achieved.

Airway. Assessment of ABCs is essential to ensure optimal oxygenation and perfusion to all vital organs, including the spinal cord. Complete cardiovascular and respiratory assessments are essential to the patient's survival and prognosis. The primary assessment begins with an evaluation of airway clearance. In an unresponsive person, an oral airway is inserted while the patient's neck is maintained in a neutral position. The patient must undergo intubation before severe hypoxia can occur, which could further damage the spinal cord.

Breathing. Assessment of breathing patterns and gas exchange is made after an airway has been secured. The level of injury dictates the degree of altered breathing patterns and gas exchange (Table 25-5). Because complete injuries above the C3 level result in paralysis of the diaphragm, patients with these injuries require ventilatory assistance.

Circulation. Assessment of cardiac output and tissue perfusion is imperative to detect life-threatening injuries and promote recovery of injured spinal cord tissue. The patient with SCI is at high risk for developing alterations in cardiac output and tissue perfusion because the cardiovascular system is subjected to a variety of serious and potential physiologic alterations, including dysrhythmias, cardiac arrest, orthostatic hypotension, emboli, and thrombophlebitis.

The patient with an SCI is assessed for adequate tissue perfusion by means of both invasive and non-

Table 25-5

Effects of Spinal Cord Injury on Ventilatory Functions

NEUROLOGIC LEVEL OF COMPLETE INJURY (VERTEBRAE)	RESPIRATORY FUNCTION	COMMENT
C1-C2	Paralysis of diaphragm	Ventilator-dependent
C3-C5	Varying degrees of diaphragm paralysis	Some diaphragm control; may need ventilatory support; weaning depends on preinjury pulmonary status
C6-T11	Varying degrees of impaired intercostal muscles and abdominal muscles	Compromised respiratory function; reduced inspiratory ability; paradoxical breathing patterns; ineffective cough, sneeze

Modified from Moore EE et al: *Surg Clin North Am* 74:295, 1995.

invasive hemodynamic monitoring techniques. Cardiac monitoring is required to detect bradycardia and other dysrhythmias that occur in response to reflex vagus activity mediated by the dominant parasympathetic nervous system, as well as changes in cardiac rhythm that result from hypothermia or hypoxia.

Once the ABCs have been evaluated and interventions for life-threatening complications have been initiated, a full physical assessment is made to determine the extent of injury.

Neurologic Status. The initial neurologic assessment may not be an accurate indication of eventual motor and sensory loss. It focuses on the rapid and accurate identification of present, absent, or impaired functioning of the motor, sensory, and reflex systems that coordinate and regulate vital functions. A detailed motor and sensory examination includes the assessment of all 32 spinal nerves for evidence of dysfunction. Carefully mapped pathways for the sensory portion of the spinal nerves, termed *dermatomes,* can assist in localizing the functional sensory level of injury. Motor function may be graded on a 0 to 5-point scale (Box 25-10). A grade of 0/5 indicates no movement, and 5/5 indicates normal movement. Initial assessment must be performed correctly and findings thoroughly documented in detail so that subsequent serial assessments can rapidly identify deterioration. Ongoing spinal cord assessments must be documented during the critical care phase.

Diagnostic Procedures. Diagnostic radiographic evaluations can identify the severity of damage to the spinal cord. Initial evaluation includes anteroposterior and lateral views for all areas of the spinal cord. Films of all seven cervical vertebrae and the top of T1 must be obtained to rule out cervicothoracic junction injury. Flexion and extension views can identify subtle ligamentous injuries. CT scan, tomograms, myelography, and MRI also may be used in the diagnostic process.

Screening for Spinal Cord Injury. About 15% of trauma patients with injury will have a cervical spine injury.[18] Screening of the spinal cord for injury becomes an integral part of the assessment for all trauma patients. The degree of trauma, alteration in mentation, intoxication, or distracting injuries will dictate the type and extent of examination required to clear the cervical spine. The Eastern Association for the Surgery of Trauma (EAST) developed guidelines for the clearance of the cervical spine (Table 25-6). On admission, the spine is palpated for obvious deformity and the patient is assessed for the subjective response of pain to palpation. If the patient has distracting injuries, such as rib fractures, is intoxicated, or has received analgesics, examination of the spinal cord may be deferred.[18] An MRI may be done to make a definitive diagnosis.

Medical Management

After assessment and diagnosis of the SCI, medical management begins. The primary treatment goal is to preserve remaining neurologic function. Medical interventions are divided into pharmacologic, surgical, and nonsurgical interventions.

Box 25-10

Muscle Strength Scale

Active movement against maximal resistance
Active movement through range of motion against resistance
Active movement through range of motion against gravity
Active movement through range of motion with gravity eliminated
Flicker or trace of contraction
No contraction; total paralysis

Table 25-6

EAST Guidelines for Cervical Spine Clearance

PATIENT POPULATION	RECOMMENDATION
Alert, awake, not intoxicated, neurologically normal, no complaints of neck pain	Neck is palpated in all directions for tenderness or pain. If physical examination is negative for pain or tenderness, plain films are not necessary.
Awake, alert, not intoxicated, with complaints of neck pain	Cervical spine x-ray films are obtained. CT scan may be obtained through suspicious areas identified on three-view cervical spine x-ray films.
Neurologic deficits referable to a spine injury	Plain films and CT images with MRI of the cervical spine.
Altered mental status and return of normal mental status not anticipated for 2 days or more (e.g., severe traumatic or hypoxic, ischemic brain injury)	Plain films and CT images. Axial CT images at 3-mm intervals with sagittal reconstruction from the base of the occiput through C2. If plain films and CT images are normal, flexion/extension lateral cervical spine fluoroscopy with static images obtained at extremes of flexion and extension.

EAST guidelines: determination of cervical spine stability in trauma patients, East Northport, NY, 2000. Eastern Association for the Surgery of Trauma, http://www.east.org.
CT, Computed tomography; *MRI,* magnetic resonance imaging; *EAST,* Eastern Association for the Surgery of Trauma.

Pharmacologic Management. Methylprednisolone has been shown to improve neurologic outcome after spinal cord injury. Patients with SCI should receive a methylprednisolone bolus followed by a continuous infusion for at least 24 hours, and preferably 48 hours, if their treatment began 3 to 8 hours after their injury.[25] Methylprednisolone directly affects the changes that occur within the spinal cord after injury, primarily by preventing posttraumatic spinal cord ischemia, improving energy metabolism, restoring extracellular calcium, and improving nerve impulse conduction.

Surgical Management. Surgical intervention provides spinal column stability in the presence of an unstable injury. Unstable injuries include disrupted ligaments and tendons, as well as a vertebral column that cannot maintain normal alignment. Identification and immobilization of unstable injuries is particularly important for the patient with incomplete neurologic deficit. Without adequate stabilization, movement and dislocation of the vertebral column could cause a complete neurologic deficit. A variety of surgical procedures may be performed to achieve decompression and stabilization. The question of when surgery should be performed remains controversial.

Nonsurgical Management. If the injury to the spinal cord is stable, nonsurgical management is the treatment of choice. Nonsurgical management for cervical and thoracolumbar injuries is discussed here.

Cervical Injury. Management of cervical injuries involves the immobilization of the fracture site and realignment of any dislocation. This is accomplished through skeletal traction that involves the use of two-point tongs, which are inserted into the skull through shallow burr holes and are connected to traction weights. Several types of cervical tongs are used. Gardner-Wells and Crutchfield tongs are the most common. These tongs can be applied at the bedside with the use of a local anesthetic.

After the procedure the patient can be immobilized on a kinetic therapy bed or a regular bed. The kinetic therapy bed is the most popular method used for cervical immobilization because it maintains spinal column alignment while providing constant turning motion to reduce pulmonary and skin breakdown. Use of cervical skeletal traction on a regular bed makes it difficult to provide adequate care to the pulmonary system and skin because of the extensive degree of immobility.

After the spinal column has been adequately realigned by means of skeletal traction, a halo traction brace often is applied. The halo vest consists of a metal ring secured to the skull with two occipital and two temporal screws. Steel bars anchor the screws to the vest to provide cervical immobilization (Figure 25-5). The halo traction brace immobilizes the cervical spine, which allows the patient to ambulate and participate in self-care.

Thoracolumbar Injury. Nonsurgical management of the patient with a thoracolumbar injury also involves immobilization. Skeletal traction may be used in high thoracic injury. For the most part, misalignment of the spinal canal does not occur in stable injuries of the thoracolumbar spine. Immobilization to allow fractures to heal is accomplished by bed rest (with bed flat) and the use of a plastic or fiberglass jacket, a body cast, or a brace.

Nursing Management

Nursing diagnoses and management for the patient with spinal cord injury are summarized in Box 25-11. The goal during the critical care phase is to prevent life-threatening complications while maximizing the function of all organ systems. **Nursing priorities are aimed at (1) preventing secondary damage to the spinal cord, (2) managing cardiovascular and pulmonary complications, and (3) coaching the patient to overcome the psychosocial challenges associated with severe neurologic deficit** (see Box 25-11). Because almost all body systems are affected by SCI, nursing management includes interventions that optimize nutrition, elimination, skin integrity, and mobility. Patients with SCI have complex psychosocial needs that necessitate a great deal of emotional support from the critical care nurse.

THORACIC INJURIES

Thoracic injuries involve trauma to the chest wall, the lungs, the heart, the great vessels, and the esophagus.

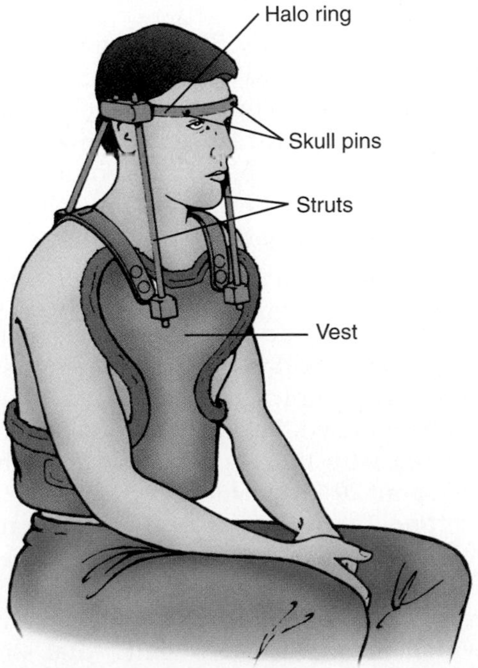

FIGURE 25-5. Halo vest. The halo traction brace immobilizes the cervical spine, which allows the patient to ambulate and participate in self-care.

Box 25-11

NURSING DIAGNOSIS PRIORITIES

Spinal Cord Injury

- Decreased Cardiac Output related to lack of sympathetic innervation, p. A-12
- Risk for Autonomic Dysreflexia related to spinal cord injury above T8
- Impaired Gas Exchange related to alveolar hypoventilation, p. A-29
- Ineffective Breathing Pattern related to impairment of innervation of diaphragm (lesion above C5), complete or mixed loss of intercostal muscle function, p. A-34
- Impaired Physical Mobility related to neuromuscular impairment, immobilization by traction, paralysis
- Risk for Impaired Skin Integrity related to immobility, traction, tissue pressure, altered peripheral circulation, and sensation
- Bowel Incontinence related to disruption of innervation to bowel and rectum, perceptual impairment, altered fluid and food intake
- Constipation related to disruption of innervation to bowel and rectum, perceptual impairment, altered fluid and food intake
- Impaired Urinary Elimination related to disruption in bladder innervation, bladder atony
- Disturbed Body Image related to actual change in body structure, function, or appearance, p. A-20
- Ineffective Coping related to situational crisis and personal vulnerability, p. A-38

Thoracic trauma most commonly is the result of a violent crime or MVC.

Mechanism of Injury

Blunt Thoracic Trauma. Blunt trauma to the chest most often is caused by MVCs or falls. Second only to head and spinal cord injury, thoracic injuries account for 20% of trauma deaths. The underlying mechanism of injury tends to be a combination of acceleration/deceleration injury and direct transfer mechanics, such as in a crush injury. Varying mechanisms of blunt trauma are associated with specific injury patterns. After head-on collisions, drivers have a higher frequency of injury than do backseat passengers because the driver comes in contact with the steering assembly. Severe thoracic injuries often are seen in patients who are unrestrained. Falls from greater than 20 feet are associated with thoracic injury. Pneumothorax is present in about 20% of major blunt trauma.[26]

Penetrating Thoracic Injuries. The penetrating object involved determines the damage sustained from penetrating thoracic trauma. Trauma from firearms raises many clinical issues such as the path of the bullet within the chest and whether vital structures are involved and identification of the bullet entrance and corresponding exit wound (if present) because sometimes the bullet remains inside.[27] Another concern are stab wounds that involve the anterior chest wall between the midclavicular lines, Louis's angle, and the epigastric region because of the proximity of the heart and/or great vessels.

Specific Thoracic Traumatic Injuries

Chest Wall Injuries

Rib Fractures. Fractures of certain ribs or multiple rib fractures can be more serious. Fractures of certain ribs are associated with more underlying, life-threatening injuries. Fractures of the first and second ribs are associated with intrathoracic vascular injuries (brachial plexus, great vessels). Right-sided fractures at the eighth rib and below are associated with liver injury.[28] Left-sided fractures at the same level are associated with spleen injury.[28] If six or more ribs are fractured, this is associated with an increased number of complications such as pneumonia and also death.[29]

The pain associated with rib fractures is aggravated by respiratory excursion. As a result, the patient often splints, takes shallow breaths, and refuses to cough, which can result in atelectasis and pneumonia. Nonsteroidal antiinflammatory drugs (NSAIDs), intercostal nerve blocks, thoracic epidural analgesia, and narcotics may all assist with pain control.[28] Epidural analgesia is associated with lower mortality in major trauma with rib fractures; however, it is infrequently employed in trauma critical care.[29] Epidural analgesia has been shown to help increase functional residual capacity (FRC), dynamic lung compliance, and vital capacity; decrease airway resistance; and increase partial pressure of oxygen (PaO_2).[30] External splints are not recommended because they further limit chest wall expansion and may add to atelectasis.[30]

Flail Chest. Flail chest, caused by blunt trauma, disrupts the continuity of chest wall structures. A flail chest occurs when two or more ribs are fractured in two or more places and are no longer attached to the thoracic cage.[31] This results in a free-floating segment of the chest wall. This segment moves independently from the rest of the thorax and results in paradoxic chest wall movement during the respiratory cycle (Figure 25-6). During inspiration the intact portion of the chest wall expands, while the injured part is sucked in. During expiration the chest wall moves in, and the flail segment moves out. Inspection of the chest reveals *paradoxic movement*. Palpation of the chest may reveal crepitus and tenderness near fractured ribs. A chest x-ray examination will show multiple rib fractures. The effects of impaired chest wall motion include decreased tidal volume and vital capacity and impaired cough, which lead to hypoventilation and atelectasis.

Ruptured Diaphragm. Diagnosis of a diaphragmatic rupture may be missed in trauma patients because of the subtle and nonspecific symptoms this injury produces. The mechanism of injury appears to be a rapid rise

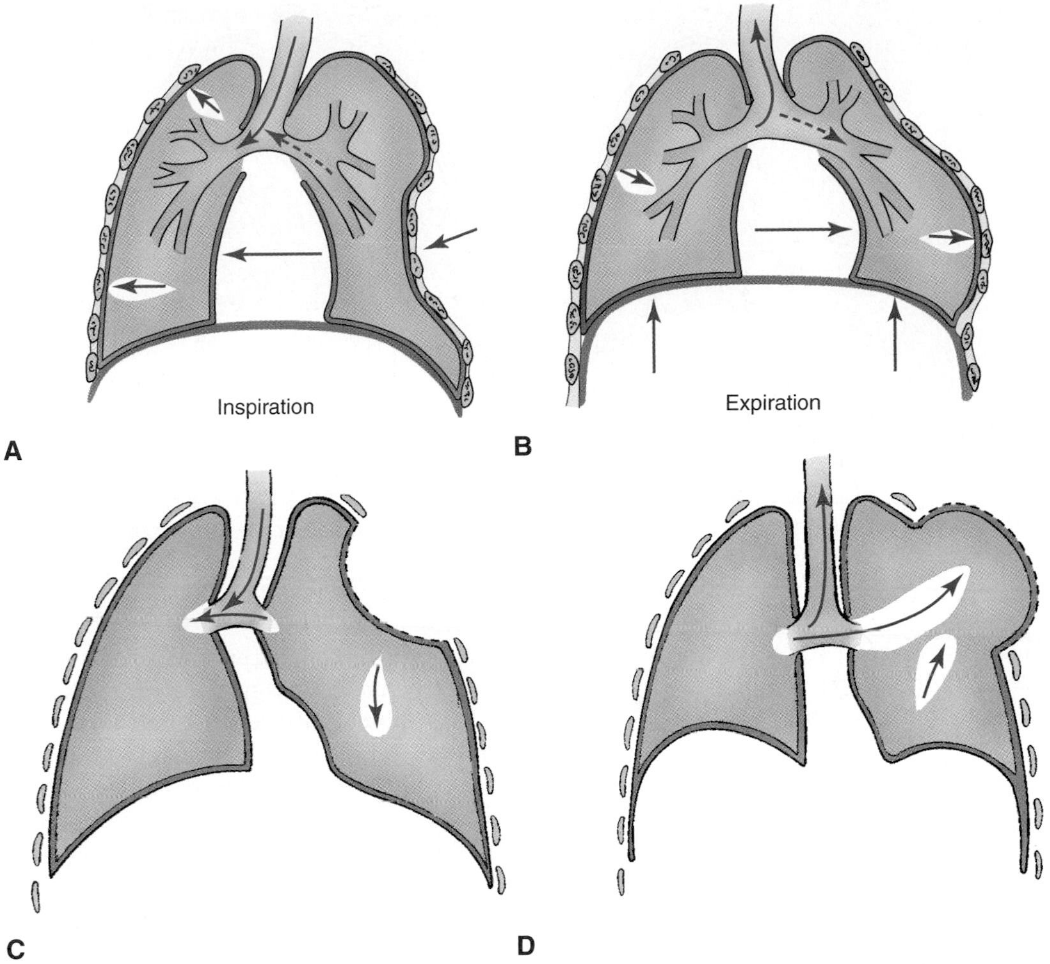

FIGURE 25-6. Flail chest. **A,** Normal inspiration. **B,** Normal expiration. **C,** Inspiration: area of lung underlying unstable chest wall sucks in on inspiration. **D,** Same area balloons out on expiration. Note movement of mediastinum toward opposite lung on inspiration.

in intraabdominal pressure as a result of compression force applied to the lower part of the chest or upper region of the abdomen. This injury can occur when a person is thrown forward over the tip of the steering wheel in a high-speed deceleration accident. The force can cause the diaphragm, which offers little resistance, to rupture or tear. Abdominal viscera then can gradually enter the thoracic cavity, moving from the positive pressure of the abdomen to the negative pressure in the thorax. Diaphragmatic rupture can be life-threatening. Massive herniation of abdominal contents into the thoracic cavity can compress the lungs and mediastinum, which then hampers venous return and leads to decreased cardiac output. In addition, herniated bowel can become strangulated and perforate.

Diaphragmatic herniation may produce significant compromise and changes in respiratory effort. Auscultation of bowel sounds in the chest or unilateral breath sounds may indicate a ruptured diaphragm. The patient may complain of shoulder pain, shortness of breath, or abdominal tenderness. Thoracoscopy may be helpful in evaluating the diaphragm in indeterminate cases.[32] A chest film may reveal the tip of a nasogastric tube above the diaphragm, a unilaterally elevated hemidiaphragm, a hollow or solid mass above the diaphragm, and a shift of the mediastinum away from the affected side. Treatment of a ruptured diaphragm includes its immediate repair.

Pulmonary Injuries

Pulmonary Contusion. A pulmonary contusion is fundamentally a bruise of the lung. Pulmonary contusion often is associated with blunt trauma and other chest injuries, such as rib fractures and flail chest, and is the most common potentially lethal chest injury.[31] Pulmonary contusions can occur unilaterally or bilaterally. A contusion manifests initially as a hemorrhage followed by alveolar and interstitial edema. The edema can remain rather localized in the contused area or can spread to other lung areas. Inflammation affects alveolar-capillary units. As more units are affected by inflammation, further pathophysiologic events can occur, including decreased compliance, increased pulmonary vascular resistance, and decreased pulmonary

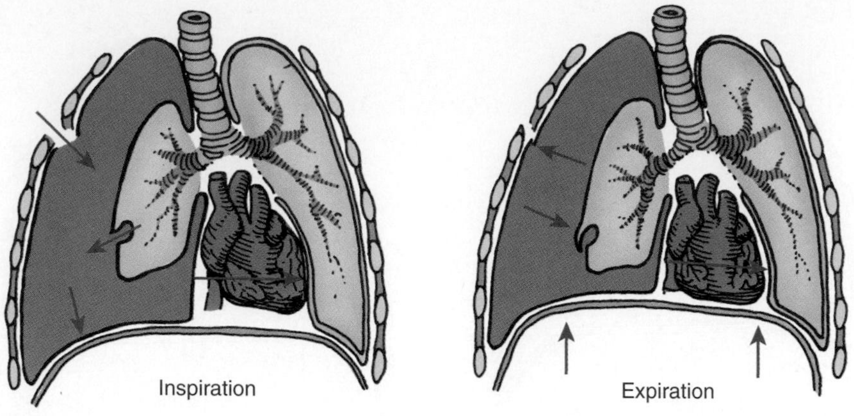

FIGURE 25-7. A tension pneumothorax usually is caused by an injury that perforates the chest wall or pleural space. Air flows into the pleural space with inspiration and becomes trapped. As pressure in the pleural space increases, the lung on the injured side collapses and causes the mediastinum to shift to the opposite side. (From Marx J et al: *Rosen's emergency medicine: concepts and clinical practice,* ed 5, St Louis, 2002, Mosby.)

blood flow. These processes result in a ventilation/perfusion imbalance, which results in hypoxemia and poor ventilation that progresses over a 24- to 48-hour period.

Clinical manifestations of pulmonary contusion may take up to 24 to 48 hours to develop. Inspections of the chest wall may reveal ecchymosis at the site of impact. Moist crackles may be noted in the contused lung. A cough may be present with blood-tinged sputum. Abnormal lung function can be detected by systemic arterial hypoxemia. The diagnosis is made primarily by chest x-ray studies consistent with pulmonary infiltrate corresponding to the area of external chest impact that is manifested within 12 to 24 hours of injury. Pulmonary contusions tend to worsen over a 24- to 48-hour period and then slowly resolve unless complications occur such as infection or acute respiratory distress syndrome [ARDS].

Tension Pneumothorax. A tension pneumothorax usually is caused by an injury that perforates the chest wall or pleural space. Air flows into the pleural space with inspiration and becomes trapped. As pressure in the pleural space increases, the lung on the injured side collapses and causes the mediastinum to shift to the opposite side (Figure 25-7). As pressure continues to build, the shift exerts pressure on the heart and thoracic aorta, which results in decreased venous return and decreased cardiac output. Tissue perfusion with oxygenated blood is further hampered because the collapsed lung cannot participate in gas exchange.

Clinical manifestations of a tension pneumothorax include dyspnea, tachycardia, hypotension, or sudden chest pain extending to the shoulders. Tracheal deviation will be noted as the trachea shifts away from the injured side. On the injured side, breath sounds can be decreased or absent. Percussion of the chest reveals a hyperresonant sound over the affected side. Diagnosis of tension pneumothorax is made by clinical assessment. There is no time for a chest film inasmuch as this potentially lethal condition must be treated immediately.[12] A large-bore (14-gauge) needle or chest tube is inserted into the affected lung. This procedure allows immediate release of air from the pleural space. A hissing sound is heard as the tension pneumothorax is converted to a simple pneumothorax.

Open Pneumothorax. An open pneumothorax, or "sucking chest wound," usually is caused by penetrating trauma. Open communication between the atmosphere and intrathoracic pressure results in immediate lung deflation. Air moves in and out of the hole in the chest, producing a sucking sound heard on inspiration. An open pneumothorax produces the same symptoms as does a tension pneumothorax. In addition, subcutaneous emphysema may be palpated around the wound. Initial management of an open pneumothorax is accomplished by promptly closing the wound at end expiration with a sterile occlusive dressing (plastic wrap or petroleum gauze) large enough to overlap the wound's edges.[33] This dressing should be taped securely on three sides. As the patient breathes in, the dressing gets sucked in to occlude the wound and prevent air from entering. A chest tube is placed as soon as possible. Surgical intervention may be required to close the wound.

Hemothorax. Blunt or penetrating thoracic trauma can cause bleeding into the pleural space, resulting in a hemothorax (Figure 25-8). A massive hemothorax results from the accumulation of more than 1500 ml in the chest cavity.[33] The source of bleeding may be the intercostal or internal mammary arteries, the lungs, the heart, or the great vessels. Lacerations to the lung parenchyma are low-pressure bleeds and therefore typically stop bleeding spontaneously.[31] Arterial bleeding from hilar vessels usually requires immediate

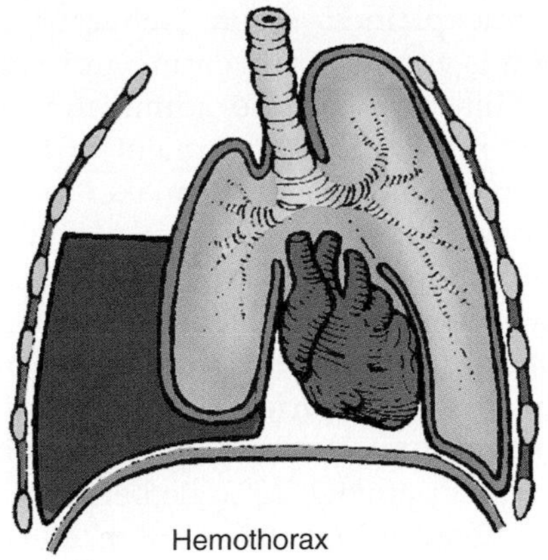

FIGURE 25-8. Blunt or penetrating thoracic trauma can cause bleeding into the pleural space to form a hemothorax.

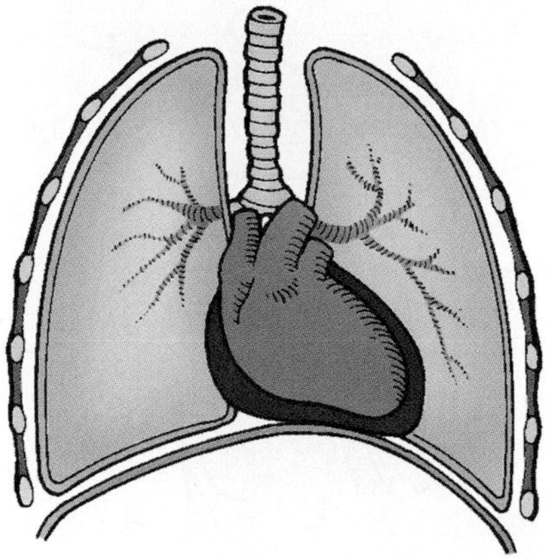

FIGURE 25-9. Cardiac tamponade is the progressive accumulation of blood in the pericardial sac.

surgical intervention.[12] In either case, increasing intrapleural pressure results in a decrease in vital capacity. Increasing vascular blood loss into the pleural space causes decreased venous return and decreased cardiac output.

Breath sounds may be diminished or absent over the affected lung. With hemothorax, the neck veins are collapsed and the trachea is at midline. Massive hemothorax can be diagnosed on the basis of clinical manifestations of hypotension associated with the absence of breath sounds and/or dullness to percussion on one side of the chest.[12] This life-threatening condition must be treated immediately. Resuscitation with IV fluids is initiated to treat the hypovolemic shock. A chest tube is placed on the affected side to allow drainage of blood. An autotransfusion device can be attached to the chest tube collection chamber. Thoracotomy may be necessary for patients who require persistent blood transfusions or who have significant bleeding (200 ml/hr for 2 to 4 hours) or when there are injuries to major cardiovascular structures.[34]

Nursing Management. **Nursing priorities for the patient with traumatic chest or pulmonary injury emphasize delivery of adequate (1) oxygenation, (2) ventilation, and (3) pain management.** Assistance with intubation and monitoring of mechanical ventilation may be required to prevent tissue hypoxia and provide adequate ventilatory support. Aggressive removal of airway secretions is important to avoid infection and improve ventilation. Hypoxemia is prevented by continuous pulse oximetry monitoring of arterial oxygen saturation (Spo_2) and arterial blood gas (ABG) analysis. Judicious administration of IV fluids and analgesia is important to improve patient comfort.

Cardiac Injuries

Penetrating Cardiac Injuries. Penetrating cardiac trauma can occur from mechanical injuries as a result of bullets, knives, or impalements. The chest wall offers little protection to the heart from penetrating trauma. The most common site of injury is the right ventricle because of its anterior position. Mortality from penetrating trauma to the heart is high. Prehospital mortality for penetrating cardiac injuries is very high, and most deaths occur within minutes after injury as a result of exsanguination or tamponade.

Cardiac Tamponade. Cardiac tamponade is the progressive accumulation of blood in the pericardial sac (Figure 25-9). With cardiac tamponade a progressive accumulation of blood, 120 to 150 ml, increases the intracardiac pressure and compresses the atria and ventricles.[33] An increase in intracardiac pressure leads to decreased venous return and decreased filling pressure, which leads to decreased cardiac output, myocardial hypoxia, cardiac failure, and cardiogenic shock.[33]

Classic assessment findings associated with cardiac tamponade are termed *Beck's triad*—presence of elevated central venous pressure with neck vein distention, muffled heart sounds, and hypotension. Pulsus paradoxus may be present. Pulseless electrical activity (PEA) in the absence of hypovolemia and tension pneumothorax is suggestive of cardiac tamponade.[12] Ultrasonography in the emergency setting may be used in penetrating cardiac injuries to identify a hemopericardium.[35] The major nursing diagnosis for this injury is Decreased Cardiac Output. Immediate treatment is required to remove the accumulation of fluid in the pericardial sac. Pericardiocentesis involves the aspiration of fluid from the pericardium by use of a large-bore needle. The inherent risk in this procedure is potential laceration of the coronary artery. Other approaches include surgical procedures, such as thoracotomy or median sternotomy. The goal of these procedures is to locate and control the source of bleeding.

Blunt Cardiac Injuries. The most common causes of blunt cardiac trauma include high-speed MVCs, direct blows to the chest, and falls. The heart, because of its mobility and its location between the sternum and thoracic vertebrae, is susceptible to blunt traumatic injury. Sudden acceleration (as from contact with a steering wheel) can cause the heart to be thrown against the sternum (Figure 25-10). Sudden deceleration can

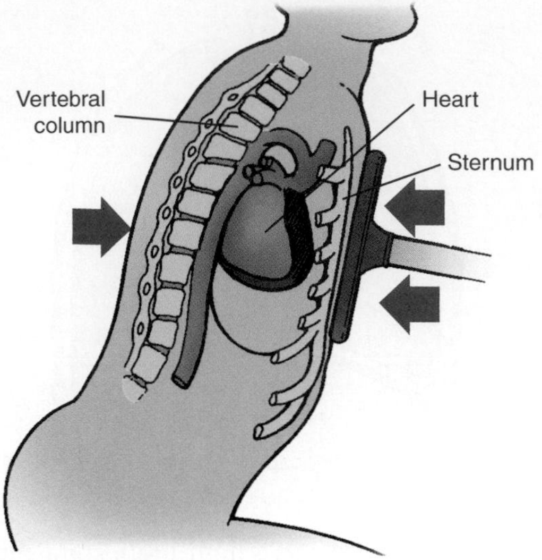

FIGURE 25-10. Blunt cardiac trauma. Sudden acceleration (as from contact with the steering wheel) can cause the heart to be thrown against the sternum.

Box 25-12

EAST Guidelines for Screening of Blunt Cardiac Injury (BCI)

- Admission ECG for all patients in whom there is suspected BCI.
- If ECG is abnormal, the patient should be admitted for continuous ECG monitoring for 24 to 48 hours.
- If the patient is hemodynamically unstable, an echocardiogram may be performed.
- Cardiac enzymes and/or cardiac troponin T are not useful in predicting which patients will have complications related to BCI.

Data from EAST guidelines: determination of cervical spine stability in trauma patients, East Northport, NY, 2000, Eastern Association for the Surgery of Trauma, http://www.east.org.
EAST, Eastern Association for the Surgery of Trauma; *ECG,* electrocardiogram.

cause the heart to be thrown against the thoracic vertebrae by a direct blow to the chest (such as blows caused by a baseball, animal kick, or fall).

Blunt cardiac injury (BCI), formerly called *myocardial contusion,* covers the spectrum of myocardial contusion, concussion, and rupture. The most often injured chambers include the right atrium and ventricle because of their anterior position in the chest.[36]

Few clinical signs and symptoms are specific for BCI. Evidence of external chest trauma, such as steering wheel imprint or sternal fractures, should raise the suspicion for blunt cardiac injury. However, the presence of a sternal fracture does not predict the incidence of BCI. The patient may complain of chest pain that is similar to anginal pain. However, it is not typically relieved with nitroglycerin.[36] The chest pain is usually caused by associated injuries. The EAST Guidelines for screening of BCI are listed in Box 25-12. An ECG may reveal dysrhythmias, ST changes, heart block, or unexplained sinus tachycardia. Medical management is aimed at preventing and treating complications. This may include administration of antidysrhythmic medications, treatment of heart failure, or insertion of a temporary pacemaker to control conduction abnormalities. Assessment of fluid and electrolyte balance is imperative to ensure adequate cardiac output and myocardial conduction.

Aortic Injury. Blunt aortic injury is one of the most lethal blunt thoracic injuries. Disruption of the aorta in blunt chest trauma is a leading cause of immediate death in trauma patients: 22% die before reaching the ED, 37% die during initial resuscitation or in the operating room, and 14% die after surgery.[37] Of the survivors, 19% develop paraplegia or paresis.[37] Injuries associated with aortic injury include a first or second rib fracture, high sternal fracture, left clavicular fracture at the level of the sternal margin, and massive hemothorax.[38] However, blunt aortic injury should be suspected in all victims of trauma with a rapid deceleration or acceleration mechanism of injury.[33]

The thoracic aorta is relatively mobile and tears at fixed anatomic points within the thorax. Sites of aortic disruption in order of frequency include the aortic isthmus, just distal to the subclavian artery (where the vessel is fixed to the chest by the ligamentum arteriosum); at the ascending aorta (where the aorta leaves the pericardial sac); at the descending aorta (where the aorta enters the diaphragm); and avulsion of the innominate artery from the aortic arch.[33]

The nurse assesses blood pressure bilaterally because a tear in the aortic arch may create a pressure gradient, resulting in blood pressure changes between upper extremities. If aortic disruption is suspected, blood pressure is also compared between upper and lower extremities. Baroreceptors are stimulated, resulting in upper extremity hypertension with relative lower extremity hypotension. Additional clinical assessment findings include a pulse deficit anywhere, unexplained hypotension, sternal pain, precordial systolic murmur, hoarseness, dyspnea, and lower extremity sensory deficits.

Initial radiograph is obtained in the upright position once it is considered safe to do so.[33] Radiograph findings suggestive of aortic injury include a widened mediastinum, obscured aortic knob, deviation of the left mainstem bronchus or nasogastric tube, and opacification of the aortopulmonary window.[38] A spiral or helical CT may be warranted if the initial radiograph is inconclusive, but definitive diagnosis is made by aortography in indeterminate cases.[38]

During the resuscitation phase for a patient with aortic disruption, blood pressure management is the primary goal to minimize injury. Patients with tears at the aortic isthmus are typically hypertensive, and minimizing stress on the vessel is achieved by maintaining the systolic blood pressure at less than 90 mm Hg by using antihypertensive agents such as sodium nitroprusside.[38] The nurse anticipates definitive surgical intervention early in the resuscitation. Surgical repair may be achieved by grafting, primary anastomosis, and bypassing.[38]

Postoperative care is directed toward BP stabilization with the goal of minimizing vessel stress while maintaining tissue perfusion, typically accomplished by use of sodium nitroprusside. Careful assessment of postoperative paraplegia is needed, because lack of blood flow to the spinal column may have occurred perioperatively. Paraplegia is closely related to duration of clamp time intraoperatively.[33] The critical care nurse monitors for signs of bowel ischemia (tube feeding intolerance, lactic acidosis) and renal failure (poor urinary output, rising creatinine level) because mesenteric and renal blood flow may have been compromised as a result of the injury or aortic clamp time.

Abdominal Injuries

Abdominal injuries often are associated with multisystem trauma. Abdominal injuries are the third leading cause of traumatic death. Injuries to the abdomen are the result of blunt or penetrating trauma. Two major, life-threatening conditions that occur after abdominal trauma are hemorrhage and hollow viscus perforation with its associated peritonitis. Death occurring after 48 hours following injury is the result of sepsis and its complications. The critical care nurse must pay particular attention to complication prevention strategies throughout the trauma cycle.

Mechanism of Injury

Blunt Trauma. Blunt abdominal injuries are common. They result most often from MVCs, falls, and assaults. In MVCs, abdominal injury is more likely to occur when a vehicle is struck from the side. In the passenger position of the front seat, hepatic injury is likely when the point of impact is on the same side as the passenger. A driver is likely to sustain injury to the spleen when the impact is on the driver's side. Pedestrians hit by motor vehicles are at risk for serious abdominal injuries. Blunt trauma to the thorax can produce injuries to the liver, the spleen, and the diaphragm.[39] Deceleration and direct forces can produce retroperitoneal hematomas. Intestinal injuries are more common sources of injury when compared to penetrating trauma injuries.[39] Blunt abdominal injuries often are hidden, requiring careful assessment and reassessment. Unrecognized abdominal trauma is a frequent cause of preventable deaths, and blunt abdominal injury deaths are more likely to be fatal than are penetrating abdominal injuries.

Penetrating Trauma. Penetrating abdominal trauma is caused most often by knives or bullets. The danger of penetrating abdominal trauma is that the outside appearance of the wound does not reflect the extent of internal injury. Commonly injured organs from knife wounds are the colon, the liver, the spleen, and the diaphragm. Gunshot wounds to the abdomen usually are more serious than are stab wounds. A bullet destroys tissue along its path. Once inside the abdomen, a bullet can travel in erratic paths and ricochet off bone. Death from penetrating injuries depends on the injury to major vascular structures and resultant intraabdominal hemorrhage.

Assessment

The initial assessment of the trauma patient, whether in the ED or the critical care unit, follows the primary and secondary survey techniques as outlined by ATLS guidelines.[12] The initial physical assessment may be unreliable given the confounding influences of alcohol, illicit drugs, analgesics, and an altered level of consciousness. Specific assessment findings associated with abdominal trauma are reviewed here.

Physical Assessment. The location of entry and exit sites associated with penetrating trauma are assessed and documented. Inspection of the patient's abdomen may reveal purplish discoloration of the flanks or umbilicus (Cullen's sign), which is indicative of blood in the abdominal wall. Ecchymosis in the flank area (Grey Turner's sign) may indicate retroperitoneal bleeding or a possible fracture of the pancreas. A hematoma in the flank area is suggestive of renal injury. A distended abdomen may indicate the accumulation of blood, fluid, or gas secondary to a perforated organ or ruptured blood vessel. Auscultation of the abdomen may reveal friction rubs over the liver or spleen and may indicate rupture. The abdomen is assessed for rebound tenderness and rigidity. Presence of these assessment findings indicates peritoneal inflammation. Referred pain to the left shoulder (Kehr's sign) may indicate a ruptured spleen or irritation of the diaphragm from bile or other material in the peritoneum. Subcutaneous emphysema palpated on the abdomen suggests free air as a result of a ruptured bowel.

Diagnostic Procedures. Insertion of a nasogastric tube and urinary catheter serves as a useful diagnostic and therapeutic aid. A nasogastric tube can decompress the stomach, and the contents can be checked for blood. Urine obtained from the urinary catheter can be tested for the presence of blood.

Serial laboratory test results may be nonspecific for the patient with abdominal trauma. A serum amylase determination can detect pancreatic injuries. Because of hemoconcentration, hemoglobin and hematocrit results may not reflect actual values. Serial values are more valuable in diagnosing abdominal injuries.

Diagnostic testing may occur simultaneously during the primary and secondary surveys. Tests may include the diagnostic peritoneal lavage (DPL), bedside ultrasonography, and chest radiograph. DPL can exclude or confirm the presence of intraabdominal injury with a high accuracy rate. After the patient's bladder has been emptied, a small incision is made in the abdomen through the skin and into the peritoneum. A small catheter is inserted (Figure 25-11). If frank blood is encountered, intraabdominal injury is obvious and the patient is taken immediately to the OR. If gross blood is not initially encountered, a liter of fluid (lactated Ringer's or 0.9% normal saline) is infused through the catheter into the abdomen. The IV bag is then placed in a dependent position, and abdominal fluid is allowed to drain into the IV bag. The drainage fluid is sent to the laboratory for analysis. Positive DPL results signal intraabdominal trauma and usually necessitate surgical intervention (Box 25-13). DPL is invasive, has been associated with complications, and cannot exclude retroperitoneal injuries.

Bedside ultrasonography has gained wide use in the United States for the detection of abdominal free fluid and hemoperitoneum. Focused Assessment with Sonography for Trauma (FAST) is noninvasive, does not involve potentially dangerous dyes, is convenient, and is cost-effective. Typically four areas are examined: the right upper quadrant (RUQ) Morrison's pouch; the pericardial sac; the left upper quadrant (LUQ) splenorenal area; and the pelvis (Douglas' pouch).[40] The primary disadvantage of FAST is the need for free intraperitoneal fluid to cause a positive study.[41] An initial negative FAST may be followed with either serial ultrasound examinations, DPL, or abdominal CT.[42]

Although this test has been shown to have good sensitivity and specificity, it is not intended to replace DPL or CT. Obese abdomens and patients with ascites may have erroneous results, and further work-up for these patients is warranted.[40] Ultrasonography is also limited in its ability to diagnose diaphragmatic, intestinal, or pancreas injuries.[41] Abdominal CT scanning is the mainstay of diagnostic evaluation in the hemodynamically stable trauma patient.[41] Abdominal CT provides information as to specific organ injury, pelvic injury, and retroperitoneal hemorrhage.

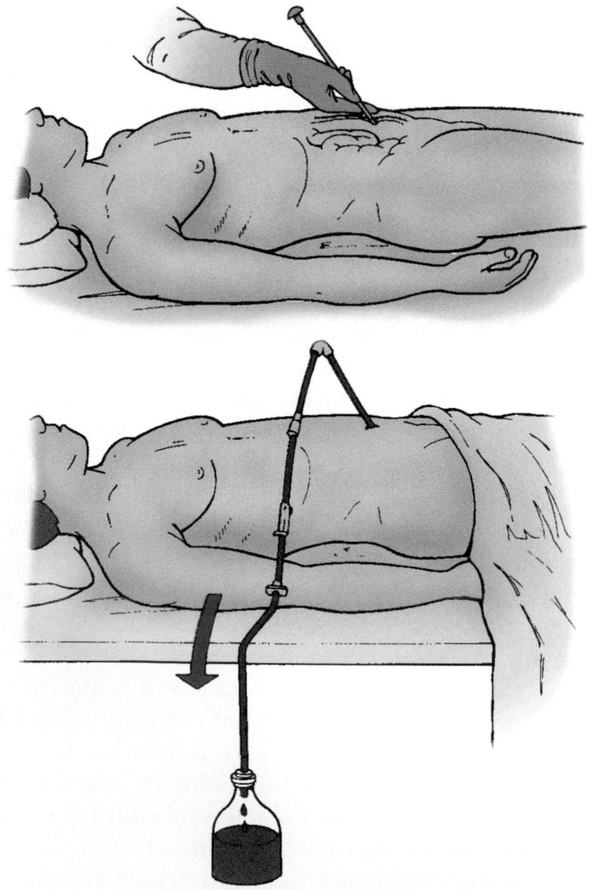

FIGURE 25-11. Diagnostic peritoneal lavage (DPL) can exclude or confirm the presence of intraabdominal injury with a high accuracy rate.

Combined Abdominal Organ Injuries

Patients with multivisceral injuries may require surgical intervention that uses somewhat nontraditional techniques, referred to as "damage control" surgery. The three phases to this treatment strategy are *initial operation, ICU resuscitation,* and *definitive reoperation* (Box 25-14).[43] The duration of this initial operation is kept to a minimum. The decision to abbreviate the initial operation is made early during surgery. Decisions that could lead the surgeon to choose an abbreviated

Box 25-13

Positive Peritoneal Lavage Results

- Red blood cell count: 100,000/mm³
- White blood cell count: 500/mm³
- Amylase: 175 units/dl
- Presence of blood, stool, bile, bacteria

Box 25-14

Damage Control Sequence

1. Initial operation
   Control contamination
   Control hemorrhage
   Intraabdominal packing
   Temporary closure
2. Intensive care unit (ICU) resuscitation
   Correct coagulopathy
   Rewarming
   Maximize hemodynamics
   Ventilatory support
   Injury identification
3. Planned reoperation
   Pack removal
   Definitive repair

laparotomy include hypothermia and coagulopathy in a patient who is hemodynamically unstable, inability to control bleeding by direct pressure, and inability to close the abdomen because of massive abdominal content edema.[43] Hypothermia induced by an open visceral cavity in conjunction with massive blood transfusion can lead to coagulopathy and continued bleeding, which results in shock and metabolic acidosis. The triad of hypothermia, coagulopathy, and acidosis creates a self-propagating cycle that can eventually lead to an irreversible physiologic insult.[43] The initial operation must be completed quickly to terminate this self-propagating cycle. Reconstruction and formal closure of the wound are not completed at this time. The patient is transferred to the ICU.

The goal of the ICU phase of this strategy is to continue aggressive resuscitation and to correct hypothermia, coagulopathy, and acidosis. Rewarming techniques, described in Table 25-7, are used to correct hypothermia. Coagulation factors and platelets may be given to correct coagulopathies. Serial lactate and base deficit measurements, as well as a mixed venous oxygen saturation (Svo_2) pulmonary artery catheter, may be used to guide fluid resuscitation, inotropic support, and oxygenation to prevent further development of acidosis.

The patient is assessed for additional complications, including ongoing hemorrhage, intraabdominal hypertension, and abdominal compartment syndrome. Abdominal compartment syndrome is defined as end-organ dysfunction secondary to intraabdominal hypertension.[43] The increased pressure can be caused by bleeding, ileus, visceral edema, or a noncompliant abdominal wall. Increased abdominal cavity pressure can impinge on diaphragmatic excursion and also can affect ventilation. Clinical manifestations of abdominal compartment syndrome include decreased cardiac output, increased pulmonary vascular resistance, increased peak pulmonary pressures, decreased urine output, and hypoxia.[44]

Intraabdominal pressure can be measured through a bladder catheter after the injection of 50 to 100 ml of normal saline.[44] Serial monitoring of bladder pressures, about every 2 to 4 hours, is useful in detecting the onset of intraabdominal hypertension and the progression to abdominal compartment syndrome. Measurements may be graded: grade I (10 to 15 mm Hg), grade II (15 to 25 mm Hg), grade III (25 to 35 mm Hg), and grade IV (greater than 35 mm Hg).[44] Surgical decompression of the abdomen may be required for abdominal pressures greater than 20 to 25 mm Hg that are associated with other assessment findings such as decreased cardiac output, hypotension, elevated peak inspiratory pressures, and decreased urine output.[44] Surgical decompression involves opening the abdomen and then temporarily closing the abdomen with a sterile perforated plastic sheet, clips, vacuum-assisted techniques, as well as many other options.[43] The open abdomen is then covered with towels or dressings, and closed suction drains are placed over the top and brought out through a plastic drape over the entire wound. The wound is closed permanently several weeks later, or it is allowed to heal by secondary intention and eventual skin grafting.

Once the patient is hemodynamically stable and the triangle of hypothermia, coagulopathy, and acidosis has been corrected, the patient is taken back to the OR for the definitive operation. This usually occurs within 48 to 72 hours of the initial operation.[43] It is during this phase that definitive repairs and wound closure are made. After surgery the patient is transported back to the ICU for continued care.

Specific Organ Injuries

Physical assessment findings, DPL, and CT scanning aid in making a diagnosis of specific abdominal organ injury. The medical and nursing management vary according to specific organ injuries. Liver, spleen, and bowel injuries, which are seen more commonly, are discussed here.

Liver Injuries. The liver is the primary organ injured in penetrating trauma and the second most often injured organ in blunt trauma. Abdominal CT is considered to be the most reliable diagnostic tool

Table 25-7
Interventions for Rewarming the Trauma Patient

	EXTERNAL REWARMING PROCEDURES	INTERNAL REWARMING PROCEDURES
Passive	Maintain a warm room temperature. Remove all wet clothing and linen. Cover the patient with blankets. Avoid bathing patient until normothermia achieved.	Administer warmed, humidified oxygen. Administer warmed intravenous fluids.
Active	Use radiant heat lamps, heating blankets/pads, hot water bottles.	Perform GI irrigation with warmed solutions. Perform extracorporeal rewarming for profound hypothermia. Use esophageal rewarming tubes.

Modified from Morris J: Environmental emergencies. In Newberry L, editor: *Sheehy's emergency nursing: principles and practice,* ed 5, St Louis, 2003, Mosby.
GI, Gastrointestinal.

to identify and assess the severity of the injury to the liver.[45] The severity of liver injuries is graded to provide a mechanism for determining the amount of trauma sustained by that organ, the care needed, and possible outcomes (Table 25-8). Nonoperative management is considered the standard of care for hemodynamically stable patients with liver injury.[45] Patients are admitted to the ICU or a step-down unit and are monitored for signs of hemorrhage. Serial serum hematocrit and hemoglobin levels and vital signs are monitored over several days.

Patients with penetrating or blunt liver trauma who are hemodynamically unstable may require surgical intervention to correct the defect. Resection of the devitalized tissue is required for massive injuries. Hemorrhage is common with liver injuries, and ligation of the hepatic arteries or veins may be required to control hemorrhage. Drains may be placed intraoperatively to drain areas of blood and to prevent hematomas.

Care of the patient with severe liver injuries can be challenging for the critical care nurse. Lack of hemodynamic stability can result from hemorrhage and hypovolemic shock, leading to fluid volume deficit, decreased cardiac output, and decreased tissue perfusion. Combinations of crystalloid and colloid IV solutions may be used to correct hypovolemia. Fresh-frozen plasma, platelets, and cryoprecipitate may be administered to correct coagulopathies. A crucial nursing responsibility is to monitor the patient's response to medical therapies. Continued hemodynamic instability (hypotension, decreased cardiac output) in spite of aggressive medical intervention may indicate continued hemorrhage, in which case an exploratory laparotomy may be required to determine and correct the source of bleeding. The patient's postoperative ICU course may be complicated by coagulopathy, acidosis, and/or hypothermia. Jaundice may occur as a sign of hepatic dysfunction, but it may also be caused by resorption of hematomas or breakdown of transfused blood.

Spleen Injuries. The spleen is the organ most commonly injured by blunt abdominal trauma and is second to the liver as a source of life-threatening hemorrhage. Spleen injuries, like liver injuries, are graded for the purpose of determining the amount of trauma sustained, the care needed, and possible outcomes (Table 25-9). Hemodynamically stable patients may be monitored in the critical care unit by means of serial hematocrit values and vital signs. Progressive deterioration may indicate the need for operative management.[45]

Patients who exhibit hemodynamic instability require operative intervention with splenectomy, partial splenectomy, or splenorrhaphy. Patients who have had a splenectomy are at risk for the development of overwhelming postsplenectomy sepsis with streptococcal pneumonia. These patients require polyvalent

Table 25-8

Liver Injury Scale

GRADE*	INJURY	DESCRIPTION
I	Hematoma	Subcapsular, <10% surface area
	Laceration	Capsular tear, <1 cm parenchymal depth
II	Hematoma	Subcapsular, 10%-50% surface area; intraparenchymal <10 cm in diameter
	Laceration	Capsular tear, 1-3 cm parenchymal depth, <10 cm in length
III	Hematoma	Subcapsular, >50% surface area or expanding; ruptured subcapsular or parenchymal hematoma; intraparenchymal hematoma >10 cm or expanding
	Laceration	>3 cm parenchymal depth
IV	Laceration	Parenchymal disruption involving 25%-75% of hepatic lobe or 1-3 Couinaud's segments within a single lobe
V	Laceration	Parenchymal disruption involving >75% of hepatic lobe or >3 Couinaud's segments within a single lobe
	Vascular	Juxtahepatic venous injuries (i.e., retrohepatic vena cava/central major hepatic veins)
VI	Vascular	Hepatic avulsion

From the American Association for the Surgery of Trauma, http://www.ast.org.
*Advance one grade for multiple injuries up to grade III.

Table 25-9

Spleen Injury Scale

GRADE*	INJURY	DESCRIPTION
I	Hematoma	Subcapsular, <10% surface area
	Laceration	Capsular tear, <1 cm parenchymal depth
II	Hematoma	Subcapsular, 10%-50% surface area; intraparenchymal <5 cm in diameter
	Laceration	Capsular tear, 1-3 cm parenchymal depth, which does not involve a trabecular vessel
III	Hematoma	Subcapsular, >50% surface area or expanding; ruptured subcapsular or parenchymal hematoma; intraparenchymal hematoma >5 cm or expanding
IV	Laceration	>3 cm parenchymal depth or involving trabecular vessels
	Laceration	Laceration involving segmental or hilar vessels producing major devascularization (>25% of spleen)
V	Laceration	Completely shattered spleen
	Vascular	Hilar vascular injury that devascularizes spleen

From the American Association for the Surgery of Trauma, http://www.ast.org.
*Advance one grade for multiple injuries up to grade III.

pneumococcal vaccine (Pneumovax) to help promote immunity against most pneumococcal bacteria. Patients with isolated spleen injuries that necessitate surgical intervention rarely are admitted to the critical care unit. Complications after splenic trauma include wound infection; sepsis; subdiaphragmatic abscess; and fistulas of the colon, pancreas, and stomach.

Intestinal Injuries. Intestinal injuries can result from blunt or penetrating trauma. The diagnosis of small intestinal injuries is difficult. Surgical intervention is usually required in the presence of multiple findings on CT scan (unexplained free fluid, pneumoperitoneum, bowel wall thickening, mesenteric fat streaking, mesenteric hematoma, or IV contrast extravasation).[41] Regardless of the mechanism of injury, intestinal contents (bile, stool, enzymes, bacteria) leak into the peritoneum and cause peritonitis. Surgical resection and repair are required. The patient's postoperative course is dictated by the amount of spillage of intestinal contents. The patient is observed for signs of sepsis and abscess or fistula formation.

Genitourinary Injuries

Trauma to the genitourinary (GU) tract seldom occurs as an isolated injury. A GU injury must be suspected in any patient with penetrating trauma to the torso; pelvic fracture; blunt trauma to the lower chest or flank; contusions, hematoma, tenderness over the flank, lower abdomen, or perineum; genital swelling or discoloration; blood at the urethral meatus; hematuria after Foley catheter placement; or difficulty with micturition.[12]

Mechanism of Injury

GU injuries, like all other traumatic injuries, can result from blunt or penetrating trauma.

Assessment

Evaluation of GU trauma begins after the primary survey has been conducted and immediately life-threatening conditions have been effectively managed. The conscious patient may complain of flank pain or colic pain. Rebound tenderness can be elicited if intraperitoneal extravasation of urine has occurred. Inspection may reveal blood at the urethral meatus. Bluish discoloration of the flanks may indicate retroperitoneal bleeding, whereas perineal discoloration may indicate a pelvic fracture and possible bladder or urethral injury. Hematuria is the most common assessment finding with GU trauma; however, the absence of gross or microscopic hematuria does not exclude a urinary tract injury.[12]

Specific Genitourinary Injuries

Renal Trauma. Most renal trauma is caused by blunt trauma, resulting in contusions or lacerations without urinary extravasation. Renal injury may be reflected by flank ecchymosis and fracture of inferior ribs or spinous processes. Gross or microscopic hematuria may be present; however, the extent of renal damage is often incongruous with the degree of hematuria.[46] Gross hematuria can be present with minor injuries and usually clears within a few hours. CT scan is the most accurate modality available for diagnosing renal injuries because it can assess the extent of parenchymal laceration, urine extravasation, surrounding hemorrhage, and the presence of vascular injury.[47] Contusions and minor lacerations can usually be treated with observation. The success of nonoperative management may be assisted and enhanced by using angiographic embolization. Nonoperative treatment of patients with major lacerations and vascular injuries may be achieved in patients who are hemodynamically stable.[47] Operative intervention may be performed in patients with renal injuries with a devascularized segment of the kidney. Postoperative and postinjury complications can include infection, hemorrhage, infarction, extravasation, calcification, acute tubular necrosis, and hypertension.

Bladder Trauma. A large percentage of bladder injuries result from pelvic fractures.[48] Physical findings may include lower abdominal bruising, distention, and pain. More definitive findings include difficulty in voiding or incomplete recovery of irrigation fluids from catheterized patients.[46] Definitive diagnosis is made by retrograde urethrogram. Bladder injuries are classified as contusions, extraperitoneal ruptures, intraperitoneal ruptures, or combined injuries. The type of injury depends on the location and strength of the blunt force and volume of urine in the bladder at the time of injury. Extraperitoneal rupture of the bladder may be managed conservatively with catheterization and antibiotics for 7 to 10 days.[47] Unresolved extravasation may require surgical intervention.

Nursing Management

Nursing diagnoses that can be applicable in caring for a patient with GU trauma include Ineffective Tissue Perfusion, Pain, Risk for Infection, and Risk for Deficient Fluid Volume.

After the patient is admitted to the critical care unit, the nurse makes an assessment according to ATLS guidelines. Once the patient's condition has stabilized, nursing management of postoperative renal trauma is similar to that for GU surgery. The primary nursing interventions include assessment for hemorrhage, maintenance of fluid and electrolyte balance, and maintenance of patency of drains and tubes. Measurement of urinary output includes drainage from the urinary catheter and the nephrostomy or suprapubic tubes. Drainage from these areas is recorded separately. Urine output is measured frequently until bloody drainage and clots have cleared. Gentle irrigation of drainage tubes may be required to clear clots and maintain the patency of the tubes.

Pelvic Fractures

More patients die from pelvic fractures than from any other skeletal injury, and survivors of this injury often suffer prolonged disability.[49] The pelvis is a ring-shaped structure composed of the hip bones, the sacrum, and the coccyx. Because the pelvis protects the lower urinary tract and major blood vessels and nerves of the lower extremities, pelvic trauma can result in life-threatening hemorrhage as well as urologic and neurologic dysfunction.

Mechanism of Injury

Blunt trauma to the pelvis can be caused by MVCs, falls, or a crushing accident. Pelvic injuries may be associated with damage to underlying tissues. Pelvic injuries often are associated with motorcycle crashes, pedestrian-vehicle collisions, direct crushing injury to the pelvis, and falls from heights greater than 12 feet.[50]

Assessment

Signs of pelvic fracture include perianal ecchymosis (scrotum or vulva) indicating extravasation of urine or blood, pain on palpation or "rocking" of the iliac crests, lower limb paresis or hypoesthesia, and hematuria. Lower extremity rotation or leg shortening is also cause for suspicion of a pelvic injury. Patients with a suspected pelvic injury should also have a rectal examination to assess for spinal cord injury or presence of occult or obvious rectal bleeding.

The diagnosis of pelvic fracture is made by an anteroposterior pelvic x-ray study with the patient in the supine position.[51] Further films may be required for definitive treatment, but the timing depends on the patient's hemodynamic stability.

Classification of Pelvic Fractures

Pelvic fractures constitute a spectrum of complexity ranging from a single, nondisplaced fracture of a pubic ramus to a life-threatening condition in which there are multiple fractures and crush injuries associated with significant hemorrhage and internal injuries. The classifications of pelvic fractures follow.

Lateral Compression (LC). The lateral compression vector of pelvic injury is the most common.[50] This type of fracture produces a shortening of the pelvis diameter and typically does not involve ligamentous injury. Although this type of fracture is forgiving to the pelvic ring vessels, localized bleeding may occur, particularly to the posterior pelvis. There are three types of LC fractures. Type I includes the posterior compression of the sacroiliac joint without ligament disruption or an oblique pubic ramus fracture. Type II includes rupture of the posterior sacroiliac ligament or internal rotation of the hemipelvis with a crush injury of the sacrum and an oblique pubic ramus fracture. Type III includes the findings of type II LC injury with additional evidence of anterior-posterior (AP) compression to the contralateral hemipelvis.

Anterior-Posterior Compression. When force is applied in the anterior-posterior direction, the pelvic diameter widens. In this case, the injury can be completely ligamentous; it manifests as an open sacroiliac joint or open pubic symphasis.[50] This type of injury is also commonly associated with vascular injury. There are three types of AP compression fractures. Type I includes disruption of the pubic symphysis with less than 2.5 cm of diastasis with insignificant posterior pelvic involvement. Type II includes the disruption of the pubic symphysis of more than 2.5 cm with tearing of associated ligaments. Type III is a complete disruption of the pubic symphysis, posterior ligament complexes, and hemipelvic involvement.

Vertical Shear. A vertical shear pelvic injury includes a complete disruption of a hemipelvis associated with a hemipelvic displacement. This type of injury typically occurs in people who fall from a great height and land on one extremity.

Open Fractures. Open pelvic fractures involve an open wound with direct communication between the site of the fracture and a laceration involving the vagina, rectum, or perineum. Mortality from these injuries is high because, unlike closed pelvic fractures that bleed into the peritoneum, open pelvic fractures result in external exsanguination.[50]

Medical Management

The priority of the medical management of pelvic fractures is to prevent or to control life-threatening hemorrhage. External exsanguination is an immediate threat to patients with an open pelvic fracture. These patients are taken directly to the OR for aggressive resuscitation, ligation, and packing to control the exsanguination.[50] Patients with an open pelvic fracture may require an exploratory laparotomy to treat intra-abdominal injuries. A diverting colostomy may be performed to prevent ongoing contamination of the pelvic wound from feces. If there are no obvious intra-abdominal injuries, the pelvis is stabilized. After the initial operation, frequent operative débridement and pelvic wound irrigations are required for several days. Once the wound is clean and granulation tissue is present, definitive closure of the wound is done using a combination of techniques including free flap closure, split-thickness skin grafts, and rotation flaps.[49]

Patients who are hemodynamically stable and have stable closed pelvic fractures are usually treated conservatively with bed rest. These patients may receive elective orthopedic stabilization within 2 to 3 days after injury.[50] Patients who remain hemodynamically unstable may undergo temporary pelvic stabilization by wrapping the pelvis with a sheet between the greater trochanter and the iliac crests. Advantages of this technique are that it is quick, does not involve specialized training, allows continued access to the patient during the resuscitation, and does not require specialized equipment.[51] Temporary external fixation is performed concurrently with resuscitation in order to reduce further bleeding of the vessels in the pelvis. These patients require more drastic means to control hemorrhage, including embolization by angiography and external pelvic fracture stabilization. Definitive management of pelvic fracture may include placement of internal or external fixation devices. Immediate external fixation is used as the primary method for controlling hemorrhage associated with closed pelvic fractures.[51] Angiography may be used to embolize bleeding vessels and achieve hemostasis in the hemodynamically unstable patient when other sources of bleeding have been excluded. Later, as the patient becomes more hemodynamically stable, internal fixation may be required.

Nursing Management

Initial assessment of the patient with a pelvic fracture in the critical care unit proceeds according to ATLS guidelines. Nursing diagnoses include Ineffective Tissue Perfusion, Acute Pain, Risk for Infection, and Risk for Injury.

Massive blood loss contributes to alteration in tissue perfusion. On the patient's admission to the critical care unit, hemodynamic instability, with abnormal coagulation factors, may be present. Interventions include intravenously administered crystalloid and colloid fluids. The nurse must ensure that an appropriate amount of blood remains cross-matched and available if needed. Adequate oxygenation is assessed by means of pulse oximetry and Svo_2 and by monitoring serial hematocrit and hemoglobin levels.

The patient is at high risk for injury secondary to neurovascular compromise, development of abdominal compartment syndrome, fat embolism syndrome (FES), and wound infection. These syndromes are discussed in further detail later in this chapter. Before the patient is moved, it is important that the nurse knows whether the physician has classified the closed pelvic fracture as *stable* or *unstable.* A stable pelvic injury implies that no further pathologic displacement of the pelvis can occur with physical turning or moving. An unstable pelvic fracture means that further pathologic displacement of the pelvis can occur with turning or moving.[49] Routine nursing assessments include neurovascular assessments of the lower extremities. Neurologic injury as a result of pelvic fracture may be transient and temporary. Open pelvic fractures may necessitate complex, time-consuming dressing changes. Aggressive pain management strategies should be employed during these dressing changes, because they can be quite painful.

Patients with open pelvic fractures usually have a prolonged critical care course, with varying degrees of complications. The patient with pelvic fracture is at risk for infection because of associated injuries and internal or external fixation devices. Nursing management of external fixation insertion sites is directed at preventing infection. Most institutions have protocols for pin care that require strict compliance.

COMPLICATIONS OF TRAUMA

In the trimodal distribution of trauma deaths, the third peak of death often occurs in the critical care unit as a result of complications days to weeks after the initial injury. Ongoing nursing assessments are imperative for early detection of complications often associated with traumatic injuries. A single complication can increase hospital length of stay, in addition to the associated costs of treating the complication.

HYPERMETABOLISM

Nutritional support is being recognized increasingly as an essential component in the care of critically ill trauma patients. Within 24 to 48 hours after traumatic injury, a predictable hypermetabolic response occurs. The metabolic response to injury mobilizes amino acids and accelerates protein synthesis to support wound healing and the immunologic response to invading organisms.[52] Stress hypermetabolism occurs after any major injury and is characterized by increases in metabolic rate and oxygen consumption. Energy requirements accelerate to promote immune function and tissue repair. The goal of early aggressive nutrition is to maintain host defenses by supporting this hypermetabolism and to preserve lean body mass.[52] Most nutrition experts advocate beginning enteral nutrition. Current guidelines recommend enteral feedings be initiated within 72 hours for patients with blunt and penetrating abdominal injuries and those with severe head injuries.[52] Enteral feeding sites can include the gastric route or any site beyond the pylorus of the stomach, including the duodenum and jejunum. Prompt feeding tube placement by the critical care nurse must be a priority, unless contraindicated. Diminished or absent bowel sounds should not be interpreted to mean that the small bowel is not working. Small bowel function and the ability to absorb nutrients remains intact, despite the presence of gastroparesis and absent bowel sounds.[53] Because access to the stomach can be obtained more quickly and easily than to the duodenum, early gastric feeding is possible.[52] Patients at risk for pulmonary aspiration due to gastric retention or gastroesophageal reflex should receive enteral feedings into the jejunum.[52] If enteral feeding is not successful, parenteral nutrition should be initiated by day 7.[52]

INFECTION

Infection remains a major source of mortality and morbidity in critical care units. The trauma patient is at risk for infection because of contaminated wounds, invasive therapeutic and diagnostic catheters, intubation and mechanical ventilation, host susceptibility, and the critical care environment. Nursing management must include interventions to decrease and eliminate the trauma patient's risk of infection.

The patient with multiple trauma is at risk for infection because of host susceptibility (including preexisting medical conditions) and the adverse effect of trauma on the immune system.

Wound contamination poses an infection risk to the trauma patient, especially with injuries resulting from deep or penetrating trauma. Exogenous bacteria (from the external environment) can enter through open wounds. Exogenous bacteria can be introduced by dirt, grass, and debris inoculated into the wound at the time of injury, or they can later be introduced during wound care. Endogenous bacteria (from the internal environment) can be released as a result of gastrointestinal or genitourinary perforation, which spills bacteria into the internal environment. Meticulous wound care is essential. The goals of wound care include minimizing infection risks, removing dead and devitalized tissue, allowing for wound drainage, and promoting wound epithelialization and contraction. Wound healing also is accomplished through interventions that promote tissue perfusion of well-oxygenated blood and that ensure adequate nutritional support for wound healing.

SEPSIS

The patient with multiple injuries is especially at risk for overwhelming infections and sepsis. The source of sepsis in the trauma patient can be invasive therapeutic and diagnostic catheters or wound contamination with exogenous or endogenous bacteria. The source of the septic nidus must be promptly evaluated. Gram stain and cultures of blood, urine, sputum, invasive catheters, and wounds are obtained (see Severe Sepsis and Septic Shock in Chapter 26).

PULMONARY

Respiratory Failure

Posttraumatic respiratory failure often leads to the development of ARDS. ARDS can be caused by direct injury to the lungs or indirect injury (see Chapter 15). The primary direct injuries in the trauma patient can include aspiration, inhalation, and pulmonary contusion.[54] The indirect injuries include sepsis, massive transfusion, fat emboli, and missed injury.[54] ARDS in the trauma patient can develop 24 to 72 hours after initial injury.

Fat Embolism Syndrome

FES can occur as a complication of orthopedic trauma. The clinical onset of FES ranges from 12 to 72 hours after injury, although 90% of patients with FES develop it within 24 hours after injury.[51] FES appears to develop as a result of fat droplets that leak from fractured bone and embolize to the lungs. The droplets are broken down into free fatty acids that are toxic to the pulmonary microvascular membranes. Pulmonary fat embolization alters pulmonary hemodynamics and pulmonary vascular permeability. The lung becomes highly edematous and hemorrhagic. The clinical presentation is almost indistinguishable from ARDS (see Chapter 15). Early stabilization of unstable extremity fractures may limit the seeding of fat droplets into the pulmonary system.[51]

PAIN

Pain in the ICU may come from many sources, including surgery, procedures, and trauma. Trauma may contribute to cellular death and/or inflammation that leads to pain.[55] Relief of pain is a major component in the care of trauma patients. An issue that often complicates pain management is the high incidence of substance abuse in patients who sustain traumatic injury. The Society of Critical Care Medicine (SCCM) proposed guidelines for the optimal use of sedatives and analgesics[56] (see Chapters 8 and 9).

RENAL COMPLICATIONS

Renal Failure

Assessment and ongoing monitoring of renal function are critical to the survival of the trauma patient. The etiology of posttraumatic renal failure is complex and may involve a variety of factors, as listed in Box 25-15.

Prevention of renal failure is the best treatment and begins with ensuring adequate renal perfusion. Serial assessments of blood urea nitrogen (BUN) and creatinine levels are commonly used to evaluate renal function. Urine output as a measurement to determine renal function can be misleading because posttraumatic renal insufficiency can manifest as nonoliguric renal failure. Progressive renal failure requires prompt diagnosis and treatment (see Acute Renal Failure in Chapter 20).

Myoglobinuria

Patients with a crush injury are susceptible to the development of myoglobinuria, with subsequent secondary renal failure. Crush injuries can compromise blood

Box 25-15

Etiologic Factors in Posttraumatic Renal Failure

- Preexisting disease
  - Hypertension
  - Diabetes
  - Chronic renal insufficiency
  - Chronic liver disease
- Prolonged shock states
- Profound acidosis
- SIRS/reperfusion injury
- Abdominal compartment syndrome
- Muscle ischemia; myoglobinuria
- Microemboli
- Nephrotoxic drugs
- Radiocontrast dye

SIRS, Systemic inflammatory response syndrome.

flow. Loss of arterial blood flow, particularly to the extremities, results in the loss of oxygen transport to distal tissues and ischemia. This initiates a cascade of events that leads to the necrosis of skeletal muscle cells. As cells die, intracellular contents—particularly potassium and myoglobin—are released. Myoglobin (muscular pigment) is a large molecule. There are three mechanisms by which circulating myoglobin can lead to the development of renal failure: decreased renal perfusion, cast formation with tubular obstruction, and direct toxic effects of myoglobin in the renal tubuoles.[57]

Dark, tea-colored urine is suggestive of myoglobinuria. Testing for myoglobin in the urine can be done but may take several days, depending on laboratory resources available for this test. The most rapid screening test is a serum creatine kinase (CK) level. Urine output and serial CK levels should be monitored.

Once myoglobinuria is diagnosed, treatment is aimed at prevention of subsequent renal failure. Aggressive administration of intravenous fluids increases renal blood flow and decreases the concentration of nephrotoxic pigments. Continuous infusion of mannitol and sodium bicarbonate ($NaHCO_3$) may be used. Mannitol and $NaHCO_3$ are thought to alkalinize the urine and prevent myoglobin crystallization in the renal tubules. Acetazolamide (Diamox) may be given to prevent metabolic alkalosis that may be caused by the continuous $NaHCO_3$ infusion. Nursing management is directed toward achievement of fluid and electrolyte balance. The patient should be assessed for hypernatremia, hyperosmolality, and volume overload. Assessment parameters may include maintaining urine output greater than or equal to 200 ml/hr and maintaining urine pH 6.0 to 7.0 and serum pH less than 7.5.[57]

Vascular Complications

Compartment Syndrome

Compartment syndrome is a condition in which increased pressure within a limited space compromises circulation, resulting in ischemia and necrosis of tissues within that space. Among those at high risk for the development of compartment syndrome are patients with lower extremity trauma, including fractures, penetrating trauma, vascular ruptures, massive tissue injuries, or venous obstruction. Clinical manifestations of compartment syndrome include obvious swelling and tightness of an extremity, paresis, and pain of the affected extremity. Diminished pulses and decreased capillary refill do not reliably identify compartment syndrome because they may be intact until after irreversible changes have occurred. Elevated intracompartmental pressures confirm the diagnosis. The treatment can consist of simple interventions, such as removing an occlusive dressing, to more complex interventions, including a fasciotomy.

Deep Vein Thrombosis

Despite improvements in the care of the trauma patient, deep vein thrombosis (DVT) and the attendant risk of pulmonary embolism are important causes of morbidity and mortality in the trauma patient with multiple injuries. Major trauma patients have a DVT risk exceeding 50%.[58] The factors that are thought to form the basis of pathophysiology of DVT are stasis (reduction of blood flow in the veins), injury (to the intimal surface of the vessel), and hypercoagulopathy. Trauma patients are at risk for developing DVT because of endothelial injury, coagulopathy, immobility, and bed rest.

Trauma patients are at the greatest risk for developing thromboembolism early in their hospitalization. Prevention is key. The Eastern Association for the Surgery of Trauma developed practice guidelines for the prevention and management of DVT.[59] They recommended that trauma patients at high risk for DVT wear sequential compression devices for prophylaxis against DVT. High-risk patients include those with spinal cord injury, lower extremity or pelvic fractures, need for surgical procedure, increasing age, central venous catheters or venous injury, and prolonged immobility or hospital stay.[58] For patients in whom the lower leg is inaccessible, foot pumps may act as an effective alternative to lower the rate of DVT formation. Low-molecular-weight heparin (e.g., enoxaparin) is recommended for DVT prophylaxis in trauma patients with the following injury patterns: (1) pelvic fractures requiring operative fixation or prolonged bed rest (more than 5 days), (2) complex lower extremity fractures requiring operative fixation or prolonged bed rest, and (3) SCI with complete or incomplete motor paralysis. The selection of DVT prophylaxis in trauma patients is often challenging because a balance between DVT risk and bleeding risk must be evaluated.

Missed Injury

Nursing assessment of the patient with multiple injuries in the critical care unit may reveal missed diseases or missed injuries. Missed "diseases" may include preexisting undiagnosed medical illnesses, such as endocrine disorders (diabetes, hypothyroidism); myocardial infarction; hypertension; respiratory insufficiency; renal insufficiency; or malnutrition.

Occasionally injuries may not be diagnosed in the pre–critical care phases. Missed injuries are commonly discovered in the first 24 to 48 hours of the hospital stay. Injuries are missed for a variety of reasons[60] as summarized in Box 25-16. In the critical care unit, a missed injury may be suspected if the patient fails to show appropriate response to medical or surgical intervention. Change in the character of drainage from wounds or catheters may represent biliary or duodenal injuries. Hypotension and a falling hematocrit level despite aggressive fluid administration may indicate an expanding hematoma. The critical care nurse must be alert to the possibility of a missed injury, especially when the patient does not appear to be responding appropriately to interventions. The physician must be notified immediately because potential complications of infection and hemorrhage may be life-threatening. Nurses play a key role in identifying missed injuries, particularly when patients regain consciousness and begin to increase their activity.

Multiple Organ Dysfunction Syndrome

Multiple organ dysfunction syndrome (MODS) is a clinical syndrome of progressive dysfunction of organ systems. Trauma patients are at high risk for systemic inflammatory response syndrome (SIRS) and MODS. Organ dysfunction can be the result of "primary MODS," which is caused by direct traumatic injury such as that which occurs with acute lung dysfunction because of pulmonary contusion. Organ dysfunction that occurs latently in the trauma patient's ICU course, "secondary MODS," results from uncontrolled systemic inflammation with resultant organ dysfunction. Trauma patients may experience both primary and secondary MODS. Treatment is aimed at controlling or eliminating the source of inflammation, maintenance of oxygen delivery and consumption, and nutritional and metabolic support for individual organs.

Box 25-16

Factors Contributing to Missed Injuries

Hemodynamic Instability

Shock states in the emergency department
Aggressive resuscitation
Emergent surgery may take precedence over thorough secondary surveys

Alterations in Consciousness

Presence of drugs or alcohol intoxication confuses physical assessments and masks physical findings
Disoriented patients are challenging to assess
Agitation makes diagnostic testing challenging
Patients with altered consciousness cannot provide a history of the injury

SPECIAL CONSIDERATIONS

Meeting the Needs of Family Members/Significant Others

The impact of traumatic injury can be devastating not only for patients but also and especially for family members and significant others. "Trauma doesn't happen to an individual; it happens to a family."[61] They are faced with a crisis situation for which they have had little time to prepare. Trauma can precipitate a crisis within the family. Families may exhibit physical and sociocultural reactions as well as a combination of emotional reactions, including anger, fear, powerlessness, confusion, and mistrust. Recovery from traumatic injury can be long and frustrating for families. There may be many peaks and valleys of good days and bad days. During this time the family may exhaust its social and financial support systems. Nurses should recognize this and facilitate supportive relationships for families.

A valuable intervention is to bring families of trauma patients together in support group experiences. Trauma family support groups can offer sharing of experiences, the opportunity to express emotions, mutual support, sharing of coping strategies, and education about hospital and community services.

Trauma in the Elderly

Trauma is a disease that affects people of all ages. The elderly are predisposed to traumatic injuries because of the inevitable consequences of aging. The ability to react to or avoid environmental hazards is impaired because of age-related deterioration of the senses and changes in motor strength, postural stability, balance, and coordination.

The elderly experience the majority of all falls that result in injuries, and these falls are likely to occur from level surfaces or steps.[62] Factors that predispose the elderly to falls are summarized in Box 25-17.[63] Because many of the falls may be caused by an underlying medical condition (e.g., syncope, myocardial infarction, dysrhythmias), management of the elderly patient who has fallen must include an evaluation of events and conditions immediately preceding the fall. The exposure of the elderly to MVC trauma is a consequence of the increasing growth of the elderly population and the growing number of elderly drivers and occupants of motor vehicles. Factors that predispose the elderly to MVCs are summarized in Box 25-18.[63] A pedestrian struck by a motor vehicle receives some of the most devastating injuries. Many deaths that occur at crosswalks are of elderly individuals. Physiologic deterioration of cerebral and motor skills and alterations in visual and auditory acuity cause elder pedestrians to walk directly into the path of oncoming vehicles.

Trauma in the elderly is associated with higher mortality even when the injuries are less severe. The elderly have a higher complications rate and a higher mortality rate, starting at 39 years of age, due to preexisting medical conditions, decreased physiologic reserves, and decreased ability to compensate for severe injury.[64] Elderly patients who do survive traumatic injury are often faced with changes in their preinjury functional status. Relatively minor trauma can be the event that changes the lifestyle of an elderly person from one of relative independence to one that requires prolonged rehabilitation or skilled nursing care. Discharge planning early in the patient's hospitalization is necessary.

The concept of "limited physiologic reserve" in the elderly trauma patient highlights the key difference between the average younger trauma patient with normal physiologic reserve and the elderly patient with underlying physiologic derangements.[65] Age-related changes that occur in virtually every organ system may not produce evidence of organ dysfunction in the resting state. However, the ability of organs to augment function in response to traumatic stress may be greatly compromised. Fluid resuscitation is an integral part of trauma resuscitation. Patients on chronic diuretic therapy may require more volume and potassium supplementation as a result of chronic volume and potassium depletion. The assessment and management of hypovolemic shock is more complex in the elderly trauma patient. The elderly have limited ability to increase their heart rate in response to blood loss, thus obscuring one of the earliest signs of hypovolemia—tachycardia.[12] Loss of physiologic reserve and the presence of preexisting medical conditions are likely to produce further conflicting hemodynamic data. The older patient's lack of physiologic reserve makes it imperative that early nutritional support be initiated.

Trauma protocols are well established for the management of young patients after injury. Clinicians increasingly are recognizing that these protocols must be individualized for the elderly trauma patient. The best outcomes in this trauma patient population have been achieved through early appropriate aggressive trauma care, including early hemodynamic monitoring in high-risk elderly trauma patients (those with a high-risk mechanism of injury, unknown cardiovascular status, or preexisting cardiac or renal disease).[66]

Box 25-17

Risk Factors for Falls in the Elderly

Acute Illness
Cerebrovascular accidents
Dysrhythmias
Syncope
Diabetes

Cognitive Impairment
Dementia

Neuromuscular Disorders
Arthritis
Lower extremity weakness
Unstable gait

Medications
Antidepressants
Benzodiazepines
Diuretics
Phenothiazines

Box 25-18

Factors That Predispose the Elderly to Motor Vehicle Crashes

- Alterations in visual and auditory acuity
- Deterioration in strength and slower reaction times
- Diminution of cerebral skills
- Diminution of motor skills
- Exacerbation of acute or chronic medical conditions
- Medications that may interfere with safe driving

evolve To test your mastery of this chapter, try the Open-Book Quiz at http://evolve.elsevier.com/Urden/priorities/

REFERENCES

1. Davis JW et al: Victims of domestic violence on the trauma service, *J Trauma* 54:352, 2003.
2. Guth AA, Pachter L: Domestic violence and the trauma surgeon, *Am J Surg* 179:134, 2000.
3. Melnick DM et al: Domestic violence and alcohol abuse in female trauma patients admitted to trauma centers, *J Trauma* 53:33, 2002.
4. Anglin D, Sachs C: Preventative care in the emergency department: screening for domestic violence in the ED, *Acad Emerg Med* 10:1118, 2003.
5. Sisley A, Jacobs LM, People G: Violence in America: a public health crisis—domestic violence, *J Trauma* 46:1105, 1999.

6. National Traffic Safety Association: *Traffic safety facts 2002: alcohol,* Washington, DC, 2003, The Association.
7. Blincoe L et al: *The economical impact of motor vehicle crashes: 2000,* Washington, DC, 2002, Department of Transportation, NHTSA.
8. Shults RA et al: Reviews of evidence regarding mechanisms to reduce alcohol-impaired driving, *Am J Prev Med* 21(4S):66, 2001.
9. Shults RA et al: Association between state level drinking and driving countermeasures and self-reported alcohol impaired driving, *Inj Prev* 8:106, 2002.
10. McCarthy MC: Trauma and critical care, *J Am Coll Surg* 190:232, 1999.
11. Nilssen O, Ries RK, Rivara FP: The CAGE questionnaire and the Michigan Alcohol Screening Test in trauma patients: comparisons of their correlations with biological markers, *J Trauma* 36:784, 1994.
12. American College of Surgeons: *Advanced trauma life support,* ed 6, Chicago, 1997, American College of Surgeons.
13. Vles J et al: Prevalence and determinants of disabilities and return to work after major trauma, *J Trauma* 58:126, 2005.
14. Eastern Association for the Surgery of Trauma: *Clinical practice guidelines: endpoints of resuscitation,* 2003, The Association, http://www.east.org.
15. Kern JW, Shoemaker WC: Meta-analysis of hemodynamic optimization in high risk patients, *Crit Care Med* 30:1686, 2002.
16. Centers for Disease Control and Prevention: *Traumatic brain injury in the United States: a report to Congress,* September 23, 2003, http://www. cdc.gov/doc.do/id/0900f3ec800101e6, accessed June 29, 2004.
17. McQuillan KA, Mitchell PH: Traumatic brain injuries. In McQuillan KA et al, editors: *Trauma nursing: from resuscitation through rehabilitation,* ed 3, Philadelphia, 2002, WB Saunders.
18. Chestnut RM: Management of brain and spinal cord injuries, *Crit Care Clin* 20(1):25, 2004.
19. Valadka AB: Injury to the cranium. In Moore EE, Feliciano DV, Mattox KL: *Trauma,* ed 5, New York, 2004, McGraw Hill.
20. Brain Trauma Foundation: *Management and prognosis of severe traumatic brain injury, part I: guidelines for the management of severe traumatic brain injury,* 2000, http://www2.braintrauma.org/guidelines/downloads/btf_guidelines_management.pdf.
21. Brain Trauma Foundation: *Guidelines for the management of severe traumatic brain injury: cerebral perfusion pressure,* 2003,http://www2.braintrauma.org/guidelines/downloads/btf_guidelines_cpp_u1.pdf.
22. Sekhon LHS, Fehlings MG: Epidemiology, demographics, and pathophysiology of acute spinal cord injury, *Spine* 26(24S):S2, 2001.
23. Wuermser LA et al: Spinal cord injury medicine. II. Acute management of traumatic and nontraumatic injury, *Arch Phys Med Rehabil* 88:3(supp 1):S55, 2007.
24. Russo-McCourt TA: Spinal cord injuries. In McQuillan KA et al, editors: *Trauma nursing: from resuscitation through rehabilitation,* ed 3, Philadelphia, 2002, WB Saunders.
25. Marion DW, Przybylski GJ: Injury to the vertebrae and spinal cord. In Moore EE, Feliciano DV, Mattox KL, editors: *Trauma,* ed 5, New York, 2004, McGraw Hill.
26. Huber-Wagner S et al: Emergency chest tube placement in trauma care—which approach is preferable? *Resuscitation* 72(2):226, 2007.
27. Denton JS, Segovia A, Filkins JA: Practical pathology of gunshot wounds, *Arch Pathol Lab Med* 130(9):1283, 2006.
28. Easter A: Management of patients with multiple rib fractures, *Am J Crit Care* 10(5):320, 2001.
29. Flagel BT et al: Half-a-dozen ribs: the breakpoint for mortality, *Surgery* 138(4):717, 2005.
30. Karmakar MK, Ho AM: Acute pain management of patients with multiple fractured ribs, *J Trauma* 54(3):615, 2003.
31. Keough V, Pudelek B: Blunt chest trauma: review of selected pulmonary injuries focusing on pulmonary contusion, *AACN Clin Issues* 12(2):270, 2001.
32. Asensio JA, Demetriades D, Rodriguez A: Injury to the diaphragm. In Moore EE, Feliciano DV, Mattox KL, editors: *Trauma,* ed 5, New York, 2004, McGraw Hill.
33. Sherwood S, Hartsock RL: Thoracic injuries. In McQuillan KA et al, editors: *Trauma nursing: from resuscitation through rehabilitation,* ed 3, Philadelphia, 2002, WB Saunders.
34. Wall MJ, Storey JH, Mattox KL: Indications for thoracotomy. In Moore EE, Feliciano DV, Mattox KL, editors: *Trauma,* ed 5, New York, 2004, McGraw Hill.
35. Ivatury RR: The injured heart. In Mattox KL, Feliciano DV, Moore EE, editors: *Trauma,* ed 4, New York, 2004, McGraw Hill.
36. Schultz JM, Trunkey DD: Blunt cardiac injury, *Crit Care Clin* 20(1):57, 2004.
37. Morgan PB, Buetchter KJ: Blunt thoracic aortic injuries: initial evaluation and management, *South Med J* 93(2):173, 2000.
38. Eastern Association for the Surgery of Trauma: *Guidelines for the diagnosis and management of blunt aortic injury,* 2000, The Association, http://www.east.org.
39. Fabian T, Crose N: Abdominal trauma, including indications for celiotomy. In Moore EE, Feliciano DV, Mattox KL, editors: *Trauma,* ed 5, New York, 2004, McGraw Hill.
40. Montonye J: Abdominal injuries. In McQuillan KA et al, editors: *Trauma nursing: from resuscitation through rehabilitation,* ed 3, Philadelphia, 2002, WB Saunders.
41. Todd SR: Critical concepts in abdominal injury, *Crit Care Clin* 20:119, 2004.
42. Eastern Association for the Surgery of Trauma: *Practice management guidelines for the evaluation of blunt abdominal trauma,* 2001, The Association, http://www.east.org.
43. Schreiber MA: Damage control surgery, *Crit Care Clin* 20:119, 2004.
44. McNelis J, Marini CP, Simms HH: Abdominal compartment syndrome: clinical manifestations and predictive factors, *Curr Opin Crit Care* 9:133, 2003.
45. Eastern Association for the Surgery of Trauma: *Practice management guidelines for the nonoperative management of blunt injury to the liver and spleen,* 2003, The Association.
46. Peterson N: Genitourinary trauma. In Moore EE, Feliciano DV, Mattox KL, editors: *Trauma,* ed 5, New York, 2004, McGraw Hill.
47. Eastern Association for the Surgery of Trauma: *Practice management guidelines for the management of genitourinary trauma,* 2003, The Association, http://www.east.org.
48. Nayduch DA: Genitourinary injuries and renal management. In McQuillan KA et al, editors: *Trauma nursing:*

from resuscitation through rehabilitation, ed 3, Philadelphia, 2002, WB Saunders.

49. Walsh C: Musculoskeletal injuries. In McQuillan KA et al, editors: *Trauma nursing: from resuscitation through rehabilitation,* ed 3, Philadelphia, 2002, WB Saunders.
50. Scalea TM, Burgess AR: Pelvic fractures. In Moore EE, Feliciano DV, Mattox KL, editors: *Trauma,* ed 5, New York, 2004, McGraw Hill.
51. Mirza A, Ellis T: Initial management of pelvic and femoral fractures in the multiply injured patient, *Crit Care Clin* 20:159, 2004.
52. Eastern Association for the Surgery of Trauma: *Practice management guidelines for nutritional support of the trauma patient*, 2003, The Association, http://www.east.org.
53. Marik PE, Zaloga GP: Early enteral nutrition in acutely ill patients: a systematic review, *Crit Care Med* 29:2264, 2001.
54. Micheals AJ: Management of post-traumatic respiratory failure, *Crit Care Clin* 29:83, 2004.
55. Hall LG, Oyen LJ, Murray MJ: Analgesic agents: pharmacology and application in critical care, *Crit Care Clin* 17:899, 2001.
56. Jacobi F et al: Clinical practice guidelines for the sustained use of sedatives and analgesics in the critically ill adult, *Crit Care Med* 30:119, 2002.
57. Malinowski DJ, Slater MS, Mullins RJ: Crush injury and rhabdomyolysis, *Crit Care Clin* 20:171, 2004.
58. Geerts WH, Heit JA: Prevention of venous thromboembolism, *Chest* 119:1325, 2001.
59. Eastern Association for the Surgery of Trauma: *Practice management guidelines for the management of venous thromboembolism in trauma patients,* 1998, The Association, http://www.east.org.
60. Sommers MS: Missed injuries: a case of trauma hide and seek, *AACN Clin Issues* 6:187, 1995.
61. Richmond TS: Trauma: beyond the hospital for patients and families, *Crit Care Nurse* 15(4):75, 1995.
62. Sterling DA, O'Connor JA, Bondies J: Geriatric falls: injury severity is high and disproportionate to mechanisms, *J Trauma* 50:116, 2001.
63. Johnson KL, Johnson SB: Geriatric trauma. In Fulmer T, Walker M, Foreman M, editors: *Critical care nursing of the elderly,* New York, 2001, Springer.
64. Victorino G, Chong TJ, Pal JD: Trauma in the elderly, *Arch Surg* 138:1093, 2003.
65. Jacobs DG: Special considerations in geriatric trauma, *Curr Opin Crit Care* 9:535, 2003.
66. Eastern Association for the Surgery of Trauma: *Practice management guidelines for geriatric trauma,* 2001, The Association, http://www.east.org.

CHAPTER

26 Shock and Multiple Organ Dysfunction Syndrome

BEVERLY CARLSON ■ LORRAINE FITZSIMMONS ■ LAURA PAGANO

OBJECTIVES

- Describe the generalized shock response and systemic inflammatory response.
- List the etiologies of hypovolemic, cardiogenic, and anaphylactic, neurogenic, and septic shock and multiple organ dysfunction syndrome (MODS).
- Explain the pathophysiology of the five forms of shock and MODS.
- Identify the clinical manifestations of the five forms of shock and MODS.
- Outline the important aspects of the medical management of hypovolemic, cardiogenic, and anaphylactic, neurogenic, and septic shock and MODS.
- Summarize the nursing priorities for managing a patient with each type of shock or MODS.

Shock is an acute, widespread process of impaired tissue perfusion that results in cellular, metabolic, and hemodynamic alterations. Ineffective tissue perfusion occurs when an imbalance develops between cellular oxygen supply and cellular oxygen demand. This imbalance can occur for a variety of reasons and eventually results in cellular dysfunction, multiple organ dysfunction syndrome (MODS), and death.[1] This chapter presents an overview of the general shock response, or shock syndrome, followed by a discussion of the different shock states and MODS.

SHOCK SYNDROME

Shock is a complex pathophysiologic process that often results in multiple organ dysfunction syndrome (MODS) and death. All types of shock eventually result in ineffective tissue perfusion and the development of acute circulatory failure. The shock syndrome is a pathway involving a variety of pathologic processes that may be categorized into four stages: initial, compensatory, progressive, and refractory. Progression through each stage varies with the patient's prior condition, duration of initiating event, response to therapy, and correction of underlying cause.[1]

Etiology

Shock can be classified as hypovolemic, cardiogenic, or distributive, depending on the pathophysiologic cause and hemodynamic profile. Hypovolemic shock results from a loss of circulating or intravascular volume. Cardiogenic shock results from the impaired ability of the heart to pump. Distributive shock results from maldistribution of circulating blood volume and can be further classified as septic, anaphylactic, or neurogenic. Septic shock is the result of microorganisms entering the body. Anaphylactic shock is the result of a severe antibody-antigen reaction. Neurogenic shock is the result of the loss of sympathetic tone.[1]

Pathophysiology

During the initial stage, cardiac output (CO) is decreased and tissue perfusion is threatened. Almost immediately, the compensatory stage begins as the body's homeostatic mechanisms attempt to maintain CO, blood pressure (BP), and tissue perfusion. The compensatory mechanisms are mediated by the sympathetic nervous system (SNS) and consist of neural, hormonal, and chemical responses. The neural response includes an increase in heart rate (HR) and contractility, arterial and venous vasoconstriction, and shunting of blood to the vital organs. Hormonal compensation includes activation of the renin response and stimulation of the anterior pituitary and adrenal medulla. Activation of the renin response results in the production of angiotensin II, which causes vasoconstriction and the release of aldosterone and antidiuretic hormone (ADH), leading to sodium and water retention. Stimulation of the anterior pituitary results in the secretion of adrenocorticotropic hormone (ACTH), which in turn stimulates the adrenal cortex to produce glucocorticoids, causing a rise in blood glucose levels. Stimulation of the adrenal medulla causes the release of epinephrine and norepinephrine, which further enhance the compensatory mechanisms.[1]

During the progressive stage, the compensatory mechanisms begin failing to meet tissue metabolic needs and the shock cycle is perpetuated. As tissue perfusion becomes ineffective, the cells switch from aerobic to anaerobic metabolism as a source of energy. Anaerobic metabolism produces small amounts of energy but large amounts of lactic acid, producing lactic acidemia. Increased vascular permeability from endothelial and epithelial hypoxia and inflammatory mediators results in intravascular hypovolemia, tissue edema, and further decline in tissue perfusion.[1,2] At the cellular level, the small amount of energy created by anaerobic metabolism is not enough to keep the cell functional and irreversible damage begins to occur. Some cells die as a result of apoptosis, an injury-activated preprogrammed cellular suicide.[3] Others die as the sodium-potassium pump in the cell membrane fails, causing the cell and its organelles to swell. Cellular energy production comes to a complete halt as the mitochondria swell and rupture. At this point the problem becomes one of oxygen utilization instead of oxygen delivery. Even if the cell were to receive more oxygen, it would be unable to use it because of damage to the mitochondria. The cell's digestive organelles swell, resulting in leakage of destructive enzymes into the cell, accelerating cell death.[1]

Every system in the body is affected by this process (Box 26-1). Cardiac dysfunction develops as a result of myocardial hypoperfusion and the release of myocardial depressant substances.[1,2] Ventricular failure eventually occurs, further perpetuating the entire process. Central nervous system (CNS) dysfunction develops as a result of cerebral hypoperfusion, leading to failure of the SNS, cardiac and respiratory depression, and thermoregulatory failure. Endothelial injury from hypoxia and inflammatory cytokines and impaired blood flow result in microvascular thrombosis. Hematologic dysfunction occurs as a result of consumption of clotting factors, release of inflammatory cytokines, and dilutional thrombocytopenia. Disseminated intravascular coagulation (DIC) may eventually develop. Pulmonary dysfunction occurs as a result of increased pulmonary capillary membrane permeability, pulmonary microemboli, and pulmonary vasoconstriction. Ventilatory failure and acute respiratory distress syndrome (ARDS) eventually develop. Renal dysfunction develops as a result of renal vasoconstriction and renal hypoperfusion, leading to acute tubular necrosis (ATN). Gastrointestinal dysfunction occurs as a result of splanchnic vasoconstriction and hypoperfusion and leads to failure of the gut organs. Disruption of the intestinal epithelium releases gram-negative bacteria into the system, which further perpetuates the entire shock syndrome.[3]

During the refractory stage, shock becomes unresponsive to therapy and is considered irreversible. As the individual organ systems die, MODS, defined as failure of two or more body systems, occurs. Death is the final outcome. Regardless of etiologic factors, death occurs from ineffective tissue perfusion because of the failure of the circulation to meet the oxygen needs of the cell.[1]

Box 26-1

Consequences of Shock

Cardiovascular
Ventricular failure
Microvascular thrombosis

Neurologic
Sympathetic nervous system dysfunction
Cardiac and respiratory depression
Thermoregulatory failure
Coma

Pulmonary
Acute respiratory failure
Acute lung injury (ALI)

Renal
Acute tubular necrosis (ATN)

Hematologic
Disseminated intravascular coagulation (DIC)

Gastrointestinal
Gastrointestinal tract failure
Hepatic failure
Pancreatic failure

ASSESSMENT AND DIAGNOSIS

The patient with a systolic blood pressure (SBP) less than 90 mm Hg and accompanied by tachycardia and altered mental status is considered to be in a shock state.[1] Clinical manifestations will differ though, according to underlying cause and the stage of the shock, and are related to both the cause of and the patient's response to shock.[1,4]

Compensatory mechanisms may produce normal hemodynamic values even when tissue perfusion is compromised.[5,6] Global indicators of systemic perfusion and oxygenation include serum lactate and base deficit levels. Inadequate cellular oxygenation with anaerobic metabolism produces an elevated serum lactate. The level and duration of this hyperlactatemia are predictive of morbidity and mortality.[6,7] The base deficit derived from arterial blood gas (ABG) values also reflects global tissue acidosis and is frequently used to assess severity of shock.[6,7] (See individual shock sections for a discussion of clinical assessment and diagnosis of the patient in shock.)

Medical Management

The major focus of the treatment of shock is the improvement and preservation of tissue perfusion. Adequate tissue perfusion depends on an adequate supply of oxygen being transported to the tissues and the cell's ability to use it. Oxygen transport is influenced by pulmonary gas exchange, cardiac output, and hemoglobin level. Oxygen utilization is influenced by the internal metabolic environment. Management of the patient in shock focuses on supporting oxygen transport and oxygen utilization.[1]

Adequate pulmonary gas exchange is critical to oxygen transport. Establishing and maintaining an adequate airway are the first steps in ensuring adequate oxygenation. Once the airway is patent, emphasis is placed on improving ventilation and oxygenation. Therapies include administration of supplemental oxygen and mechanical ventilatory support.[1]

An adequate CO and hemoglobin level are crucial to oxygen transport. CO depends on HR, preload, afterload, and contractility. A variety of fluids and drugs are used to manipulate these parameters. The types of fluids used include both crystalloids and colloids. The categories of drugs used include vasoconstrictors, vasodilators, positive inotropes, and antidysrhythmics.[1]

Indicated for decreased preload related to intravascular volume depletion, fluid administration can be accomplished by use of either a crystalloid or colloid solution, or both. Crystalloids are balanced electrolyte solutions that may be hypotonic, isotonic, or hypertonic. Examples of crystalloid solutions used in shock situations are normal saline and lactated Ringer's solution. Colloids are protein- or starch-containing solutions. Examples of colloid solutions are blood and blood components and pharmaceutical plasma expanders, such as hetastarch, dextran, and mannitol.[1]

The choice of fluid is the subject of much debate and depends on the situation.[1,8-11] Advantages of colloids include faster restoration of intravascular volume and use of smaller amounts. Colloids are believed to stay in the intravascular space as opposed to crystalloids, which readily leak into the extravascular space. Disadvantages include expense, allergic reactions, and difficulties in typing and cross-matching blood. Colloids also can leak out of damaged capillaries and cause a variety of additional problems, particularly in the lungs. Blood should be used to augment oxygen transport if the patient's hemoglobin level is low, although controversy exists as to what threshold value should be used.[2,10]

Vasoconstrictor agents are used to increase afterload by increasing the systemic vascular resistance (SVR) and improving the patient's blood pressure level. Vasodilator agents are used to decrease preload or afterload, or both, by decreasing venous return and SVR. Positive inotropic agents are used to increase contractility. Antidysrhythmic agents are used to influence HR.[1] Box 26-2 provides examples of each of these agents.

Sodium bicarbonate is no longer recommended in the treatment of shock-related lactic acidosis.[1,5,10,12] No overall benefit has been found, and risks associated with its use are significant. These include shifting of the oxyhemoglobin dissociation curve to the left, rebound increase in lactic acid production, development of hyperosmolar state, fluid overload resulting from excessive sodium, and rapid cellular electrolyte shifts.[5,10,12]

The patient also should be started on a nutritional support therapy.[1] The type of nutritional supplementation initiated varies according to the cause of shock and should be tailored to the individual patient's need, as indicated by the underlying condition and

Box 26-2
Agents Used in the Treatment of Shock

Vasoconstrictors
Epinephrine (Adrenalin)
Norepinephrine (Levophed)
α-Range dopamine (Intropin)
Metaraminol (Aramine)
Phenylephrine (Neo-Synephrine)
Ephedrine
Vasopressin (Pitressin)

Vasodilators
Nitroprusside (Nipride, Nitropress)
Nitroglycerin (Nitrol, Tridil)
Hydralazine (Apresoline)
Labetalol (Normodyne, Trandate)

Inotropes
β-Range dopamine (Intropin)
Dobutamine (Dobutrex)
Epinephrine (Adrenalin)
Isoproterenol (Isuprel)
Norepinephrine (Levophed)

Antidysrhythmics
Lidocaine (Xylocaine)
Adenosine (Adenocard)
Procainamide (Pronestyl)
Labetalol (Normodyne, Trandate)
Verapamil (Calan, Isoptin)
Esmolol (Brevibloc)
Diltiazem (Cardizem)
Amiodarone (Cordarone)

laboratory data. The enteral route is preferred over the parenteral.[13,14]

Nursing Management

The nursing management of a patient in shock is a complex and challenging responsibility. It requires an in-depth understanding of the pathophysiology of the disease and the anticipated effects of each intervention, as well as a solid understanding of the nursing process. (Individual shock sections contain separate discussions of specific interventions for the patient in shock.)

The psychosocial needs of the patient and family dealing with shock are extremely important. These needs, which differ with each patient and family, are based on situational, familial, and patient-centered variables. **Nursing priorities in managing the patient with shock are directed toward (1) providing information on patient status, (2) explaining procedures and routines, (3) supporting the family, (4) encouraging the expression of feelings, (5) facilitating problem solving and decision making, (6) involving the family in the patient's care, and (7) establishing contacts with necessary resources.**[15-17]

Collaborative management of the patient with shock is outlined in Box 26-3.

HYPOVOLEMIC SHOCK

Hypovolemic shock occurs from inadequate fluid volume in the intravascular space. The lack of adequate circulating volume leads to decreased tissue perfusion and initiation of the general shock response. Hypovolemic shock is the most commonly occurring form of shock.[18]

Box 26-3

Collaborative Management

Shock

- Support oxygen transport.
  - Establish a patent airway.
  - Initiate mechanical ventilation.
  - Administer oxygen.
  - Administer fluids (crystalloids, colloids, blood and other blood products).
  - Administer vasoactive medications.
  - Administer positive inotropic medications.
  - Ensure sufficient hemoglobin and hematocrit.
- Support oxygen use.
  - Identify and correct cause of lactic acidosis.
  - Ensure adequate organ and extremity perfusion.
  - Initiate nutritional support therapy.
- Identify underlying cause of shock and treat accordingly.
- Maintain surveillance for complications.
- Provide comfort and emotional support.

Etiology

Hypovolemic shock can result from either absolute or relative hypovolemia. Absolute hypovolemia occurs when there is a loss of fluid from the intravascular space. This can result from an external loss of fluid from the body or when there is an internal shifting of fluid from the intravascular space to the extravascular space. Fluid shifts can result from loss in intravascular integrity, increased capillary membrane permeability, or decreased colloidal osmotic pressure. Relative hypovolemia occurs when vasodilation produces an increase in vascular capacitance relative to circulating volume (Box 26-4).[18]

Pathophysiology

Hypovolemia results in a loss of circulating fluid volume. A decrease in circulating volume leads to a decrease in venous return, which, in turn, results in a decrease in end-diastolic volume or preload. Preload is

Box 26-4

Etiologic Factors in Hypovolemic Shock

Absolute

Loss of Whole Blood
Trauma or surgery
Gastrointestinal bleeding

Loss of Plasma
Thermal injuries
Large lesions

Loss of Other Body Fluids
Severe vomiting or diarrhea
Massive diuresis

Loss of Intravascular Integrity
Ruptured spleen
Long bone or pelvic fractures
Hemorrhagic pancreatitis
Hemothorax or hemoperitoneum
Arterial dissection or rupture

Relative

Vasodilation
Sepsis
Anaphylaxis
Loss of sympathetic stimulation

Increased Capillary Membrane Permeability
Sepsis
Anaphylaxis
Thermal injuries

Decreased Colloidal Osmotic Pressure
Severe sodium depletion
Hypopituitarism
Cirrhosis
Intestinal obstruction

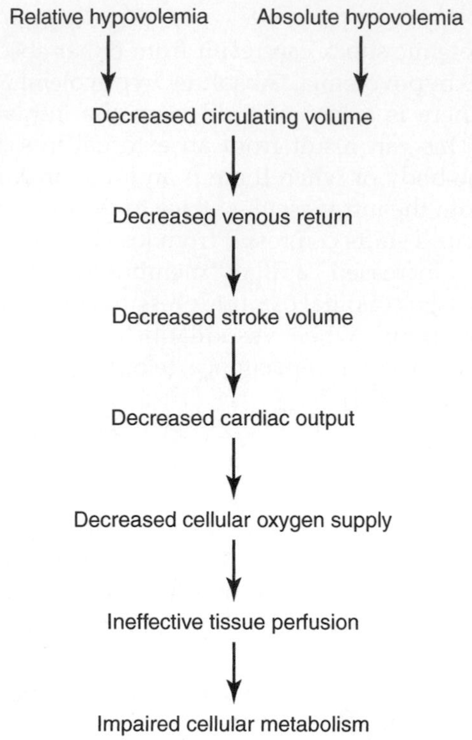

FIGURE 26-1. The pathophysiology of hypovolemic shock.

a major determinant of stroke volume (SV) and CO. A decrease in preload results in a decrease in SV and CO. The decrease in CO leads to inadequate cellular oxygen supply and ineffective tissue perfusion (Figure 26-1).[18]

ASSESSMENT AND DIAGNOSIS

The clinical manifestations of hypovolemic shock vary, depending on the severity of fluid loss and the patient's ability to compensate for it. Clinical classes have been developed by the American College of Surgeons to describe the levels of severity of hypovolemic shock. Class I indicates a fluid volume loss up to 15% or an actual volume loss up to 750 ml. Compensatory mechanisms maintain CO, and the patient appears symptom-free other than slight anxiety.[2,18]

Class II hypovolemic shock occurs with a fluid volume loss of 15% to 30% or an actual volume loss of 750 to 1500 ml. Falling CO activates more intense compensatory responses. The HR increases to over 100 beats/min in response to increased SNS stimulation. The pulse pressure (PP) narrows as the diastolic blood pressure increases because of vasoconstriction. Respiratory rate (RR) increases to 20 to 30 breaths/min, and depth increases in an attempt to improve oxygenation. ABG specimens drawn during this phase reveal respiratory alkalosis and hypoxemia, as evidenced by a low arterial partial pressure of carbon dioxide ($Paco_2$) and a low arterial partial pressure of oxygen (Pao_2), respectively. Urine output (UO) starts to decline to 20 to 30 ml/hr as renal perfusion decreases. Urine sodium decreases while urine osmolality and specific gravity increase as the kidneys start to conserve sodium and water. The patient's skin becomes pale and cool, with delayed capillary refill because of peripheral vasoconstriction. Jugular veins appear flat as a result of decreased venous return.[2,18]

Hypovolemic shock that is Class III occurs with a fluid volume loss of 30% to 40% or an actual volume loss of 1500 to 2000 ml. This level of severity produces the progressive stage of shock as compensatory mechanisms become overwhelmed and ineffective tissue perfusion develops. Systolic BP decreases. The HR increases to over 120 beats/min, and dysrhythmias develop as myocardial ischemia ensues. Respiratory distress occurs as the pulmonary system deteriorates. ABG values during this phase reveal respiratory and metabolic acidosis and hypoxemia, as evidenced by a high $Paco_2$, low bicarbonate (HCO_3^-), and low Pao_2, respectively. Decreased renal perfusion results in the development of oliguria. Blood urea nitrogen (BUN) and serum creatinine levels start to rise as the kidneys begin to fail. The patient's skin becomes ashen, cold, and clammy, with marked delayed capillary refill. The patient appears confused as cerebral perfusion decreases and level of consciousness (LOC) deteriorates.[2,6,18]

Class IV hypovolemic shock is usually refractory in nature. It occurs with a fluid volume loss of greater than 40% or an actual volume loss of more than 2000 ml. The compensatory mechanisms of the body completely deteriorate, and organ failure occurs.[6] Severe tachycardia and hypotension ensue. Peripheral pulses are absent, and because of marked peripheral vasoconstriction, capillary refill does not occur. The skin appears cyanotic, mottled, and extremely diaphoretic. Urine output ceases. The patient becomes lethargic and unresponsive, and a variety of clinical manifestations associated with failure of the different body systems develop.[2,6,18]

Assessment of the hemodynamic parameters of a patient in hypovolemic shock varies by stage, but commonly reveals a decreased CO and cardiac index (CI). Loss of circulating volume leads to a decrease in venous return to the heart, which results in a decrease in the preload of the right and left ventricles. This is evidenced by a decline in the right atrial pressure (RAP) and pulmonary artery occlusion pressure (PAOP). Vasoconstriction of the arterial system results in an increase in the afterload of the heart as evidenced by an increase in the SVR. This vasoconstriction may produce a falsely elevated systolic BP when measured by arterial catheter. Mean arterial pressure (MAP) is more accurate in this low-flow state.[6]

MEDICAL MANAGEMENT

Treatment of the patient in hypovolemic shock requires an aggressive approach. The major goals of therapy

Box 26-5

NURSING DIAGNOSIS PRIORITIES

Hypovolemic Shock

- Deficient Fluid Volume related to active blood loss
- Deficient Fluid Volume related to interstitial fluid shift
- Decreased Cardiac Output related to alterations in preload, p. A-12
- Imbalanced Nutrition: Less Than Body Requirements related to increased metabolic demands or lack of exogenous nutrients, p. A-28
- Risk for Infection, p. A-46
- Anxiety related to threat to biologic, psychologic, and/or social integrity, p. A-9
- Compromised Family Coping related to critically ill family member, p. A-11

are to correct the cause of the hypovolemia and to restore tissue perfusion. This approach includes identifying and stopping the source of fluid loss and vigorously administering fluid to replace circulating volume. Fluid administration can be accomplished with use of either a crystalloid or a colloid solution, or a combination of both. The type of solution used usually depends on the type of fluid lost, the degree of hypovolemia, and the severity of hypoperfusion.[18,19]

Aggressive fluid resuscitation in the trauma patient with uncontrolled hemorrhage is a subject of debate. Research is evaluating the benefit of limited or hypotensive (SBP >70 mm Hg) volume resuscitation, which is postulated to lessen bleeding and improve survival.[19-22]

Nursing Management

Prevention of hypovolemic shock is one of the primary responsibilities of the nurse in the critical care area. Preventive measures include the identification of patients at risk and frequent assessment of the patient's fluid balance. Accurate monitoring of intake and output and daily weights are essential components of preventive nursing care. Early identification and treatment result in decreased mortality.

Management of the patient in hypovolemic shock requires continuous evaluation of intravascular volume, tissue perfusion, and response to therapy. The patient in hypovolemic shock may have any number of nursing diagnoses, depending on the progression of the process (Box 26-5). **Nursing priorities are directed toward (1) minimizing fluid loss, (2) administering volume replacement, (3) promoting comfort and emotional support, and (4) maintaining surveillance for complications.**

Measures to minimize fluid loss include limiting blood sampling, observing lines for accidental disconnection, and applying direct pressure to bleeding sites. Measures to facilitate the administration of volume replacement include insertion of large-bore peripheral intravenous (IV) catheters, rapid administration of prescribed fluids, and positioning the patient with the legs elevated, trunk flat, and head and shoulders above the chest. In addition, monitoring the patient for clinical manifestations of fluid overload or complications related to blood product administration is critical to preventing further problems.[18]

CARDIOGENIC SHOCK

Cardiogenic shock is the result of failure of the heart to effectively pump blood forward. It can occur with dysfunction of either the right or the left ventricle, or both. The lack of adequate pumping function leads to decreased tissue perfusion and circulatory failure. It occurs in approximately 6% to 10% of the patients with an acute myocardial infarction (MI) and is the leading cause of death in patients hospitalized with MI.[23-25] The mortality rate for cardiogenic shock has decreased with the advent of early revascularization therapy and is currently around 50 to 60%.[23,26,27]

Etiology

Cardiogenic shock can result from primary ventricular ischemia, structural problems, and dysrhythmias.[1,23,25] The most common cause is acute MI resulting in the loss of 40% or more of the functional myocardium. The damage to the myocardium may occur after one massive MI (usually anterior wall), or it may be cumulative as a result of several smaller MIs or a small MI in a patient with preexisting ventricular dysfunction.[1,23] Structural problems of the cardiopulmonary system and dysrhythmias also may cause cardiogenic shock if they disrupt the forward motion of the blood through the heart (Box 26-6).[1,23,25]

Pathophysiology

Cardiogenic shock results from the impaired ability of the ventricle to pump blood forward, which leads to a decrease in SV and an increase in the blood left in the ventricle at the end of systole. The decrease in SV results in a decrease in CO, which leads to decreased cellular oxygen supply and ineffective tissue perfusion.[19,25] Typically, myocardial performance spirals downward as compensatory vasoconstriction increases myocardial afterload and low blood pressure worsens myocardial ischemia. Recent research suggests that an alternate physiologic sequence may occur at some point in this process in a subset of patients. Evidence of a systemic inflammatory response has been noted in a number of patients with cardiogenic shock.[26,28,29] Activation of inflammatory cytokines may induce systemic vasodilation, normalization of the CO, and defective cellular oxygen use. It is unknown whether

Box 26-6

Etiologic Factors in Cardiogenic Shock

Primary Ventricular Ischemia
Acute myocardial infarction
Cardiopulmonary arrest
Open heart surgery

Structural Problems
Septal rupture
Papillary muscle rupture
Free wall rupture
Ventricular aneurysm
Cardiomyopathies
- Congestive
- Hypertrophic
- Restrictive

Intracardiac tumor
Pulmonary embolus
Atrial thrombus
Valvular dysfunction
Acute myocarditis
Cardiac tamponade
Myocardial contusion

Dysrhythmias
Bradydysrhythmias
Tachydysrhythmias

this process contributes to the genesis or the outcome of cardiogenic shock.[26,29] As left ventricular contractility falls, an increase in end-systolic volume results in the backup of blood into the pulmonary system and the subsequent development of pulmonary edema. Pulmonary edema causes impaired gas exchange and decreased oxygenation of the arterial blood, which further impair tissue perfusion (Figure 26-2). Death due to cardiogenic shock may result from multiple organ failure or cardiopulmonary collapse.[25,26,28,29]

Assessment and Diagnosis

A variety of clinical manifestations occur in the patient in cardiogenic shock, depending on etiologic factors in pump failure, the patient's underlying medical status, and the severity of the shock state. Some clinical manifestations are caused by failure of the heart as a pump, whereas many relate to the overall shock response (Box 26-7).

Initially the clinical manifestations relate to the decline in CO. These signs and symptoms include SBP less than 90 mm Hg; decreased sensorium; cool, pale, moist skin; and UO less than 30 ml/hr. The patient also may complain of chest pain. Tachycardia develops to compensate for the fall in CO. A weak, thready pulse develops, and heart sounds may reveal a diminished

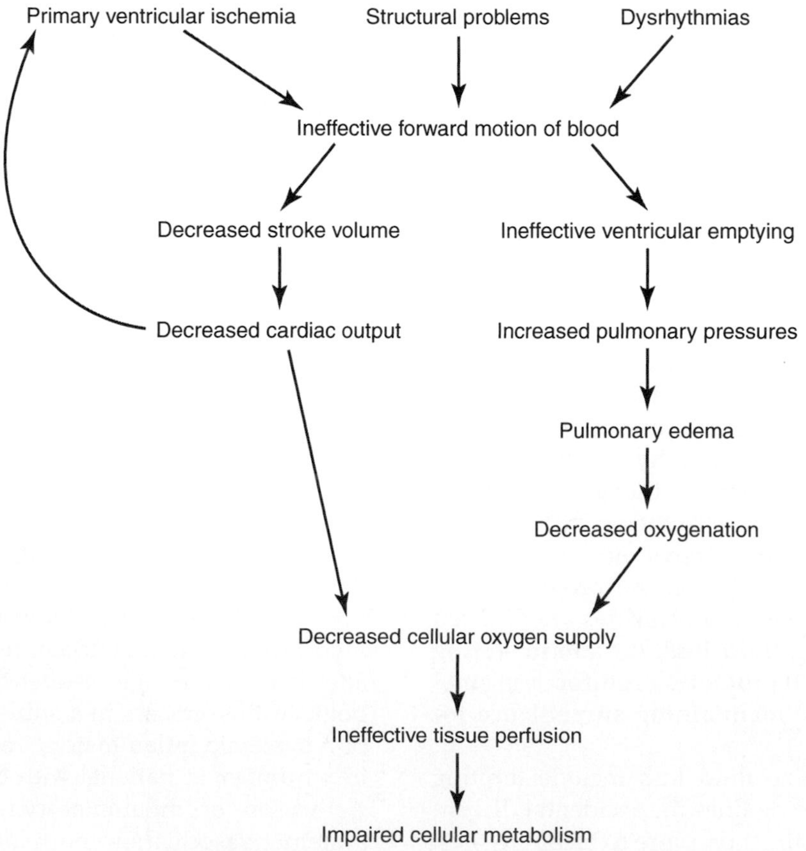

FIGURE 26-2. The pathophysiology of cardiogenic shock.

S_1 and S_2 as a result of the decrease in contractility. Respiratory rate increases to improve oxygenation. ABG values at this time indicate respiratory alkalosis as evidenced by a decrease in $Paco_2$. Urinalysis findings demonstrate a decrease in urine sodium and an increase in urine osmolality and specific gravity as the kidneys start to conserve sodium and water. The patient also may experience a variety of dysrhythmias, depending on the underlying problem.[25]

As the left ventricle fails, auscultation of the lungs may disclose crackles and rhonchi, indicating the development of pulmonary edema. Hypoxemia occurs as evidenced by a fall in Pao_2 and Sao_2 as measured by ABG values. Heart sounds may reveal an S_3 and S_4. Jugular venous distention is evident with right-sided failure.[25]

Assessment of the hemodynamic parameters of a patient in cardiogenic shock reveals a decreased CO with a CI less than 2.2 L/min/m^2 in the presence of elevated PAOP over 15 to 18 mm Hg.[23,25] Increased filling pressures are necessary to rule out hypovolemia as the cause of circulatory failure. The increase in PAOP reflects an increase in the left ventricular end-diastolic pressure (LVEDP) and end-diastolic volume (LVEDV) resulting from decreased SV. With right ventricular failure, the RAP also will increase. Compensatory vasoconstriction results in an increase in the afterload of the heart as evidenced by an increase in the SVR. Echocardiography confirms the diagnosis of cardiogenic shock and rules out other causes of circulatory failure.[23,25]

As compensatory mechanisms fail and ineffective tissue perfusion develops, a variety of other clinical manifestations appear. Myocardial ischemia progresses as evidenced by continued increases in HR, dysrhythmias, and chest pain. Pulmonary function deteriorates, which leads to respiratory distress. ABG values during this phase reveal respiratory and metabolic acidosis and hypoxemia as indicated by a high $Paco_2$, low HCO_3^-, and low Pao_2, respectively. Renal failure occurs as exhibited by the development of anuria and increases in BUN and serum creatinine levels. Cerebral hypoperfusion manifests as decreasing LOC.[25]

Box 26-7

Clinical Manifestations of Cardiogenic Shock

- Systolic blood pressure <90 mm Hg
- Heart rate >100 beats/min
- Weak, thready pulse
- Diminished heart sounds
- Change in sensorium
- Cool, pale, moist skin
- Urine output <30 ml/hr
- Chest pain
- Dysrhythmias
- Tachypnea
- Crackles
- Decreased cardiac output
- Cardiac index <2.2 L/min/m^2
- Increased pulmonary artery occlusion pressure
- Increased right atrial pressure
- Increased systemic vascular resistance

Medical Management

Treatment of the patient in cardiogenic shock requires an aggressive approach. The major goals of therapy are to treat the underlying cause, enhance the effectiveness of the pump, and improve tissue perfusion. This approach includes identifying the etiologic factors of pump failure and administering pharmacologic agents to enhance CO. Inotropic agents are used to increase contractility and maintain adequate BP and tissue perfusion. Diuretics are used for preload reduction. Once blood pressure has been stabilized, vasodilating agents are used for preload and afterload reduction. Antidysrhythmic agents should be used to suppress or control dysrhythmias that can affect CO.[23,25] Intubation and mechanical ventilation may be necessary to support oxygenation.

Intraaortic balloon pump (IABP) support should be instituted if drug therapy does not quickly reverse the shock state.[26,27] The IABP is a temporary measure to decrease myocardial workload by improving myocardial supply and decreasing myocardial demand. It achieves this goal by improving coronary artery perfusion and reducing left ventricular afterload. See Chapter 13 for further discussion on IAPB therapy.

Once the cause of pump failure has been identified, measures should be taken to correct the problem if possible. If the problem is related to an acute MI, early revascularization by coronary angioplasty or coronary artery bypass surgery provides significant survival benefit.[23,26,27] Thrombolytic agents may be used in select patients. Therapies to decrease myocardial demand should include activity restrictions, analgesics, and sedatives.[25] When conventional therapies fail, extracorporeal membrane oxygenation (ECMO) and/or a ventricular assist device (VAD) may be used to support the patient in acute cardiogenic shock.[30-32] These mechanical circulatory assist devices provide an external means to sustain effective organ perfusion, allowing time for the patient's ventricle to heal or for cardiac transplantation to take place.

Nursing Management

Prevention of cardiogenic shock is one of the primary responsibilities of the nurse in the critical care area. Preventive measures include the identification of patients at risk and frequent assessment and management of the patient's cardiopulmonary status. The

Box 26-8

NURSING DIAGNOSES PRIORITIES

Cardiogenic Shock

- Ineffective Cardiopulmonary Tissue Perfusion related to acute myocardial ischemia
- Decreased Cardiac Output related to alterations in contractility, p. A-13
- Decreased Cardiac Output related to alterations in heart rate, p. A-13
- Imbalanced Nutrition: Less Than Body Requirements related to increased metabolic demands or lack of exogenous nutrients, p. A-28
- Risk for Infection, p. A-46
- Disturbed Body Image related to functional dependence on life-sustaining technology, p. A-21
- Compromised Family Coping related to critically ill family member, p. A-11

patient in cardiogenic shock may have any number of nursing diagnoses, depending on the progression of the process (Box 26-8). **Nursing priorities are directed toward (1) limiting myocardial oxygen demand, (2) enhancing myocardial oxygen supply, (3) promoting comfort and emotional support, and (4) maintaining surveillance for complications.**

Measures to limit myocardial oxygen demand include administering analgesics, sedatives, and agents to control afterload and dysrhythmias; positioning the patient for comfort; limiting activities; providing a calm and quiet environment and offering support to reduce anxiety; and teaching the patient about the condition. Measures to enhance myocardial oxygen supply include administering supplemental oxygen, monitoring the patient's respiratory status, and administering prescribed medications.

Effective nursing management of cardiogenic shock requires precise monitoring and management of HR, preload, afterload, and contractility. This is accomplished through accurate measurement of hemodynamic variables and controlled administration of fluids and inotropic and vasoactive agents. Close assessment and management of respiratory function is also essential to maintain adequate oxygenation.

Patients who require IABP therapy need to be observed frequently for complications. Complications include emboli formation, infection, rupture of the aorta, thrombocytopenia, improper balloon placement, bleeding, improper timing of the balloon, balloon rupture, and circulatory compromise of the cannulated extremity.[33]

Anaphylactic Shock

Anaphylactic shock, a type of distributive shock, is the result of an immediate hypersensitivity reaction. It is a life-threatening event that requires prompt intervention. The severe antibody-antigen response leads to decreased tissue perfusion and initiation of the general shock response.[34-36]

Etiology

Anaphylactic shock is caused by an antibody-antigen response. Almost any substance can cause a hypersensitivity reaction. These substances, known as *antigens,* can be introduced by injection or ingestion or through the skin or respiratory tract. A number of antigens have been identified that can cause a reaction in a hypersensitive person. This list includes foods, food additives, diagnostic agents, biologic agents, environmental agents, drugs, and venoms (Box 26-9).[35,36]

Pathophysiology

The antibody-antigen response (immunologic stimulation) or the direct triggering (nonimmunologic activation) of the mast cells results in the release of biochemical mediators. These mediators include histamine, eosinophil chemotactic factor of anaphylaxis (ECF-A), neutrophil chemotactic factor of anaphylaxis (NCF), platelet activating factor (PAF), proteinases, heparin, serotonin, leukotrienes (also known as *slow-reacting substance of anaphylaxis*), and prostaglandins. The activation of the biochemical mediators causes vasodilation, increased capillary permeability, bronchoconstriction, excessive mucus secretion, coronary vasoconstriction, inflammation, cutaneous reactions, and constriction of the smooth muscle in the intestinal wall, bladder, and uterus. Coronary vasoconstriction causes severe myocardial depression. Cutaneous reactions cause stimulation of nerve endings followed by itching and pain.[34-36]

ECF-A promotes chemotaxis of eosinophils, thus facilitating the movement of eosinophils into the area. During allergic reactions, eosinophils phagocytose the antibody-antigen complex and other inflammatory debris and release enzymes that inhibit vasoactive mediators, such as histamine and leukotrienes. In addition, secondary mediators are produced that either enhance or inhibit the already released biochemical mediators. For example, bradykinin, a secondary mediator, increases capillary permeability and facilitates vasodilation.[35]

Peripheral vasodilation results in relative hypovolemia and decreased venous return. Increased capillary membrane permeability results in the loss of intravascular volume, worsening the hypovolemic state. Decreased venous return results in decreased end-diastolic volume and SV. The decline in SV leads to a fall in CO and ineffective tissue perfusion. Death may result from airway obstruction or cardiovascular collapse, or both (Figure 26-3).[34-37]

Box 26-9

Etiologic Factors in Anaphylactic Shock

Foods
Eggs and milk
Fish and shellfish
Nuts and seeds
Legumes and cereals
Citrus fruits
Chocolate
Strawberries
Tomatoes
Avocados
Bananas
Other

Food Additives
Food coloring
Preservatives

Diagnostic Agents
Iodinated contrast dye
Sulfobromophthalein (Bromsulphalein) (BSP)
Dehydrocholic acid (Decholin)
Iopanoic acid (Telepaque)

Biologic Agents
Blood and blood components
Insulin and other hormones
Gamma globulin
Seminal plasma
Enzymes
Vaccines and antitoxins

Environmental Agents
Pollens, molds, and spores
Sunlight
Animal hair
Latex

Drugs
Antibiotics
Aspirin
Narcotics
Dextran
Vitamins
Local anesthetic agents
Muscle relaxants
Barbiturates
Other

Venoms
Bees and wasps
Snakes
Jellyfish
Spiders
Deer flies
Fire ants

Assessment and Diagnosis

Anaphylactic shock is a severe systemic reaction that can affect any number of organ systems. A variety of clinical manifestations occur in the patient in anaphylactic shock, depending on the extent of multisystem involvement. The symptoms usually start to appear within minutes of exposure to the antigen, but they may not occur for up to 1 hour (Box 26-10).[34] Symptoms may also reappear following a 1- to 12-hour window of resolution. These late-phase reactions may be similar to the initial anaphylactic response, milder, or more severe.[34,35]

The cutaneous effects may appear first and include pruritus, generalized erythema, urticaria, and angioedema. Commonly seen on the face and in the oral cavity and lower pharynx, angioedema develops as a result of fluid leaking into the interstitial space. The patient may appear restless, uneasy, apprehensive, and anxious and may complain of being warm. Respiratory effects include the development of laryngeal edema, bronchoconstriction, and mucus plugs. Clinical manifestations of laryngeal edema include inspiratory stridor, hoarseness, a sensation of fullness or a lump in the throat, and dysphagia. Bronchoconstriction causes dyspnea, wheezing, and chest tightness.[34-36] In addition, gastrointestinal and genitourinary manifestations may develop as a result of smooth muscle contraction. These include vomiting, diarrhea, cramping, and abdominal pain.[34]

As the anaphylactic reaction progresses, hypotension and reflex tachycardia develop. This occurs in response to massive vasodilation and loss of circulating volume. Jugular veins appear flat as right ventricular end-diastolic volume is decreased. The eventual outcome is circulatory failure and ineffective tissue perfusion.[34-36] The patient's level of consciousness may deteriorate to unresponsiveness.[34]

Assessment of the hemodynamic parameters of a patient in anaphylactic shock reveals a decreased CO and CI. Venous vasodilation and massive volume loss lead to a decrease in preload, which results in a decline in the RAP and PAOP. Vasodilation of the arterial system results in a decrease in the afterload of the heart, as evidenced by a decrease in the SVR.[35]

Medical Management

Treatment of anaphylactic shock requires an immediate and direct approach. The goals of therapy are to remove the offending antigen, reverse the effects of the biochemical mediators, and promote adequate tissue perfusion. When the hypersensitivity reaction

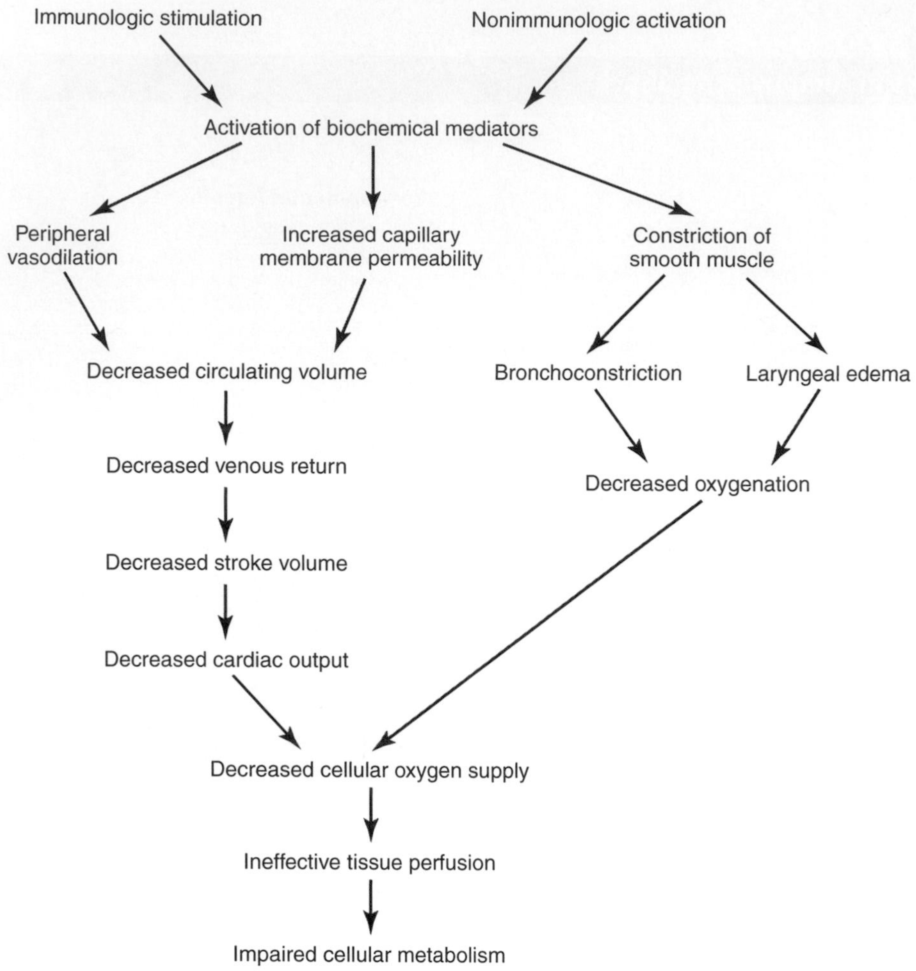

FIGURE 26-3. The pathophysiology of anaphylactic shock.

Box 26-10

Clinical Manifestations of Anaphylactic Shock

Cardiovascular
Hypotension
Tachycardia

Respiratory
Lump in throat
Dysphagia
Hoarseness
Stridor
Wheezing
Rales and rhonchi

Cutaneous
Pruritus
Erythema
Urticaria
Angioedema

Neurologic
Restlessness
Uneasiness
Apprehension
Anxiety
Decreased level of consciousness

Gastrointestinal
Nausea
Vomiting
Diarrhea

Genitourinary
Incontinence
Vaginal bleeding

Subjective Complaints
Sensation of warmth
Dyspnea
Abdominal cramping and pain
Itching

Hemodynamic Parameters
Decreased cardiac output (CO)
Decreased cardiac index (CI)
Decreased right atrial pressure (RAP)
Decreased pulmonary occlusion pressure (PAOP)
Decreased systemic vascular resistance (SVR)

occurs as a result of administration of medications, dye, blood, or blood products, the infusion should be immediately discontinued. Many times it is not possible to remove the antigen because it is unknown or has already entered the patient's system.[34-36]

Reversal of the effects of the biochemical mediators involves the preservation and support of the patient's airway, ventilation, and circulation. This is accomplished through oxygen therapy, intubation, mechanical ventilation, and administration of drugs and fluids.[35]

Epinephrine is given to promote bronchodilation and vasoconstriction and to inhibit further release of biochemical mediators. In mild cases of anaphylaxis, 0.3 to 0.5 mg (0.3 to 0.5 ml) of a 1:1000 dilution of epinephrine is administered by either intramuscular or subcutaneous route and repeated every 5 to 15 minutes until anaphylaxis is resolved.[34-37] Evidence suggests that intramuscular administration into the lateral thigh achieves maximum absorption.[38] For anaphylactic shock with hypotension, epinephrine is administered intravenously. The IV dose is 0.3 to 0.5 mg (3 to 5 ml) of a 1:10,000 dilution administered over at least 3 to 10 minutes and repeated every 15 minutes if needed. If hypotension persists, a continuous infusion of epinephrine administered at 1 mcg/min with titration up to 10 mcg/min as needed is recommended.[35,36] It must be noted that patients receiving β-blockers may have a limited response to epinephrine. Intravenous glucagon administered at 5 to 15 mcg/min is recommended for inotropic and vasoactive support for these patients.[34,36]

Diphenhydramine (Benadryl), 1 to 2 mg/kg (maximum 50 mg) IV every 4 to 8 hours, is used to block the histamine response.[34-36] Corticosteroids also may be given with the goal of preventing a delayed reaction and stabilizing capillary membranes.[34-36] Fluid replacement is accomplished by use of either a crystalloid or colloid solution. In addition, positive inotropic agents and vasoconstrictor agents may be necessary to reverse the effects of myocardial depression and vasodilation.[34-36]

Nursing Management

Prevention of anaphylactic shock is one of the primary responsibilities of the nurse in the critical care area. Preventive measures include the identification of patients at risk and cautious assessment of the patient's response to the administration of drugs, blood, and blood products. A complete and accurate history of the patient's allergies is an essential component of preventive nursing care. In addition to a list of the allergies, a detailed description of the type of response for each one should be obtained.

The patient in anaphylactic shock may have any number of nursing diagnoses, depending on the progression of the process (Box 26-11). **Nursing priorities are directed toward (1) facilitating ventilation, (2) administering volume replacement, (3) promoting comfort and emotional support, and (4) maintaining surveillance for complications.**

> **Box 26-11**
>
> **NURSING DIAGNOSES PRIORITIES**
>
> **Anaphylactic Shock**
>
> - Deficient Fluid Volume related to relative loss, p. A-17
> - Decreased Cardiac Output related to alterations in preload, p. A-12
> - Decreased Cardiac Output related to alterations in afterload, p. A-12
> - Ineffective Breathing Pattern related to decreased lung expansion, p. A-34
> - Impaired Gas Exchange related to ventilation/perfusion mismatching or intrapulmonary shunting, p. A-29
> - Imbalanced Nutrition: Less Than Body Requirements related to increased metabolic demands or lack of exogenous nutrients, p. A-28
> - Risk for Infection, p. A-46
> - Ineffective Coping related to situational crisis and personal vulnerability, p. A-38
> - Compromised Family Coping related to critically ill family member, p. A-11

Measures to facilitate ventilation include positioning the patient to assist with breathing and instructing the patient to breathe slowly and deeply. Airway protection through prompt administration of prescribed medications is essential. Measures to facilitate the administration of volume replacement include inserting large-bore peripheral intravenous catheters, rapidly administering prescribed fluids, and positioning the patient with the legs elevated, trunk flat, and head and shoulders above the chest. Measures to promote comfort include administering medications to relieve itching, applying warm soaks to skin, and if necessary, covering the patient's hands to discourage scratching. In addition, observing the patient for clinical manifestations of a delayed reaction is critical to preventing further problems.

NEUROGENIC SHOCK

Description

Neurogenic shock, another type of distributive shock, is the result of the loss or suppression of sympathetic tone. The lack of sympathetic tone leads to decreased tissue perfusion and initiation of the general shock response. Neurogenic shock is the rarest form of shock.

Etiology

Neurogenic shock can be caused by anything that disrupts the SNS. The problem can occur as the result of interrupted impulse transmission or blockage of sympathetic outflow from the vasomotor center in

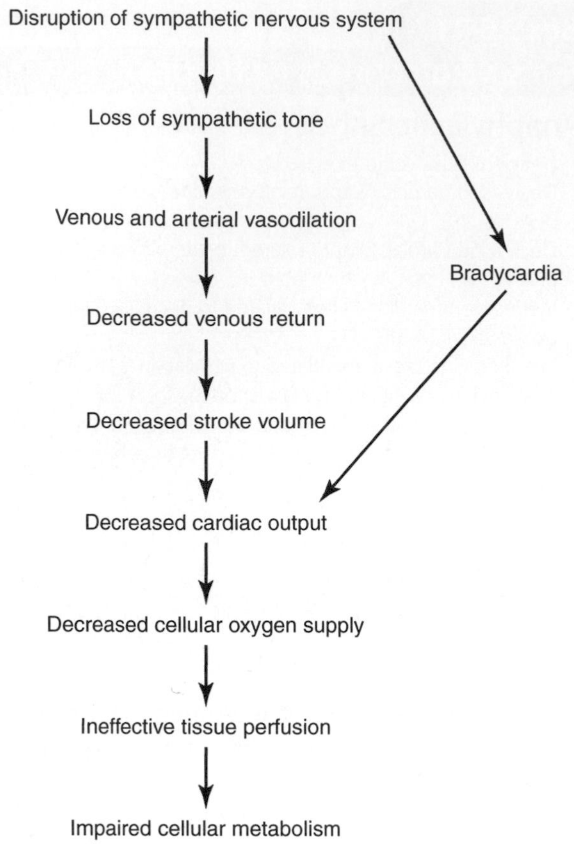

FIGURE 26-4. The pathophysiology of neurogenic shock.

the brain.[39,40] The most common cause is spinal cord injury. Neurogenic shock may mistakenly be referred to as *spinal shock*. The later condition refers to loss of neurologic activity below the level of spinal cord injury, but does not necessarily involve ineffective tissue perfusion.[40]

Pathophysiology

Loss of sympathetic tone results in massive peripheral vasodilation, inhibition of the baroreceptor response, and impaired thermoregulation. Arterial vasodilation leads to a decrease in SVR and a fall in blood pressure. Venous vasodilation leads to relative hypovolemia and pooling of blood in the venous circuit. The decreased venous return results in a decrease in end-diastolic volume or preload causing a decrease in SV and CO. The fall in blood pressure and CO leads to inadequate or ineffective tissue perfusion. Loss of sympathetic tone and inhibition of the baroreceptor response result in bradycardia.[41] The slow HR worsens CO, which further compromises tissue perfusion. Impaired thermoregulation occurs because of loss of vasomotor tone in the cutaneous blood vessels that dilate and constrict to maintain body temperature. The patient becomes poikilothermic, or dependent on the environment for temperature regulation (Figure 26-4).

Assessment and Diagnosis

The patient in neurogenic shock characteristically presents with hypotension, bradycardia, and warm, dry skin.[40,41] The decreased blood pressure results from massive peripheral vasodilation. The decreased HR is caused by inhibition of the baroreceptor response and unopposed parasympathetic control of the heart.[41] Hypothermia develops from uncontrolled heat loss peripherally. The warm, dry skin occurs as a consequence of pooling of blood in the extremities and loss of vasomotor control in surface vessels of the skin that control heat loss.[39]

Assessment of the hemodynamic parameters of a patient in neurogenic shock reveals a decreased CO and CI. Venous vasodilation leads to a decrease in preload, which results in a decline in the RAP and PAOP. Vasodilation of the arterial system causes a decrease in the afterload of the heart as evidenced by a decrease in the SVR.[39]

Medical Management

Treatment of neurogenic shock requires a careful approach. The goals of therapy are to treat or remove the cause, prevent cardiovascular instability, and promote optimal tissue perfusion. Cardiovascular instability can occur from hypovolemia, bradycardia, and hypothermia. Specific treatments are aimed at preventing or correcting these problems as they occur.

Hypovolemia is treated with careful fluid resuscitation. The minimal amount of fluid is administered to ensure adequate tissue perfusion. Volume replacement is initiated for SBP lower than 90 mm Hg, urine output less than 30 ml/hr, or changes in mental status that indicate decreased cerebral tissue perfusion. The patient is carefully observed for evidence of fluid overload. Vasopressors are used as necessary to maintain blood pressure and organ perfusion.[39,40]

Bradycardia should be treated with atropine when necessary.[40] Hypothermia is treated with warming measures and environmental temperature regulation.

Nursing Management

Prevention of neurogenic shock is one of the primary responsibilities of the nurse in the critical care area. This includes the identification of patients at risk and constant assessment of the neurologic status. Vigilant immobilization of spinal cord injuries and slight elevation of the head of bed of the patient after spinal anesthesia are essential components of preventive nursing care. Early identification allows for early treatment and decreased mortality.

The patient in neurogenic shock may have any number of nursing diagnoses, depending on the progression of the process (Box 26-12). **Nursing priorities are directed toward (1) treating hypovolemia, (2) main-**

Box 26-12

NURSING DIAGNOSES PRIORITIES

Neurogenic Shock

- Deficient Fluid Volume related to relative loss, p. A-17
- Decreased Cardiac Output related to sympathetic blockade, p. A-14
- Hypothermia related to exposure to cold environment, trauma, or damage to the hypothalamus, p. A-26
- Imbalanced Nutrition: Less Than Body Requirements related to increased metabolic demands or lack of exogenous nutrients, p. A-28
- Risk for Infection, p. A-46
- Anxiety related to threat to biologic, psychologic, or social integrity, p. A-9
- Compromised Family Coping related to critically ill family member, p. A-11

taining normothermia, (3) monitoring for dysrhythmias, (4) providing comfort and emotional support, and (5) maintaining surveillance for complications.

Venous pooling in the lower extremities promotes the formation of deep vein thrombosis (DVT), which can result in a pulmonary embolism. All patients at risk for DVT should be started on prophylaxis therapy. DVT prophylactic measures include monitoring of calf and thigh measurements, passive range-of-motion exercises, application of antiembolic stockings and/or sequential pneumatic stockings, and administration of prescribed anticoagulation therapy.

Severe Sepsis and Septic Shock

Sepsis occurs when microorganisms invade the body and initiate a systemic inflammatory response. This host response often results in perfusion abnormalities with organ dysfunction (severe sepsis) and eventually hypotension (septic shock).[12] The primary mechanism of this type of shock is the maldistribution of blood flow to the tissues.[5,43,44] Severe sepsis is estimated to occur in 650,000 to 750,000 patients annually in the United States,[45,46] with an estimated mortality rate for septic shock at 45%.[5]

Specific terms are used to describe the continuum of conditions the patient with an infection may experience. In 1991, at the American College of Chest Physicians/Society of Critical Care Medicine (ACCP/SCCM) Consensus Conference, definitions were developed to describe and differentiate these conditions (Box 26-13).[42] A second conference in 2001 reinforced and clarified these definitions.[47] This discussion focuses on severe sepsis and septic shock.

Box 26-13

Definitions for Sepsis and Organ Failure

Infection Microbial phenomenon characterized by an inflammatory response to the presence of microorganisms or the invasion of normally sterile host tissue by those organisms.

Bacteremia Presence of viable bacteria in the blood.

Systemic inflammatory response syndrome (SIRS) Systemic inflammatory response to a variety of severe clinical insults. The response is manifested by two or more of the following conditions: (1) temperature >38° C or <36° C; (2) heart rate >90 beats/min; (3) respiratory rate >20 breaths/min or $Paco_2$ <32 mm Hg; and (4) white blood cell count >12,000/mm^3, <4,000/mm^3, or >10% immature (band) forms.

Sepsis Systemic response to infection, manifested by two or more of the following conditions as a result of infection: (1) temperature >38° C or <36° C; (2) heart rate >90 beats/min; (3) respiratory rate >20 breaths/min or $Paco_2$ <32 mm Hg; and (4) white blood cell count >12,000/mm^3, <4,000/mm^3, or >10% immature (band) forms.

Severe sepsis Sepsis associated with organ dysfunction, hypoperfusion, or hypotension. Hypoperfusion and perfusion abnormalities may include, but are not limited to, lactic acidosis, oliguria, or an acute alteration in mental status.

Septic shock Sepsis-induced shock with hypotension despite adequate fluid resuscitation, along with the presence of perfusion abnormalities that may include, but are not limited to, lactic acidosis, oliguria, or an acute alteration in mental status. Patients who are receiving inotropic or vasopressor agents may not be hypotensive at the time that perfusion abnormalities are measured.

Sepsis-induced hypotension A systolic blood pressure <90 mm Hg or a reduction of ≥40 mm Hg from baseline in the absence of other causes for hypotension.

Multiple organ dysfunction syndrome (MODS) Presence of altered organ function in an acutely ill patient such that homeostasis cannot be maintained without intervention.

From American College of Chest Physicians/Society of Critical Care Medicine Consensus Conference Committee: *Crit Care Med* 20:864, 1992.
$Paco_2$, Arterial partial pressure of carbon dioxide.

Etiology

Sepsis is caused by a wide variety of microorganisms including gram-negative and gram-positive aerobes, anaerobes, fungi, and viruses. The source of these microorganisms is varied. Exogenous sources include the hospital environment and members of the health care team. Endogenous sources include the patient's skin, gastrointestinal (GI) tract, respiratory tract, and genitourinary tract.[43] In recent years, the incidence of chest-related infections has risen dramatically and the lungs have replaced the intraabdominal organs as the most common site of infection producing severe sepsis and septic shock.[48,49] Gram-negative bacteria are responsible for more than half of the cases of septic shock, though the proportionate incidence of gram-positive septicemia is rising dramatically.[49] Sepsis and septic shock are associated with a wide variety of intrinsic and extrinsic precipitating factors (Box 26-14). All of these factors interfere directly or indirectly with the body's anatomic and physiologic defense mechanisms. Several of the intrinsic factors are not modifiable or are very difficult to control. Several of the extrinsic factors may be required for diagnosis and management. All critically ill patients are therefore at risk for the development of septic shock.

Box 26-14

Precipitating Factors Associated With Septic Shock

Intrinsic Factors

Extreme of age
Coexisting diseases
- Malignancies
- Burns
- Acquired immunodeficiency syndrome (AIDS)
- Diabetes
- Substance abuse
- Dysfunction of one or more of the major body systems

Malnutrition

Extrinsic Factors

Invasive devices
Drug therapy
Fluid therapy
Surgical and traumatic wounds
Surgical and invasive diagnostic procedures
Immunosuppressive therapy

Pathophysiology

The syndrome encompassing severe sepsis and septic shock is a complex systemic response that is initiated when a microorganism enters the body and stimulates the inflammatory/immune system. Shed protein fragments and the release of toxins and other substances from the microorganism activate the plasma enzyme cascades (complement, kallikrein/kinin, coagulation, and fibrinolytic factors), as well as platelets, neutrophils, monocytes, and macrophages. Once activated, these systems and cells release a variety of mediators, or cytokines, that initiate a chain of complex interactions.[43,50-53] This host response is normally a protective mechanism controlled by feedback mechanisms. In severe sepsis and septic shock, the host response is altered and often exaggerated and uncontrolled.[51,54]

Once the mediators are activated, a variety of physiologic and pathophysiologic events occur that affect clotting, the distribution of blood flow to the tissues and organs, capillary membrane permeability, and the metabolic state of the body. Subsequently, a systemic imbalance between cellular oxygen supply and demand develops that results in cellular hypoxia, damage, and death (Figure 26-5).[2]

Hallmarks of severe sepsis are endothelial damage and coagulation dysfunction.[50,53-55] Tissue factor is released from endothelial cells and monocytes in response to stimulation by the inflammatory cytokines.[48,50,53] Release of tissue factor initiates the coagulation cascade producing widespread microvascular thrombosis and further stimulation of the systemic inflammatory

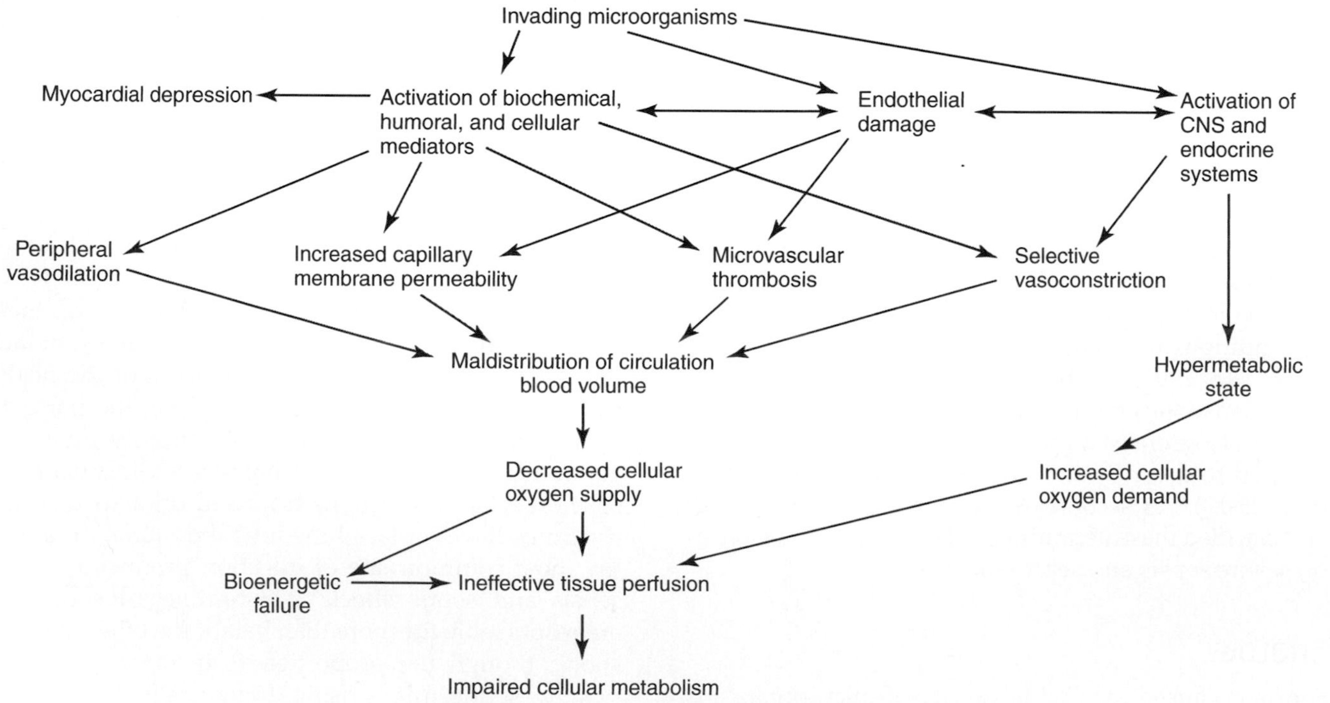

FIGURE 26-5. The pathophysiology of septic shock.

pathways.[43,53] Diffuse endothelial damage impairs endogenous anticlotting mechanisms.[43,51,53] Mediator-induced suppression of fibrinolysis slows clot breakdown. Eventual consumption of coagulation factors may produce bleeding and hemorrhage.[53,55]

Significant alterations in cardiovascular hemodynamics are also produced by the activation of inflammatory cytokines and endothelial damage.[5,51,53] Massive peripheral vasodilation results in the development of relative hypovolemia. Increased capillary permeability produces loss of intravascular volume to the interstitium, which accentuates the reduction in preload and cardiac output. These changes coupled with the microvascular thrombosis produce maldistribution of circulating blood volume, decreased tissue perfusion, and inadequate oxygen delivery to the cells. Impaired ventricular contractility results from cytokine activity and hypoxic myocyte dysfunction.[2,5]

Activation of the central nervous and endocrine systems also occurs as part of the response to invading microorganisms. This activation leads to stimulation of the SNS and the release of ACTH. These events trigger the release of epinephrine, norepinephrine, glucocorticoids, aldosterone, glucagon, and renin, resulting in the development of a hypermetabolic state and contributing to vasoconstriction of the renal, pulmonary, and splanchnic beds. Selective vasoconstriction in the splanchnic bed may contribute to hypoperfusion of the gastric mucosa. The resulting gut injury propagates the inflammatory response.[44,56] Activation of the CNS also causes the release of endogenous opiates that are believed to cause vasodilation and to further decrease myocardial contractility.[57]

A number of metabolic alterations occur as a result of CNS and endocrine system activation. The hypermetabolic state increases cellular oxygen demand and contributes to cellular hypoxia. Lactic acid is produced as a result of anaerobic metabolism. Glucocorticoids, ACTH, epinephrine, and glucagon are all catabolic hormones that are released as part of this response. These hormones favor the use of fats and proteins over glucose for energy production.[57]

The hypermetabolic state also increases the cellular metabolic needs. Increased glucose requirements in conjunction with the high level of catabolic hormones result in the limited ability of the cells to use glucose as a substrate for energy production. This causes glucose intolerance, hyperglycemia, relative insulin resistance, and the use of fat for energy (lipolysis).[43] The relative insulin resistance causes the body to produce more insulin, which inhibits the use of fat as an energy substrate. This promotes the use of protein as an energy substrate and catabolism of protein stores in the visceral organs and skeletal muscles.[57]

Metabolic derangements in severe sepsis and septic shock may also include an inability of the cells to use oxygen even if blood flow is adequate. Mitochondrial dysfunction is thought to be the underlying mechanism.[58] This bioenergetic failure may play an important role in the development of multiple organ dysfunction.[5,58] In addition, the exaggerated inflammatory response in severe sepsis also results in apoptosis, a programmed cell death or cellular suicide.[54]

These complex and interrelated pathophysiologic changes in severe sepsis and septic shock produce a pathologic imbalance between cellular oxygen demand and cellular oxygen supply/consumption. If unabated, this situation ultimately results in tissue ischemia, multiple organ dysfunction syndrome (MODS), and death.[49]

Assessment and Diagnosis

Effective treatment of severe sepsis and septic shock is dependent on timely recognition. The diagnosis of severe sepsis is based on the identification of three conditions: known or suspected infection, two or more of the clinical indications of the systemic inflammatory response, and evidence of at least one organ dysfunction. Clinical indications of systemic inflammatory response and sepsis were included in the original ACCP/SCCM consensus definitions and are listed in Box 26-13. The second consensus conference expanded this list to facilitate prompt clinical recognition (Box 26-15).[47]

Signs of individual organ dysfunction are discussed in the MODS section. The two most common organs to demonstrate dysfunction in severe sepsis are the heart and the lungs. The patient with persistent hypotension requiring vasopressor therapy despite adequate volume resuscitation is demonstrating cardiovascular dysfunction. Pulmonary dysfunction is manifested by PaO_2/FIO_2 ratio less than 300, indicative of acute lung injury (ALI).[50] Signs indicating septic shock are hypotension despite adequate fluid resuscitation and the presence of perfusion abnormalities such as lactic acidosis, oliguria, or acute change in mentation.

The patient in severe sepsis or septic shock may present with a variety of clinical manifestations that may change dynamically as the condition progresses (Box 26-16). During the initial stage, massive vasodilation occurs in both the venous and arterial beds. Dilation of the venous system leads to a decrease in venous return to the heart, which results in a decrease in the preload of the right and left ventricles. This is evidenced by a decline in the RAP and PAOP. Dilation of the arterial system results in a decrease in the afterload of the heart as evidenced by a decrease in the SVR. The patient's skin becomes pink, warm, and flushed as a result of the massive vasodilation. Myocardial contractility is decreased, as evidenced by a decline in the left ventricular stroke work index (LVSWI).[59]

The HR rises in response to increased SNS, metabolic, and adrenal gland stimulation. If circulating volume

Box 26-15

Expanded List of Diagnostic Criteria for Sepsis

General Variables

Core temperature >38.3° or <36° C
Heart rate >90 beats/min
Tachypnea
Altered mental status
Significant edema or positive fluid balance >20 ml/kg over 24 hours
Hyperglycemia (>120 mg/dl) in absence of diabetes

Inflammatory Variables

WBC count >12,000/mm^3, <4,000/mm^3, or >10% immature forms
Elevated plasma C-reactive protein
Elevated plasma procalcitonin

Hemodynamic Variables

Systolic BP <90 mm Hg or decrease >40 mm Hg
Mean arterial pressure <70 mm Hg
Svo_2 >70%
CI >3.5 L/m/m^3

Tissue Perfusion Variables

Serum lactate >1 mmol/L
Decreased capillary refill or mottling

Organ Dysfunction Variables

Pao_2/Fio_2 <300
Urine output <0.5 ml/kg/hour
Creatinine increase >0.5 mg/dl
INR >1.5 or aPTT >60 sec
Ileus
Platelet count <100,000/mm^3
Hyperbilirubinemia (plasma total bilirubin >4 mg/dl)

Modified from Levy MN et al: *Crit Care Med* 31:1250, 2003.
WBC, White blood cells; *BP,* blood pressure; *Svo_2,* mixed venous oxygen saturation; *CI,* cardiac index; *Pao_2,* arterial partial pressure of oxygen; *Fio_2,* fraction of oxygen in inspired air; *INR,* International Normalized Ratio; *aPTT,* activated partial thromboplastin time.

Box 26-16

Clinical Manifestations of Septic Shock

- Increased heart rate
- Decreased blood pressure
- Wide pulse pressure
- Full, bounding pulse
- Pink, warm, flushed skin
- Increased respiratory rate (early)/decreased respiratory rate (late)
- Crackles
- Change in sensorium
- Decreased urine output
- Increased temperature
- Increased cardiac output and cardiac index
- Decreased systemic vascular resistance
- Decreased right atrial pressure
- Decreased pulmonary artery occlusion pressure
- Decreased left ventricular stroke work index
- Decreased Pao_2
- Decreased $Paco_2$ (early)/increased $Paco_2$ (late)
- Decreased HCO_3^-
- Increased mixed venous oxygen saturation (Svo_2)

Pao_2, Arterial partial pressure of oxygen; *$Paco_2$,* arterial partial pressure of carbon dioxide; *Svo_2,* mixed venous oxygen saturation.

and preload are adequate, this results in a normal to high CO and CI in spite of the impaired contractility. The PP widens as the diastolic blood pressure decreases because of the vasodilation, and the SBP increases because of the elevated CO. A full, bounding pulse develops. The net result of these changes is a relatively normal blood pressure in severe sepsis. However, as the reduction in preload and afterload becomes overwhelming and contractility fails, hypotension ensues resulting in septic shock.[59]

In the lungs, ventilation/perfusion mismatching develops as a result of pulmonary vasoconstriction and the formation of pulmonary microemboli. Hypoxemia occurs, and the RR increases to compensate for the lack of oxygen. Crackles develop as increased pulmonary capillary membrane permeability leads to pulmonary edema.[43,60]

Level of consciousness starts to change as a result of decreased cerebral perfusion, immune mediator activation, hyperthermia, and lactic acidosis. This septic encephalopathy is demonstrated by acute onset of impaired cognitive functioning, or delirium, which may fluctuate during its course.[43,60] The patient may appear disoriented, confused, combative, or lethargic.[60]

Arterial blood gas values initially reveal respiratory alkalosis, hypoxemia, and metabolic acidosis. This is demonstrated by a low Pao_2, low $Paco_2$, and low HCO_3^-, respectively. The respiratory alkalosis is caused by the patient's increased RR. As pathologic pulmonary changes progress and the patient becomes fatigued, effectiveness of respirations decreases and the $Paco_2$ increases, resulting in respiratory acidosis.[60] The metabolic acidosis is the result of lack of oxygen to the cells and the development of lactic acidemia. Serum lactate levels rise over 2 mmol/L secondary to anaerobic metabolism. The mixed venous oxygen saturation (Svo_2) may increase because of maldistribution of the circulating blood volume and impaired cellular metabolism.[59] The white blood cell (WBC) count is elevated as part of the immune response to the invading microorganisms. In addition, the WBC differential reveals an increase in immature neutrophils (shift to the left). This occurs because the body has to mobilize increasing numbers of WBCs to fight the infection. Serum glucose also increases as part of the hypermetabolic response and the development of insulin resistance. The patient's temperature is elevated in response to pyrogens released from the invading microorganisms,

Box 26-17

Severe Sepsis Bundles

Sepsis resuscitation bundle:

1. Serum lactate measured
2. Blood cultures obtained before antibiotics administered
3. Improve time to broad-spectrum antibiotics
4. In the event of hypotension or lactate >4 mmol/L (36 mg/dl)
    a. Deliver an initial minimum of 20 ml/kg of crystalloid (or colloid equivalent)
    b. Apply vasopressors for ongoing hypotension
5. In the event of persistent hypotension despite fluid resuscitation or lactate >4 mmol/L (36 mg/dl)
    a. Achieve central venous pressure of ≥8 mm Hg
    b. Achieve central venous oxygen saturation of ≥70%

Sepsis management bundle:

1. Administer low-dose steroids
2. Administer drotrecogin alfa (activated)
3. Maintain adequate glycemic control
4. Prevent excessive inspiratory plateau pressures

From Hurtado FJ, Nin N:, *Crit Care Clin* 22:521, 2006.

immune mediator activation, and increased metabolic activity.[59] Urine output declines because of decreased perfusion of the kidneys. As impaired tissue perfusion develops, a variety of other clinical manifestations appear indicating the development of MODS.

Medical Management

Treatment of the patient in severe sepsis or septic shock requires a multifaceted approach (see Evidence-Based Collaborative Practice: Severe Sepsis). The goals of treatment are to reverse the pathophysiologic responses, control the infection, and promote metabolic support. This approach includes supporting the cardiovascular system and enhancing tissue perfusion, identifying and treating the infection, limiting the systemic inflammatory response, restoring metabolic balance, and initiating nutritional therapy. In addition, dysfunction of the individual organ systems must be prevented. Guidelines for the management of severe sepsis and septic shock have been developed under the auspices of the Surviving Sepsis Campaign (SSC), an international effort of 11 organizations to improve patient outcomes.[10] From these guidelines a group or "bundle" of selected interventions was identified as having the most impact on patient outcome (Box 26-17). The "sepsis resuscitation bundle" should be implemented within the first 6 hours while the "sepsis management bundle" should be implemented within the first 24 hours. For more information regarding these interventions, go to the Surviving Sepsis Campaign website (http://www.survivingsepsis.org).[61]

The patient in severe sepsis or septic shock requires immediate resuscitation of the hypoperfused state. Specific interventions are aimed at increasing cellular oxygen supply and decreasing cellular oxygen demand. These treatments include administration of fluids, vasopressors, and positive inotropic agents. Early goal-directed therapy during the first 6 hours of resuscitation improves survival[61-63] and is recommended in the SSC guidelines.[10] This therapy includes aggressive fluid resuscitation to augment intravascular volume and increase preload until a central venous pressure (CVP) of 8 to 12 mm Hg (12 to 15 mm Hg in mechanically ventilated patients) is achieved. Crystalloids or colloids may be used. Administration of vasopressors, either norepinephrine or dopamine as first-choice agent, should be used as necessary to maintain a MAP of at least 65 mm Hg. These agents reverse the massive peripheral vasodilation and increase SVR. Vasopressin may be considered only for patients refractory to high doses of the first-choice agents.[10,61-63] Arterial line placement is recommended for any patient requiring vasopressor therapy. Intermittent or continuous monitoring of central venous or mixed venous oxygen saturation ($Scv{O_2}$ or $Sv{O_2}$) allows evaluation of the effectiveness of oxygen delivery. If the $Scv{O_2}$ is less than 70%, administration of packed red cells is recommended to achieve a hematocrit of at least 30%.[59,61-63] Inotropic stimulation with dobutamine (administered to a maximum of 20 mcg/kg/min) is recommended as necessary to counteract myocardial depression and maintain adequate CO and $Scv{O_2}$ greater than 70%.[10,59] The dobutamine infusion should be reduced or discontinued if a tachycardia greater than 120 beats/min develops.[59,63]

Intubation and mechanical ventilatory support are also usually required to optimize oxygenation and ventilation for the patient in severe sepsis or septic shock. Ventilation with lower than traditional tidal volumes (6 ml/kg versus 12 ml/kg) in patients with ALI and ARDS decreases mortality.[64] SSC guidelines recommend the goal of 6 ml/kg of predicted body weight for patients with severe sepsis or septic shock with ALI or ARDS.[10] Increased $Pa{CO_2}$ may result from this therapy and is acceptable if tolerated. Ventilator settings should be adjusted to provide the patient with a $Pa{O_2}$ greater than 70 mm Hg and a pH within the normal range. Patients receiving mechanical ventilation should be maintained in a semirecumbent position with the head of the bed raised to 45 degrees to decrease the incidence of ventilator-acquired pneumonia.[10] Prone positioning should be considered in the septic patient with ARDS requiring high levels of oxygen.[10] Sedation protocols using either intermittent bolus or continuous infusion using a standardized sedation scale and specific goals are recommended for all patients requiring mechanical ventilation. Daily interruption of sedative infusions to allow wakefulness and reevaluation of sedation needs reduces duration of mechanical ventilation and is recommended.[10,65] Neuromuscular

EVIDENCE-BASED COLLABORATIVE PRACTICE

American Association of Critical-Care Nurses Practice Alert: Severe Sepsis

Expected Practice:

- Assess all patients and immediately notify physician when a patient presents with risk factors for sepsis, which includes documented or suspected infection and 2 or more of the following SIRS criteria.
  - Heart rate >90 beats per minute
  - Temperature < 36° C (96.8 F) or >38° C (100.4 F)
  - Respiratory rate > 20 breaths per minute or $PaCO_2$ <32 mm Hg or mechanical ventilation
  - White blood cell count > 12,000/mm^3 or < 4000mm^3 or <10% mature neutrophils
- Obtain serum lactate measurements.
- Obtain blood cultures as well as cultures from all potential sites of infection prior to initiating broad-spectrum antibiotics.
  - Evaluate for and remove other potential sources of infection (ie, obviously infected invasive devices).
- Administer fluids to maintain mean arterial pressure at > 65 mm Hg, central venous pressure (CVP) 8-12 mm Hg and central venous or mixed venous oxygen saturation >70%.
- Administer vasopressors if necessary to achieve a mean arterial blood pressure of 65 mm Hg if fluid replacement is not successful.
- Obtain cortisol stimulation test and start continuous low-dose steroid infusion.
- Maintain cardiac output at normal physiologic levels.
- Maintain blood glucose levels at < 150 mg/dL.
- Consider administration of human recombinant activated protein C (drotrecogin alfa activated) for patients at risk for dying and presenting with septic shock, sepsis with multiple organ failure and sepsis induced acute respiratory distress syndrome.

Supporting Evidence:

- More than 750,000 cases of severe sepsis occurred annually (year 2000) and mortality ranges from 28%-50% with an overall hospital mortality of about 30%.[1] Sepsis (infection and 2 of the 4 SIRS criteria) can rapidly progress to severe sepsis (infection + organ dysfunction + SIRS criteria) to septic shock (persistent tissue hypoxia with vasopressors on board) within 24 hours.[1-4] Treatment should be initiated regardless of where the patient is located within the hospital. A prospective randomized study of 263 emergency department patients diagnosed with severe sepsis or septic shock showed that patients treated aggressively with a goal direction towards tissue oxygenation within the first 6 hours of presentation had a 16% improvement in mortality. Another small retrospective study showed a decrease in mortality in patients identified with signs of severe sepsis and treated within the first 6 hours.[3,5,6] (Level V)
- Serum lactate levels can be elevated in the setting of a normal or increased cardiac output. The measurement of serum lactate can reflect occult decreases in global tissue perfusion and as such may be an indicator of organ dysfunction. The presence and the clearance rate of lactate are associated with increases in patient morbidity and mortality.[3,7] (Level IV)
- Early administration of appropriate antibiotics decreases mortality in patients with Gram positive and negative bacteremias. Empiric broad spectrum antibiotics should be initiated prior to identification of the infecting organism and reassessed after 48-72 hours based on culture results and clinical data.[8]
- According to the Surviving Sepsis Campaign guidelines, during the first 6 hours of treatment the goal is to achieve and maintain a CVP of 8-12 mm Hg or 12-15 mm Hg for patients receiving mechanical ventilation and a MAP of at least 65 mm Hg with fluid resuscitation.[7] Dobutamine is identified as the medication of choice to increase cardiac output to normal levels or to improve lactate clearance when cardiac output is not being measured. Two large clinical trials did not show a benefit from increasing CO above physiologic normal levels in order to increase oxygen delivery to the tissues.[9–11] Available data do not support the use of low dose dopamine for renal protection.[12] (Level V evidence)
- Colloids have not been shown to be of more benefit than crystalloid for fluid resuscitation. One large randomized controlled trial compared 4% albumin with normal saline in the treatment of patients requiring volume resuscitation found no significant difference in mortality between the groups. Several literature reviews have concluded that choice of fluids does not appear to change outcomes.[13,14] (Level V)
- In the setting of hypotension fluid replacement should be optimized before vasopressors are started. No high-level evidence exists to identify the most appropriate vasopressor to use for the treatment of septic shock and selection is based on multiple clinical parameters. However, in the Surviving Sepsis Campaign Guidelines for the Management of Severe Sepsis and Septic Shock norepinephrine or dopamine are identified as the initial vasopressors of choice to increase vascular tone and blood pressure.[7]
- Two meta analyses concluded that administration of high dose corticosteroids are of no benefit or may be detrimental to patients with septic shock.[15,16] (Level VI) In vasopressor dependent shock, the addition of low-dose exogenous cortisol has been shown to improve the uptake of the patients own and the exogenously administered sympathetic stimulants when serum cortisol levels are low.[17] (Level IV)
- Maintaining glucose levels within normal range (80-110 mg/dL) but at least <150 mg/dL has been shown to decrease morbidity and mortality in a surgical population but did not focus on septic patients. Maintaining glucose levels <150 mg/dL showed reduced morbidity but not mortality in critically ill medical patients with sepsis.[18-19] (Level V)

SIRS, Systemic inflammatory response syndrome; *$Paco_2$,* arterial partial pressure of carbondioxide; *MAP,* mean arterial pressure; *CO,* cardiac output.

EVIDENCE-BASED COLLABORATIVE PRACTICE

American Association of Critical-Care Nurses Practice Alert: Severe Sepsis—*cont'd*

- In a large double blind study, human recombinant activated protein C (drotrecogin alfa activated) decreased mortality by 6% in patients with severe sepsis and decreased mortality by 13% for patients at high risk for death (ie, patients having an APACHE II score of 25 or greater).[20,21] (Level V)

What You Should Do:

- Educate all nursing staff on the risk factors and clinical signs of sepsis.
- Create an interdisciplinary team including but not limited to physicians, pharmacist, respiratory care practitioner, nursing and dietitian to develop protocols or guidelines for the initial identification and management of the patient presenting with signs of sepsis. Consider development of a rapid response team to facilitate prompt identification and treatment of patients with sepsis.

AACN Grading of Evidence System

Level I: Manufacturer's recommendations only
Level II: Theory based, no research data to support recommendations; recommendations from expert consensus group may exist
Level III: Laboratory data, no clinical data to support recommendations
Level IV: Limited clinical studies to support recommendations
Level V: Clinical studies in more than one or two patient populations and situations to support recommendations
Level VI: Clinical studies in a variety of patient populations and situations to support recommendations.

Need More Information or Help?

- Talk with a clinical practice specialist for additional information/assistance at www.aacn.org then select PRN.

References

1. Angus DC, Linde-Zwirble WT, Lidicker J, et al. Epidemiology of severe sepsis in the United States: analysis of incidence, outcome, and associated costs of care. Crit Care Med. 2001; 29:1303-1310.
2. Ahrens T, Tuggle D. Surviving severe sepsis: early recognition and treatment. Crit Care Nurse. October 2004; 24(suppl): 2-13.
3. Rivers E, Bryant N, Havstad S, et al. Early goal-directed therapy in the treatment of severe sepsis and septic shock. N Engl J Med. 2001; 345:1368-77.
4. Rivers E, McIntyre L, Morro DC, Kandis KR. Early and innovative interventions for severe sepsis and septic shock: taking advantage of a window of opportunity. Can Med Assoc J. 2005; 173:1054-1065.
5. McIntyre LA, Fergusson DA, Cebert PC, et al. Are delays in the recognition and initial management of patients with severe sepsis associated with hospital mortality? Crit Care Med. 2003; 31(suppl):A75.
6. Engoren, M. The effect of prompt physician visits on intensive care unit mortality and cost. Crit Care Med. 2005; 33:727-733.
7. Dellinger RP, Carlet JM, Masur H, et al. Surviving Sepsis Campaign guidelines for management of severe sepsis and septic shock. Crit Care Med. 2004; 32:858-870.
8. Bochud P-Y, Bonten M, Marchetti O, Calandra, T. Antimicrobial therapy for patients with severe sepsis and septic shock: an evidence-based review. Crit Care Med. 2004; 32(11 suppl):S495-S512.
9. Hayes MA, Timmins AC, Yau EH, et al. Elevation of systemic oxygen delivery in the treatment of critically ill patients. N Engl J Med. 1994; 330:1717-1722.
10. Gattinoni L, Brazzi L, Pelosi P, et al. A trial of goal-oriented hemodynamic therapy in critically ill patients. N Engl J Med. 1995; 333:1025-1032.
11. Beale RJ, Hollenberg SM, Vincent JL, Parrillo JE. Vasopressor and inotropic support in septic shock: an evidence-based review. Crit Care Med. 2004; 32(11suppl): S455-S465.
12. Bellomo R, Chapman M, Finfer S, et al. Low-dose depominc in patients with early renal dysfunction: a placebo-controlled randomized trial. Lancet. 2000; 356:2139-2143.
13. Finfer S, Bellomo R, Boyce N, et al. A comparison of albumin and saline for fluid resuscitation in the intensive care unit. N Engl J Med. 2004; 350:2247-2256.
14. Vincent JL, Herwig G. Fluid resuscitation in severe sepsis and septic shock: An evidence-based review. Crit Care Med. 2004; 32(11 suppl):S451-S454.
15. Lefering R, Neugebaruer EA. Steroid controversy in sepsis and septic shock: a meta analysis. Crit Care Med. 1995;23:1294-1303.
16. Cronin L, Cook DJ, Carlet J, et al, Corticosteroid treatment for sepsis: a critical appraisal and meta-analysis of the literature. Crit Care Med. 1995:1430-1439.
17. Annane D, Sebille V, Charpentier C, et al. Effect of treatment with low doses of hydrocortisone and fludrocortisone on mortality in patients with septic shock. JAMA. 2002; 288:862-871.
18. Van den Berghe G, Wouters, et al. Intensive insulin therapy in the critically ill patients. N Engl J Med. 2001; 345:1359-1367.
19. Van den Berghe G, Wilmer A, Hermans G, et al. Intensive insulin therapy in the medical ICU. N Engl J Med. 2006; 354:449-461.
20. Bernard GR, Vincent JL, Laterre PF, et al. Recombinant human protein C worldwide evaluation in severe sepsis (PROWESS) study group: efficacy and safety of recombinant human activated protein C for severe sepsis. N Engl J Med. 2001; 344:699-709.
21. Bernard GR, Margolis BD, Shanies HM, et al. Extended evaluation of recombinant human activated protein C United States trial (ENHANCE USA): a single-arm phase 3B multicenter study of drotrecogin alfa (activated) in severe sepsis. Chest. 2004; 125:2206-2216.

blocking agents should be avoided, if possible, to prevent prolonged blockade following discontinuation.[10]

A key measure in the treatment of septic shock is finding and eradicating the cause of the infection. At least two blood cultures plus urine, sputum, and wound cultures should be obtained to find the location of the infection before antibiotic therapy is initiated.[10,63] Antibiotic therapy should be started within 1 hour of recognition of severe sepsis. If the microorganism is unknown, antiinfective therapy with one or more agents known to be effective against likely pathogens should be initiated. Once the microorganism is identified, an antibiotic more specific to the microorganism should be started.[10,63] Surgical intervention to debride infected or necrotic tissue or to drain abscesses also may be necessary to facilitate removal of the septic source.[10,66] Intravascular devices potentially the source of the infection should be removed following establishment of alternative vascular access.[66]

Recombinant human activated protein C (rhAPC) administration has been demonstrated to improve survival in patients with severe sepsis.[10,48,51] Drotrecogin alfa (activated) (Xigris) is indicated for adult patients with severe sepsis who have a high risk of death. Patients with sepsis-induced ARDS or multiple organ failure or with septic shock meet these criteria.[10] Although its specific mechanisms for improving survival are not fully understood, drotrecogin alfa has anticoagulant, profibrinolytic, and antiinflammatory properties.[10,48,51] Guidelines for patient selection and appropriate administration of this agent must be strictly followed for safe and effective use. It is administered intravenously at an infusion rate of 24 mcg/kg/hr for a total infusion duration of 96 hours. Interruption of the infusion is necessary for invasive procedures. The most common serious side effect of drotrecogin alfa is bleeding. Contraindications for use include active internal bleeding, recent hemorrhagic stroke (within 3 months) or intracranial/intraspinal surgery (within 2 months); severe head trauma, trauma with an increased risk of life-threatening bleeding, or presence of an epidural catheter; and intracranial neoplasm/mass lesion or evidence of cerebral herniation.[67] Studies of numerous other drugs believed to block or alter the effects of immune mediators have failed to demonstrate effectiveness or have been associated with unacceptable adverse effects.[55,63]

Intravenous corticosteroids reduce mortality in catecholamine-dependent septic shock patients with relative adrenal insufficiency.[68] The patient in septic shock who requires vasopressor therapy despite adeuate fluid replacement should receive intravenous hydrocortisone at a stress-dose of 200 to 300 mg/day in divided doses or continuous infusion for 7 days without waiting for ACTH stimulation results.[10,68] Doses greater than 300 mg/day may be harmful and should not be used.

Continuous infusion of insulin and glucose to maintain blood glucose less than 150 mg/dl improves outcomes[60] and is recommended by SSC guidelines following initial stabilization. Platelets should be administered when counts are less than 5000/mm^3.[10] Stress ulcer prophylaxis using histamine$_2$ (H_2) receptor blockers and DVT prophylaxis are recommended for all patients with severe sepsis or septic shock. Treatment of lactic acidemia with bicarbonate therapy is not beneficial and is not recommended if pH is equal to or greater than 7.15. Low-dose dopamine infusion for renal protection is not beneficial and should not be used either.[10,63]

The initiation of nutritional therapy is critical in the management of the patient in severe sepsis or septic shock. The goal is to improve the patient's overall nutritional status, enhance the immune system, and promote wound healing. A daily caloric intake of 25 to 30 kcal/kg usual body weight is recommended. The enteral route is preferred. The ideal nutritional supplement for the patient in septic shock should be high in protein because of the metabolic derangements that develop in the hypermetabolic state. The amount of protein calories given depends on the patient's nitrogen balance. In early sepsis, the mix of nonprotein calories may be divided evenly between carbohydrates and fats. In the later stages, significant alterations in fat metabolism occur and the lipid content should be limited to 10% to 15% of the total nonprotein calories. The lipid emulsion should contain long-chain fatty acid triglycerides for their protein-sparing effects.[57]

Nursing Management

Prevention of severe sepsis and septic shock is one of the primary responsibilities of the nurse in the critical care area. These measures include the identification of patients at risk and reduction of their exposure to invading microorganisms. Hand washing, aseptic technique, and an understanding of how microorganisms can invade the body are essential components of preventive nursing care. Early identification allows for early treatment and decreased mortality.[43] Box 26-18 depicts a simple screening tool for identifying patients with severe sepsis.

The patient in septic shock may have any number of nursing diagnoses, depending on the progression of the process (Box 26-19). **Nursing priorities are directed toward (1) early identification of the sepsis syndrome, (2) administering prescribed fluids, vasoactive agents, antibiotics, rhAPC, and other drugs, (3) preventing complications of critical illness and therapeutic interventions, (4) providing comfort and emotional support, and (5) maintaining surveillance for complications.** Continual observation to detect subtle changes that indicate the progression of the septic process is also very important.

Box 26-18

Screening Patients for Severe Sepsis

A patient who meets the following 3 criteria has a positive screen suggestive of severe sepsis:

A. INFECTION—Does your patient have **one or more** of the following infection criteria?

- ❑ DOCUMENTED OR SUSPECTED—Does the patient have positive culture results (from blood, sputum, urine, etc.)?
- ❑ ANTI-INFECTIVE THERAPY—Is the patient receiving antibiotic, antifungal, or other anti-infective therapy?
- ❑ PNEUMONIA—Is there documentation of pneumonia (x-ray, etc.)?
- ❑ WBCs—Have WBCs been found in normally sterile fluid (urine, CSF, etc.)?
- ❑ PERFORATED VISCUS—Does the patient have a perforated hollow organ (bowel)?

? DID YOU CHECK ANY BOXES ABOVE?

B. SIRS—Does your patient have **two or more** of the following SIRS criteria?

- ❑ TEMPERATURE—Is the patient's temperature ≥ 38° C (≥ 100.4° F) or ≤ 36° C (≤ 96.8° F)?
- ❑ HEART RATE—Is the patient's heart rate ≥ 90 bpm?
- ❑ RESPIRATORY RATE—Is the patient's respiratory rate ≥ 20 breaths/min?
- ❑ WBC COUNT—Is the patient's WBC count ≥ 12,000/mm^3, ≤ 4000/mm^3, or are there >10% immature neutrophils (left shift)?

? DID YOU CHECK TWO OR MORE BOXES ABOVE?

C. ACUTE ORGAN DYSFUNCTION—Does your patient have **one or more** of the following organ dysfunction criteria?

- ❑ CARDIOVASCULAR—Does the patient have a systolic BP ≤ 90 mm Hg or mean arterial pressure ≤ 70 mm Hg (for at least 1 hour despite fluid resuscitation) or require vasopressor support?
- ❑ RESPIRATORY—Does the patient have a PaO2/FiO2 ratio ≤ 250, PEEP > 7.5 or require mechanical ventilation?
- ❑ RENAL—Does the patient have low urine output (e.g., < 0.5 ml/kg/hr for 1 hour despite adequate fluid resuscitation), increased creatinine (> 50% increase from baseline) or require acute dialysis?
- ❑ HEMATOLOGIC—Does the patient have a low platelet count (< 100,000/mm^3) or PT/PTT > upper limit of normal?
- ❑ METABOLIC—Does the patient have a low pH with high lactate (e.g., pH < 7.30 and plasma lactate ≥ upper limit of normal)?
- ❑ HEPATIC—Are the patient's liver enzymes ≥ 2x upper limit of normal?
- ❑ CNS—Does the patient have altered consciousness or a reduced Glasgow Coma score?

? DID YOU CHECK ANY BOXES ABOVE?

IF YOU CHECKED:

A) INFECTION + B) SIRS + C) ORGAN DYSFUNCTION = POSITIVE SCREEN SUGGESTIVE OF SEVERE SEPSIS

From Eli Lilly and Company, 2004. *WBC,* White blood cell; *CSF,* cerebral spinal fluid; *SIRS,* systemic inflammatory response syndrome; *BP,* blood pressure; *Pao_2,* arterial partial pressure of oxygen; *Fio_2,* fraction of oxygen in inspired air; *PEEP,* positive end-expiratory pressure; *PT,* prothrombin time; *PTT,* partial thromboplastin time; *CNS,* central nervous system.

Multiple Organ Dysfunction Syndrome

MODS results from progressive physiologic failure of two or more separate organ systems. It is defined as the "presence of altered organ function in an acutely ill patient such that homeostasis cannot be maintained without intervention."[42] Lack of consensus regarding definitions for organ dysfunction, the number of organs involved, and the duration of organ dysfunction have hampered an accurate account of organ dysfunction in critically ill patients. Failure of two or more organs is associated with an estimated 45% to 55% mortality. This may increase to 80% when three or more organ systems fail, and 100% if three or more organ systems fail for more than 4 days.[69] Patient outcome is directly related to the number of organs that fail.

Although various patient populations are at risk for organ dysfunction, trauma patients are particularly vulnerable because they often experience no-flow-reflow (or ischemia-reperfusion) events secondary to hemorrhage, blunt trauma, or sympathetic induced vasoconstriction.[70] Other high-risk patients include those who have experienced infection, a shock episode, various ischemia-reperfusion events, acute pancreatitis, sepsis, burns, aspiration, multiple blood transfusions, or surgical complications.[71,72] Patients age 65 years and older are at increased risk secondary to their decreased organ reserve and comorbidities.[73]

Box 26-19

NURSING DIAGNOSIS PRIORITIES

Septic Shock

- Deficient Fluid Volume related to relative loss, p. A-17
- Decreased Cardiac Output related to alterations in preload, p. A-12
- Decreased Cardiac Output related to alterations in afterload, p. A-12
- Decreased Cardiac Output related to alterations in contractility, p. A-13
- Impaired Gas Exchange related to ventilation/perfusion mismatching or intrapulmonary shunting, p. A-29
- Imbalanced Nutrition: Less Than Body Requirements related to increased metabolic demands or lack of exogenous nutrients, p. A-28
- Risk for Infection, p. A-46
- Anxiety related to threat to biologic, psychologic, or social integrity, p. A-9
- Compromised Family Coping related to critically ill family member, p. A-11

Etiology

Organ dysfunction may be a direct consequence of the insult (primary MODS) or can manifest latently and involve organs not directly affected in the initial insult (secondary MODS). Patients can experience both primary and secondary MODS.[42]

Primary MODS "directly results from a well-defined insult in which organ dysfunction occurs early and is directly attributed to the insult itself"[42] and accounts for only a small fraction of MODS cases. Direct insults initially cause localized inflammatory responses. Examples of primary MODS include the immediate consequences of posttraumatic pulmonary failure, thermal injuries, acute tubular necrosis, or invasive infections.[74] These cellular or microcirculatory events may lead to a loss of critical organ function induced by failure of delivery of oxygen and substrates, coupled with the inability to remove end-products of metabolism.[74,75] Primary MODS generally results in one of three patient outcomes: recovery, a stable hypermetabolic state, or death.[72]

Secondary MODS is a consequence of widespread systemic inflammation that results in dysfunction of organs not involved in the initial insult.[42,76] Secondary MODS develops latently after an initial insult. The early impairment of organs normally involved in immunoregulatory function, such as the liver and GI tract, intensify the host response to the insult. This intensified host response may be determined by factors such as age, comorbidities, and gene transcription.[77] It is postulated that the initial insult "primes" the inflammatory system in such a way that a mild second "hit" may perpetuate a hyperinflammatory response.

Systemic Inflammatory Response Syndrome

Systemic inflammatory response syndrome (SIRS) is a common initiating event in the development of secondary MODS. SIRS pertains to the widespread inflammation occurring in patients with a variety of insults. Clinical conditions and manifestations associated with SIRS are listed in Box 26-20. SIRS is present when two or more clinical manifestations are present in the high-risk patient. Manifestations of SIRS must represent an acute alteration from the patient's normal baseline and must not be related to other causes (e.g., neutropenia from chemotherapy). Organ dysfunction or failure, such as acute lung injury, acute renal failure, and MODS, is a complication of SIRS.[42,74,76,78,79] The findings of a recent epidemiology study suggest that SIRS occurs in one third of all hospitalized patients, in more than 50% of all patients in critical care units, and in about 80% of all patients in surgical critical care units.[80]

When SIRS is a result of infection, the term *sepsis* is used. Severe sepsis is sepsis with either hypoperfusion or systemic manifestations of hypoperfusion. Septic shock is sepsis-induced hypotension despite fluid resuscitation. Therefore SIRS, sepsis, severe sepsis, and septic shock represent a hierarchical continuum of the inflammatory response to infection.[81] Although infection and shock remain the most common precipitating factors, any disease that can induce a major inflammatory response is capable of initiating the events that lead to MODS.[74] Noninfectious stimuli (inflammation, perfusion deficit, or dead tissue) also initiate similar cellular consequences. Interruption of tissue perfusion may ensue as a result of mismatched oxygen supply and demand setting the stage for activation of SIRS and MODS.[72]

Box 26-20

Clinical Conditions and Manifestations Associated With Systemic Inflammatory Response Syndrome

Clinical Conditions
- Infection
- Infection of vascular structures (heart and lungs)
- Pancreatitis
- Ischemia
- Multiple trauma with massive tissue injury
- Hemorrhagic shock
- Immune-mediated organ injury
- Exogenous administration of tumor necrosis factor or other cytokines
- Aspiration of gastric contents
- Massive transfusion
- Host defense abnormalities

Clinical Manifestations
- Temperature >38° C or <36° C
- Heart rate >90 beats/min
- Respiratory rate >20 breaths/min or $Paco_2$ <32 mm Hg
- WBC >12,000 cells/mm^3 or <4000 cells/mm^3 or >10% immature (band) forms

SIRS, Systemic inflammatory response syndrome; *$Paco_2$,* arterial partial pressure of carbon dioxide.

When SIRS is not contained, several consequences occur that lead to organ dysfunction, including intense, uncontrolled activation of inflammatory cells; direct damage of vascular endothelium; disruption of immune cell function; persistent hypermetabolism; and maldistribution of circulatory volume to organ systems.[74,78,82] During hypermetabolism, changes occur in cellular anabolic and catabolic function, resulting in autocatabolism. Autocatabolism manifests as a severe decrease in lean body mass, severe weight loss, anergy, and increased cardiac output and flow-dependent oxygen consumption (VO_2) secondary to profound alterations in carbohydrate, protein, and fat metabolism and production.[83] Concurrently, GI, hepatic, and immunologic dysfunction may occur, which intensifies the SIRS. Clinical consequences may affect gut function, wound healing, muscles wasting, host response, respiratory function, and continued promotion of the hypermetabolic response.[83]

Consequently, inflammation becomes a systemic self-perpetuating process that is inadequately controlled and results in organ dysfunction.[60,74,84] However, not all patients develop MODS from SIRS. The development of MODS appears to be associated with failure to control the source of inflammation or infection, persistent hypoperfusion, VO_2, and/or the continued presence of necrotic tissue.[74]

Pathophysiology

Secondary MODS results from altered regulation of the patient's acute immune and inflammatory responses. Dysregulation, or failure to control the host inflammatory response, leads to the excessive production of inflammatory cells and biochemical mediators that cause widespread damage to vascular endothelium and organ damage.[53,72,78] The critically ill patient's compromised immune state also fosters an environment conducive to organ failure.

The definitive clinical course of secondary MODS has not been completely identified. One theory suggests that organ dysfunction may occur in a sequential or progressive pattern. This pattern generally begins with the lungs, the most commonly affected major organs, then the liver, the gut, and finally the kidneys. A late component is cardiac and, at times, bone marrow dysfunction. Neurologic and coagulopathic impairment may occur at any time during this progression.[85] Organs may fail simultaneously, for example, renal dysfunction may occur concurrently with hepatic dysfunction. After the initial insult and resuscitation, patients develop persistent hypermetabolism, a metabolic consequence of sustained systemic inflammation and physiologic stress, followed closely by pulmonary dysfunction, manifested as ALI.

A significant predictor of mortality in MODS is a change in organ system dysfunction over the initial 3 days. Worsening neurologic, renal, and hematologic function are specific to an increased mortality.[86] The development of renal and hepatic failure is a preterminal event in MODS, with death most common approximately 14 to 21 days after the initial insult.[72] Patients with decreased physiologic organ reserve may manifest signs and symptoms of organ dysfunction earlier than previously healthy patients.[73,78] Survivors may develop generalized polyneuropathy and a chronic form of pulmonary disease from ALI, complicating recovery. These patients often require prolonged, expensive rehabilitation.

The inflammatory and immune responses implicated in SIRS and MODS are evoked by certain cells and biochemicals that, in turn, affect cellular activity.[53] As outlined in Box 26-21, mediators associated with SIRS and MODS can be classified as inflammatory cells, biochemical mediators, or plasma protein systems. Activation of one mediator often leads to activation of another. The biologic activity of inflammatory cells, biochemical mediators, and plasma protein systems and how they work in concert to cause SIRS and MODS are not yet totally defined.[53]

Box 26-21

Inflammatory Mediators Associated With Systemic Inflammatory Response Syndrome and Multiple Organ Dysfunction Syndrome

Inflammatory Cells
Neutrophils
Macrophages/monocytes
Mast
Lymphocytes
Endothelial

Biochemical Mediators
Reactive oxygen species
- Superoxide radical
- Hydroxyl radical
- Hydrogen peroxide

Tumor necrosis factor
Interleukins
Platelet activating factor
Arachidonic acid metabolites
- Prostaglandins
- Leukotrienes
- Thromboxanes

Proteases

Plasma Protein Systems
Complement
Kinin
Coagulation

Assessment and Diagnosis

Secondary MODS is a systemic disease with organ-specific manifestations. Organ dysfunction is influenced by numerous factors, including organ host defense function, response time to the injury, metabolic requirements, organ vasculature response to vasoactive drugs, and organ sensitivity to damage and physiologic reserve. The responses of the GI, hepatobiliary, cardiovascular, pulmonary, renal, and coagulation systems are discussed in the following text. Clinical manifestations of organ dysfunction are outlined in Box 26-22.

Gastrointestinal Dysfunction

The GI tract plays an important role in MODS. GI organs normally have immunoregulatory functions. The GI tract contains about 70% to 80% of the immunologic tissue of the entire body. Consequently, GI dysfunction amplifies SIRS and gut damage, which may lead to bacterial translocation and endogenous endotoxemia.[84,87-89]

Three specific mechanisms link the GI tract and latent organ dysfunction. First, hypoperfusion and/or shocklike states damage the normal GI mucosa barrier by decreasing mesenteric blood flow, leading to hypo-

Box 26-22

Clinical Manifestations of Organ Dysfunction

Gastrointestinal
Abdominal distention
Intolerance to enteral feedings
Paralytic ileus
Upper/lower gastrointestinal bleeding
Diarrhea
Ischemic colitis
Mucosal ulceration
Decreased bowel sounds
Bacterial overgrowth in stool

Liver
Jaundice
Increased serum bilirubin (hyperbilirubinemia)
Increased liver enzymes (AST, ALT, LDH, alkaline phosphatase)
Increased serum ammonia
Decreased serum albumin
Decreased serum transferrin

Gallbladder
Right upper quadrant tenderness/pain
Abdominal distention
Unexplained fever
Decreased bowel sounds

Metabolic/Nutritional
Decreased lean body mass
Muscle wasting
Severe weight loss
Negative nitrogen balance
Hyperglycemia
Hypertriglyceridemia
Increased serum lactate
Decreased serum albumin, serum transferrin, and prealbumin
Decreased retinol-binding protein

Immune
Infection
Decreased lymphocyte count
Anergy

Pulmonary
Tachypnea
ALI pattern of respiratory failure
- Dyspnea
- Patchy infiltrates
- Refractory hypoxemia
- Respiratory acidosis
- Abnormal oxygen (O_2) indices

Pulmonary hypertension

Renal
Increased serum creatinine/BUN levels
Oliguria, anuria, or polyuria consistent with prerenal azotemia or ATN
Urinary indices consistent with prerenal azotemia or ATN

Cardiovascular
Hyperdynamic
Decreased pulmonary capillary occlusion pressure (PAOP)
Decreased systemic vascular resistance (SVR)
Decreased right atrial pressure (RAP)
Decreased left ventricular stroke work index (LVSWI)
Increased O_2 consumption
Increased cardiac output (CO)/cardiac index (CI)/heart rate

Hypodynamic
Increased SVR
Increased RAP
Increased LVSWI
Decreased O_2 delivery/consumption
Decreased CO/CI

Central Nervous System
Lethargy
Altered level of consciousness
Fever
Hepatic encephalopathy

Coagulation/Hematologic
Thrombocytopenia
DIC pattern

AST, Aspartate transaminase (SGOT); *ALT,* alanine transaminase (SGPT); *LDH,* lactate dehydrogenase; *ALI,* acute long injury; *BUN,* blood urea nitrogen; *ATN,* acute tubular necrosis; *DIC,* disseminated intravascular coagulation.

perfusion of the villi, mucosal edema, ischemic necrosis, sloughing of the mucosa, and malabsorption. The GI tract is extremely vulnerable to oxygen metabolite-induced reperfusion injury. Endothelial injury and GI lesions occur in response to mediator-induced tissue damage. In addition, ischemic events and the absence of feedings can disrupt the normal metabolism of the gastric/intestinal lumen and the normal protective function of the gut barrier.[78,87-89]

Second, the translocation of normal GI bacteria via a "leaky gut" into the systemic circulation initiates and perpetuates an inflammatory focus in the critically ill patient. The GI tract harbors organisms that present an inflammatory focus when translocated from the gut into the portal circulation and inadequately cleared by the liver. Hepatic macrophages respond to the presence of enteric organisms by producing tissue-damaging amounts of tumor necrosis factor (TNF). Bacterial translocation has been associated with paralytic ileus and drugs commonly used in the critically ill patient, including antibiotics, antacids, and histamine blockers.[72,77,87]

The third mechanism linking the GI tract and organ dysfunction is colonization. The oropharynx of the critically ill patient becomes colonized with potentially pathogenic organisms from the GI tract. Pulmonary aspiration of colonized sputum presents an inflammatory focus. Antacids, H_2 antagonists, and antibiotics also increase colonization of the upper GI tract.[72,78,80]

Hepatobiliary Dysfunction

The liver plays a vital role in host homeostasis related to the acute inflammatory response. In addition, the liver responds to SIRS by selectively changing carbohydrate (CHO), fat, and protein metabolism. Consequently, hepatic dysfunction after a critical insult threatens the patient's survival.[90]

The liver normally controls the inflammatory response by several mechanisms. Kupffer cells, which are hepatic macrophages, detoxify substances that might normally induce systemic inflammation, as well as vasoactive substances that cause hemodynamic instability. Failure to detoxify gram-negative bacteria translocated from the GI tract causes endotoxemia, perpetuates SIRS, and may lead to MODS. In addition, the liver produces proteins and antiproteases to control the inflammatory response; however, hepatic dysfunction limits this response.[72,90]

The liver and gallbladder are extremely vulnerable to ischemic injury. Ischemic hepatitis occurs after a prolonged period of physiologic shock and is associated with centrilobular hepatocellular necrosis.[36] The degree of hepatic damage is related directly to the severity and duration of the shock episode. Terms such as *shock liver* and *posttraumatic hepatic insufficiency* have been used to describe ischemic hepatitis. Both anoxic and reperfusion injury damage hepatocytes and the vascular endothelium.[91] Patients at high risk for ischemic hepatitis after a hypotensive event include those with a history of cardiac failure and/or cardiac dysrhythmias. Clinical manifestations of hepatic insufficiency are evident 1 to 2 days after the insult. Jaundice and transient elevations in serum transaminase and bilirubin levels occur. Hyperbilirubinemia results from hepatocyte anoxic injury and an increased production of bilirubin from the hemoglobin catabolism. Ischemic hepatitis may either resolve spontaneously or progress to fulminant hepatic failure. Although ischemic hepatitis is not a life-threatening complication, it can contribute to patient morbidity and mortality as a component of MODS.[91] Researchers have recently proposed that serum bilirubin is a valid indicator of hepatic dysfunction in MODS because it significantly differentiates MODS survivors from nonsurvivors.[90,92,93] For further discussion on fulminant hepatic failure, see Chapter 22.

Acalculous cholecystitis manifests 3 to 4 weeks after an insult. Its pathogenesis is unclear but may be related to ischemic reperfusion injury, positive end-expiratory pressure (PEEP) greater than 5 cm H_2O, volume depletion, total parenteral nutrition, narcotics, and cystic duct obstruction as a result of hyperviscous bile.[94] Visceral hypotension and vasoactive medication use may decrease perfusion of the gallbladder mucosa contributing to ischemia. Bacterial invasion may stimulate activation of factor XII and initiate the coagulation pathway.[94] Clinical manifestations of acalculous cholecystitis may mimic acute cholecystitis with gallstones. Patients may demonstrate vague symptoms, however, including right upper quadrant pain and tenderness. Critical to the detection of acalculous cholecystitis is the recognition of abdominal distention, unexplained fever, loss of bowel sounds, and a sudden deterioration in the patient's condition. About 50% of patients with acalculous cholecystitis have gallbladder gangrene, and 10% have gallbladder perforation. Consequently, a cholecystectomy may be performed.[95]

Hypermetabolism accompanies SIRS and is commonly referred to as the "metabolic response to injury." During hypermetabolism and SIRS, the liver perpetuates select changes in metabolism including increased gluconeogenesis, glucogenesis, lipogenesis, and increased production of acute phase reactant proteins. Concurrently, the liver decreases synthesis of proteins, particularly albumin and transferrin. This metabolic response is partially mediated by interleukin-1 (IL-1), TNF, select amino acid (AA) metabolites, and the stress hormones.[72,90,96]

Pulmonary Dysfunction

The lungs, a frequent and early target organ for mediator-induced injury, are usually the first organs affected in secondary MODS. Acute pulmonary dysfunction in secondary MODS manifests as ALI. Patients who develop MODS generally develop ALI; however, not all patients with ALI develop secondary MODS. ALI patients who develop SIRS/sepsis concurrently with acute respiratory failure are at the greatest risk for MODS.[86]

ALI generally occurs 24 to 72 hours after the initial insult and manifests in four phases.[96] In summary, patients initially exhibit a low-grade fever, tachycardia, dyspnea, and mental confusion. As dyspnea, hypoxemia, and the work of breathing increase, intubation and mechanical ventilation are required. Pulmonary function is acutely disrupted, resulting in refractory hypoxemia secondary to intrapulmonary shunting, decreased pulmonary compliance, altered airway mechanics, and radiographic evidence of noncardiogenic pulmonary edema.[78,83]

Mediators associated with ALI include inflammatory cells, such as polymorphonuclear cells, macrophages, monocytes, endothelial cells, and mast cells; and biochemical mediators, such as AA metabolites, toxic oxygen metabolites, proteases, TNF, PAF, and interleukins.[78] Intense mediator activity damages the pulmonary vascular endothelium and the alveolar epithelium, resulting in surfactant deficiency, mild pulmonary hypertension, and increased lung water (noncardiogenic pulmonary edema) resulting from increased pulmonary capillary permeability. Pulmonary hypertension and hypoxic pulmonary vasoconstriction occur secondary to loss of the vascular bed.[72,78,81,97] For further discussion on ALI, see Chapter 15.

Renal Dysfunction

Acute renal failure is a common manifestation of MODS. The kidney is highly vulnerable to reperfusion injury. Consequently, renal ischemic-reperfusion injury may be a major cause of renal dysfunction in MODS. The patient may demonstrate oliguria or anuria secondary to decreased renal perfusion and relative hypovolemia. The condition may become refractory to diuretics, fluid challenges, and dopamine. Additional signs and symptoms include azotemia, decreased creatinine clearance, abnormal renal indices, and fluid and electrolyte imbalances. Prerenal oliguria may progress to acute tubular necrosis, necessitating hemodialysis or other renal therapies.[83,98] The frequent use of nephrotoxic drugs during critical illness also intensifies the risk of renal failure. Researchers have proposed that the serum creatinine is a valid indicator of renal function because it significantly differentiates MODS survivors from nonsurvivors.[99] For further discussion on acute renal failure, see Chapter 20.

Cardiovascular Dysfunction

The initial cardiovascular response in SIRS/sepsis is myocardial depression; decreased right atrial pressure and SVR; and increased venous capacitance, VO_2, CO, and HR. Despite an increased CO, myocardial depression occurs and is accompanied by decreased SVR, increased HR, and ventricular dilation. These compensatory mechanisms help maintain CO during the early phase of SIRS/sepsis. An inability to increase CO in response to a low SVR may indicate myocardial failure or inadequate fluid resuscitation and is associated with increased mortality. VO_2 may be twice normal and may be flow dependent. Mediators implicated in the hyperdynamic response include bradykinin, select AA metabolites, PAF, endogenous opioids, and β-adrenergic stimulators.[82,85]

As MODS progresses, cardiac failure develops. Cardiac dysfunction is characterized by ventricular dilation, decreased diastolic compliance, and decreased systolic contractile function. Cardiovascular function becomes vasopressor dependent. Cardiac failure may be caused by immune mediators, TNF, acidosis, or myocardial depressant factor (MDF), a substance secreted by the pancreas. TNF has a myocardial-depressant effect and is associated with myocardial depression during septic shock.[100] Myocardial depression is exacerbated by myocardial hypoperfusion from a low CO state and persistent lactic acidosis. Cardiogenic shock and biventricular failure occur and lead to death.[78,85] For further discussion on cardiac failure see Chapter 12.

Coagulation System Dysfunction

Anemia and coagulation abnormalities are common hematologic findings in the SIRS/MODS patient.[85] Coagulation system dysfunction manifests as DIC. DIC is a complex, consumptive coagulopathy that occurs in patients with a variety of disorders, including sepsis, tissue injury, and shock, and is an overstimulation of the normal coagulation process. DIC results in simultaneous microvascular clotting and hemorrhage in organ systems, leading to thrombosis and fibrinolysis in life-threatening proportions. Clotting factor derangement leads to further inflammation and further thrombosis. Microvascular damage leads to further organ injury. Cell injury and damage to the endothelium activate the intrinsic or extrinsic coagulation pathways.[60,78] Low platelet counts, elevated D-dimer concentrations, and fibrinogen degradation products are clinical indicators of DIC.[79] For further discussion on DIC, see Chapter 27.

Medical Management

The MODS patient requires interdisciplinary collaboration in clinical management. Medical management includes the identification and treatment of infection, maintenance of tissue oxygenation, administration of nutritional/metabolic support, and support for individual organs.[42,78,77] The use of investigational therapies may be part of the patient's clinical management.

Identification and Treatment of Infection

Identification and treatment of the underlying source of inflammation or infection are the most important aspects to reducing mortality. Medical and surgical intervention to remove sources of infection or contamination may limit the inflammatory response and improve chance of recovery.[78] Therefore surgical procedures such as early fracture stabilization, removal of infected organs or tissue, and burn excision are helpful. Appropriate antibiotics are needed if the focus cannot be removed surgically.[78,101] Other timely interventions such as prevention of skin ulceration and early nutritional support are measures to assist in improving outcomes.[78,43] Regardless of the identification of potential risk factors, clinical markers, bacterial contaminants, and investigative approaches for detection and prevention, treatment remains largely supportive and little improvement in the mortality rate has been appreciated.[101]

Maintenance of Tissue Oxygenation

Normally, under steady state conditions, VO_2 is relatively constant and independent of oxygen delivery (DO_2) unless delivery becomes severely impaired. The relationship is termed *supply-independent oxygen consumption.* VO_2 is about 25% of DO_2. Consequently a percentage of oxygen is not used (physiologic reserve).

SIRS/MODS patients often develop supply-dependent oxygen consumption in which VO_2 becomes dependent on DO_2, rather than demand, at a normal or high DO_2. When VO_2 does not equal demand, a tissue oxygen debt develops, subjecting organs to failure.[72,78]

Hypoperfusion and resultant organ hypoxemia often occur in patients at high risk for MODS, subjecting essential organs to failure. Therefore effective fluid resuscitation and early recognition of flow-dependent VO_2 is essential. Patients at risk for MODS require pulmonary artery catheterization, frequent measurements of DO_2 and VO_2, and arterial lactate levels to guide therapy. Arterial lactate levels provide information regarding the severity of impaired perfusion and the presence of lactic acidosis[83] and differ significantly in MODS survivors and nonsurvivors. Failure to maintain adequate oxygenation to vital organs results in organ dysfunction. Despite adequate DO_2, VO_2 may not meet the needs of the body during MODS.

Patients with ALI and sepsis frequently manifest supply-dependent oxygen consumption and are unable to use oxygen appropriately despite normal delivery.[72,73,78,102] Interventions that decrease oxygen demand and increase oxygen delivery are essential. Decreasing oxygen demand may be accomplished by sedation, mechanical ventilation, temperature and pain control, and rest. DO_2 may be increased by maintaining normal hematocrit and PaO_2 levels, using PEEP, increasing preload or myocardial contractility to enhance CO, or reducing afterload to increase CO. Many critical care clinicians advocate the maintenance of a supranormal DO_2 to increase VO_2; however, this therapeutic measure has not significantly improved survival, except in select groups of trauma patients.[75,101]

Nutritional/Metabolic Support

Hypermetabolism in SIRS/MODS results in profound weight loss, cachexia, and loss of organ function. The goal of nutritional support is the preservation of organ structure and function. Although nutritional support may not alter the course of organ dysfunction, it prevents generalized nutritional deficiencies and preserves gut integrity. The enteral route is preferable to parenteral support.[78,103-107] Enteral feedings are given distal to the pylorus to prevent pulmonary aspiration. Enteral feedings may limit bacterial translocation. In addition to early nutritional support, the pharmacologic properties of enteral feeding formulas may limit SIRS for select critical care populations. Supplementation of enteral feedings with glutamine and arginine may be beneficial. Enteral feedings with omega-3 fatty acids may lessen the development of SIRS.[72,77,103-107] Guidelines for nutritional support are outlined in Evidence-Based Collaborative Practice: Nutritional Support During Systemic Inflammatory Response Syndrome for Trauma Patients. For further discussion on nutritional support, see Chapter 6.

EVIDENCE-BASED COLLABORATIVE PRACTICE

Nutritional Support During Systemic Inflammatory Response Syndrome for Trauma Patients

- Patients are to receive 25 to 30 kcal/kg/day, with 3 to 5 g/kg/day as glucose.
- The respiratory quotient is monitored and maintained under 0.9.
- Long-chain polyunsaturated fatty acids (less than 1.5 g/kg/day) and amino acids (1.5 mg/kg/day) are given.
- Fat emulsions are limited to 0.5 to 1 g/kg/day to prevent iatrogenic immunosuppression associated with lipids and fat overload syndromes.
- Plasma transferrin and prealbumin levels are used to monitor hepatic protein synthesis. Efficient protein use must be assessed via nitrogen balance studies.

From Orr PA, Case KO, Stevenson JJ: *J Infus Nurs* 25:45, 2002.

Nursing Management

Preventive measures include a multitude of assessment strategies to detect early organ manifestations of this syndrome. Patients who continue to experience sites of inflammation, septic foci, and inadequate tissue perfusion may be at higher risk. Hand hygiene, aseptic technique, and an understanding of how microorganisms can invade the body are essential components of preventive nursing care.

Nursing management of the patient with acute MODS incorporates a variety of nursing diagnoses (Box 26-23). **Nursing priorities are directed toward (1) preventing development of infections, (2) facilitating tissue oxygen delivery and limiting tissue oxygen demand, (3) facilitating nutritional support, (4) providing comfort and emotional support, and (5) maintaining surveillance for complications.**

Patients are assessed closely for inflammation and infection. Subtle expressions of infection warrant investigation. Nursing measures include strict adherence to standards of practice to prevent infection. Practices related to infection control with invasive hemodynamic monitoring, urinary catheters, endotracheal tubes, intracranial pressure monitoring devices, total parenteral nutrition (TPN), and wound care must be stringent to prevent further infection. Measures to limit tissue oxygen consumption include (1) administering analgesics and sedatives, (2) positioning the patient for comfort, (3) limiting activities, (4) offering support to reduce anxiety, (5) providing a calm and quiet environment, and (6) teaching the patient about the

Box 26-23

NURSING DIAGNOSIS PRIORITIES

Multiple Organ Dysfunction Syndrome

- Decreased Cardiac Output related to alterations in preload, p. A-12
- Decreased Cardiac Output related to alterations in afterload, p. A-12
- Decreased Cardiac Output related to alterations in contractility, p. A-13
- Impaired Gas Exchange related to ventilation/perfusion mismatching or intrapulmonary shunting, p. A-29
- Ineffective Renal Tissue Perfusion related to decreased renal blood flow, p. A-42
- Ineffective Cardiopulmonary Tissue Perfusion related to decreased coronary blood flow, p. A-35
- Imbalanced Nutrition: Less Than Body Requirements related to increased metabolic demands or lack of exogenous nutrients, p. A-28
- Risk for Infection, p. A-46
- Acute Pain related to transmission and perception of cutaneous, visceral, muscular, or ischemic impulses, p. A-3
- Acute Confusion related to sensory overload, sensory deprivation, and sleep pattern disturbance, p. A-3
- Anxiety related to threat to biologic, psychologic, or social integrity, p. A-9
- Compromised Family Coping related to critically ill family member, p. A-11

condition. Measures to enhance tissue oxygen supply include administering supplemental oxygen, monitoring the patient's respiratory status, and administering prescribed fluids and medications.

REFERENCES

1. Kumar A, Parrillo JE: Shock: classification, pathophysiology, and approach to management. In Parrillo JP, Dellinger RP, editors: *Critical care medicine: principles of diagnosis and management in the adult*, ed 2, St Louis, 2002, Mosby.
2. Hameed SM, Aird WC, Cohn SM: Oxygen delivery, *Crit Care Med* 31:S658, 2003.
3. Szabó C: Mechanisms of cell necrosis, *Crit Care Med* 33(12 suppl): S530, 2005.
4. Kellum JA, Pinsky MR: Use of vasopressor agents in critically ill patients, *Curr Opin Crit Care* 8:236, 2002.
5. Dellinger RP: Cardiovascular management of septic shock, *Crit Care Med* 31:946, 2003.
6. Wilson M, Davis DP, Coimbra R: Diagnosis and monitoring of hemorrhagic shock during the initial resuscitation of multiple trauma patients: a review, *J Emerg Med* 24:413, 2003.
7. Casaletto JJ: Differential diagnosis of metabolic acidosis, *Emerg Med Clin North Am* 23:771, 2005.
8. Vincent JL, Weil MH: Fluid challenge revisited, *Crit Care Med* 34:1333, 2006.
9. Berlot G, Bacer B, Gullo A: Controversial aspects of the prehospital trauma care, *Crit Care Clin* 22:457, 2006.
10. Dellinger RP et al: Surviving Sepsis Campaign guidelines for management of severe sepsis and septic shock, *Crit Care Med* 32:858, 2004.
11. Vincent JL, Navickis RJ, Wilkes MM: Morbidity in hospitalized patients receiving human albumin: a meta-analysis of randomized, controlled trials, *Crit Care Med* 32:2029, 2004.
12. Cariou A, Vinsonneau C, Dhainaut JF: Adjunctive therapies in sepsis: an evidence-based review, *Crit Care Med* 32(11 suppl):S562, 2004.
13. Bistrian BR, McCowen KC: Nutritional and metabolic support in the adult intensive care unit: key controversies, *Crit Care Med* 34:1525, 2006.
14. Baudouin SV, Evans TW: Nutritional support in critical care, *Clin Chest Med* 24:633, 2003.
15. Jansen MP, Schmitt NA: Family-focused interventions, *Crit Care Nurs Clin North Am* 15:347, 2003.
16. Fox-Wasylyshyn SM, El-Masri MM, Williamson KM: Family perceptions of nurses' roles toward family members of critically ill patients: a descriptive study, *Heart Lung* 34:335, 2005.
17. Kirchhoff KT, Song MK, Kehl K: Caring for the family of the critically ill patient, *Crit Care Clin* 20:453, 2004.
18. Kelley DM: Hypovolemic shock: an overview, *Crit Care Nurs Q* 28:2, 2005.
19. Holmes CL, Walley KR: The evaluation and management of shock, *Clin Chest Med* 24:775, 2003.
20. Revell M, Greaves I, Porter K: Endpoints for fluid resuscitation in hemorrhagic shock, *J Trauma* 54:S63, 2003.
21. Solomonov E et al: The effect of vigorous fluid resuscitation in uncontrolled hemorrhagic shock after massive splenic injury, *Crit Care Med* 28:749, 2000.
22. Stern SA: Low-volume fluid resuscitation for presumed hemorrhagic shock: helpful or harmful? *Curr Opin Crit Care* 7:422, 2001.
23. Ashby DT, Stone GW, Moses JW: Cardiogenic shock in acute myocardial infarction, *Catheter Cardiovasc Interv* 59:34, 2003.
24. Goldberg RJ et al: Recent magnitude of and temporal trends (1994-1997) in the incidence and hospital death rates of cardiogenic shock complicating acute myocardial infarction: the second National Registry of Myocardial Infarction, *Am Heart J* 141:65, 2001.
25. Hollenberg SM, Parrillo JP: Cardiogenic shock. In Parrillo JP, Dellinger RP, editors: *Critical care medicine: principles of diagnosis and management in the adult*, ed 2, St Louis, 2002, Mosby.
26. Hochman JS: Cardiogenic shock complicating acute myocardial infarction: expanding the paradigm, *Circulation* 107:2998, 2003.
27. Menon V, Fincke R: Cardiogenic shock: a summary of the randomized SHOCK trial, *Congest Heart Fail* 9:35, 2003.
28. Geppert A et al: Multiple organ failure in patients with cardiogenic shock is associated with high plasma levels of interleukin-6, *Crit Care Med* 30:1987, 2002.
29. Lim N et al: Do all nonsurvivors of cardiogenic shock die with a low cardiac index? *Chest* 124:1885, 2003.
30. Shannon D et al: Mechanical circulatory support devices, *AACN Adv Crit Care* 17:368, 2006.
31. Magliato KE et al: Biventricular support inpatient with profound cardiogenic shock: a single center experience, *ASAIO J* 49:475, 2003.

32. Samuels LE; Darzé ES: Management of acute cardiogenic shock, *Cardiol Clin* 21:43, 2003.
33. Tremper RS: Intra-aortic balloon pump therapy—a primer for perioperative nurses, *AORN J* 84:34, 2006.
34. Lieberman P: Anaphylaxis, *Med Clin North Am* 90:77, 2006.
35. Haupt MT: Anaphylaxis and anaphylactic shock. In Parrillo JP, Dellinger RP, editors: *Critical care medicine: principles of diagnosis and management in the adult*, ed 2, St Louis, 2002, Mosby.
36. Tang A: A practical guide to anaphylaxis, *Am Fam Physician* 38:1325, 2003.
37. McLean APC et al: Adrenaline in the treatment of anaphylaxis: what is the evidence? *BMJ* 327:1332, 2003.
38. Sicherer SH: Advances in anaphylaxis and hypersensitivity reactions to foods, drugs, and insect venom, *J Allergy Clin Immunol* 111:S829, 2003.
39. Cottingham CA: Resuscitation of traumatic shock, *AACN Adv Crit Care* 17:317, 2006.
40. Karlet MC: Acute management of the patient with spinal cord injury, *Int J Trauma Nurs* 7:43, 2001.
41. Bilello JF et al: Cervical spinal cord injury and the need for cardiovascular intervention, *Arch Surg* 138:1127, 2003.
42. American College of Chest Physicians/Society of Critical Care Medicine Consensus Conference Committee: Definitions for sepsis and organ failure and guidelines for the use of innovative therapies in sepsis, *Crit Care Med* 20:864, 1992.
43. Kleinpell RM, Graves BT, Ackerman MH: Incidence, pathogenesis, and management of sepsis, *AACN Adv Crit Care*, 17:385, 2006.
44. Beale RJ et al: Vasopressor and inotropic support in septic shock: an evidence-based review, *Crit Care Med* 32(11 suppl):S455, 2004.
45. Angus DC et al: Epidemiology of severe sepsis in the United States: analysis of incidence, outcome, and associated costs of care, *Crit Care Med* 29:1303, 2001.
46. Martin GS et al: The epidemiology of sepsis in the United States from 1979 through 2000, *N Engl J Med* 348:1546, 2003.
47. Levy MN et al.: 2001 SCCM/ESICM/ACCP/ATS/SIS international sepsis definitions conference, *Crit Care Med* 31:1250, 2003.
48. Bernard GR: Drotrecogin alfa (activated) (recombinant human activated protein C) for the treatment of severe sepsis, *Crit Care Med* 31(1 suppl):S85, 2003.
49. Balk RA: Optimum treatment of severe sepsis and septic shock: evidence in support of the recommendations, *Dis Mon* 50:168, 2004.
50. Ahrens T, Vollman K: Severe sepsis management: are we doing enough? *Crit Care Nurs* 23(suppl):2, 2003.
51. Janice Tazbir J: Sepsis and the role of activated protein C, *Crit Care Nurse* 24:40, 2004.
52. Groeneveld AB et al: Circulating inflammatory mediators predict shock and mortality in febrile patients with microbial infection, *Clin Immunol* 106:106, 2003.
53. Sommers MS: The cellular basis of septic shock, *Crit Care Nurs Clin North Am* 15:13, 2003.
54. Sharma S, Kumar A: Septic shock, multiple organ failure, and acute respiratory distress syndrome, *Curr Opin Pulm Med* 9:199, 2003.
55. Angus DC, Crowther MA: Unraveling severe sepsis: why did OPTIMIST fail and what's next? *JAMA* 290:256, 2003.
56. Tamion F et al: Gastric mucosal acidosis and cytokine release inpatients with septic shock, *Crit Care Med* 31:2237, 2003.
57. Mizock BA: Metabolic derangements in sepsis and septic shock, *Crit Care Clin* 16:319, 2000.
58. Brealey D et al: Association between mitochondrial dysfunction and severity and outcome of septic shock, *Lancet* 360:219, 2002.
59. Ahrens T: Hemodynamics in sepsis, *AACN Adv Crit Care* 17:435, 2006.
60. Kleinpell RM: The role of the critical care nurse in the assessment and management of the patient with severe sepsis, *Crit Care Nurs Clin North Am* 15:27, 2003.
61. Hurtado FJ, Nin N: The role of bundles in sepsis care, *Crit Care Clin* 22:521, 2006.
62. Otero RM et al. Early goal-directed therapy in severe sepsis and septic shock revisited: concepts, controversies, and contemporary findings, *Chest* 130:1579, 2006.
63. Powers J, Jacobi J: Pharmacologic treatment related to severe sepsis, AACN *Adv Crit Care* 17:423, 2006.
64. The ARDS Network: Ventilation with lower tidal volumes as compared with traditional tidal volumes for acute lung injury and the acute respiratory distress syndrome, *N Engl J Med* 342:1301, 2000.
65. Kress JP et al: Daily interruption of sedative infusions in critically ill patients undergoing mechanical ventilation, *N Engl J Med* 342:1471, 2000.
66. Gullo A, Bianco N, Berlot G: Management of severe sepsis and septic shock: challenges and recommendations, *Crit Care Clin* 22:489, 2006.
67. Dellinger RP, Parrillo JE: Mediator modulation therapy of severe sepsis and septic shock: does it work? *Crit Care Med* 32:282, 2004.
68. Jacobi J: Corticosteroid replacement in critically ill patients, *Crit Care Clin* 22:245, 2006.
69. Baldwin KM, Morris SE: Shock, multiple organ dysfunction syndrome, and burns in adults. In McCance KL, Huether SE, editors: *Pathophysiology: the biologic basis for disease in adults and children*, ed 5, St Louis, 2006, Mosby.
70. Deitch EA, Dayal SD: Intensive care unit management of the trauma patient, *Crit Care Med* 34:2294, 2006.
71. Motoyama T et al: Possible role of increased oxidant stress in multiple organ failure after systemic inflammatory response syndrome, *Crit Care Med* 31:1048, 2003.
72. Awad SS: State-of-the-art therapy for severe sepsis and multisystem organ dysfunction, *Am J Surg* 186(5A):23S, 2003.
73. Epstein CD et al: Oxygen transport and organ dysfunction in the older trauma patient, *Heart Lung* 31:315, 2002.
74. Fry DE: Systemic inflammatory response and multiple organ dysfunction syndrome: biologic domino effect. In Baue AE, Faist E, Fry DE, editors: *Multiple organ failure: pathophysiology, prevention, and therapy*, New York, 2000, Springer-Verlag.
75. Lee CC et al: A current concept of trauma-induced multiorgan failure, *Ann Emerg Med* 38:170, 2001.

76. Levy MM et al: 2001 SCCM/ESICM/ACCP/ATS/SIS international sepsis definitions conference, *Crit Car Med* 31:1250, 2003.
77. Biffle WL, Moore EE: Role of the gut in multiple organ failure. In Grenvik A et al, editors: *Textbook of critical care,* ed 4, Philadelphia, 2000, Saunders.
78. Meeran H, Messent M: The systemic inflammatory response syndrome, *Trauma* 3:89, 2001.
79. Jacobi J: Pathophysiology of sepsis, *Am J Health Syst Pharm* 59:S3, 2002.
80. Brun-Breson C: The epidemiology of the systemic inflammatory response, *Intensive Care Med* 26:S64, 2000.
81. Khadaroo RG, Marshall JC: ARDS and the multiple organ dysfunction syndrome. Common mechanisms of a common systemic process, *Crit Care Clin* 18:127, 2002.
82. Baldwin KM, Morris SE: Shock, multiple organ dysfunction syndrome, and burns in adults. In McCance KL, Huether SE, editors: *Pathophysiology: the biologic basis for disease in adults and children,* ed 5, St Louis, 2006, Mosby.
83. Majetschak M, Waydhas C: Infection, bacteremia, sepsis, and the sepsis syndrome: metabolic alterations, hypermetabolism, and cellular alterations. In Baue AE, Faist E, Fry DE, editors: *Multiple organ failure: pathophysiology, prevention, and therapy,* New York, 2000, Springer-Verlag.
84. Rote NS: Inflammation. In McCance KL, Huether SE, editors: *Pathophysiology: the biologic basis for disease in adults and children,* ed 5, St Louis, 2006, Mosby.
85. Evans TW, Smithies M: ABC of intensive care: organ dysfunction, *Br Med J* 318:1606, 1999.
86. Russell JA et al: Changing pattern of organ dysfunction in early human sepsis is related to mortality, *Crit Care Med* 28:3405, 2000.
87. Deitch EA: Gut failure: its role in the multiple organ failure syndrome. In Deitch EA, editor: *Multiple organ failure: pathophysiology and basic concepts of therapy,* New York, 1990, Thieme Medical.
88. Crouser ED: Gastrointestinal tract dysfunction in critical illness: pathophysiology and interaction with acute lung injury in adult respiratory distress syndrome/multiple organ dysfunction syndrome, *New Horizons* 2:476, 1994.
89. Cole L: Early enteral feeding after surgery, *Crit Care Nurs Clin North Am* 11:227, 1999.
90. Dhainaut JF et al: Hepatic response to sepsis: interaction between coagulation and inflammatory processes, *Crit Care Med* 29: S42, 2002.
91. Wong F: Liver and kidney diseases, *Clin Liver Dis* 6:981, 2002.
92. Baue AE: Liver: multiple organ dysfunction and failure. In Baue AE, Faist E, Fry DE, editors: *Multiple organ failure: pathophysiology, prevention, and therapy,* New York, 2000, Springer-Verlag.
93. Marshall JC et al: Multiple organs dysfunction score: a reliable descriptor of a complex clinical outcome, *Crit Care Med* 23:1638, 1995.
94. Puc MM et al: Ultrasound is not a useful screening tool for acute acalculous cholecystitis in critically ill trauma patients, *Am Surg* 68:65, 2002.
95. Proctor DD: Critical issues in digestive diseases, *Clin Chest Med* 24:623, 2003.
96. McMahon K: Multiple organ failure: the final complication of critical illness, *Crit Care Nurs* 15:23, 1995.
97. Zallen G et al: Circulating postinjury neutrophils are primed for the release of proinflammatory cytokines, *J Trauma* 46:42, 1999.
98. Huether S: Alterations of renal and urinary tract function. In McCance KL, Huether SE, editors: *Pathophysiology: the biologic basis for disease in adults and children,* ed 5, St Louis, 2006, Mosby.
99. Mullins RJ: Renal function and dysfunction in multiple organ failure. In Baue AE, Faist E, Fry DE, editors: *Multiple organ failure: pathophysiology, prevention, and therapy,* New York, 2000, Springer-Verlag.
100. Kumar A et al: Myocardial dysfunction in septic shock. II. Role of cytokines and nitric oxide, *J Cardiothorac Vasc Anesth* 15:485, 2001.
101. Richards M, Thursky K, Buising K: Epidemiology, prevalence, and sites of infections in intensive care unit, *Semin Resp Crit Care Med* 24:3, 2003.
102. Hauser CJ: Is supranormal oxygen delivery beneficial? In Deitch EA, Vincent JL, Windsor ACJ, editors: *Sepsis and multiple organ dysfunction: a multiple disciplinary approach,* London, 2001, Harcourt International.
103. McQuiggan MM, Moore FA: Nutrition support in blunt and penetrating torso trauma. In Pichard C, Kudsk KA, editors: *From nutrition support to pharmacologic nutrition in the ICU,* Berlin, 2000, Springer-Verlag.
104. Fitzsimmons L, Hadley SA: Nutritional management of the metabolically stressed patient, *Crit Care Nurs Q* 17:1, 1994.
105. Cheever KH: Early enteral feeding of patients with multiple trauma, *Crit Care Nurse* 19:40, 1999.
106. McClave SA, Mallampalli A: Nutrition in the ICU. I. Enteral feeding—when and why? *J Crit Illness* 16:197, 2001.
107. Alexander JW: Is early enteral feeding of benefit? *Int Care Med* 25:129, 1999.

CHAPTER

27 Hematologic and Oncologic Issues

BARBARA MAYER

OBJECTIVES

- Describe the etiology and pathophysiology of disseminated intravascular coagulation, heparin-induced thrombocytopenia, and tumor lysis syndrome.
- Identify the clinical manifestations of disseminated intravascular coagulation, heparin-induced thrombocytopenia, and tumor lysis syndrome.
- Explain the treatment of disseminated intravascular coagulation, heparin-induced thrombocytopenia, and tumor lysis syndrome.
- Discuss the nursing priorities for managing the patient with disseminated intravascular coagulation, heparin-induced thrombocytopenia, and tumor lysis syndrome.

Understanding the pathology of a disease, the areas of assessment on which to focus, and the usual medical management allows the critical care nurse to more accurately anticipate and plan nursing interventions. This chapter focuses on hematologic and oncologic disorders commonly seen in the critical care environment.

DISSEMINATED INTRAVASCULAR COAGULATION

Disseminated intravascular coagulation (DIC) is a syndrome that arises as a complication of serious or life-threatening conditions. Although not likely to be seen often, it can seriously hamper diagnosis and treatment efforts in the critically ill patient. An understanding of the etiology and pathophysiologic mechanisms of DIC can assist in anticipation of the occurrence of the syndrome, recognition of signs and symptoms, and prompt intervention. Also known as consumptive coagulopathy, DIC is characterized by both bleeding and thrombosis that result from depletion of clotting factors, platelets, and red blood cells. It is always a complication of another critical, life-threatening condition and, if not treated quickly, will result in multiple organ failure and death.[1]

ETIOLOGY

There are many clinical events that can prompt the development of DIC in the critically ill patient, although the true underlying trigger may not be clearly identifiable (Box 27-1). There are, however, some commonly known conditions associated with the development of DIC.

Sepsis, particularly that caused by gram-negative organisms, can be identified as the culprit in as many as 20% of cases, making it the most common cause of DIC. In this instance, endotoxins serve as a trigger for activation of tissue factor and the extrinsic coagulation pathway. Metabolic acidosis and hypoperfusion associated with shock syndromes can result in increased formation of free radicals and damage to tissues. Again, tissue factor is activated, resulting in DIC. Massive trauma or burns can also be frequently associated with DIC. Direct tissue damage activates the extrinsic coagulation pathway, whereas damage to endothelial surfaces activates the intrinsic pathway.[2] Obstetric emergencies such as abruptio placentae, retained placenta, or incomplete abortion are also associated with the development of DIC. Tissue factor is notably concentrated in the placenta, so damage or disruption of this structure can activate coagulation pathways, resulting in coagulopathy.[3]

PATHOPHYSIOLOGY

Regardless of etiology, the common thread in the development of DIC is damage to the endothelium, resulting in activation of the coagulation mechanism (Figure 27-1). The extrinsic coagulation pathway plays a major role in the development of DIC. Direct damage to the endothelium results in the release of tissue factor and activation of this pathway. However, it is the secondary surge of thrombin formation as a result of activation of the intrinsic coagulation pathway that leads to the massive disruption of the delicate balance that is hemostasis. Excessive thrombin formation results in rapid consumption of coagulation factors and depletion of regulatory substances—protein C, protein S, and antithrombin.[1,4] With no checks and balances, thrombi continue to form along damaged epithelial walls, resulting in occlusion of the vessels. As occlusion reaches a critical level, tissue ischemia ensues, leading to further tissue damage perpetuating the process. Eventually, end-organ function is affected by the ischemia and failure is evident.[1,5]

In response to the formation of clots, the fibrinolytic system is activated. As plasmin breaks down the fibrin clots, fibrin split products are released and act as anticoagulants as well.[2,3] Coupled with depletion of circulating clotting factors, activation of fibrinolysis results in excessive bleeding. The end result is shock and further tissue ischemia, aggravating end-organ dysfunction and failure. Death is imminent if this destructive cycle is not interrupted.[5]

Box 27-1

Etiology of Disseminated Intravascular Coagulation

Obstetric Complications
Abruptio placentae
Retained dead fetus
Septic abortion
Amniotic fluid embolism
Toxemia

Infections
Gram-negative sepsis
Meningococcemia
Rocky Mountain spotted fever
Histoplasmosis
Aspergillosis
Malaria

Neoplasms
Carcinomas of pancreas, prostate, lung, and stomach
Acute promyelocytic leukemia

Massive Tissue Injury
Traumatic
Burns
Extensive surgery

Miscellaneous
Acute intravascular hemolysis
Snakebite
Giant hemangioma
Shock
Heat stroke
Vasculitis
Aortic aneurysm
Liver disease

From Cotran RS, Kumar V, Collins T: *Robbins pathologic basis of disease,* ed 6, Philadelphia, 1999, WB Saunders.

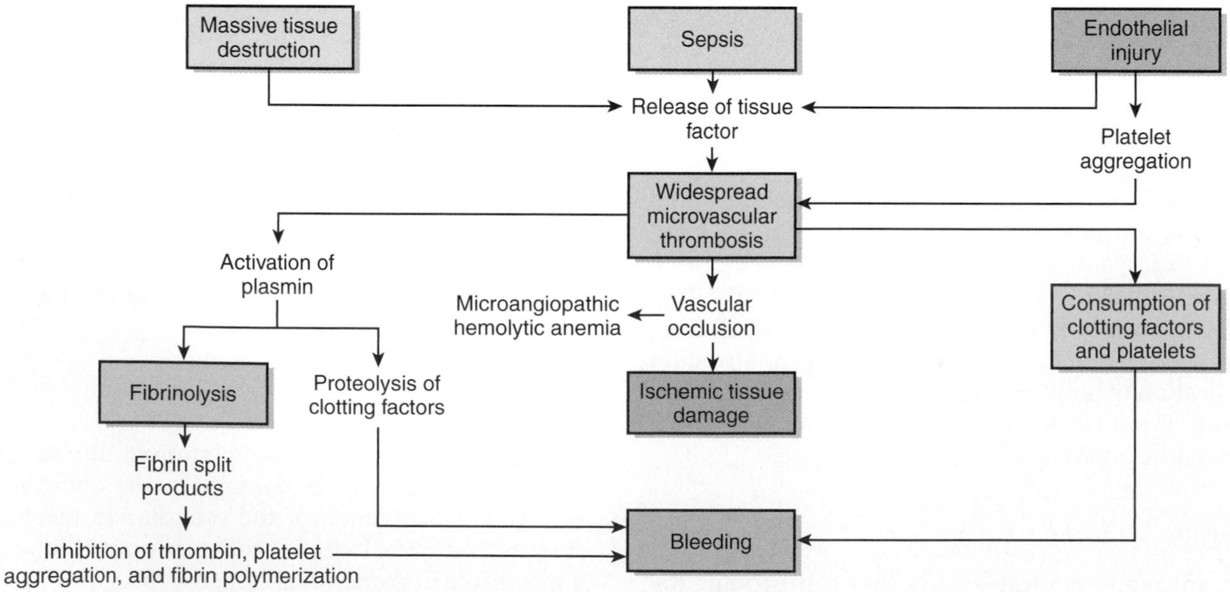

FIGURE 27-1. Pathophysiology of disseminated intravascular coagulation. (From Cotran RS, Kumar V, Collins T: *Robbins pathologic basis of disease,* ed 6, Philadelphia, 1999, WB Saunders.)

Assessment and Diagnosis

Favorable outcomes in the presence of DIC are dependent on accurate and timely diagnosis of the condition. Realization of the role the underlying pathologic condition plays, recognition of clinical manifestations, and assessment of appropriate laboratory values are key steps in this process.

Clinical Manifestations

Clinical manifestations are related to the two primary pathophysiologic mechanisms present in DIC: the formation of thrombi and bleeding. Thrombi in peripheral capillaries can lead to cyanosis, notably in the fingers, toes, ears, and nose. In severe, untreated cases this peripheral ischemia may progress to gangrene.[2,4,6] As the condition progresses, ischemia worsens and end organs are affected. The result of this more central ischemia can be respiratory insufficiency and failure, acute tubular necrosis (ATN), bowel infarct, and cerebrovascular accident (CVA). The tissue damage that results perpetuates the anomalies present in DIC.

As coagulation factors are depleted, bleeding from intravenous (IV) and other puncture sites is noted. Ecchymoses may result from even routine interventions such as the use of a manual blood pressure (BP) cuff, bathing, or turning.[2] Bloody drainage may also be noted from surgical sites, drains, and urinary catheters. With progression of DIC, the patient is at risk for severe gastrointestinal or subarachnoid hemorrhage.[2] Table 27-1 lists many of the common signs and symptoms of DIC.

Laboratory Findings

Laboratory tests used to diagnose DIC essentially assess the following four basic characteristics of DIC: (1) increased coagulant activity, (2) increased fibrinolytic activity, (3) impaired regulatory function, and (4) the presence of end-organ failure.

Continuous activation of the coagulation pathways results in consumption of coagulation factors. Because of this, the prothrombin time, (PT), activated partial thromboplastin time (aPTT), and the international normalized ratio (INR) will all be elevated. Although the platelet count may fall within normal ranges, serial examination will reveal a declining trend in values. An unexpected drop of at least 50% in the platelet count, particularly in the presence of known contributing factors and associated signs and symptoms, is highly indicative of DIC.[7] In addition, fibrinogen levels drop as more and more clots are formed. Thrombi formation in small vessels narrows the vessel lumen, forcing red blood cells to squeeze through. This results in damage and fragmentation of these cells, which can be seen on microscopic examination of blood samples. Damaged, fragmented red blood cells are called *schistocytes*.[1,2,8]

In response to the excess clotting activity, the fibrinolytic process accelerates, resulting in increasing levels of by-products. This is reflected in marked elevation of fibrin degradation products (FDPs). Another key laboratory test used to evaluate the degree of clot dissolution, and therefore the severity of the coagulopathy, is the D-dimer level.[7] D-dimers are exclusively indicative of clot degradation because, unlike FDPs, which also result from breakdown of free circulating fibrin, D-dimers only result from dissolution of clots.[7] With progression of the coagulopathy, normal regulatory mechanisms are disrupted. This disruption is reflected in decreasing levels of inhibitory factors such as protein C, factor V, and antithrombin III.[1,2]

Finally, unchecked DIC, resulting in occlusion of vessels and tissue ischemia, leads to end-organ dysfunction. Respiratory failure, indicated by abnormal arterial blood gas (ABG) levels; liver failure, indicated by increasing liver enzyme levels; and renal impairment, indicated by rising blood urea nitrogen (BUN) and creatinine (Cr) levels, are common findings in advanced DIC.

No single laboratory study can confirm the diagnosis of DIC, but there are several key results that are strong indicators the condition is present (Table 27-2). The International Society of Thrombosis and Hemostasis emphasizes early detection of DIC through observation of abnormal trends in laboratory values.[4]

Table 27-1

Common Signs and Symptoms of Disseminated Intravascular Coagulation

SYSTEM	SIGNS RELATED TO HEMORRHAGE	SIGNS RELATED TO THROMBI
Integumentary	Bleeding from gums, venipunctures, and old surgical sites, epistaxis, ecchymoses	Peripheral cyanosis, gangrene
Cardiopulmonary	Hemoptysis	Dysrhythmias, chest pain, acute myocardial infarction, pulmonary embolus, respiratory failure
Renal	Hematuria	Oliguria, acute tubular necrosis, renal failure
Gastrointestinal	Abdominal distention, hemorrhage	Diarrhea, constipation, bowel infarct
Neurologic	Subarachnoid hemorrhage	Altered level of consciousness, cerebrovascular accident

Table 27-2

Key Laboratory Studies in Disseminated Intravascular Coagulation

TEST	VALUE
Prothrombin time (PT)	>12.5 seconds
Platelets	<50,000/mm^3, or at least 50% drop from baseline
Activated partial thromboplastin time (aPTT)	>40 seconds
D-Dimer	>250 ng/ml
Fibrin degradation products (FDPs)	>40 mcg/ml
Fibrinogen	<100 mg/dl

Medical Management

Without question, the primary intervention in DIC is prevention. Being aware of those conditions that commonly contribute to the development of DIC and treating them vigorously and without delay is the best defense against this devastating condition.[1,2,4,6,8] However, once DIC is identified, maintaining organ perfusion and slowing consumption of coagulation factors is paramount to achieving a favorable outcome.[2]

Multiple organ dysfunction syndrome (MODS) is frequently a result of DIC and only serves to exacerbate the underlying pathologic condition. Therefore it is essential to prevent end-organ ischemia and damage by supporting blood pressure and circulating volume. Administration of IV fluids, inotropic agents, and if overt hemorrhaging is evident, infusion of packed red blood cells would be appropriate to replace blood volume and essential oxygen-carrying red blood cells.

In the presence of severe platelet depletion (<50,000/mm^3) and severe hemorrhage, platelet transfusions are often indicated.[1,4] However, caution must be used when administering platelets because antiplatelet antibodies may be formed. These antibodies may then become activated during future platelet transfusions, and they elicit DIC.[2]

Replacement of clotting factors in the patient with DIC is thought by some to perpetuate the coagulopathy; however, there is little scientific evidence to support this is theory.[7] Fibrinogen levels less than 100 mg/dl indicate the appropriateness of administering cryoprecipitate. Prolonged PT indicates the need for fresh frozen plasma.[1,2,4]

Slowing consumption of coagulation factors by inhibiting the processes involved in clot formation is also a strategy in treating DIC. The use of heparin, particularly low-molecular-weight heparin (LMWH), to prevent formation of future clots is controversial. It is contraindicated in those patients with DIC accompanying recent surgery or gastrointestinal (GI) or central nervous system (CNS) bleeding. However, it has been found to be beneficial in obstetric emergencies such as retained placenta or incomplete abortion, severe arterial occlusions, or MODS caused by microemboli.[1,2] To interfere with excessive fibrinolysis, inhibitors such as aminocaproic acid may be used in conjunction with heparin.[1]

The use of recombinant human protein C is gaining popularity in treating DIC, especially in the presence of severe sepsis. Protein C acts as an anticoagulant and works to restore normal inhibition of coagulation pathways. However, it has been associated with an increased incidence of intracerebral bleeding and must be used with caution in patients with severely decreased platelets.[2,4]

Thrombin production in DIC surpasses that of antithrombins and other regulatory factors that would normally be present to inactivate thrombin and all of its subsequent actions. The use of antithrombin III has just recently been approved in the United States. Ongoing research is yielding very promising results in the treatment of DIC. Another promising avenue of research concerns the use of protease inhibitors. Normally, protease molecules inhibit the conversion of fibrinogen to fibrin in the coagulation mechanism. In DIC, this normal inhibitory mechanism is impaired. The introduction of protease inhibitors through IV infusion may therefore be advantageous in arresting DIC.[2]

Nursing Management

Nursing management of the patient with DIC incorporates a variety of nursing diagnoses (Box 27-2). Assessment and monitoring are the primary weapons in the critical care nurse's arsenal where DIC is concerned. Knowing the diseases and conditions that are most often associated with DIC and understanding the pathophysiologic mechanisms involved enable the critical care nurse to anticipate its development and intervene quickly. **Nursing priorities are directed toward (1) supporting the patient's vital functions, (2) initiating bleeding precautions, (3) providing comfort and emotional support, and (4) maintaining surveillance for complications.**

Box 27-2

NURSING DIAGNOSIS PRIORITIES

Disseminated Intravascular Coagulation

- Deficient Fluid Volume related to active blood loss.
- Decreased Cardiac Output related to alterations in preload, p. A-12
- Risk for Infection, p. A-46
- Anxiety related to threat to biologic, psychologic, and/or social integrity, p. A-9
- Compromised Family Coping related to critically ill family member, p. A-11

Frequent assessments should include parameters for neurologic status, renal function, cardiopulmonary function, and skin integrity indicating impaired tissue or organ perfusion. Particular parameters to include are mental status, BUN and Cr levels, urine output, vital signs, hemodynamic values, cardiac rhythm, arterial blood gas and pulse oximetry values, skin breakdown, ecchymoses, or hematomas.[1]

The critical care nurse must recognize and support the patient's vital physiologic functions. Administration of IV fluids, blood products, and inotropic agents to provide adequate hemodynamic support and tissue oxygenation is essential in preventing or combating end-organ damage. Close monitoring of vital signs, hemodynamic parameters, intake and output, and appropriate laboratory values will assist the critical care nurse in administering and titrating appropriate agents.

Awareness of the patient's bleeding potential necessitates adjustments to normal nursing interventions. Avoid unnecessary venipunctures that may result in bleeding, bruising, or hematomas by drawing blood from and administering medications through existing arterial or venous lines. Avoid the use of manual or automatic blood pressure cuffs whenever possible. If tracheal or oral suctioning is necessary, the use of low-level suction is recommended.[1] Meticulous skin care is advised, keeping the skin moist and using specialty mattresses and beds as appropriate to prevent breakdown. Finally, use gentle care when bathing or turning the patient to avoid bruising or hematomas.

The development of DIC in the already critically ill patient can cause a great deal of stress in both the patient and his or her significant others. It is imperative to provide psychosocial support throughout this crisis. Calm reassurance and uncomplicated explanations of the care the patient is receiving can help allay much of the anxiety experienced. Be sure to answer all questions and provide information in terms best understood by all. When English is not the primary language, the use of an interpreter can enhance understanding and help avoid misconceptions. Providing spiritual support as requested may also be of assistance.

Collaborative management of the patient with DIC is outlined in Box 27-3.

Box 27-3

Collaborative Management

Disseminated Intravascular Coagulation

- Identify and eliminate the underlying cause.
- Provide hemodynamic support to prevent end-organ ischemia.
  - Intravenous fluids
  - Positive inotropic agents
- Administer blood and blood components.
  - Fresh frozen plasma
  - Platelets
  - Cryoprecipitate
  - Antithrombin III
- Administer medications.
  - Heparin
  - Aminocaproic acid
  - Protein C
  - Antithrombin III
- Initiate bleeding precautions.
- Maintain surveillance for complications.
  - Hypovolemic shock
  - Peripheral ischemia
  - Central ischemia
  - Multiple organ dysfunction syndrome (MODS)
- Provide comfort and emotional support.

HEPARIN-INDUCED THROMBOCYTOPENIA

Another form of thrombocytopenia seen in critical care patients is heparin-induced thrombocytopenia (HIT). There are two distinct types of HIT. The most common form is type 1 HIT. Seen in up to 30% of patients receiving heparin therapy, this nonautoimmune condition manifests within a few days of initiation of therapy. Platelet depletion is moderate, counts usually are less than 100,000/mm^3, and the condition is transient, often resolving spontaneously. Discontinuation of heparin is not required. The second form is type II HIT, which is less commonly encountered but has more severe consequences.[9-11] This discussion is limited to type 2 HIT.

ETIOLOGY

Type 2 HIT is an immune-mediated response to the administration of heparin therapy. It has been observed in 3% to 5% of patients treated with unfractionated heparin and has also occurred after exposure to LMWH though to a lesser degree. The disorder is characterized by severe thrombocytopenia during heparin therapy. Diagnostically it is identified by a platelet count less than 100,000/µl or at least a 50% decrease from the baseline platelet count from the initiation of therapy. Onset is usually 5 to 14 days from the first exposure to heparin, but the onset can be within hours of a reexposure to heparin.[10-13] Depending on the source, mortality rates can be as high as 30%.[10,11,13]

PATHOPHYSIOLOGY

The thrombocytopenia that occurs with type 2 HIT is related to the formation of heparin-antibody complexes. These complexes release a substance known as platelet factor 4 (PF4). PF4 attracts heparin molecules, forming immunogenic complexes that adhere to platelet and endothelial surfaces (Figure 27-2). Activation of platelets stimulates the release of thrombin and the subsequent formation of platelet clumps.[9]

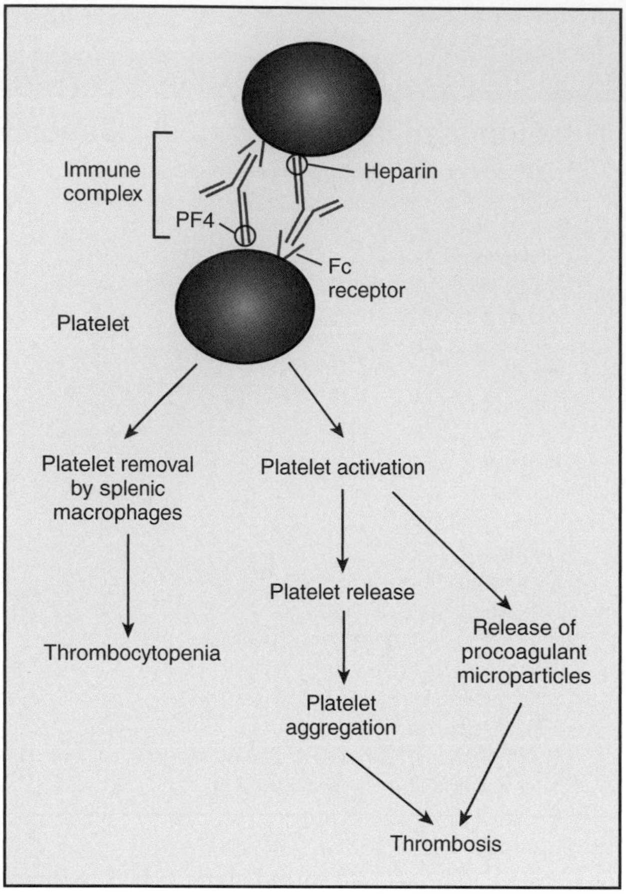

FIGURE 27-2. Pathophysiology of heparin-induced thrombocytopenia. First, heparin binds to platelet factor 4 (PF4), forming a highly reactive antigenic complex on the surface of platelets. Susceptible patients then develop an antibody (IgG) to the heparin/PF4 antigenic complex. Once produced, the IgG then activates the platelets via their Fc receptors. Thrombocytopenia develops as the reticuloendothelial system consumes activated platelets, platelet microaggregates, and IgG-coated platelets. (Courtesy GlaxoSmithKline, Philadelphia, Pa.)

Thus patients with type 2 HIT are at a greater risk of developing thrombosis rather than bleeding. Vessel occlusion can result in the need for limb amputation, stroke, acute myocardial infarction, and even death.[9-11, 13,14] The resultant formation of thrombi is the primary distinguishing factor of HIT from other forms of thrombocytopenia and gives it its more descriptive name, "white clot syndrome."[9]

Assessment and Diagnosis

HIT can be associated with severe consequences. Rapid recognition of risk factors and subsequent development of signs and symptoms is essential in treating this condition.

Clinical Manifestations

Common signs and symptoms are listed in Table 27-3. The clinical manifestations of HIT are related to the formation of thrombi and subsequent vessel occlusion. Most thrombotic events are venous, although both venous and arterial thrombosis can occur.[13] Thrombotic events typically include deep vein thrombosis, pulmonary embolism, limb ischemia thrombosis, thrombotic stroke, and myocardial infarction.[13] The presence of blanching and the loss of peripheral pulses, sensation, or motor function in a limb is indicative of peripheral vascular thrombi. Neurologic signs and symptoms, such as confusion, headache, and impaired speech can signal the onset of cerebral artery occlusion and stroke. Acute myocardial infarction may be heralded by dyspnea, chest pain, pallor, and alterations in blood pressure. Thrombi in the pulmonary vasculature may result as evidenced by pleuritic pain, rales, and dyspnea.[9,12,14]

Table 27-3

Common Signs and Symptoms and Laboratory Data Seen With Heparin-Induced Thrombocytopenia

SYSTEM	SIGNS AND SYMPTOMS
Cardiac	Chest pain, diaphoresis, pallor, alterations in blood pressure, dysrhythmias
Vascular	Arterial—Pain, pallor, pulselessness, paresthesia, paralysis
	Venous—Pain, tenderness, unilateral leg swelling, warmth, erythema, a palpable cord, pain upon passive dorsiflexion of the foot, and spontaneous maintenance of the relaxed foot in abnormal plantar flexion (Homans' sign)
Pulmonary	Dyspnea, pleuritic pain, rales, chest pain, chest wall tenderness, back pain, shoulder pain, upper abdominal pain, syncope, hemoptysis, shortness of breath, wheezing
Renal	Thirst, decreased urine output, dizziness, orthostatic hypotension
Gastrointestinal	Abdominal pain, vomiting, bloody diarrhea, abnormal bowel sounds
Neurologic	Confusion, headache, impaired speech patterns, hemiparesis or hemiplegia, vision disturbances, dysarthria, aphasia, ataxia, vertigo, nystagmus, sudden decrease in consciousness
Laboratory	Platelets <50,000/mm^3 or sudden drop of 30%-50% from baseline; positive HIPA, SRA, ELISA

HIPA, Heparin-induced platelet aggregation; *SRA,* serotonin release assay; *ELISA,* enzyme-linked immunosorbent assay.

Laboratory Findings

The key indicator in identifying the development of HIT is the platelet count. General consensus in the literature states that a platelet count of less than 50,000/mm^3 or a sudden drop of 30% to 50% from the patient's baseline following initiation of heparin therapy is highly indicative of HIT.[9,12,13]

More recently, two types of assays are available to assist in confirming the diagnosis of HIT: (1) functional assays, based on platelet aggregation or the release of granular contents such as serotonin, and (2) assays that identify the HIT antigen. Functional assays are highly sensitive in detecting the presence of the HIT. The two most common functional assays are heparin-induced platelet aggregation (HIPA) and serotonin release assay (SRA). The enzyme-linked immunosorbent assay (ELISA) actually identifies the presence of the HIT antigen.[9]

Medical Management

Early identification is critical to managing the effects of type 2 HIT. Recommendations of the College of American Pathologists include obtaining a baseline platelet count before initiation of therapy and routine monitoring during the highest risk period, 5 to 10 days following intiation.[13] When a decrease in the platelet count is detected, heparin therapy should be discontinued immediately and the patient should be tested for the presence of heparin antibodies.[9,11,13,14]

If the original indication for heparin still exists or new thromboses occur, an alternative form of anticoagulation is usually necessary.[9,12,13]

Direct thrombin inhibitors (DTIs) are being used with increasing frequency to treat HIT. DTIs bind directly to the thrombin molecule; thereby inhibiting its action.[9] The Food and Drug Administration (FDA) has approved two such drugs for use in the United States: lepirudin and argatroban. Warfarin, although commonly used to treat deep vein thrombosis, is not indicated as a sole agent in treating HIT because of its prolonged onset of action.[9,13] Studies have shown that the use of warfarin without concomitant use of DTIs can significantly increase the incidence of thrombosis in patients with HIT. The optimal duration of anticoagulation in patients with HIT is not known.[13]

Nursing Management

Nursing management of the patient with HIT incorporates a variety of nursing diagnoses (Box 27-4). **Nursing priorities are directed toward (1) ensuring all heparin is discontinued, (2) maintaining surveillance for complications, and (3) providing comfort and emotional support.** The critical care nurse plays a pivotal role in prevention and detection of heparin-induced thrombocytopenia. Initial assessment is crucial to identifying those patients at risk for developing HIT. Ascertaining past medical history that includes previous heparin therapy, deep vein thrombosis, or cardiovascular surgery, including the use of cardiopulmonary bypass, will alert the nurse to potential problems. Patients with HIT remain at high risk of thrombotic complications for several days or weeks after cessation of heparin. Vigilant monitoring, early recognition of signs and symptoms, and prompt notification of the physician are key roles of the critical care nurse. Ensuring that all heparin has been removed from the patient's hemodynamic pressure monitoring system and avoiding the use of heparin flushes to maintain the patency of other intravenous lines is also essential.[13] Finally, prevention of subsequent episodes in patients sensitized to heparin is necessary. Patient and family education is essential. The use of medical alert bracelets and listing heparin allergies in the medical record will be necessary to avoid this serious complication in the future.

Collaborative management of the patient with Type 2 HIT is outlined in Box 27-5.

Box 27-4

NURSING DIAGNOSIS PRIORITIES

Heparin-Induced Thrombocytopenia

- Ineffective Cardiopulmonary Tissue Perfusion related to decreased coronary blood flow, p. A-35
- Ineffective Peripheral Tissue Perfusion related to decreased peripheral blood flow, p. A-41
- Ineffective Renal Tissue Perfusion related to decreased renal blood flow, p. A-42
- Ineffective Gastrointestinal Tissue Perfusion related to decreased gastrointestinal blood flow, p. A-40
- Ineffective Cerebral Tissue Perfusion related to decreased cerebral blood flow, p. A-36
- Powerlessness related to lack of control over current situation or disease progression, p. A-44
- Deficient Knowledge related to lack of previous exposure to information (see Patient Education: Heparin-Induced Thrombocytopenia), p. A-18

PATIENT EDUCATION

Heparin-Induced Thrombocytopenia

- Pathophysiology of disease
- Purpose of heparin
- Measures to avoid future exposure to heparin
  - Identify different types of heparin (unfractionated and low-molecular-weight)
  - Encourage purchase of medical alert bracelet or similar type of warning device
  - Tell any new health care provider about heparin allergy and previous reaction

TUMOR LYSIS SYNDROME

Tumor lysis syndrome (TLS) refers to a variety of metabolic disturbances that may be seen with the treatment of cancer. A potentially lethal complication of various forms of cancer treatment, TLS occurs when large numbers of neoplastic cells are rapidly killed, resulting in the release of large amounts of potassium, phosphate, and uric acid into the systemic circulation. It is most commonly seen in patients with lymphoma, leukemia, or multiple metastatic conditions.[15-17]

Box 27-5

Collaborative Management

Heparin-Induced Thrombocytopenia

- Stop all heparin exposure.
  - Unfractionated and low-molecular-weight heparins by any route
  - Heparin flushes
  - Heparin-coated vascular access devices
- Begin therapy with an alternative anticoagulant.
  - Lepirudin
  - Argatroban
- Maintain surveillance for complications.
  - Deep vein thrombosis
  - Pulmonary emboli
  - Acute limb ischemia
  - Cerebrovascular accident
  - Acute myocardial infarction
- Administer antifibrinolytic therapy (as indicated) if thrombosis occurs.
- Prepare patient for surgical embolectomy (as indicated) if thrombosis occurs.
- Provide comfort and emotional support.

ETIOLOGY

Though most often associated with the use of chemotherapeutic and biologic agents and radiation in the treatment of malignant disorders, TLS can in rare instances occur spontaneously. The development of TLS has been linked to other pathophysiologic conditions such as elevated white blood cell (WBC) counts, large tumors or multiple organ involvement, and renal insufficiency.[16,18]

PATHOPHYSIOLOGY

The primary mechanism involved in the development of TLS is the destruction of massive numbers of malignant cells, either by chemotherapy or radiation. This mass destruction results in the release of large amounts of potassium, phosphorus, and nucleic acids, leading to severe metabolic disturbances, such as hyperuricemia, hyperkalemia, hyperphosphatemia, and hypocalcemia (Table 27-4). Death in TLS is most often due to complications of renal failure or cardiac arrest.[15]

Hyperuricemia

Tumor cells undergo rapid growth and development, and therefore large amounts of nucleic acids are present within them. When therapy is initiated, tumor cell destruction causes the release of nucleic acids, which are metabolized into uric acid. Metabolic acidosis ensues, resulting in crystallization of the uric acid in the distal tubules of the kidney, leading to obstruction of flow. Glomerular filtration rates drop as the kidneys are unable to clear the increasing amounts of uric acid. Consequently, renal insufficiency and eventually acute renal failure occur. For further discussion on acute renal failure, see Chapter 20.

Table 27-4

Characteristic Electrolyte Abnormalities Encountered in Tumor Lysis Syndrome and Their Clinical Consequences

ELECTROLYTE	PATHOPHYSIOLOGY	CLINICAL CONSEQUENCE	TREATMENT OPTIONS
Potassium	Rapid expulsion of intracellular K^+ into the circulation due to cell lysis.	Adverse skeletal and cardiac manifestations (e.g., ventricular dysrhythmia, weakness, paresthesias)	Insulin/glucose, sodium bicarbonate, inhaled β-agonist, K-binding resins, dialysis, calcium gluconate
Phosphate	Release of intracellular PO_4^- due to cell lysis. May be compounded by renal dysfunction.	Muscle cramps, tetany, dysrhythmias, seizures	Dialysis, phosphate binders
Calcium	Precipitation of the calcium phosphate complex because of the rapid increase in the phosphorus concentration.	Muscle cramps, tetany, dysrhythmias, seizures, renal failure (acute nephrocalcinosis)	Calcium gluconate (treatment should be reserved for those with neuromuscular irritability)
Uric acid	Cell lysis leads to increased levels of purine nucleic acids into the circulation that are metabolized to uric acid.	Renal failure (uric acid nephropathy)	Hydration, dialysis, xanthine oxidase inhibitors, alkalization of urine, urate oxidase

From Davidson MB et al: *Am J Med* 116:546, 2004.

Hyperuricemia associated with TLS can be potentiated by several other factors, including elevated levels before the initiation of therapy. Other causes of increased uric acid production are elevated WBC counts, destruction of WBCs, and enlargement of the lymph nodes, spleen, or liver.[15-17]

Hyperkalemia

In addition to release of nucleic acids, destruction of tumor cells also results in the release of potassium. Renal insufficiency related to hyperuricemia prevents adequate excretion of potassium, and levels rise. The resultant hyperkalemia may have a profound effect on intracellular and extracellular fluid levels.[15] Left untreated, hyperkalemia can have devastating consequences, including cardiac arrest and death.[15,17]

Hyperphosphatemia and Hypocalcemia

Phosphorus levels also rise as a consequence of tumor cell destruction. Calcium ions then bind with the excess phosphorus, creating calcium phosphate salts and hypocalcemia. These salts precipitate in the kidney tubules, worsening renal insufficiency. Hypocalcemia causes tetany and cardiac dysrhythmias, which can result in cardiac arrest and death.[15,17]

Assessment and Diagnosis

Detection and recognition of TLS is accomplished through assessment of clinical manifestations, evaluation of laboratory findings, and other diagnostic tests. Table 27-5 provides a summary of common findings in TLS.[15-17]

Clinical Manifestations

Clinical manifestations are related to the metabolic disturbances associated with TLS. The patient history will reveal an unexplained weight gain following initiation of chemotherapy or radiation treatments. The weight gain is associated with fluid retention due to electrolyte disturbances. Other early signs heralding the onset of TLS include diarrhea, lethargy, muscle cramps, nausea and vomiting, paresthesias, and weakness.

Laboratory Findings

Laboratory findings will demonstrate electrolyte disturbances such as elevated potassium and phosphorus levels and a decreased calcium level. Uric acid levels will also rise. Elevations in BUN and creatinine and a decreased creatinine clearance are also indicative of TLS. Metabolic acidosis will be evident by the presence of decreased pH, bicarbonate levels, and $Paco_2$ on arterial blood gas values.

Other Diagnostic Tests

Physical examination will reveal positive Chvostek's and Trousseau's signs related to hypocalcemia. Hyperactive deep tendon reflexes are indicative of both hyperkalemia and hypocalcemia.[15] Potassium and calcium disturbances also result in changes that can be noted on the ECG such as peaked or inverted T waves, altered QT intervals, widened QRS complexes, and dysrhythmias.[15-17]

Table 27-5

Common Findings in Tumor Lysis Syndrome

DIAGNOSTIC PARAMETER	FINDINGS
Clinical	Weight gain, edema, diarrhea, lethargy, muscle cramps, nausea and vomiting, paresthesia, weakness, oliguria, uremia, seizures
Laboratory	↑ Potassium, phosphorus, uric acid, BUN, Cr ↓ Calcium, creatinine clearance, pH, bicarbonate, $Paco_2$
Diagnostic	Positive Chvostek's and Trousseau's signs, hyperactive deep tendon reflexes, dysrhythmias, ECG changes

BUN, Blood urea nitrogen; *Cr*, creatinine; *$Paco_2$*, partial pressure of carbon dioxide; *ECG*, electrocardiogram.

Medical Management

Medical interventions are aimed at maintaining adequate hydration, treating metabolic imbalances, and preventing life-threatening complications (see Table 27-4).[17] Administration of IV fluids may be necessary early on if inadequate hydration exists. The administration of isotonic saline (0.9% normal saline [NS]) reduces serum concentrations of uric acid, phosphate, and potassium.[17] The use of nonthiazide diuretics and/or low-dose dopamine to maintain adequate urine output may also be required.[19] If renal failure is present, hemodialysis should be considered.[17]

Levels of electrolytes and arterial blood gases are closely monitored. Dietary restrictions of potassium and phosphorus may be necessary. Hyperuricemia can be treated with administration of sodium bicarbonate and allopurinol. If potassium levels rise dangerously, Kayexalate may be given orally or, if the patient is unable to tolerate oral medications due to nausea and vomiting, rectal instillation may be used. If the patient is oliguric, glucose and insulin infusions may be given to facilitate lowering the potassium levels. Phosphorus-binding antacids can be used when hyperphosphatemia is present. Stool softeners may be necessary to treat constipation often associated with the administration of these antacids. Finally, calcium gluconate may be required to replace calcium.[15,19]

NURSING MANAGEMENT

Nursing management of the patient with TLS incorporates a variety of nursing diagnoses (Box 27-6). **Nursing priorities are directed toward (1) monitoring the patient's fluid and electrolytes, (2) providing comfort and emotional support, and (3) maintaining surveillance for complications.** Assessment and continued monitoring of the patient is an important role of the critical care nurse when caring for the patient with TLS. Recognizing critical laboratory changes or development of symptoms and notifying the physician in a timely manner are essential. Insertion of a urinary catheter and maintenance of the IV site are necessary in monitoring and ensuring adequate intake and output. Frequent vital signs and daily weight should also be monitored.

Nursing interventions are also aimed at preventing complications. Instituting seizure precautions will be necessary, especially if calcium levels are disrupted. Insertion of a nasogastric tube if nausea or vomiting is present is appropriate. Dietary adjustments will also be necessary, such as potassium and phosphorus restrictions in the presence of elevated serum levels and providing additional fiber to combat diarrhea associated with the administration of antacids.

Education of the patient and family is also a primary role of the critical care nurse. All treatments and interventions should be explained before carrying them out and questions answered at a level understandable to the patient and family. Before discharge, potential risk factors and identification of early signs and symptoms should be reviewed.

Collaborative management of the patient with TLS is outlined in Box 27-7.

Box 27-6

NURSING DIAGNOSIS PRIORITIES

Tumor Lysis Syndrome

- Excess Fluid Volume related to renal dysfunction, p. A-24
- Decreased Cardiac Output related to alterations in contractility, p. A-12
- Anxiety related to threat to biologic, psychologic, and/or social integrity, p. A-9
- Ineffective Coping related to situational crisis and personal vulnerability, p. A-38

Box 27-7

Collaborative Management

Tumor Lysis Syndrome

- Facilitate adequate renal function.
  - Volume hydration with 0.9% NS
  - Nonthiazide diuretics
  - Low-dose dopamine
- Treat hyperkalemia.
  - Kayexalate
  - Glucose and insulin
- Treat hyperuricemia.
  - Sodium bicarbonate
  - Allopurinol
- Treat hyperphosphatemia.
  - Dietary restrictions
  - Phosphorus-binding antacids
- Treat hypocalcemia.
  - Calcium gluconate
- Maintain surveillance for complications.
  - Acute renal failure
  - Cardiac dysrhythmias
- Provide comfort and emotional support.

NS, Normal saline.

evolve To test your mastery of this chapter, try the Open-Book Quiz at http://evolve.elsevier.com/Urden/priorities/

REFERENCES

1. Levi M: Disseminated intravascular coagulation: What's new? *Crit Care Clin* 21:449, 2005.
2. Geiter H: Disseminated intravascular coagulation, *Dimens Crit Care Nurs* 22:108, 2003.
3. Lapointe LA, VonRueden KT: Coagulopathies in trauma patients, *AACN Clin Issues Crit Care Nurs* 13:192, 2002.
4. Toh CH, Dennis M: Disseminated intravascular coagulation: old disease, new hope, *BMJ* 327:974, 2003.
5. Vincent JL, De Backer D: Does disseminated intravascular coagulation lead to multiple organ failure? *Crit Care Clin* 21:469, 2005.
6. Slofstra SH, Spek CA, ten Cate H: Disseminated intravascular coagulation, *Hematol J* 4:295, 2003.
7. McCance KL: Structure and function of the hematologic system. In McCance KL, Huether SE, editors: *Pathophysiology: the biologic basis for disease in adults and children,* ed 5, St Louis, 2006, Mosby.
8. Bick RL: Disseminated intravascular coagulation current concepts of etiology, pathophysiology, diagnosis, and treatment, *Hematol Oncol Clin North Am* 17:149, 2003.
9. Housholder-Hughes SD, Bennett J: *The nurses' role in managing HIT: preventing life- and limb-threatening thrombosis*, Aliso Viejo, Calif, 2003, American Association of Critical Care Nurses.
10. Arepally GM, Ortel TL: Heparin-induced thrombocytopenia, *N Eng J Med* 355:809, 2006.
11. Cooney MF: Heparin-induced thrombocytopenia, *Crit Care Nurse* 26(6):30, 2006.
12. Jang IK, Hursting MJ: When heparins promote thrombosis: review of heparin-induced thrombocytopenia, *Circ* 111:2671, 2005.
13. Warkentin TE, Greinacher A, editors: *Heparin-induced thrombocytopenia*, ed 3, New York, 2004, Marcel Dekker.
14. Menajovsky LB: Heparin-induced thrombocytopenia: clinical manifestations and management strategies, *Am J Med* 118(suppl 8A):21S, 2005.

15. Robison J: Tumor lysis syndrome. In Chernecky CC, Berger BJ, editors, *Advanced and critical care oncology nursing,* Philadelphia, 1998, WB Saunders.
16. Cantril CA, Haylock PJ: Tumor lysis syndrome, *Am J Nurs* 104(4):49, 2004.
17. Davidson MB et al: Pathophysiology, clinical consequences, and treatment of tumor lysis syndrome, *Am J Med* 116:546, 2004.
18. Otto SE: *Oncology nursing clinical reference,* St. Louis, 2004, Mosby.
19. Gobel BH: Management of tumor lysis syndrome: prevention and treatment, *Semin Oncol Nurs* 3(suppl 3):12, 2002.

APPENDIX A

Nursing Management Plans of Care

NURSING MANAGEMENT PLAN
Activity Intolerance

Definition: Insufficient physiologic or psychologic energy to endure or complete required or desired daily activities.

Activity Intolerance Related to Cardiopulmonary Dysfunction

DEFINING CHARACTERISTICS
- Chest pain with activity
- Electrocardiographic changes with activity
- Heart rate elevations 15 beats/min above baseline with activity for patients on β-blockers or calcium channel blockers
- Heart rate elevations above baseline 5 minutes after activity
- Breathlessness with activity
- Spo_2 <92% with activity
- Postural hypotension when moving from supine to upright position
- Patient reports fatigue with activity

OUTCOME CRITERIA
- Heart rate elevations are less than 20 beats/min above baseline with activity and are less than 10 beats/min above baseline with activity for patients on β-blockers or calcium channel blockers.
- Heart rate returns to baseline 5 minutes after activity.
- Chest pain with activity is absent.
- Patient reports tolerance to activity.

NURSING INTERVENTIONS AND *RATIONALE*
1. Encourage active or passive range-of-motion exercises while the patient is in bed *to keep joints flexible and muscles stretched.*
2. Teach patient to refrain from holding breath while performing exercises and *to avoid the Valsalva maneuver.*
3. Encourage performance of muscle-toning exercises at least 3 times daily, because a toned muscle uses less oxygen when performing work than an untoned muscle.
4. Progress ambulation to increase tolerance to activity.
5. Teach patient to take pulse *to determine activity tolerance:* Take pulse for full minute *before exercise* and then for 10 seconds and multiply by 6 *at exercise peak.*

Activity Intolerance Related to Prolonged Immobility or Deconditioning

DEFINING CHARACTERISTICS
- Systolic blood pressure (SBP) drop >20 mm Hg; heart rate increase >20 beats/min with postural change
- Syncope with postural change
- Patient reports light-headedness with postural change

OUTCOME CRITERIA
- SBP drop is less than 10 mm Hg; heart rate increase is less than 10 beats/min with postural change.
- Syncope or light-headedness is absent with postural change.

NURSING INTERVENTIONS AND *RATIONALE*
1. Instruct the patient in how to perform straight leg raises, dorsiflexion/plantar flexion, and quadriceps-setting and gluteal-setting exercises *to increase muscular and vascular tone.*
2. Consult with physician regarding the administration of fluids to ensure that the patient is hydrated to 24-hour fluid requirements per body surface area (BSA) *to increase preload and thus stroke volume and cardiac output.*
3. Reposition patient incrementally *to avoid syncope:*
   - Head of bed to 45 degrees, and hold until symptom-free.
   - Head of bed to 90 degrees, and hold until symptom-free.
   - Dangle until symptom-free.
   - Stand until symptom-free, and ambulate.
4. Collaborate with physician regarding patient's activity level *to ensure patient's safety.*

NURSING MANAGEMENT PLAN
Acute Confusion

Definition: Abrupt onset of a cluster of global, transient changes and disturbances in attention, cognition, psychomotor activity, level of consciousness, and/or sleep/wake cycle.

Acute Confusion Related to Sensory Overload, Sensory Deprivation, and Sleep Pattern Disturbance

DEFINING CHARACTERISTICS

Early Symptoms

- Sudden onset of global cognitive function impairment (from hours to days)
- Restlessness, agitation, and combative behavior
- Drowsiness (can lead to loss of consciousness)
- Slurring of speech, inappropriate statements or "word salad," mumbling, or inappropriate gestures
- Short attention span (needs questions repeated); inability to learn new material
- Disordered sleep/wake cycle
- Disorientation to person, time, place, and situation
- Difficulty in separating dreams from reality (may experience bizarre dreams or nightmares)
- Anger at staff for continued questions about his or her orientation

Later Symptoms

- Symptoms that tend to fluctuate throughout the day and night
- Continuations of early symptoms, which may be more frequent or of longer duration
- Illusions
- Hallucinations
- Extreme agitation (e.g., attempts to climb out of bed, pull out catheters, rip off dressings)
- Calling out in loud voice, swearing, or attempting to bite or hit people who approach patient

NURSING INTERVENTIONS AND *RATIONALE*

1. Determine and document the patient's dominant spoken language, his or her literacy, and the language(s) in which he or she is literate. *Sometimes people are not literate in their spoken language, or less commonly, they are literate only in their second language.*
2. Determine and document patient's premorbid degree of orientation, cognitive capabilities, and any sensory-perceptual deficits. *Assuming that the patient was or was not fully oriented before critical care admission bases the nurse's assessment on possibly erroneous assumptions.*

Sensory Overload

1. Initiate each nurse-patient encounter by calling the patient by name and identifying yourself by name. *This fosters reality orientation and assists the patient in filtering irrelevant or impersonal conversation.*
2. Assess the patient's immediate physical environment from his or her viewpoint, and explain equipment, its sounds, and its therapeutic purpose. Demonstrate audible and visual alarms, and explain possible alarm conditions. *This decreases alienation of the patient from the technologic environment and reduces the inherent sense of fear and urgency accompanying alarm conditions.*
3. For each procedure performed, provide "preparatory sensory information" (i.e., explain procedures in relation to the sensations the patient will experience, including duration of sensations). *Preparatory sensory information enhances learning and lessens anticipatory anxiety.*
4. Limit noise levels. Certainly, audible alarms cannot and must not be silenced, and many critical, albeit noisy, activities must take place in the critical care area. It has been shown, however, that noise levels produced by clinical personnel exceed those levels designated as "acceptable" and are often greater than those generated by technologic devices. Staff conversations must be kept soft enough that they are inaudible to the patient whenever possible. Critical care personnel are to assume that everything said at or around a patient's bedside is intended for that patient's awareness and that it will be interpreted as pertaining to him or her. *As in the discussion that follows, conversations about the patient but not to him or her foster depersonalization and delusions of reference.*
5. Enforce nighttime noise limits.
6. Readjust alarm limits on physiologic monitoring devices as the patient's condition changes (improves or deteriorates) *to lessen unnecessary alarm states.*
7. Consider use of headphones and compact disk or digital music player with patient's favorite and/or subliminal or classical music. *This can effectively filter out assaultive noise of the critical care environment and supplant it with familiar, soothing sounds and rhythms.*
8. Modify lighting. Day/night cycles need to be simulated with environmental lighting. At no time should overhead fluorescent lights be turned on abruptly without warning the patient, assisting him or her out of the supine position, and/or shielding his or her eyes with gauze or a face cloth. *Continuous bright lighting sustains anxiety and promotes circadian rhythm desynchronization.*
9. To the extent possible, shield patients from viewing urgent and emergent events in the critical care unit. Resuscitation efforts, albeit difficult to conceal, engender fear in the patient and a sense of instability and vulnerability (e.g., "I'm next"). When such an event occurs, the nurse needs to elicit the patient's cognitive and emotional reaction; thoughts, impressions, and feelings need to be shared and misconceptions clarified. A useful approach for the nurse in this interchange is that of emphasizing the differences between the patient at hand and the one resuscitated (e.g., "He was considerably older," "He was more unstable," "He had serious lung disease").
10. Ensure patients' privacy, their modesty, and, at the very least, their dignity. Physical exposure and nudity, although seemingly pale in importance compared with such priorities as physiologic assessment and stabilization, are primal indignities in all individuals. Patients must be

Continued

NURSING MANAGEMENT PLAN—*cont'd*
Acute Confusion—*cont'd*

Acute Confusion Related to Sensory Overload, Sensory Deprivation, and Sleep Pattern Disturbance—*cont'd*

kept minimally exposed. When, in the course of assessment and intervention, it becomes necessary to expose the patient, the nurse is to first verbally apologize for this necessity. *To be naked is to feel vulnerable; to be vulnerable is to feel fearful. In this regard, fear is an emotion concomitant to critical care that is preventable through nursing intervention.*

Sensory Deprivation

1. Provide reality orientation in four spheres (personal, place, time, and situation) at more frequent intervals than when testing. Convey this information in the context of routine conversation. *Sample statements:* "Mr. Clark, this is Tuesday morning and you're in University Hospital. Your heart surgery was yesterday morning, and you're doing well. My name is Joe, and I'm your nurse today." *The patient is made to feel patronized by repetitions such as, "Do you know where you are?"* Given the effects of general anesthesia, narcotic analgesics, sedatives, and sleep, it is expected that some degree of disorientation will exist normally.
2. Ensure the patient's visual access to a calendar.
3. Apprise the patient of daily news events and the weather.
4. Touch patients for the express purpose of communicating caring. Hold their hands, stroke their brows, rub the skin on an aspect of the arms. *Touch is the universal language of caring. In the setting of critical care, in which there is considerable physical body manipulation, it is useful and important to contrast assaultive touch with comforting touch.* Touch can be used as a technique for distraction from painful stimuli when used in conjunction with uncomfortable procedures. (IMPORTANT: See discussion of the use of touch in management of the patient experiencing hallucinations.)
5. Foster liberal visitation by family and significant others. Encourage significant others to touch the patient as consistent with their individual comfort level and cultural norms.
6. Structure and identify opportunities for the patient to exercise decision-making skills, however small. Although not so designated, patients with sensory alterations experience a type of "cognitive deprivation" as well.
7. Assist patients with finding meaning in their experiences. Explain the therapeutic purpose of all they are asked to do for themselves and all that is done with them and for them. Avoid statements such as "Will you turn to that side for me?" or "I need you to swallow this medication." *These statements implicitly convey that the maneuver has some value for the nurses versus the patient.* Similarly, use "thank you" judiciously. *This simple salutation, when used indiscriminately, suggests something was done to benefit the nurses and not the patient.* Patients need to find meaning and to identify their roles in the experience of critical illness and critical care. The sensations that constitute this experience and those that do not are made bearable and intelligible when attached to a larger picture of their condition, treatment, and progress.

Hallucinations

1. Approach the patient with a calm, matter-of-fact demeanor. The goal of this interaction is for the nurse to demonstrate external control. This helps decrease the anxiety and fear that generally accompany hallucinations and allows the patient to feel safe. Anxiety is transferable.
2. Address the patient by name. This is a useful presentation of reality because self-identity is the last sphere of orientation to vanish.
3. In responding to the patient's description of the hallucination, do not deny, argue, or attempt to disprove the existence of the perceived event. *Statements such as "There are no voices coming from that air vent" or "Look, I'm brushing my hand across the wall, and there are no bugs" confuse the patient further, because the hallucination, although frightening, is his or her perceived reality.*
4. Express to the patient that your experiences are dissimilar, and acknowledge how frightening his or hers must be. *Sample statements:* "I don't hear (see, etc.) what you do, but I know how frightening such an experience must be to you. I'm Joe, your nurse, and I'm going to stay with you until the voices (etc.) go away." Remain with any patient who is experiencing a hallucination. *Feelings of fear and anxiety often accelerate when a patient is left alone. He or she needs someone to represent a nonthreatening reality. In addition, validating the patient's feelings demonstrates acceptance and sensitivity to the experience and promotes trust.*
5. Do not explore the content of the hallucination with the patient by asking about its nature or character. The nurse is the patient's link with reality. Pursuit of a detailed description of a hallucination may signify to the patient that the nurse accepts his or her sensory distortion as factual. This may further confuse the patient and distance him or her more from reality. (An exception is the patient who the nurse suspects is experiencing auditory hallucinations [i.e., hearing "voice commands"]. To ascertain that the voices are not telling the patient to harm himself or herself, it is appropriate for the nurse to ask simply and concretely, "What are the voices saying?") The nurse can help bridge the gap between the patient's misperception and reality by addressing the feelings (e.g., fear, anxiety) and/or meanings (e.g., danger, death) engendered by the hallucination. Determining how the misperception affects the patient emotionally, acknowledging those feelings, and using a calm, controlled, matter-of-fact approach will provide the trust and comfort the patient needs to tolerate this frightening experience. In other words, deal with the intent more than the content of the hallucination. The resultant decrease in anxiety will enable the patient to focus more accurately on his or her immediate environment.
6. Talk concretely with the patient about things that are really happening. *Sample statements:* "How does your

NURSING MANAGEMENT PLAN—*cont'd*

chest incision feel this afternoon, Mr. Clark?" "Your sister Kate was here to see you, but you were sleeping. She went down to the cafeteria and will be back." "Your secretions are a little easier for you to cough up today." ***Interpretation of reality-based stimuli by the nurse encourages the patient to focus on actual circumstances and discourages a preoccupation with sensory misperceptions.***

7. There may be circumstances in which it is appropriate for the nurse simply to distract the patient by changing the topic. This tactic is useful in situations of escalating anxiety and confusion or when all else fails. Topics need to consist of basic themes that are universally understood and culturally congruent, such as music, food, or weather. They may also be topics of special interest to the patient, such as hobbies, crafts, or sports. Topics that evoke strong emotions, such as politics, religion, or sexuality, are to be avoided with most patients. ***This is especially true of the patient with reality distortions; sometimes hallucinations and delusions are expressions of repressed conflicts associated with religious, sexual, or aggressive issues. Pursuit of such subjects could increase confusion and anxiety.***
8. Consider the following regarding the use of touch. Touch presents a nonthreatening external reality and can therefore be useful in the management of patients with sensory alterations. However, for the patient experiencing hallucinations (as well as delusions and illusions), touch can be readily misinterpreted as, for instance, aggression or pain, or it can actually provide the basis for a tactile illusion. Therefore avoid the use of touch as an intervention strategy for any patient who demonstrates escalating anxiety or paranoid, suspicious, or mistrustful thoughts.
9. Auditory hallucinations
   - *Patient behaviors:* Head cocked as if listening to an unseen presence; lips moving.
   - *Therapeutic nurse responses:* "Mr. Clark, you appear to be listening to something." If the patient acknowledges voices, respond, "I don't hear any voices, but I know this is troubling you. The voices will go away. Nothing is going to harm you. I'm Joe, your nurse, and I'll be here with you."
   - *Nontherapeutic nurse responses:* "Tell me about your conversations with these voices." "To whom do these voices belong—anyone you know?"
10. Visual hallucinations
    - *Patient behaviors:* Staring into space as if focused on an unseen object; startled movements and anxious facial expression.
    - *Therapeutic nurse responses:* "Mr. Clark, something seems to be troubling you. Tell me what it is." If patient states he visualizes people, images, or the devil in his environment and implies a sense of danger, respond, "There are only nurses and doctors here, Mr. Clark. I know this must be upsetting, but these images will go away. We're here with you in the hospital. Nothing will happen to you."
    - *Nontherapeutic nurse responses:* "Describe the people you see. What are they wearing?" "What does the devil mean in your life? What about God?"

Delusions

1. Explain all unseen noises, voices, and activity simply and clearly. ***They readily feed a delusional system.*** *Sample statements:* "That is Dr. Smith. He's come to see you and other patients here in the hospital." "The voices and activity you hear are from the bedside of the patient behind this curtain. He's being helped by one of the nurses."
2. Avoid the "negative challenge" of the patient's delusions (e.g., "Nobody here stole your belongings," "Doctors and nurses do not harm people"). Similarly, avoid defending the referents of the patient's belief (e.g., "Nurses are good," "Doctors mean well"). ***Remember, a delusion is a belief, albeit false, that cannot be changed with logic. To attempt this change is to challenge the patient's belief system and thereby escalate his or her anxiety, further blurring the boundaries between reality and the patient's internally based "logic."***
3. For the patient with persecutory delusions who refuses food, fluids, or medications because of a belief that they have been poisoned or are tainted, permit the refusal unless it is a life-threatening event. Try again in 20 minutes; allow the patient to choose an alternative selection of food, or to read the label on the unit's medication. Coercion, show of force, or engagement in complicated, logical justifications will only heighten the patient's suspiciousness and possibly reinforce the delusional belief. ***When the patient feels more in control, he or she need not rely on the "paradoxical" quality of the delusion to equip him or her with a false sense of power. His or her power instead is derived from making reality-based decisions.***
4. Staff members should be particularly careful not to engage in unnecessary laughter or whispering within view of the delusional patient. ***The delusional patient is hypervigilant, scanning the environment for evidence to corroborate or confirm his or her belief that staff members are colluding against him or her; clearly, laughter and whispers easily suggest this belief, this delusion of reference. This rationale pertains to the patient experiencing hallucinations and/or illusions as well.***
5. Observe the principles detailed in the third intervention of Hallucinations

Illusions

1. As with the management of delusions, the nurse simply and briefly interprets a reality-based stimulus for the patient in a calm, matter-of-fact manner. ***Seen and unseen noises, voices, activity, and people can provide the stimulus for a sensory misinterpretation, an illusion.***
2. There should be minimal stimulation in the patient's immediate environment. Nursing interventions detailed previously under Sensory Overload are especially relevant here.
3. The theme of the nurse's verbal approach to the patient experiencing illusions is similar to that outlined for hallucinations and delusions: address the feeling and meaning associated with the experience, not the content of the sensory misinterpretation.
   - *Patient behaviors:* Eyes darting, startled movements, frightened facial expression. "I know who you are. You're the devil come to take me to hell."

Continued

NURSING MANAGEMENT PLAN—*cont'd*

Acute Confusion—*cont'd*

Acute Confusion Related to Sensory Overload, Sensory Deprivation, and Sleep Pattern Disturbance—*cont'd*

- *Therapeutic nurse response:* "I'm Joe, your nurse. I know this experience is troubling for you. You're in the hospital, and no one here will harm you."
- *Nontherapeutic nurse responses:* "There are no such things as devils and angels." "Do you think the devil would be dressed in white?" *The first nontherapeutic nurse response carries a parental tone (i.e., "You know better than that."), thus infantilizing the patient and adding to his or her feelings of powerlessness over the environment. The second nontherapeutic response reflects obvious logic, which is not in the patient's sensory domain; therefore it cannot be processed and only adds to his or her confused state.*

4. Observe the principles detailed in the fifth intervention of Hallucinations.

NURSING MANAGEMENT PLAN
Acute Pain

Definition: Unpleasant sensory and emotional experience arising from actual or potential tissue damage or described in terms of such damage (International Association for the Study of Pain); sudden or slow onset of any intensity from mild to severe with an anticipated or predictable end and a duration of less than 6 months.

Acute Pain Related to Transmission of Perception of Cutaneous, Visceral, Muscular, or Ischemic Impulses

DEFINING CHARACTERISTICS

Subjective
- Patient verbalizes presence of pain.
- Patient rates pain on scale of 0 to 10 using a visual analog scale.

Objective
- Increase in blood pressure (BP), heart rate (HR), and respiratory rate (RR)
- Pupillary dilation
- Diaphoresis, pallor
- Skeletal muscle reactions (grimacing, clenching fists, writhing, pacing, guarding or splinting of affected part)
- Apprehension, fearful appearance
- May not exhibit any physiologic change

OUTCOME CRITERIA

NOTE: Outcome is highly variable, depending on individual patient and pain circumstance factors.
- Patient verbalizes that pain is reduced to a tolerable level or is totally relieved.
- Patient's pain rating is lower on scale of 1 to 10.
- BP, HR, and RR return to baseline 5 minutes after administration of intravenous (IV) narcotic or 20 minutes after administration of intramuscular (IM) narcotic.

NURSING INTERVENTIONS AND *RATIONALE*

Modification of Variables That Heighten the Patient's Experience of Pain
1. Explain to the patient that frequent, detailed, and seemingly repetitive assessments will be conducted to allow the nurse to better understand the patient's pain experience, not because the existence of pain is in question.
2. Explain the factors responsible for pain production in the individual. Estimate the expected duration of the pain if possible.
3. Explain diagnostic and therapeutic procedures to the patient in relation to sensations the patient should expect to feel.
4. Reduce the patient's fear of addiction by explaining the difference between drug tolerance and drug addiction. Drug tolerance is a physiologic phenomenon in which a drug does begins to lose effectiveness after repeated doses; drug dependence is a psychologic phenomenon in which narcotics are used regularly for emotional, not medical, reasons.
5. Instruct the patient to ask for pain medication when pain is beginning and not to wait until it is intolerable.
6. Explain that the physician will be consulted if pain relief is inadequate with the present medication.
7. Instruct patient in the importance of adequate rest, especially when it reduces pain *to maintain strength and coping abilities and to reduce stress.*

Pharmacologic Interventions (in Collaboration With Physician)

POSTSURGICAL OR POSTTRAUMATIC CUTANEOUS, MUSCULAR, OR VISCERAL PAIN
1. Medicate with narcotic maximally to break the pain cycles as long as level of consciousness and vital signs are stable: check patient's previous response to similar dosage and narcotic. NOTE: First dose received postoperatively is usually reduced by one half *to evaluate patient's individual response to medication.*
2. Provide continuous analgesia, as required by continuous pain.
   - Establish optimal analgesic dose that brings optimal pain relief.
   - Offer pain medication at prescribed regular intervals rather than making patient ask for it *to maintain more steady blood levels.*
   - Consider waking patient to avoid loss of opiate blood levels during sleep.
3. If administering medication on as-necessary (PRN) basis, give it when the patient's pain is just beginning, rather than at its peak. Advise patient to intercept pain, not endure it, or several hours and higher doses of narcotics may be necessary to relieve pain, leading to a cycle of undermedication and pain alternating with overmedication and drug toxicity.
4. Perform rehabilitation exercises (turn, deep breathe, leg exercises, ambulate) shortly before peak of drug effect *because this will be the optimal time for the patient to increase activity with the least risk of increasing pain.*
5. When making the transition from one drug to another or from IM or IV to oral (PO) medication, the use of an equianalgesic chart is helpful. Equianalgesic means *approximately* the same pain relief. Many consider the IM and IV dose of medications equianalgesic; however, others recommend using one half the IM dose for the IV dose. To effectively use analgesics, each patient requires an individual choice of drug, dose, time interval, and route. The patient's response should be closely monitored to determine if the right analgesic choice was made.
6. Assess effectiveness of pain medication.
   - Reevaluate pain 5 minutes after IV and 20 minutes after IM medication administration, observe patient's behavior, and ask patient to rate pain on scale of 1 to 10.
   - Collaborate with physician to add or delete other medications that potentiate the action of analgesics, such as antiemetics, hypnotics, sedatives, or muscle relaxants.
   - Observe for indicators of undertreatment: report of pain not relieved; observed restlessness, sleeplessness, irritability, and anorexia; decreased activity level.

Continued

NURSING MANAGEMENT PLAN—*cont'd*
Acute Pain—*cont'd*

Acute Pain Related to Transmission of Perception of Cutaneous, Visceral, Muscular, or Ischemic Impulses—*cont'd*

- Observe for indicators of overtreatment: hypotension or bradycardia; respiratory rate <10/ min; excessive sedation.

7. If IV patient-controlled analgesia (PCA) is used, do the following. (NOTE: PCA allows patients to administer small doses of their prescribed medication when they feel the need. Constant levels of the drug in the bloodstream mean lower doses can be used to obtain analgesia. Pain control is improved because the patient is in control and experiences less fear of unrelieved pain. Reduced net narcotic use is noted, as is less sedation. Critical care patients appropriate for PCA are those who are alert, such as burn patients, trauma patients without head injury, and some postoperative patients.)
   - Instruct the patient in what the drug is, the dose, and how often it can be self-administered by pushing the button to activate the PCA machine. For example, "When you have pain, instead of asking the nurse to bring medication, push the button that activates the machine and a small dose of the pain medicine will be injected into your IV line. You can keep your pain under control by administering additional medicine as soon as your pain begins to return or increases. Also, push the button before undertaking a painful activity, such as ambulation. Try to balance your pain relief against sleepiness, and don't activate the machine if you start to feel sleepy. If your pain medicine seems to stop working despite pushing the button several times, call the nurse to check your IV. If you are not receiving adequate pain relief, the nurse will call your doctor."
   - Monitor vital signs, especially BP and RR, every hour for the first 4 hours, and assess postural HR and BP before initial ambulation.
   - Monitor respirations every 2 hours while patient is on patient-controlled analgesia.
   - If patient's respirations decrease to <10/min or if patient is overly sedated, anticipate IV administration of naloxone.
8. If epidural narcotic analgesia is used, do the following. (NOTE: The delivery of narcotics, such as morphine or fentanyl, by epidural route to specific receptors in the spinal cord selectively blocks pain impulses to the brain for up to 24 hours. Effective analgesia can be obtained without many of the negative side effects or serum narcotic concentrations.)
   - Keep patient's head elevated 30 to 45 degrees after injection *to prevent respiratory depressant effects.*
   - Observe closely for respiratory depression up to 24 hours after injection. Monitor respiratory rate every 15 minutes for 1 hour; every 30 minutes for 7 hours; and every hour for the remaining 16 hours.
   - Assess for adequate cough reflex.
   - Avoid use of other central nervous system (CNS) depressants, such as sedatives.
   - Observe for reports of pruritus, nausea, and vomiting.
   - Anticipate administration of naloxone for respiratory depression (and smaller doses of naloxone for pruritus).
   - Assess for and treat urinary retention.
   - Assess epidural catheter site for local infection. Keep catheter taped securely *to prevent catheter migration.*

PERIPHERAL VASCULAR ISCHEMIC PAIN (HYPOTHETIC VASCULAR OCCLUSION OF LEG)

1. Correctly identify and differentiate ischemic pain from other types of pain. (NOTE: Ischemic pain is usually a burning, aching pain made worse by exercise and lessened or relieved by rest. Eventually the pain occurs at rest. Coldness and pallor of extremity may be noted, especially if the limb is elevated above the heart level. Rubor and mottling of the skin may be evident from prolonged tissue anoxia and inability of damaged vessels to constrict. Eventually cyanosis and gangrenous tissue will be evident. Chronic ischemia leads to visible changes in the limb, such as flaking skin, brittle nails and hair, leg ulcers, and cellulitis).
2. Administer pain medications, and evaluate their effectiveness as previously described. Remember that the pain of ischemia is chronic and continuous and can make the patient irritable and depressed.
3. Treat the cause of the ischemic pain, and institute measures to increase circulation to the affected part.

Nonpharmacologic Interventions

1. Treat contributing factors; provide explanations (see Pharmacologic Interventions).
2. Apply comfort measures.
   - Use relaxation techniques, such as back rubs, massage, warm baths, music, and aromatherapy. Use blankets and pillows *to support the painful part and reduce muscle tension.* Encourage slow, rhythmic breathing.
   - Encourage progressive muscle relaxation techniques.
     (1) Instruct patient to inhale and tense (tighten) specific muscle groups and then relax the muscles as exhalation occurs.
     (2) Suggest an order for performing the tension/relaxation cycle (e.g., start with facial muscles and move down body, ending with toes).
   - Encourage guided imagery.
     (1) Ask patient to recall an experienced image that is very pleasurable and relaxing and involves at least two senses.
     (2) Have patient begin with rhythmic breathing and progressive relaxation and then travel mentally to the scene.
     (3) Have the patient slowly experience the scene (how it looks, sounds, smells, feels).
     (4) Ask patient to practice this imagery in private.
     (5) Instruct patient to end the imagery by counting to three and saying, "Now I'm relaxed." If person does not end the imagery and falls asleep, the purpose of the technique is defeated.

NURSING MANAGEMENT PLAN
Anxiety

Definition: Vague uneasy feeling of discomfort or dread accompanied by an autonomic response (the source often nonspecific or unknown to the individual); a feeling of apprehension caused by anticipation of danger. It is an alerting signal that warns of impending danger and enables the individual to take measures to deal with threat.

Anxiety Related to Threat to Biologic, Psychologic, and/or Social Integrity

DEFINING CHARACTERISTICS

Subjective

- Verbalizes increased muscle tension
- Expresses frequent sensation of tingling in hands and feet
- Relates continuous feeling of apprehension
- Expresses preoccupation with a sense of impending doom
- Reports difficulty falling asleep
- Repeatedly expresses concerns about changes in health status and outcome of illness

Objective

- Psychomotor agitation (fidgeting, jitteriness, restlessness)
- Tightened, wrinkled brow
- Strained (worried) facial expression
- Hypervigilance (scans environment)
- Startles easily
- Distractibility
- Sweaty palms
- Fragmented sleep patterns
- Tachycardia
- Tachypnea

OUTCOME CRITERIA

- Patient effectively uses learned relaxation strategies.
- Patient demonstrates significant decrease in psychomotor agitation.
- Patient verbalizes reduction in tingling sensations in hands and feet.
- Patient is able to focus on the tasks at hand.
- Patient expresses positive, future-based plans to family and staff.
- Patient's heart rate and rhythm remain within limits commensurate with physiologic status.

NURSING INTERVENTIONS AND *RATIONALE*

1. Instruct the patient in the following simple, effective relaxation strategies:
   - If not contraindicated for cardiovascular reasons, tense and relax all muscles progressively from toes to head.
   - Perform slow deep-breathing exercises.
   - Focus on a single object or person in the environment.
   - Listen to soothing music or relaxation tapes with eyes closed.

   Progressive toe-to-head relaxation releases the muscular tension that may be a stress-related effect resulting from the threat or change in the patient's health status and outcome of illness. Deep-breathing exercises provide slow, rhythmic, controlled breathing patterns that relax the patient and distract him or her from the effects of his or her illness and hospitalization. Focusing on a single object or person helps the patient dismiss myriad disorienting stimuli from his or her visual-perceptual field, which can have a dizzying, distorted effect. A clear sensorium allows him or her to feel more in control of his or her environment. Music or words expressed in soft, low tones tend to produce soothing, relaxing effects that counteract or inhibit escalating anxiety and provide respites from the patient's situational crisis. Closed eyes eliminate distracting visual stimuli and promote a more restful environment.
2. Actively listen to and accept the patient's concerns regarding the threats from his or her illness, outcome, and hospitalization. *Active listening and unconditional acceptance validate the patient as a worthwhile individual and assure him or her that his or her concerns, no matter how great, will be addressed. Knowledge that he or she has an avenue for ventilation will assuage anxiety.*
3. Help the patient distinguish between realistic concerns and exaggerated fears through clear, simple explanations. *Sample statements:* "Your lab results show that you're doing OK right now." "The shortness of breath you're experiencing is not unusual." "The pain you described is expected, and this medication will relieve it." *A patient who is informed about his or her progress and is reassured about expected symptoms and management of care will be better equipped to maintain a more realistic perspective of his or her illness and its outcome. Thus anxiety emanating from imagined or exaggerated fears will likely be assuaged or averted.*
4. Provide simple clarification of environmental events and stimuli that are not related to the patient's illness and care. *Sample statements:* "That loud noise is coming from a machine that is helping another patient." "The visitor behind the curtain is crying because she's had an upsetting day." "That gurney is here to take another patient to x-ray." *Clarification of events and stimuli that are unrelated to the patient helps to disengage him or her from the extant anxiety-provoking situations surrounding him or her, thus avoiding further anxiety and apprehension.*
5. Assist the patient in focusing on building on prior coping strategies to deal with the effects of his or her illness and care. *Sample statements:* "What methods have helped you get through difficult times in the past?" "How can we help you use those methods now?" (See plan for Ineffective Coping for interventions that assist patients with using coping strategies effectively.) *Use of previously successful coping strategies in conjunction with newly learned techniques arms the patient with an arsenal of weapons against anxiety, providing him or her with greater control over the situational crisis and decreased feelings of doom and despair.*
6. Give the patient permission to deny or suppress the effects of his or her illness and hospitalization with which he or she cannot cope or control. *Sample statements:* "It's perfectly okay to ignore things you can't handle right now." "How can we help ease your mind during this time?" "What are some things or tasks that may help distract you?" *Adaptive denial can be helpful in reducing feelings of anxiety in patients with life-threatening illness.*

NURSING MANAGEMENT PLAN
Autonomic Dysreflexia

Definition: Life-threatening, uninhibited sympathetic response of the nervous system to a noxious stimulus after a spinal cord injury at T7 or above.

Autonomic Dysreflexia Related to Excessive Autonomic Response to Noxious Stimuli (e.g., Distended Bladder, Distended Bowel, Skin Irritation)

DEFINING CHARACTERISTICS

Major

- Paroxysmal hypertension (sudden periodic elevated blood pressure [BP] greater than 20 mm Hg above patient's normal BP); for many spinal cord injury patients, a normal BP may be only 90/60 mm Hg
- Bradycardia (most common; heart rate <60 beats/min) or tachycardia (heart rate >100 beats/min)
- Diaphoresis (above the injury)
- Facial flushing
- Pallor (below the injury)
- Pounding headache (a diffuse pain in different portions of the head and not confined to any nerve distribution area)

Minor

- Nasal congestion
- Engorgement of temporal and neck vessels
- Conjunctival congestion
- Chills without fever
- Pilomotor erection (goose bumps) below the injury
- Blurred vision
- Chest pain
- Metallic taste in mouth
- Horner syndrome (constriction of the pupil, partial ptosis of the eyelid, enophthalmos, and sometimes loss of sweating over the affected side of the face)

OUTCOME CRITERIA

- BP has returned to patient's norm.
- Heart rate is greater than 60 or less than 100 beats/min (or within patient's norm).
- Headache is absent.
- Nasal stuffiness, sweating, and flushing above level of injury are absent.
- Chills, goose bumps, and pallor below level of injury are absent.
- Patient verbalizes causes, prevention, symptoms, and treatment of condition.

NURSING INTERVENTIONS AND *RATIONALE*

1. Place the patient on cardiac monitor, and assess for bradycardia, tachycardia, or other dysrhythmias. *Disturbances of cardiac rate and rhythm can occur because of autonomic dysfunction associated with dysreflexia.*
2. Do not leave the patient alone. One nurse monitors the BP and patient status every 3 to 5 minutes while another provides treatment.
3. Place the patient's head of bed to upright position *to decrease BP and promote cerebral venous return.*
4. Remove any support stockings or abdominal binder to reduce venous return.
5. Investigate for and remove offending cause of dysreflexia:

BLADDER

- If indwelling catheter not in place, catheterize patient immediately.
- Lubricate catheter with lidocaine jelly before insertion.
- Drain 500 ml of urine, and recheck BP.
- If BP still elevated, drain another 500 ml of urine.
- If BP declines after the bladder is empty, serial BP must be monitored closely *because the bladder can go into severe contractions, causing hypertension to recur.*
- Collaborate with physician regarding the instillation of 30 ml tetracaine through the catheter *to decrease the flow of impulses from the bladder.*
- If indwelling catheter is in place, check for kinks or granular sediment that may indicate occlusion.
- If catheter is plugged, irrigate it gently with no more than 30 ml of sterile normal saline solution. If the bladder is in tetany, fluid will go in but will not drain out. Atropine is sometimes administered *to relieve bladder tetany.*
- If unable to irrigate catheter, remove it and prepare to reinsert a new catheter: proceed with its lubrication, drainage, and observation as outlined above.

BOWEL

- Using glove lubricated with anesthetic ointment, check rectum for fecal impaction.
- If impaction is felt, *to decrease flow of impulses from bowel,* insert anesthetic ointment into rectum 10 minutes before manual removal of impaction.
- A low, hypertonic enema or a suppository may be given to assist bowel evacuation.

SKIN

- Loosen clothing or bed linens as indicated.
- Inspect skin for pimples, boils, pressure sores, and ingrown toenails, and treat as indicated.

6. If symptoms of dysreflexia do not subside, have available the intravenous (IV) solutions and antihypertensive drugs of the physician's choosing (e.g., hydralazine, nifedipine, phentolamine, diazoxide, sodium nitroprusside). Administer medications, and monitor their effectiveness. Assess BP and pulse.
7. Instruct patient about causes, symptoms, treatment, and prevention of dysreflexia.
8. Encourage patient to carry medical bracelet or informational card to present to medical personnel in the event dysreflexia may be developing.

NURSING MANAGEMENT PLAN

Compromised Family Coping

Definition: Usually supportive primary person (family member or close friend) provides insufficient, ineffective, or compromised support, comfort, assistance, or encouragement that may be needed by the patient to manage or master adaptive tasks related to his or her health challenge.

Compromised Family Coping Related to Critically Ill Family Member

DEFINING CHARACTERISTICS

- Disruption of usual family functions and roles
- Inability to accept or deal with crisis situation; use of defense mechanisms (e.g., denial, anger); unrealistic expectations of patient's outcome and care provided; judgmental toward health care providers
- Nonrecognition that family is in state of crisis
- Inappropriate emotional outbursts; arguments among family and with others; inability to respond to each other's feelings or support each other
- Misinterpretation of information; short attention span with repeated questions about information already provided; members not sharing information with each other
- Inability to make decisions regarding changes in family structure or about course of care for ill member; noncooperation among family members
- Expressions of grief, hopelessness, powerlessness, and isolation; do not seek or respond to support services
- Hesitancy to spend time with ill person in the critical care unit or inappropriate behavior when visiting (may upset patient)
- Neglect of own personal health; fatigue, apathy; refusal of offers for respite time

OUTCOME CRITERIA

- The family will express an understanding of course/prognosis of illness, therapies, and alternative measures.
- The family will diminish or resolve conflicts and cooperate in decision making.
- The family will develop trust and mutual support for each member and form a cohesive unit.
- The family will support ill person in making decisions (if capable) or respect prior wishes regarding provision of health care.
- Family efforts will be directed toward a purpose and readjust to changes in life patterns and role function. Members will accept responsibility for changes.
- The family will identify and use effective coping strategies.
- The family will identify and use available resources as needed to facilitate resolution of the crisis.
- The family will have a sense of control and confidence in meeting personal and collective needs.

NURSING INTERVENTIONS AND *RATIONALE*

1. Identify family's perception of the crisis situation. Determine family structure; role developmental phase; and ethnic, cultural, and belief factors that may affect communication with family and the plan of care. Identify strengths of the family. *All initial nursing interventions should be directed toward resolving the crisis situation. Understanding and using family theory principles will facilitate this process and individualize care.*
2. Provide honest and accurate information in language persons can understand. Give updated information as appropriate. Listen! *This facilitates open communication among family and health care providers, projects a caring attitude and concern for them and patient, and assists family in making decision and being involved with the plan and goals of care.*
3. Encourage liberal visitation with patient. Before the visit, prepare family members for what they will observe in a technical environment. Inform them about patient's appearance, behaviors, etc. that may be distressing to them. Explain the etiology of patient responses to stimuli (e.g., pain, trauma, surgery, medication), and explain that these behaviors are being monitored and are usually temporary. Encourage them to touch the patient and let the patient know of their presence. *This prevents a strong emotional reaction to an unfamiliar and frightening situation, involves family as support to each other and to the patient, demonstrates the nurse's concern for them as persons, and facilitates satisfaction with care being provided for their loved one.*
4. Identify and support effective coping behaviors. *This aids in the family's sense of control and resolution of helplessness/powerlessness.*
5. Observe for signs of fatigue and the need for emotional/spiritual support and respite from hospital waiting routine. Encourage family to verbalize feelings. Provide information on available resources. Alert interdisciplinary team members (social, psychologic, spiritual) to family needs. Provide pager device (if available), or obtain phone numbers when family leaves the hospital premises. *This provides support and comfort, facilitates hope, resolves sense of isolation, gives sense of security, and diminishes guilt feelings for attending to personal needs.*
6. Instruct family in simple caregiving techniques, and encourage participation in patient's care. *This facilitates giving a sense of "normalcy" to experience, self-confidence, and assurance that good care is being provided.*
7. Serve as advocate for patient and family. Teach family how to negotiate with the health care delivery system, and include them in health care team conferences when appropriate. *This facilitates informed decision making, promotes control and satisfaction, and permits mutual goal-setting.*
8. Consider nonbiologic or nonlegal family relationships. Encourage contact with patient and participation in care. *This facilitates holistic care and support of emotional ties and demonstrates respect for the family unit and relationships.*
9. Provide emotional support and compassion when patient's condition worsens or deteriorates. *The use of touch and expression of concern for the patient and family convey comfort and trust in the health care provider and respect and assurance that the family's loved one will receive appropriate care and attention.*

NURSING MANAGEMENT PLAN
Decreased Cardiac Output

Definition: Inadequate blood pumped by the heart to meet the metabolic demands of the body.

Decreased Cardiac Output Related to Alterations in Preload

DEFINING CHARACTERISTICS

- Cardiac output (CO) <4.0 L/min
- Cardiac index (CI) <2.5 L/min/m^2
- Heart rate (HR) >100 beats/min
- Urine output <30 ml/hr or 0.5 ml/kg/hr
- Decreased mentation, restlessness, agitation, confusion
- Diminished peripheral pulses
- Blue, gray, or dark purple tint to tongue and sublingual area
- Systolic blood pressure (SBP) <90 mm Hg
- Subjective complaints of fatigue

Reduced Preload

- Right atrial pressure (RAP) <2 mm Hg
- Pulmonary artery occlusion pressure (PAOP) <5 mm Hg

Excessive Preload

- RAP >6 mm Hg
- PAOP >12 mm Hg

OUTCOME CRITERIA

- CO 4-8 L/min
- CI 2.5-4 L/min/m^2
- RAP 2-8 mm Hg
- PAOP 5-12 mm Hg

NURSING INTERVENTIONS AND *RATIONALE*

1. Collaborate with physician regarding the administration of oxygen to maintain oxygen saturation (Spo_2) >92% *to prevent tissue hypoxia.*
2. Maintain surveillance for signs of decreased tissue perfusion and acidosis *to facilitate the early identification and treatment of complications.*
3. Monitor fluid balance and daily weights *to facilitate regulation of the patient's fluid balance.*

For Reduced Preload Secondary to Volume Loss

1. Collaborate with physician regarding the administration of crystalloids, colloids, blood, and blood products *to increase circulating volume.*
2. Limit blood sampling, observe intravenous lines for accidental disconnection, apply direct pressure to bleeding sites, and maintain normal body temperature *to minimize fluid loss.*
3. Position patient with legs elevated, trunk flat, and head and shoulders above the chest *to enhance venous return.*
4. Encourage oral fluids (as appropriate), administer free water with tube feedings, and replace fluids that are lost through wound or tube drainage *to promote adequate fluid intake.*
5. Maintain surveillance for signs of fluid volume excess and adverse effects of blood and blood product administration *to facilitate the early identification and treatment of complications.*

For Reduced Preload Secondary to Venous Dilation

1. Collaborate with physician regarding the administration of vasoconstrictors *to increase venous return.*
2. Maintain surveillance for adverse effects of vasoconstrictor therapy *to facilitate the early identification and treatment of complications.*
3. If patient is hyperthermic, administer tepid bath, hypothermia blanket, and/or ice bags to axilla and groin *to decrease temperature and promote vasoconstriction.*

For Excessive Preload Secondary to Volume Overload

1. Collaborate with physician regarding the administration of the following:
   - Diuretics to remove excessive fluid.
   - Vasodilators to decrease venous return.
   - Inotropes to increase myocardial contractility.
2. Restrict fluid intake and double concentrate intravenous drips *to minimize fluid intake.*
3. Position patient in semi-Fowler's or high-Fowler's position *to reduce venous return.*
4. Maintain surveillance for signs of fluid volume deficit and adverse effects of diuretic, vasodilator, and inotropic therapies *to facilitate the early identification and treatment of complications.*

For Excessive Preload Secondary to Venous Constriction

1. Collaborate with physician regarding the administration of vasodilators *to promote venous dilation.*
2. Maintain surveillance for adverse effects of vasodilator therapy *to facilitate the early identification and treatment of complications.*
3. If patient is hypothermic, wrap patient in warm blankets or administer hyperthermia blanket *to increase temperature and promote vasodilation.*

Decreased Cardiac Output Related to Alterations in Afterload

DEFINING CHARACTERISTICS

- CO <4 L/min
- CI <2.5 L/min/m^2
- HR >100 beats/min
- Urine output <30 ml/hr
- Decreased mentation, restlessness, agitation, confusion
- Diminished peripheral pulses
- Blue, gray, or dark purple tint to tongue and sublingual area
- SBP <90 mm Hg
- Subjective complaints of fatigue

Reduced Afterload

- Pulmonary vascular resistance (PVR) <100 dynes/sec/cm^{-5}
- Systemic vascular resistance (SVR) <800 dynes/sec/cm^{-5}

NURSING MANAGEMENT PLAN—*cont'd*

Excessive Afterload
- PVR >250 dynes/sec/cm^{-5}
- SVR >1200 dynes/sec/cm^{-5}

OUTCOME CRITERIA
- CO 4-8 L/min
- CI 2.5-4 L/min/m^2
- PVR 80-250 dynes/sec/cm^{-5}
- SVR 800-1200 dynes/sec/cm^{-5}

NURSING INTERVENTIONS AND *RATIONALE*
1. Collaborate with physician regarding the administration of oxygen to maintain an Spo_2 >92% *to prevent tissue hypoxia.*
2. Maintain surveillance for signs of decreased tissue perfusion and acidosis *to facilitate the early identification and treatment of complications.*

For Reduced Afterload
1. Collaborate with physician regarding the administration of vasoconstrictors *to promote arterial vasoconstriction and prevent relative hypovolemia.* If decreased preload is present, implement plan for Decreased Cardiac Output Related to Alterations in Preload.
2. Maintain surveillance for adverse effects of vasoconstrictor therapy *to facilitate the early identification and treatment of complications.*
3. If patient is hyperthermic, administer tepid bath, hypothermia blanket, and/or ice bags to axilla and groin *to decrease temperature and promote vasoconstriction.*

For Excessive Afterload
1. Collaborate with physician regarding the administration of vasodilators *to promote arterial vasodilation.*
2. Collaborate with physician regarding initiation of intra-aortic balloon pump *to facilitate afterload reduction.*
3. Promote rest and relaxation and decrease environmental stimulation *to minimize sympathetic stimulation.*
4. Maintain surveillance for adverse effects of vasodilator therapy *to facilitate the early identification and treatment of complications.*
5. If patient is hypothermic, wrap patient in warm blankets or administer hyperthermia blanket *to increase temperature and promote vasodilation.*
6. If patient is in pain, treat pain *to reduce sympathetic stimulation.* Implement plan for Acute Pain Related to Transmission of Perception of Cutaneous, Visceral, Muscular, or Ischemic Impulses.

Decreased Cardiac Output Related to Alterations in Contractility

DEFINING CHARACTERISTICS
- CO <4 L/min
- CI <2.5 L/min/m^2
- HR >100 beats/min
- Urine output <30 ml/hr
- Decreased mentation, restlessness, agitation, confusion
- Diminished peripheral pulses
- Blue, gray, or dark purple tint to tongue and sublingual area
- SBP <90 mm Hg
- Subjective complaints of fatigue
- Right ventricular stroke work index (RVSWI) <7 g/m^2/beat
- Left ventricular stroke work index (LVSWI) <35 g/m^2/beat

OUTCOME CRITERIA
- CO 4-8 L/min
- CI 2.5-4 L/min/m^2
- RVSWI 7-12 g/m^2/beat
- SVSWI 35-85 g/m^2/beat

NURSING INTERVENTIONS AND *RATIONALE*
1. Collaborate with physician regarding the administration of oxygen to maintain an Spo_2 >92% *to prevent tissue hypoxia.*
2. Maintain surveillance for signs of decreased tissue perfusion and acidosis *to facilitate the early identification and treatment of complications.*
3. Ensure preload is optimized. If preload is reduced or excessive, implement plan for Decreased Cardiac Output Related to Alterations in Preload.
4. Ensure afterload is optimized. If afterload is reduced or excessive, implement plan for Decreased Cardiac Output Related to Alterations in Afterload.
5. Ensure electrolytes are optimized. Collaborate with physician regarding the administration of electrolyte replacement therapy *to enhance cellular ionic environment.*
6. Collaborate with physician regarding the administration of inotropes *to enhance myocardial contractility.*
7. If myocardial ischemia present, implement plan for Ineffective Cardiopulmonary Tissue Perfusion.

Decreased Cardiac Output Related to Alterations in Heart Rate or Rhythm

DEFINING CHARACTERISTICS
- CO <4 L/min
- CI <2.5 L/min/m^2
- HR >100 beats/min or <60 beats/min
- Urine output <30 ml/hr or 0.5 ml/kg/hr
- Decreased mentation, restlessness, agitation, confusion
- Diminished peripheral pulses
- Blue, gray, or dark purple tint to tongue and sublingual area
- SBP <90 mm Hg
- Subjective complaints of fatigue
- Dysrhythmias

Continued

NURSING MANAGEMENT PLAN—*cont'd*

Decreased Cardiac Output—*cont'd*

Decreased Cardiac Output Related to Alterations in Heart Rate or Rhythm—*cont'd*

OUTCOME CRITERIA

- CO 4-8 L/min
- CI 2.5-4 L/min/m^2
- Absence of dysrhythmias or return to baseline
- HR >60 beats/min or <100 beats/min

NURSING INTERVENTIONS AND *RATIONALE*

1. Collaborate with physician regarding the administration of oxygen to maintain an Spo_2 >92% *to prevent tissue hypoxia.*
2. Ensure electrolytes are optimized. Collaborate with physician regarding the administration of electrolyte therapy *to enhance cellular ionic environment and avoid precipitation of dysrhythmias.*
3. Collaborate with physician and pharmacist regarding patient's current medications and their effect on heart rate and rhythm *to identify any prodysrhythmic or bradycardic side effects.*
4. Maintain surveillance for signs of decreased tissue perfusion and acidosis *to facilitate the early identification and treatment of complications.*
5. Monitor ST segment continuously *to determine changes in myocardial tissue perfusion.* If myocardial ischemia is present, implement plan for Ineffective Cardiopulmonary Tissue Perfusion.

For Lethal Dysrhythmias or Asystole

1. Initiate advanced cardiac life support (ACLS) interventions, and notify physician immediately.

For Nonlethal Dysrhythmias

1. Collaborate with physician regarding administration of antidysrhythmic therapy, synchronized cardioversion, and/or overdrive pacing *to control dysrhythmias.*
2. Maintain surveillance for adverse effects of antidysrhythmic therapy *to facilitate the early identification and treatment of complications.*

For Heart Rate Less Than 60 Beats/Min

1. Collaborate with physician regarding the initiation of temporary pacing *to increase heart rate.*

Decreased Cardiac Output Related to Sympathetic Blockade

DEFINING CHARACTERISTICS

- Decreased CO and CI
- SBP <90 mm Hg or below patient's baseline
- Decreased RAP and PAOP
- Decreased SVR
- Bradycardia
- Cardiac dysrhythmias
- Postural hypotension

OUTCOME CRITERIA

- CO and CI are within normal limits.
- SBP is greater than 90 mm Hg or returns to baseline.
- RAP and PAOP are within normal limits.
- SVR is within normal limits.
- Sinus rhythm is present.
- Dysrhythmias are absent.
- Fainting or dizziness with position change is absent.

NURSING INTERVENTIONS AND *RATIONALE*

1. Implement measures to prevent episodes of postural hypertension:
   - Change patient's position slowly to allow the cardiovascular system time to compensate.
   - Apply antiembolic stockings to promote venous return.
   - Perform range-of-motion exercises every 2 hours to prevent venous pooling.
   - Collaborate with the physician and physical therapist regarding the use of a tilt table to progress the patient from supine to upright position.
2. Collaborate with the physician regarding the administration of the following:
   - Crystalloids and/or colloids to increase the patient's circulating volume, which increases stroke volume and subsequently cardiac output.
   - Vasopressors if fluids are ineffective to constrict the patient's vascular system, which increases resistance and subsequently blood pressure.
3. Monitor cardiac rhythm for bradycardia and/or dysrhythmias, *which can further decrease cardiac output.*
4. Avoid any activity that can stimulate the vagal response *because bradycardia can result.*
5. Treat symptomatic bradycardia and symptomatic dysrhythmias according to unit's emergency protocol or ACLS guidelines.

NURSING MANAGEMENT PLAN

Decreased Intracranial Adaptive Capacity

Definition: Intracranial fluid dynamic mechanisms that normally compensate for increases in intracranial volumes are compromised, resulting in repeated disproportionate increases in intracranial pressure (ICP) in response to a variety of noxious and nonnoxious stimuli.

Decreased Intracranial Adaptive Capacity Related to Failure of Normal Intracranial Compensatory Mechanisms

DEFINING CHARACTERISTICS

- ICP >15 mm Hg, sustained for 15 to 30 minutes
- Headache
- Vomiting, with or without nausea
- Seizures
- Decrease in Glasgow Coma Scale score of 2 or more points from baseline
- Alteration in level of consciousness, ranging from restlessness to coma
- Change in orientation: disoriented to time and/or place and/or person
- Difficulty or inability to follow simple commands
- Increasing systolic blood pressure of more than 20 mm Hg with widening pulse pressure
- Bradycardia
- Irregular respiratory pattern (e.g., Cheyne-Stokes, central neurogenic hyperventilation, ataxic, apneustic)
- Change in response to painful stimuli (e.g., purposeful to inappropriate or absent response)
- Signs of impending brain herniation:
  - Hemiparesis or hemiplegia
  - Hemisensory changes
  - Unequal pupil size (1 mm or more difference)
  - Failure of pupil to react to light
  - Disconjugate gaze and inability to move one eye beyond midline if third, fourth, or sixth cranial nerves involved
  - Loss of oculocephalic or oculovestibular reflexes
  - Possible decorticate or decerebrate posturing

OUTCOME CRITERIA

- ICP is less than or equal to15 mm Hg.
- Cerebral perfusion pressure (CPP) is greater than 60 mm Hg.
- Clinical signs of increased ICP as previously described are absent.

NURSING INTERVENTIONS AND *RATIONALE*

1. Maintain adequate CPP.
   - Collaborate with physician regarding the administration of volume expanders, vasopressors, or antihypertensives *to maintain the patient's blood pressure within normal range.*
   - Implement measures to reduce ICP.

   (a) Elevate head of bed 30 to 45 degrees *to facilitate venous return.*

   (b) Maintain head and neck in neutral plan (avoid flexion, extension, or lateral rotation) *to enhance venous drainage from the head.*

   (c) Avoid extreme hip flexion.

   (d) Collaborate with the physician regarding the administration of steroids, osmotic agents, and diuretics and need for drainage of cerebrospinal fluid (CSF) if a ventriculostomy is in place.

   (e) Assist patient with turning and moving self in bed (instruct patient to exhale while turning or pushing up in bed) *to avoid isometric contractions and Valsalva maneuver.*
2. Maintain patent airway and adequate ventilation, and supply oxygen *to prevent hypoxemia and hypercarbia.*
3. Monitor arterial blood gas (ABG) values and maintain $Pa{O_2}$ >80 mm Hg, $Pa{CO_2}$ at 25 to 35 mm Hg, and pH at 7.35 to 7.45 *to prevent cerebral vasodilation.*
4. Avoid suctioning beyond 10 seconds at a time; hyperoxygenate and hyperventilate before and after suctioning.
5. Plan patient care activities and nursing interventions around patient's ICP response. Avoid unnecessary additional disturbances, and allow patient up to 1 hour of rest between activities as frequently as possible. *Studies have shown the direct correlation between nursing care activities and increases in ICP.*
6. Maintain normothermia with external cooling or heating measures as necessary. Wrap hands, feet, and male genitalia in soft towels before cooling measures *to prevent shivering and frostbite.*
7. With physician's collaboration, control seizures with prophylactic and as-necessary (PRN) anticonvulsants. *Seizures can greatly increase the cerebral metabolic rate.*
8. Collaborate with the physician regarding the administration of sedatives, barbiturates, or paralyzing agents *to reduce cerebral metabolic rate.*
9. Counsel family members to maintain calm atmosphere and avoid disturbing topics of conversation (e.g., patient condition, pain, prognosis, family crisis, financial difficulties).
10. If signs of impending brain herniation are present, implement the following:
    - Notify the physician at once.
    - Be sure head of bed is elevated 45 degrees and patient's head is in neutral plane.
    - Administer mainline intravenous (IV) infusion slowly to keep-open rate.
    - Drain CSF as ordered if a ventriculostomy is in place.
    - Prepare to administer osmotic agents and/or diuretics.
    - Prepare patient for emergency computed tomography (CT) head scan and/or emergency surgery.

NURSING MANAGEMENT PLAN
Deficient Fluid Volume

Definition: Decreased intravascular, interstitial, and/or intracellular fluid. This refers to dehydration, water loss alone without change in sodium.

Deficient Fluid Volume Related to Absolute Loss

DEFINING CHARACTERISTICS

- Cardiac output (CO) <4 L /min
- Cardiac index (CI) <2.2 L /min
- Pulmonary artery occlusion pressure (PAOP) and/or right atrial pressure (RAP) less than normal or less than baseline
- Tachycardia
- Narrowed pulse pressure
- Systolic blood pressure (SBP) <100 mm Hg
- Urinary output <30 ml/hr
- Pale, cool, moist skin
- Apprehensiveness

OUTCOME CRITERIA

- CO is greater than 4 L/min, and CI is less than 2.2 L /min.
- PAOP and RAP are normal or back to baseline level.
- Heart rate is normal or back to baseline.
- SBP is greater than 90 mm Hg.
- Urinary output is greater than 30 ml/hr.

NURSING INTERVENTIONS AND *RATIONALE*

1. Secure airway, and administer high-flow oxygen.
2. Place patient in supine position with legs elevated *to increase preload.* For patient with head injury, consider using low-Fowler's position with legs elevated.
3. For fluid repletion, use the 3:1 rule, replacing three parts of fluid for every unit of blood lost.
4. Administer crystalloid solutions using the fluid challenge technique: infuse precise amounts of fluid (usually 5 to 20 ml/min) over 10-minute periods; monitor cardiac loading pressure serially *to determine successful challenging.* If the pulmonary PAOP elevates more than 7 mm Hg above beginning level, the infusion should be stopped. If the PAOP rises only to 3 mm Hg above baseline or falls, another fluid challenge should be administered.
5. Replete fluids first before considering use of vasopressors, because vasopressors increase myocardial oxygen consumption out of proportion to the reestablishment of coronary perfusion in the early phases of treatment.
6. When blood replacement is indicated, replace it with fresh packed red cells and fresh frozen plasma *to keep clotting factors intact.*
7. Move or reposition patient minimally to decrease or limit tissue oxygen demands.
8. Evaluate patient's anxiety level, and intervene through patient education or sedation *to decrease tissue oxygen demands.*
9. Maintain surveillance for signs and symptoms of fluid overload.

Deficient Fluid Volume Related to Decreased Secretion of Antidiuretic Hormone (ADH)

DEFINING CHARACTERISTICS

- Confusion and lethargy
- Decreased skin turgor
- Thirst
- Weight loss over short period
- Decreased PAOP
- Decreased RAP
- Urinary output >6 L/day
- Serum sodium >148 mEq/L
- Serum osmolality >295 mOsm/kg
- Urine osmolality <100 mOsm/kg
- Urine specific gravity <1.005

OUTCOME CRITERIA

- Weight returns to baseline.
- Urinary output is greater than 30 ml/hr and less than 200 ml/hr.
- Serum osmolality is 280 to 295 mOsm/kg.
- Urine specific gravity is 1.010 to 1.030.

NURSING INTERVENTIONS AND *RATIONALE*

1. Record intake and output every hour, noting color and clarity of urine *because color and clarity are an indication of urine concentration.*
2. Monitor ECG rhythm continuously for dysrhythmias *caused by electrolyte imbalance.*
3. Collaborate with physician regarding administration of vasopressin or desmopressin *to replace ADH.*
   - Monitor patient for adverse effects of medications (i.e., headache, chest pain, abdominal pain) *caused by vasoconstriction.*
   - Report adverse effects to physician immediately.
4. Collaborate with physician regarding intravenous fluid and electrolyte replacement therapy *to restore fluid balance, correct dehydration, and maintain electrolyte balance.*
   - Administer hypotonic saline to replace free water deficit.
5. Provide oral fluids low in sodium such as water, coffee, tea, or orange juice *to decrease sodium intake.*
6. Weigh patient daily (at same time, in same amount of clothing, and preferably with same scale) *to ensure accuracy of readings.*
7. Reposition patient every 2 hours to prevent skin integrity issues caused by dehydration.
8. Provide mouth care every 4 hours to prevent breakdown of oral mucous membranes.
9. Collaborate with physician regarding administration of medications to prevent constipation *caused by dehydration.*
10. Maintain surveillance for symptoms of hypernatremia (muscle twitching, irritability, seizures), hypovolemic shock (hypotension, tachycardia, decreased PAP and PAOP), and deep vein thrombosis (calf pain, tenderness, swelling).

NURSING MANAGEMENT PLAN—*cont'd*

Deficient Fluid Volume Related to Relative Loss

DEFINING CHARACTERISTICS

- PAOP, RAP less than normal or less than baseline
- Tachycardia
- Narrowed pulse pressure
- SBP <100 mm Hg
- Urinary output <30 ml/hr
- Increased hematocrit level

OUTCOME CRITERIA

- PAOP and RAP are normal or back to baseline.
- SBP is greater than 90 mm Hg.
- Urinary output is greater than 30 ml/hr.
- Hematocrit level is normal.

NURSING INTERVENTIONS AND *RATIONALE*

1. Collaborate with the physician regarding the administration of intravenous (IV) fluid replacements (usually normal saline solution or lactated Ringer's solution) at a rate sufficient to maintain urinary output greater than 30 ml/hr. Colloid solutions are avoided in the initial phases (but can be used later) because of the possibility of increased edema formation *as a result of the increased capillary permeability.*

NURSING MANAGEMENT PLAN
Deficient Knowledge

Definition: Absence or deficiency of cognitive information related to a specific topic.

Deficient Knowledge Related to Cognitive/Perceptual Learning Limitations (e.g., sensory overload, sleep deprivation, medications, anxiety, sensory deficits, language barrier)

DEFINING CHARACTERISTICS
- Verbalized statement of inadequate knowledge of skills
- Verbalization of inadequate recall of information
- Verbalization of inadequate understanding of information
- Evidence of inaccurate follow-through of instructions
- Inadequate demonstration of a skill
- Lack of compliance with prescribed behavior

OUTCOME CRITERIA
- Patient participates actively in necessary and prescribed health behaviors.
- Patient verbalizes adequate knowledge or demonstrates adequate skills.

NURSING INTERVENTIONS AND *RATIONALE*
1. Determine specific cause of patient's cognitive or perceptual limitation.
2. Provide uninterrupted rest period before teaching session *to decrease fatigue and encourage optimal state for learning and retention.*
3. Manipulate environment as much as possible to provide quiet and uninterrupted learning sessions.
   - Ensure that lights are bright enough *to see teaching aids but not too bright.*
   - Schedule care and medications *to allow uninterrupted teaching periods.*
   - Move patient to quiet, private room for teaching if possible.
4. Adapt teaching sessions and materials to patient's and family's levels of education and ability to understand.
   - Provide printed material appropriate to reading level.
   - Use terminology understood by the patient.
   - Provide printed materials in patient's primary language *if possible.*
   - Use interpreters during teaching sessions *when necessary.*
5. Teach only present-tense focus during periods of sensory overload.
6. Determine potential effects of medications on ability to retain or recall information.
   - Avoid teaching critical content while patient is taking sedatives, analgesics, or other medications that affect memory.
7. Reinforce new skills and information in several teaching sessions. Use several senses when possible in teaching session (e.g., see a film, hear a discussion, read printed information, and demonstrate skills related to self-injection of insulin).
8. Reduce patient's anxiety.
   - Listen attentively, and encourage verbalization of feelings.
   - Answer questions as they arise in a clear and succinct manner.
   - Elicit patient's concerns, and address those issues first.
   - Give only correct and relevant information.
   - Continually assess response to teaching session, and discontinue if anxiety increases or physical condition becomes unstable.
   - Provide nonthreatening information before more anxiety-producing information is presented.
   - Plan for several teaching sessions so information can be divided into small, manageable packages.

Deficient Knowledge Related to Lack of Previous Exposure to Information

DEFINING CHARACTERISTICS
- Verbalized statement of inadequate knowledge or skills
- New diagnosis or health problem requiring self-management or care
- Lack of prior formal or informal education about the specific health problem
- Demonstration of inappropriate behaviors related to management of health problem

OUTCOME CRITERIA
- Patient verbalizes adequate knowledge about or performs skills related to disease process, its causes, factors related to onset of symptoms, and self-management of disease or health problem.
- Patient actively participates in health behaviors required for performance of a procedure or in those behaviors enhancing recovery from illness and preventing recurrence or complications.

NURSING INTERVENTIONS AND *RATIONALE*
1. Determine existing level of knowledge or skill.
2. Assess factors that affect the knowledge deficit.
   - Learning needs, including patient's priorities and the necessary knowledge and skills for safety
   - Learning ability of patient, including language skills, level of education, ability to read, preferred learning style
   - Physical ability to perform prescribed skills or procedures; consider effect of limitations imposed by treatment such as bed rest, restriction of movement by intravenous or other equipment, or effect of sedatives or analgesics
   - Psychologic effect of stage of adaptation to disease
   - Activity tolerance and ability to concentrate
   - Motivation to learn new skills or gain new knowledge

NURSING MANAGEMENT PLAN—*cont'd*

3. Reduce or limit barriers to learning:
   - Provide consistent nurse-patient contact to encourage development of trusting and therapeutic relationship.
   - Structure environment to enhance learning; control unnecessary noise, interruptions.
   - Individualize teaching plan to fit patient's current physical and psychologic status.
   - Delay teaching until patient is ready to learn.
   - Conduct teaching sessions during period of day when patient is most alert and receptive.
   - Meet patient's immediate learning needs as they arise (e.g., give brief explanation of procedures when they are performed).
4. Promote active participation in the teaching plan by the patient and family.
   - Solicit input during development of plan.
   - Develop mutually acceptable goals and outcomes.
   - Solicit expression of feelings and emotions related to new responsibilities.
   - Encourage questions.
5. Conduct teaching sessions, using the most appropriate teaching methods.
6. Repeat key principles, and provide them in printed form *for reference at a later time.*
7. Give frequent feedback to patient when practicing new skills.
8. Use several teaching sessions when appropriate. New information and skills should be reinforced several times after initial learning.
9. Initiate referrals for follow-up if necessary.
   - Health educators
   - Home health care
   - Rehabilitation programs
   - Social services
10. Evaluate effectiveness of teaching plan, based on patient's ability to meet preset goals and objectives *to determine need for further teaching.*

NURSING MANAGEMENT PLAN

Disturbed Body Image

Definition: Confusion in mental picture of one's physical self.

Disturbed Body Image Related to Actual Change in Body Structure, Function, or Appearance

DEFINING CHARACTERISTICS

- Actual change in appearance, structure, or function
- Avoidance of looking at body part
- Avoidance of touching body part
- Hiding or overexposing body part (intentional or unintentional)
- Trauma to nonfunctioning part
- Change in ability to estimate spatial relationship of body to environment
- Verbalization of the following:
  - — Fear of rejection or reaction by others
  - — Negative feeling about body
  - — Preoccupation with change or loss
  - — Refusal to participate in or to accept responsibility for self-care of altered body part
- Personalization of part or loss with a name
- Depersonalization of part or loss by use of impersonal pronouns
- Refusal to verify actual change

OUTCOME CRITERIA

- Patient verbalizes the specific meaning of the change to him or her.
- Patient requests appropriate information about self-care.
- Patient completes personal hygiene and grooming daily with or without help.
- Patient interacts freely with family or other visitors.
- Patient participates in the discussions and conferences related to planning his or her medical and nursing management in the critical care unit and transfer from the unit.
- Patient talks with trained visitors (support-group representatives) at least twice about his or her loss.

NURSING INTERVENTIONS AND *RATIONALE*

1. Evaluate patient's mental, physical, and emotional state; recognize assets, strengths, response to illness, coping mechanisms, past experience with stress, and support system.
2. Appraise the response of family and significant others. *Body image is derived from the "reflected appraisals" of family and significant others.*
3. Determine the patient's goals and readiness for learning.
4. Provide the necessary information to help the patient and family adapt to the change. Clarify misconceptions about future limitations.
5. Permit and encourage the patient to express the significance of the loss or change; note nonverbal behavior responses.
6. Allow and encourage the patient's expression of anxiety. *Anxiety is the most predominant emotional response to a body image disturbance.*
7. Recognize and accept the use of denial as an adaptive defense mechanism when used early and temporarily.
8. Recognize maladaptive denial as that which interferes with the patient's progress and/or alienates support systems. Use confrontation.
9. Provide an opportunity for the patient to discuss sexual concerns.
10. Touch the affected body part *to provide the patient with sensory information about altered body structure and/or function.*
11. Encourage and provide movement of altered body part *to establish kinesthetic feedback. This enables the person to know his or her body as it now exists.*
12. Prepare the patient to look at the body part. Call the body part by its anatomic name (e.g., stump, stoma, limb) as opposed to "it" or "she." *The use of impersonal pronouns increases a sense of fantasy and depersonalization of the body part.*
13. Allow the patient to experience excellence in some aspect of physical functioning—walking, turning, deep breathing, healing, self-care—and point out progress and accomplishment. *This helps to balance the patient's sense of dysfunction with function.*
14. Avoid false reassurance. Acknowledge the difficulty of incorporating the altered body part or function into one's body image. *This evidences the nurse's sensitivity and promotes trust.*
15. Talk with the patient about his or her life, generativity, and accomplishments. *Patients with disturbances in body image frequently see themselves in a distortedly "narrow" sense. Encouraging a wider focus of themselves and their life reduces this distortion.*
16. Help the patient explore realistic alternatives.
17. Recognize that incorporating a body change into one's body image takes time. Avoid setting unrealistic expectations and *thereby inadvertently reinforcing a low self-esteem.*
18. Suggest the use of additional resources such as trained visitors who have mastered situations similar to those of the patient. Refer the patient to a psychiatrist if needed.

NURSING MANAGEMENT PLAN—*cont'd*

Disturbed Body Image Related to Functional Dependence on Life-Sustaining Technology (e.g., ventilator, dialysis, intraaortic balloon pump, halo traction)

DEFINING CHARACTERISTICS

- Actual change in function requiring permanent or temporary replacement
- Refusal to verify actual loss
- Verbalization of the following: feelings of helplessness, hopelessness, powerlessness, fear of failure to wean from technology

OUTCOME CRITERIA

- Patient verifies actual change in function.
- Patient does not refuse or fight technologic intervention.
- Patient verbalizes acceptance of expected change in lifestyle.

NURSING INTERVENTIONS AND *RATIONALE*

1. Evaluate patient's response to the technologic intervention.
2. Assess responses of family and significant others. *Body image is derived from the "reflected appraisals" of family and significant others.*
3. Provide information needed by patient and family.
4. Promote trust, security, comfort, and privacy.
5. Recognize anxiety. Allow and encourage its expression. *Anxiety is the most predominant emotion accompanying body image alterations.* Implement plan for Anxiety.
6. Assist patient with recognizing his or her own functioning and performance in the face of technology. For example, assist patient with distinguishing spontaneous breaths from mechanically delivered breaths. *The activity will assist in weaning patient from the ventilator when feasible. To establish realistic, accurate body boundaries, a patient needs help to separate himself or herself from the technology that is supporting his or her functioning. Any participation or function on the part of the patient during periods of dependency is helpful in preventing and/or resolving an alteration in body image.*
7. Plan for discontinuation of the treatment (e.g., weaning from ventilator). Explain procedure that will be followed, and be present during its initiation.
8. Plan for transfer from the critical care environment.
9. Document care, ensuring an up-to-date management plan is available to all involved caregivers.

NURSING MANAGEMENT PLAN

Dysfunctional Ventilatory Weaning Response

Definition: Inability to adjust to lowered levels of mechanical ventilator support that interrupts and prolongs the weaning process.

Dysfunctional Ventilatory Weaning Response (DVWR) Related to Physical, Psychologic, or Situational Factors

DEFINING CHARACTERISTICS

Mild DVWR

- Responds to lowered levels of mechanical ventilator support with the following:
  - — Restlessness
  - — Slightly increased respiratory rate from baseline
  - — Expressed feelings of increased need for oxygen; breathing discomfort; fatigue; warmth
  - — Queries about possible machine malfunction
  - — Increased concentration on breathing

Moderate DVWR

- Responds to lowered levels of mechanical ventilator support with the following:
  - — Slight baseline increase in blood pressure <20 mm Hg
  - — Slight baseline increase in heart rate <20 beats per minute (beats/min)
  - — Baseline increase in respiratory rate <5 breaths/min
  - — Hypervigilance to activities
  - — Inability to respond to coaching
  - — Inability to cooperate
  - — Apprehension
  - — Diaphoresis
  - — Eye-widening ("wide-eyed look")
  - — Decreased air entry on auscultation
  - — Color changes: pale, slight cyanosis
  - — Slight respiratory accessory muscle use

Severe DVWR

- Responds to lowered levels of mechanical ventilator support with the following:
  - — Agitation
  - — Deterioration in arterial blood gas values from current baseline
  - — Baseline increase in blood pressure >20 mm Hg
  - — Baseline increase in heart rate >20 beats/min
  - — Respiratory rate increases significantly from baseline
  - — Profuse diaphoresis
  - — Full respiratory accessory muscle use
  - — Shallow, gasping breaths
  - — Paradoxic abdominal breathing
  - — Discoordinated breathing with the ventilator
  - — Decreased level of consciousness
  - — Adventitious breath sounds, audible airway secretions
  - — Cyanosis

OUTCOME CRITERIA

- Airway is clear.
- Underlying disorder is resolving.
- Patient is rested, and pain is controlled.
- Nutritional status is adequate.
- Patient has feelings of perceived control, situational security, and trust in the nurses.
- Patient is able to adapt to selected levels of ventilator support without undue fatigue.

NURSING INTERVENTIONS AND *RATIONALE*

1. Communicate interest and concern for the patient's well-being, and demonstrate confidence in ability to manage weaning process *to instill trust in the patient.*
2. Use normalizing strategies (e.g., grooming, dressing, mobilizing, social conversation) *to reinforce the patient's self-esteem and feeling of identity.*
3. Identify parameters of the patient's usual functioning before the weaning process begins *to facilitate early identification of problems.*
4. Identify the patient's strengths and resources that can be mobilized *to enhance the patient's coping and maximize weaning effort.*
5. Note concerns that adversely affect the patient's comfort and confidence, and manage them discretely *to facilitate the patient's ease.*
6. Praise successful activities, encourage a positive outlook, and review the patient's positive progress to date *to increase the patient's perceived self-efficacy.*
7. Inform the patient of his or her situation and weaning progress *to permit the patient as much control as possible.*
8. Teach the patient about the weaning process and how he or she can participate in the process.
9. Negotiate daily weaning goals with the patient *to gain cooperation.*
10. Position the patient with the head of the bed elevated *to optimize respiratory efforts.*
11. Coach the patient in breath control by regular demonstrations of slow, deep, rhythmic patterns of breathing *to assist with dyspnea.*
12. Remain visible in the room, and reassure the patient that help is immediately available if needed *to reduce the patient's anxiety and fearfulness.*
13. Encourage the patient to view weaning trials as a form of training, regardless of whether the weaning goal is achieved *to avoid discouragement.*
14. Encourage the patient to maintain emotional calmness by reassuring, being present, comforting, talking down if emotionally aroused, and reinforcing the idea that he or she can and will succeed.
15. Monitor the patient's status frequently *to avoid undue fatigue and anxiety.*
16. Provide regular periods of rest by reducing activities, maintaining or increasing ventilator support, and providing oxygen as needed before fatigue advances.
17. Provide distraction (e.g., visitors, radio, television, conversation) when the patient's concentration starts to create tension and increases anxiety.

NURSING MANAGEMENT PLAN—*cont'd*

18. Ensure adequate nutritional support, sufficient rest and sleep time, and sedation or pain control *to promote the patient's optimal physical and emotional comfort.*
19. Start weaning early in the day *when the patient is most rested.*
20. Restrict unnecessary activities and visitors who do not cooperate with weaning strategies *to minimize energy demands on the patient during the weaning process.*
21. Coordinate necessary activities to promote adequate time for rest and relaxation.
22. Monitor the patient's underlying disease process *to ensure it is stabilized and under control.*
23. Advocate for additional resources (e.g., sedation, analgesia, rest) needed by the patient *to maximize comfort status.*
24. Develop and adhere to an individualized plan of care *to promote the patient's feelings of control.*

NURSING MANAGEMENT PLAN

Excess Fluid Volume

Definition: Increased isotonic fluid retention.

Excess Fluid Volume Related to Increased Secretion of Antidiuretic Hormone (ADH)

DEFINING CHARACTERISTICS

- Headache
- Decreased sensorium
- Weight gain over short period
- Intake greater than output
- Increased pulmonary artery occlusion pressure (PAOP)
- Increased right atrial pressure (RAP)
- Urine output <30 ml/hr
- Serum sodium <120 mEq/L
- Serum osmolality <275 mOsm/kg
- Urine osmolality greater than serum osmolality
- Urine sodium >200 mEq/L
- Urine specific gravity >1.03

OUTCOME CRITERIA

- Weight returns to baseline.
- Urine output is greater than 30 ml/hr.
- Serum sodium is 135 to 145 mEq/L.
- Urine specific gravity is 1.005 to 1.030.

NURSING INTERVENTIONS AND *RATIONALE*

1. Monitor electrocardiogram (ECG) rhythm continuously for dysrhythmias *caused by electrolyte imbalance.*
2. Restrict patient's fluids to 500 ml less than output per day *to decrease fluid retention.*
3. Provide patient chilled beverages high in sodium content such as tomato juice or broth *to increase sodium intake.*
4. Collaborate with physician regarding administration of demeclocycline, lithium, and/or narcotic agonists *to inhibit renal response to ADH.*
5. Collaborate with physician regarding administration of hypertonic saline and furosemide *for rapid correction of severe sodium deficit and diuresis of free water.*
   - Administer hypertonic saline at a rate of 1 to 2 ml/kg/hr until the patient's serum sodium level is increased no greater than 1 to 2 mEq/L/hr.
6. Weigh patient daily (at same time, in same amount of clothing, and preferably with same scale) *to ensure accuracy of readings.*
7. Provide frequent mouth care to prevent breakdown of oral mucous membranes.
8. Initiate seizure precautions because patient is at high risk as a result of hyponatremia.
   - Pad side rails of bed to protect patient from injury.
   - Remove any objects from immediate environment that could injure patient in the event of a seizure.
   - Keep appropriate-size oral airway at bedside to assist with postseizure airway management.
9. Collaborate with physician regarding administration of medications to prevent constipation *caused by decreased fluid intake and immobility.*
10. Maintain surveillance for symptoms of hyponatremia (headache, abdominal cramps, weakness) and congestive heart failure (dyspnea, rales, increased central venous pressure [CVP] and PAOP).

Excess Fluid Volume Related to Renal Dysfunction

DEFINING CHARACTERISTICS

- Weight gain that occurs during a 24- to 48-hour period
- Dependent pitting edema
- Ascites in severe cases
- Fluid crackles on lung auscultation
- Exertional dyspnea
- Oliguria or anuria
- Hypertension
- Engorged neck veins
- Decrease in urinary osmolality as renal failure progresses
- RAP >12 cm of H_2O
- PAOP >18 mm Hg

OUTCOME CRITERIA

- Weight returns to baseline.
- Edema or ascites is absent or reduced to baseline.
- Lungs are clear to auscultation.
- Exertional dyspnea is absent.
- Blood pressure returns to baseline.
- Heart rate returns to baseline.
- Neck veins are flat.
- Mucous membranes are moist.

NURSING INTERVENTIONS AND *RATIONALE*

1. Promote skin integrity of edematous areas by frequent repositioning and elevation of areas where possible. Avoid massaging pressure points or reddened areas of skin *because this results in further tissue trauma.*
2. Plan patient care to provide rest periods *to not heighten exertional dyspnea.*
3. Weigh patient daily (at same time, in same amount of clothing, and preferably with same scale).
4. Instruct the patient about the correlation between fluid intake and weight gain, using commonly understood fluid measurements; for example, ingesting 4 cups (1000 ml) of fluid results in an approximate 2-pound weight gain in the anuric patient.

NURSING MANAGEMENT PLAN
Hyperthermia

Definition: Body temperature elevated above normal range.

Hyperthermia Related to Increased Metabolic Rate

DEFINING CHARACTERISTICS
- Increased body temperature above normal range
- Seizures
- Flushed skin
- Increased respiratory rate
- Tachycardia
- Skin warm to touch
- Diaphoresis

OUTCOME CRITERIA
- Temperature is within normal range.
- Respiratory rate and heart rate are within patient's baseline range.
- Skin is warm and dry.

NURSING INTERVENTIONS AND *RATIONALE*
1. Monitor temperature every 15 minutes to 1 hour until within normal range and stable and then every 4 hours *to maintain close surveillance for temperature fluctuations and evaluate effectiveness of interventions.*
   - Use temperature taken from pulmonary artery catheter or bladder catheter if available *because these methods closely reflect core body temperature.*
   - Use tympanic membrane temperature if core body temperature devices are unavailable.
   - Use rectal temperature if none of the methods listed above are available.
2. Collaborate with physician regarding administration of antithyroid medications *to block the synthesis and release of thyroid hormone.*
3. Collaborate with physician regarding the use of cooling blanket *to facilitate heat loss via conduction.*
   - Wrap hands, feet, and genitalia to protect them from maceration during cooling and decrease chance of shivering.
   - Avoid rapidly cooling the patient and overcooling the patient because this initiates the heat-conserving response (i.e., shivering).
4. Place ice packs in patient's groin and axilla *to facilitate heat loss via conduction.*
5. Maintain patient on bed rest *to decrease the effects of activity on the patient's metabolic rate.*
6. Provide tepid sponge baths *to facilitate heat loss via evaporation.*
7. Decrease the patient's room temperature *to facilitate radiant heat loss.*
8. Place fan near patient to circulate cool air *to facilitate heat loss via convection.*
9. Provide patient with nonrestrictive gown and lightweight bed coverings *to allow heat to escape from the patient's trunk.*
10. Collaborate with physician and respiratory therapist on the administration of oxygen to maintain Spo_2 greater than 90% *because patient has increased oxygen consumption secondary to increased metabolic rate.*
11. Collaborate with physician regarding use of antipyretic medications *to facilitate patient comfort.*
12. Collaborate with physician regarding use of intravenous and oral fluids *to maintain adequate hydration of the patient.*

NURSING MANAGEMENT PLAN
Hypothermia

Definition: Body temperature below normal range.

Hypothermia Related to Decreased Metabolic Rate

DEFINING CHARACTERISTICS
- Reduction in body temperature below normal range
- Shivering
- Pallor
- Piloerection
- Hypertension
- Skin cool to touch
- Tachycardia
- Decreased capillary refill

OUTCOME CRITERIA
- Temperature is within normal range.
- Heart rate is within patient's baseline range.
- Skin is warm and dry.
- Capillary refill is normal.

NURSING INTERVENTIONS AND *RATIONALE*
1. Monitor temperature every 15 minutes to 1 hour until within normal range and stable and then every 4 hours *to maintain close surveillance for temperature fluctuations and evaluate effectiveness of interventions.*
   - Use temperature taken from pulmonary artery catheter or bladder catheter if available *because these methods closely reflect core body temperature.*
   - Use tympanic membrane temperature *if core body temperature devices are unavailable.*
   - Use rectal temperature if none of the methods listed above are available.
2. Collaborate with physician regarding administration of thyroid medications *to replace lacking thyroid hormone.*
3. Collaborate with physician regarding the use of fluid-filled heating blanket *to facilitate rewarming via conduction.*
4. Initiate forced air-warming therapy *to facilitate convective heat gain.*
5. Provide patient with warm blankets *to facilitate heat transfer to the patient.*
6. Increase the patient's room temperature *to decrease radiant heat loss.*
7. Replace wet patient gown and bed linen promptly *to decrease evaporative heat loss.*
8. Warm intravenous fluids and blood products *to facilitate rewarming via conduction.*

Hypothermia Related to Exposure to Cold Environment, Trauma, or Damage to the Hypothalamus

DEFINING CHARACTERISTICS
- Core body temperature below 35° C (95° F)
- Skin cold to touch
- Slurred speech, incoordination
- At temperature below 33° C (91.4° F):
  — Cardiac dysrhythmias (atrial fibrillation, bradycardia)
  — Cyanosis
  — Respiratory alkalosis
- At temperatures below 32° C (89.6° F):
  — Shivering replaced by muscle rigidity
  — Hypotension
  — Dilated pupils
- At temperatures below 28° to 29° C (82.4° to 84.2° F):
  — Absent deep tendon reflexes
  — (3 to 4 breaths/min to apnea)
  — Ventricular fibrillation possible
- At temperatures below 26° to 27° C (78.8° to 80.6° F):
  — Coma
  — Flaccid muscles
  — Fixed, dilated pupils
  — Ventricular fibrillation to cardiac standstill
  — Apnea

OUTCOME CRITERIA
- Core body temperature is greater than 35° C (95° F).
- Patient is alert and oriented.
- Cardiac dysrhythmias are absent.
- Acid-base balance is normal.
- Pupils are normoreactive.

NURSING INTERVENTIONS AND *RATIONALE*
1. Monitor core body temperature continuously.
2. Collaborate with the physician regarding the need for intubation and mechanical ventilation.
   - Heated air or oxygen can be added *to help rewarm the body core.*
   - Do not hyperventilate the hypothermic patient because carbon dioxide production is low and this action may induce severe alkalosis and precipitate ventricular fibrillation.
3. Maintain cardiopulmonary resuscitation (CPR) and advanced cardiac life support (ACLS) until core body temperature is up to at least 29.5° C (85.1° F) before determining that patients cannot be resuscitated. *Electrical defibrillation is usually successful in terminating ventricular fibrillation if the temperature is greater than 28° C (82.4° F).*

NURSING MANAGEMENT PLAN—*cont'd*

4. Administer cardiac resuscitation drugs sparingly *because as the body warms, peripheral vasodilation occurs. Drugs that remain in the periphery are suddenly released, leading to a "bolus effect" that may cause fatal dysrhythmias.*
5. Monitor arterial blood gas (ABG) values *to direct further therapy,* and ensure that the pH, Pao_2, and $Paco_2$ are corrected for temperature.
6. Rewarm patient rapidly *because the pathophysiologic changes associated with chronic hypothermia have not had time to evolve.*
   - Institute rapid, active rewarming by immersion in warm water (38° to 43° C) (100.4° to 109.4° F).
   - Apply thermal blanket at 36.6° to 37.7° C (97.9° to 99.9° F). Some researchers suggest rewarming only the torso or trunk first, leaving the extremities exposed to room temperature. *This is to prevent early peripheral vasodilation with abrupt redistribution of intravascular volume. This also prevents colder blood trapped in the extremities from returning to the body core before the heart is rewarmed.*
   - Perform rapid core rewarming with heated (37° to 43° C) (98.6° to 109.4° F) intravenous (IV) infusion, hemodialysis, peritoneal dialysis, and colonic or gastric irrigation fluids.
7. Monitor peripheral circulation because gangrene of the fingers and toes is a common complication of accidental hypothermia.

NURSING MANAGEMENT PLAN

Imbalanced Nutrition: Less Than Body Requirements

Definition: Intake of nutrients insufficient to meet metabolic needs.

Imbalanced Nutrition: Less than Body Requirements Related to Lack of Exogenous Nutrients and Increased Metabolic Demand

DEFINING CHARACTERISTICS

- Unplanned weight loss of 20% of body weight within the past 6 months
- Serum albumin <3.5 g/dl
- Total lymphocytes <1500/mm^3
- Anergy
- Negative nitrogen balance
- Fatigue; lack of energy and endurance
- Nonhealing wounds
- Daily caloric intake less than estimated nutritional requirements
- Presence of factors known to increase nutritional requirements (e.g., sepsis, trauma, multiple organ dysfunction syndrome [MODS])
- Maintenance of nothing by mouth (NPO) status for >7-10 days
- Long-term use of 5% dextrose intravenously
- Documentation of suboptimal calorie counts
- Drug or nutrient interaction that might decrease oral intake (e.g. chronic use of bronchodilators, laxatives, anticonvulsives, diuretics, antacids, narcotics)
- Physical problems with chewing, swallowing, choking, and salivation and presence of altered taste, anorexia, nausea, vomiting, diarrhea, or constipation

OUTCOME CRITERIA

- Patient exhibits stabilization of weight loss or weight gain of $^1/_2$ pound daily.
- Serum albumin level is greater than 3.5 g/dl.
- Total lymphocyte count is greater than 1500/mm^3.
- Patient has positive response to cutaneous skin antigen testing.
- Patient is in positive nitrogen balance.
- Wound healing is evident.
- Daily caloric intake equals estimated nutritional requirements.
- Increased ambulation and endurance are evident.

NURSING INTERVENTIONS AND *RATIONALE*

1. Inquire if patient has any food allergies and food preferences *to ensure the food provided to the patient is not contraindicated.*
2. Monitor patient's caloric intake and weight daily *to ensure adequacy of nutritional interventions.*
3. Collaborate with dietitian regarding patient's nutritional and caloric needs *to determine the appropriateness of the patient's diet to meet those needs.*
4. Monitor patient for signs of nutritional deficiencies *to facilitate evaluation of extent of nutritional deficit.*
5. Provide patient with oral care before eating *to ensure optimal consumption of diet.*
6. Assist patient with eating as appropriate *to ensure optimal consumption of diet.*
7. Collaborate with physician regarding the administration of parenteral and enteral nutrition as needed.

NURSING MANAGEMENT PLAN
Impaired Gas Exchange

Definition: Excess or deficit in oxygenation and/or carbon dioxide elimination at the alveolar-capillary membrane.

Impaired Gas Exchange Related to Alveolar Hypoventilation

DEFINING CHARACTERISTICS
- Abnormal arterial blood gas (ABG) values (decreased $Pa{O_2}$, increased $Pa{CO_2}$, decreased pH, decreased $Sa{O_2}$)
- Somnolence
- Neurobehavioral changes (restlessness, irritability, confusion)
- Tachycardia or dysrhythmias
- Central cyanosis

OUTCOME CRITERIA
- ABG values are within patient's baseline.
- Central cyanosis is absent.

NURSING INTERVENTIONS AND *RATIONALE*
1. Initiate continuous pulse oximetry, or monitor $Sp{O_2}$ every hour.
2. Collaborate with physician on the administration of oxygen to maintain an $Sp{O_2}$ greater than 90%.
   - Administer supplemental oxygen via appropriate oxygen-delivery device *to increase driving pressure of oxygen in the alveoli.*
   - If supplemental oxygen alone is not effective, administer continuous positive airway pressure (CPAP) or mechanical ventilation with positive end-expiratory pressure (PEEP) *to open collapsed alveoli and increase the surface area for gas exchange.*
3. Prevent hypoventilation.
   - Position patient in high-Fowler's position or semi-Fowler's position *to promote diaphragmatic descent and maximal inhalation.*
   - Assist with deep-breathing exercises and/or incentive spirometry with sustained maximal inspiration 5 to 10 times per hour *to help reinflate collapsed portions of the lung.* See plan for Ineffective Breathing Pattern Related to Decreased Lung Expansion for further instructions.
   - Treat pain, if present, *to prevent hypoventilation and atelectasis.* Implement plan for Acute Pain Related to Transmission of Perception of Cutaneous, Visceral, Muscular, or Ischemic Impulses.
4. Assist physician with intubation and initiation of mechanical ventilation as indicated.

Impaired Gas Exchange Related to Ventilation/Perfusion Mismatching or Intrapulmonary Shunting

DEFINING CHARACTERISTICS
- Abnormal ABG values (decreased $Pa{O_2}$, decreased $Sa{O_2}$)
- Somnolence
- Neurobehavioral changes (restlessness, irritability, confusion)
- Central cyanosis

OUTCOME CRITERIA
- ABG values are within patient's baseline.
- Central cyanosis is absent.

NURSING INTERVENTIONS AND *RATIONALE*
1. Initiate continuous pulse oximetry, or monitor $Sp{O_2}$ every hour.
2. Collaborate with physician on the administration of oxygen to maintain an $Sp{O_2}$ greater than 90%.
   - Administer supplemental oxygen via appropriate oxygen-delivery device *to increase driving pressure of oxygen in the alveoli.*
   - If supplemental oxygen alone is not effective, administer continuous positive airway pressure (CPAP) or mechanical ventilation with positive end-expiratory pressure (PEEP) *to open collapsed alveoli and increase the surface area for gas exchange.*
3. Position patient to optimize ventilation/perfusion matching.
   - For patient with unilateral lung disease, position with the good lung down *because gravity will improve perfusion to this area, and this will best match ventilation with perfusion.*
   - For patient with bilateral lung disease, position with the right lung down *because this lung is larger than the left and affords a greater area for ventilation and perfusion,* or change position every 2 hours, favoring positions that improve oxygenation.
   - Avoid any position that seriously compromises oxygenation status.
4. Perform procedures only as needed, and provide adequate rest and recovery time in between *to prevent desaturation.*
5. Collaborate with the physician regarding the administration of the following:
   - Sedatives *to decrease ventilator asynchrony and facilitate patient's sense of control.*
   - Neuromuscular blocking agents *to prevent ventilator asynchrony and decrease oxygen demand.*
   - Analgesics *to treat pain if present.* Implement plan for Acute Pain Related to Transmission of Perception of Cutaneous, Visceral, Muscular, or Ischemic Impulses.
6. If secretions are present, implement plan for Ineffective Airway Clearance Related to Excessive Secretions or Abnormal Viscosity of Mucus.

NURSING MANAGEMENT PLAN
Impaired Spontaneous Ventilation

Definition: Decreased energy reserves results in an individual's inability to maintain breathing adequate to support life.

Impaired Spontaneous Ventilation Related to Respiratory Muscle Fatigue or Metabolic Factors

DEFINING CHARACTERISTICS

- Dyspnea and apprehension
- Increased metabolic rate
- Increased restlessness
- Increased use of accessory muscles
- Decreased tidal volume
- Increased heart rate
- Abnormal arterial blood gas (ABG) values (decreased Pao_2, increased $Paco_2$, decreased pH, decreased Sao_2)
- Decreased cooperation

OUTCOME CRITERIA

- Metabolic rate and heart rate are within patient's baseline.
- Patient experiences eupnea.
- ABG values are within patient's baseline.

NURSING INTERVENTIONS AND RATIONALE

1. Collaborate with the physician regarding the application of pressure support to the ventilator *to assist patient in overcoming the work of breathing imposed by the ventilator and endotracheal tube.*
2. Carefully snip excess length from the proximal end of the endotracheal tube *to decrease dead space and thereby decrease the work of breathing.*
3. Collaborate with the physician and dietitian to ensure that at least 50% of the diet's nonprotein caloric source is in the form of fat versus carbohydrates *to prevent excess carbon dioxide production.*
4. Collaborate with the physician and respiratory therapist regarding the best method of weaning for individual patients *because each situation is different and a variety of weaning options are available.*
5. Collaborate with the physician and physical therapist regarding a progressive ambulation and conditioning plan *to promote overall muscle conditioning and respiratory muscle functioning.*
6. Determine the most effective means of communication for the patient *to promote independence and reduce anxiety.*
7. Develop a daily schedule, and post it in patient's room *to coordinate care and facilitate patient's involvement in the plan.*
8. Treat pain, if present, *to prevent respiratory splinting and hypoventilation.* Implement plan for Acute Pain Related to Transmission of Perception of Cutaneous, Visceral, Muscular, or Ischemic Impulses.
9. Ensure that patient receives at least 2- to 4-hr intervals of uninterrupted sleep in a quiet, dark room. Collaborate with the physician and respiratory therapist regarding the use of full ventilatory support at night *to provide respiratory muscle rest.*
10. Place patient in semi-Fowler's position or in a chair at the bedside *for best use of ventilatory muscles and to facilitate diaphragmatic descent.*
11. Explain the weaning procedure to the patient before the trial *so that patient will understand what to expect and how to participate.*
12. Monitor patient during the weaning trial for evidence of respiratory muscle fatigue *to avoid overtiring the patient.*
13. Provide diversional activity during the weaning trial *to reduce the patient's anxiety.*
14. Collaborate with physician and respiratory therapist regarding the removal of the ventilator and artificial airway when patient has been successfully weaned.

NURSING MANAGEMENT PLAN
Impaired Swallowing

Definition: Abnormal functioning of the swallowing mechanism associated with deficits in oral, pharyngeal, or esophageal structure or function.

Impaired Swallowing Related to Neuromuscular Impairment, Fatigue, and Limited Awareness

DEFINING CHARACTERISTICS

Evidence of Difficulty Swallowing

- Drooling
- Difficulty handling oral secretions
- Absence of gag, cough, and/or swallow reflex
- Moist, wet, gurgling voice quality
- Decreased tongue and mouth movements
- Presence of dysarthria
- Difficulty handling solid foods:
  - — Uncoordinated chewing or swallowing
  - — Stasis of food in the oral cavity
  - — Wet-sounding voice or change in voice quality
  - — Sneezing, coughing, or choking with eating
  - — Delay in swallowing of more than 5 seconds
  - — Change in respiratory patterns
- Difficulty handling liquids:
  - — Momentary loss of voice or change in voice quality
  - — Nasal regurgitation of liquids
  - — Coughing with drinking

Evidence of Aspiration

- Hypoxemia
- Productive cough
- Frothy sputum
- Wheezing, crackles, or rhonchi
- Temperature elevation

OUTCOME CRITERIA

- Evidence of swallowing difficulties is absent.
- Evidence of aspiration is absent.

NURSING INTERVENTIONS AND *RATIONALE*

1. Collaborate with physician and speech therapist regarding swallowing evaluation and rehabilitation program *to decrease the incidence of aspiration.*
2. Collaborate with physician and dietitian regarding a nutritional assessment and nutritional plan *to ensure that the patient is receiving enough nutrition.*
3. Place the patient in an upright position with the head midline and the chin slightly down *to keep food in the anterior portion of the mouth and to prevent it from falling over the base of the tongue into the open airway.*
4. Provide patient with single-textured soft foods (e.g., cream cereals) that maintain their shape *because these foods require minimal oral manipulation.*
5. Avoid particulate foods (e.g., hamburger) and foods containing more than one texture (e.g., stew) *because these foods require more chewing and oral manipulation.*
6. Avoid dry foods (e.g., popcorn, rice, crackers) and sticky foods (e.g., peanut butter, bananas) *because these foods are difficult to manipulate orally.*
7. Provide patient with thick liquids (e.g., fruit nectar, yogurt) *because thick liquids are more easily controlled in the mouth.*
8. Thicken thin liquids (e.g., water, juice) with a thickening preparation or avoid them *because thin liquids are easily aspirated.*
9. Place foods in the uninvolved side of the mouth *because oral sensitivity and function are greatest in this area.*
10. Avoid the use of straws *because they can deposit the liquid too far back in the mouth for the patient to handle.*
11. Serve foods and liquids at room temperature *because the patient may be overly sensitive to heat or cold.*
12. Offer solids and liquids at different times *to avoid swallowing solids before being properly chewed.*
13. Provide oral hygiene after meals *to clear food particles from the mouth that could be aspirated.*
14. Collaborate with physician and pharmacist regarding oral medication administration *to adjust medication regimen to prevent aspiration and choking and to ensure all prescribed medications are swallowed.*
15. Crush tablets (if appropriate) and mix with food that is easily formed into a bolus, use thickened liquid medications (if available), and/or embed small capsules into food *to facilitate oral medication administration.*
16. Inspect mouth for residue after all medication administration *to ensure medication has been swallowed.*
17. Educate patient and family on the swallowing problem, rehabilitation program, and emergency measures for choking.

NURSING MANAGEMENT PLAN
Impaired Verbal Communication

Definition: Decreased, delayed, or absent ability to receive, process, transmit, and use a system of symbols.

Impaired Verbal Communication Related to Cerebral Speech Center Injury

DEFINING CHARACTERISTICS
- Inappropriate or absent speech or responses to questions
- Inability to speak spontaneously
- Inability to understand spoken words
- Inability to follow commands appropriately through gestures
- Difficulty or inability to understand written language
- Difficulty or inability to express ideas in writing
- Difficulty or inability to name objects

OUTCOME CRITERION
- Patient is able to make basic needs known.

NURSING INTERVENTIONS AND *RATIONALE*
1. Consult with physician and speech pathologist *to determine the extent of the patient's communication deficit (e.g., whether fluent, nonfluent, or global aphasia is involved).*
2. Have the speech therapist post a list of appropriate ways to communicate with the patient in the patient's room *so that all nursing personnel can be consistent in their efforts.*
3. Assess the patient's ability to comprehend, speak, read, and write.
   - Ask questions that can be answered with a "yes" or a "no." If a patient answers "yes" to a question, ask the opposite (e.g., "Are you hot?" "Yes." "Are you cold?" "Yes."). *This may help determine whether in fact the patient understands what is being said.*
   - Ask simple, short questions, and use gestures, pantomime, and facial expressions to give the patient additional clues.
   - Stand in the patient's line of vision, giving a good view of your face and hands.
   - Have the patient try to write with a pad and pencil. Offer pictures and alphabet letters at which to point.
   - Make flash cards with pictures or words depicting frequently used phrases (e.g., glass of water, bedpan).
4. Maintain an uncluttered environment, and decrease external distractions *that could hinder communication.*
5. Maintain a relaxed and calm manner, and explain all diagnostic, therapeutic, and comfort measures before initiating them.
6. Do not shout or speak in a loud voice. *Hearing loss is not a factor in aphasia, and shouting will not help.*
7. Have only one person talk at a time. *It is more difficult for the patient to follow a multisided conversation.*
8. Use direct eye contact, and speak directly to the patient in unhurried, short phrases.
9. Give one-step commands and directions, and provide cues through pictures and gestures.
10. Try to ask questions that can be answered with a "yes" or a "no," and avoid topics that are controversial, emotional, abstract, or lengthy.
11. Listen to the patient in an unhurried manner, and wait for his or her attempt to communicate.
    - Expect a time lag from when you ask the patient something until the patient responds.
    - Accept the patient's statement of essential words without expecting complete sentences.
    - Avoid finishing the sentence for the patient if possible.
    - Wait approximately 30 seconds before providing the word the patient may be attempting to find (except when the patient is very frustrated and needs something quickly, such as a bedpan).
    - Rephrase the patient's message aloud *to validate it.*
    - Do not pretend to understand the patient's message if you do not.
12. Encourage the patient to speak slowly in short phrases and to say each word clearly.
13. Ask the patient to write the message, if able, or draw pictures if only verbal communication is affected.
14. Observe the patient's nonverbal clues for validation (e.g., answers "yes" but shakes head "no").
15. When handing an object to the patient, state what it is *because hearing language spoken is necessary to stimulate language development.*
16. Explain what has happened to the patient, and offer reassurance about the plan of care.
17. Verbally address the problem of frustration over inability to communicate, and explain that both the nurse and the patient need patience.
18. Maintain a calm, positive manner, and offer reassurance (e.g., "I know this is very hard for you, but it will get better if we work on it together").
19. Talk to the patient as an adult. Be respectful, and avoid talking down to the patient.
20. Do not discuss the patient's condition or hold conversations in the patient's presence without including him or her in the discussion. *This may be the reason some aphasic patients develop paranoid thoughts.*
21. Do not exhibit disapproval of emotional utterances or spontaneous use of profanity; instead, offer calm, quiet reassurance.
22. If the patient makes an error in speech, do not reprimand or scold but try to compliment the patient by saying, "That was a good try."
23. Delay conversation if the patient is tired. *The symptoms of aphasia worsen if the patient is fatigued, anxious, or upset.*
24. Be prepared for emotional outbursts and tears from patients who have more difficulty in expressing themselves than with understanding. The patient may become depressed, refuse treatment and food, ignore relatives, and push objects away. Comfort the patient with statements such as, "I know it's frustrating and you feel sad, but you are not alone. Other people who have had strokes have felt the way you do. We will be here to help you get through this."

NURSING MANAGEMENT PLAN
Ineffective Airway Clearance

Definition: Inability to clear secretions or obstructions from the respiratory tract to maintain a clear airway.

Ineffective Airway Clearance Related to Excessive Secretions or Abnormal Viscosity of Mucus

DEFINING CHARACTERISTICS

- Abnormal breath sounds (displaced normal sounds, adventitious sounds, diminished or absent sounds)
- Ineffective cough with or without sputum
- Tachypnea, dyspnea
- Verbal reports of inability to clear airway

OUTCOME CRITERIA

- Cough produces thin mucus.
- Lungs are clear to auscultation.
- Respiratory rate, depth, and rhythm return to baseline.

NURSING INTERVENTIONS AND *RATIONALE*

1. Assess sputum for color, consistency, and amount.
2. Assess for clinical manifestations of pneumonia.
3. Provide for maximal thoracic expansion by repositioning, deep breathing, splinting, and pain management *to avoid hypoventilation and atelectasis.* If hypoventilation is present, implement plan for Ineffective Breathing Pattern Related to Decreased Lung Expansion.
4. Maintain adequate hydration by administering oral and intravenous fluids (as ordered) *to thin secretions and facilitate airway clearance.*
5. Provide humidification to airways via oxygen-delivery device or artificial airway *to thin secretions and facilitate airway clearance.*
6. Administer bland aerosol every 4 hours *to facilitate expectoration of sputum.*
7. Collaborate with the physician regarding the administration of the following:
   - Bronchodilators *to treat or prevent bronchospasms and facilitate expectoration of mucus.*
   - Mucolytics and expectorants *to enhance mobilization and removal of secretions.*
   - Antibiotics *to treat infection.*
8. Assist with directed coughing exercises *to facilitate expectoration of secretions.* If patient is unable to perform cascade cough, consider using huff cough (patients with hyperactive airways), end-expiratory cough (patient with secretions in distal airway), or augmented cough (patient with weakened abdominal muscle), instructing patient as follows:
   - Cascade cough
     (1) Take a deep breath, and hold it for 1 to 3 seconds.
     (2) Cough out forcefully several times until all air is exhaled.
     (3) Inhale slowly through the nose.
     (4) Repeat once.
     (5) Rest, and then repeat as necessary.
   - Huff cough
     (1) Take a deep breath, and hold it for 1 to 3 seconds.
     (2) Say the word "huff" while coughing out several times until air is exhaled.
     (3) Inhale slowly through the nose.
     (4) Repeat as necessary.
   - End-expiratory cough
     (1) Take a deep breath, and hold it for 1 to 3 seconds.
     (2) Exhale slowly.
     (3) At the end of exhalation, cough once.
     (4) Inhale slowly through the nose.
     (5) Repeat as necessary, or follow with cascade cough.
   - Augmented cough
     (1) Take a deep breath, and hold it for 1 to 3 seconds.
     (2) Perform one or more of the following maneuvers to increase intraabdominal pressure:
       — Tighten knees and buttocks.
       — Bend forward at the waist.
       — Place a hand flat on the upper abdomen just under the xiphoid process, and press in and up abruptly during coughing.
       — Keep hands on the chest wall, and press inward with each cough.
     (3) Inhale slowly through the nose.
     (4) Rest and repeat as necessary.
9. Suction nasotracheally or endotracheally as necessary *to assist with secretion removal.*
10. Reposition patient at least every 2 hours, or use continuous lateral rotation therapy *to mobilize and prevent stasis of secretions.*
11. Allow rest periods between coughing sessions, suctioning, or any other demanding activities *to promote energy conservation.*

NURSING MANAGEMENT PLAN
Ineffective Breathing Pattern

Definition: Inspiration and/or expiration that does not provide adequate ventilation.

Ineffective Breathing Pattern Related to Decreased Lung Expansion

DEFINING CHARACTERISTICS
- Abnormal respiratory patterns (hypoventilation, hyperventilation, tachypnea, bradypnea, obstructive breathing)
- Abnormal arterial blood gas (ABG) values (increased $Paco_2$, decreased pH)
- Unequal chest movement
- Shortness of breath, dyspnea

OUTCOME CRITERIA
- Respiratory rate, rhythm, and depth return to baseline.
- Use of accessory muscles is minimal or absent.
- Chest expands symmetrically.
- ABG values return to baseline.

NURSING INTERVENTIONS AND *RATIONALE*
1. Treat pain, if present, *to prevent hypoventilation and atelectasis.* Implement plan for Acute Pain Related to Transmission and Perception of Cutaneous, Visceral, Muscular, or Ischemic Impulses.
2. Position patient in high-Fowler's or semi-Fowler's position *to promote diaphragmatic descent and maximal inhalation.*
3. Assist with deep-breathing exercises and incentive spirometry with sustained maximal inspiration 5 to 10 times per hour, instructing patient as follows, *to help reinflate collapsed portions of the lung.*
   - Deep breathing
     - — Sit up straight or lean forward slightly while sitting on edge of bed or chair (if possible).
     - — Take in a slow, deep breath.
     - — Pause slightly, or hold breath for at least 3 seconds.
     - — Exhale slowly.
     - — Rest, and repeat.
   - Incentive spirometry
     - — Exhale normally.
     - — Place lips around the mouthpiece, and close mouth tightly around it.
     - — Inhale slowly and as deeply as possible, noting the maximal volume of air inspired.
     - — Hold maximal inhalation for 3 seconds.
     - — Take the mouthpiece out of mouth, and slowly exhale.
     - — Rest, and repeat.
4. Assist physician with intubation and initiation of mechanical ventilation as indicated.

Ineffective Breathing Pattern Related to Musculoskeletal Fatigue or Neuromuscular Impairment

DEFINING CHARACTERISTICS
- Unequal chest movement
- Shortness of breath, dyspnea
- Use of accessory muscles
- Tachypnea
- Thoracoabdominal asynchrony
- Abnormal ABG values (increased $Paco_2$, decreased pH)
- Nasal flaring
- Assumption of three-point position

OUTCOME CRITERIA
- Respiratory rate, rhythm, and depth return to baseline.
- Use of accessory muscles is minimal or absent.
- Chest expands symmetrically.
- ABG values return to baseline.

NURSING INTERVENTIONS AND *RATIONALE*
1. Prevent unnecessary exertion *to limit drain on patient's ventilatory reserve.*
2. Instruct patient in energy-saving techniques *to conserve patient's ventilatory reserve.*
3. Assist with pursed-lip and diaphragmatic breathing techniques *to facilitate diaphragmatic descent and improved ventilation.*
   - Diaphragmatic breathing
     - — Sit in the upright position.
     - — Place one hand on the abdomen just above the waist and the other on the upper chest.
     - — Breathe in through the nose, and feel the lower hand push out; the upper hand should not move.
     - — Breathe out through pursed lips, and feel the lower hand move in.
4. Position patient in high-Fowler's or semi-Fowler's position *to promote diaphragmatic descent and maximal inhalation.*
5. Assist physician with intubation and initiation of mechanical ventilation as indicated.

NURSING MANAGEMENT PLAN
Ineffective Cardiopulmonary Tissue Perfusion

Definition: Decrease in oxygen resulting in the failure to nourish the tissues at the capillary level.

Ineffective Cardiopulmonary Tissue Perfusion Related to Decreased Coronary Blood Flow

DEFINING CHARACTERISTICS

- Angina for more than 30 minutes
- ST-segment elevation on 12-lead electrocardiogram (ECG)
- Elevated troponin I
- Elevated CK-MB enzymes
- Apprehension
- Shortness of breath

OUTCOME CRITERIA

- Systolic blood pressure (SBP) is greater than 90 mm Hg.
- Mean arterial pressure (MAP) is greater than 60 mm Hg.
- Heart rate is less than 100 beats/min.
- Pulmonary artery (PA) pressures are within normal limits or back to baseline.
- Cardiac index (CI) is greater than 2.2 L/min/m^2.
- Urine output is greater than 0.5 ml/kg/hr or greater than 30 ml/hr.
- 12-lead ECG is normalized without new Q waves.
- Angina is absent.
- CK-MB enzymes and troponin I levels are within normal range.

NURSING INTERVENTIONS AND *RATIONALE*

1. Collaborate with the physician regarding the administration of thrombolytic therapy or percutaneous transluminal coronary angioplasty (PTCA) *to restore myocardial blood flow.*
2. Collaborate with the physician regarding the administration of aspirin, antiplatelet therapy, and heparin *to prevent recurrent thrombosis and inhibit platelet function.*
3. Collaborate with the physician regarding the administration of β-blockers *to decrease myocardial oxygen demand and prevent recurrent ischemia.*
4. Collaborate with the physician regarding the administration of angiotensin-converting enzyme (ACE) inhibitors *to block the conversion of angiotensin I to angiotensin II, a potent vasoconstrictor.*
5. Collaborate with physician regarding the administration of sublingual nitroglycerin (NTG) and/or intravenous (IV) NTG infusion *to augment coronary blood flow and reduce cardiac work by decreasing preload and afterload.*
6. Collaborate with physician regarding the administration of morphine *to control pain.*
7. Collaborate with physician regarding the administration of oxygen at 2 L/min to achieve Spo_2 greater than 90% *to maximize myocardial oxygen supply.*
8. Maintain the patient on bed rest with bedside commode privileges *to minimize myocardial oxygen demand.*
9. Monitor patient's hemodynamic and cardiac rhythm status.
   - Select electrocardiographic (ECG) monitoring leads based on infarct location and rhythm to obtain the best rhythm for monitoring.
   - Evaluate cardiac rhythm for presence of dysrhythmias, which are common complications of myocardial ischemia.
   - Collaborate with physician regarding the administration of antidysrhythmic medications.
   - Assess serum electrolyte (potassium and magnesium) levels and arterial blood gas (ABG) values.
   - Collaborate with physician regarding the administration of electrolytes to correct any imbalances.
   - Monitor ST segment continuously to determine changes in myocardial tissue perfusion.
   - Monitor patient's blood pressure at least every hour because many conditions (drugs, dysrhythmias, myocardial ischemia) may cause hypotension (SBP <90 mm Hg).
   - Treat symptomatic dysrhythmias according to unit's emergency protocol or advanced cardiac life support (ACLS) guidelines.
10. Instruct patient to avoid the Valsalva maneuver because forced expiration against a closed glottis causes sudden and intense changes in systolic blood pressure and heart rate.

NURSING MANAGEMENT PLAN

Ineffective Cerebral Tissue Perfusion

Definition: Decrease in oxygen resulting in the failure to nourish the tissues at the capillary level.

Ineffective Cerebral Tissue Perfusion Related to Decreased Blood Flow

DEFINING CHARACTERISTICS

- Decreased level of consciousness
- Hemiparesis or hemiplegia
- Visual changes
- Aphasia
- Dysphagia
- Facial droop
- Cognitive deficits
- Ataxia

OUTCOME CRITERIA

- Neurologic deficits are absent.
- Blood pressure is within ordered parameters.

NURSING INTERVENTIONS AND *RATIONALE*

1. Collaborate with physician regarding the administration of thrombolytic therapy *to facilitate lysis of the clot and restoration of blood flow to affected area.*
2. Monitor the patient for alterations in blood pressure, oxygenation, temperature, rhythm, and glucose levels.
3. Collaborate with physician regarding the administration of vasodilators for hypertension *to maintain the patient's blood pressure within desired range.* Use caution in lowering blood pressure *because hypotension decreases cerebral blood flow.*
   - Patients receiving thrombolytic therapy: Keep systolic blood pressure (SBP) less than 185 mm Hg and diastolic blood pressure (DPB) less than 110 mm Hg.
   - Patients not receiving thrombolytic therapy: Keep SBP less than 220 mm Hg and DBP less than 140 mm Hg.
4. Collaborate with physician regarding the administration of intravenous fluids and vasoconstrictors for hypotension *because hypotension decreases cerebral blood flow.*
5. Collaborate with physician regarding the administration of oxygen to maintain Spo_2 greater than 95% *to prevent hypoxemia and potential worsening of the neurologic injury.*
6. Collaborate with physician regarding administration of acetaminophen for elevated temperature *because hyperthermia is associated with increased morbidity in the stroke patient.*
7. Collaborate with the physician regarding the treatment of dysrhythmias *due to increased sympathetic nervous system stimulation.*
8. Collaborate with the physician regarding the administration of insulin for hyperglycemia *because elevated blood glucose level has been linked to an increase in the area of infarct.*
9. Collaborate with the speech therapist regarding the patient's ability to swallow before initiating oral feedings *to ensure patient is not at risk for aspirating.*
10. Collaborate with the physical therapist to assess the patient's ability to ambulate safely *to ensure the patient is not at risk for falling* and ability to perform activities of daily living *to facilitate discharge home.*
11. Maintain surveillance for complications such as increased intracranial pressure, seizures, and acute respiratory failure.

Ineffective Cerebral Tissue Perfusion Related to Hemorrhage

DEFINING CHARACTERISTICS

Intracerebral Hemorrhage

- Alteration in level of consciousness
- Nausea and vomiting
- Headache
- Seizures
- Hypertension
- Focal neurologic deficits

Subarachnoid Hemorrhage

- Sudden onset of severe headache, nausea, and/or vomiting
- Symptoms of meningeal irritation:
  —Nuchal rigidity and pain
  —Back pain
  —Bilateral leg pain
  —Kernig's sign: resistance to full extension of the leg at the knee when the hip is flexed
  —Brudzinski's sign: flexion of the hip and knee during passive neck flexion
- Photophobia and visual changes
- Sudden loss of consciousness
- Altered level of consciousness
- Seizures
- Focal neurologic deficits

OUTCOME CRITERIA

- Patient is oriented to time, place, person, and situation.
- Pupils are equal and normoreactive.
- Blood pressure is within patient's norm.
- Motor function is bilaterally equal.
- Headache, nausea, and vomiting are absent.
- Patient verbalizes importance of and displays compliance with reduced activity.

NURSING INTERVENTIONS AND *RATIONALE*

1. Assess for indicators of increased intracranial pressure (ICP) and brain herniation (see plan for Decreased Intracranial Adaptive Capacity Related to Failure of Normal Intracranial Compensatory Mechanisms).
2. Collaborate with the physician regarding the administration of anticonvulsant medications *to prevent the onset of seizures or to control seizures.*
3. Collaborate with physician regarding the administration of vasodilators for hypertension *to avoid further bleeding.* Use caution in lowering blood pressure *because hypotension decreases cerebral blood flow.*

NURSING MANAGEMENT PLAN—*cont'd*

4. Initiate precautions *to prevent rebleeding.*
   - Ensure bed rest in a quiet environment *to lessen external stimuli.*
   - Maintain a darkened room *to lessen symptoms of photophobia.*
   - Restrict visitors, and instruct them to keep conversation as nonstressful as possible.
   - Administer prescribed sedatives as prescribed *to reduce anxiety and to promote rest.*
   - Administer analgesics as prescribed *to relieve or lessen headache.*
   - Provide a soft, high-fiber diet and stool softeners *to prevent constipation,* which can lead to straining and increased risk of rebleeding.
   - Assist with activities of daily living (feeding, bathing, dressing, toileting).
   - Avoid any activity that could lead to increased ICP; ensure that patient does not flex hips beyond 90 degrees and avoids neck hyperflexion, hyperextension, or lateral hyperrotation *that could impede jugular venous return.*

NURSING MANAGEMENT PLAN

Ineffective Coping

Definition: Inability to form a valid appraisal of the stressors, inadequate choices of practiced responses, and/or inability to use available resources.

Ineffective Coping Related to Situational Crisis and Personal Vulnerability

DEFINING CHARACTERISTICS

- Verbalization of inability to cope (e.g., "I can't take this anymore," "I don't know how to deal with this.")
- Ineffective problem solving (problem lumping) (e.g., "I have to eliminate salt from my diet. They tell me I can no longer mow the lawn. This hospitalization is costing a mint. What about my kids' future? Who's going to change the oil in the car? This is an incredible amount of time away from work.")
- Ineffective use of coping mechanisms
  - Projection: blames others for illness or pain
  - Displacement: directs anger and/or aggression toward family (e.g., "Get out of here. Leave me alone."); cursing, shouting, or demanding attention; striking out or throwing objects
  - Denial: of severity of illness and need for treatment
- Noncompliance (e.g., activity restriction; refusal to allow treatment or to take medications)
- Suicidal thoughts (verbalizes desire to end life)
- Self-directed aggression (e.g., disconnects or attempts to disconnect life-sustaining equipment; deliberately tries to harm self)
- Failure to progress from dependent to more independent state (refusal or resistance to care for self)

OUTCOME CRITERIA

- Patient verbalizes beginning ability to cope with illness, pain, and hospitalization ("I'm trying to do the best I can," "I want to help myself get better").
- Patient demonstrates effective problem solving (lists and prioritizes problems from most to least urgent).
- Patient uses effective behavioral strategies to manage the stress of illness and care.
- Patient demonstrates interest or involvement in illness or environment.
  - Requests medications when anticipating pain
  - Questions course of treatment, progress, and prognosis
  - Asks for clarification of environmental stimuli and events
  - Seeks out supportive individuals in his or her environment
  - Uses coping mechanisms and strategies more effectively to manage situational crisis
  - Demonstrates significant reduction in impulsive, angry, or aggressive outbursts (projection, shouting, cursing) directed toward family
  - Verbalizes future-based plans, with cessation of self-directed aggressive acts and suicidal thoughts
  - Willingly complies with treatment regimen
  - Begins to participate in self-care

NURSING INTERVENTIONS AND RATIONALE

1. Actively listen and respond to patient's verbal and behavioral expressions. *Active listening signifies unconditional respect and acceptance of the patient as a worthwhile individual. It builds trust and rapport, guides the nurse toward problem areas, encourages the patient to express concerns, and promotes compliance.*
2. Offer effective coping strategies to help the patient better tolerate the stressors related to his or her illness and care. Give permission to vent feelings in a safe setting. Sample statements: "I don't blame you for feeling angry or frustrated." "Others who are ill like you have expressed similar feelings." "I will listen to anything you want to share with me." "We don't have to talk; I'd like to sit here with you." "It's perfectly OK to cry." *Individuals who are provided with opportunities to express their feelings will be better able to release pent-up emotions and derive a greater sense of relief and comfort. Thus they are less likely to resort to overly impulsive, aggressive acts, which may harm self or others.*
3. Inform the family that the patient needs to displace anger occasionally but that you will be working with the patient to help him or her release his or her feelings in a more constructive, effective way. *Family members who are well-informed are better equipped to cope with their loved one's emotional anguish and outbursts. They are less likely to waste energy on feelings of guilt, fear, anger, or despair and can use their strength to help the patient in more constructive ways. The knowledge that their loved one is being cared for emotionally, as well as physically, will offer family members a greater sense of comfort and understanding. They will feel nurtured and respected by the nurse's attempt to include them in the process.*
4. With the patient, list and number problems from the most to least urgent. Assist him or her in finding immediate solutions for most urgent problems; postpone those that can wait; delegate some to family members; and help him or her to acknowledge problems that are beyond his or her control. *Listing and numbering problems in an organized fashion help to break them down into more manageable "pieces" so that the patient is better able to identify solutions for those that are solvable and to suppress those that are less relevant or not amenable to interventions.*
5. Identify individuals in the patient's environment who best help him or her to cope, as well as those who do not. Validate your observations with the patient. Sample statements: "I notice you seemed more relaxed during your daughter's visit." "After the clergy left, you were able to sleep a bit longer than usual; would you like to see him more often?" "Your grandson was a bit upset today; I'll be glad to talk to him if you like." *Supportive persons can invoke a calming effect on the patient's physiologic and psychologic states. Conversely, well-meaning but nonsupportive individuals can have a deleterious effect on the patient's ability to cope and must be carefully screened and counseled by the nurse.*
6. Teach the patient effective cognitive strategies to help him or her better manage the stress of critical illness and care. Help him or her construct pleasant thoughts,

NURSING MANAGEMENT PLAN—*cont'd*

situations, or images that can simultaneously inhibit unpleasant realities (e.g., a day at the beach, a walk in the park, drinking a glass of wine, or being with a loved one). *Pleasant thoughts and images constructed during critical illness and care tend to inhibit or reduce the intensity of the unpleasant, stressful effects of the experience.*

7. Assist the patient in using coping mechanisms more effectively so he or she can better manage his or her situational crisis.
   - Suppression of problems beyond his or her control
   - Compensation for illness and its effects; focusing on his or her strengths, interests, family, and spiritual beliefs
   - Adaptive displacement of anger, fear, or frustration through healthy, verbal expressions to staff. *Effective use of coping mechanisms helps to assuage the patient's painful feelings in a safe setting. Thus the patient is strengthened and need not resort to the use of more ineffective defenses to eliminate anxiety.*
8. Initiate a suicidal assessment if the patient verbalizes the desire to die, states that life is not worth living, or exhibits self-directed aggression. *Sample statement:* "We know that this is a bad time for you. You're saying repeatedly that you want to die. Are you planning to harm yourself?" If the response is "yes," remain with the patient, alert staff members, and provide for psychiatric consultation as soon as possible. Continue to express concern to the patient and protect him or her from harm. *Suicidal thoughts as a result of ineffective coping or exhaustion of coping devices are not an uncommon occurrence in critically ill patients. If the mood state is distressing enough, a patient may seek relief by attempting a self-destructive act. Although the patient may not imminently have the energy to succeed in his or her attempt, voicing a specific plan signifies a depressed mood state and depletion of coping strategies. Thus immediate intervention is needed, because the attempt may be successful when the patient's energy is restored.*
9. Encourage the patient to participate in self-care activities and treatment regimen in accordance with his or her level of progress. Offer praise for his or her efforts toward self-care. *Patients who take an active role in their own treatment and progress are less apt to feel like helpless or powerless victims. This greater sense of control over their illness and environment will guide them more swiftly toward becoming as independent as possible.*

NURSING MANAGEMENT PLAN
Ineffective Gastrointestinal Tissue Perfusion

Definition: Decrease in oxygen resulting in the failure to nourish the tissues at the capillary level.

Ineffective Gastrointestinal Tissue Perfusion Related to Decreased Gastrointestinal Blood Flow

DEFINING CHARACTERISTICS
- Abdominal pain
- Melena
- Abdominal distention
- Hyperactive to absent bowel sounds
- Guarding
- Fever
- Hypotension
- Tachycardia
- Altered mental status
- Urine output <30 ml/hr

OUTCOME CRITERIA
- Bowel sounds are normal.
- Abdominal pain, distention, and guarding are absent.
- Urinary output is greater than 30 ml/hr.
- Vital signs are at baseline.
- Mentation is normal.

NURSING INTERVENTIONS AND *RATIONALE*
1. Collaborate with physician regarding the administration of crystalloids, colloids, blood, and blood products *to maintain adequate circulating volume.* Implement plan for Deficient Fluid Volume Related to Absolute Loss.
2. Collaborate with physician regarding pain management. Implement plan for Acute Pain Related to Transmission of Perception of Cutaneous, Visceral, Muscular, or Ischemic Impulses.
3. Collaborate with physician regarding the administration of oxygen to maintain Spo_2 greater than 92% *to prevent hypoxemia and potential worsening of the gastrointestinal injury.*
4. Collaborate with physician regarding the administration of electrolyte replacement therapy *to maintain adequate electrolyte balance.*
5. Collaborate with dietitian regarding administration of nutrition *because patient will be unable to eat.* Implement plan for Imbalanced Nutrition: Less Than Body Requirements.
6. Maintain surveillance for complications such as gastrointestinal hemorrhage, hypovolemic shock, and septic shock.
7. Collaborate with physician regarding preparation for surgery *to remove infarcted bowel.*

NURSING MANAGEMENT PLAN

Ineffective Peripheral Tissue Perfusion

Definition: Decrease in oxygen resulting in the failure to nourish the tissues at the capillary level.

Ineffective Peripheral Tissue Perfusion Related to Decreased Peripheral Blood Flow

DEFINING CHARACTERISTICS

- Weak and/or unequal peripheral pulses
- Delayed capillary refill
- Ischemic pain from extremity
- Cool skin on extremity
- Pale extremity
- Paresthesias from extremity

OUTCOME CRITERIA

- Peripheral pulses are full and equal bilaterally.
- Capillary refill is equal bilaterally.
- Ischemic pain is absent.
- Skin temperature is equal in both extremities.
- Skin is pink and warm in both extremities.
- Paresthesias are absent.

NURSING INTERVENTIONS AND *RATIONALE*

1. Collaborate with physician regarding the administration of antiplatelet, anticoagulant, and/or thrombolytic therapy.
2. Collaborate with physician regarding pain management. Implement plan for Acute Pain Related to Transmission of Perception of Cutaneous, Visceral, Muscular, or Ischemic Impulses.
3. Ensure patient is adequately hydrated *to decrease blood viscosity.*
4. Maintain affected extremity in dependent position if possible *to enhance blood flow.*
5. Keep affected extremity warm and protect it from injury. *Do not apply heat directly to the affected extremity because this can result in injury.*
6. Maintain surveillance for pain, pallor, pulselessness, paresthesia, paralysis, and poikilothermy *as indicators of abrupt change in blood flow.*
7. Maintain surveillance for tissue breakdown and arterial ulcers *as indicators of injury.*
8. Prepare patient for possible surgery or interventional procedure to restore blood flow.

NURSING MANAGEMENT PLAN
Ineffective Renal Tissue Perfusion

Definition: Decrease in oxygen resulting in the failure to nourish the tissues at the capillary level.

Ineffective Renal Tissue Perfusion Related to Decreased Renal Blood Flow

DEFINING CHARACTERISTICS

- Anuria or oliguria
- Decreased urinary creatinine clearance
- Increased serum creatinine
- Increased blood urea nitrogen (BUN)
- Electrolyte abnormalities: potassium, sodium
- Increased pulmonary artery occlusion pressure (PAOP) and right atrial pressure (RAP) secondary to fluid overload
- Sinus tachycardia
- Metabolic acidosis
- Crackles on lung auscultation
- Engorged neck veins
- Fluid weight gain
- Pitting edema
- Mental status changes
- Anemia

OUTCOME CRITERIA

- Cardia output (CO) is greater than 4.0 L/min.
- Cardiac index (CI) is greater than 2.2 L/min/m^2.
- PAOP and RAP are within normal limits for patient.
- Electrolyte levels are within normal range.
- Serum creatinine and BUN levels are within normal range.
- Acid-base balance is normal.
- Level of consciousness is normal.
- Lungs are clear on auscultation.
- Urinary output is within normal limits, or patient is stable on dialysis.
- Hemoglobin and hematocrit values are stable.

NURSING INTERVENTIONS AND *RATIONALE*

1. Monitor intake and output, urine output, and patient weight.
2. Collaborate with physician regarding the administration of crystalloids, colloids, blood, and blood products *to increase circulating volume and maintain MAP greater than 70 mm Hg.*
3. Collaborate with physician regarding the administration of inotropes *to enhance myocardial contractility and increase CI to greater than 2.5 L/min/m^2.*
4. Collaborate with physician regarding the administration of diuretics to the oliguric patient *to flush out cellular debris and increase urine output.*
5. Minimize the patient's exposure to nephrotoxic drugs *to decrease damage to kidneys.*
6. Monitor blood levels of drugs cleared by kidneys *to avoid accumulation.*
7. Monitor patient for signs of electrolyte imbalance *due to impaired electrolyte regulation.*
8. Maintain surveillance for signs and symptoms of fluid overload.
9. Monitor patient's clinical status and response to dialysis therapy *to ensure the patient is receiving safe and effective dialytic therapy.*

NURSING MANAGEMENT PLAN
Insomnia

Definition: Time-limited disruption of sleep (natural, periodic suspension of consciousness) amount and quality.

Insomnia Related to Fragmented Sleep

DEFINING CHARACTERISTICS

- Decreased sleep during one block of sleep time
- Daytime sleepiness
- Decreased sleep
  - — Less than one half of normal total sleep time
  - — Decreased slow-wave, or rapid-eye-movement (REM), sleep
- Anxiety
- Fatigue
- Restlessness
- Disorientation and hallucinations
- Combativeness
- Frequent awakenings

OUTCOME CRITERIA

- Patient's total sleep time approximates patient's normal.
- Patient can complete sleep cycles of 90 minutes without interruption.
- Patient has no delusions or hallucinations.
- Patient has reality-based thought content.

NURSING INTERVENTIONS AND *RATIONALE*

1. Assess normal sleep pattern on admission and any history of sleep disturbance or chronic illness that may affect sleep or sedative/hypnotic use. Promote normal sleep activity while patient is in critical care unit. Assess sleep effectiveness by asking patient how his or her sleep in the hospital compares with sleep at home. ***The best treatment for sleep pattern disturbance is prevention.***
2. Promote comfort, relaxation, and a sense of well-being. Treat pain; change, smooth, or refresh bed linens at bedtime; and provide oral hygiene. Eliminate stressful situations before bedtime. Use relaxation techniques, imagery, music, massage, or warm blankets. Other interventions may include having a close family member sit beside the bed and providing the patient with his or her own garments or coverings. Individual patients may prefer quiet or may prefer the background noise of the television or music to best promote sleep. Provide a comfortable room temperature.
3. Minimize noise, particularly that of the staff and noisy equipment. Reduce the level of environmental stimuli. Dim lights at night.
4. Foods containing tryptophan (e.g., milk, turkey) may be appropriate ***because these promote sleep.***
5. Plan nap times to assist in approximating the patient's normal 24-hour sleep time.
6. Minimize awakenings ***to allow for at least 90-minute sleep cycles.*** Continually assess the need to awaken the patient, particularly at night. Distinguish between essential and nonessential nursing tasks. Organize nursing management to allow for maximal amount of uninterrupted sleep while ensuring close monitoring of the patient's condition. Whenever possible, monitor physiologic parameters without waking the patient. Coordinate awakenings with other departments, such as respiratory therapy, laboratory, and x-ray, ***to minimize sleep interruptions.***
7. Be aware of the effects of commonly used medications on sleep. ***Many sedative and hypnotic medications decrease REM sleep.*** Sedative and analgesic medications should not be withheld, but rather, drugs that minimally disrupt sleep are to be used to complement comfort measures, with dosages reduced gradually as the medication is no longer necessary. Do not abruptly withdraw REM-suppressing medications ***because this can result in "REM rebound."***
8. Document amount of uninterrupted sleep per shift, especially sleep episodes lasting longer than 2 hours. This can be effectively documented as part of the 24-hour flow sheet and reported routinely, shift to shift. ***Sleep pattern disturbance is diagnosed, treated, and resolved more efficiently when formally documented in this manner.***

NURSING MANAGEMENT PLAN
Powerlessness

Definition: Perception that one's own action will not significantly affect an outcome; a perceived lack of control over a current situation or immediate happening.

Powerlessness Related to Lack of Control Over Current Situation and/or Disease Progression

DEFINING CHARACTERISTICS

Severe

- Verbal expressions of having no control or influence over situation
- Verbal expressions of having no control or influence over outcome
- Verbal expressions of having no control over self-care
- Depression over physical deterioration that occurs despite patient's compliance with regiments
- Apathy

Moderate

- Nonparticipation in care or decision making when opportunities are provided
- Expressions of dissatisfaction and frustration about inability to perform previous tasks and/or activities
- Lack of progress monitoring
- Expressions of doubt about role performance
- Reluctance to express true feelings, fearing alienation from caregivers
- Passivity
- Inability to seek information about care
- Dependence on others that may result in irritability, resentment, anger, and guilt
- No defense of self-care practices when challenged

Low

- Passivity

OUTCOME CRITERIA

- Patient verbalizes increased control over situation by wanting to do things his or her way.
- Patient actively participates in planning care.
- Patient requests needed information.
- Patient chooses to participate in self-care activities.
- Patient monitors progress.

NURSING INTERVENTIONS AND *RATIONALE*

1. Evaluate the patient's feelings and perception of the reasons for lack of power and sense of helplessness.
2. Determine as far as possible the patient's usual response to limited control situations. Determine through ongoing assessment the patient's usual locus of control (i.e., believes that influence over his or her life is exerted by luck, fate, powerful persons [external locus of control] or that influence is exerted through personal choices, self-effort, self-determination [internal locus of control]).
3. Support patient's physical control of the environment by involving him or her in care activities; knock before entering room if appropriate; ask permission before moving personal belongings. Inform the patient that, although an activity may not be to his or her liking, it is necessary. *This gives the patient permission to express dissatisfaction with the environment and the regimen.*
4. Personalize the patient's care using his or her preferred name. *This supports the patient's psychologic control.*
5. Provide therapeutic rationale for all the patient is asked to do for himself or herself and for all that is being done for and with him or her. Reinforce the physician's explanations; clarify misconceptions about the illness situation and treatment plans. *This supports the patient's cognitive control.*
6. Include the patient in care planning by encouraging participation and allowing choices wherever possible (e.g., timing of personal care activities; deciding when pain medicines are needed). Point out situations in which no choices exist.
7. Provide opportunities for the patient to exert influence over himself or herself and his or her body, thereby affecting an outcome. For example, share with the patient the nurse's assessment of his or her breath sounds and explain that they can be improved by self-initiated deep-breathing exercises. *Feedback that the patient has been successful in helping clear his or her lungs reinforces the influence he or she does retain.*
8. Encourage family to permit patient to do as much independently as possible *to foster perception of personal power.*
9. Assist the patient in establishing realistic short-term and long-term goals. *Setting unrealistic or unattainable goals inadvertently reinforces the patient's perception of powerlessness.*
10. Document care to provide for continuity *so that the patient can maintain appropriate control over the environment.*
11. Assist the patient in regaining strength and activity tolerance as appropriate, *thus increasing a sense of control and self-reliance.*
12. Increase the sensitivity of the health team members and significant others to the patient's sense of powerlessness. Use power over the patient carefully. Use the words "must," "should," and "have to" with caution *because they communicate coercive powers and imply that the objects of "musts" and "shoulds" are of benefit to the nurse versus the patient.*
13. Plan with the patient for transfer from the critical care unit to the intermediate unit and eventually to home.

NURSING MANAGEMENT PLAN
Risk for Aspiration

Definition: At risk for entry of gastrointestinal secretions, oropharyngeal secretions, solids, or fluids into tracheobronchial passages.

RISK FACTORS

- Impaired laryngeal sensation or reflex
- Reduced level of consciousness
- Extubation
- Impaired pharyngeal peristalsis or tongue function
  - — Neuromuscular dysfunction
  - — Central nervous system dysfunction
  - — Head or neck injury
- Impaired laryngeal closure or elevation
  - — Laryngeal nerve dysfunction
  - — Artificial airways
  - — Gastrointestinal tubes
- Increased gastric volume
  - — Delayed gastric emptying
  - — Enteral feedings
  - — Medication administration
- Increased intragastric pressure
  - — Upper abdominal surgery
  - — Obesity
  - — Pregnancy
  - — Ascites
- Decreased lower esophageal sphincter pressure
  - — Increased gastric acidity
  - — Gastrointestinal tubes
- Decreased antegrade esophageal propulsion
  - — Trendelenburg or supine position
  - — Esophageal dysmotility
  - — Esophageal structural defects or lesions

OUTCOME CRITERIA

- Breath sounds are normal, or there is no change in patient's baseline breath sounds.
- Arterial blood gas (ABG) values remain within patient's baseline.
- There is no evidence of gastric contents in lung secretions.

NURSING INTERVENTIONS AND *RATIONALE*

1. Assess gastrointestinal function *to rule out hypoactive peristalsis and abdominal distention.*
2. Position patient with head of bed elevated 30 degrees *to prevent gastric reflux through gravity.* If head elevation is contraindicated, position patient in right lateral decubitus position *to facilitate passage of gastric contents across the pylorus.*
3. Maintain patency and functioning of nasogastric suction apparatus *to prevent accumulation of gastric contents.*
4. Provide frequent and scrupulous mouth care *to prevent colonization of the oropharynx with bacteria and inoculation of the lower airways.*
5. Ensure that endotracheal/tracheostomy cuff is properly inflated *to limit aspiration of oropharyngeal secretions.*
6. Treat nausea promptly; collaborate with physician on an order for antiemetic *to prevent vomiting and resultant aspiration.*

Additional Interventions for Patient Receiving Continuous or Intermittent Enteral Tube Feedings

7. Position patient with head of bed elevated 45 degrees *to prevent gastric reflux.* If a head-down position becomes necessary at any time, interrupt the feeding 30 minutes before the position change.
8. Check placement of feeding tube either by auscultation or radiographically at regular intervals (e.g., before administering intermittent feedings and after position changes, suctioning, coughing episodes, or vomiting) *to ensure proper placement of the tube.*
9. Monitor patient for signs of delayed gastric emptying *to decrease potential for vomiting and aspiration.*
   - For large-bore tubes, check residuals of tube feedings before intermittent feedings and every 4 hours during continuous feedings. Consider withholding feedings for residuals greater than 150% of the hourly rate (continuous feeding) or greater than 50% of the previous feeding (intermittent feeding).
   - For small-bore tubes, observe abdomen for distention, palpate abdomen for hardness or tautness, and auscultate abdomen for bowel sounds.

NURSING MANAGEMENT PLAN
Risk for Infection

Definition: At increased risk for being invaded by pathogenic organisms.

RISK FACTORS

- Inadequate primary defenses (broken skin, traumatized tissue, decreased ciliary action, stasis of body fluids, change in pH secretions, altered peristalsis)
- Inadequate secondary defenses (decreased hemoglobin, leukopenia, suppressed inflammatory/immune response)
- Immunocompromise
- Inadequate acquired immunity
- Tissue destruction and increased environmental exposure
- Chronic disease
- Invasive procedures
- Malnutrition
- Pharmacologic agents (antibiotics, steroids)

OUTCOME CRITERIA

- Total lymphocyte count is greater than $1000/mm^3$.
- White blood cell count is within normal limits.
- Temperature is within normal limits.
- Blood, urine, wound, and sputum cultures are negative.

NURSING INTERVENTIONS AND *RATIONALE*

1. Perform proper hand hygiene before and after patient care *to reduce the transmission of microorganisms.*
2. Use aseptic technique for insertion and manipulation of invasive monitoring devices, intravenous (IV) lines, and urinary drainage catheters *to maintain sterility of environment.*
3. Stabilize all invasive lines and catheters *to avoid unintentional manipulation and contamination.*
4. Use aseptic technique for dressing changes *to prevent contamination of wounds or insertion sites.*
5. Change any line placed under emergent conditions within 24 hours *because aseptic technique is usually breached during an emergency.*
6. Collaborate with the physician to change any dressing that is saturated with blood or drainage *because these are mediums for microorganism growth.*
7. Minimize use of stopcocks and maintain caps on all stopcock ports *to reduce the ports of entry for microorganisms.*
8. Avoid the use of nasogastric tubes, nasoendotracheal tubes, and nasopharyngeal suctioning in the patient with a suspected cerebrospinal fluid leak *to decrease the incidence of central nervous system infection.*
9. Change ventilator circuits with humidifiers no more often than every 48 hours *to avoid introducing microorganisms into the system.*
10. Provide the patient with a clean manual resuscitation bag *to avoid cross-contamination between patients.*
11. Provide meticulous mouth care at least every 4 hours, and suction oropharyngeal subglottic secretions (in patients with artificial airways) *to avoid accumulation.*
12. Cleanse in-line suction catheters with sterile saline according to the manufacturer's instructions *to avoid accumulation of secretions within the catheter.*
13. Maintain the head of the bed elevated at 30 to 45 degrees in patient artificial airways *to decrease the incidence of aspiration.*
14. Use disposable sterile scissors, forceps, and hemostats *to reduce the transmission of microorganisms.*
15. Maintain a closed urinary drainage system *to decrease incidence of urinary infections.*
16. Keep the urinary drainage tubing and bag below the level of the patient's bladder *to prevent the backflow of urine.*
17. Assess the urinary drainage tubing for kinks *to prevent stasis of urine.*
18. Protect all access device sites from potential sources of contamination (nasogastric reflux, draining wounds, ostomies, sputum).
19. Refrigerate parenteral nutrition solutions and opened enteral nutrition formulas *to inhibit bacterial growth.*
20. Maintain daily surveillance of invasive devices for signs and symptoms of infection.
21. Notify physician of elevated temperature or if any signs or symptoms of infection are present.

Additional Interventions for Patient Receiving Immunosuppressive Drugs

22. Obtain blood, urine, and sputum cultures for temperature elevations greater than 38° C (100.4° F) *inasmuch as elevation likely is caused by bacteremia or bladder or pulmonary infection.*
23. Auscultate breath sounds at least every 6 hours. *Pulmonary infection is the most common type of infection, and changes in breath sounds might be an early indication.*
24. Inspect wounds at least every 8 hours for redness, swelling, and/or drainage, *which may indicate infection.*
25. Inspect overall skin integrity and oral mucosa for signs of breakdown, *which place the patient at risk for infection.*
26. Notify physician of new-onset cough. *Even a nonproductive cough may indicate pulmonary infection.*
27. Monitor white blood cell count daily, and report leukocytosis or sudden development of leukopenia, *which may indicate an infectious process.*
28. Protect patient from exposure to any staff or family member with contagious lesion (e.g., herpes simplex) or respiratory infections.
29. Collaborate with dietitian regarding the patient's nutritional status and need for augmentation of nutritional intake as necessary *to prevent debilitation and increased susceptibility to infection.*
30. Collaborate with physician to remove invasive lines and catheters as soon as possible *to decrease potential portals of entry.*
31. Teach patient the clinical manifestations of infection. *A knowledgeable patient will seek medical attention promptly, which will result in earlier treatment and a decreased risk that infection will become life-threatening.*

NURSING MANAGEMENT PLAN

Situational Low Self-Esteem

Definition: Development of a negative perception of self-worth in response to a current situation.

Situational Low Self-Esteem Related to Feelings of Guilt About Physical Deterioration

DEFINING CHARACTERISTICS

- Inability to accept positive reinforcement
- Lack of follow-through
- Nonparticipation in therapy
- Not taking responsibility for self-care (i.e., self-neglect)
- Self-destructive behavior
- Lack of eye contact

OUTCOME CRITERIA

- Patient verbalizes feelings of self-worth.
- Patient maintains positive relationships with significant others.
- Patient manifests active interest in appearance by completing personal grooming daily.

NURSING INTERVENTIONS AND *RATIONALE*

1. Evaluate the meaning of health-related situation. How does the patient feel about himself or herself, the diagnosis, and the treatment? How does the present fit into the larger context of his or her life?
2. Assess the patient's emotional level, interpersonal relationships, and feeling about himself or herself. Recognize the patient's uniqueness (how the hair is worn, preference for name used).
3. Help the patient discover and verbalize feelings and understand the crisis by listening and providing information.
4. Assist the patient with identifying strengths and positive qualities that increase the sense of self-worth. Focus on past experiences of accomplishment and competency. Help the patient with positive self-reinforcement. Reinforce the obvious love and affection of family and significant others.
5. Assess coping techniques that have been helpful in the past. Help the patient decide how to handle negative or incongruent feedback about the situation.
6. Encourage visits from family and significant others. Facilitate interactions, and ensure privacy. Help family members entering the critical care unit by explaining what they will see. Increase visitors' comfort with equipment; offer chairs and other courtesies.
7. Encourage the patient to pursue interest in individual or social activities, even though difficult in the critical care unit.
8. Reflect caring, concern, empathy, respect, and unconditional acceptance in nurse-patient relationships.
9. Remember that for the patient the nurse is a significant other who provides important appraisals of the patient and who can facilitate the change process.
10. Help the family support the patient's self-esteem.
11. Provide for continuity of nurse assignment to ensure consistent contacts that can *facilitate support of the patient's self-esteem.*

NURSING MANAGEMENT PLAN
Unilateral Neglect

Definition: Lack of awareness and attention to one side of the body.

Unilateral Neglect Related to Perceptual Disruption

DEFINING CHARACTERISTICS
- Neglect of involved body parts and/or extrapersonal space
- Denial of existence of the affected limb or side of body
- Denial of hemiplegia or other motor and sensory deficits
- Left homonymous hemianopia
- Difficulty with spatial-perceptual tasks
- Left hemiplegia

OUTCOME CRITERIA
- Patient is safe and free from injury.
- Patient is able to identify safety hazards in the environment.
- Patient recognizes disability and describes physical deficits present (e.g., paralysis, weakness, numbness).
- Patient demonstrates ability to scan the visual field to compensate for loss of function or sensation in affected limb(s).

NURSING INTERVENTIONS AND *RATIONALE*
1. Adapt environment to patient's deficits *to maintain patient safety.*
   - Position the patient's bed with the unaffected side facing the door.
   - Approach and speak to the patient from the unaffected side. If the patient must be approached from the affected side, announce your presence as soon as entering the room *to avoid startling the patient.*
   - Position the call light, bedside stand, and personal items on the patient's unaffected side.
   - If the patient will be assisted out of bed, simplify the environment *to eliminate hazards* by removing unnecessary furniture and equipment.
   - Provide frequent reorientation of the patient to the environment.
   - Observe the patient closely, and anticipate his or her needs. In spite of repeated explanation, the patient may have difficulty retaining information about the deficits.
   - When patient is in bed, elevate his or her affected arm on a pillow *to prevent dependent edema and support the hand in a position of function.*
2. Assist the patient with recognizing the perceptual defect.
   - Encourage the patient to wear any prescriptive corrective glasses or hearing aids *to facilitate communication.*
   - Instruct the patient to turn the head past midline *to view the environment on the affected side.*
   - Encourage patient to look at the affected side and to stroke the limbs with the unaffected hand. Encourage handling of the affected limbs *to reinforce awareness of the affected side.*
   - Instruct the patient to look for the affected extremity when performing simple tasks *to know where it is at all times.*
   - After pointing to them, have the patient name the affected parts.
   - Encourage the patient to use self-exercises (e.g., lifting the affected arm with the unaffected hand).
   - If the patient is unable to discriminate between the concepts of "right" and "left," use descriptive adjectives such as "the weak arm," "the affected leg," or "the good arm" to refer to the body. Use gestures, not just words, to indicate right and left.
3. Collaborate with the patient, physician, and rehabilitation team *to design and implement a beginning rehabilitation program for use during the critical care unit stay.*
   - Use adaptive equipment (braces, splints, slings) as appropriate.
   - Teach the patient the individual components of any activity separately, and then proceed to integrate the component parts into a completed activity.
   - Instruct the patient to attend to the affected side, if able, and to assist with the bath or other tasks.
   - Use tactile stimulation to reintroduce the arm or leg to the patient. Rub the affected parts with different textured materials to stimulate sensations (warm, cold, rough, soft).
   - Encourage activities that require the patient to turn the head toward the affected side, and retrain the patient to scan the affected side and environment visually.
   - If the patient is allowed out of bed, cue him or her with reminders to scan visually when ambulating. Assist and remain in constant attendance *because the patient may have difficulty maintaining correct posture, balance, and locomotion.* There may be vertical-horizontal perceptual problems, with the patient leaning to the affected side to align with the perceived vertical. Provide sitting, standing, and balancing exercises before getting the patient out of bed.
   - Assist patient with oral feedings.
     - —Avoid giving patient any very hot food items that could cause injury.
     - —Place the patient in an upright sitting position if possible.
     - —Encourage the patient to feed himself or herself; if necessary, guide the patient's hand to the mouth.
     - —If the patient is able to feed himself or herself, place one dish at a time in front of the patient. When the patient is finished with the first, add another dish. Tell the patient what he or she is eating.
     - —Initially place food in patient's visual field; then gradually move the food out of the field of vision and teach the patient to scan the entire visual field.
     - —When the patient has learned to visually scan the environment, offer a tray of food with various dishes.

NURSING MANAGEMENT PLAN—*cont'd*

- —Instruct the patient to take small bites of food and to place the food in the unaffected side of the mouth.
- —Teach the patient to sweep out pockets of food with the tongue after every bite ***to eliminate retained food in the affected side of the mouth.***
- —After meals or oral medications, check the patient's oral cavity for pockets of retained material.

4. Initiate patient and family health teaching.
   - Assess to ensure that both the patient and the family understand the nature of the neurologic deficits and the purpose of the rehabilitation plan.
   - Teach the proper application and use of any adaptive equipment.
   - Teach the importance of maintaining a safe environment, and point out potential environmental hazards.
   - Instruct family members how to facilitate relearning techniques (e.g., cueing, scanning visual fields).

APPENDIX

B Physiologic Formulas for Critical Care

HEMODYNAMIC FORMULAS

Mean Arterial Pressure (MAP)

$$MAP = \frac{SBP + (2 \times DBP)}{3}$$

SBP = Systolic blood pressure (measured via arterial line or blood pressure cuff)
DBP = Diastolic blood pressure (measured via arterial line or blood pressure cuff)
Normal range: 70 to 100 mm Hg

Cardiac Index (CI)

$$CI = \frac{CO}{BSA}$$

CO = Cardiac output (measured via pulmonary artery catheter)
BSA = Body surface area (calculated value)
Normal range: 2.5 to 4.0 L/min/m^2

Stroke Volume (SV)

$$SV = \frac{CO \times 1000}{HR}$$

CO = Cardiac output (measured via pulmonary artery catheter)
HR = Heart rate (measured via bedside electrocardiogram)
Normal range: 60 to 100 ml/beat

Stroke Volume Index (SVI)

$$SVI = \frac{CI \times 1000}{HR}$$

CI = Cardiac index (calculated value)
HR = Heart rate (measured via bedside electrocardiogram)
Normal range: 33 to 47 ml/m^2/beat

Systemic Vascular Resistance (SVR)

$$SVR = \frac{MAP - RAP}{CO} \times 80$$

MAP = Mean arterial pressure (measured via arterial line or calculated value)
RAP = Right atrial mean pressure (measured via pulmonary artery catheter)
CO = Cardiac output (measured via pulmonary artery catheter)
Normal range: 800 to 1200 dynes/sec/cm^{-5}

Pulmonary Vascular Resistance (PVR)

$$PVR = \frac{PAMP - PAOP}{CO} \times 80$$

PAMP =Pulmonary artery mean pressure (measured via pulmonary artery catheter)
PAOP = Pulmonary artery occlusion pressure or "wedge" pressure (measured via pulmonary artery catheter)
CO = Cardiac output (measured via pulmonary artery catheter)
Normal range: less than 250 dynes/sec/cm^{-5}

Left Ventricular Stroke Work Index (LVSWI)

LVSWI = (MAP − PAOP) × SVI × 0.0136
MAP = Mean arterial pressure (measured via arterial line or calculated value)
PAOP = Pulmonary artery occlusion pressure or "wedge" pressure (measured via pulmonary artery catheter)
SVI = Stroke volume index (calculated value)
Normal range: 50 to 62 g-m/m^2/beat

Right Ventricular Stroke Work Index (RVSWI)

$$RVSWI = (PAMP - RAP) \times SVI \times 0.0136$$

PAMP = Pulmonary artery mean pressure (measured via pulmonary artery catheter)
RAP = Right atrial mean pressure (measured via pulmonary artery catheter)
SVI = Stroke volume (calculated value)
Normal range: 7.9 to 9.7 g-m/m^2/beat

Corrected QT Interval (QTc)

$$QTc = \frac{QT}{\sqrt{RR}}$$

QT = QT interval
RR = R-to-R interval
Upper limit: 0.44 second

Body Mass Index (BMI)

$$\text{Body Mass Index} = \text{Weight (kg)}/\text{Height (m)}^2$$

Body Surface Area (BSA)

To calculate (Figure A-1):

1. Obtain patient's height and weight.
2. Mark height on the left scale and weight on the right scale.
3. Draw a straight line between the two points marked on each scale.

The number where the line crosses the middle scale is the BSA value.

PULMONARY FORMULAS

Shunt Equation (Qs/Qt)

$$\frac{Qs}{Qt} = \frac{Cco_2 - Cao_2}{Cco_2 - Cvo_2}$$

Cco_2 = Pulmonary capillary oxygen content (calculated value)
Cao_2 = Arterial oxygen content (calculated value)
Cvo_2 = Venous oxygen content (calculated value)
Normal range: less than 5%

Pulmonary Capillary Oxygen Content (Cco_2)

$$Cco_2 = (Hgb \times 1.34 \times Sco_2) + (Pco_2 \times 0.003)$$

Hgb = Hemoglobin (measured via laboratory sample or arterial blood gas)
Sco_2 = Pulmonary capillary oxygen saturation
Pco_2 = Partial pressure of oxygen in capillary blood

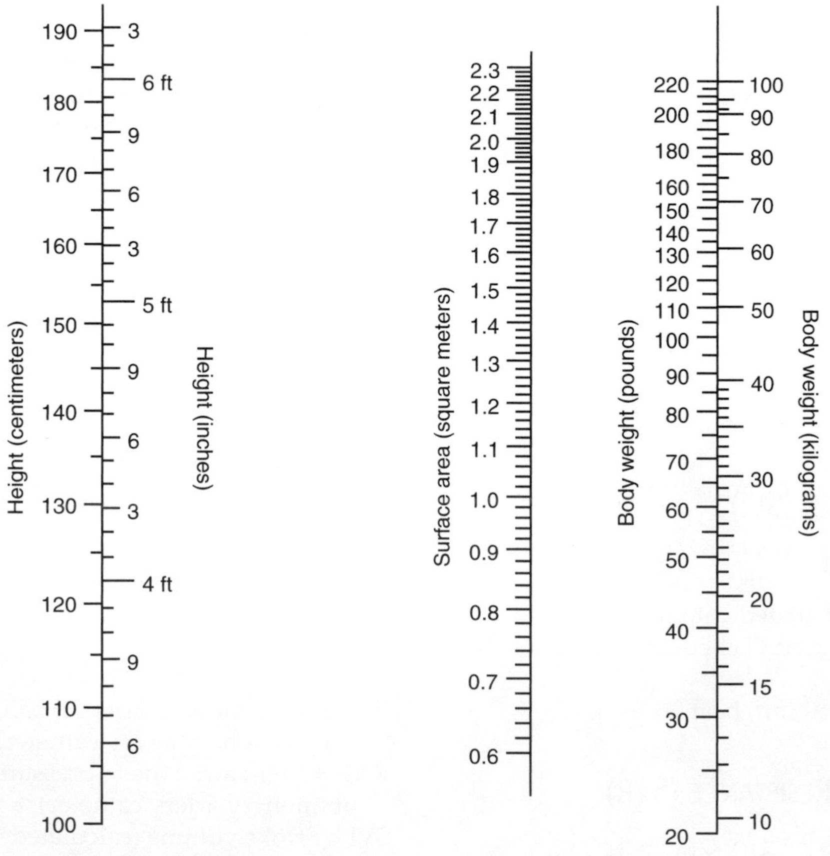

FIGURE A-1. Body surface area (BSA) nomogram.

Arterial Oxygen Content (Co2)

$$Cao_2 = (Hgb \times 1.34 \times Sao_2) + (0.003 \times Pao_2)$$

Hgb = Hemoglobin (measured via laboratory sample or arterial blood gas)
Sao_2 = Arterial oxygen saturation (measured via arterial blood gas)
Pao_2 = Partial pressure of oxygen in arterial blood (measured via arterial blood gas)
Normal range: 17 to 20 ml/dl

Venous Oxygen Content (Cvo_2)

$$Cvo_2 = (Hgb \times 1.34 \times Svo_2) + (0.003 \times Pvo_2)$$

Hgb = Hemoglobin (measured via laboratory sample or arterial blood gas)
Svo_2 = Mixed venous oxygen saturation (measured via mixed venous blood gas)
Pvo_2 = Partial pressure of oxygen in mixed venous blood (measured via mixed venous blood gas)
Normal range: 12 to 15 ml/dl

Alveolar Pressure of Oxygen (PAO_2)

$$PAO_2 = FIO_2 \times (Pb - PH_2O) - Paco_2/RQ$$

FIO_2 = Fraction of inspired oxygen (obtained from oxygen settings)
Pb = Barometric pressure (assumed to be 760 mm Hg at sea level)
PH_2O = Water pressure in the lungs (assumed to be 47 mm Hg)
$Paco_2$ = Partial pressure of carbon dioxide in arterial blood (measured via arterial blood gas)
RQ = Respiratory quotient (assumed to be 0.8)
Normal range: 60 to 100 mm Hg

Arterial/Inspired Oxygen Ratio

$$Pao_2/FIO_2 \text{ ratio} = \frac{Pao_2}{FIO_2}$$

Pao_2 = Partial pressure of oxygen in arterial blood (measured via arterial blood gas)
FIO_2 = Fraction of inspired oxygen (obtained from oxygen settings)
Normal range: greater than 300

Arterial/Alveolar Oxygen Ratio

$$Pao_2/PAO_2 = \frac{Pao_2}{PAO_2}$$

Pao_2 = Partial pressure of oxygen in arterial blood (measured via arterial blood gas)
PAO_2 = Partial pressure of oxygen in alveoli (calculated value)
Normal range: greater than 0.75 (75%)

Alveolar-Arterial Gradient

$P(A\text{-}a)O_2 = PAO_2 - Pao_2$
PAO_2 = Partial pressure of oxygen in alveoli (calculated value)
Pao_2 = Partial pressure of oxygen in arterial blood (measured via arterial blood gas)
Normal range: 25 to 65 mm Hg

Dead Space Equation (Vd/Vt)

$$Vd = \frac{Paco_2 - Petco_2}{Vt\ Paco_2}$$

$Paco_2$ = Partial pressure of carbon dioxide in arterial blood (measured via arterial blood gas)
$Petco_2$ = Partial pressure of carbon dioxide in exhaled gas (measured via end-tidal CO_2 monitor)
Normal range: 2 to 0.4 (20% to 40%)

Static Compliance (C_{ST})

This value is calculated for mechanically ventilated patients.

$$C_{ST} = \frac{Vt}{PP} - PEEP$$

Vt = Tidal volume (obtained from ventilator)
PP = Plateau pressure (measured via ventilator)
PEEP = Positive end-expiratory pressure (obtained from ventilator)
Normal value: 60-100 ml/cm H_2O

Dynamic Compliance (C_{DY})

Also called *characteristic,* this value is calculated for mechanically ventilated patients.

$$C_{DY} = \frac{Vt}{PIP} - PEEP$$

Vt = Tidal volume (obtained from ventilator)
PIP = Peak inspiratory pressure (obtained from ventilator)
PEEP = Positive end-expiratory pressure (obtained from ventilator)
Normal value: 40 to 80 ml/cm H_2O

NEUROLOGIC FORMULAS

Cerebral Perfusion Pressure (CPP)

$$CCP = MAP - ICP$$

MAP = Mean arterial pressure (measured via arterial line or blood pressure cuff)

ICP = Intracranial pressure (measured via ICP monitoring device)
Normal range: 60 to 150 mm Hg

Arteriojugular Oxygen Difference ($AjDO_2$)

$$AjDO_2 = (SaO_2 - SjvO_2) \times 1.34 \times Hgb$$

SaO_2 = arterial oxygen saturation (measured via arterial blood gas)
$SjvO_2$ = jugular venous oxygen saturation (measured jugular blood gas or jugular venous catheter)
Hgb = hemoglobin (measured via laboratory sample or arterial blood gas)
Normal range: 5 to 7.5 ml/dl

ENDOCRINE FORMULA

Serum Osmolality

$$\text{Serum Osmolality} = 2\,(Na^+ + K^+) + \frac{\text{Glucose}}{18} + \frac{\text{BUN}}{2.8}$$

Na^+ = Sodium
K^+ = Potassium
BUN = Blood urea nitrogen
Normal range: 275 to 295 mOsm/kg of water

RENAL FORMULA

Renal Clearance

$$\text{Clearance} = [U] \times \frac{V}{[P]}$$

[U] = Concentration of substance in urine
V = Time
[P] = Concentration of substance in plasma
Normal range: dependent on substance measured

NUTRITIONAL FORMULAS*

Estimate of Caloric Needs

Step 1. Calculate basal energy expenditure (BEE). This is the energy needed for basic life processes, such as respiratory function and maintenance of body temperature.

$$\text{Women: BEE} = 795 + 7.18 \times \text{Weight (kg)}$$

$$\text{Men: BEE} = 879 + 10.20 \times \text{Weight (kg)}$$

*Data from Deitch EA: *Crit Care Clin* 11:735, 1995; Owen OE et al: *Am J Clin Nutr* 4:1, 1986; Owen OE et al: *Am J Clin Nutr* 46:875, 1987; and Garrel DR, Jobin N, de Jonge LH: *Nutr Clin Pract* 11:99, 1996.

TYPE OF STRESS	MULTIPLY VALUE FROM STEP 2 BY:
Fever	1 + 0.13/° C elevation above normal (or 0.07/° F)
Pneumonia	1.2
Major injury	1.3
Severe sepsis	1.5
Burn 15%-30% BSA	1.5
Burn 31%-49% BSA	1.5-2.0
Burn 50% or greater BSA	1.8-2.1

BSA, Body surface area.

Step 2. Multiply by an appropriate stress factor to meet needs of ill or injured patient (see the following table). If patient has more than one stress present (e.g., burn and pneumonia), use only the stress factor for the *highest level* of stress.

Estimate of Protein Needs

Protein needs vary with degree of malnutrition and stress (see the following table).

Example of Calculation of Caloric and Protein Needs

A 28-year-old female patient has a fracture of the left femur and burns of 40% of her body surface area (BSA) after a motor vehicle crash. Her height is 1.65 m (5 ft 5 in), and her weight is 59.1 kg (130 lb).

Energy needs
1. BEE = 795 + 7.18 × 59.1 = 1219 calories/day
2. Energy needs for injury = 1219 calories × 1.75 = 2133 calories/day

Protein needs
Protein needs = 59.1 kg × 1.75 g = 103 g/day

CONDITION	MULTIPLY DESIRABLE BODY WEIGHT (kg) BY:
Healthy individual	0.8-1.0 g protein
Well-nourished elective surgery patient	
Malnourished or catabolic state	1.2 to 2+ g protein
• Sepsis	
• Major injury	
Burns	
• 15%-30% BSA	1.5 g protein
• 31%-49% BSA	1.5-2.0 g protein
• 50% or greater BSA	2.0-2.5 g protein

BSA, Body surface area.

Index

Page numbers followed by f, figures; t, tables; and b, boxes

E

N

O

P

U